Pharmacology
in Nursing
Practice, Fourth Edition

Gordon E. Johnson
Maureen Osis
Kathryn J. Hannah

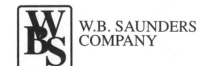

W.B. SAUNDERS COMPANY

A Harcourt Canada Health Sciences Company

Toronto Montreal Fort Worth New York Orlando
Philadelphia San Diego London Sydney Tokyo

Canadian Cataloguing in Publication Data

Johnson, G.E. (Gordon E.)
    Pharmacology in nursing practice

4th ed.
Previous editions published under the title: Pharmacology and
the Nursing Process.
Includes index.
ISBN 0-920513-23-9

I. Pharmacology. 2. Drugs. 3. Nursing. I. Osis, M. (Maureen)
II. Hannah, Kathryn J. (Kathryn Jane), 1944–   . III. Title.
IV. Title: Pharmacology and the nursing process.

RM300.J65 1998   615'.1'024613   C98-930222-9

Editing/Production Coordination: Francine Geraci
Proofreading: Gail Copeland
Design/Desktop Publishing: C.J. Design
Cover Photo: Barbara Bellingham/Masterfile
Printing and Binding: Webcom Limited

Harcourt Canada
55 Horner Avenue, Toronto, ON, Canada M8Z 4X6
Customer Service
Toll-Free Tel.: 1-800-387-7278
Toll-Free Fax: 1-800-665-7307

This book was printed in Canada.

2 3 4 5 6   04 03 02 01 00

Dedication and Acknowledgments

Gordon E. Johnson would like to thank his wife Mary-Jane and daughter Rebecca for their efforts in proofreading this text and in preparing the index. He would also like to dedicate this book to his granddaughter, Christina, to all other patients who are living with cystic fibrosis and to their valiant caregivers. Hopefully, in a few years, Christina and others like her will be able to breathe easier, eat without fear and enjoy the luxury of growing old.

Maureen Osis would like to express her gratitude to her family — Imants, Andrew, Lara and Sean — for their patience, encouragement and support during the writing of this book.

Gordon and Maureen must also say thank you to their editor, Francine Geraci, who laboured long hours to ensure the successful completion of this work. We hope our relationship with Francine will continue in the years to come.

Gordon E. Johnson
Director
Saskatchewan Drug Research Institute
University of Saskatchewan

Maureen Osis
Osis Consulting
Calgary, Alberta

Preface

Nursing education is a continual process. Beginning when the neophyte first enters nursing school or college, it continues long after graduation. Recognizing this point, we have attempted to meet the needs of nurses at all levels of education who are interested in learning about the use of drugs. Obviously, some chapters will appeal more to some readers than to others. Undergraduates may find most interest in the material pertaining to the systemic study of drugs. Staff nurses, charged with the daily care of the ill, may be more concerned with the specifics of clinical practice related to the use of drugs in particular conditions. We hope that all readers will appreciate our approach to the study of pharmacology.

Pharmacology is not the study of individual drugs. Rather, it involves an understanding of the interaction between drugs and the physiological, psychological and pathological processes occurring in the body. Therefore, we have discussed the physiology and pathology of the pertinent organ systems before presenting the drugs. Only by following this system will nurses understand the actions of drugs currently in use and be prepared for new drugs as they appear on the market.

Our title, *Pharmacology in Nursing Practice*, was selected because it reflects our approach to the use of drugs. Following the prescription of a drug by a physician, nurses must assess the risk versus benefit of the drug, implement the medication order, assist in teaching the patient and family and monitor the results of treatment. Accordingly, each chapter describes the nursing management of the patient with respect to the drugs being discussed.

No book can pretend to be a comprehensive text on drug therapy. This text seeks to provide a synopsis of each topic, together with a list of recommended readings at the end of each chapter. If nurses require more information on individual drugs, there are many excellent references available, including the *Compendium of Pharmaceuticals and Specialties,* the *American Medical Association Drug Evaluations,* and *Davis's Drug Guide for Nurses.*

Contents

A Statement on Drug Doses

This text contains numerous drug dosages. Unless otherwise stated, these are intended for the average adult patient. Pediatric and geriatric doses have been provided when available. Although every effort has been made to ensure that the doses listed are correct, nurses must check with the latest information from the manufacturer if any doubt exists concerning the dosage of a drug.

Abbreviations Used in This Book

In order to reduce the size of the book, it has been necessary to abbreviate many measurements and terms. The list that follows will assist the nurse with regard to quantities and abbreviations.

ac	Before meals
ACE	Angiotensin-converting enzyme
ACEI	Angiotensin-converting enzyme inhibitor
ADL	Activities of daily living
ALP	Alkaline phosphatase
AP	Arterial pressure
aPTT	Activated partial prothrombin time
AST	Aspartate transaminase
ATC	Around the clock
BCE	Before common era
bid	Twice daily
BP	Blood pressure
CBC	Complete blood count
CHF	Congestive heart failure
CI	Cardiac index
CIBD	Chronic inflammatory bowel disease
CNS	Central nervous system
CO	Cardiac output
COPD	Chronic obstructive pulmonary disease
CrCl	Creatinine clearance
CV	Cardiovascular
CVP	Central venous pressure
D5W	Dextrose 5% in water
dL	Decilitre(s)
FPG	Fasting plasma glucose
g	Gram(s)
GI	Gastrointestinal
h	Hour(s)
HCT	Hematocrit
HR	Heart rate

hs	At bedtime
hx	History
IGT	Impaired glucose tolerance
IM	Intramuscular
I/O	Intake/output (fluids)
IU	International units
IV	Intravenous
L	Litre(s)
LOC	Level of consciousness
μg	Microgram(s)
MAOI	Monoamine oxidase inhibitor
mEq	Milliequivalent(s)
mg	Milligram(s)
MI	Myocardial infarction
min	Minute(s)
mL	Millilitre(s)
mmol	Millimole(s)
N/G	Nasogastric
NPO	Nil per os (nothing by mouth)
NS	Normal saline
NSAID	Nonsteroidal anti-inflammatory drug
OGTT	Oral glucose tolerance test
P	Pulse
pc	After meals
PO	Per os (orally)
prn	Pro re nata (as necessary)
pt(s)	Patient(s)
PT	Prothrombin time
PWP	Pulmonary wedge pressure
od	Once daily
q4h	Every 4 hours
q6h	Every 6 hours
q8h	Every 8 hours
qh	Every hour
qid	Four times daily
qod	Every other day
R	Respiration
RBC	Red blood (cell) count
ROM	Range of motion
r/t	Related to
SGOT	Serum glutamic-oxaloacetic transaminase
s/s	Signs and symptoms
stat	Immediately
T	Temperature
TCA	Tricyclic antidepressant
tid	Three times daily
tx	Treatment, therapy
U	Unit(s)
VS	Vital signs
WBC	White blood (cell) count

Commonly Used Equivalencies

Source: Miller and Keane (1983), *Encyclopedia and Dictionary of Medicine, Nursing and Allied Health,* 3rd ed. Reprinted with permission.

Metric Doses with Approximate Apothecary Equivalents* — Liquid Measure

These approximate dose equivalents represent the quantiles usually prescribed, under identical conditions, by physicians trained, respectively, in the metric or in the apothecary system of weights and measures. In labelling dosage forms in both the metric and the apothecary systems, if one is the approximate equivalent of the other, the approximate figure shall be enclosed in parentheses.

When prepared dosage forms such as tablets, capsules, pills, etc. are prescribed in the metric system, the pharmacist may dispense the corresponding approximate equivalent in the apothecary system, and vice versa, as indicated in the following table.

Metric	Approx. Apothecary Equivalents
1000 mL	1 quart
750 mL	1.5 pints
500 mL	1 pint
250 mL	8 fluid ounces
200 mL	7 fluid ounces
100 mL	3.5 fluid ounces
50 mL	1.75 fluid ounces
30 mL	1 fluid ounce
15 mL	4 fluid drams
10 mL	2.5 fluid drams
8 mL	2 fluid drams
5 mL	1.25 fluid drams
4 mL	1 fluid dram
3 mL	45 minims
2 mL	30 minims
1 mL	15 minims
0.75 mL	12 minims
0.6 mL	10 minims
0.5 mL	8 minims
0.3 mL	5 minims
0.25 mL	4 minims
0.2 mL	3 minims
0.1 mL	1.5 minims
0.06 mL	1 minim
0.05 mL	0.75 minim
0.03 mL	0.5 minim

Caution: For the conversion of specific quantities in a prescription that requires compounding, or in converting a pharmaceutical formula from one system of weights or measures to the other, exact equivalents must be used.

Metric Doses with Approximate Apothecary Equivalents* — Weight

Metric	Approx. Apothecary Equivalents
30 g	1 ounce
15 g	4 drams
10 g	2.5 drams
7.5 g	2 drams
6 g	90 grains
5 g	75 grains
4 g	60 grains
3 g	45 grains
2 g	30 grains
1.5 g	22 grains
1 g	15 grains
0.75 g	12 grains
0.6 g	10 grains
0.5 g	7.5 grains
0.4 g	6 grains
0.3 g	5 grains
0.25 g	4 grains
0.2 g	3 grains
0.15 g	2.5 grains
0.12 g	2 grains
0.1 g	1.5 grains
75 mg	1.25 grains
60 mg	1 grain
50 mg	0.75 grain
40 mg	0.67 grain
30 mg	0.5 grain
25 mg	0.375 grain
20 mg	0.33 grain
15 mg	0.25 grain
12 mg	0.2 grain
10 mg	0.17 grain
8 mg	0.125 grain
6 mg	0.1 grain
5 mg	0.08 grain
4 mg	0.07 grain
3 mg	0.05 grain
2 mg	0.03 grain
1.5 mg	0.025 grain
1.2 mg	0.02 grain
1 mg	0.016 grain
0.8 mg	0.0125 grain
0.6 mg	0.01 grain
0.5 mg	0.008 grain
0.4 mg	0.007 grain
0.3 mg	0.005 grain
0.25 mg	0.004 grain
0.2 mg	0.003 grain
0.15 mg	0.0025 grain
0.12 mg	0.002 grain
0.1 mg	0.0017 grain

Note: A millilitre (mL) is the approximate equivalent of a cubic centimetre (cc).

*Adopted by the latest *Pharmacopeia, National Formulary, and New and Nonofficial Remedies,* and approved by the U.S. Federal Food and Drug Administration.

Pharmacotherapeutics of Nursing

Unit 1 provides the foundation for understanding and applying pharmacotherapeutics in nursing practice. One major assumption of this text is that nursing relies on a systematic, rational, disciplined way of thinking called the *nursing process*. Another important assumption is that critical thinking leads to clinical nursing judgment, including a knowledge of which data to observe, the ability to derive meaning from those observations and appropriate decision making for optimal benefit and minimal risk for patients and families.

Chapter 1 provides an understanding of the integration of the science of pharmacology into nursing practice. The reader is encouraged to pay special attention to this chapter and to return to it occasionally for review. Of particilar interest is the information on patient teaching.

Chapter 2 presents essential drug regulations and standards as legislated in Canada and the United States. It offers a framework for understanding nursing accountability and the importance of patient consent to drug therapy.

Chapter 3 reviews some issues in drug development and drug use in contemporary society. In many settings, nurses can make an important contribution in reducing drug misuse. It is hoped that this chapter will stimulate the reader's interest in accepting such a role.

Nursing Therapeutics

Topics Discussed
- Nursing role and relationship in pharmacotherapeutics
- Application of pharmacology in nursing therapeutics
- Phases of nursing process in relationship to pharmacotherapeutics
- Nursing role in patient/family education, health education and compliance
- Individual variation in response to drug therapy and the essential component of monitoring

Pharmacotherapeutics, the use of drugs to prevent, modify or cure disease, is among the most frequently used medical treatments. Historically, physicians have been responsible both for diagnosing disease and for prescribing — preparing medications as well as administering them as treatment. With increased knowledge, complexity and specialization came the development of the health care team. Specifically, with regard to medications, a trio of health professionals have become the essential agents of drug therapy: the physician diagnoses the illness and prescribes the medications, which the pharmacist dispenses and the nurse administers. Expectations of society and increasing nursing expertise have expanded the nurse's role even further, from simple administration to participatory collaboration. Today, the professional nurse is expected to contribute to the design, implementation and evaluation of the patient's drug regimen.

Nursing pharmacotherapeutics requires the application of knowledge from a variety of sources. For example, the nurse studies drug actions, effects and adverse reactions (pharmacology), factors that affect drug-taking behaviour and capability to learn self-medication (sociology and psychology) and techniques of administration by various routes (nursing science). Mastering this knowledge can be both challenging and rewarding. This chapter introduces the first steps in this process.

Chapter 1 is based on the belief of the authors that to survive the rapid changes of the future, nurses will need to rely on more than specific knowledge and psychomotor skills. The profession will best serve its societal goal through competent decision making and complex problem solving, achieved through critical thinking.

The contribution of Alfaro-Lefevre (1995) is integrated throughout the text and particularly in this chapter. Alfaro-Lefevre's definition and description of critical thinking provide the framework for nursing pharmacotherapeutics:

> Unlike the "mindless" thinking we do when going about our daily routines, critical thinking is purposeful, goal-directed thinking that aims to make judgments based on evidence (fact), rather than conjecture (guesswork). Based on principles of science and the scientific method (e.g., maintaining a questioning attitude, following an organized approach to discovery, and making sure information is reliable), critical thinking requires developing strategies that maximize human potential (e.g., tapping on individual strengths) and compensate for problems caused by human nature (e.g., the powerful influence of personal perceptions, values and beliefs). (Alfaro-Lefevre, 1995:9)

The concept of critical thinking is not new, having been described by Glaser as early as the 1940s and more recently researched and developed by Paul (1993). Critical thinking occurs on three levels — basic, complex and committed — and is the outcome of five components: specific knowledge base, experience, competencies, attitudes and standards (Alfaro-Lefevre, 1995:168).

Critical thinking leads to clinical nursing judg-

Figure 1.1
Essential elements and relationships of the nursing process

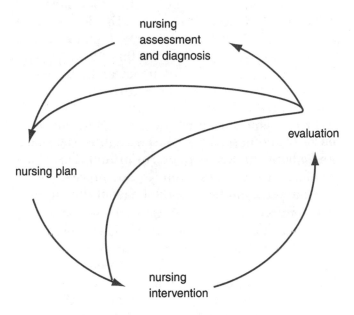

Figure 1.2
The nursing process and pharmacotherapeutics

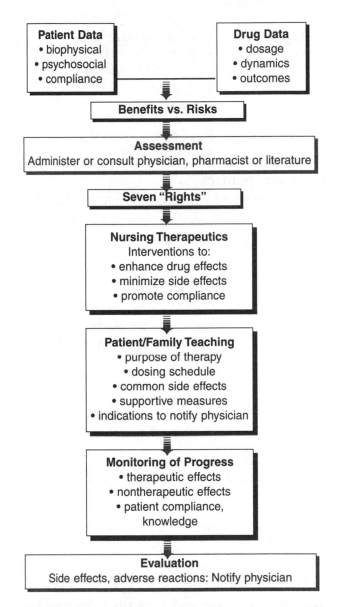

ment. It includes decisions regarding what to observe in the patient's situation, determining the meaning of those observations, and deciding what interventions to take for optimal benefit and minimal risk to the patient and his or her family (Alfaro-Lefevre, 1995:169).

The Nursing Process

This text is organized on the premise that the practice of professional nursing relies on a systematic, rational, disciplined way of thinking called the *nursing process*. Traditionally, the nursing process has included the five components of *assessment, analysis, planning, intervention* (or *implementation*) and *evaluation*. The interrelationship of the phases of the nursing process are illustrated in Figure 1.1.

The nursing process offers a structure for identification of priorities and activation of resources for care. It is action oriented, yet its most telling feature is judgment, for in professional practice problems rarely have ready solutions.

This concept of seeking individual solutions to clinical problems is the most appropriate feature of the nursing process when applied to pharmaco-

therapeutics. It has been said that every instance of therapy is a miniature experiment, and this remains true today in spite of advances in medical science. Finding the right drug in the right dose for the right patient is a challenge shared by physicians, pharmacists and nurses.

Nurses can contribute through each phase of the nursing process. For the purposes of this text, emphasis will be placed on assessment and analysis, intervention through administration and therapeutics, and evaluation or monitoring. The nursing process for pharmacotherapeutics is visually depicted in Figure 1.2 and explained in the follow-

Table 1.1
Relationship between nursing process and critical thinking skills

Nursing Process	Critical Thinking Skill
Assessment	• Identifying assumptions • Identifying an organized and comprehensive approach to discovery • Checking accuracy and reliability of data • Distinguishing relevant from irrelevant • Recognizing inconsistencies • Distinguishing normal from abnormal
Analysis/ Diagnosis	• Clustering related information • Identifying patterns • Identifying missing information • Drawing valid conclusions • Considering different conclusions • Identifying factual and potential problems and supporting conclusions with evidence
Planning	• Identifying causes and setting priorities • Determining realistic, client-centred goals • Determining specific interventions
Evaluating/ Monitoring	*Note:* All skills for assessment are also used for monitoring. • Correcting our thinking

Source: Adapted from Alfaro-Lefevre, 1995.

ing section. The relationship between the nursing process and the skills of clinical thinking is depicted in Table 1.1.

Assessment

The term assessment refers to the information gathering and observations conducted prior to medication administration. The major purpose is threefold: (a) to identify risk factors that might affect the safety and/or effectiveness of drug therapy, (b) to provide baseline data for evaluation and (c) to assess patient/family education needs or ability for self-medication.

Assessment includes the collection of biophysical and psychosocial data as well as information and observations that indicate the patient's ability and willingness to participate in the treatment plan.

As illustrated in Figure 1.2, the assessment phase begins by considering the completeness of the drug order. A legal order must be written by a practitioner licensed to prescribe medications and must be legible and complete. The order must specify the full name of the drug, the dosage, and the route and time (or frequency) of administration. Nurses are expected to be familiar with the usual dosage range and frequency and must consult the prescriber if the order varies from the recommendations.

It is essential that the nurse understand the goal of drug therapy before administering a medication to a patient. It is important to know why a particular patient is receiving a specific drug in order to plan and implement supportive nursing interventions that will promote the desired outcome. The goal is particularly relevant when the order is *prn* (*pro re nata,* or as necessary) because administration occurs at the discretion of the nurse. Furthermore, it is impossible to evaluate the therapeutic effectiveness of a drug if the desired outcome is not known. Do not make assumptions; if the goal of therapy is unclear, consult the physician.

Simultaneously, the nurse determines any patient factors (e.g., age, weight, disease, previous response to drugs) that may affect therapeutic safety or require precautions for administration. It is not the nurse's responsibility to know all medical contraindications or precautions for drug treatment; this is the primary responsibility of the prescriber. However, the nurse should recognize pertinent information such as potential or actual allergy or previous negative responses to drug treatment. A distinction does exist between absolute contraindication and a warning for caution in using a drug. One contraindication to receiving a particular drug is a pre-existing condition that precludes the use of the drug. In contrast, one precaution to drug therapy is a pre-existing condition that may increase the risk for an adverse reaction but is still warranted owing to the circumstances.

Usually, the nurse collects the patient's drug history and current drug regimen, including prescription and nonprescription (over-the-counter, or OTC) drugs, herbal and home remedies, and alcohol and caffeine use. This information is applied by the health care team to detect and prevent adverse drug interactions.

Physical status is thoroughly assessed in order to provide baseline measures for evaluating the patient's response to the medication. Physical examination and laboratory reports are important. The factors of body mass/weight, liver and kidney function, age and pathology are described later. Equally important is the assessment of the patient's emotional, psychological and social status. Cultural attitudes and beliefs about drugs may influence the decision to accept a treatment plan. Drug taking is a psychosocial as well as a biophysical experience. This information is very useful in designing a teaching plan. Finally, the patient's understanding of the medication, its purpose and effects is explored to determine learning needs.

Analysis and Nursing Diagnosis

The final element of the assessment component of the nursing process is to make a concluding statement or hypothesis about the data gathered. The diagnosis focuses on identification of actual and potential health problems for this particular patient and leads to the development of short- and long-term goals. Generally, the diagnostic statement consists of three parts: the problem (P), etiology (E) and the signs/symptoms (S). In addition to this PES format, the statement must address concerns that fall within the realm of nursing practice.

The standardization of terms used for nursing diagnoses is still under development, most notably through the North American Nursing Diagnosis Association (NANDA).

Intervention

Administration. Traditionally, the administration of medications was given the highest priority. Nurses and agencies placed great emphasis on the task of giving drugs and getting the pills out on time. Although this task is important, it is essential to recognize that it is only one component in the nursing management of drug therapy.

The nurse is professionally and legally responsible to calculate doses correctly and administer medications accurately. For over forty years, nurses have used the seven "rights" listed in Box 1.1 as a guide to prevent error.

> **Box 1.1**
> **Seven rights of medication administration**
>
> ✔ Right patient
> ✔ Right drug
> ✔ Right dose
> ✔ Right route
> ✔ Right time
> ✔ Right technique
> ✔ Right approach

The first five rights are self-explanatory, but the last two may be less familiar. The *right technique* refers to the correct use of psychomotor skills for the prescribed route of administration; for example, maintaining medical asepsis with oral medications or covering an intravenous solution with aluminum foil to prevent exposure of the medication to light. The *right approach* refers to the interpersonal and psychosocial skills associated with preparing a patient for administration; for example, comforting a child who is about to receive an injection. Implementing the teaching plan also requires the right approach.

The rights of medication administration provide a framework for reducing the incidence of medication errors. Chapter 2 discusses the most common causes for errors and suggests strategies to prevent their occurrence. Legal obligations are also explored.

Note: The skills of administration are beyond the scope of this book; only unique precautions related to specific drugs are included, as appropriate, throughout this text.

Value of nursing therapeutics. Although pharmacotherapeutics has a scientific foundation, there are multiple factors related to the patient, the drug and the context that can affect an individual's response to drug therapy. These variables will be discussed in detail in subsequent chapters. This is noted to emphasize the importance of nursing therapeutics which can enhance drug action, reduce adverse effects and substitute for drug therapy.

Nursing interventions for drug therapy are derived from all the domains of nursing practice and may involve promoting or restoring health, preventing illness and alleviating suffering. Considerable research has been conducted in defining and validating nursing interventions. Actions such as supporting, teaching, facilitating, monitoring and promoting have been defined for many patient situations.

Patient teaching. Instructing the patient and family regarding drug treatment is a shared responsibility of the nurse, pharmacist and physician. All three professionals must collaborate to complement and validate the information provided by the others, although it is often the nurse who is most involved.

Patient teaching promotes independence through self-medication and self-monitoring. With the increasing emphasis on early discharge from hospital settings and the growth of community and self-care, patient and family education have gained importance in contemporary nursing. By alerting the individual to potential adverse effects or precautions, the nurse is promoting safety; for example, explaining the dangers of combining alcohol with some analgesics or driving after taking a depressant drug. A major goal of teaching is to ensure safe adherence to the treatment plan within the therapeutic relationship.

This text will assist the reader to identify relevant information that should be communicated about specific drugs. The nursing process provides a suitable structure to patient/family teaching, as illustrated in Figure 1.3. The type of information that can be included in all drug teaching plans is outlined in Box 1.2. The actual skills required for effective teaching can be learned through other sources, and selected references are identified in the Instructor's Manual accompanying this text. Some general principles and roles of health care professionals are outlined here.

Principles of health education. Health education includes all approaches (written and verbal) used to inform the public regarding choices of behaviours that affect health. The main principle is that complete and accurate information should be presented in language that is readily understood. Self-care has been broadly defined as all the things that people do to protect, maintain or improve their own health. The self-care movement has made a significant impact on the roles and

---

Box 1.2
General information that can be included in most teaching plans

- ✔ Name of drug
- ✔ Reasons for taking the drug
- ✔ How much to take, when and how
- ✔ What to do if a dose is missed
- ✔ Actions to take or to avoid while taking the medication
- ✔ Common side effects
- ✔ Indications for notifying physician
- ✔ Follow-up visits

---

relationships between health care professionals and the public. Today's patient and family expect to have sufficient information to make choices, and this requires interdisciplinary collaboration. The roles of various health care providers are similar and should be complementary. Table 1.2 illustrates these roles.

Factors that affect compliance. Compliance is the extent to which the care plan or medical orders are followed. It is determined by many factors. How many times have you intended to follow your physician's instructions — such as, "Take all

---

Table 1.2
Roles in health education for self-care

Pharmacist
- Asks questions to determine if self-medication is appropriate/safe and to detect possible interactions
- Recommends products
- Instructs regarding side effects and adverse reactions
- Assists with follow-up

Physician
- Asks questions to confirm diagnosis and to determine appropriate treatment
- Instructs regarding expected outcomes
- Monitors progress

Nurse
- In clinics, homes, offices, advises regarding self-limiting daily health problems
- Instructs regarding choices of behaviours
- Instructs regarding effects of drugs
- Monitors responses

Figure 1.3   Nursing process and patient teaching

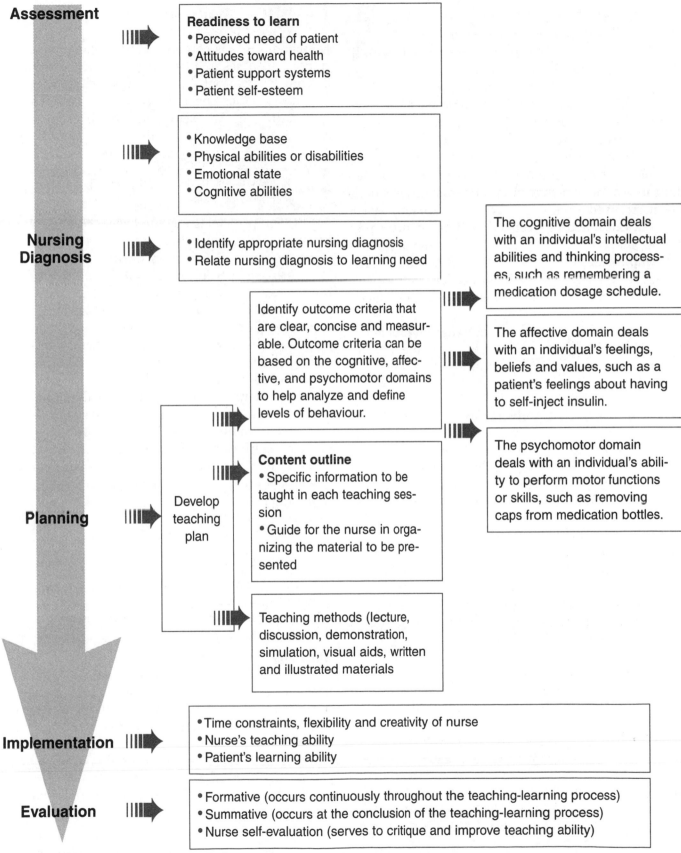

Source: Adapted from Williams B, Baer C. *Essentials of Clinical Pharmacology in Nursing.* 2nd ed. Philadelphia: Springhouse; 1994. Reproduced with permission.

of this medication" — only to find that two tablets are left a week after your symptoms ended? Most of us intend to do the right thing, but sometimes we don't know the "right" thing to do!

The three main factors that influence how well and correctly we follow instructions are knowledge, skill and attitude. With regard to knowledge, we cannot take a drug correctly if we do not have complete and accurate instructions. As well, we need certain skills to take drugs correctly. A good example might be eye drops, which must be properly instilled. Further, our personal attitudes about drugs may influence how we use, misuse or abuse them. An individual who views taking medications as "weakness" may prefer to suffer through a cold rather than take any remedy. In contrast, the person who believes that "we can put a human on the moon, so we should be able to cure the common cold" may rely on drugs to alleviate all symptoms and may expect the proverbial "magic bullet" — a single remedy that, once taken, fixes the problem. For self-medication to work well, individuals need accurate knowledge, a certain amount of skill and a realistic attitude.

Monitoring and Evaluation

By law, the nurse is required to keep a written record of the actual administration of all drugs. For high-quality care, this documentation should also include evidence of progress towards the therapeutic outcome as well as any indications of side effects or adverse reactions. The Clinical Challenge on the page opposite provides an example.

The real challenge in monitoring is that it requires the ability to evaluate and, if necessary, change our own thinking. Many personal and situational factors may impede this component of the nursing process. Lack of motivation, time limitations, reluctance to question our decisions and actions are but a few examples.

The risk for the individual receiving drug therapy is that side effects may be overlooked or minimized as part of the treatment. For example, if a drug causes dizziness, it does not follow that this side effect must be accepted without efforts to reduce or eliminate it. The older patient is at greater risk because many side effects may be overlooked as age-related changes; frequently health care professionals can be heard saying, "Well, what can you expect at her age?"

Ethical Decisions and Patients' Rights

Ethical distress is becoming a more common experience for nurses in all settings. Advanced technology has brought with it dilemmas regarding reproduction, genetics, invasive treatments, and extension of life. The American and Canadian Nurses' Associations have each published a Code of Ethics for professional nursing practice. Inherent in the practice of nursing is respect for individuals and families without regard to race, religion, gender, socioeconomic status or politics.

Ethical principles include *beneficence* (duty to do good), *nonmaleficence* (duty to do no harm), *integrity* (being true to one's word), *veracity* (telling the truth), *fidelity* (faithfulness), *justice* (considering the needs of the individual with the needs of others), and *client autonomy* (respecting individual right to self-determination). In some situations these principles may appear contradictory, for example, if telling the truth may do harm. They do, however, provide a useful guide.

Consumers' groups have developed and published documents espousing patients' rights. While not legally binding, these documents provide guidance to health care professionals. Some rights, such as the right to be informed of possible consequences of accepting or refusing treatment, have been supported in law.

Learning to Think

As you develop critical thinking skills for nursing pharmacotherapeutics, you will proceed from a basic to a complex level. At the basic level, you will ask, "What is the right answer?" You will know that you have proceeded to a more complex level when you begin to answer, "It depends."

Your ability to learn to think critically will be influenced by environmental factors such as tolerance for risk taking, encouragement for creativity, and many individual characteristics. Are you curious and insightful, humble, honest, open minded, and willing to exert a conscious effort to work in a planful manner (Alfaro-Lefevre, 1995:10)?

Read the Clinical Challenge on the next page, then consider the questions posed in Figure 1.4.

Clinical Challenge

Mrs. H., a 75-year-old woman, is admitted to hospital for investigation and possible abdominal surgery. During the initial examination, the physician diagnoses a urinary tract infection and orders an antibiotic. Mrs. H. is already on other medications for treatment of chronic problems including hypertension.

During the nursing assessment, Mrs. H.'s husband mentions that his wife reacted severely to a drug, possibly an antibiotic, several years ago. This information was not mentioned to the physician. You ask further questions about the previous illness and the type of reaction, and conclude the possibility of drug allergy. Old records confirm that the ordered medication was the offending agent.

Mrs. H. is currently taking a diuretic and antihypertensive drug to treat her hypertension. She is experiencing dizzy spells and weakness when she gets out of bed or stands up suddenly.

What is your next action?

Figure 1.4
Steps in nursing pharmacotherapeutics

Patient Data
1. Any patient factors that affect drug actions or outcomes? (Biophysical, psychosocial or compliance factors? Contraindications?)

Drug Data
2. Is drug order complete? State generic and trade names. Potential interactions?
3. Is dose within the recommended range? Defend schedule.

Outcomes
4. Summarize usual therapeutic effects. Why is patient receiving this drug?
5. Describe the nontherapeutic effects (side effects or adverse reactions) that may occur with this drug.

Assessment/Benefits vs. Risks
6. Summarize your opinion on the benefits and hazards of this drug for this patient. Any actions required? Precautions?

Follow the Rights
7. Any policies, procedures or techniques for administration?

Nursing Therapeutics
8. Name 2–4 nursing actions that will enhance drug effectiveness or reduce side effects.

Teaching Plan
9. Design a teaching plan for patient and family (purpose of drug, schedule, common side effects, supportive measures and indications for notifying physician).

Monitor Progress
10. List the observations to note progress toward goal of therapy. Any side effects or adverse reactions? Actions required?

Response to Clinical Challenge

Assessment

For Mrs. H., the short-term goal is her safety. Long-term goals may relate to substitution of drug and successful treatment of infection, patient/family education regarding causes and prevention of urinary tract infections, and preventive approaches such as wearing a medical-alert bracelet to avoid future treatment with the offending drug.

The following nursing diagnosis can be written: "High risk for injury due to probable drug allergy." The physician should be contacted.

In this clinical example, the nurse must analyze the benefit versus the risk of drug therapy for a specific patient and respond appropriately. If Mrs. H.'s reaction had been mild, or if there had been no defining evidence that this drug caused the previous reaction, then the drug may still have been ordered, but the nurse would have the responsibility for increased vigilance in monitoring the therapy.

Monitoring

The record of Mrs. H.'s blood pressure readings will indicate the degree of success of the drug therapy (diuretic and antihypertensive). Communicating that Mrs. H. experiences dizziness may result in modification of the drug therapy. The physician may lower the dose of one or both drugs, eliminate one drug, or substitute another drug that may not cause her the same degree of hypotension. Using patient data and a knowledge of pharmacology, the nurse writes the following diagnosis: "Potential for injury related to ortho-static hypotension associated with drug therapy as evidenced by dizziness, weakness, and BP variation in lying/sitting/standing positions."

Evaluation leads to adaptation of the care plan. Actions may include:

- teach Mrs. H. to change position slowly
- assist Mrs. H. to rise from bed and chair
- monitor blood pressure lying/sitting/standing
- daily until stable
- discuss with physician.

Case studies such as this Clinical Challenge are a useful means for applying and improving your critical thinking skills. Many chapters of this text begin with a Clinical Challenge; possible responses are given at each chapter's end.

Setting Learning Priorities

In clinical practice, nurses must set priorities for use of their time. The intensity of observation for adverse drug reactions is related to the risk presented by the actual drug therapy and the individual patient. Further chapters will describe specific risk factors, but the comparison of two patients will quickly illustrate the major principles.

Consider Miss V., who is 91 years old, takes three prescribed drugs and an occasional laxative, has poor vision but good hearing, and can generally manage her own medications at home. Now consider Mr. M., who is 75 years old with moderate heart disease, takes five prescribed drugs and over-the-counter antacids and laxatives, sometimes forgets to take his pills, and occasionally uses alcohol. Mr. M. is at greater risk because of underlying disease and polypharmacy (multiple-drug therapy).

Box 1.3 presents a sample outline for patient teaching with respect to general drug therapy.

Further Reading

Alfaro-Lefevre R. *Critical Thinking in Nursing.* Philadelphia: W.B. Saunders; 1995.

Barnes L. The illiterate client. *Am J Maternal Child Nurs* 1992;17(2):99.

Canadian Nurses Association. *Code of Ethics for Nursing.* Ottawa: CNA; 1991.

Ericksen J. Putting ethics into education. *Can Nurse* 1993;89(5):18–20.

Foster P, et al. Helping students learn to make ethical decisions. *Holistic Nurs Pract* 1993;7(3): 28–35.

Jackson L. Understanding, eliciting and negotiating clients' multicultural health beliefs. *Nurse Practitioner: Am J Primary Health Care* 1993;18(4):30, 32, 37–38.

Lilley L, Guacci G. Unfamiliar drug uses. *Am J Nurs* 1995;95(1):15.

Nursing interventions. *Nurs Clin North Am* (suppl) 1992 (June).

Osis M. *Dosage Calculations in SI Units.* 3rd ed. St. Louis: Mosby-Year Book; 1995.

Paul R. *Critical Thinking: How to Prepare Students for a Rapidly Changing World.* Santa Rosa, CA: Foundation for Critical Thinking; 1993.

Pike S. Ethics, the law and clinical decision. *Can Nurse* 1993;89(5):39–40.

Ross F. Patient compliance — whose responsibility? *Soc Sci Medicine* 1991;32(1):89–94.

Box 1.3
Patient teaching: General drug therapy

✔ **What can you do to remember to take your medicine?**
Use a calendar to check off each dose, or put pills into a compartmentalized dosette.

✔ **What should you do if you miss a dose of your medicine?**
When you notice that you have missed a dose, look at the time and calculate which is closer — the time of the dose that you missed, or the next dose that you will take. For example, you usually take your blood pressure pills at 8 a.m. and 6 p.m., and it is now noon. As it is four hours since the missed time and six hours until the next time, take the dose.

However, if you did not notice until 2 p.m. (six hours since the missed dose and only four hours until the next dose), skip the dose and carry on with your usual routine. Do not double any doses. If uncertain, contact your pharmacist for advice.

✔ **Where should you store your medicines?**
Keep all medicines out of the reach of children and in their original container. Store in a tight container, in a cool, dry place. If you need to take a supply of pills with you for travel, be certain to label them. (Note: The bathroom is not the ideal place to keep medicines!)

✔ **When you stop taking a medicine, what should you do with the remaining supply?**
Ideally, to prevent contaminating the public water supply, take your pills to your pharmacy for disposal. Never use expired medications.

✔ **What should you do if you think you are experiencing side effects from your medicines?**
Call your pharmacist and check whether your problem could be medication related. Make a note of the problem and when it occurs. Discuss with your physician. Do not take another pill to cure the side effect. Expect side effects if you combine prescription and OTC drugs or medications with alcohol.

✔ **Where should you get your medicines?**
Purchasing all your medications at the same pharmacy has several advantages. For one thing, you get to know the pharmacist and will feel more comfortable asking questions. More importantly, the pharmacist also gets to know you and the complete profile of your medications. Pharmacists are valuable community resources to advise on how and when to take drugs, and to warn of side effects or dangerous combinations (e.g., what might happen if you take a certain drug with alcohol). Select your pharmacist as carefully as you select your physician. Don't bother driving around town looking for "bargains"; minor savings are not worth the risk to your health.

✔ **What should you ask the doctor or pharmacist?**
Each time you take a product for self-medication, you should know:
  – the name of the drug
  – the effects you can expect
  – when to take the drug
  – the indications for stopping the drug, or calling the doctor or pharmacist.

✔ **How can you make over-the-counter drugs safer?**
  – Use the same pharmacy.
  – Ask questions before you purchase an OTC drug.
  – Read the label carefully.
  – Do not combine drugs or alcohol without advice.
  – Discuss side effects with physician or pharmacist.
  – Follow instructions carefully.
  – Dispose of expired-date products.
  – Ask — ask — ASK!

Legal Implications of the Pharmacologic Aspects of Nursing Practice*

Topics Discussed

● Definition of drug, prescription, order, proprietary medicine, over-the-counter (OTC) medication, narcotic preparation, procedure, protocol, policy
● Accountability, liability, negligence, competence, battery, assault
● Canadian and U.S. drug regulations and the restrictions they impose on drug use in each country
● Drug standards and legislation
● Sources and prevention of medication errors

Clinical Challenge

Consider this clinical challenge as you read through this chapter. The response to the challenge appears on page 21.

Ms. F., a 23-year-old woman, is admitted through emergency with a severe migraine headache. During the nursing assessment, the patient states that she has felt sick for the past 2 weeks and may be pregnant. On the chart the order reads: *Ergotamine tartrate 1 tab SL. Repeat q30 min up to 3 tabs.* Unfamiliar with the drug, the nurse refers to the *CPS,* which states that the drug is contraindicated in pregnancy.

What are the professional and legal responsibilities of the nurse? If she gives the drug, is she incompetent, negligent or both?

This chapter describes the laws governing drug use in Canada and the United States and explains their relationship to the profession of nursing.

A *drug* is defined as "any substance used in the diagnosis, treatment, mitigation, or prevention of a disease, disorder, or abnormal physical state and in restoring, correcting, or modifying organic function in man or animal" (Health & Welfare Canada, 1983).

By this definition, it is clear that drugs are potent chemicals, capable of causing as much harm as good. Their use must therefore be controlled. The availability of drugs is governed by their safety and efficacy, their potential for abuse and the amount of professional consultation required for their appropriate use.

Drugs are a very diverse group of compounds. At one end of the spectrum, acetylsalicylic acid (ASA) can provide relief of minor pain and be purchased over the counter. At the other end is

*By A.J. Remillard, PharmD and M. Osis, MSc

lysergic acid diethylamide (LSD), a substance with no known medicinal use and available only to research institutions on authorization from the Health Protection Branch in Canada or the Food and Drug Administration in the United States.

Physicians, pharmacists and nurses are important in controlling and monitoring drug use. The extent of their involvement depends on the safety of the products concerned. Safe drugs are widely available and require minimal supervision. Drugs with a greater potential for abuse are usually available only on prescription, and require the assistance of a health professional to ensure their safe and effective use.

Federal laws in both Canada and the United States regulate the availability of drugs. Provincial or state laws may supplement federal laws and further restrict the distribution of a drug. For example, federal laws in Canada do not classify digoxin as a prescription product. However, various provincial acts have placed digoxin on the prescription list within their respective provincial borders. Provincial or state laws may not remove a drug from the prescription list if it has been placed there by federal authority.

In general, there are two categories of medications: those that require a prescription and those that do not. *Prescription* drugs themselves represent a diversified group, ranging from those prescribed and refilled over the telephone (e.g., antihypertensive drugs) to those requiring a written *order* with no allowance for refills (e.g., potent narcotics).

Canadian Drug Regulations

Drug Laws
Drug laws evolved for the purpose of ensuring the safe and effective use of drugs. They control both the quality of drugs placed on the market and their use in the community. In Canada, the Food and Drug Act and the Narcotic Control Act (1961) form the basis of drug laws. The Health Protection Branch, which is part of the Department of National Health and Welfare, is responsible for administering these acts.

The Inland Revenue Act of 1875 was the first drug act introduced in Canada. It dealt specifically with the adulteration of alcohol. In 1953, after many revisions, the Food and Drug Act became law. This act presently controls the manufacture, distribution and sale of all drugs except narcotics.

The Opium Act of 1908 prohibited the unauthorized importation and possession of opium gum and the smoking of opium. This was the first act of the present-day Narcotic Control Act (1961), which controls the manufacture, distribution and sale of narcotic drugs.

Nonprescription Drugs
Nonprescription drugs can be obtained without a medical prescription. In Canada there are three groups of nonprescription medications.

The first group includes *proprietary medicines* and may be purchased in any retail outlet. They are effective for the treatment of self-limited minor illness, injury or discomfort. Generally, the directions for proper use are clearly indicated on the package, and the advice of a health professional is not required. Examples of proprietary medicines are some minor pain relievers, medicated shampoos and cough drops.

The second group of drugs includes those available mainly in pharmacies and commonly referred to as *over-the-counter (OTC) medications*. These agents are also intended for the treatment of self-limiting problems but may require the advice of a health professional to ensure their proper use. Examples of such drugs include laxatives, cough and cold medicines, and vitamins.

The third group is the smallest. It consists of medications available only in the pharmacy, to be used only upon the advice and recommendation of a physician. Insulin, nitroglycerin and muscle relaxants are examples of such medicines. Also included in this category are medications that can be purchased only if the pharmacist dispenses the drug personally after consulting with the patient. These drugs must be placed so as to limit public access. Examples include analgesic compounds containing low doses of codeine (e.g., 222s).

Prescription Drugs (Schedule F)
Many drugs require a prescription, which is an order given by a practitioner directing that a stated amount of a drug be dispensed for the person named in the order. Drugs for humans are available on prescription if the conditions they treat require the diagnosis and medical management of a physician or dentist.

All prescription drugs are listed in Schedule F of the Food and Drug Regulations and must be identified by the symbol **Pr** on their labels. More than two hundred drugs, representing a wide diversity of classes including antibiotics, antihypertensives, hormones and psychotropic medications, are listed in this schedule. Schedule F is frequently revised as new drugs are developed. Nonprescription drugs may be transferred to Schedule F if new hazards are uncovered.

Controlled Drugs (Schedule G)

Controlled drugs are listed in Schedule G of the Food and Drug Act. These have mood-modifying effects and can be habit forming. Like drugs listed in Schedule F, chemicals placed in Schedule G also require a prescription. However, greater control is exercised over their use because of their potential for abuse. The symbol ⓒ must appear on labels and all professional advertisements. Schedule G includes some narcotic analgesics (e.g., nalbuphine, butorphanol), amphetamines and related stimulants, and barbiturates (e.g., phenobarbital, amobarbital, secobarbital).

Narcotic Drugs

Narcotic drugs are controlled by the Narcotic Control Act and its regulations. This class of drugs includes derivatives of the coca leaf (cocaine), opiates and opium derivatives (morphine, codeine, hydromorphone, methadone and meperidine), phencyclidine, and cannabis (marijuana). Drugs classified legally as narcotics have potent psychotropic and addictive properties. This has led to stringent restrictions on their availability. The letter **N** must appear on all labels and professional advertisements.

Among the narcotics, only codeine can be purchased without a prescription. To qualify for nonprescription status, codeine must be combined with at least two additional drugs and contain no more than 8 mg of codeine per tablet, or 20 mg per 28 mL of oral solution. These codeine-containing products are known as *narcotic preparations*.

Restricted Drugs (Schedule H)

These substances have no recognized medicinal properties, have hallucinogenic properties and are dangerous. There are about twenty-three chemicals listed in Schedule H of the Food and Drug Act. Examples include LSD, peyote and mescaline.

Distribution of Drugs

As one progresses from nonprescription drugs to narcotic drugs, the distribution of these agents becomes more restrictive. Schedule F medications (prescription drugs) can be obtained by written or oral (i.e., verbal telephone order) prescription and may be refilled as often as indicated by the physician. Schedule G drugs (controlled drugs) can also be prescribed in written or oral format, but may be refilled only if indicated on a written prescription. Narcotic agents can be dispensed only according to a written prescription and cannot be refilled (i.e., they require a new written prescription every time).

Hospital and retail pharmacies are required by law to keep records of all narcotics received and dispensed. Although there are some federal regulations on the distribution of controlled drugs, the provinces dictate how much record keeping is necessary.

United States Drug Regulations

The Food, Drug and Cosmetic Act contains the basic laws relating to food and drugs in the United States and is enforced by the Food and Drug Administration. The Controlled Substances Act is enforced by the Drug Enforcement Administration, which is part of the United States Justice Department.

Drug Laws

The Import Drugs Act of 1848 was the first federal statute enacted to ensure drug quality. The act was initiated when adulterated quinine from Mexico was administered to American army troops suffering from malaria. The Food and Drug Act of 1906 required that drugs marketed for interstate commerce meet minimal standards of strength, purity, quality and proper labelling.

Revision of the act in 1938 was precipitated by the death of many patients who had used elixir of sulfanilamide containing toxic ethylene glycol. The Federal Food, Drug and Cosmetic Act required that drugs entering interstate commerce and sold in the United States must also meet standards of safety for human use.

The Durham-Humphrey Amendment of 1951 determined whether a drug should be available as a prescription or nonprescription product. The Kefauver-Harris Amendment of 1962, which came about as a result of the thalidomide tragedy, required that products provide proof of safety and efficacy. This applied to all products entering the market after 1938. This amendment also enforced tighter control, testing and marketing of new drugs.

The Comprehensive Drug Abuse Prevention and Control Act of 1970 regulates the manufacture, distribution and dispensing of controlled substances.

Nonprescription Drugs

Nonprescription or over-the-counter (OTC) medicines must be safe and effective. Safety is defined as a low potential for adverse drug effects causing harm that may result from abuse under conditions of widespread availability. Efficacy implies reasonable expectation of clinically significant relief in the majority of the population.

All nonprescription drugs in the United States can be purchased at any retail outlet. At present there are no categories of OTC that are restricted to pharmacy-only sales. For many years there have been attempts to create a "third class of drugs" that could be sold only in a pharmacy without the prescriber's order. However, the authority to create such a class of agents would require amendments to the Food, Drug and Cosmetic Act by the U.S. Congress. In 1985 the state of Florida took the initiative and found a way to overcome the federal law restriction. Pharmacists in that state may, after extensive consultation with the consumer, dispense medications from a limited formulary. The formulary lists medications previously requiring a prescription. Some examples include antihistamines, lindane, keratolytics and anthelmintics.

Prescription Drugs

As a result of the Durham-Humphrey Amendment, a class of agents was developed requiring the use of a prescription. A drug is placed on the prescription list if it is (a) habit-forming, (b) not safe for self-medication because of its toxicity, potential for harmful effects or method of administration, or (c) a "new drug" that has not been shown to be safe and is restricted to prescription-only status by the FDA when it approves the New Drug Application.

The purpose of these restrictions is to ensure the safe use of drugs by the general public and adequate supervision by a licensed practitioner. Prescription drugs, also known as legend drugs, require that their label bear the following statement: "Caution — Federal law prohibits dispensing without a prescription." Examples of legend or prescription drugs include antibiotics, antihypertensives and steroid medications.

Controlled Drugs

The Controlled Substances Act of 1971 supersedes most previous narcotic and drug abuse control laws. The act categorizes drugs into five schedules according to their potential for abuse.

Schedule I. Drugs in this schedule have a high potential for abuse and for the most part no accepted medical use in the United States. Schedule I contains certain opiates and opium derivatives, such as heroin. It also contains the hallucinogens LSD, cannabis, peyote and mescaline. The FDA has authorized the use of marijuana for treatment of glaucoma, and vomiting secondary to cancer chemotherapy.

Controlled substances require symbols located in the upper right-hand corner of the label. Schedule I drugs are identified by the symbols **C** or **I**.

Schedule II. Drugs in this category also have a high potential for abuse. In contradistinction to the chemicals listed in Schedule I, drugs in Schedule II have a currently accepted medical use. These are agents that, if abused, may lead to severe psychological or physical dependence. Schedule II includes opiates and opium derivatives (morphine, codeine, methadone and meperidine), derivatives of coca leaves (cocaine), and certain central nervous system stimulants (amphetamines, methylphenidate). All drugs in this class are labelled **C** or **II**.

Schedule III. Drugs in Schedule III have an accepted medical use and perhaps a lower potential for abuse than those in Schedules I or II. This category contains narcotic and non-narcotic drugs not listed in other schedules. Examples are glutethimide and nalorphine. Schedule III agents are labelled **C** or **III**.

Table 2.1
Drug schedules in Canada and the United States

Canadian category	Symbol on labels	U.S. category	Symbol on labels	Examples		
Schedule F (Food & Drug Regulations)	Pr	Prescription (Legend)	*	Antibiotics Antihypertensives Hormonal products	Can. only: U.S. only:	Benzodiazepines Nalbuphine Butorphanol
Schedule H (Food & Drug Act)	—	†Schedule I	Ⓒor I	Peyote LSD Mescaline	U.S. only:	Heroin Cannabis
Narcotics (Narcotic Control Act)	N	Schedule II	Ⓒor II	Morphine Codeine Methadone	Can. only: U.S. only:	Heroin Cannabis Pentazocine Amphetamine Short-acting barbiturates
Controlled (Schedule G, Food & Drug Act)	◇Ⓒ	Schedule III	Ⓒor III	Butalbital preparations Chlorphentermine	Can. only:	Amphetamine All barbiturates Nalbuphine Butorphanol
—	—	Schedule IV	Ⓒor IV	Benzodiazepines Phenobarbital Pentazocine		
Mostly OTC (restricted to pharmacy)		Schedule V	Ⓒor V	Low-dose codeine preparations		

* All labels must bear the warning, "Caution: Federal law prohibits dispensing without a prescription"
† Comprehensive Drug Abuse Prevention and Control Act

Schedule IV. Schedule IV drugs have a lower potential for abuse than those of Schedule III. However, abuse of these agents may still lead to limited physical or psychological dependence. This group includes long-acting barbiturates (phenobarbital), certain hypnotics (chloral hydrate) and minor tranquilizers (all benzodiazepines and meprobamate). All are labelled Ⓒ or **IV**.

Schedule V. Drugs in Schedule V have the lowest potential for abuse of all controlled substances. They include preparations containing limited quantities of certain narcotics for antitussive and antidiarrheal purposes. Although some items in Schedule V are considered OTC but are restricted to pharmacies only, most states have placed these drugs on the prescription list.

Table 2.1 lists Canadian and U.S. drug schedules.

Distribution

All prescription or legend drugs can be dispensed by oral (i.e., telephone) or written prescription with no restriction on the number of refills or repeats. Many states include Schedule V drugs under the same regulations. Schedule III and IV drugs can be obtained by written or oral prescription. The prescription cannot be filled or refilled six months after the date of issue, and the maximum number of repeats allowed is six. Schedule II agents can be dispensed only with a written prescription and no refills are allowed.

Nursing Practice and the Drug Laws

We have reviewed the many drug acts and regulations that constitute the drug laws in Canada and the United States. The next issue is how these apply to nursing practice. Nursing practice is regu-

Table 2.2
Legal concepts and nursing practice

Accountability	• Answerability (usually to an authority) for one's conduct or performance, responsibility for one's own actions
Liability	• Obligation according to law and determined by the individual's education, experience and circumstances
Negligence	• Civil negligence is acting below the professional standard of care the nurse owes to the patient; failure to exercise the care (or skill) that a reasonable, prudent person with similar experience and education would exercise, resulting in injury, loss or damage • Criminal negligence is defined by the Criminal Code of Canada and refers to doing anything or omitting to do anything that is one's duty to do and showing wanton or reckless disregard for the lives or safety of others
Competence	• Capable, suitable or proper performance; ability to perform to an accepted reasonable standard • Incompetence means just the opposite: not qualified or not able to do an act
Battery	• A civil wrong referring to intentionally touching a person without consent
Assault	• Threat to do physical harm to another coupled with a apparent ability to carry out the threat • Civil assault may result in payment of damages, whereas criminal assault can result in fines or imprisonment

lated not only by drug standards and legislation, but also by individual state or provincial nursing practice acts. The four areas deserving review are consent to drug therapy, drug prescribing or ordering, drug administration and drug dispensing.

Consent to Drug Therapy

In Canada, every adult of sound mind has a right to determine what may be done with his or her body. Every treatment, medical or nursing, requires a client's consent with the exception of those emergency situations where nurses and physicians act to preserve life or health. Each health care provider is responsible for ensuring that the individual gives valid consent to any *procedures* or therapies offered by that provider. Consent may be implied, such as when a patient reaches out to accept a pill or rolls over to receive an injection. In some situations, consent for drug therapy should be given verbally or formally in a written agreement. For consent to be legally valid, the following conditions must be met:

• The individual must have the *capacity* to give consent (factors include age, mental status and level of consciousness).
• Consent must be *voluntary* and is not be obtained through force, coercion or misrepresentation.
• Consent must be for the *specific treatment* and

cannot be extended to other treatments.
• Consent must be *informed,* i.e., the patient must be given, in language he or she understands, an honest and reasonable explanation of the treatment and the general risks of having and of not having such treatment. Alternatives to treatment should also be explored so that the patient can make a reasoned decision.

All competent adults have the right to refuse medications. Should a patient refuse any drug, the nurse should explore the reason for the refusal and respond appropriately. The patient may be experiencing a side effect that requires attention, or may not like the form or taste of the medication. Generally, the nurse will encourage the patient to accept drug therapy. In some situations, the nurse may have to force administration. However, this usually occurs only after the patient has been certified mentally incompetent by a physician. Such situations require careful professional judgment. Remember that in law, intentionally touching an individual without his or her consent can result in a charge of battery or assault. (See Table 2.2.)

Prescribing Drugs

Historically, the physician prescribed, the pharmacist dispensed and the nurse administered medications. Prescribing of medications has been exclusively a medical function. However, some provinces or states may permit limited prescribing by nurse practitioners.

Some agencies have established procedures allowing nurses to administer medication without a physician's order, for example, in emergency situations or to treat minor symptoms associated with self-limiting problems such as headaches or nasal congestion. In the latter case, the medications administered are usually nonprescription products.

Nurses may also be guided by approved institutional *protocols,* whereby clinical algorithms provide the nurse with the basis for clinical practice and decision making. The protocol specifies the sequence of tests, treatments or actions that are appropriate according to the patient's symptoms or prior test/treatment results. For example, a heparin protocol is presented in Chapter 44. However, nurses should implement a previously approved protocol only on the order of a physician.

Drug Administration

Drug administration is an important role for the nurse. Three conditions must be met before a nurse may safely administer medication. These are: (a) the medication order must be valid, (b) the physician and nurse must be licensed, and (c) the nurse must know the purpose, actions, effects and major side effects of the drug.

A valid order leaves no room for doubt. It must include the name of the medication, its dose, the route and frequency of administration and the prescriber's signature. The law requires that a nurse check a drug order with the prescribing physician when faced with a question, doubt or apparent error in the order. The nurse has a moral, ethical and legal responsibility to ensure that the order is appropriate for the patient. It is the right of a nurse to refuse to give a medication if he or she feels it is inappropriate. The physician assumes full responsibility if he or she administers the medication personally.

The following example illustrates the importance of validating orders and the shared responsibility between physicians and nurses for patient safety. A young man is admitted to a medical unit due to unstable diabetes. The physician telephones an order for regular insulin, and the novice nurse believes that the order is for 50 units of insulin stat. This order does not seem to be correct, and

the nurse verifies it with a drug reference text and a discussion with a colleague and a pharmacist. Recognizing the potential danger to this patient, the nurse contacts the physician, who clarifies that the order is for 15 units.

In the course of drug administration, society and the law expect nurses to perform to a reasonable standard consistent with that of other nurses with similar education and experience. In order for nurses to fulfill their responsibilities within the nursing process for management of drug therapy, they must have a thorough understanding of the pharmacology of the drugs being administered. Nurses use this knowledge to guide the assessment of patients, to plan and implement the administration of medication, to focus the evaluation of a patient's response to drug treatment and to identify areas of emphasis for patient teaching.

In the administration of all medications, nurses must be aware of, and have an obligation to follow, the policies and procedures of the specific clinical setting. A *policy* is a regulatory statement made by an agency defining what can and cannot be done. While policy statements cannot contradict legislation, they can limit or expand nursing practice within that setting. Procedures describe a series of recommended actions for the completion of a specific task or function. In other words, procedures outline how a policy will be followed. Unlike a protocol, which allows for some independent decision making within guidelines, a procedure must be followed completely.

Although there are relatively few legislated regulations regarding the nursing management of drug therapy, there are some concepts that apply generally to nursing practice and, in some situations, specifically to medication administration. (See Table 2.2 on the previous page.)

Administration of intravenous medication. Medication can be directly administered into a vein through large-volume infusions or by direct push — the administration of small-volume, undiluted medications directly into the vein or into intravenous tubing. Administration of large-volume infusions has become common nursing practice in many hospital and community settings. In contrast, because of the potential risk, direct push is considered an advanced competency carried out by nurses certified in the technique and following the policy and procedure of the clinical setting.

Because direct intravenous push is potentially more risky, the policy statements of the institution that allow a specially trained nurse to administer drugs in this manner must carefully delineate the roles of nurses and physicians, and present guidelines for this procedure. They should include a list of drugs and routes of administration to be used only by physicians and a list of criteria for permitting nurses to give medicines intravenously.

As with other routes of administration, the nurse must know the pharmacology of the drug, including the expected therapeutic and nontherapeutic effects. In addition, the nurse must know the rate of administration, incompatibilities with other drugs or the intravenous fluid, and the monitoring parameters for potential adverse effects.

Drug Dispensing

In the hospital, the nurse must be careful to differentiate between drug administration and drug dispensing to avoid violation of the Pharmacy Practice Act. The act states that dispensing of medication is a function of a licensed pharmacist. It is generally agreed that it is legal for a nurse to take one dose of a drug for a particular patient from a pharmacy-prepackaged, properly labelled medication container at the nurses' station, since this constitutes drug administration. On the other hand, it is not legal for a nurse to fill or refill a container from the nurses' station, or any other container, with the drug specified because such an act is dispensing and may be performed legally only by a pharmacist.

The following acts are specifically *prohibited* by Canadian federal laws and apply to the nurse's handling of all prescription drugs:

• Compounding or dispensing the designated drugs except by authorized parties for legal distribution and administration.
• Distributing the drugs to any person who is not licensed or authorized by law to receive them.

Although the Pharmacy Act is clear in defining who is authorized to dispense, any experienced nurse who has worked in remote areas or where pharmacy service is limited can testify to the lack of adequate provisions for the act. Most will agree

that in a situation where a pharmacist is not immediately available, a nurse may provide sufficient medications as ordered by the physician to cover those times when the services of a pharmacist are not available.

Consistent with drug laws, the physician may prescribe, dispense and administer medications. When a nurse is faced with a situation where he or she has to dispense a limited quantity of medication, it would seem reasonable to have the prescribing physician check that the proper drug has been given out and that the dose and instruction on the label are correct. This procedure would not contravene the Pharmacy Act. If this situation occurred frequently, it would be in the best interest of the nurse to become familiar with the basic aspects of pharmacy distribution, such as dispensing and labelling.

In remote areas, a registered nurse may have to assume responsibility for the pharmacy. In such cases, written policies need to be developed by administration, nursing and medical representatives of the institution for legal protection of nurse and patient. It may be advisable to have these policies approved by the respective provincial or state professional associations in nursing and pharmacy. Once the policies have been adopted, the nurse should receive additional preparation and education in pharmacy practice, such as inventory and storage control, method of labelling drugs, and method of narcotic control. A periodic visit by a licensed pharmacist is recommended to ensure that all procedures and operations accord with accepted standards of practice.

Controlled and narcotic substances. Every practising nurse encounters situations that require knowledge of, or familiarity with, controlled or narcotic substances. Federal and provincial or state laws dealing with those substances are complex, but it is important for nurses to know their responsibilities and limitations under the regulation.

The Narcotic Control Act in Canada and the Controlled Substances Act in the United States were enacted to improve the administration and regulation of the manufacturing, distribution and dispensing of these substances. They provide a closed system of distribution for legitimate handling of the drugs. The purpose of this system is to reduce the widespread diversion of these drugs from legitimate channels to the illicit market.

Only authorized persons can be in possession of a narcotic or controlled substance. Legal possession by a nurse is limited to the following situations:

• When a drug is administered to a patient on the order of a physician. The nurse is then acting as an agent for the practitioner.
• When the nurse is acting as the official custodian of narcotics in the hospital or clinic.
• When the nurse is a patient for whom a physician has prescribed narcotics.

Federal and provincial or state laws make the possession of controlled or narcotic substances a crime except for the above specified cases. The laws make no distinction between registered and practical nurses in regard to possession of controlled drugs. Violating or failing to comply with the act is punishable by fine, imprisonment, or both.

Nursing procedure and controlled substances. Unlike simple prescription drugs, certain rules for controlled drugs have been accepted in most hospitals. A prn order (pro re nata, or "as required") for narcotics must be rewritten every seventy-two hours. A standing order (i.e., a drug dose administered by the nurse for the physician without first obtaining a signed order) is not permitted for narcotic drugs. In an emergency situation, a verbal order is permitted if the nurse documents the nature of the emergency in the chart and the physician validates the order within twenty-four hours.

When a narcotic drug is administered to a patient, the nurse must record the date, time of administration, patient's name, physician's name, and signature of the nurse. When a dose of a narcotic is refused by the patient, it should be disposed of in the presence of a witness. If a dose of the drug is contaminated or wasted, the nurse should make an entry in the records book explaining how the dose was disposed of, and the entry should be signed by a witness.

All controlled substances stored at nursing stations must be kept in locked cabinets so that only authorized personnel have access to them.

Policies and procedures for the secure distribu-tion and accounting of narcotic and controlled substances must be written by the health agency (province, state, board, hospital). These should reflect national standards of practice, such as the "Guidelines for the Secure Distribution of Narcotic and Controlled Drugs in Hospitals" written by a joint committee of the Bureau of Dangerous Drugs, the Canadian Hospital Association, the Canadian Nurses Association and the Canadian Society of Hospital Pharmacists in January, 1990.

Sources of drug errors. The American Society of Hospital Pharmacists defines a medication error as:

> The administration of the wrong medication or dose of medication, drug, diagnostic agent, or treatment requiring the use of such agents to the wrong patient or at the wrong time or the failure to administer such agents at the specified time or in the manner prescribed or normally considered as acceptable practice.

The literature indicates that the average rate of error within institutions is approximately eleven percent. Fortunately, not all such errors cause harm to the patient, but all errors must be addressed seriously. The most frequent cause of error (at least seventy percent of the time) is due to failure to follow policy or procedure. For example, it is standard procedure to check the identification of the patient before giving any medication but with frequent interruptions or workload factors or complacency, nurses may overlook this important step.

As many as twenty percent of errors are caused by communication problems such as improper abbreviations, incomplete or illegible orders, or failure to verify verbal orders. Telephone orders constitute a special problem because the order may be misunderstood and the nurse may not read the order back to the physician to verify that it is correct. Also, nurses must ensure that the order is signed by the physician within twenty-four hours. Telephone orders should be limited to emergencies or urgent situations.

Many drug distribution systems have been developed to minimize drug errors. Use of computer systems or sending the physician's orders directly to the pharmacy prevents errors that may occur during transcribing. Similarly, the use of a computer-generated medication administration record, which is sent from the pharmacy to the nursing unit, reduces the risk of error. Unfortunately, in some agencies, ward secretaries or clerks transcribe orders and nurses write orders on cards for administration. Such systems increase the risk for error. It is a common requirement that all transcribed orders be countersigned by a nurse, who then shares liability for any errors that occur.

Product liability. Although manufacturers are liable for injury caused by defects in their products, nurses should be alert to defects in the drugs they administer. Detection of chemical defects is beyond the nurse's responsibility, but detection of observable physical defects is not. Nurses should be keenly aware of the proper physical characteristics of the drugs they administer. Discolouration or improper consistency of tablets, capsules, liquids, or precipitates, or foreign bodies in parenteral fluids, should be considered suspect and be referred to the pharmacist.

Drug information sources. Many good reference books provide excellent drug information. They are helpful for double-checking doses, rates of administration, drug interactions and side effects. They can be used to clarify orders and avoid drug errors. However, they should never be used as a substitute for contacting the prescribing physician. The most popular texts are the *Compendium of Pharmaceuticals and Specialties (CPS)* in Canada and the *Physician's Desk Reference (PDR)*, the *American Hospital Formulary Service (AHFS)* and the *U.S. Pharmacopeial Drug Information (USP DI)* in the United States. All these reference sources are reviewed and revised annually.

The *CPS* and *PDR* are similar; both contain a list of drug monographs plus a limited product-recognition section with coloured illustrations of medications. The *CPS* is compiled and produced by the Canadian Pharmaceutical Association for the benefit of all health professionals. It can be purchased only through the Association or at health-professional book stores. The *PDR* is published by the Medical Economics Company, Inc. and is intended primarily for physicians, although it is available at most public book stores.

The *AHFS* is published by the American Society of Hospital Pharmacy; it is updated with four supplements yearly. The volume contains monographs on every drug available in the United States. The *USP DI*, published by the United States Pharmacopeial Convention, comprises drug monographs from both the United States and Canada. It also is updated throughout the year with supplements.

Conclusion

The nursing profession is a challenging and interesting career. Along with the responsibilities of providing safe and effective nursing care, the nurse also has a major responsibility in the administration of medications. The nurse must be familiar not only with the ethical and moral issues surrounding the administration of drugs, but the legal issues as well.

Response to Clinical Challenge

Ms. F. has given important information during the admission nursing assessment. The nurse should notify the physician in the emergency department, discuss the possibility of pregnancy and expect a change in medication order. Failure to take this action could be called negligence (see Table 2.2). Any nurse who does not recognize that such action is needed may be judged incompetent — that is, not capable of performing his or her duties.

Further Reading

Fennell K. Prescriptive authority for nurse-midwives: a historical review. *Nurs Clin North Am* 1991; 26(2):511–522.

Health & Welfare Canada. *Health Protection and Drug Laws.* Ottawa: Canadian Government Publishing Centre; 1983.

Keatings M, Smith O. *Ethical and Legal Issues in Canadian Nursing.* Toronto: W.B. Saunders; 1995.

Pike S. Ethics, the law and clinical decisions. *Can Nurse* 1993;89(5):39–40.

Strauss S, Sherman M. A capsulated history of drug laws in the U.S. *U.S. Pharmacist* 1985;10:11.

Drugs and Society

Topics Discussed
● Definition of chemical name, generic/nonproprietary name, trade/proprietary name; placebo
● Drug classification and nomenclature
● Drug misuse and abuse
● Psychosocial factors in drug use
● Drug development and testing
● Nursing practice and drug research
● Contemporary issues in drug development, marketing and use
● Sources of drug information

As long ago as 1000 BCE, humankind was using drugs that affected the heart, central nervous system, skin, gastrointestinal tract and respiratory system. Examples included cardiac glycosides, alcohol, cocaine, antiseptics, laxatives, belladonna alkaloids and the powerful poison curare. While this may seem an impressive list, notice what is missing: anesthetics were discovered only in 1842. Imagine having surgery prior to this time.

There are many reasons we use drugs today: prevention of illness with immunization, cure of infections with antibiotics, relief of symptoms with analgesics and antipsychotics, and management of chronic conditions with insulin and thyroid products are among the most important uses. Drugs are also useful for diagnostic purposes; for example, radioactive iodine is used to confirm hyperthyroidism, and phentolamine hydrochloride aids in the diagnosis of pheochromocytoma (an adrenal tumour). Drug treatment deserves both skepticism and respect. The Greeks must have understood this paradox when they named these chemicals *pharmakon,* a word meaning both "drug" and "poison."

Many people engage in self-medication for a variety of common problems. In some instances, this results in safe, efficient and cost-effective care. In other situations, self-medication can cause harm because of misdiagnosis, improper use of a drug or use of the wrong agent, and interactions between drugs or between drugs and food.

This chapter provides a brief overview of the social, rather than chemical, issues related to drug therapy and a discussion of contemporary issues.

Drug Nomenclature

Have you ever wandered through a library and marvelled at how this vast amount of information is organized? The classification of drugs is almost as overwhelming. If you are a botanist you might like a *taxonomic* grouping based on the plants and animals from which the drugs are obtained. If chemistry is your field, you might prefer a *chemical* classification, which groups drugs according to structural similarities. (Interestingly, these drugs may not have similar pharmacologic actions or properties.) The pharmacologist identifies drugs by their mechanisms of actions (pharmacologic classification). Those who prescribe drugs are most interested in the clinical indication for their use (*therapeutic* classification). Nurses will find both pharmacologic and therapeutic classifications helpful. Table 3.1 shows the various ways in which digoxin is classified.

What's In a Name?
The naming of drugs is confusing to the novice in pharmacology because a drug can have several names. Drugs are named according to their molecular formula, their scientific name, and the drug marketing people's perception of a "catchy" trade name. One drug can have several aliases. The

Table 3.1
Classifications of digoxin

Classification	Term	Rationale
Taxonomic	Digitalis	• A group of drugs found in plants and the venom of certain toads
Chemical	Glycoside	• A chemical with a steroid portion which is the pharmacologically active part and a sugar portion
Pharmacologic	Cardiotonic	• Most significant action is on the myocardium
Therapeutic	Antidysrhythmic	• Indicated for treatment of tachydysrhythmias (rapid, irregular heartbeat)

chemical name is the true scientific name which precisely describes the chemical composition and molecular structure; for example, 2-methy-2-propyl-1,3-propanedioldicarbamate. (Say that fast three times!) The *generic name,* also called the *nonproprietary name,* is an abbreviated version of the scientific name. It is simpler and not owned by any particular proprietor; for example, meprobamate. (Can you find me-pro-bamate in the previous chemical name?) The *trade, brand* or *proprietary name* is owned by a proprietor. It is a proper noun that is copyrighted; for example, Wallace calls their brand of meprobamate Miltown®, whereas Wyeth-Ayerst has named their brand Equanil®.

The term "generic" has gained attention recently because of the debate regarding the use of brand versus generic products. This is a complex issue that lies beyond the scope of this text. By definition, the products must be chemically equivalent. However, they can vary in the method of preparation, and in the presence of special agents such as preservatives, bufferings or coatings which may affect bioavailability (the degree to which the drug becomes available to the target tissue). Brand name companies argue that their products are better; companies that produce generics argue that their products are equally effective and cheaper.

Drug Misuse and Abuse

The distinction between the terms "misuse" and "abuse" seems to be a fine one. The first refers to the inappropriate use of legal drugs, while the second commonly means patterns of illicit drug use. Drug misuse encompasses a range of situations in which drugs are erroneously used through lack of knowledge or competence, or through unrealistic attitudes regarding the expected benefits. Misuse includes overutilization, underutilization, or inappropriate use of legal drugs and is generally due to the two poorly informed components of the health care system: professionals and the public. Although the desired outcomes of this type of drug use are intended to be beneficial, unfortunately in many instances the results do not warrant the associated risks (including expense).

In contrast to misuse, drug abuse refers to the self-administration of a chemical substance to an extent that significantly impairs the user's physical or mental health or ability to function in a social context. Abuse involves use of a drug in any manner that deviates from culturally acceptable medical and social uses. The term "addiction" has previously been used to denote the overwhelming

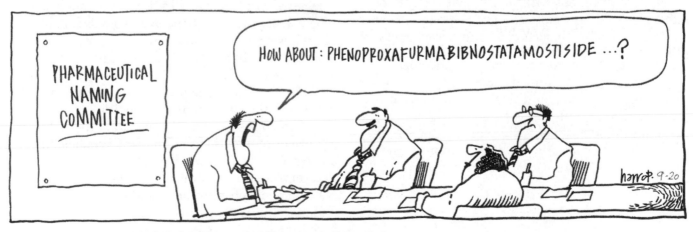

Table 3.2
Definitions of drug dependence

Psychological dependence	A state of emotional reliance on a drug in order to maintain well-being; may range from a mild desire to intense craving. Exhibited pattern of behaviour is individual
Physical dependence	An altered physiological state caused by drug use in which withdrawal symptoms occur if the drug is stopped. Serious and fatal symptoms can result from withdrawal. For example, after prolonged use of the benzodiazepines, withdrawal can cause serious psychological and physical reactions including agitation, aggressive or psychotic behaviour and seizures
Functional dependence	Reliance on a drug such as insulin to survive, or acquired dependence on drug action in the body system

involvement with obtaining and using a drug for its psychic effects rather than for medically or socially approved reasons. More recently, the World Health Organization (WHO) has suggested the less judgmental term "dependence," which is defined as a state of reliance upon a drug that is harmful to physical or mental health, social well-being or economic functioning. This may include psychological or physical dependence, as well as functional dependence. Table 3.2 lists definitions and examples.

Patterns of Drug Misuse
Drug misuse can occur because of:

- overdose: unintentional
- underdose: unintentional
- omission: intentional; possible factors include financial costs, attitudes regarding drug use (drugs mean illness, loss of independence)
- self-selection, self-medication: e.g., using the wrong medication
- duplication: by self-selection of OTCs or combinations of prescriptions from multiple doctors
- pill swapping
- knowledge deficit: poor initial instructions; sensory changes that may affect ability to read labels, hear instructions; complex dosage schedules
- iatrogenic (physician-caused) problems: excessive dosages, prescribing additional drugs to treat other drug-induced problems
- expired medications
- poor initial evaluation: e.g., telephone prescriptions, automatic refills without reevaluation

Drug Abuse in Health Professionals
The abuse of medications is not limited to a particular age or socioeconomic group. When health professionals become drug dependent, the results are doubly serious: in addition to personal risk, there is risk to clients. Acknowledging that this problem is often denied or ignored, many professional groups have developed programs to offer diagnosis, support and treatment. Abuse and dependence on drugs, alcohol or both can be successfully treated but must first be recognized and acknowledged.

Psychosocial Factors in Drug Use

Drugs have symbolic meaning to every patient. Some see them as magic cures, others view drug taking as a sign of weakness or loss of independence. Social and cultural factors as well as the treatment setting influence the outcome of drug therapy. One psychological phenomenon that deserves a brief discussion is the placebo effect.

Placebos
The use of placebos is one of the oldest medical practices and is still commonly used today. The term placebo is derived from the Latin, "I shall please." A *placebo* is any therapeutic procedure, including medications and surgery, that does not have specific activity for the condition being treated. Placebo response is the effect of any such procedure or medication, and may be psychological or biological. For example, it is theorized that placebos relieve pain by stimulating the body to release its own endorphins (opiate-like substances that produce analgesia).

Table 3.3
The placebo: Principles and clinical application

Principles	Clinical application
• Individuals show therapeutic improvement with placebos for a wide variety of conditions including acne, hypertension, depression and postoperative pain	Some so-called active drugs may in fact work only because of the placebo response, not due to the drug's action
• In most studies, approximately 30%–35% of patients treated with placebos will respond	Thirty percent of patients with abdominal surgery report relief of pain with a placebo
• No well-defined personality type has been found to be a placebo reactor. In fact, different people will respond to placebos at different times, with up to 90% of individuals reporting positive effects over time. In general, reactors may be more outgoing, anxious, and concerned with physical complaints. Placebo response is unrelated to age, sex, education, race, or social class	Everyone might be a placebo responder in certain circumstances
• The mechanism of the placebo effect is not well understood but relates to the patient's knowledge, desire for improvement, past experience with drugs, and the relationship with the doctor (or therapist or nurse). It may be that placebos work because the individual wants them to	There is a common myth that placebo responders are weak willed and easily suggestible, yet perhaps just the opposite is true: they may be strong, independent people who "cure themselves"
• Placebo response may be either positive or negative	ASA is an effective analgesic, but some people do not believe it works because it is available without prescription
• The use of placebos presents an ethical dilemma: e.g., they can be used: to "prove" that pain is not "real," to punish a malingerer, or to satisfy a doctor's need to treat when other means fail	"Real" postoperative pain may be relieved by placebos
• Placebos carry risks. They foster deception in doctor-patient and nurse-patient relationships. Given that the relationship is therapeutic, it should not be jeopardized	Patients have the right to be informed; should they be told that a placebo is being used? Placebos have caused adverse drug reactions (including anaphylaxis!) How would you react if told you were taking a placebo?

In one study, 97 preoperative patients were divided into two groups: one received a routine visit from the anesthetist, the other received more intensive contact that included an explanation of the nature, causes and course of postoperative pain. The second group required almost fifty percent less analgesic and went home 2.7 days earlier than the first. The question may be posed: Is the response to a placebo the chemical basis of mental events, or the mental basis of chemical events? The psychological response to any drug is influenced by the setting and the relationship between the patient and the health care provider. Clear, direct communication with the patient can be as important as the drug administered.

Table 3.3 summarizes important principles regarding the placebo.

Development of New Drugs

The development of a new drug may require years of expert testing and research with thousands of chemical components. Table 3.4 on the next page lists the usual stages of drug testing.

Limitations of Testing

Initial clinical trials, following extensive testing on animals, are conducted on normal, male, adult volunteers. Thus, responses in children, all adult women and all older adults are not known in early phases of testing. The small number of patients are carefully selected. Trials are time limited. Adverse reactions that develop with long duration of drug treatment are not detected. As a case in point, the antipsychotics were heralded in the 1950s as the great new discovery that would revolutionize psychiatry — until tardive dyskinesia began occurring about a decade later.

Table 3.4
Stages in the development of a new drug

Stage	Explanation
Preclinical testing	• Tests in animals determine toxicity, pharmacokinetics, potential uses
IND (investigational new drug) status	• May have limited application to humans
Clinical testing:	• May take several years
Phase I	• Tests in normal volunteers evaluate drug metabolism and general effects
Phase II	• Tests in small sample of pts establish dosage ranges, therapeutic effects
Phase III	• Tests in larger sample of pts determine safety and effectiveness
New drug application	• Selected medical centres and qualified MDs use drug in selected pts under
Phase IV	closely monitored conditions; drug is released for general marketing
Postmarketing surveillance	• Voluntary reporting of effects and adverse reactions

Orphan Drugs

Some drugs, although useful in the treatment of specific diseases, may be abandoned without government help before their development is completed because they have a limited market (i.e., they are useful only for rare diseases). These products are called *orphan drugs*. An example is clofazimine for the treatment of leprosy.

Canada does not recognize orphan drugs. However, in the United States the manufacturer of a designated orphan drug that is the first to be approved for a specific rare disease or condition has several years for exclusive marketing regardless of the patent status of the drug.

Nursing and Drug Research

Clinical trials for drug evaluation may be conducted in all settings. Nurses may participate in many ways that ensure the accuracy of the findings and fulfill ethical obligations to patients and families. The nurse may help identify potential candidates for the trial, explain the protocol to patients and families, ensure that informed consent is obtained and administer medications according to protocol. Agency policies govern whether further certification is required for nurses, physicians or pharmacists giving these drugs. Monitoring and documenting response is another important contribution.

With respect to the research process for drug trials, the term placebo has a specialized meaning. In this context, the placebo is a pharmacologically inert substance given in place of the active drug to compare therapeutic and adverse responses. Experimental study designs use two groups of subjects divided into the control group, which may receive a placebo or have an alternative treatment, and the experimental group, which does receive the trial drug. A double-blind drug trial also controls for bias in that neither the physician/nurse nor the patient/family knows whether the trial drug or the placebo is being used.

Contemporary Issues in Drug Development, Marketing and Use

There are many issues concerning drug development, marketing and use in society. As a detailed discussion is beyond the scope of this text, a few comments must suffice. Current literature provides further information on these concerns.

One important issue relates to the rights of consumers: should all people have equal access to medications, and should all available medications be marketed and provided by health insurance? A related issue is the concern of cost efficiency; for example, one antibiotic may be efficacious and inexpensive, whereas another may produce equal outcomes at greater cost. Economic accountability is a modern-day responsibility for all health care providers, and nurses are expected to develop awareness of the cost implications of therapeutic interventions. The relative benefits, risks and costs of drugs are determined at all levels of the health care system, as shown in Table 3.5.

Another issue that has not been adequately addressed by the pharmaceutical industry centres on gender and age issues in drug research.

Table 3.5
Benefit/risk/cost decision in drug therapy

Health care agent	Decision
Drug manufacturer	Research a specific chemical?
Federal regulatory agency	Allow a drug on the market?
Provincial/State government	Include drug in health insurance plan?
Hospital/Agency	Include drug in formulary?
Physician	Select drug to treat patient?
Pharmacist	Interactions with other drugs?
Nurse	Equipment for administration?
Patient	Follow or question health professional's advice?

Continued vigilance is necessary to determine specific risks related to gender and age.

The right to prescribe medications has been traditionally protected by physicians. Nurse practitioners in many states have been granted specific prescribing rights. There are many questions to be answered regarding extending this role to other health care professionals. Should physical therapists prescribe analgesics and anti-inflammatories? Should pharmacists prescribe the medication following the diagnosis by the physician? What knowledge base would nurses require to assume this role in a variety of clinical settings?

A final word on an important issue, namely the commonplace use of herbal remedies. Not to be confused with the application of herbal medicines by trained health care providers, the use of health food products to treat minor ailments or more serious conditions is not based on scientific research. The inherent risks are similar to those previously discussed with self-medication. Is this herb or health food product effective and safe? Is it being taken for a condition that is misdiagnosed? Is more effective treatment being ignored?

Sources of Drug Information

Learning about the many new drugs entering the market annually, along with new uses for old products, can be overwhelming without a systematic approach. It is very difficult to know everything about every drug you administer, monitor, or take. Memorizing pharmacological information is a little like memorizing a large telephone book. The most effective approach is to master the information that is required and determine quick sources of further information that will be accessible when needed. Box 3.1 suggests a method for learning about drugs.

Box 3.1
Learning about new drugs and drug uses

✔ **First**
Before becoming overwhelmed, make a list of the drug categories that are most commonly used in your setting. For example, in many hospitals the most frequently used groups include antibiotics, diuretics, sedatives, narcotic analgesics and cardiac drugs.

✔ **Second**
Learn one drug in each group. It is then much easier to understand other drugs in the same family.

✔ **Third**
Seek out reliable sources of drug information, including written information and competent personnel.

✔ **Fourth**
Use a systematic approach when studying new drugs. Chapter 1 outlined such an approach. Recall that one characteristic of critical thinking is to have an organized and systematic approach to solving problems and making decisions.

Further Reading

Canadian Public Health Association. *Benefit, risk and cost management of drugs. Report of the CPHA National Advisory Panel on Risk-Benefit Management of Drugs*. Ottawa: CPHA; 1993.

French S. The placebo effect: magic pills. *Nurs Times* 1990;86(17):28.

Holloway M. Trends in pharmacology: treatment for addiction. *Scientific American* 1991 (March):94–103.

Solari-Twadell P. Recreational drugs: societal and professional issues. *Nurs Clin North Am* 1991; 26(2):499–510.

Trevelyn J. Herbal medicine. *Nurs Times* 1993; 89(43):36–38.

General Principles of Pharmacology

Unit 2 introduces the reader to the meaning of the word drug and the general principles underlying the use of drugs. The unit is divided into five chapters. Chapter 4 discusses the physical and chemical properties of drugs and their influence on drug absorption. In Chapter 4, we also present the various routes by which drugs may be administered. Chapter 5 describes the distribution of drugs throughout the body and their elimination, primarily by metabolism in the liver and/or excretion by the kidneys. We also take this opportunity to discuss the nature of the interaction of drugs with their receptors. In Chapter 6, we discuss the nature of these drug-receptor interactions to prepare nurses for the subsequent chapters in the book that describe the particular types of drug receptors stimulated or blocked by drugs. Chapter 7 deals with drug interactions. Chapter 8, the final chapter of this unit, describes the effects of aging on drug action. As patients age, they often respond differently to drugs. Nurses must recognize this and be prepared to deal with the special needs of the elderly.

Although Unit 2 contains little information on any one group of drugs or the treatment of any disease, it forms the core of this book with direct links to all other chapters. The general principles of pharmacology, outlining as they do drug absorption, distribution and metabolism, together with a discussion of how drugs actually work, apply to all subsequent units of this book.

Routes of Administration and Drug Absorption

Topics Discussed
● Definition of drug, pharmacology, pharmacodynamics, pharmacotherapeutics, therapeutic objective; ionized, nonionized; first-pass metabolism
● Drug solubility
● Routes of administration
● Bioavailability

A drug is a chemical that affects living processes. Pharmacology is the study of the effects of drugs on the body, including the absorption, distribution, metabolism and elimination of drugs. The study of pharmacology also encompasses the mechanisms of action, therapeutic uses and adverse effects of drugs. To understand the material that follows in

this book, the reader should become familiar with the terms shown in Box 4.1.

Solubility of Drugs

If a drug is to be absorbed and distributed throughout the body, it must be in solution in the body. The absorption of a drug involves moving it from a solution in the fluids of the gastrointestinal tract to a solution in the blood plasma. It is important, therefore, to understand the factors that control the solubility of drugs.

Most drugs are either weak acids or weak bases. Acetylsalicylic acid, barbiturates and non-steroidal anti-inflammatory drugs (NSAIDs) are examples of acidic drugs. Narcotics, tricyclic antidepressants and phenothiazine antipsychotics are examples of basic drugs.

When acidic or basic drugs dissolve in the body fluids, they form both ionized and nonionized drug

---

Box 4.1
Basic definitions

Drug	Any chemical that affects living organisms. When used in medicine, a drug is usually defined as any substance used to diagnose, treat, mitigate or prevent a disease state or to restore, correct or modify organic function in humans or animals
Pharmacology	The science dealing with the origin, nature and effects of drugs on living tissue (i.e., the study of how drugs produce their biologic effects)
Clinical pharmacology	The study of drugs in humans
Pharmacodynamics	The study of how drugs work (i.e., their mechanisms of action)
Pharmacotherapeutics	The application of drugs in the prevention, treatment or diagnosis of disease
Pharmacognosy	The study of natural drug sources (e.g., plants, animals, minerals)
Toxicology	The study of poisons and adverse effects of drugs on living organisms
Therapeutic objective	The goal of producing the maximum benefit with the minimum harm

molecules. Ionized means that the drug carries an electrical charge, negative for acidic drugs and positive for bases.

Ionized drug molecules are soluble in water and insoluble in fat. This means that they easily remain in solution in the aqueous fluids of the body, such as the gastrointestinal juices or the plasma, but they have great difficulty diffusing across lipid membranes, such as the gastrointestinal tract or the blood-brain barrier.

Nonionized drug molecules are more lipid soluble and dissolve less readily in water than their ionized counterparts. Although nonionized drug molecules are only sparingly soluble in water, they still remain in solution in the body because of the large volume of water available to dissolve them. The total body water of an average 70-kg person is approximately 41 L, and this large volume of water is capable of diluting nonionized drug molecules to the point where they remain in solution.

Figure 4.1 depicts the effects of ionization on the ability of a drug to cross a lipid membrane. From this figure, it can be seen that only the nonionized molecules can diffuse back and forth across a lipid membrane. It also shows that a balance exists between the ionized and nonionized molecules on each side of the lipid membrane. The ratio of ionized to nonionized molecules on either side is determined by the pH of the fluid. In the stomach, for example, acids are mainly nonionized and bases are ionized. Once drugs move into the intestine, more acidic molecules become ionized and more basic molecules change from ionized to nonionized. As will be discussed later, this has considerable significance in determining drug absorption from each site.

The relevance of this information will become apparent as we review the routes of drug administration and the factors that control drug absorption and distribution.

Routes of Drug Administration

Drugs may be injected, ingested, inhaled or insufflated (blown into a body cavity). In addition, they may be applied to the skin or instilled into the ear, nose or eye. Drugs may be used for their local effects or for their systemic actions. The following pages discuss the absorption of drugs following their parenteral, oral or rectal administration.

Figure 4.1
Diffusion of a drug across a lipid membrane

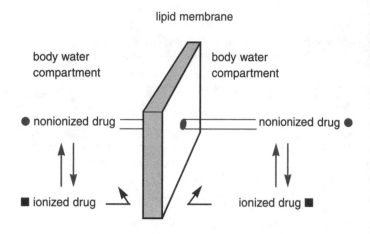

Table 4.1 presents the advantages and disadvantages of some common routes of drug administration.

Parenteral Administration

Intravenous injection and infusion. Drug absorption is immediate and blood levels are predictable following intravenous (IV) injection. However, because intravenous administration produces an immediate effect, an incorrect calculation of the dose can lead to instant toxicity.

Intravenous injections should be given slowly to allow the drug to be diluted in the blood before it reaches the heart. If drugs are administered rapidly, high concentrations reach the heart quickly. This can lead to cardiac arrhythmias. Nurses should also be concerned about the rapid intravenous administration of drug that has been diluted in a large volume of fluid because this can cause fluid overload.

Intramuscular injection. Drugs injected into muscle are absorbed through blood capillaries. Capillaries have pores and drug molecules easily pass through these pores into the blood. Once in the bloodstream, the drug molecules are rapidly carried away from the muscle and moved to other parts of the body.

Most intramuscular (IM) injections involve the administration of a drug in solution. In this

Table 4.1
Comparison of routes of administration

Route of drug administration	Advantages	Disadvantages
Intravenous	• immediate effect • predictable blood levels • rapid modification of dose • preferred route for patients in shock • large volumes can be given	• incorrect calculation can lead to immediate toxicity • rapid injection can lead to arrhythmias • oily solutions are contraindicated
Intramuscular	• drug is absorbed from solutions within the muscle in 10–30 min	• blood flow to muscle mass must be adequate for absorption • only small volumes can be given • IM injections are contraindicated if patient is taking an anticoagulant • IM injections may interfere with some lab tests (injection into muscle causes destruction of some muscle cells and increases enzyme levels)
Oral	• easiest route of administration • retrievable route • safest route	• drug must pass through several cellular membranes before it takes effect • greatest variability in drug absorption • patient's emotional status can affect absorption • food in the stomach reduces the rate of absorption

situation, both the ionized and nonionized drug molecules are absorbed quickly through capillary pores. Absorption is usually complete within ten to thirty minutes.

Some drugs are administered in suspension. When given this way, drugs are absorbed slowly because they must first be dissolved in muscle fluids before they can be absorbed. Drug suspensions are used to produce sustained effects. These products are often called "depot" drugs. Examples are Depo-Medrol and Depo-Provera. In both cases, these products have prolonged effects as their active ingredients are gradually absorbed from the muscle mass.

Increasing muscle circulation can hasten intramuscular drug absorption. Massaging a muscle or walking after an injection can increase the rate of absorption. The nurse, for example, might suggest that the patient walk after an injection of iron to speed its absorption and alleviate discomfort.

Inactivity, disuse and pathology can have the opposite effect. Paraplegic or bedridden individuals absorb drugs more slowly from the dorsogluteal and vastus lateralis sites. The ventrogluteal site is recommended for these individuals.

Some drugs are poorly absorbed from muscle because of their chemical or physical properties. Chlordiazepoxide, for example, is poorly soluble in the extracellular fluids bathing muscle. Although it is injected as a solution, the drug rapidly comes out of solution at pH 7.4. Its rate of absorption then depends on the rate at which the drug is redissolved. As a result, chlordiazepoxide is poorly and erratically absorbed when injected intramuscularly.

Subcutaneous injection. Drugs are absorbed more slowly when injected subcutaneously (SC), compared with intramuscular injections. Subcutaneous injections are, however, usually more acceptable for patients and they produce reliable rapid absorption. Irritant drugs often cause too much pain when injected subcutaneously, and only relatively small volumes of fluid can be tolerated. Subcutaneous injections are not advised in cases involving shock because reduced peripheral circulation severely decreases the rate of drug absorption.

Intradermal injection. Intradermal (ID) injections are usually used when a local effect is desired, as in local anesthetics or testing for sensitivity (e.g., tuberculin testing or allergy testing). Injections are made into the dermis. A short needle and a small-barrelled syringe are necessary for intradermal injections. Frequent sites for intradermal injections include the back and the medial surface of the forearm. With the bevel up, insert the point of the needle just below the skin. The fluid is injected to form a small visible wheal.

Transdermal Administration

The application of drugs directly on the skin, for example in ointments or patches, provides for the slow, continuous absorption of medications over relatively prolonged periods of time. This route can be used for drugs that are lipid soluble and will pass through the keratin layer of the skin (the stratum corneum). It is particularly suitable for drugs that are extensively destroyed in the gastrointestinal tract or by first-pass metabolism (see Chapter 5).

The recent introduction of nicotine patches to help patients withdraw from cigarette smoking is an excellent example of a drug applied to the skin. Other examples of drugs administered transdermally include hyoscine (for motion sickness), nitroglycerin (for prevention of angina pectoris), estradiol (for hormone replacement) and fentanyl (for pain relief).

Oral Administration

Oral dosage forms. Most drugs are given orally. This is the safest, most convenient and most economical route of administration. There are some risks to giving drugs orally, including aspiration and gastric irritation. Drugs can be administered in solutions, suspensions, capsules, compressed tablets, coated tablets and sustained-release tablets and capsules. (See Box 4.2.)

Sites of oral drug absorption. Acidic drugs, such as acetylsalicylic acid and nonsteroidal anti-inflammatory compounds, are mainly nonionized in the gastric juices. As a result, they can be absorbed from the stomach. A few drugs, such as ethanol, do not dissociate into ionized and nonionized forms and they, too, can be absorbed from the stomach.

Most basic drugs are highly ionized in the acidic pH of the stomach and are not absorbed from this organ. Basic drugs can usually be identified by the fact that their generic names end with the letters "amine" or "ine." Thus amphetamine, meperidine, codeine and chlorpromazine are bases and will not be absorbed from the stomach.

Most basic drugs are absorbed from the intestine because in the pH of the intestinal fluids (approximately 6) many ionized molecules are converted to their nonionized form. Drug absorption occurs mainly in the duodenum, but it can also take place in the jejunum and ileum.

Acidic drugs can also be absorbed from the small bowel. Although they are mainly ionized in the intestine, there are usually sufficient nonionized drug molecules to permit absorption. Once nonionized molecules leave the intestine to enter the blood, more ionized molecules are converted to their nonionized forms in the intestine to maintain a constant ionized/nonionized ratio. The newly formed nonionized drug molecules are then absorbed, and the entire process is repeated until drug absorption is complete.

The surface of the small intestine contains many folds (plicae circulares) and projections (microvilli and villi) that provide a much larger surface for drug absorption than is afforded by the gastric mucosa. These evolutionary adaptations have resulted in the typical adult having an intestinal surface area that is roughly equivalent to that of a doubles tennis court. As a result, drugs that can be absorbed from both the stomach and intestine (such as acids and liquids that do not ionize) are absorbed faster from the intestine.

Ethanol can be used to illustrate this principle. Most nurses have encountered its notorious effects after imbibing it on an empty stomach: it passes quickly into the duodenum, from whence it is rapidly absorbed. If consumed with food, ethanol is retained in the stomach because the pyloric sphincter closes in response to the presence of food. Taken under these conditions, ethanol's effects are less dramatic, because it is absorbed more slowly through the gastric mucosa.

Most drugs are poorly absorbed from the large intestine. The surface area here is much smaller than that provided by the small intestine. As a result, if a drug is not absorbed by the time it reaches the large intestine, it usually exits the body in the feces.

Box 4.2
Oral dosage forms

Solutions	• Usually absorbed quickly
Suspensions	• Absorbed more slowly because the drug must first be dissolved in the gastro-intestinal tract
Gelatin capsules	• Usually disintegrate rapidly in the stomach; then the drug must disperse through the stomach and/or intestine and dissolve before absorption can occur
Compressed or coated tablets	• Disintegrate and disperse more slowly; thus, absorption takes longer
Enteric-coated tablets	• Protect the drug from the stomach or vice versa. The coating placed on the tablet is acid resistant, and the tablet does not disintegrate in the stomach. Disintegration occurs when the drug reaches the duodenum. *Examples:* To protect the gastric mucosa, ASA can be incorporated into an enteric-coated tablet; erythromycin is destroyed by gastric acid, but is protected in an enteric-coated tablet
Sustained-release tablets, capsules	• Release the drug over a period of several hours. They decrease the number of times a day a patient must take a medication, reduce fluctuations in drug levels in the body, and maintain therapeutic concentrations of the drug in the body for longer periods of time. Drugs with short durations of action (see Chapter 5) benefit from sustained-release formulations. Drugs that act for a long period of time do not require sustained-release formulations to prolong their durations of action

---

Factors influencing drug absorption after oral administration. The stability of drugs in the stomach can dramatically affect drug absorption. Some drugs are not stable in acid and are rapidly destroyed in the gastric juices. Penicillin G and erythromycin are two examples. In the case of penicillin G, the drug is taken on an empty stomach to speed its transfer to the duodenum. Erythromycin is usually given in an enteric-coated tablet to protect it from the gastric secretions.

Food in the stomach can also alter drug absorption. As described before, most basic drugs are absorbed only from the intestine. Even acidic drugs, which can be absorbed from the stomach, are more rapidly absorbed from the intestine. Taking a drug with food increases the time the compound is held in the stomach and reduces its rate of absorption. Drugs that are unstable in acid should not be taken with food. The longer they are retained in the stomach the greater the amount that will be destroyed. On the other hand, drugs that irritate the stomach and are stable in an acidic pH are best taken with meals. The presence of food will decrease irritation of the gastric mucosa and improve patient compliance.

Some drugs are destroyed by gastric acid or enzymes. Many penicillin products are unstable in an acid pH and are destroyed in the stomach (see Chapter 10). Obviously, these drugs should not be taken orally. Insulin is destroyed by stomach enzymes and therefore must be injected.

First-pass metabolism refers to the metabolism of a drug in the tissues of the gastrointestinal tract and the liver as the compound passes through these tissues for the first time. Because first-pass metabolism occurs before a drug is circulated throughout the body, it can significantly reduce the percentage of an oral dose reaching the systemic circulation. Some drugs are rapidly destroyed by intestinal tissue or by the hepatic cells on their first pass through the liver in the portal circulation. Only 10% to 20% of the absorbed dose of the beta blocker propranolol, for example, escapes metabolism the first time it passes through the liver.

Crushing a tablet can also affect drug absorption. Box 4.3 on the next page summarizes the factors a nurse must consider before deciding to crush a tablet.

Box 4.3
Oral administration of tablets

Before crushing a tablet, nurses should consult a pharmacist and consider the following principles.

Do *not* crush a tablet if the medication:

✘   has an enteric coating (designed to be protect the drug from the stomach). These products are often identified by the suffixes **EC** or **Entab**

✘   is formulated for delayed absorption (slow release or extended release). Note: Slow release beads may be added to food that is not chewed (pudding, jello) because they will still maintain their slow absorption properties. Sustained-release products may be identified by the codes:

      Dur — duration   **SA** — sustained action
      Slo   **Span**
      SR — sustained release

✘   has a bitter taste

✘   has a local anesthetic effect

✘   will decompose due to exposure to light, air, moisture

✘   is formulated to be absorbed in the mouth

✘   has a narrow therapeutic margin; crushing may increase absorption and produce toxicity

---

Sublingual Administration

Sublingual administration may be an alternative to the oral route if a drug is either destroyed in the stomach or completely inactivated as it passes through the liver for the first time. To be effective sublingually, a drug must be absorbed very quickly. Otherwise, its presence in the mouth will result in the accumulation of saliva that must be swallowed, carrying the drug with it. It is also imperative that a drug be nonirritating if it is to be held under the tongue. Few drugs are both rapidly absorbed and nonirritating and, as a result, the number of drugs given sublingually is small.

Nitrates, such as nitroglycerin, are given sublingually to circumvent extensive first-pass inactivation (see Chapter 5) that occurs if they are given orally. Ergotamine can be given sublingually to treat migraine headaches. The drug can produce nausea and vomiting, which are often already present as a result of the migraine headache. For this reason, ergotamine is more effective if taken sublingually. Otherwise, patients who swallow ergotamine tablets for the treatment of migraine headaches often see the drug a second time as it passes their teeth in the reverse direction.

Rectal Administration

Drugs may be given rectally for either a local or a systemic effect. With respect to local use, a variety of anti-inflammatory substances and topical anesthetics may be inserted or squirted into the rectum to soothe inflamed tissues and/or freeze hemorrhoids.

Drugs can be given rectally when it is difficult, if not impossible, to administer them orally, as in the case of migraine headaches with accompanying nausea and vomiting, mentioned above. Ergotamine can be given in suppository form in this situation. Young children or babies may be unable to swallow a drug. Rectal administration is advisable in these cases. Some drugs may be absorbed more slowly from a suppository and provide a benefit for several hours. For example, arthritis sufferers can insert indomethacin suppositories (an anti-inflammatory analgesic) in the evening to obtain a long-term effect.

Drug absorption from suppositories is erratic. The rate-limiting factor in absorption appears to be extracting the drug from the suppository mass and dissolving it in the rectal or colonic secretions.

Bioavailability

The term bioavailability refers to the amount of administered drug that reaches the systemic circulation. Bioavailability is the most important concept of drug absorption because it reflects the concentration of drug that can potentially reach its site of action. Two factors can reduce oral bioavailability: poor absorption and first-pass metabolism (see Chapter 5).

Bioavailability may vary considerably from one brand of a drug to another. Generic drugs have become very popular during the past twenty years. Often these products, which are intended as "copy cats" of the major innovators' brands, are substituted for the original product because they cost less. Before a generic drug is approved for sale, its bioavailability is compared with that of the brand name product. It is important to determine if its absorption characteristics — which include the speed at which it is absorbed, the peak concentration produced in the plasma of the patient and the total percentage of the dose absorbed — are equivalent to those of the brand name drug. If all these parameters are equivalent to the standard brand name drug, the two products are considered to be bioequivalent.

Further Reading

Benet LZ, Kroetz DL, Sheiner LB. Pharmacokinetics: The dynamics of drug absorption, distribution and elimination. In: Hardman JG, Limbird LE (eds.), *Goodman and Gilman's The Pharmacological Basis of Therapeutics,* 9th ed. New York: Pergamon; 1996:3–28.

Gram TE. Drug absorption and distribution. In: Craig CR, Stitzel RE (eds.), *Modern Pharmacology.* 4th ed. Boston: Little, Brown; 1994:19–32.

Drug Distribution and Elimination

Topics Discussed
- Definition of therapeutic window, minimum effective concentration, maximum tolerated level, biotransformation
- Drug distribution in the body
- Factors influencing blood levels of drugs
- Drug elimination
- Pharmacokinetics, drug half-life and steady state

Drug Distribution in the Body

Chapter 4 discussed drug absorption. Following their absorption, drugs are distributed throughout the body. Three factors control drug distribution. They are tissue perfusion, plasma protein binding and lipid solubility.

Tissue perfusion determines the initial distribution of a drug, with richly perfused organs receiving most of the drug molecules. Once carried to an organ, most drugs must diffuse out of the blood into the tissues, if they are to have an effect. Their ability to leave the blood may be limited by plasma protein binding. Only unbound molecules can diffuse through capillary pores. Drug molecules bound to plasma albumin cannot diffuse into the interstitial water and are, at that moment, pharmacologically inert.

Once in interstitial water some drug molecules may cross cell membranes. Their ability to do so depends on their lipid solubility. Lipid-soluble drugs cross cell membranes easily. Water-soluble drugs experience greater difficulty. As a result, lipid-soluble or nonionized drug molecules are distributed throughout the total body water.

Water-soluble or ionized molecules usually are restricted in their distribution to the plasma and interstitial water compartments, which together make up the extracellular water compartment.

With this brief discussion as a background, we will now consider in greater detail the factors controlling drug distribution, beginning with tissue perfusion.

Tissue Perfusion

Richly perfused organs receive more drug initially than poorly perfused tissues. Figure 5.1 illustrates the distribution of the lipid-soluble drug thiopental in the dog.

Liver and muscle, as well as heart, kidneys, brain and adrenals, are richly perfused and receive more drug than poorly perfused fat or bone during the initial distribution of a drug in the body. Even thiopental, a very fat-soluble drug, cannot be found in high concentration in adipose tissue during the first thirty minutes after absorption. Thereafter, however, its concentration in fat continues to climb and eventually exceeds the levels in the more richly perfused tissues. This is explained by the fact that thiopental is retained by fat. Acting like a sponge, fat takes up most of the drug brought to it in the circulation. As a result, thiopental is removed from the richly perfused tissues, for which it has little affinity, and concentrated in fat cells.

From this example, it is possible to derive a principle. Drugs are distributed initially to those tissues that are richly perfused. Thereafter, a redistribution occurs with the drugs accumulating in tissues for which they have affinity. Thiopental was used as an example of a fat-soluble drug accumulating in adipose tissue. But fat is not the only

Figure 5.1
Distribution of thiopental in the dog

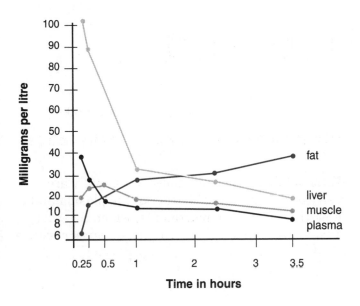

Note the high levels found initially in the liver and muscle and the subsequent redistribution to fat.

Source: Brodie BB. Distribution and fate of drugs: Therapeutic implications. In: Binns TB, *Absorption and Distribution of Drugs.* E&S Livingstone; 1964. Reproduced with permission.

tissue that can retain a drug. Any tissue that has an affinity for a particular drug can retain it in high concentrations. A further example is the binding of tetracycline antibiotics to calcium, which is concentrated in bones and teeth.

Plasma protein binding

Effect of plasma protein binding on drug distribution. Under normal circumstances the plasma proteins, such as albumin, do not leave the blood, and drug molecules bound to them do not diffuse into tissues. Phenylbutazone, warfarin and salicylate are 98% bound to albumin. If the total plasma level of phenylbutazone is 10 mg/mL, 9.8 mg/mL are bound to albumin and 0.2 mg/mL are free in solution in the plasma (Figure 5.2). Only drug molecules free in solution diffuse through the capillary endothelium and equilibrate between the plasma water and the interstitial water.

Unless the capacity of the plasma proteins to bind a drug is saturated, the ratio of bound/free drug remains constant. As the free level of a drug

Figure 5.2
Diffusion of a drug that is 98% bound to plasma proteins across a capillary

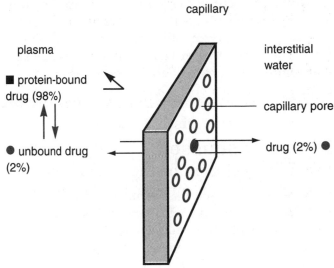

falls, due to metabolism, renal excretion, or both, more drug leaves the albumin to become free in the plasma before diffusing out of the vascular system.

Saturation of plasma protein binding sites with drugs. Plasma contains a finite concentration of albumin. If enough drug is given, it is possible to occupy all the binding sites on albumin and thereby saturate the plasma proteins. When this occurs, the free level of drug in the plasma will increase suddenly. In this event the pharmacologic activity of the drug increases as more molecules diffuse into the tissues.

Nurses are aware that disease can affect plasma protein concentrations. Patients with cirrhosis, for example, can have lower plasma protein concentrations. In these patients, drugs may more easily saturate plasma protein binding sites, and subsequently show increased effects.

Elderly patients may also have lower plasma albumin. Saturation of protein binding sites and increased concentrations of free drug are more likely in this age group. If this happens, the elderly patient will experience an increased drug effect (see Chapter 8).

Drug competition for plasma protein binding. Drugs can compete for the available plasma protein binding sites. For example, both warfarin and salicylate are bound extensively to plasma albumin. If a patient, previously stabilized on warfarin, is given acetylsalicylic acid (ASA), bleeding may occur because the salicylate provided in the ASA displaces some of the warfarin from its binding sites on plasma albumin. As a result, more warfarin is able to enter the liver, where it blocks prothrombin synthesis, thereby decreasing the clotting mechanism of the blood.

Barriers to Drug Distribution

To summarize the information presented so far, drugs are carried throughout the body in the blood. Richly perfused tissues initially receive more drug than organs with poorer blood supply. Thereafter, drugs may redistribute in accordance with their affinities for particular tissues. Plasma protein binding prevents a drug from leaving the blood vessels. Drug molecules that are not bound to plasma proteins can leave the blood vessels and enter the interstitial water of all tissues — with one exception, the brain.

Blood-brain barrier. The distribution of drugs into the brain is unique. Brain capillary endothelial cells differ from most other areas of the body by the absence of pores. In addition, glial connective tissue, called astrocytes, is attached closely to the basement membrane of the capillary endothelium. Together these structural modifications are referred to as the blood-brain barrier. Figure 5.3 shows the relatively tight endothelial cellular junction that prevents nonlipid-soluble (ionized) molecules from leaving the blood and entering the brain. Lipid-soluble (nonionized) drug molecules, not bound to plasma proteins, diffuse easily through the blood-brain barrier and enter the brain.

The rate at which a drug enters the brain is largely determined by the drug's lipid solubility. Stated simply, lipid-soluble drugs cross the blood-brain barrier easily; drugs that are poorly lipid soluble cannot enter the brain. This explains why some drugs have major beneficial or adverse effects in the brain and others do not.

Drug diffusion across the placenta. The mature placenta contains a network of maternal

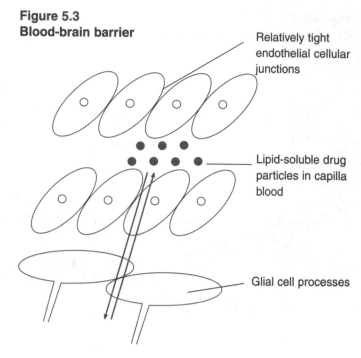

Figure 5.3
Blood-brain barrier

Relatively tight endothelial cellular junctions

Lipid-soluble drug particles in capilla blood

Glial cell processes

Source: Morgan JP. *Alcohol and Drug Abuse: Curriculum Guide for Pharmacology Faculty.* Rockville, MD: U.S. Department of Health & Human Services; 1985:8. Reproduced with permission.

blood sinuses that interface with villi that carry the fetal capillaries. The membranes that separate the fetal capillary blood from maternal blood resemble membranes elsewhere in the body. Lipid-soluble drugs diffuse readily from the maternal to the fetal circulation. Water-soluble molecules experience greater difficulty. However, if taken for a sufficient period of time, most drugs, regardless of their physical or chemical properties, will cross the placenta. In contradistinction to the blood-brain barrier, there is no placental barrier to the diffusion of drugs. Some drugs cross more easily than others, but almost any drug can reach the fetus. Only drugs with very high molecular weights, such as insulin or heparin, will not cross the placenta.

Figure 5.4 depicts the distribution of a drug from the maternal to the fetal circulation. In this figure, the drug is administered to the mother. Once in the mother's circulation, it distributes throughout her body. The drug also crosses the placenta and distributes throughout fetal tissues. The drug, or its metabolite(s), leaves the fetus by re-entering the mother.

Figure 5.4
Drug distribution in the maternal–placental–fetal unit

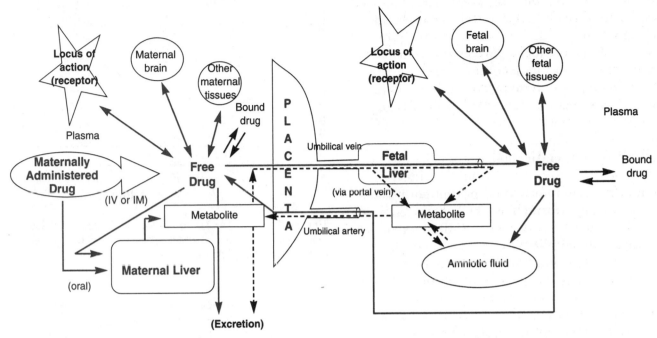

Source: Mirkin BL. Drug distribution in pregnancy. In: Boreus L (ed.), *Fetal Pharmacology.* New York: Raven Press; 1972:22. Reproduced with permission.

Factors Influencing the Blood Levels of Drugs

Several factors influence the blood level of a drug. The dose of the drug obviously affects its blood level. Higher doses produce higher blood levels. Bioavailability also influences the concentration of the drug in the blood. If two drugs are given in identical doses to the same individual, the one with the greater bioavailability will produce the higher blood concentrations.

Volume of distribution is also an important factor in influencing the blood level of a drug. If one drug is distributed throughout the total body water, it will have a lower concentration in the blood than an equivalent dose of a drug that is distributed only in the extracellular fluid. Drugs bound to plasma proteins will have higher blood levels than drugs not bound to albumin.

Big patients have larger body water compartments than small patients. Equal doses of any drug will produce higher blood levels in the smaller individual.

Finally, the elimination rate of drugs influ- ences significantly the concentration of drugs in the blood. If a drug is eliminated quickly, its plasma concentration will fall rapidly. The major routes of drug elimination are renal excretion, hepatic metabolism and biliary excretion. These will be discussed below.

It is often important to measure the concentration of a drug in plasma or serum because this value reflects its concentration at the site of action. It is essential, for example, to know the concentration of cardiac drugs, such as digoxin, in the heart. However, one cannot measure directly digoxin's concentration in the heart. Instead, a blood sample is drawn and digoxin's serum concentration is measured on the assumption that the concentration in the serum is in equilibrium with the concentration in the heart and reflects digoxin's level in the heart.

The plasma or serum concentration of a drug can best be thought of as a "window" to look at the level of a drug in the affected tissue. If the concentration of the drug in the serum is low, then its level in the tissue will also be low, and little effect will be seen. If the concentration of drug in serum is high, its level will also be high in the tissue concerned, and drug-induced toxicities may be seen. It has been possible to establish serum concentrations for many drugs that correlate with the safe and effective levels of these compounds in the tissues concerned.

In the United States, it is common practice to report serum or plasma levels of drugs in micrograms or nanograms of drug per millilitre of fluid. In Canada and many other parts of the world, serum levels are routinely reported in Système international (SI) units, which present the concentration of drug in millimoles, micromoles, or nanomoles of drug per litre of fluid. In this text both systems are used, with the serum or plasma levels of a drug reported first in SI units followed (in brackets) by its concentration in micrograms or nanograms per millilitre.

For digoxin, serum levels range from 1.0–2.6 nanomoles/L (0.5–2 nanograms/mL). Concentrations below 1.0 nanomoles/L (0.5 nanogram/mL) usually do not increase cardiac function. Levels above 2.6 nanomoles/L (2 nanograms/mL) can be expected to produce cardiac and other toxicities. The range between the minimum effective level and maximum tolerated level is referred to as the *therapeutic window*.

The *minimum effective concentration (MEC)* is a term that indicates the lowest concentration of a drug in the blood that is able to produce the desired therapeutic effect. The *maximum tolerated level* is the highest plasma concentration a patient can tolerate and still remain on the medication. Figure 5.5 depicts the dose-response curve for a drug, and Figure 5.6 describes both the minimum effective concentration and the maximum tolerated level.

Drug Elimination

Renal excretion

Filtration, secretion and reabsorption. The kidney is a major organ for the elimination of drugs. It can filter, secrete and reabsorb drugs (Figure 5.7). Every minute about 1300 mL of blood enters the glomeruli (tuft of capillaries in the nephron surrounded by the Bowman's capsule). Of this volume, about 120 mL of plasma and dissolved substances are filtered into the renal tubules. Ninety-nine percent of this filtrate is reabsorbed.

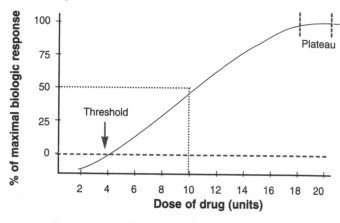

Figure 5.5
Dose-response curve

Threshold is the dose of drug required to produce a measurable response. Plateau occurs when increasing drug dose does not increase biologic response.

The kidneys conserve water, electrolytes and glucose. They excrete waste products.

Most drugs are passively filtered with the plasma. However, drugs that are bound to plasma proteins are not filtered. This explains why highly bound drugs remain in the body longer.

When the filtrate is reabsorbed in the tubules, drug molecules may also be reabsorbed. Lipid-soluble drugs (nonionized drug molecules) are readily reabsorbed across the tubule membranes back into the capillaries and recirculated throughout the body. Thus, a drug molecule may be absorbed and distributed throughout the body, act at its target site, be excreted into the glomerular filtrate and be reabsorbed and redistributed to act again.

Figure 5.6
Plasma level profiles: Minimum effective concentration (A) and maximum tolerated level (B)

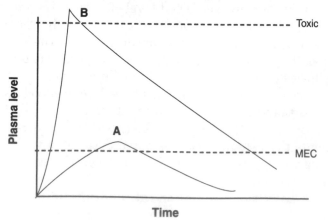

Table 5.1 summarizes the mechanisms by which the kidney handles drugs.

Effect of plasma protein binding on drug elimination. Plasma protein binding often reduces the rate of drug elimination. Under normal conditions, plasma proteins are not filtered by renal glomeruli, and drugs eliminated by glomerular filtration have longer half-lives if they are bound to plasma albumin. Likewise, many drugs eliminated by liver metabolism will have longer half-lives in the body if they are bound to plasma proteins because they cannot easily diffuse into the liver to be metabolized.

There are, of course, always exceptions to the basic rule that plasma protein binding reduces the rate of drug elimination. Drugs secreted by the renal tubules are not influenced by plasma protein binding. Whereas it is true that only free molecules are secreted, tubular secretion proceeds so rapidly that new molecules quickly dissociate from plasma proteins to maintain a constant ratio of bound to free molecules. The newly freed molecules are themselves then secreted.

Renal clearance. The capacity of the kidney to excrete a drug can be expressed as a renal clearance value. This is obtained by dividing the amount of drug excreted in the urine by its plasma concentration. For example, if drug A has a plasma level of 1.5 nanograms per millilitre and the kidney excretes 180 nanograms per minute, the renal clearance of drug A is 180/1.5 = 120 mL/min. This

**Figure 5.7
Excretion of drugs by the kidney**

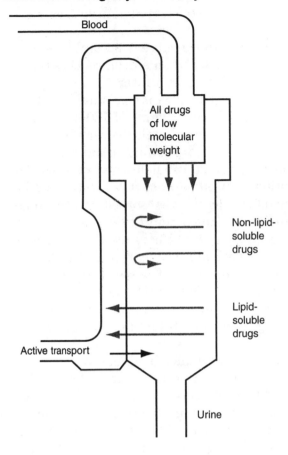

Blood

All drugs of low molecular weight

Non-lipid-soluble drugs

Lipid-soluble drugs

Active transport

Urine

Source: Brodie BB. Distribution and fate of drugs: therapeutic implications. In: Binns TB, *Absorption and Distribution of Drugs.* E&S Livingstone; 1964. Reproduced with permission.

**Table 5.1
Actions of the kidney**

Glomerular filtration	In the healthy adult, the glomeruli produce about 120 mL of filtrate every minute, of which 99% is reabsorbed as it passes through the renal tubules. Free drug molecules (not bound to plasma proteins) easily pass into the filtrate
Tubular reabsorption	When drug molecules are in the filtrate, they may be excreted in the urine or they may be reabsorbed back into the capillaries. Recall that lipid-soluble drugs (nonionized drug molecules) easily diffuse through cell membranes and are reabsorbed from the kidney
Tubular secretion	Drugs secreted through the renal tubules into the tubular lumen are cleared quickly by the kidneys (e.g., the penicillins, which have half-lives of about 1 h). It is possible to saturate the kidney's capacity to secrete drugs, and two drugs are sometimes used together, with one competing with the other for the renal secretory mechanism. (E.g., probenecid and penicillin G are often used together; both are secreted by the same transport mechanism. The secretion of probenecid reduces the amount of penicillin G that can be secreted. Thus, penicillin G stays in the body for a longer period of time and is better able to fight an infection)

is the volume of plasma that contains the amount of drug excreted. In theory, in this example, 120 mL of plasma were cleared of drug A every minute.

The renal clearance value is helpful in determining what happens when a drug reaches the kidney. The renal glomeruli filter 120 mL of plasma every minute. Thus, it may be stated on the basis of a renal clearance value of 120 mL/min that drug A is filtered through the renal glomeruli and that no net reabsorption has occurred as it passes down the renal tubules. The expression "net reabsorption" is used because it is always possible that some of the drug is reabsorbed, but this quantity is equalled by the amount that is secreted.

If a drug has a renal clearance value considerably below 120 mL/min, it means that the drug is either not filtered well as it passes through the renal glomeruli or it is filtered and extensively reabsorbed in the tubules. The only factor that stops a drug from being filtered is plasma protein binding.

Renal clearance values in excess of 120 mL/min indicate that the drug undergoes filtration and tubular secretion. The renal plasma flow is about 650 mL/min. Penicillin has a renal clearance value of about 600 mL/min. This means that almost all drug molecules carried to the kidney in the blood are eliminated.

Drugs with high renal clearance values depend heavily on the kidney for their elimination from the body. If, for example, a drug has a renal clearance value of 120 mL/min or more, the kidney is an important organ for its elimination. This drug will accumulate if normal doses are given repeatedly to an individual with kidney failure. Drugs with low renal clearance values must be eliminated by other means, usually liver metabolism. It is not necessary to modify their doses in patients with renal impairment. However, it may be necessary to reduce the dose in patients with liver disease because a diseased liver may be unable to eliminate drugs (see Biotransformation, below).

Newborns have immature kidneys and cannot excrete drugs as rapidly as babies a few months old. Aminoglycoside antibiotics (e.g., gentamicin, tobramycin) and digoxin are among the drugs eliminated more slowly by the neonate. Thus, newborns must receive lower doses of these drugs to prevent their accumulation in the body to toxic levels.

As a person ages, renal blood flow falls, reduced glomerular filtration becomes apparent, and a decreased capacity to secrete chemicals occurs (see Chapter 8). To compensate for these changes, elderly patients must receive lower doses of many drugs that are eliminated by the kidneys. Failure to do so can result in overdose.

Biotransformation

Many drugs are changed chemically in the body. This process is called *biotransformation*. It is also referred to as metabolism. (In this book, the terms biotransformation and metabolism will be used interchangeably.) Most tissues have the capacity to metabolize drugs. The liver is the major organ involved in drug metabolism, with the lungs, kidneys, intestinal mucosa and placenta also playing a role for certain compounds. Drugs reach the liver via the portal vein (from the digestive tract) and the hepatic artery (from the aorta). Each minute a total volume of 1500 mL of blood passes through the liver: about one-third of the blood is arterial and two-thirds is venous.

Lipophilic drugs, that is, those compounds that are fat soluble, cannot be eliminated by the kidney. After being filtered they are reabsorbed into the blood. In response to the inability of the kidney to eliminate lipophilic agents (including endogenous materials such as steroids), the body evolved a system of enzymes to metabolize these chemicals. Drug metabolism or biotransformation involves the conversion of lipophilic chemicals into compounds with increased water solubility, thereby facilitating their elimination by the kidneys.

Drug metabolism should not be equated with drug inactivation. Although most drugs are inactivated by metabolism, a significant number maintain their activity and some drugs are even activated by metabolism. For example, more than sixty years ago it was found that the body metabolized the dye Prontosil, converting it into the active sulfonamide, sulfanilamide. Drug metabolism is best thought of as a polarization process during which fat-soluble drugs are made more polar or more water soluble.

Several factors can influence the rate of drug metabolism. Age is one. Neonates have a reduced capacity to metabolize drugs. Elderly patients may also experience difficulty in metabolizing drugs.

Genetic factors also control drug metabolism. Identical twins often metabolize drugs at identical rates. Fraternal twins metabolize drugs at different rates.

The activity of drug-metabolizing enzymes can be increased or decreased by the administration of certain drugs and by exposure to various chemicals in the environment.

Biliary Excretion

Some drugs, or their metabolites, are removed from the plasma by the liver and secreted into the bile, before being passed into the duodenum. The concentrations of these drugs may be several hundred times higher in bile than in plasma. Little is known of the means by which the liver secretes drugs into bile or why it selects some drugs and neglects others.

Once passed into the intestines in the bile, some drugs, or their metabolites, are reabsorbed into the blood. This is called enterohepatic recirculation. Anyone who has taken phenolphthalein, the active ingredient in ExLax and many other laxatives, has experienced the consequence of enterohepatic recirculation. Phenolphthalein acts as a laxative because it irritates the colon. When the drug is taken, its desired effect is seen within 12 to 16 h. However, unbeknownst to the patient, some of the phenolphthalein is absorbed into the circulatory system. Following glucuronide conjugation in the liver, the drug is returned to the intestinal tract in the bile. Upon reaching the depths of the intestinal tract the glucuronide is cleaved from the parent drug by bacterial enzymes, freeing the phenolphthalein to work its wonders again.

Pharmacokinetics

Pharmacokinetics refers to the dynamics of drug absorption, distribution and elimination. Thus, most of the information provided in Chapters 4 and 5 can be classified under the term pharmacokinetics. The study of pharmacokinetics has taken on increasing importance over the years with the realization that the intensity of drug action is most frequently related to the concentration of the drug at the site of action. We have already discussed drug absorption, distribution and elimination, all factors that control the concentration of a drug at

its site of action. Only two additional topics relating to pharmacokinetics remain to be discussed. These are half-life and steady state.

Half-Life

Pharmacologists routinely determine the plasma or serum levels of drugs. Figure 5.8 plots the serum concentrations of a drug following its injection. From the figure, it is apparent that immediately following the injection of a drug, its blood levels fall dramatically (alpha phase). This initial fall results from the distribution of the drug out of the vascular system and into the various body compartments. If a drug is extensively bound to plasma proteins, its ability to leave the blood will be reduced and the initial fall in plasma or serum levels will be minimal.

The second phase in the blood concentration–time curve (beta phase) reflects the rate at which the drug is eliminated from the body. *Half-life* is the time taken to eliminate half the drug from the

Figure 5.8
Disappearance of a drug from the plasma after intravenous injection

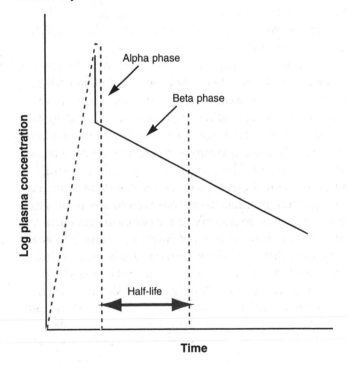

Source: Morgan JP. *Alcohol and Drug Abuse: Curriculum Guide for Pharmacology Faculty.* Rockville, MD: U.S. Department of Health & Human Sciences; 1985:17. Reproduced with permission.

body. If the plasma concentration is 10 mg/mL at time 0 and 5 mg/mL 4 h later, the half-life of the drug is 4 h. By the same token, it should take 4 h for the plasma concentration to fall from 5 mg/mL to 2.5 mg/mL.

Steady State

Drugs are often administered on a regular basis for long periods of time. During the first few doses of a drug its concentration in the body usually increases. Eventually, however, the level of the drug in the body stops increasing and reaches a steady concentration (Figure 5.9). At this point, the amount of drug being absorbed equals the quantity being eliminated. This is referred to as *steady state*. If the patient is treated with 250 mg of a drug every 6 h and absorbs 100% of the dose, steady state is reached when 250 mg is eliminated every 6 h.

Steady state is usually reached within five half-lives for a drug. A drug with a half-life of 6 h is given once every 6 h, it will reach steady state in 30 h. In contrast, a drug with a half-life of 30 h will require more than one week before it reaches steady-state concentrations.

Two basic approaches can be used to attain steady state. The first is to give the patient the maintenance dose every half-life. This is the approach just described and depicted in Figure 5.9. Its disadvantage is that it takes a relatively long time to attain steady state. Alternatively, the patient can be given an initial dose that is twice the maintenance dose. By administering this loading dose and following it with the maintenance dose every half-life, it is possible to establish the desired steady state concentration quickly and maintain it. Following from the example given in the previous paragraph, an initial loading dose of 500 mg would see 250 mg eliminated in 6 h and 250 mg retained in the body. Subsequent maintenance doses of 250 mg every 6 h would replace the amount lost in that time interval and maintain the patient in steady state.

**Figure 5.9
Steady state**

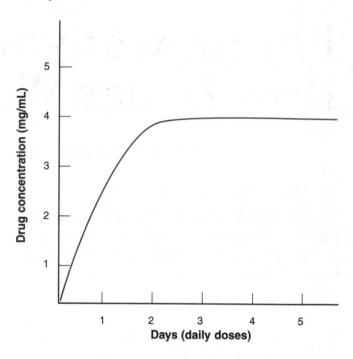

Further Reading

Benet LZ, Kroetz DL, Sheiner LB. Pharmacokinetics: the dynamics of drug absorption, distribution and elimination. In: Hardman JG, Limbird LE (eds.), *Goodman and Gilman's The Pharmacological Basis of Therapeutics*. 9th ed. New York: Pergamon; 1996:3–28.

Berndt WO, Stitzel RE. Excretion of drugs. In: Craig CR, Stitzel RE (eds.), *Modern Pharmacology*. 4th ed. Boston: Little, Brown; 1994:47–53.

Boreus LO. Principles of pediatric pharmacology. *Mon Clin Pharmacol* 1985;6:60.

Gram TE. Drug absorption and distribution. In: Craig CR, Stitzel RE (eds.), *Modern Pharmacology*. 4th ed. Boston: Little, Brown; 1994:19–32.

Gram TE. Metabolism of drugs. In: Craig CR, Stitzel RE (eds.), *Modern Pharmacology*. 4th ed. Boston: Little, Brown; 1994:33–46.

Pucino F, Beck CL, Seifert RL, Strommen GL, Sheldon PA, Silbergleit IL. Pharmacogenetics. *Pharmacotherapy* 1985;5:314–326.

Reynolds J. Pharmacokinetic considerations in critical care. *Nurs Clin North Am* 1993;5(2):227–235.

Roberts RJ. Pharmacologic principles in therapeutics in infants. In: Roberts RJ (ed.), *Drug Therapy in Infants*. Philadelphia: W.B. Saunders; 1984.

CHAPTER 6

Pharmacodynamics: How Drugs Work

Topics Discussed
- Definition of pharmacodynamics, drug receptor, agonist, antagonist, down-regulation, up-regulation, maximal efficacy
- Drug receptors
- Drug effects not mediated through receptors
- Dose-response effects
- Adverse effects of drug therapy

Pharmacodynamics is the study of how drugs act and produce their effects. The pharmacodynamic action of the antiulcer drug cimetidine, for example, is its ability to block H_2 receptors in the stomach, thereby decreasing gastric acid secretion. It is most important for nurses to understand the mechanism of action of each drug they give. They should understand, for example, how the same drug can produce such diverse effects as insomnia, hypertension and urinary retention. It is only by knowing the drug's mechanism of action that nurses will understand how one drug can produce all these effects.

Drug Receptors

Agonists and Antagonists

Most drugs stimulate or block drug receptors. A *drug receptor* is a specialized macromolecule located on a cell membrane or within a cell. Although the exact nature of each drug receptor is not known, it is recognized that each type of receptor shows amazing specificity for the drug or drugs with which it unites. For example, narcotic receptors in the brain show an affinity for both natural and synthetic narcotics, but they are not affected by non-narcotic analgesics, such as ASA.

Because most drugs work by interacting with specific receptors, they affect only those tissues that have those receptors. Tissues that are devoid of particular receptors are not affected by drugs requiring those receptors to act. It is for this reason that a drug affects some tissues and not others. Corticosteroids, for example, have major effects on the brain, retina, intestine, lung, heart, smooth muscle, kidney, liver, testes and skeletal muscle, because these tissues have glucocorticoid receptors. They have no effect on the bladder, seminal vesicles, prostate and uterus because these tissues do not have glucocorticoid receptors.

If a drug has affinity for a receptor, and stimulates the receptor, the drug is called an *agonist*. The ability to stimulate a drug receptor is called intrinsic activity. Thus, agonist drugs have both affinity for a receptor and intrinsic activity. Morphine is an agonist. It binds to specific narcotic receptors in the central nervous system and stimulates them to produce euphoria, pain relief and respiratory depression.

Drugs that have affinity for a receptor but no intrinsic activity are called *antagonists*. These drugs occupy a receptor but, because they have no intrinsic activity, they will not stimulate it. However, during the time these drugs occupy the receptor, they block any chemical with intrinsic activity from binding to the receptor and stimulating it. Antagonists, therefore, prevent effects from occurring. They may be used to block the effects of other drugs or to prevent endogenous chemicals from working.

Antihistamines are antagonists. During an allergic reaction, histamine is released from mast cells. The released histamine stimulates histaminergic receptors to produce many of the effects of the allergic reaction. Antihistamines have affinity for histaminergic receptors. They bind to the receptors and prevent histamine from stimulating them. As a result, antihistamines stop many of symptoms of an allergic reaction.

Drug receptor interactions are usually reversible. As the concentration of the drug in the body falls, its effects gradually diminish as fewer and fewer drug molecules are available either to stimulate or to block the drug receptor.

Specificity of Drug Receptors

Both the affinity of a drug for its receptor and its intrinsic activity depend on its chemical structure. Changing the structure of a drug, even slightly, can increase or decrease its affinity for a receptor and modify its pharmacologic effect significantly. Epinephrine has affinity for beta$_2$ receptors and dilates bronchioles. The structure of norepinephrine is only slightly different from epinephrine, yet it has no affinity for beta$_2$ receptors and will not dilate bronchioles.

Chemists have exploited the exquisite structural requirements of particular receptors to modify the chemical structures of drugs so that they will affect only certain subclasses of receptors. The beta blocker propranolol blocks both beta$_1$ and beta$_2$ receptors. This is a mixed blessing. Although blocking beta$_1$ receptors is important for propranolol to lower blood pressure and reduce the number of anginal attacks, antagonizing beta$_2$ effects increases the number of adverse effects patients experience. Once the structural requirements of the beta$_1$ and beta$_2$ receptors were identified, chemists were able to synthesize the so-called cardioselective beta blockers that preferentially bind to, and block, beta$_1$ receptors.

Effects of Agonists and Antagonists on Drug Receptor Density

Drug receptor density can be affected by chronic drug therapy. Long-term treatment with an agonist reduces the number of drug receptors. This is called *down-regulation*. When this occurs, the effects of the drug diminish. This can also be called *tissue tolerance* or *desensitization*. An example of this type of drug receptor interaction is seen when asthmatic patients receive constant therapy with

a beta$_2$ agonist to dilate their bronchioles. As therapy continues, the effect of the drug is diminished because of a reduced density of beta$_2$ receptors.

Chronic therapy with an antagonist increases the density of drug receptors (*up-regulation*). Long-term treatment with a beta blocker causes up-regulation of beta receptors. If the beta blocker is subsequently stopped, patients can experience cardiac dysrhythmias through stimulation of these receptors.

Antagonists can be classified as competitive or noncompetitive. Most antagonists used in medicine are competitive antagonists. These drugs bind reversibly to their receptors and compete with agonists for receptor binding. Because competitive antagonists bind reversibly to receptors, their effects can be overcome by giving larger doses of the agonist. Examples of competitive antagonists include beta blockers, anticholinergics, antihistamines and histamine$_2$ receptor blockers.

There are very few examples of noncompetitive antagonists used in medicine. These drugs bind irreversibly to receptors and reduce their number. Noncompetitive antagonists decrease the maximal response to an agonist. If a large amount of noncompetitive antagonist is given, it will block completely all effects of the agonist. Because noncompetitive antagonists bind irreversibly to receptors, their effects cannot be overcome with an agonist.

Drug Effects Not Mediated through Receptors

Although most drugs work by either stimulating or blocking receptors, not all drugs depend on receptors for their effects. Antacids, for example, work simply by neutralizing gastric acid. Cathartics, which work either by irritating the bowel or by drawing water from the blood into the feces by osmosis, also do not work by affecting receptors. Some drugs, such as certain anticancer drugs, produce their effects by affecting enzymes. It will become apparent throughout this book which drug effects depend on drug receptor interactions and which do not.

Dose-Response Effects

Pharmacology is a dose-dependent science. The intensity of the effect depends on the dose of the

Figure 6.1
Time course of action of a single dose of a drug

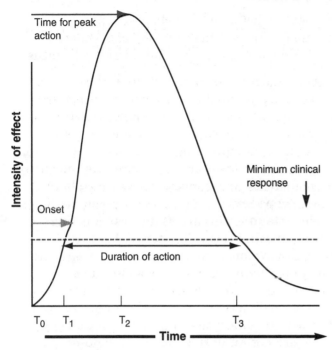

The drug is administered at T_0. The time interval between T_0 and T_1 represents the time of onset of action of the drug. Peak action occurs at T_2. The time interval between T_0 and T_2 represents the time for peak action. At T_3, the drug response falls below the minimum required for clinical effectiveness. The time interval between T_1 and T_3 represents the duration of action of the drug.

drug and its concentration at the receptor site. Figure 6.1 illustrates the concepts of onset of action, peak effect, and duration of action.

Figure 6.2 presents a typical dose-response curve for two drugs. At low doses of each drug, an increase in the dose produces only a small increase in effect. However, subsequent increases in dose produce a sharp increase in effect. Thereafter, additional increases in dose produce little or no increase in effect because the drug has attained its *maximal efficacy* or *effectiveness*.

The concept of maximal efficacy is very important because it describes the maximum effect of a drug. Morphine has greater maximal efficacy than codeine. Codeine can never produce the same degree of pain relief afforded by high doses of morphine, regardless of how much codeine is given.

Returning to Figure 6.2, we can see that drug A is more potent than drug B because it produces the same effect as drug B, but at lower doses. In contrast to maximal efficacy, which dictates the overall clinical effectiveness of a drug, potency is

Figure 6.2
Typical dose-response curves

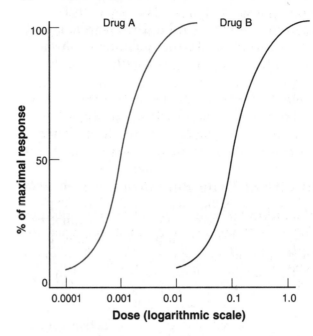

far less important. The fact that one drug can produce the same effect as another, but at a lower dose, does not mean that it is a better drug. The better drug is the one that can deliver the effect wanted, regardless of the dose needed, with fewer undesirable actions. Knowing the relative potencies of two drugs is useful when equating the effect of a new drug to that of an older agent. It is also helpful in managing patients who are switched from one drug to another.

Adverse Effects of Drugs

All drugs have the potential to produce adverse effects. In controlled clinical trials even patients on placebos (i.e., tablets or capsules containing no active ingredients) complain of adverse effects. The expression "side effect" is often used to mean adverse effect. In this text, we prefer the use of adverse effect or adverse drug reactions (ADR), because these terms accurately reflect the unwanted effect of a drug on the body.

Types of Adverse Drug Effects or Reactions

Adverse effects or adverse drug reactions include all unintended or undesired consequences of drug therapy. They can be broadly classified into two groups. Group 1 involves those effects that can be predicted by the pharmacology of the drug and account for approximately 70% to 80% of all adverse drug reactions. In higher doses, beta blockers produce bradycardia. Bradycardia is a predictable effect because beta blockers reduce sympathetic nervous system stimulation of the heart.

Group 2 adverse effects cannot be predicted from the major pharmacologic action of a drug. Angiotensin-converting enzyme (ACE) inhibitors dilate arterioles and are used to lower blood pressure. However, these drugs sometimes induce coughing. This adverse effect cannot be predicted from the main pharmacologic action of the drug. Other examples of adverse effects that cannot be predicted beforehand include a positive Coombs test in patients taking methyldopa, the development of a systemic lupus erythematosus-like effect in patients taking high doses of hydralazine, and an attack of angioedema produced by some ACE inhibitors. These types of adverse effects account for only 20% to 30% of all reactions. However, they are frequently the most difficult to predict, and sometimes they are not dependent on the dose of the drug given.

Drug-Induced Allergic Reactions

Drug-induced allergic reactions can be classified in group 2 because an allergic reaction is not a manifestation of the pharmacodynamics of the drug. Penicillin provides an excellent example of this principle. All penicillins inhibit bacterial cell wall synthesis and kill many common bacteria. These drugs also produce a high incidence of allergic reactions. None of these allergic reactions can be attributed to the ability of penicillins to block bacterial cell wall synthesis.

Allergic reactions are immune responses to drugs and result from the formation of antigen-antibody complexes. They can be classified as either early onset or late onset. For example, anaphylaxis is an immediate, severe, life-threatening response. Its symptoms are due to the release of histamine. They include rash, bronchospasm, laryngeal edema, abdominal pain and severe hypotension. Serum sickness has a less acute onset and may even take days to appear. Its symptoms include fever, lymphadenopathy and skin rashes.

Factors Predisposing Patients to Adverse Drug Reactions

A variety of factors can predispose a patient to adverse reactions. These include age, genetics, renal or hepatic pathology and nutritional status.

Age. Older patients are at greater risk for experiencing an adverse reaction to a drug (see Chapter 8). They have reduced renal function, lower body water compartments and increased sensitivities to many drugs. As a result, they often are given lower doses of drugs to reduce the possibility of adverse drug reactions. The golden rule for elderly patients is, "Start low and go slow."

Neonates are also at greater risk for drug-induced toxicities (see Chapter 8). Because neonates have immature livers and kidneys, they cannot eliminate drugs at the same rate as children and adults. As a result, it is not possible to extrapolate directly from a milligram-per-kilogram adult dose to obtain the correct dose for a baby. Babies are not miniature adults, and doses of drugs should be selected to reflect the reduced ability of a baby to eliminate a drug.

Genetics. The genetic makeup of a patient also is important for many adverse drug reactions, and the field of pharmacogenetics has become most significant. In essence, the response of patients to drug therapy is frequently controlled by their genetic characteristics. For example, the antimalarial drug primaquine (Chapter 21) can produce hemolysis in certain patients. This effect is due to a genetic deficiency of glucose-6-phosphate dehydrogenase.

Another example involves the prolonged effect of the skeletal muscle relaxant succinylcholine (Chapter 31) in certain patients. In most individuals, succinylcholine has a fleeting effect once the infusion is stopped. In a few patients, however, succinylcholine continues to paralyze muscles long after treatment is finished. These individuals have an atypical plasma cholinesterase, the enzyme responsible for the hydrolysis and inactivation of succinylcholine. As a result, these individuals cannot destroy the drug quickly.

Many other examples of the influence of pharmacogenetics on drug action will be presented throughout the course of this text. The moral of the story is that patients should be very careful how they pick their parents!

Reduced renal or hepatic function. As explained in Chapter 5, most drugs are eliminated by renal excretion or hepatic metabolism. As a result, drug accumulation frequently occurs in patients with either kidney or liver pathologies. Nurses should remember this and be prepared for an increased incidence of drug adverse reactions in these individuals.

Malnutrition. Patients who fail to eat a balanced diet, and who are low in vitamin K, are more likely to experience bleeding on oral anticoagulants. Hypokalemic patients treated with digoxin are more likely to experience digoxin toxicities (Chapter 32). These are two examples of the effects of an improper diet on the actions of drugs. Other examples will be provided as we proceed through this text.

Further Reading

Ross EM. Pharmacodynamics: mechanisms of drug action and the relationship between drug concentration and effect. In: Hardman JG, Limbird LE (eds.), *Goodman and Gilman's The Pharmacological Basis of Therapeutics*. 9th ed. New York: Pergamon Press; 1996:29–42.

Fleming WW. Mechanisms of drug action. In: Craig CR, Stitzel RE (eds.), *Modern Pharmacology*. 4th ed. Boston: Little, Brown; 1994:9–18.

Drug Interactions

Topics Discussed
- Definition of chelate, synergistic, antagonistic
- Pharmaceutical incompatibility
- Sites and mechanisms of drug interaction

Patients in hospital as well as outpatients frequently receive many medications. The average hospitalized patient, for example, receives six to ten drugs. Over-the-counter (OTC) products are also often taken by patients receiving prescription drugs. In view of the widespread acceptance of polypharmacy (the concurrent use of more than one medication), nurses should recognize the possible interactions that may occur when patients are given more than one drug. This is not easy!

Several textbooks have been written listing all known drug interactions. Many of these have little clinical significance. It is important for health professionals to differentiate those interactions that can affect the patient from those that have little clinical importance. Although nurses are not expected to know all reported drug interactions, they should know the more common ones that pose risks to patients. Nurses should also understand the sites in the body where interactions can occur. This chapter provides an overview of drug interactions and indicates where in the body two drugs can interact.

Pharmaceutical Incompatibility

Before we discuss drug interactions within the body, it is important to address the possibility that interactions may occur before the drugs enter the body. Nurses recognize that some drugs cannot be mixed in the same solution because of pharmaceutical incompatibilities. For example, aminoglycoside antibiotics (e.g., amikacin, gentamicin, netilmicin and tobramycin) and antipseudomonal penicillins (e.g., carbenicillin, ticarcillin, azlocillin, mezlocillin and piperacillin) cannot be mixed in the same bottle prior to infusion because aminoglycosides are inactivated by interacting with these penicillins. With the ever-increasing number of drugs on the market, it is very difficult for the nurse to remain abreast of all pharmaceutical incompatibilities. For nurses, the general rule is: "If you do not know whether two drugs are compatible when mixed in the same solution, do *not* mix."

Sites of Drug Interaction in the Body

Drug interactions may occur at five possible sites within the body. These involve:

- drug absorption in the gastrointestinal tract
- drug binding to plasma protein
- drug excretion by the kidneys
- drug metabolism by the liver
- drug action on the target tissue.

Drug Interactions Involving Drug Absorption

Drugs must be dissolved before absorption can proceed. If one drug affects the dissolution of another, it may influence its absorption. We saw in Chapter 4 that most drugs are either weak acids or weak bases. Nonsteroidal anti-inflammatory drugs (NSAIDs) are an example of acids, and narcotics are an example of bases. Basic drugs depend on the acidic pH of the stomach for dissolution.

Raising the pH in the stomach decreases the ability of the gastric juices to dissolve drugs such as narcotics, antidepressants and antipsychotics. If a basic drug is not dissolved in the stomach, it cannot be absorbed from the intestines.

Drugs that increase gastric pH, like antacids and H_2 blockers, reduce the capacity of the stomach secretions to dissolve some basic drugs. Sodium bicarbonate, for example, decreases the ability of gastric secretions to dissolve tetracycline and reduces tetracycline absorption.

Drug absorption may also be affected by direct physical or chemical interactions in the intestine. An example of a physical interaction can be found in the ability of mineral oil to reduce the absorption of fat-soluble vitamins. Fat-soluble vitamins are readily soluble in mineral oil. If mineral oil is taken, it will coat the surface of the gastrointestinal tract and dissolve fat-soluble vitamins taken by patients. Because mineral oil is not absorbed, neither are the vitamins dissolved in it.

Chemical interaction is illustrated by referring to the interaction between tetracyclines and calcium, iron or aluminum. These three ions are capable of interacting chemically with most tetracycline antibiotics to form insoluble compounds called chelates which cannot be absorbed. Thus, patients taking tetracyclines should not take products containing calcium, aluminum or iron. In practical terms, this means antacids, products containing milk, and iron-containing products.

Drug Interactions Involving Drug Distribution

Following absorption, drugs are distributed throughout the body in the blood. When drugs are carried in plasma they may be either bound to plasma proteins or free in solution in plasma water.

Plasma proteins are large molecules and usually cannot leave the vascular compartment. As a result, drug molecules bound to plasma proteins cannot leave the blood vessels and enter the intercellular and intracellular water. Thus, while a drug molecule remains bound to a plasma protein, it is pharmacologically inactive. Although some drugs bind to plasma globulins, most drug binding involves albumin.

Two characteristics mark plasma protein binding:

- the finite capacity of plasma proteins to bind drugs, and
- the reversible nature of the binding.

Because there is a limit to the number of protein molecules in plasma, and one protein molecule usually binds only one drug molecule, it is possible, with high levels of a drug, to exceed the capacity of plasma proteins to bind it.

Drug binding is reversible. A molecule that is bound at one moment to plasma proteins may be free the next. When a drug molecule leaves its binding site on a plasma protein, it is replaced by another molecule that had been free.

Drugs can compete for plasma protein binding sites. If a patient has been stabilized on one drug and a second is added that competes with the first for plasma protein binding, it may displace some of the original drug on albumin. The result is an increase in both the free level of the original drug and its effect in the body. Acetylsalicylic acid (ASA) can displace warfarin on plasma protein binding sites. When this happens, the newly freed warfarin molecules are free to enter the liver and reduce further the formation of prothrombin. Thus, the interaction of two drugs at plasma protein binding sites usually leads to an increase in the effect of one, or both, of the drugs.

Drug Interactions Involving Renal Excretion of Drugs

The three drug elimination processes that take place in the kidney are filtration, reabsorption and secretion. As we saw in Chapter 5, the kidney filters all drugs not bound to plasma proteins through its renal glomeruli. Following filtration, lipid-soluble drugs are extensively reabsorbed into the blood by the renal tubules. Some drugs are actively secreted by the renal tubules and appear in the urine in high concentration.

Drugs that are filtered and secreted are eliminated very quickly by the kidneys. Compounds that are filtered, not reabsorbed and not secreted are also eliminated rapidly, but not as quickly as those drugs that are also secreted. For drugs that are filtered and extensively reabsorbed, renal excretion proceeds very slowly.

Drug interactions affecting renal filtration. Drugs may interact with each other to affect renal filtration, secretion or reabsorption. Drug molecules free in plasma water are filtered through the renal glomeruli. Drug molecules bound to plasma proteins are normally not filtered. If two drugs compete for plasma protein binding, the free levels of each will increase. This, in turn, will increase the number of molecules that can be filtered by the renal glomeruli.

Drug interactions affecting renal secretion. The secretion of drugs from the blood, through the renal tubules, into the developing urine is an active process that can be saturated by high drug concentrations. When this happens, drug secretion reaches its maximum and the concentration of drug in the blood and body suddenly increases.

The kidney has one transport mechanism for acidic drugs and another transport process for bases. If two acids, each of which is secreted, are administered concomitantly, they compete for the same transport mechanism. When this happens, the renal secretion of each drug is reduced. The same holds true for basic drugs. If two bases that are secreted are administered together, they too will compete with each other. The result is that less of each is secreted by the renal tubules and their rates of elimination from the body are reduced.

Probenecid and penicillins are acids that are secreted by the renal tubules. The renal clearance rates for penicillins often exceed 600 mL/min. As a result, penicillins are rapidly eliminated by the kidneys, and they have short half-lives (approximately 1 h) in the body. Probenecid is sometimes given with a penicillin to reduce the rate at which the antibiotic is secreted by the kidney and to increase its half-life and duration of action in the body. The presence of penicillin in the body also reduces the rate of probenecid secretion. However, this point has little clinical significance.

Drug interactions affecting tubular reabsorption. Reabsorption occurs passively as drug molecules diffuse across the renal tubules into the blood. The amount of drug reabsorbed by the renal tubules into the blood depends on the lipid solubility of the drug molecules. Because lipid solubility of a drug is determined by the percentage of the drug in its nonionized form (see Chapters 4 and 5),

reabsorption depends on the ratio of ionized to nonionized drug molecules. If a drug is highly ionized, it will not be reabsorbed. If, on the other hand, most of the drug molecules are nonionized, drug reabsorption will take place.

The major factor controlling the degree of ionization in the tubular lumen is the pH of the developing urine inside the tubular lumen. A change in the pH of this fluid affects the ionization of acidic and basic drugs.

If a drug is an acid, raising the pH of the developing urine with a chemical such as sodium bicarbonate will increase the percentage of the drug in the ionized form. Sodium bicarbonate is often administered to patients who have ingested toxic amounts of acetylsalicylic acid to increase its rate of elimination from the body. Acidifying the urine has just the opposite effect on acidic drugs. Administering a drug such as ammonium chloride or ascorbic acid, which will lower the pH in the urine, increases the percentage of acidic drug molecules in the nonionized form. The result of this is to increase the number of molecules that will diffuse back into the blood.

The reverse is true for basic drugs. Acidifying the urine increases the percentage of molecules in the ionized form and decreases renal tubular reabsorption. Adding a drug that will raise the pH in the renal tubular lumen will have the opposite effect. The percentage of molecules in the nonionized form will increase and tubular reabsorption will be facilitated.

Drug Interactions Involving Hepatic Metabolism of Drugs

Many drugs can either increase or decrease the drug-metabolizing capacity of the liver. Some of the most important drug interactions result from drug-induced changes in the ability of the liver to metabolize drugs.

Increases in drug metabolism. Many drugs increase the drug-metabolizing ability of the liver. These include the antituberculosis drug rifampin and the antiepileptic drugs phenobarbital, phenytoin, carbamazepine and primidone. The antifungal drug griseofulvin can also increase the capacity of the body to metabolize drugs.

Because protein synthesis is needed for the induction of drug metabolism, a time span of two to three weeks is required between the time of starting the inducer and the maximum increase in drug metabolism. By the same token, two to three weeks are necessary after stopping the inducer before drug metabolic enzymes return to pretreatment levels, with the resultant gradual increase in the plasma concentration of the affected drug(s).

In choosing examples of compounds that can increase drug metabolism, one cannot ignore phenytoin, phenobarbital and other enzyme-inducing anticonvulsants. These drugs can increase the metabolism of a wide variety of other drugs. For example, they enhance the metabolic elimination of hydrocortisone (cortisol). Phenobarbital has been reported to precipitate acute asthma in steroid-dependent patients. Phenobarbital also reduces the response to prednisolone in rheumatoid arthritis.

The interactions of phenobarbital and phenytoin are not restricted to glucocorticoids. Long-term treatment with enzyme-inducing anticonvulsants increases the incidence of cyclic disturbances and of contraceptive failure. Pregnancies have been reported after the coadministration of an enzyme-inducing antiepileptic and an oral contraceptive.

Decreases in drug metabolism. Commonly prescribed inhibitors of drug metabolism include erythromycin, cimetidine, sodium valproate, dextropropoxyphene, oral contraceptives, propranolol, some tricyclic antidepressants, phenothiazines and sulfonamides. The extent of their effect is unpredictable, but they usually increase circulating drug levels by an average of twenty percent. Once the inhibitor is stopped, drug metabolism gradually returns to normal.

An example of one drug inhibiting the metabolism of another can be found in the interaction between isoniazid and phenytoin. Isoniazid can inhibit the metabolism of phenytoin. When isoniazid is administered to epileptic patients on long-term therapy with phenytoin, the frequency of drowsiness and intoxication is increased several-fold.

Drug Interactions on the Target Tissue

Pharmacodynamic interactions are the easiest to note and probably represent the most common form of drug interaction. Two drugs may interact in a tissue to produce either a synergistic or antagonistic effect. If the response is synergistic, the two drugs act together to give an effect greater than either alone. If the effect is antagonistic, one drug blocks the effects of the other.

Most drugs act through specific receptors. Interactions occur frequently when two drugs act on the same receptor. An excellent example is blocking the effects of $beta_2$ agonists on the bronchioles with a nonselective beta blocker, or inhibiting the effects of a cholinergic drug with an anticholinergic compound.

Drugs may also interact at the tissue level by affecting different, but complementary, systems. Beta agonists stimulate $beta_2$ receptors and dilate bronchioles. Theophylline also dilates bronchioles, although not through beta stimulation. If theophylline is given together with a $beta_2$ agonist, the degree of bronchodilatation is often greater with the two drugs than with either agent alone.

The treatment of hypertension provides another example of the principle that two drugs that produce their effects by different mechanisms may interact to produce an effect greater than either alone. A diuretic lowers blood pressure by decreasing blood volume and dilating arterioles. A beta blocker owes its antihypertensive actions to its ability to reduce cardiac output. If the two are used together, the combined antihypertensive effect is greater than when either agent is employed alone.

A drug interaction may also entail the administration of one drug that affects tissue sensitivity to another. The interaction between a thiazide or loop diuretic and digoxin serves as an excellent example of this type of interaction. These diuretics increase potassium excretion, often leading to hypokalemia. The sensitivity of the heart to digoxin-induced cardiac arrhythmias is increased by hypokalemia. Therefore, although the diuretics are often indicated in patients requiring digoxin, care must be taken to prevent a diuretic-induced hypokalemia. Failure to do so will predispose the heart to digoxin-induced cardiac arrhythmias.

Regardless of the type of interaction produced, it is important to remember that one drug may affect the actions of another drug directly, or indirectly, on the target tissue. Care must be taken to consider this fact when using more than one medication in a patient.

CHAPTER 8

Drug Therapy across the Lifespan

Topics Discussed
- Definition of teratogenic
- Drugs and the fetus
- Pediatric pharmacology
- Drugs and the elderly patient

The therapeutic and adverse effects of drugs can be influenced by age and developmental stage. For example, the immature systems of the newborn and the aging systems of the elderly may alter pharmacokinetics. This chapter highlights significant alterations across the lifespan: important information for the assessment, monitoring and education of patients and families, from birth to old age.

Drugs and the Fetus

One study of 168 pregnant women showed that they had consumed an average of 11 drugs during pregnancy and 7 during labour and delivery. This included over-the-counter (OTC) drugs, such as laxatives and antacids. Drugs produce significant effects on the fetus because almost all drugs can transfer through the placental barrier, which is in fact not a barrier at all!

Some drugs are *teratogenic,* that is, they are able to cause birth defects. Generally, drugs cause most significant effects during the first trimester (first three months of pregnancy) because this is the stage of organ development. However, drugs can affect the fetus throughout its entire development. In addition to medications, pregnant women should avoid alcoholic beverages because alcohol is a drug that can produce serious adverse effects on the development of the child. Unfortunately, many women may not even be aware that they are pregnant during the first four to six weeks.

The United States Food and Drug Administration (FDA) has developed categories to indicate the risk of drugs during pregnancy. As indicated in Table 8.1, the risk is not always clear. An excellent principle to following during pregnancy is to take drugs only if they are absolutely required.

Pediatric Pharmacology

Pediatrics refers to all patients from birth to age 16 and is traditionally divided into the following subgroups: neonate, first four weeks of life; infant, to 1 year; children, 1 to 12 years; and adolescent, 12 to 16 years.

A major challenge in prescribing for pediatric patients is that the majority of drugs are not tested in children. When clinical need dictates their use, a minor experiment is occurring. Vigilance in the assessment and monitoring of pediatric patients has primary importance in nursing management for safe and effective drug therapy for this population.

Drugs and the Neonate

There are significant potential pharmacokinetic alterations in the newborn as a result of the incomplete development of many body systems. Absorption of orally administered drugs may be enhanced or reduced by such factors as reduced gastric acid, absence of intestinal flora, and altered transit time through the intestine. Gastrointestinal membranes are not completely developed and

Table 8.1
FDA pregnancy risk categories

Category	Description
Category A	Controlled studies in women did not demonstrate risk to the fetus in the first trimester or throughout pregnancy
Category B	Either animal studies have demonstrated an adverse effect in the fetus but controlled studies in women have not confirmed the effect, or animal studies have not demonstrated a risk and there are no controlled studies in pregnant women
Category C	Because controlled studies in women are lacking, the pregnancy risk is unknown, and animal studies may or may not demonstrate an adverse effect on the fetus. Drug therapy may be used if the potential benefit justifies the potential risk to the fetus
Category D	Evidence of fetal risk is demonstrated but the potential benefit justifies the potential risk to the fetus
Category X	Human or animal studies demonstrate fetal abnormalities. The risk of using the drug in pregnant women clearly outweighs possible benefits

may allow, or block, the transport of some substances. First-pass metabolism is reduced, thus improving the bioavailability of some drugs. Absorption from intramuscular injections is erratic owing to smaller muscle mass and circulation. In contrast, topically applied drugs have increased absorption through the skin.

Distribution is altered owing to a higher amount of body water (65% to 75% of body weight) and less fat than the adult. Lower levels of plasma protein, plus competition from endogenous chemicals, reduce drug binding to plasma proteins. As a consequence, the free levels of drugs are increased.

Biotransformation in the liver is reduced because of immature enzyme systems. Drug conjugation is particularly reduced. As a result, many drugs, such as chloramphenicol, have a greatly reduced rate of inactivation. The renal excretion of drugs is also reduced in the neonate because of a lower glomerular filtration rate.

The consequences of these alterations may be generally summarized by stating that neonates should receive smaller doses than would be expected on a body-weight basis. In addition, the onset of action, time to peak effect and duration of action for drugs may differ from those seen in the adult. Accurate calculation and administration of dosages is the first step to providing effective drug treatment in the neonate.

Newborns may also receive drugs inadvertently through the breast milk. Drugs diffuse from the plasma into milk passively. Usually the concentration in milk is low. However, for some drugs, such as lithium, breastfeeding is absolutely contraindicated. All nursing mothers should ascertain the safety of taking drugs.

Drugs and the Infant/Child

Liver and kidney function rapidly increase during the first few months of life, and most body systems mature by the age of one year. Generally, infants and children can handle drug doses calculated on the basis of body weight or body surface area (through the use of a nomogram). An unexpected increase in metabolic rate or rapid turnover of body water can increase the required dosage for some drugs. For example, a child with a seizure disorder may require higher doses of the anticonvulsant phenytoin to achieve therapeutic blood levels.

Pharmacodynamics can also be affected in this age group because receptor development and sensitivity can vary with age.

Administration techniques and educational strategies must be adapted for the infant and child. Skillful approaches can help alleviate the fear associated with injections. Involving the parents is essential.

Some adverse reactions are unique to children because of developmental factors. Table 8.2 on the next page lists some examples.

Table 8.2
Adverse drug effects that are unique or increased in children

Drug Class	Adverse Effect
ASA	Acute intoxication with acidosis; Reye's syndrome
Chloramphenicol	Grey-baby syndrome
Corticosteroids	Reduced growth; reduced height caused by early closure of epiphyseal bone
Phenobarbital	Hyperactivity
Phenothiazines	Sudden infant death syndrome (SIDS)
Tetracyclines	Staining of teeth; impaired bone growth
Vitamin K	Kernicterus

Drugs and the Elderly Patient

The elderly patient has arbitrarily been defined as someone who is 65 years of age or older. This is unfortunate, because aging is not exclusively linked to a calendar. Aging is a dynamic process that is influenced by many factors, such as genetics; lifelong nutrition; presence and frequency of disease, trauma, injury and surgeries; and clinical and social factors, including stress and socioeconomic status.

Elderly patients often respond differently to drugs. Older people often suffer from one or more chronic diseases that require concurrent medications. Because organ function and pharmacologic responses are more variable among older patients, the effects of standard doses are difficult to predict. Increased drug use, decreased predictability of response and increased susceptibility to adverse reactions complicate drug therapy in the elderly.

Nurses must consider elderly patients to be "brittle" and manage them with great care. Physiological functions, such as conduction velocity, basal metabolic rate, cardiac index, glomerular filtration rate, renal plasma flow and maximum breathing capacity, decline with age. These changes may modify the response of older patients to drugs, and they must be considered in selecting the correct drug and the right dose. With the exception of most antibiotics, the motto in selecting a dose of a drug for an elderly patient should be "start low and go slow."

This section will discuss some of the problems encountered in treating elderly patients with drugs. It will summarize the pharmacokinetic changes seen in the elderly and some of the general problems encountered in determining the correct dose for the elderly patient.

Some Reasons for Prescribing Difficulties

Prescribing drugs for the elderly patient can be difficult. A number of factors, such as atrophy of disuse, malnutrition, multimorbidity, and difficulties in the diagnostic process, combine to make prescribing for older patients particularly complex.

With advancing age, patients are faced with an increasing number of predominantly chronic diseases and disabilities (see Figure 8.1). Many elderly patients suffer from four or more different conditions, with as many as nine different pathologic conditions frequently identified in persons 70 years and older. It is also not uncommon for a patient to be seen by several different physicians and to patronize multiple pharmacies. The problem may be compounded by the fact that many disabilities

Figure 8.1
Incidence of chronic disease with advancing age

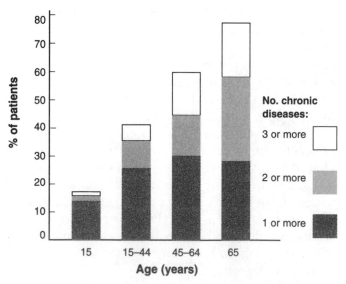

Source: Lamy PP. Modifying drug dosage in elderly patients. In: Covington TR, Walker JI (eds.), *Current Geriatric Therapy.* Philadelphia: W.B. Saunders; 1984. Reproduced with permission.

remain unknown to the primary provider. The consequence of this situation is that one physician may be unaware of what another has prescribed and may thus duplicate drug orders or increase the interaction potential between drugs. Further, failure of the patient to patronize a single pharmacy precludes the maintenance of a comprehensive patient drug profile, thus prohibiting effective drug utilization review by the pharmacist.

Pharmacokinetic Changes in the Elderly

Drug absorption. The amount of drug that reaches the systemic circulation (bioavailability) following oral drug administration depends upon the gastrointestinal absorption and metabolism during the drug's first pass through the GI mucosa and the liver (first-pass metabolism).

Extensive changes take place in the GI tract with advancing age, but its general anatomic and physiologic integrity is generally well maintained. That fact notwithstanding, there is often a decrease in acid secretion in the stomach. Achlorhydria occurs much more frequently in older patients. If this occurs, the ratio of nonionized/ionized molecules of weakly acidic drugs will decrease. It has been suggested that this may reduce the amount of drug absorbed from the stomach.

Because of an increase in gastric pH and a reduction in stomach secretions, it is speculated that poorly soluble drugs, such as ampicillin, digoxin and griseofulvin, may not be as well absorbed in older people. The older patient may have dry mucous membranes or dentures, and tablets may stick to the cheek or the esophagus. Adequate water with tablets is essential. Many aging people have difficulty swallowing (dysphagia). It is tempting to crush pills and add them to food. This must not be done for any products that are designed for sustained release or that have an enteric coating.

Little is known concerning the role of intestinal motility of drug absorption. One assumes that decreased motility may increase the rate of absorption, particularly of poorly soluble drugs, because they stay in contact with absorbing surfaces longer. However, this point remains to be demonstrated. Absorption from muscles may be somewhat slower, if muscle mass has decreased and if the individual is inactive.

Drug distribution. Both body weight and body composition change with advancing age. Total body water decreases by 15% to 20%, and extracellular fluid by 35% to 40% between the ages of 25 and 65. The significance of this is recognized when it is remembered that drugs are dissolved in body fluids. The smaller the volume of distribution for any drug, the greater its concentration. This is one reason to administer lower doses of most drugs to elderly patients.

Changes in organ blood flow with aging may also affect drug distribution. Cardiac output may decrease and peripheral vascular resistance can increase with age. Hepatic and renal blood flow are decreased and an increased fraction of the cardiac output is distributed to the brain, heart and skeletal muscle. Although many of these changes are at least partly the result of prior illness, the average elderly patient will probably have altered blood flow compared with younger patients.

Because drug distribution and end-organ effect are dependent upon the free drug concentration, changes in plasma protein binding may be important. Although total protein levels are not changed, the albumin/globulin ratio is reduced in elderly patients. Drugs bound predominantly to albumin may have an increase in the fraction of free (pharmacologically active) drug in the plasma. In contrast, many drugs including antidepressants, antipsychotic drugs and beta blockers, bind mainly to alpha$_1$-acid glycoprotein, a protein that is often increased in the presence of chronic diseases that occur frequently in the elderly population. Hence, the free drug concentration in elderly patients may be relatively increased in the case of drugs bound to albumin or decreased in the case of those bound to alpha$_1$-acid glycoprotein.

Drug elimination. Reduced renal function is probably the single most important factor responsible for altered drug levels and, therefore, increased drug action in the elderly. Many changes in renal structure and function occur with advancing age. Renal blood flow, glomerular filtration rate and tubular function all decline with aging. Between the ages of 20 and 90 years, there is an average decline of 35% in glomerular filtration rate. Serum creatinine values are often used to reflect the state of renal function. An increase in serum creatinine is interpreted to indicate a decreased glomerular filtration rate (GFR). In the elderly, however, renal function may fall without producing a commensurate increase in serum creatinine because of a decrease in endogenous creatinine production.

In addition to the physiological decline in renal function, the elderly patient is particularly liable to renal impairment due to dehydration, congestive heart failure, hypotension and urinary retention, or to intrinsic renal involvement (e.g., diabetic nephropathy or pyelonephritis).

Most drugs that are either filtered or secreted have age-related decreases in excretion that correlate with altered renal function. Altered drug secretion generally parallels decreases in glomerular filtration. Many drugs that are eliminated primarily by the kidney must undergo a dosage reduction to prevent their accumulation in the body of the elderly patient to toxic levels. Drugs with significant toxicity that have diminished renal excretion with age include aminoglycoside antibiotics, amantadine, lithium, digoxin, procainamide and cimetidine.

Hepatic metabolism of drugs. The liver continues to function well in the elderly, reasonably fit individual without liver disease. Liver and body weight correlate with each another, both starting to decline in the fifth or sixth decade of life. A majority of elderly persons may well have more than one abnormality in liver function, but serious deterioration of liver function is not consistent with the effects of primary aging and is induced only by a large loss of functioning liver cells.

Although in vitro studies in animals suggest that both basal activity and inducibility of the hepatic microsomal mixed-function oxidase enzymes may be reduced with age, these alterations have not been demonstrated clearly in humans. It is difficult to generalize with respect to the effects of aging on the metabolism of drugs. It is true that hepatic extraction and clearance can change with age. For some drugs it has been possible to demonstrate a reduced rate of metabolism. However, there is no uniform change in the hepatic plasma clearance of drugs with age.

The consequences of a reduction in liver metabolism of drugs depend on the drug concerned. If the drug is inactivated by metabolism, a reduction in hepatic metabolism should increase the duration of action of the drug. If bioavailability depends on the quantity of the drug able to escape first-pass metabolism, a reduction in liver metabolism should be reflected in increased initial serum levels of the drug and possibly also a longer half-life. If, on the other hand, a drug is activated by first-pass metabolism in the liver, it may have a reduced effect in the elderly patient.

Much research on the pharmacokinetics of drugs in older adults has been conducted over the past two decades, but our need for further knowledge in this area continues. There are many limitations to what we know. For example, we can be fairly confident in our understanding of changes in renal drug excretion and altered volume of distribution of drugs in this target group and can use this knowledge to adjust drug dosing. What we lack is adequate proof of therapeutic range and pharmacodynamic responses. Studies on a single-dose administration of drug X, when given to "healthy" 75-year-old males, cannot be generalized to chronic administration of the same drug to a 75-year-old female with multiple pathology. Consequently, careful clinical monitoring of every older patient is an important contribution to safe drug therapy.

Pharmacodynamic Changes in the Elderly

Drug receptor sensitivity may be reduced in the elderly. As humans age and are less able to balance catabolism with anabolism, it would appear logical to expect that their ability to manufacture drug receptors would also be reduced. However, there is little substantive evidence to support this contention. We do, however, have isolated reports of elderly patients demonstrating reduced responses to drugs that would suggest an altered drug receptor interaction.

Elderly patients seem less sensitive to bronchodilator effects of beta agonists or the antianginal or antihypertensive actions of beta blockers. This observation has led to the speculation that aging is associated with a reduction in the number of beta receptors and/or a reduction in the affinity of beta receptors for both agonist and antagonist. However, the evidence to support this hypothesis is not strong.

It has also been suggested that elderly patients may demonstrate increased sensitivity to the oral anticoagulant warfarin. At equal plasma concentrations of warfarin, elderly subjects showed greater inhibition of vitamin K-dependent clotting factor synthesis than young subjects, while plasma half-life, volume of distribution and protein binding were not altered. In addition, the rate of clotting factor degradation was not changed with age. Although these results suggest that hepatocyte sensitivity to warfarin may be increased with age, the mechanism of the altered response is not established. Receptors, enzyme activity, membrane transport mechanisms or substrate availability may all be involved.

Elderly patients are also known to have an increased sensitivity to psychotherapeutic drugs. Impairment of psychomotor function by benzodiazepines, for example, occurs at lower concentrations in the elderly than in young patients. Central nervous system adverse effects, including confusion, disorientation, agitation or sedation from tricyclic antidepressants, phenothiazines, anticholinergic drugs, barbiturates, levodopa and cimetidine are more common in the elderly.

Although pharmacokinetic parameters are altered with age in some cases, adverse effects may be more frequent in the elderly even when free drug concentrations are similar to those in the young. Increased receptor sensitivity has not been firmly established, and it is likely that these altered effects in the elderly are due to a combination of increased tissue sensitivity, decreased ability to compensate for altered central nervous system function, and altered pharmacokinetic characteristics causing increased or prolonged tissue exposure.

Adverse Drug Reactions

Adverse drug reactions (ADRs) refer to the unintended consequences of drug therapy. It is estimated that 10% to 15% of the elderly population will have an ADR. Adverse drug reactions are two to seven times more frequent in the over-60 age group. For example, in hospital the incidence of ADRs is estimated at 3% to 8% in those under 60, but increases to 11% to 21% for those over 60. Approximately 16% of admissions to psychogeriatric units are due to ADRs. Drug-induced illness accounts for 5% to 30% of hospital admissions for those over 65.

Two significant adverse reactions for older individuals are drug-induced confusion and drug-related falls. The former may be induced by a variety of drug groups, including central nervous system depressants, psychotropics, anticholinergics and digoxin. This confusion or disorientation may be dismissed as old age or misdiagnosed as dementia. Equally serious is the risk of falls and injury that can be caused by orthostatic hypotension from antihypertensives, oversedation from centrally acting depressants, or bathroom urgency resulting from diuretic therapy.

Table 8.3
Index of risk for adverse drug reactions

Factor	Risk
Age	The greater the age, the greater the risk of medication errors and ADRs
Gender	Females experience more ADRs
Number of drugs	Elderly are likely to receive several drugs, "one pill for every ill." Drugs are often used to treat side effects of other drugs
Socioeconomics	Lack of resources (e.g., inability to purchase drugs or to seek medical attention promptly) often means diseases may progress before help is obtained
Support system	Living alone may make patients more prone to errors. Lack of family and friends generally leads to poor health behaviours
Multiple pathology	ADRs may complicate existing disease. ADRs may masquerade as common diseases
Multiple providers	Fragmented services and lack of monitoring often result from multiple providers
Sensory impairment	Deficits in sight, hearing, etc. can create difficulty in following instructions
Level of disability	Severe disability may result in errors, inability to follow instructions or self-monitor

Drug therapy represents a significant dilemma for older adults and their caregivers. It is truly a double-edged sword. Although many older patients benefit from their drugs, others experience severe adverse effects. Table 8.3 on the previous page provides an index of risk factors for adverse drug reactions.

Further Reading

Anderson P. Medication use while breast feeding a neonate. *Neonat Pharmacol Q* 1993;2(2):3–14.

Burke M. Safety: injuries and adverse drug reactions. In: Burke M (ed.), *Care of the Frail Elderly.* St. Louis: Mosby; 1992.

Conn V. Older adults: factors that predict the use of OTC medications. *J Adv Nurs* 1991;16:1190–1196.

Conover E. Hazardous exposures during pregnancy. *J Obstet Gynecol Neonat Nurs* 1994;23(6):524–532.

Kadzma D. Drug response: not all bodies are created equal. *Am J Nurs* 1992;92(12):48–50.

LeSage J. Polypharmacy in geriatric patients. *Nurs Clin North Am* 1991;26(2):272–290.

Levin R. Advances in pediatric drug therapy of asthma. *Nurs Clin North Am* 1991;26(2):263–272.

Romonko L, Pereles L. An evaluation of pharmacy assessment for geriatric patients. *Can J Hosp Pharm* 1992;45(1):15–20.

Stolley J, et al. Iatrogenesis in the elderly. *J Gerontol Nurs* 1991;17:112–23, 136–137.

Walker M. Pharmacology and drug therapy in critically ill elderly patients. *AACN Clin Iss Crit Care Nurs* 1992;3(1):137–148.

Wink D. Giving infants and children drugs: precision + caution = safety. *MCN: Am J Maternal Child Nurs* 1991;16(6):317–321.

Chemotherapy of Infectious Diseases

Perhaps no area of pharmacology and therapeutics is more important to the nurse than the treatment of infections. Although anti-infective therapy has been marked by one breakthrough after another over the past forty years, it is now facing a new threat — the appearance of drug resistance. Infections previously considered easily treated with drugs have developed resistance, some with alarming speed. If we are to maintain effective control of life-threatening or debilitating infections, changes must take place over the next few years. These include the development of new drugs.

However, developing new drugs is not the only answer to the current problem. If we use our new drugs in the same way as we have prescribed our older agents, resistance will also develop to them. The answer lies in changing our attitude to drug use. Anti-infectives should be used only when they are needed. Nurses must work with other members of the health team to ensure that anti-infectives are used appropriately. For this reason, we have chosen to discuss this topic first.

Unit 3 discusses the use of drugs to eradicate pathogenic bacteria, fungi, viruses, protozoans and helminths from the body. It begins with a review of the general considerations essential for the safe and effective use of anti-infectives and moves on to discuss the pharmacotherapeutics of individual groups of drugs used routinely in the treatment of infectious disease.

CHAPTER 9

General Considerations in the Use of Anti-infective Drugs

Topics Discussed
- Definition of antibiotic, antibacterial, bacteriostatic, bactericidal, synergy
- Mechanism of action
- Resistance
- Superinfection
- Selecting the right antibiotic
- Prophylactic use of antibiotics
- Nursing management

Antibiotics vs. Antibacterials

Nurses frequently hear the words "antibiotic" and "antibacterial," and they must often wonder if there is really any difference between the two. In a strict sense, there is. But practically, the two types of drug can be considered the same.

Antibiotics, such as penicillin G and gentamicin, are chemicals that are produced by microorganisms that either destroy, or suppress the growth of, other microorganisms. *Antibacterials,* such as the sulfonamides or quinolones, are not produced by microbes. Instead, they are synthesized by chemists. Setting that distinction aside, it is virtually impossible to tell these two types of drug apart. Neither their clinical uses nor their adverse effects depend on whether they are naturally derived or synthetic. Thus, the terms "antibiotic" and "antibacterial" are commonly considered interchangeable, and both mean anti-infective.

Bacteriostatics vs. Bactericidals

Bacteriostatic antibiotics, such as erythromycin or chloramphenicol, inhibit bacterial cell replication but do not kill the organism. In other words, they stop bacterial growth and allow the host's immune factors to eliminate the infection. The growth and division of bacterial cells is an essential component of the infectious process. In ideal circumstances, bacterial cells can double in number every 20 minutes. Any process that hinders bacterial growth will affect the progress of an infection. If, for example, a bacteriostatic drug can slow the multiplication of bacteria so that they double every two or three hours, this may have a considerable impact in helping the defence systems of the host to overcome the infection. Bacteriostatic drugs may not be adequate if the host's immunity is suppressed, or if the infection is in an area of poor immunologic surveillance, such as the CSF (cerebral spinal fluid).

Bactericidal antibiotics kill bacteria. These drugs rely less on host immunity for eradicating bacterial infections. Examples of bactericidal drugs include the penicillins, cephalosporins, and most aminoglycosides.

Some drugs, such as the sulfonamides and tetracyclines, can have either bacteriostatic or bactericidal actions, depending on their concentration and the specific bacteria involved in the infection.

Mechanism of Action

A clinically useful antibiotic is a drug that inhibits microbial growth in vivo and is harmless to the host. The ideal anti-infective drug is *selectively* toxic to the invading organisms. The degree to which an antibiotic demonstrates selective toxicity is determined, in part, by its mechanism of action. If a drug inhibits a bacterial enzyme or a structure that is not found in humans, it should have selective toxicity for the microbe. Penicillins and cephalosporin block cell wall formation (see below). Because cell walls are present in most bacteria, but not in humans, these drugs are selectively toxic to many bacteria.

Enzymes catalyze the processes responsible for the growth and duplication of bacteria, and antibiotics inhibit those enzymes. The chapters that follow will discuss the ways in which individual drugs or groups of drug inhibit enzymatic steps crucial to cell growth and duplication. At this time, it will suffice to provide an overview of the actions of these drugs.

Antibiotics can interfere with one or more of the following processes:

1. Cell wall synthesis. All living cells, including bacterial and mammalian cells, have cell membranes. However, the situation in which bacterial membranes find themselves differs significantly from those encountered by mammalian membranes. Mammalian membranes surround cells containing an isotonic internal environment. Thus, there is no physical pressure on these membranes. In contrast, bacterial cells are hypertonic. If they are to survive and multiply in an isotonic mammalian environment, bacteria must protect themselves from the lower pressure in the host. Bacterial cell walls, external to the cell membrane, serve that purpose. They protect bacterial cells from the isotonic environment of the host and prevent their osmotic rupture. During bacterial growth and division, new cell walls must be formed. If bacteria cannot form new walls, they rupture. Antibiotics, such as the penicillins and cephalosporins, inhibit cell wall synthesis and make growing bacteria vulnerable to osmotic rupture.

2. Maintenance of cell membrane integrity. Bacterial cell membranes maintain the intracellular contents of the microbe, both by controlling passive diffusion and by providing the mechanisms of active transport. Drugs that disorganize the cytoplasmic membrane of the bacteria produce a leakage of the intracellular contents of the microbe and death. Unfortunately, drugs can also affect mammalian cell membranes. This is particularly obvious in the kidney, where these drugs are concentrated. As a result, many of these drugs are used only topically for superficial infections.

3. Nucleic acid structure and function. The quinolone antibiotics (e.g., norfloxacin, ciprofloxacin) inhibit the replication of bacterial DNA by interfering with the action of DNA gyrase during bacterial growth and reproduction.

4. Protein synthesis. A number of antimicrobial agents act by binding to bacterial ribosomes and interfering with protein synthesis. These agents include aminoglycosides, tetracyclines, chloramphenicol and erythromycin. Because the precise biosynthetic steps involved in bacterial protein synthesis differ from those in mammalian cells, it is possible for antibiotics to inhibit protein synthesis in bacteria without affecting the formation of protein in the host.

5. Production and function of folic acid. Most bacteria must synthesize their folic acid, whereas humans can rely on dietary sources. Sulfonamides inhibit the formation of folic acid, and trimethoprim inhibits dihydrofolate reductase, the enzyme required to activate folic acid.

Figure 9.1 on the next page summarizes the sites of action of antimicrobial drugs.

Resistance

Over the past few years, concern has increased over the dramatic increase in acquired resistance to many anti-infective drugs. Most, if not all, microorganisms are capable of developing resistance to the action of anti-infective drugs.

Mutation can account for the development of antibiotic resistance in microorganisms. However, mutation is a rare, spontaneous occurrence that is not usually inducible by antibiotics, and it is not an important mechanism of drug resistance. Changes attributed to mutation include alterations of cell walls or cell membrane components that prevent the entry of drugs into bacterial cells, or changes of the target or binding site for antimicrobials inside the cell.

Figure 9.1
Antimicrobial sites of bacterial or bacteriostatic action on microorganisms

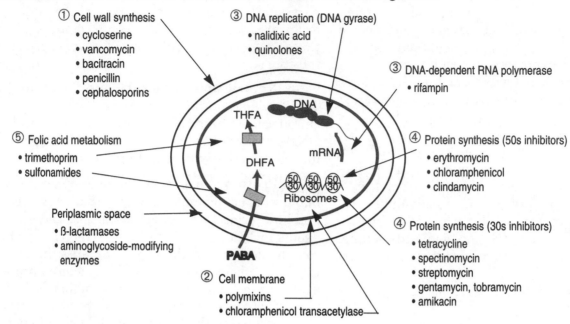

The five general mechanisms are: (1) inhibit synthesis of cell wall, (2) damage cell membrane, (3) modify nucleic acid/DNA metabolism, (4) modify protein synthesis (at ribosomes), and (5) modify energy metabolism within the cytoplasm (at folate cycle).

Source: Principles of antimicrobial use. In: Wingard LB, Brody TM, Larner J, Schwartz A (eds.). *Human Pharmacology: Molecular to Clinical.* St. Louis: Mosby; 1991. Reproduced with permission.

Inheritance is the most common way for microbes to acquire resistance to antimicrobial drugs. Inheritable resistance is induced by exposure to antibiotics, and it is transferred from one microbe to another in a microbial population by genetic agents called resistance plasmids (R plasmids). Plasmids are extrachromosomal genetic elements in bacteria. The main function of plasmids is to allow bacterial evolution under varying environmental conditions. R plasmids can encode for resistance to as many as six or seven antimicrobial drugs, and are the major threat to continued antibiotic effectiveness.

R plasmids are probably produced from the collection of foreign genes that are not normally part of a microbe's chromosomes. These genes may have come from a variety of unrelated bacterial or fungal sources, and they must have experienced strong selective pressures to be assembled into R plasmids.

R plasmid-coded activities can result in the synthesis of:

• products in cell walls or cell membranes that prevent antibiotics from entering microorganisms
• microbial enzymes that modify the site of drug action, in which case the antibiotic can enter the cell but not bind to its receptor
• microbial enzymes that destroy antibiotics
• substitute microbial enzymes that are resistant to antibiotics and replace antibiotic-sensitive essential enzymes.

Dissemination of Antibiotic Resistance

R plasmid-coded activities can be transferred from one bacterium to another by conjugation, transduction, or transformation.

Conjugation is a most important mechanism for the dissemination of antibiotic resistance. This can occur because most R plasmids possess the sex-factor necessary to initiate conjugation between resistance-positive and resistance-negative bacteria. This conjugation leads to a direct transfer of complete R plasmids from one bacterial cell to another.

The emergence of *Haemophilus* and gonococci that produce beta-lactamase is a major therapeutic problem. The gene for the production of this enzyme is carried on small plasmids. At least some of the gonococcal plasmids are similar in size to the *H. influenzae* gene, and a *Haemophilus* plasmid has been transferred to gonococci by conjugation in vitro. Likewise, many gonococcal strains carry a conjugative plasmid that enables sexual transfer to other *Neisseria* and to *Escherichia coli*. It is thus likely that beta-lactamase-producing gonococci initially obtained their plasmid from a *Haemophilus* species and may maintain the potential to transfer it to penicillin-sensitive species such as *Neisseria meningitidis*.

Transduction occurs by the intervention of a bacteriophage (a virus that infects bacteria) that can carry bacterial DNA incorporated within its protein coat. If this genetic material includes a gene for drug resistance, a newly infected bacterial cell may become resistant to the drug and thus capable of passing the trait on to its offspring. Transduction is limited to smaller R plasmids that can be accommodated in a bacteriophage chromosome. Transduction is particularly important in the transfer of antibiotic resistance among strains of *Staphylococcus aureus*, where some phages can carry plasmids that code for penicillinase, while others transfer genetic information for resistance to erythromycin, tetracycline, or chloramphenicol.

Transformation is the direct DNA transfer of R plasmids between microorganisms. It is used extensively now in the genetic engineering of new biological drugs with *E. coli*. The importance of transformation in the transfer of antibiotic resistance remains unknown.

Superinfection

Within many body tissues, notably the skin and the mucous membranes of the gastrointestinal, genitourinary and respiratory tracts, a finely balanced ecosystem exists where multitudes of microorganisms are held in check. Drug treatment disturbs this balance, and otherwise innocent organisms that are resistant to the drug multiply and produce tissue damage. This phenomenon is referred to as *superinfection*.

Several variables appear to influence the development of superinfections. They are more often seen in children younger than two years of age and in adults over fifty. The length of antimicrobial treatment is also critical, since the incidence of superinfections is uncommon when a drug is given for less than a week. Finally, the microbiological activity of the antimicrobial is important in that antibiotics with broad-spectrum activity, such as ampicillin and tetracyclines, cause a greater suppression of normal flora and thereby increase the risk of superinfections.

Because these infections occur with some frequency and can complicate recovery, health care providers and clients should know how to watch for warning signs.

Selecting the Right Antibiotic

Choosing the right drug for the right bug is not always easy. It involves clinical judgment, together with a knowledge of the likely infecting organism and the spectrum of activity of the various antibiotics. The expression "spectrum of activity" refers to the range of bacteria or fungi that are sensitive to a particular anti-infective drug. Penicillin G, for example, is primarily active against gram-positive bacteria and is classified as a narrow-spectrum antibiotic. Third-generation cephalosporins, by way of contrast, are effective against a range of gram-positive and gram-negative bacteria. These drugs are therefore classified as broad-spectrum antibiotics.

The physician must first decide whether to give any antibiotic. Many doctors automatically associate fever with a treatable infection and order an antibiotic. This practice is irrational and dangerous, because the diagnosis may be masked if cultures are not obtained prior to therapy. Furthermore, all antibiotics can cause serious toxicity. In addition, using antimicrobials in this fashion can lead to the selection of resistant microorganisms.

This is not to say, however, that antibiotics should always be withheld until the physician is sure that treatment is definitely warranted. Physicians cannot always wait for definitive proof of a treatable infection before starting therapy. Severe infections often demand immediate treatment, and empiric antibiotic treatment may well be warranted.

When they are given empirically, the drugs

chosen should cover all the most likely pathogens. Thus, it is not uncommon to find physicians prescribing broad-spectrum antibiotics or combinations of antimicrobials. Empiric therapy requires a knowledge of the most likely infecting microorganisms and their sensitivities to anti-infective drugs. The clinical picture may provide the most important clues to the offending pathogen. In this situation, the physician must know the microorganisms most likely to cause a specific infection. Whenever the physician is faced with starting empiric therapy on a presumptive bacteriological diagnosis, cultures of blood and other fluids should be taken before beginning the antibiotic(s). These cultures, when grown in a laboratory, may identify the microorganism responsible for the infection and, following tests of its sensitivity to various antibiotics, can guide the physician in the selection of the best drug for that particular bug.

Once the physician has identified the infecting microbe, treatment can become definitive. At this time, a narrow-spectrum, low-toxicity regimen is often ordered to complete the course of treatment.

Combination Antibiotic Therapy

Although antibiotic therapy often involves using drug combinations, the decision to use more than one drug should be considered carefully. Obviously, using two or more antibacterials may increase the risk of drug-induced toxicities. Although the effects of combination therapy can increase the overall antibacterial effect (synergy), this is not always the case. There are conditions when the effects of one drug antagonize the actions of the other. There are also situations when the effect of the two drugs is no different than giving one of the antibacterials alone. Obviously, combination antibiotic therapy should be used only when the two drugs produce a synergistic effect.

Synergy is best demonstrated by discussing the use of trimethoprim with sulfamethoxazole. Sulfamethoxazole inhibits the formation of folic acid, whereas trimethoprim blocks an enzyme, dihydrofolate reductase, that is essential in the activation of folic acid. Together, trimethoprim and sulfamethoxazole produce an antibacterial effect that is greater than either drug used alone. Combining a penicillin (e.g., ticarcillin) with an aminoglycoside antibiotic (e.g., tobramycin) provides another example of a synergistic effect. The inhibition of cell wall synthesis by the penicillin permits better penetration of the cell wall by the aminoglycoside and more effective inhibition of protein synthesis.

Antagonism can be illustrated by referring to the use of a penicillin and a tetracycline. Tetracyclines exert their bacteriostatic effects by inhibiting protein synthesis. Penicillins block cell wall synthesis, but their bactericidal effect depends on bacteria to be actively multiplying. When a penicillin and a tetracycline are used together, the tetracycline inhibits cell synthesis and growth and thereby prevents the penicillin from demonstrating its bactericidal activity.

Combined antibiotic therapy may be justified for the treatment of mixed bacterial infections. Some infections are caused by two or more microorganisms. These include intra-abdominal, hepatic and brain abscesses and many of the genital tract infections. In these situations it may be necessary to give different antibiotics with different antimicrobial spectra to obtain the required activity.

Two or more antibiotics may also be given to prevent the emergence of resistant microorganisms. This method of treatment has received extensive use in cases of tuberculosis, where the concomitant use of two or more antitubercular drugs reduces significantly the development of drug resistance by *Mycobacterium tuberculosis*.

Prophylactic Use of Antibiotics

Antibiotics are frequently prescribed to prevent rather than to treat infections. It has been estimated that this practice represents 30% to 50% of all antibiotic prescriptions and accounts for some of the most flagrant misuses of antibacterials.

This fact notwithstanding, there are certainly well-defined conditions in which the prophylactic use of antibiotics is essential. Generally, it can be stated that if a single drug is effective in preventing infection by a *specific microorganism* or to clear an infection immediately or soon after it has been established, then its prophylactic use is often successful. This differs significantly from the situation where the aim of prophylaxis is to prevent colonization or infection by *any or all microorganisms* present in the patient's environment. In this situation, prophylaxis frequently fails.

Chemoprophylaxis has been used to protect healthy people from acquiring specific microorganisms to which they are exposed. The use of antibiotics to prevent gonorrhea or syphilis after contact with an infected individual or giving rifampin, minocycline or sulfadiazine to prevent meningococcal disease are examples of this form of chemoprophylaxis.

Antibiotics can also be used prophylactically to prevent secondary bacterial infection in patients who are ill with other diseases. Neutropenic patients may have a reduced incidence of bacterial infections if treated with trimethoprim plus sulfamethoxazole. The newer fluoroquinolones, such ciprofloxacin, also show promise as prophylactic agents for neutropenic patients.

Antibiotics should be used prophylactically to prevent endocarditis in patients with valvular or other structural lesions of the heart who are undergoing dental, surgical or other procedures that produce a high incidence of bacteremia. Endocarditis is caused from the bacterial colonization of the endocardium, particularly the cardiac valves. Any procedure that injures a mucous membrane where there are large numbers of bacteria (such as in the oropharnyngeal or gastrointestinal tract) will produce transient bacteremia. Streptococci from the mouth, enterococci from the gastrointestinal or genitourinary tract and staphylococci from the skin have a high potential to produce endocarditis. Chemoprophylaxis directed against these microorganisms is recommended.

Nursing Management

Understanding the general considerations that have been discussed in this chapter is important for nurses working in various clinical settings including hospitals, community health, and occupational health. In particular, understanding the mechanisms of drug resistance and an appreciation of factors that promote the development of resistance are essential concepts for nursing practice. Nurses, through education of the public, can help promote effective use of antibiotics and help reduce unnecessary drug use. Box 9.1 contains a sample patient teaching.

Using the algorithm for the nursing management of drug therapy, the nurse begins with the assessment of risk versus benefit by collecting patient data and understanding the relevant pharmacology. Table 9.1 on the next page summarizes the nursing process.

Further Reading

Chambers HF, Sande MA. Antimicrobial agents. In: Hardman JG, Limbird LE (eds.). *Goodman and Gilman's The Pharmacological Basis of Therapeutics.* 9th ed. New York: Pergamon; 1996:1029–1058.

Beam TR. Principles of anti-infective use. In: Smith CM, Reynard AM (eds.). *Textbook of Pharmacology.* Philadelphia: W.B. Saunders; 1991:805–816.

Snyder IS, Finch RG. Introduction to chemotherapy. In: Craig CR, Stitzel RE (eds.). *Modern Pharmacology.* 4th ed. Boston: Little, Brown; 1994:537–544.

Box 9.1
Patient/family education for anti-infectives

This information applies to all drug groups used for the chemotherapy of infectious diseases. Instruct the patient/family to:

✔ Always ask the name of the drug and inform health care provider if any previous problems have occurred with antibiotic therapy
✔ Take all the medication, even if symptoms abate
✔ Take drug as prescribed, e.g., with or without food as ordered and with a full glass of water to dissolve medication and increase absorption
✔ Report occurrence of new symptoms and side effects for assessment and instructions
✔ Call the physician if a rash occurs (or if symptoms of superinfection appear)
✔ Contact physician if symptoms do not improve
✔ Do not save any remaining medication if drug is discontinued for any reason; take drug to pharmacy for disposal
✔ Never use any left-over antibiotic for a new illness or share drug with anyone else
✔ Store medication as instructed (e.g., most liquid preparations should be refrigerated)
✔ If you forget a dose, take as soon as you remember. Do not double any dose. Continue with regular schedule

Table 9.1
Nursing management for anti-infective drugs

Assessment of risk vs. benefit	Patient data	• *Host factors:* Defence mechanisms, particularly immune system; other diseases (e.g., reduced renal function may cause toxicity, as most anti-infectives are excreted by the kidneys); hx allergy • *Age:* Infants and elderly pts may have reduced defences and increased risk for drug toxicity • *Pregnancy and lactation:* Risks to fetus and infant
	Drug data	• Site and type of infection (drugs selected based on location of infection and causative microorganism); culture and sensitivity results
Implementation	Rights of administration	• Check right time of administration of oral anti-infectives: food may/may not interfere with absorption • For IV route, check solution, concentration, rate and compatibility with other medications • For IM route, check reconstitution instructions and administer deep into large muscle mass
	Nursing therapeutics	• Assess local/systemic signs/symptoms of infection (vary with systems involved) • Monitor VS, lab values (hematology, urinalysis) • Enhance host defences (nutrition, rest, fluids, hygiene)
	Patient/family teaching	• The principles of pt/family education have been previously described (Figure 1.3, page 7). Specific education for the proper use of anti-infectives should include the content in Box 9.1 (page 67) • Allergic reactions are the most significant adverse effects of the anti-infectives. It is important to understand the mechanisms of allergic responses and to review the signs/symptoms with the pt and family. Pts with drug allergies should carry an information card or wear a bracelet or locket engraved with this information at all times
Outcomes	Monitoring of progress	*Continually monitor:* • Clinical response indicating tx success (reduction in signs/symptoms) • Nontherapeutic reactions (side effects and adverse reactions) • Laboratory values (serum drug levels, cultures, hematology values)

C H A P T E R   1 0

The Penicillins

Topics Discussed
- Mechanism of action
- Antibacterial spectra
- Pharmacokinetics
- Therapeutic uses
- Adverse effects
- Nursing management

Drugs Discussed
amdinocillin (am-din-oh-**sill**-in)
amoxicillin (ah-mok-sih-**sill**-in)
ampicillin (am-pih-**sill**-in)
bacampicillin (bah-kam-pih-**sill**-in)
benzylpenicillin potassium (**ben**-zil-pen-ih-**sill**-in)
carbenicillin indanyl sodium (kar-ben-ih-**sill**-in **in**-dan-il)
cloxacillin (clok-sah-**sill**-in)
dicloxacillin (dye-clok-sah-**sill**-in)
flucloxacillin (flew-clok-sah-**sill**-in)
mezlocillin (mez-loe-**sill**-in)
nafcillin sodium (naf-**sill**-in)
penicillin G potassium
penicillin V
phenoxymethyl penicillin (feen-ox-ee-**meth**-il)
piperacillin (pye-per-ah-**sill**-in)
pivampicillin (piv-am-pih-**sill**-in)
procaine benzylpenicillin (**pro**-cane)
procaine penicillin G
ticarcillin (tye-kar-**sill**-in)

Clinical Challenge
Consider this clinical challenge as you read through this chapter. The response to the challenge appears on page 81.

Jane is admitted to hospital for treatment of cellulitis of her right leg. Her vital signs indicate pyrexia and mild tachycardia with normal BP. The physician orders a regimen of IV penicillin for 3 days with a plan to initiate oral therapy at that time.

While starting the IV, you explain the plan to Jane, who says she cannot take penicillin because she is allergic to it. You determine that she received an antibiotic last year, thinks it was penicillin, and developed diarrhea.

What is your next action?

In 1928, Sir Alexander Fleming noted the lysis of bacteria growing in the vicinity of a contaminating mould. Perhaps no discovery in pharmacology has had such an impact on subsequent therapy. Ten years later, Sir Howard Florey and colleagues were able to isolate, from cultures of *Penicillium notatum,* a crude preparation of penicillin capable of killing several important pathogenic bacteria.

Since the introduction of penicillin G (benzylpenicillin), several derivatives have been synthesized (Table 10.1, on the next page). The obvious differences between the various penicillins should not obscure the fact that they also have many similarities. All penicillins have the same basic chemical structure, mechanism of action and major adverse effects. This chapter will discuss the

Table 10.1
Properties of some commonly used penicillins

Name	Stability in acid	Spectrum of action	Sensitivity to penicillinase	Routes of administration
Penicillin G (benzylpenicillin penicillin)	poor	narrow	sensitive	oral, parenteral
Penicillin V (phenoxymethyl penicillin)	good	narrow	sensitive	oral
Penicillinase-resistant penicillins				
Cloxacillin	good	narrow	resistant	oral, parenteral
Dicloxacillin	good	narrow	resistant	oral, parenteral
Flucloxacillin	good	narrow	resistant	oral
Nafcillin	variable	narrow	resistant	parenteral
Expanded-spectrum penicillins				
Ampicillin	fair	broad	sensitive	oral, parenteral
Amoxicillin	good	broad	sensitive	oral
Carbenicillin	poor	broad	sensitive	parenteral
Piperacillin	poor	broad	sensitive	parenteral
Ticarcillin	poor	broad	sensitive	parenteral

pharmacology of penicillins, emphasizing both their similarities and differences.

Penicillin products are often referred to as beta-lactam antibiotics. Figure 10.1 presents the basic structure of the penicillin nucleus, pointing out the beta-lactam ring. Penicillins and cephalosporins (see Chapter 11) owe their antibacterial activity to the presence of the beta-lactam ring. The R group is important in determining stability in an acid medium, as well as susceptibility to the penicillinases, produced by most *Staphylococcus aureus* and some other bacteria.

Mechanism of Action

Bacterial cells are encased both by cell membranes and by cell walls. The cell wall lies on the outside of the bacterium and is essential to its survival. The cell membrane, found just inside the cell wall, encloses the bacterium.

Bacterial cytoplasm is hypertonic. This fact is important because it explains the necessity for a healthy cell wall. Without a rigid wall, the cell membrane cannot withstand the internal hypertonic medium. If the cell wall is damaged, the high pressure within the bacterium causes the membrane first to bulge and finally to rupture, killing the bacterium.

Penicillins bind to a group of bacterial enzymes, collectively called the penicillin-binding proteins (PBPs) on the outer surface of the cell membrane, to block cell wall formation. These molecules are called PBPs because penicillins must bind to them to produce antibacterial effects. By binding to PBPs, penicillins prevent the crosslinking of molecules essential in building cell walls. As the old walls gradually deteriorate and are not replaced by new material, they become thinner. Eventually, they are not strong enough to support the cell membranes, which then rupture, killing the bacteria. Figure 10.2 describes the consequences of a penicillin's interrupting cell wall synthesis.

Antibacterial Spectra

Synthesis of Semisynthetic Penicillins

When natural antibiotics have their potential antibacterial properties limited by poor absorption, enzymatic inactivation, narrow antibacterial spectra, etc., they are often modified chemically to produce derivatives that have the required types of activities (Figure 10.3).

The first major successes of the semisynthetic approach were seen in the penicillin field. The first penicillin introduced into therapeutic use was benzylpenicillin (penicillin G). This was a natural product of the penicillin mould; that is, the

Figure 10.1
Structural formulas of representative penicillins

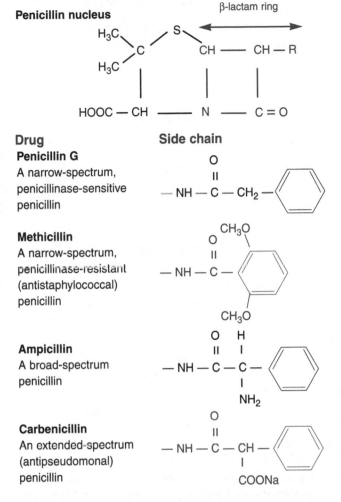

Penicillin nucleus

The unique structure of individual penicillins is determined by the side chain coupled to the penicillin nucleus at the position labelled R. This side chain influences acid stability, pharmacokinetic properties, penicillinase resistance and ability to bind specific penicillin-binding proteins.

Source: Drugs that weaken the bacterial cell wall. 1: Penicillins. In: Lehne RA, Moore LA, Crosby LJ, Hamilton DB (eds.), *Pharmacology for Nursing Care.* 2nd ed. Philadelphia: W.B. Saunders; 1994:928. Reproduced with permission.

Figure 10.2
Consequences of interrupted cell wall synthesis, as caused by penicillins and cephalosporins

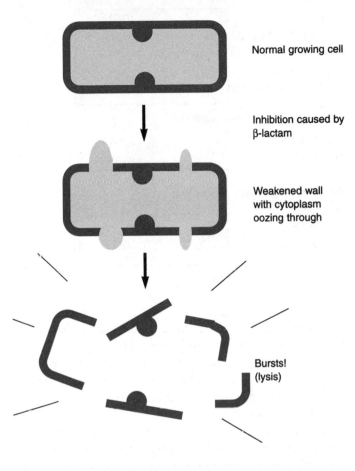

Source: Richmond MH. Beta-lactam antibiotics: the background to their use as therapeutic agents. Frankfurt: Hoeschst AG;1981:70. Reproduced with permission.

Figure 10.3
Production of semisynthetic antibacterials

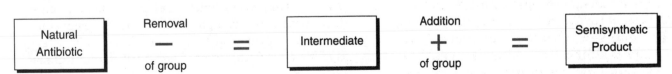

A group on the natural antibiotic is first removed and then replaced by another, which enhances activity.

Source: Richmond MH. Beta-lactam antibiotics: the background to their use as therapeutic agents. Frankfurt: Hoeschst AG; 1981:14. Reproduced with permission.

Figure 10.4
Phenoxymethyl penicillin (penicillin V)

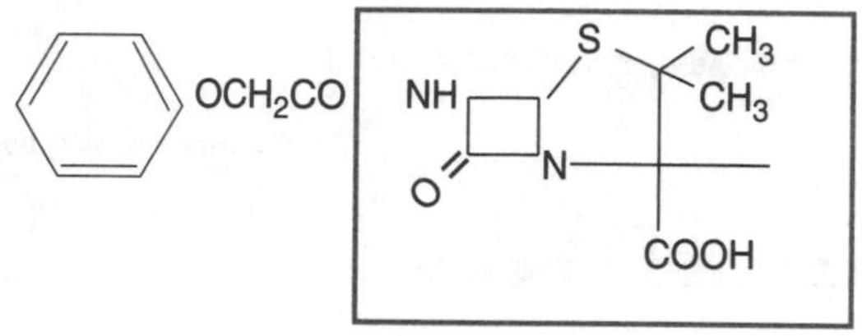

Phenoxymethyl penicillin
(penicillin V)

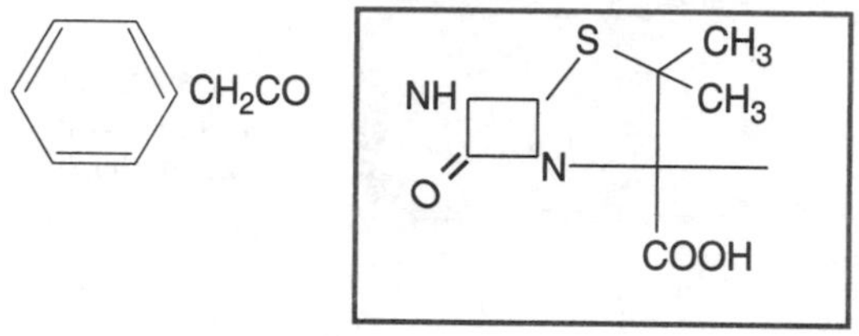

Benzylpenicillin
(penicillin G)

Figure 10.5
Route from benzylpenicillin to a semisynthetic derivative via 6-amino-penicillanic acid (6-APA)

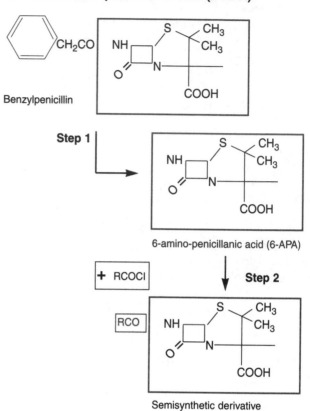

Benzylpenicillin

Step 1

6-amino-penicillanic acid (6-APA)

+ RCOCl

Step 2

RCO

Semisynthetic derivative

The presence of the phenoxymethyl side chain, in place of the benzyl group of penicillin G, confers acid stability and oral absorption on the compound.

Source: Richmond MH. Beta-lactam antibiotics: the background to their use as therapeutic agents. Frankfurt: Hoeschst AG; 1981:15. Reproduced with permission.

The benzyl group may be removed either by acid or by an enzyme. The new side chain is put on chemically.

Source: Richmond MH. Beta-lactam antibiotics: the background to their use as therapeutic agents. Frankfurt: Hoeschst AG; 1981:15. Reproduced with permission.

antibiotic was not modified chemically after it had been produced in the primary fermentation. It was soon found that if one fed the fermentation mould with precursors that differed from those normally used, small modifications of the penicillin structure could be obtained.

One of these — phenoxymethyl penicillin, or penicillin V — was introduced soon after penicillin G (Figure 10.4). It had the advantage that it was more stable to acid than penicillin G and, as a result, was better absorbed when taken orally.

However, as explained below, there was still need for penicillin activity against penicillinase-producing *Staphylococcus aureus* and gram-negative bacteria, a feature that was not part of the spectrum of benzylpenicillin (penicillin G) and phenoxymethyl penicillin (penicillin V). The break-

through in this field came about when it was realized that benzylpenicillin or phenoxymethyl penicillin could be treated chemically to generate the penicillin nucleus, 6-amino-penicillanic acid (Figure 10.5).

This molecule could be treated in turn with other chemical reagents to make semisynthetic derivatives of the penicillin nucleus. This approach led to the development of methicillin, which is resistant to penicillinase, and ampicillin, a penicillin that is active against many gram-negative bacteria. Methicillin must be injected to be effective, and it has been replaced with penicillinase-resistant penicillins that are well absorbed orally. The synthesis of methicillin is important, however, because it led to the production of the penicillinase-resistant penicillins that are currently used.

Table 10.2
Antibacterial spectra of the various penicillin groups

	Narrow-spectrum penicillins		Expanded-spectrum penicillins	
	Penicillin G Penicillin V (Penicillinase- sensitive penicillins)	Cloxacillin Dicloxacillin (Penicillinase- resistant penicillins)	Ampicillin Amoxicillin Bacampicillin Pivampicillin	Azlocillin Carbenicillin Mezlocillin Piperacillin Ticarcillin
Staphylococcus aureus (pen.-sens.)	+	+	+	+
Staphylococcus aureus (pen.-resis.)	–	+	–	–
Streptococcus pyogenes	+	+	+	+
Streptococcus pneumoniae	+	+	+	+
Enterococcus spp.	–	–	+	–
Clostridium perfringens	+	+	+	+
Neisseria gonorrhoeae	+	±	+	+
Neisseria meningitidis	+	±	+	+
Haemophilus influenzae	–	–	±	+
Escherichia coli	–	–	±	±
Klebsiella spp.	–	–	–	±
Proteus spp. (indole-negative)	–	–	±	+
Proteus spp. (indole-positive)	–	–	–	±
Serratia spp.	–	–	–	±
Salmonella spp.	–	–	+	+
Shigella spp.	–	–	±	+
Pseudomonas aeruginosa	–	–	–	+
Bacteroides fragilis	–	–	–	±
Other *Bacteroides* spp.	+	±	+	±
Chlamydiae spp.	–	–	–	–
Mycobacteria pneumoniae	–	–	–	–

Legend: + = Sensitive; – = Resistant; ± = Some strains resistant. Consult text for details on the use of each group of drugs.

Narrow-Spectrum Penicillins

Table 10.2 presents the antibacterial spectra of the major penicillin groups. Any discussion of the penicillins must begin with a review of penicillin G. This drug is extremely effective for the treatment of nonpenicillinase-producing cocci, gram-positive bacilli, and spirochetes. However, as implied above, penicillin G has three major limitations:

• Its instability in an acid medium. Much of an oral dose is destroyed in the stomach, reducing the percentage of the dose absorbed.
• Its inactivation by penicillinase-producing (beta-lactamase-producing) staphylococci, eliminating its use in many staphylococcal infections.
• Its narrow spectrum of activity, covering mainly only cocci, gram-positive bacilli, and spirochetes.

Newer semisynthetic penicillins have overcome some of penicillin G's limitations. Their rational use depends on understanding how they differ from penicillin G.

Penicillin V (phenoxymethyl penicillin) has the same antibacterial spectrum as penicillin G, but is more stable in the stomach and is better absorbed. Penicillin V is recommended in place of penicillin G for oral administration. Like penicillin G, it is not resistant to penicillinase and does not have an expanded spectrum of activity.

Penicillinase-Resistant Penicillins

Although both penicillin G and penicillin V were initially effective against most strains of *Staphylococcus aureus*, resistance built up rapidly (Figure 10.6). Within five or six years of the introduction of

Figure 10.6
Emergence of penicillin-resistant strains of *Staphylococcus aureus* following the widespread introduction of benzylpenicillin (penicillin G) for therapy

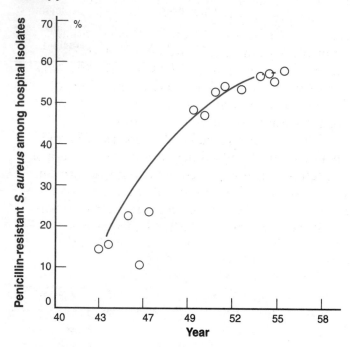

Source: Richmond MH. Beta-lactam antibiotics: the background to their use as therapeutic agents. Frankfurt: Hoeschst AG;1981: 49. Reproduced with permission.

Figure 10.7
Effect of beta-lactamase on the penicillin nucleus

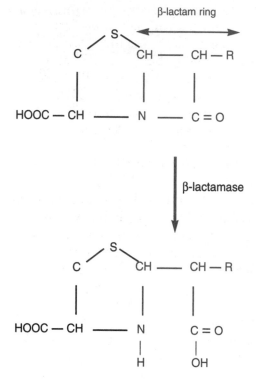

Source: Drugs that weaken the bacterial cell wall. 1: Penicillins. In: Lehne RA, Moore LA, Crosby LJ, Hamilton DB. *Pharmacology for Nursing Care.* 2nd ed. Philadelphia: W.B. Saunders; 1994:929.

penicillin G into common use, approximately 50% to 60% of all isolates of *S. aureus* made in hospitals throughout the world were resistant to them.

S. aureus resistance developed rapidly because of the ability of the bacterium to secrete enzymes called penicillinases. Penicillinases are a subgroup of enzymes called beta-lactamases that rupture the beta-lactam ring, thereby inactivating penicillins (Figure 10.7). Bacteria produce a variety of beta-lactamases; some are specific for penicillins or other beta-lactam antibiotics (e.g., cephalosporins), and some act on several kinds of beta-lactam antibiotics. Only those beta-lactamases that act selectively on penicillin are referred to as penicillinases.

S. aureus is not the only bacterium to secrete penicillinases. These enzymes are also synthesized by other gram-positive bacteria, as well as gram-negative microorganisms. Gram-positive organisms produce large amounts of the enzyme, and then release them into the surrounding medium. In contrast, gram-negative bacteria produce

relatively small amounts of penicillinase, and secrete them into the space between the cell membrane and the cell wall.

The genes that code for the synthesis of beta-lactamases are located on plasmids (Chapter 9) and chromosomes. Genes that are present on plasmids are transferred from one bacterium to another, thereby spreading penicillin resistance.

Nafcillin (Nafcil®, Nallpen®, Unipen®), cloxacillin (Bactopen®, Cloxapen®, Orbenin®, Tegopen®), dicloxacillin (Dycill®, Dynapen®, Pathocil®) and flucloxacillin (Fluclox®) are usually resistant to *Staphylococcus aureus*-secreted penicillinase. Although they are active against many penicillin-G-sensitive bacteria, the penicillinase-resistant drugs are not as effective as penicillins G or V. They should be used primarily to treat staphylococcal infections and are considered to have a very narrow spectrum of use.

In the last few years, staphylococcal strains resistant to the so-called penicillinase-resistant penicillins have emerged. These staphylococci are called methicillin-resistant staphylococci. However, this term should not lull one into the mistaken belief that only methicillin no longer works. All penicillinase-resistant penicillins are ineffective. This resistance appears to be due to the production of altered penicillin-binding proteins (PBPs) to which the penicillinase-resistant penicillins are unable to bind. Vancomycin is the drug of choice for the treatment of infections caused by the so-called methicillin-resistant staphylococci.

Expanded-Spectrum Penicillins

Group I — Aminopenicillins.

A major limitation to the use of penicillin G, penicillin V and the penicillinase-resistant penicillins is their lack of effect against most gram-negative bacteria. This can be explained on the basis of the different makeup of the cell envelope of gram-positive and gram-negative bacteria.

The cell envelope of gram-positive bacteria has only two layers — the cytoplasmic membrane and the surrounding cell wall. Although the cell wall is thick, it does not present a barrier to drug diffusion. Penicillins can readily pass through it to affect the PBPs on the outer surface of the cell membrane. It is their action on the outer surface of the cell membrane that inhibits the formation of the cell wall.

The cell envelope of gram-negative bacteria is more complex and has three layers. In addition to the inner cell membrane and surrounding cell wall, gram-negative bacteria have a second cell membrane that surrounds the cell wall. This outer membrane presents a barrier to the diffusion of many penicillins. Only those penicillins that can pass through the small pores in the outer membrane are able to cross and reach PBPs on the inner cytoplasmic membrane. The first drug to achieve this was ampicillin.

Ampicillin (Ampicin®, Ampilean®, Omnipen®, Polycillin®, Penbritin®, Principen®) and amoxicillin (Amoxil®, Larotid®, Polymox®, Trimox®) have inhibitory activity at low concentrations for all strains of *Streptococcus pyogenes*, *S. faecalis* (enterococci), *S. pneumoniae* and penicillin-G-sensitive *Staphylococcus aureus*. Neither drug is resistant to penicillinase secreted by *S. aureus*. However, it is not their activity against penicillin-G-sensitive bacteria that sets ampicillin and

amoxicillin apart from the narrow-spectrum antibiotics. Rather, it is their activity against most strains of *Escherichia coli*, *Haemophilus influenzae*, *Proteus mirabilis*, *Salmonella* and *Shigella*. However, resistant beta-lactamase-producing strains of these organisms are now prevalent in some areas of the world, and in this situation ampicillin or amoxicillin are not effective. Other Enterobacteriaceae (e.g., *Klebsiella*, *Enterobacter*, *Serratia*, indole-positive *Proteus*, *Providencia*), *Pseudomonas aeruginosa* and most *Acinetobacter* are resistant to the aminopenicillins.

Bacampicillin (Penglobe®, Spectrobid®) and pivampicillin (Pondocillin®) are inactive esters of ampicillin. Once absorbed, however, they are converted to ampicillin in the body and are called *prodrugs*. Because they are inactive in the gastrointestinal (GI) tract, both bacampicillin and pivampicillin do not produce the diarrhea that is characteristic of ampicillin.

Group II — Antipseudomonal penicillins.

Azlocillin (Azlin®), carbenicillin (Geopen®, Pyopen®), mezlocillin (Mezlin®), piperacillin (Pipracil®) and ticarcillin (Ticar®) are effective in higher concentrations against most strains of *Pseudomonas aeruginosa* and indole-positive and indole-negative *Proteus* species, which is their primary use. However, their spectrum of activity also covers many other bacteria (Table 10.2). They should be used primarily with an aminoglycoside antibiotic such as gentamicin, tobramycin, amikacin or netilmicin to treat infections caused by *Pseudomonas* and *Proteus*. As explained in Chapter 9, the inhibition of cell wall synthesis by the penicillin permits better penetration of the cell wall by the aminoglycoside and more effective inhibition of protein synthesis.

Group III — Amidino penicillins.

Amdinocillin, or mecillinam (Coactin®), has a different spectrum of activity from other beta-lactam antibiotics, in that it is active primarily against gram-negative organisms and relatively ineffective against gram-positive organisms. Amdinocillin pivoxil, also known as pivmecillinam (Selexid®), is a prodrug of amdinocillin or mecillinam that is converted to the microbiologically active amdinocillin or mecillinam during absorption from the gastrointestinal tract. Amdinocillin pivoxil is indicated in the treatment of acute and chronic urinary tract (UT) infections caused by sensitive strains of *E. coli*, *Klebsiella*, *Enterobacter* and *Proteus* species.

Group IV — Penicillins combined with a beta-lactamase inhibitor.

Beta-lactamase inhibitors are drugs that inhibit bacterial beta-lactamases. By combining a beta-lactamase inhibitor with a penicillinase-sensitive penicillin, it is possible to expand the antimicrobial spectrum of the penicillin.

Amoxicillin has been combined with potassium clavulanate (Augmentin®, Clavulin®) in 2:1 or 4:1 fixed-ratio dosage forms. Amoxicillin is susceptible to hydrolysis by beta-lactamase enzymes; therefore, bacteria that secrete beta-lactamases are resistant to the antibiotic. Potassium clavulanate, or clavulanic acid, inhibits beta-lactamases secreted by some microorganisms. By inhibiting these beta-lactamases, clavulanic acid protects amoxicillin from hydrolysis and enables it to act against microorganisms that would normally be resistant to the antibiotic. Thus, clavulanic acid increases the spectrum of activity of amoxicillin to include beta-lactamase-producing *Haemophilus influenzae*, *H. ducreyi*, *Neisseria gonorrhoeae*, *Staphylococcus aureus* and *Branhamella catarrhalis*. Concentrations attained in the urine will inhibit many beta-lactamase-producing strains of *Escherichia coli*, *Klebsiella*, *Proteus* and *Citrobacter*.

In regions where the incidence of penicillinase-producing *Neisseria gonorrhoeae* reaches 5% to 10%, Augmentin® or Clavulin® should be considered one of the alternatives to the penicillins. The combination of amoxicillin and potassium clavulanate appears suitable for the treatment of complicated urinary tract infections, otitis media, sinusitis and respiratory tract infections caused by beta-lactamase-producing strains of the previously mentioned bacteria.

Ampicillin has also been combined with sulbactam, another beta-lactamase inhibitor, in the product Unasyn®. The addition of sulbactam does not alter the susceptibility of ampicillin-sensitive strains and extends the in vitro activity of ampicillin to include many beta-lactamase-producing strains (but not methicillin-resistant staphylococci) and many anaerobic bacteria (including the *Bacteroides fragilis* group).

Piperacillin plus tazobactam (Zosyn®) and ticarcillin plus clavulanic acid (Timentin®) are other combinations of penicillins plus beta-lactamase inhibitors. The addition of tazobactam or clavulanic acid to the respective antipseudomonal penicillins extends the spectrum of the penicillin to include staphylococci and a wide variety of anaerobes and gram-negative bacteria, including multiple-drug-resistant organisms such as *Acinetobacter* and some ceftazidime-resistant strains of *Klebsiella pneumoniae*. These combinations do not have any more activity against *Pseudomonas aeruginosa* than either piperacillin or ticarcillin used alone.

Pharmacokinetics

Most penicillins are not completely absorbed following ingestion because they are at least partially destroyed by stomach acid. Approximately one-third of an oral dose of penicillin G is absorbed from the gastrointestinal tract, primarily from the duodenum. For maximum absorption, it should be taken either one hour before or two to three hours after a meal to facilitate rapid transport from the stomach to the duodenum. Under these conditions, peak blood levels are reached in about forty-five minutes.

Because penicillin G is poorly absorbed from the gastrointestinal tract, it should normally be administered intramuscularly. When injected intramuscularly, penicillin G attains peak blood levels within fifteen minutes. Procaine penicillin G or benzathine penicillin G are absorbed more slowly following intramuscular injection; peak blood levels are seen two to four hours after administration of procaine penicillin G, with concentrations falling to almost zero twenty-four hours later. Benzathine penicillin G produces very low serum levels of the antibiotic for three to four weeks after administration and must be used only to treat extremely sensitive bacteria. Figure 10.8 compares the blood levels of penicillin G following its oral and intramuscular administration.

Penicillin V is more stable than penicillin G in an acid pH and is better absorbed. As it has the same antibacterial spectrum as penicillin G, penicillin V is preferred for oral administration. It should be given on an empty stomach.

The penicillinase-resistant penicillins vary in their absorption following oral administration.

Figure 10.8
Blood concentration of various forms of penicillin G after oral or intramuscular administration

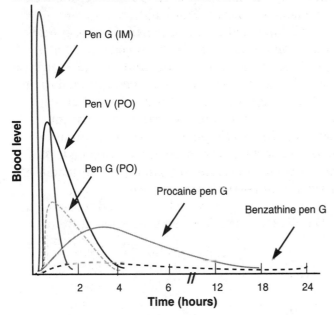

Source: Pratt WB. *Chemotherapy of Infection.* New York: Oxford; 1977. Reproduced with permission.

Methicillin is not stable in the stomach and must be injected. Nafcillin is absorbed quite erratically and should not be given orally. All other penicillinase-resistant penicillins can be taken orally. Cloxacillin has been the drug of choice for many physicians. It is prepared in both oral and parenteral dosage forms, provides effective therapeutic levels, and is usually marketed at a reasonable cost. Although dicloxacillin and flucloxacillin produce higher blood levels following oral administration, they have not been shown to be clinically more effective than cloxacillin.

Both ampicillin and amoxicillin may be given orally. Ampicillin is not completely absorbed and should be taken on an empty stomach to reduce acid inactivation. Amoxicillin enjoys the major advantage of being stable in an acid pH. It is usually preferred because it is well absorbed when given orally, both in the presence and absence of food. As a result, amoxicillin is usually taken three times daily with meals, as opposed to ampicillin, which is ingested four times daily on an empty stomach. Because of its improved absorption, amoxicillin causes less severe diarrhea than ampicillin and is better accepted by many patients.

Carbenicillin, ticarcillin and piperacillin must be injected to produce a systemic effect. Although carbenicillin is not absorbed when given orally, its indanyl sodium derivative (Geocillin®, Geopen Oral®) can be given by mouth for the treatment of urinary tract infections caused by *Pseudomonas*. The circulating levels of antibiotic following carbenicillin indanyl sodium are too low to treat a systemic infection.

The penicillins are distributed widely throughout the body but their passage into joint, ocular and cerebrospinal fluids is poor in the absence of inflammation. In the patient with inflamed meninges, however, they will enter the cerebrospinal fluid. It is this factor that enables penicillin G to treat meningitis caused by sensitive organisms.

All penicillins are rapidly excreted by the kidney. They undergo renal tubular secretion and, with renal clearance values of approximately 600 mL/min, have half-lives in the vicinity of one hour. Probenecid (Benemid®) reduces penicillin excretion and is sometimes used to reduce the rate of elimination of a penicillin and prolong its duration of action in the body.

Therapeutic Uses

Narrow-Spectrum Penicillins

Penicillin G (benzylpenicillin) is preferred for infections caused by frequently encountered gram-positive bacteria and susceptible gram-negative cocci. The major exceptions to this statement involve staphylococci and, in some cases, enterococci. Penicillin G is also the drug of choice for infections caused by certain gram-negative bacilli (e.g., *Spirillum minus, Streptobacillus moniliformis, Leptotrichia buccalis*), *Actinomycetes* and spirochetes.

As explained above, procaine penicillin G and benzathine penicillin G provide tissue depots of penicillin from which the drug is released slowly. Procaine penicillin G is absorbed over hours. The absorption of antibiotic from benzathine penicillin G is even slower, with the release of drug taking place over a period of several days. Administered intramuscularly, these products are used to treat infections, such as early syphilis, late latent syphilis and endocarditis due to penicillin-susceptible streptococci, where prolonged blood levels are needed and the frequent dosing requirements of aqueous penicillin G are undesirable.

Neither procaine penicillin G nor benzathine penicillin G should be given when high, sustained concentrations of penicillin G are needed. In this situation, aqueous penicillin G is the product that should be used.

Penicillin V is more stable than penicillin G in the acid medium of the stomach. As a result, it provides higher blood levels following ingestion, and its absorption is not affected by food. Penicillin V is preferred to penicillin G when oral treatment is indicated.

Penicillinase-Resistant Penicillins

The penicillinase-resistant penicillins currently on the market are nafcillin (Nafcil®, Nallpen®, Unipen®), cloxacillin (Bactopen®, Cloxapen®, Orbenin®, Tegopen®), dicloxacillin (Dycill®, Dynapen®, Pathocil®) and flucloxacillin (Fluclox®). Because these drugs offer no advantages over penicillin G, except in staphylococcal infections, they are recommended only for infections known or suspected to be caused by penicillinase-producing staphylococci. However, resistant strains of staphylococci have emerged to this entire group of drugs. These bacteria are commonly referred to as methicillin-resistant staphylococci because methicillin was the first drug in this group to be marketed. It is important to understand that the expression "methicillin-resistant staphylococci" means resistance to all penicillinase-resistant penicillins. When methicillin-resistant strains of *Staphylococcus aureus* or *S. epidermidis* are known or suspected to be present, vancomycin is the drug of choice (Chapter 17).

Parenteral nafcillin, oxacillin and methicillin are alternative choices for serious staphylococcal infections. Methicillin has been associated with the development of interstitial nephritis, thus the other agents are preferred. Orally, cloxacillin, dicloxacillin and flucloxacillin are alternative choices for mild to moderate infections.

Expanded-Spectrum Penicillins

Group I — Aminopenicillins. Ampicillin (Omnipen®, Penbritin®, Polycillin®, Principen®) and amoxicillin (Amoxil®, Larotid®, Polymox®, Trimox®) are the major aminopenicillins used today. Bacampicillin (Penglobe®, Spectrobid®) and pivampicillin (Pondocillin®) are inactive esters of ampicillin. Once absorbed, they are converted to ampicillin. Bacampicillin and pivampicillin should produce less diarrhea than ampicillin because they remain inactive until absorbed.

With few exceptions, the antibacterial spectra of ampicillin and amoxicillin are comparable. These antibiotics usually are the drugs of choice for infections caused by enterococci, although penicillin G is often preferred in enterococcal endocarditis. The aminopenicillins are also considered among the drugs of choice for nonpenicillinase-producing strains of *Haemophilus influenzae* and Enterobacteriaceae, particularly *Proteus mirabilis* and community-acquired *Escherichia coli*.

Ampicillin is available for oral and parenteral use. Amoxicillin is preferred over ampicillin for oral administration. Its absorption is more complete than that of ampicillin and it is less likely to produce diarrhea, particularly in children. Furthermore, food does not affect the absorption of amoxicillin.

Ampicillin is combined with sulbactam, and amoxicillin with clavulanic acid. Both sulbactam and clavulanic acid are beta-lactamase inhibitors that increase the spectrum of activity of the two penicillins (see Group IV, below).

Group II — Antipseudomonal penicillins. Ticarcillin (Ticar®), piperacillin (Pipracil®) and mezlocillin (Mezlin®) are the most frequently used antipseudomonal penicillins. Despite their broad antibacterial spectra (Table 10.2, page 73), they are preferred only as parenteral therapy over other antibiotics in the treatment of infections caused by or suspected of being caused by *Pseudomonas aeruginosa* or susceptible gram-negative bacilli that frequently are resistant to other penicillins and cephalosporins.

Pseudomonal infections are frequently nosocomial in origin, serious in severity and difficult to treat. They commonly infect compromised patients (e.g., febrile, neutropenic cancer patients; burn patients; cystic fibrosis patients). Emergence of bacterial strains is a serious problem, particularly if an antipseudomonal penicillin is used alone. Therefore, patients are often treated with an antipseudomonal penicillin, together with an aminoglycoside antibiotic (e.g., gentamicin [Garamycin®], tobramycin [Nebcin®], netilmicin [Netromycin®]). As previously explained, the antipseudomonal penicillin damages cell formation and permits increased concentrations of the amino-glycoside to enter the bacterium and modify protein synthesis.

Carbenicillin indanyl sodium (Geocillin®, Geopen Oral®) is the only antipseudomonal penicillin taken orally. It is used only for the treatment of urinary tract infections, including chronic bacterial prostatitis, because it does not produce high enough blood levels of carbenicillin to be effective systemically.

Tazobactam is a beta-lactamase inhibitor that is combined with piperacillin (Zosyn®). When used with piperacillin, tazobactam extends the spectrum of activity of piperacillin (see Group IV, below). The same rationale led to the earlier combination of ticarcillin with clavulanic acid to yield the product Timentin®.

Group III — Amidino penicillins.

Amdinocillin pivoxil or pivmecillinam (Selexid®) is a prodrug of amdinocillin that is converted during absorption from the gastrointestinal tract to the microbiologically active amdinocillin. As explained above, amdinocillin, or mecillinam, is active primarily against gram-negative organisms and relatively ineffective against gram-positive bacteria.

Amdinocillin pivoxil is indicated in the treatment of acute and chronic urinary tract infections caused by sensitive strains of *E. coli, Klebsiella, Enterobacter* and *Proteus* species.

Group IV — Penicillins combined with a beta-lactamase inhibitor.

Clavulanic acid, sulbactam and tazobactam inhibit many beta-lactamases produced by gram-positive and gram-negative bacteria. Clavulanic acid is combined with amoxicillin (Augmentin®, Clavulin®), sulbactam with ampicillin (Unasyn®), clavulanic acid with ticarcillin (Timentin®) and tazobactam with piperacillin (Zosyn®). The effect of these combinations is to protect the penicillin from the destructive effects of the beta-lactamases and to allow the drug to act against microorganisms that would normally be resistant.

Thus, clavulanic acid increases the spectrum of activity of amoxicillin to include beta-lactamase-producing *Haemophilus influenzae, H. ducreyi, Neisseria gonorrhoeae, Staphylococcus aureus,* and *Branhamella catarrhalis*. Concentrations attained in the urine will inhibit many beta-lactamase producing strains of *Escherichia coli, Klebsiella, Proteus* and *Citrobacter*.

Although combining clavulanic acid or potassium clavulanate with amoxicillin produces an effective antibiotic, the product is more expensive than amoxicillin used alone, and it is reasonable to ask when it should be used in place of amoxicillin. The combination should not displace amoxicillin or penicillin G for the treatment of gonococcal urethritis in regions of the world in which beta-lactamase-producing *Neisseria gonorrhoeae* are nonendemic. In regions where the incidence of penicillinase-producing *N. gonorrhoeae* reaches 5% to 10%, one of the combination should be considered as one alternative to the penicillins. The penicillinase-resistant penicillins are still indicated for gram-positive soft-tissue infections, unless resistant gram-negative rods are also present. The combination of amoxicillin and clavulanic acid appears suitable for the treatment of complicated urinary tract infections, otitis media, sinusitis, and respiratory tract infections caused by beta-lactamase-producing strains of the previously mentioned bacteria.

Sulbactam is combined with ampicillin in a parenteral product used to treat intra-abdominal, gynecologic and skin and soft-tissue infections causes by susceptible bacteria. Its broad antimicrobial spectrum, which includes beta-lactamase-producing gram-positive and gram-negative aerobic and anaerobic bacteria, could make this combination useful for these infections, which are frequently polymicrobial. Ampicillin plus sulbactam has also been effective for the treatment of bone, joint, lower respiratory tract (LRT) and urinary tract infections and uncomplicated gonorrhea, as well as for prophylaxis during gastrointestinal and obstetric/gynecologic surgery.

Combining potassium clavulanate with ticarcillin does not alter the susceptibility of ticarcillin-sensitive strains. It does, however, extend the activity to include beta-lactamase-producing strains of many Enterobacteriaceae. Ticarcillin plus potassium clavulanate is indicated for serious lower respiratory tract, urinary tract, bone and joint, and skin and soft-tissue infections and septicemia caused by susceptible beta-lactamase-producing strains of various gram-negative bacilli and *Staphylococcus aureus*. Because of its broad antibacterial spectrum against gram-positive and

Table 10.3
Allergic reactions to penicillins

Immediate allergic reactions (occur 2–30 min after administration)	• Urticaria • Flushing • Diffuse pruritus • Hypotension or shock • Laryngeal edema • Wheezing
Accelerated urticarial reactions (1–71 h)	• Urticaria or pruritus • Wheezing or laryngeal edema • Local inflammatory reactions
Late allergic reactions (>72 h)	• Morbilliform eruptions (occasionally occur as early as 18 h after initiation of tx) • Urticarial eruption • Erythematous eruptions • Recurrent urticaria and arthralgia • Local inflammatory reactions
Some relatively unusual late reactions	• Immunohemolytic anemia • Drug fever • Acute renal insufficiency • Thrombocytopenia

gram-negative aerobic and anaerobic bacteria, including many beta-lactamase-producing strains, ticarcillin plus potassium clavulanate is used in the treatment of mixed infections such as intra-abdominal and gynecologic infections.

Piperacillin plus tazobactam has been approved by the U.S. Food and Drug Administration for intravenous treatment of intra-abdominal, pelvic and skin-structure infections and for community-acquired pneumonia of moderate severity.

Adverse Effects

Allergic reactions are the major concern with the penicillins. These may occur in 1% to 5% of patients. Patients allergic to one penicillin should be considered allergic to all penicillins. Allergic reactions vary from skin eruptions to anaphylactic shock and death. Anaphylaxis is more common when parenteral administration is used. Table 10.3 summarizes allergic reactions to the penicillins.

Skin testing for the presence of IgE-mediated hypersensitivity to penicillin is indicated for patients with a history suggesting penicillin allergy and who have serious infections for which non-cross-reacting alternative antimicrobial agents are either unavailable or undesirable. Skin testing with penicilloyl polylysine (PPL [Pre-Pen®]), penicillin G, and a minor determinant mixture of penicilloic and penilloic acids (MDM) is a highly efficient procedure for detecting IgE-antipenicillin antibodies and, thereby, identifying patients at risk for allergic reactions. One common approach is to perform prick (scratch) tests with PPL (6×10^{-5} M), penicillin G (10 000 U/mL, 10^{-2} M) and MDM (10^{-2} M). If no positive reactions are observed, intradermal skin tests are performed using these reagents at the same concentrations used for prick testing. Penicilloyl polylysine and penicillin G are commercially available, but minor determinants are not. Presently, MDM must be freshly prepared. In the absence of an MDM determinant, some physicians will perform skin testing with PPL and penicillin G alone. This will detect approximately 93% of patients at risk for acute allergic reaction to penicillin therapy. Unfortunately, some of the patients missed may be at risk for severe, life-threatening anaphylactic reaction. Attention must also be drawn to the fact that the test itself may cause allergic reactions, and

Table 10.4
The penicillins: Drug interactions

Drug	Interaction
Aminoglycosides	• Aminoglycosides cannot be mixed with antipseudomonal penicillins. If any of these penicillins are mixed in the IV infusion as an aminoglycoside, they will impair the antibacterial activity of the latter
Bacteriostatic antibiotics	• Penicillin antibiotics kill bacteria by preventing cell wall formation. Bacteriostatic antibiotics, such as tetracyclines or erythromycin, reduce cell division and the need for new cell wall formation. They may, therefore, reduce the effectiveness of a penicillin antibiotic
Oral contraceptives	• Oral contraceptives may have decreased effect if ampicillin or penicillin V are administered. The incidence of this reaction is low and unpredictable
Probenecid	• Probenecid reduces the renal secretion of all penicillins. When given together with a penicillin, probenecid increases the half-life of the penicillin

nurses should therefore have epinephrine on hand.

Given orally, the penicillins may produce gastrointestinal upset, nausea, vomiting, and diarrhea. Ampicillin is particularly notorious for the burning diarrhea it causes. Amoxicillin is better tolerated. As troublesome as it may be, the diarrhea seen a few days after starting ampicillin should not be confused with the potentially fatal complication of pseudomembranous colitis. This condition is caused by the proliferation of *Clostridium difficile,* secondary to suppression of normal intestinal flora, and can occur later in a course of therapy.

Carbenicillin and ticarcillin are formulated as their disodium salts. Large doses can contribute significantly to the sodium load in patients with impaired sodium excretory mechanism (e.g., those with renal, cardiac or liver disease). Although azlocillin, mezlocillin and piperacillin are prepared as the monosodium salts, they too can contribute significantly to the sodium load of patients. These drugs can also produce hypokalemia. In addition, they interfere with platelet function and may cause bleeding. The antipseudomonal penicillins are chemically incompatible with aminoglycoside antibiotics (such as amikacin, gentamicin, netilmicin and tobramycin) and must not be mixed in the same injection fluid with any of the latter drugs.

Table 10.4 lists the clinically significant drug interactions for the penicillins.

Nursing Management

The nursing management of the patient receiving any of the penicillins is essentially the same (Table 10.5, pages 82–83). Unique features related to the various penicillins are included in Table 10.6 (pages 84–91).

Response to Clinical Challenge

Principles
Diarrhea is not caused by drug allergy (see Table 10.3), but rather by disturbance of the normal flora in the intestine. It can result from penicillin given by any route but is more common with oral forms. Generally, diarrhea is a minor side effect that causes discomfort but no significant harm.

Actions
1. Determine the actual drug and dose previously received
2. Discuss patient's reaction to this drug (duration and severity of the diarrhea)
3. Explain to patient the difference between a side effect and an allergic reaction
4. Administer the penicillin
5. Monitor for diarrhea and treat symptomatically (rest, fluids, avoidance of irritating foods, e.g., milk)

Table 10.5
Nursing management for the penicillins

Assessment of risk vs. benefit	Patient data	• *History:* Assess for allergy; if potential exists, discuss skin testing with physician • Assess to establish baseline VS, general state of health, indicators of present infection • Assess for other diseases (e.g., reduced renal function may cause toxicity as penicillins are excreted mainly by kidneys) • *Age:* Infants and elderly pts may have reduced defences and increased risk for drug toxicity • *Pregnancy and lactation:* Risks to fetus and infant
	Drug data	• *Allergy:* Allergic responses are more frequent with the penicillins than any other drug group (see Table 10.3) • *Site and type of infection:* Drugs selected based on location of infection and causative microorganism • Culture and sensitivity results • High dose or prolonged tx may cause blood dyscrasias
Implementation	Rights of administration	• Applying the "rights" helps prevent errors of administration
	Right route	• The penicillins are given orally and parenterally. Always ensure that the preparation is appropriate for the route
	Right time	• Absorption of many oral forms is reduced by food and therefore must be given 1 h ac or 2–3 h after pc. Amoxicillin, amoxicillin/clavulanate, bacampicillin and penicillin V may be taken with food • To ensure an effective blood level, the penicillins are given at regularly spaced intervals ATC. The penicillins have short half-lives • If giving penicillins with bacteriostatic antibiotics, separate by at least 1 h
	Right dose	• The order may specify a single dose (in U or mg) or state the dose by weight (U or mg/kg) in equally divided doses • Always refer to manufacturer's literature or label for instructions for reconstitution of powdered drugs. Use the correct amount of the proper diluent; mix well and allow any foam to settle before drawing up dose. Use only clear solutions
	Right drug	• Confusion may occur because of the use of generic and trade names and with the combination products. Always read labels carefully and check if uncertain. Note that administration of some penicillins results in concurrent administration of sodium or potassium salts
	Right technique	• Many of the penicillins are irritating and/or painful by the IM and IV route. Injections should be given deep into large muscle mass with careful procedure to avoid nerves and arteries. Except for the long-acting form, massage the site to hasten dispersal and reduce pain. Some penicillins can be mixed with lidocaine, a local anesthetic, to reduce pain. Care must be taken not to use lidocaine that includes epinephrine, a powerful vasoconstrictor

Table 10.5 (continued)
Nursing management for penicillins

Implementation (cont'd)	Right technique (cont'd)	• IV administration requires knowledge of compatibility with diluents and IV solutions, correct dilution, rate of administration and compatibility with other medications. Always refer to manufacturer's instructions for this route. Check IV sites frequently and change site every 48 h to minimize risk of phlebitis. When agency policy allows, some penicillins are given by direct IV to reduce irritation to vein
	Nursing therapeutics	• Enhance host defences (nutrition, rest, fluids, hygiene) • Note that allergy can occur at any time. Be alert for signs/symptoms and be prepared with emergency tx measures • Administer drugs ATC to ensure effective blood levels
	Patient/family teaching	• Educate for proper use of anti-infectives (Chapter 9) • Review signs/symptoms of adverse effects with pt and family. Individuals with drug allergies should carry an information card or wear a bracelet or locket engraved with this information at all times • Advise that penicillins reduce the effectiveness of oral contraceptives • Review signs/symptoms of superinfection with patient and advise to report immediately
Outcomes	Monitoring of progress	*Continually monitor:* • Clinical response indicating tx success (reduction in signs/symptoms) • Kidney function, intake/output, blood work. Treat side effects symptomatically

Further Reading

Mandell GL, Petri WA Jr. Penicillins, cephalosporins, and other beta-lactam antibiotics. In: Hardman JG, Limbird LE (eds.). *Goodman and Gilman's The Pharmacological Basis of Therapeutics.* 9th ed. New York: Pergamon; 1996:1073–1102.

Penicillins. Section 13, Systemic anti-infectives. In: *AMA Drug Evaluations Subscriptions;* 1994.

Table 10.6
The penicillins: Drug doses

Drug Generic name (Trade names)	Dosage	Nursing alert
A. Narrow-Spectrum Penicillins		
penicillin G potassium; benzylpenicillin potassium	**Oral:** *Adults/children > 12 years:* 1.6–3.2 million U (1–2 g) daily in divided doses q6h; *children < 12 years:* 40 000–80 000 U (25–50 mg) per kg/day in divided doses q6–8h	• Administer 1 h ac or 2 h pc • Dosage varies with infectious agent • Incidence of adverse reactions less with oral than parenteral route • Most common reactions incl. nausea, vomiting, epigastric distress, diarrhea
penicillin G sodium, potassium; benzylpenicillin sodium, potassium	**IM/IV:** *Adults:* 1.2–24 million U/day. Daily dosage can be given intermittently in equally divided doses at 4-h intervals (range, 2–6 h) or by constant IV infusion. Large doses (10–20 million U od) should be given IV. *Children:* 100 000–250 000 U/kg/day in divided doses q4h. For tx of infants, refer to detailed information from manufacturer For prophylaxis of bacterial endocarditis in pts with rheumatic or congenital heart lesions before dental or URT surgery or instrumentation: *Adults* (IV/IM): 2 million U of aqueous penicillin G 30–60 min prior to procedure and 1 million U 6 h later. *Children* (IV/IM): 50 000 U/kg aqueous penicillin G 30–60 min prior to procedure and 25 000 U/kg 6 h later	• 1 mg = 1600 U: Contains 1.7 mEq potassium or 2 mEq sodium for each million U. Monitor electrolytes if high doses given • May be reconstituted with sterile water for injection, D5W, or normal saline • **IM:** Inject slowly deep into muscle mass; massage well. May be diluted with 1%–2% lidocaine (without epinephrine) to minimize pain • **IV:** Refer to manufacturer's package insert (or agency parenteral manual) for appropriate dilution, list of compatible diluents and IV solutions, rate of administration, stability of drug, compatibility with other drugs. Observe site and change q48h to prevent phlebitis • Dosage reduction required if renal function is impaired • May cause false positive Clinitest® for urine glucose
procaine penicillin G; procaine benzylpenicillin	**IM:** *Adults/children:* 600 000–1.2 million U/day in 1–2 doses; 10 days–2 weeks tx is usually sufficient. *Newborn infants,* 50 000 U/kg/day Certain pts with infective endocarditis caused by penicillin-sensitive streptococci (e.g., most viridans streptococci, *S. bovis*) have been successfully treated with procaine penicillin G 1.2 million U qid for 2 weeks plus streptomycin 500 mg bid for 2 weeks For uncomplicated penicillin-susceptible gonococcal infections, a total dose of 4.8 million U, injected at 2 sites, with probenecid 1 g PO	• Reaction to procaine may occur; CNS symptoms include disorientation, anxiety • Never give IV; can cause embolism

Table 10.6 (continued)
The penicillins: Drug doses

Drug Generic name (Trade names)	Dosage	Nursing alert
benzathine penicillin G; benzathine benzylpenicillin	**IM:** The following dosages are recommended by the American Heart Association for group A streptococcal URT infections (e.g., pharyngitis): *Adults/children weighing > 27 kg,* 1.2 million U as a single dose; *infants/children weighing ≤ 27 kg,* 600 000 U as a single dose. Alternatively, the manufacturers' recommended dosages for group A streptococcal URT infections (e.g., pharyngitis) are: *Adults,* 1.2 million U in a single dose; *older children,* a single injection of 900 000 U; *infants/children weighing < 27 kg,* a single dose of 300 000–600 000 U; *neonates,* a single dose of 50 000 U/kg For prevention of recurrent attacks of rheumatic fever, 1.2 million U q 4 weeks	• Never give IV; do not massage injection site
penicillin V; phenoxymethyl penicillin (Ledercillin VK, Pen-Vee K, Pfizerpen VK, Uticillin, V-Cillin K, Veetids)	**Oral:** *Adults:* 125–500 mg q6h [qid]. For pts with creatinine clearances of ≤ 10 mL/min, maximum dose is 250 mg q6h. *Children:* 25–50 mg/kg/day in divided doses q6–8h. Duration of tx for streptococcal pharyngitis should be 10 days To prevent recurrent attacks of rheumatic fever, 250 mg bid To prevent bacterial endocarditis in pts with rheumatic or congenital heart lesions before dental surgery or URT surgery or instrumentation: *Adults,* 2 g 1 h prior to surgery, then 1 g 6 h later. *Children > 27 kg* (oral), use full adult dose; *children < 27 kg,* use 1 g 1 h before procedure, then 500 mg 6 h later	• Administer with full glass of water; fruit juice or carbonated beverages inactivate drug; may be taken with food • Advise pt that drug may decrease effectiveness of oral contraceptives

B. Penicillinase-Resistant Penicillins

Drug	Dosage	Nursing alert
cloxacillin sodium (Bactopen, Cloxapen, Orbenin, Tegopen)	**Oral:** *Adults:* 250–500 mg q6h. *Children ≤ 20 kg:* 50–100 mg/kg/day in 4 equal doses, administered q6h	• Food interferes with absorption: give 1 h ac or 2 h pc • Give with full glass of water; fruit juice or carbonated beverages inactivate drug
dicloxacillin (Dycill, Dynapen, Pathocil)	**Oral:** *Adults/children weighing ≥ 40 kg:* 125 mg q6h for mild to moderate URT infections or localized skin/soft-tissue infections. For more severe infections, 1–2 g/day in equally divided doses q6h (max. daily dose, 4 g). *Children < 40 kg:* 12.5–25 mg/kg daily in equally divided doses q6h	• Take on empty stomach 1 h ac or 2 h pc with full glass of water; acidic beverages inactivate drug • In long-term tx, assess renal, hepatic and hematopoietic function *(cont'd on next page)*

Table 10.6 (continued)
The penicillins: Drug doses

Drug Generic name (Trade names)	Dosage	Nursing alert
flucloxacillin (Fluclox)	**Oral:** *Adults:* 250–500 mg q6h. *Children < 12 years and ≤ 40 kg:* 125–250 mg q6h or 25–50 mg/kg/day in divided doses q6h. *Infants ≤ 6 months:* 25 mg/kg/day in divided doses q6h. These dosages should not exceed the recommended adults' dosage. *NB:* Upper dosage levels should be reserved for serious infections	• Take on empty stomach • Dosages must be reduced in renal disease
nafcillin sodium (Nafcil, Nallpen, Unipen)	**IM/IV:** *Adults,* 2–9 g/day in equally divided doses q4–6h; up to 12 g/day can be given for severe infections. *Children:* 100–200 mg/kg/day in equally divided doses q4–6h. Nafcillin is generally not recommended for newborns	• Parenteral product contains 2.9 mEq Na/g; monitor electrolytes • **IV:** Refer to manufacturer's package insert (or agency parenteral manual) for appropriate dilution, list of compatible diluents and IV solutions, rate of administration, stability of drug, compatibility with other drugs. Observe site and change q48h to prevent phlebitis

C. Expanded-Spectrum Penicillins — I. Aminopenicillins

Drug Generic name (Trade names)	Dosage	Nursing alert
ampicillin sodium (Amcill, Ampicin, Ampilean, Omnipen, Penbritin, Polycillin, Principen)	**Oral:** *Adults:* 2–4 g/day in equally divided doses q6–8h; *children,* 50–100 mg/kg/day in equally divided doses q6–8h	• Give 1 h ac or 2 h pc • May cause false positive Clinitest® for urine glucose
ampicillin sodium (Omnipen-N, Polycillin-N, Totacillin-N)	**IV/IM:** Ampicillin can be administered by IM injection, direct IV injection, or IV drip. The IV route is generally preferred. *Adults:* 2–12 g/day in equally divided doses q6–8h; max. daily dose in equally divided doses q4h should be used for meningitis. *Children,* 100–200 mg/kg/day in equally divided doses q6–8h; for meningitis caused by ampicillin-sensitive *H. influenzae* type B, up to 400 mg/kg/day in equally divided doses q4h For tx of infants, refer to manufacturer's dosage information In the presence of severe renal impairment (CrCl, ≤ 10 mL/min), the dosage interval should be increased to 12 h	• **IV:** Refer to manufacturer's package insert (or agency parenteral manual) for appropriate dilution, list of compatible diluents and IV solutions, rate of administration, stability of drug, compatibility with other drugs (e.g., drug cannot be diluted in dextrose solutions). Reconstituted drug in vial is stable for only 1 h. Observe site and change q48h to prevent phlebitis • Clinitest® for urine glucose may be false positive

Table 10.6 (continued)
The penicillins: Drug doses

Drug Generic name (Trade names)	Dosage	Nursing alert
amoxicillin trihydrate (Amoxil, Larotid, Polymox, Trimox)	**Oral:** *Adults/children weighing > 20 kg:* 750 mg–1.5 g/day; *children < 20 kg:* 20–40 mg/kg/day. These daily doses are administered in divided portions at 8-h intervals. The larger doses are used in more severe infections. In the presence of severe renal impairment (CrCl ≤ 10 mL/min), the adult dose probably should not exceed 500 mg q12h To prevent bacterial endocarditis in pts with rheumatic or congenital heart lesions before dental surgery or URT surgery or instrumentation: *Adults,* 3 g 1 h before procedure, then 1.5 g 6 h after initial dose. *Children,* 50 mg/kg 1 h before procedure, then 25 mg/kg 6 h after initial dose	• Give with food; reduces GI distress and does not interfere with absorption • Storage requirements vary; check label
bacampicillin HCl (Penglobe, Spectrobid)	**Oral:** *Adults:* 800 mg–1.6 g/day in equally divided doses q12h. In cases of severe renal impairment (CrCl ≤ 10 mL/min), adult dose probably should not exceed 800 mg q14h	• Prodrug of ampicillin (do not confuse with ampicillin; dose and interval differ)
pivampicillin (Pondocillin)	**Oral:** *Adults/children > 10 years,* 500 mg bid, double in severe infections. For gonococcal urethritis: *Adults,* 1.5 g as a single dose with 1 g probenecid concurrently; *children > 1 year,* 25 mg/kg/day. *Infants < 1 year,* 40–60 mg/kg/day	• Prodrug of ampicillin (do not exchange for ampicillin; dose and interval differ)

C. Expanded-Spectrum Penicillins — II. Antipseudomonal Penicillins

mezlocillin (Mezlin)	**IM:** For uncomplicated UT infections: *Adults,* 1.5–2 g q6h (100–125 mg/kg/day) **IV** (direct injection over a 3- to 5-min period or by intermittent infusion over 30 min): For uncomplicated UT infections: *Adults,* 1.5–2 g q6h (100–125 mg/kg/day). For complicated UT infections: *Adults,* 3 g q6h (150–200 mg/kg/day) For severe lower respiratory tract, intra-abdominal, gynecologic, and skin/skin structure infections or septicemia: *Adults,* 4 g q6h or 3 g q4h (225–300 mg/kg/day)	• Contains 1.85 mEq Na/g • Monitor CBC and platelet counts; drug may cause bleeding with high doses or other blood dyscrasias. High serum levels may cause seizures • Irritating and/or painful by IM/IV routes. No more than 2 g should be injected at one time • IV: Refer to manufacturer's package insert (or agency parenteral manual) for appropriate dilution, list of compatible diluents and IV solutions, rate of administration, stability of drug, compatibility with other drugs. Observe site and change q48h to prevent phlebitis. May be given direct IV (if agency policy allows) *(cont'd on next page)*

Table 10.6 (continued)
The penicillins: Drug doses

Drug Generic name (Trade names)	Dosage	Nursing alert
C. Expanded-Spectrum Penicillins — II. Antipseudomonal Penicillins (cont'd)		
mezlocillin (cont'd) (Mezlin)	For life-threatening infections: Dosage may be increased to 4 g q4h (max., 24 g/day). Usual duration of tx is 7–10 days but may be longer for some infections For tx of pts with impaired renal function or children: Consult manufacturer's recommended dosages	
piperacillin sodium (Pipracil)	**IM:** For uncomplicated UT infections and most community-acquired pneumonia: *Adults,* 6–8 g (100–125 mg/kg) daily in equally divided doses q6–12h. No more than 2 g should be injected at one time. **IV** (by direct injection over a 3- to 5-min period or by intermittent infusion over a 20- to 30-min period): For uncomplicated UT infections and most community-acquired pneumonia: *Adults,* 6–8 g (100–125 mg/kg) daily in equally divided doses q6–12h For complicated UT infections: *Adults,* 8–16 g (125–200 mg/kg) daily in equally divided doses q6–8h For severe LRT, intra-abdominal, gynecologic, skin/soft-tissue infections or septicemia: *Adults,* 12–18 g (200–300 mg/kg) daily in equally divided doses q4–6h Max. daily adult dosage is usually 24 g/day. Usual duration of tx is 7–10 days but may be longer for some infections For impaired renal function: Consult manufacturer's recommended dosages	• Contains 1.85 mEq Na/g of piperacillin. Monitor electrolytes: may cause hypernatremia and hypokalemia • Irritating and/or painful by IM/IV routes. Injection should not exceed 2 g. Lidocaine (0.5% or 1% without epinephrine) may be added to reduce pain. Inject deep into muscle mass and massage well • **IV:** Refer to manufacturer's package insert (or agency parenteral manual) for appropriate dilution, list of compatible diluents and IV solutions, rate of administration, stability of drug, compatibility with other drugs. May be given slowly by direct IV (if agency policy allows) • Observe site and change q48h to prevent phlebitis • Often given with gentamicin. Administer at separate sites
ticarcillin disodium (Ticar)	**IM:** This route is used primarily for uncomplicated UT infections. No more than 2 g should be injected at one time. IV tx in higher doses should be used for serious UT and systemic infections For uncomplicated UTIs: *Adults,* 4 g/day in divided doses q6h; *children weighing < 40 kg,* 50–100 mg/kg/day in divided doses q6–8h	• See manufacturer's literature for appropriate dilution of drug, list of compatible diluents and IV solutions, and drug stability in these solutions • Contains 5.2 mEq Na/g of ticarcillin. Use cautiously for sodium-restricted patients, and monitor electrolytes • Irritating and/or painful by IM/IV routes. Injection should not exceed 2 g. Lidocaine (0.5% or 1% without epinephrine) may be

Table 10.6 (continued)
The penicillins: Drug doses

Drug Generic name (Trade names)	Dosage	Nursing alert
ticarcillin (cont'd) (Ticar)	**IV:** This is the preferred route for serious UT and systemic infections. Ticarcillin disodium can be administered by slow injection or by intermittent or continuous infusion For severe systemic infections (e.g., septicemia, respiratory tract, skin/soft-tissue, intra-abdominal, and female pelvic and GU infections): *Adults,* 200–300 mg/kg/day in divided doses q4–6h; *children weighing < 40 kg,* 200–300 mg/kg/day in divided doses q4–6h (daily dose should not exceed that used for adults); *for Infants,* consult manufacturer's dosage recommendations For uncomplicated UT infections: *Adults,* 4 g/day in divided doses q6h; *children weighing < 40 kg,* 50–100 mg/kg/day in divided doses q6–8h For UT infections with complications: *Adults/children,* 150–200 mg/kg/day in divided doses q4–6h For renal insufficiency: *Adults/children weighing > 40 kg,* consult manufacturer's literature	added to reduce pain. Inject deep into muscle mass and massage well • **IV:** Refer to manufacturer's package insert (or agency parenteral manual) for appropriate dilution, list of compatible diluents and IV solutions, rate of administration, stability of drug, compatibility with other drugs. May be given slowly by direct IV (if agency policy allows) • Observe site and change q48h to prevent phlebitis
carbenicillin indanyl sodium (Geocillin, Geopen Oral)	**Oral:** For UT infections: *Adults,* 1–2 tablets, each containing the equivalent of 382 mg carbenicillin, q6h; *children,* clinical data insufficient to recommend a dose. Avoid giving this drug to pts with severe renal impairment (CrCl ≤ 10 mL/min)	• For most effective blood levels, give ATC, on empty stomach with full glass of water

C. Expanded-Spectrum Penicillins — III. Amidino Penicillins

amdinocillin pivoxil, pivmecillinam (Selexid)	**Oral:** *Adults/children weighing > 40 kg:* For uncomplicated cystitis and urethritis, 400–800 mg/day in 2–3 equal divided doses. In acute uncomplicated cystitis, tx should be continued for at least 3 days or at least 48 h after signs/symptoms of infection have disappeared. For chronic recurrent UTIs, 400 mg tid or qid. Continue tx until urine is sterile	• May be taken with food • Unusual side effects incl. headache, giddiness, lethargy

(cont'd on next page)

Table 10.6 (continued)
The penicillins: Drug doses

Drug Generic name (Trade names)	Dosage	Nursing alert
C. Expanded-Spectrum Penicillins — IV. Penicillins Combined with a Beta-Lactamase Inhibitor		
amoxicillin plus clavulanic acid (Augmentin, Clavulin)	**Oral:** *For adults and children weighing > 40 kg,* usual dose is amoxicillin 250 mg/potassium clavulanate 125 mg (1 Augmentin-250 or Clavulin-250 tablet) q8h; for more severe infections and infections of the respiratory tract, amoxicillin 500 mg/potassium clavulanate 125 mg (1 Augmentin-500 or Clavulin-500 F tablet) q8h. *For children weighing < 40 kg,* usual dose is 20 mg/kg/day (based on amoxicillin component) in divided doses q8h; for otitis media, sinusitis, lower respiratory infections, and other more severe infections, 40 mg/kg/day (based on amoxicillin component) in divided doses q8h	• May be given with food to reduce GI side effects • Check order and tablet strength (e.g., Augmentin-250 means tablet must contain 250 mg amoxicillin) [*NB:* Since both Augmentin-250 and Augmentin-500, and Clavulin-250 and Clavulin-500 F tablets contain the same amount of clavulanic acid (i.e., 125 mg as the potassium salt), 2 Augmentin-250 tablets are not equivalent to 1 Augmentin-500 tablet, and 2 Clavulin-250 tablets are also not equivalent to 1 Clavulin-500 F tablet]
ampicillin plus sulbactam (Unasyn)	Ampicillin/sulbactam can be administered by IM injection deep into a large muscle mass, IV by slow injection (over at least 10–15 min) or, after dilution with 50–100 mL of a compatible diluent, by IV infusion over 15–30 min **IV/IM** (deep): *Adults:* 1.5 g (1 g ampicillin + 0.5 g sulbactam) to 3 g (2 g ampicillin + 1 g sulbactam) q6h. Total dose of sulbactam should not exceed 4 g/day. Safety in children < 12 years has not been established, and dosage recommendations are unavailable For pts with impaired renal function: Consult manufacturer's recommended dosage.	• Irritating and/or painful by IM/IV routes. Lidocaine (0.5% or 1% without epinephrine) may be added to reduce pain • Inject deep into muscle mass and massage well • **IV:** Refer to manufacturer's package insert (or agency parenteral manual) for appropriate dilution, list of compatible diluents and IV solutions, rate of administration, stability of drug, compatibility with other drugs. May be given slowly by direct IV (if agency policy allows) • Observe site and change q48h to prevent phlebitis
piperacillin plus tazobactam (Zosyn)	**IV:** Piperacillin/tazobactam should be administered by intermittent infusion over 30 min. *For adults,* manufacturer's recommended total daily dose is piperacillin 12 g/tazobactam 1.5 g, given as 3.375 g q6h. Duration of tx is usually 7–10 days, but length of tx depends on the pt's condition and severity of infection *For adults with renal insufficiency, the recommended daily doses are as follows:* For pts on hemodialysis, manufacturer recommends a maximum dose of 2.25 g q8h plus an additional dose of 0.75 g following each dialysis period	• Read label carefully prior to reconstitution and administration. Drug order specifies amount of piperacillin to give; the amount of tazobactam is determined by the manufacturer's preparation • Monitor serum sodium • See package insert for appropriate dilution of drug, list of compatible diluents and IV solutions, and stability of drug in these solutions

Table 10.6 (continued)
The penicillins: Drug doses

Drug Generic name (Trade names)	Dosage	Nursing alert
ticarcillin plus clavulanic acid (Timentin)	**IV:** Ticarcillin/potassium clavulanate should be administered by intermittent infusion over 30 min. For systemic and urinary tract infections: *Adults of average weight (60 kg),* ticarcillin 3 g/potassium clavulanate 100 mg, i.e., 3.1 g Timentin q4–6h; *for pts weighing < 60 kg,* 200–300 mg/kg/day (based on ticarcillin component) in divided doses q4–6h. *For infants/children < 12,* dosages have not been established, but some experts suggest 200–300 mg/kg/day (based on ticarcillin component) in divided doses q4–6h For adults with renal insufficiency: Consult manufacturer's literature	• Monitor IV site and change q48h to prevent phlebitis • Monitor serum potassium (contains 0.15 mEq/100 mg clavulanate) • See manufacturer's literature for appropriate dilution of drug, list of compatible diluents and IV solutions, and stability of drug in these solutions

CHAPTER 11

The Cephalosporins

Topics Discussed
- Mechanism of action
- Pharmacokinetics
- Antibacterial spectra
- Resistance
- Therapeutic uses
- Adverse effects
- Nursing management

Drugs Discussed
cefaclor (**sef**-ah-klor)
cefadroxil (sef-ah-**drox**-ill)
cefamandole (sef-a-**man**-dole)
cefazolin (sef-**az**-oh-lin)
cefixime (seh-**fix**-eem)
cefmetazole (sef-**met**-ah-zole)
cefonicid (se-**fon**-ih-sid)
cefoperazone (sef-oh-**per**-ah-zone)
ceforanide (se-**for**-ah-nide)
cefotaxime (sef-oh-**tax**-eem)
cefotetan (sef-oh-**tee**-tan)
cefoxitin (seh-**fox**-ih-tin)
cefpodoxime (sef-poe-**dox**-eem)
cefprozil (sef-**proe**-zill)
ceftazidime (sef-**tay**-zih-deem)
ceftizoxime (sef-tih-**zox**-eem)
ceftriaxone (sef-try-**ax**-own)
cefuroxime (sef-yoor-**ox**-eem)
cephalexin (sef-ah-**lex**-in)
cephalothin (sef-**ah**-loe-thin)
cephapirin (sef-ah-**pir**-in)
cephradine (**sef**-re-deen)
loracarbef (lor-ah-**kar**-beff)

Clinical Challenge

Consider this clinical challenge as you read through this chapter. The response to the challenge appears on page 98.

Marieka is 9 years old and weighs 25 kg. She is admitted to hospital for treatment of pneumonia. The physician orders a regimen of IM cephalosporin antibiotic given q8h.

When you bring her injection, Marieka says, "I don't want any more needles. They hurt too much!"

What is your next action?

Perhaps no group of drugs has had so mundane a beginning as the cephalosporins. Imagine a group of antibiotics springing out of a bed of sewage. Yet, that is exactly the story. In 1945 the Italian scientist Giuseppe Brotzu isolated a strain of *Cephalosporium acremonium* from sea water near the sewage outlet in Cagliari, Sardinia. This strain secreted a substance that was inhibitory to a group of other organisms, including *Staphylococci,* *Salmonellae, Pasteurellae, Brucellae, Vibrios* and *Shigellae.* Over the next ten to fifteen years, scientists made the very long step from the septic tank to the patient's body and developed the cephalosporin antibiotics, capable of killing a wide range of pathogenic bacteria.

Before discussing the cephalosporins in greater detail, we should list some of their desirable properties.

• They are bactericidal. In this respect, cephalosporins are similar to the penicillins.
• They are relatively resistant to hydrolysis by beta-lactamases produced by *Staphylococcus aureus*. These are the enzymes most commonly called penicillinases when they attack penicillins.
• They possess an expanded spectrum of activity that includes both bacteria killed by penicillin G and several species of penicillin-G-resistant bacilli, including *Escherichia coli*, *Klebsiella pneumoniae* and *Proteus mirabilis*. Their spectrum of activity has been expanded further by the arrival of second- and third-generation cephalosporins.
• They have a high therapeutic index. The expression *therapeutic index* is used to describe the safety of a drug when it is used in therapeutically effective doses. If the dose required to produce toxic effects is several times the dose needed for therapeutic effects, the drug is said to have a high therapeutic index. With the exception of allergic reactions, which can be produced by any amount of a cephalosporin in a sensitive individual, most toxicities are seen only when high doses of these drugs are used.

Mechanism of Action

Cephalosporins, like the penicillins, are beta-lactam antibiotics (Figure 11.1). Accordingly, it should come as no surprise that they, too, inhibit cell formation. Cephalosporins bind to one or more of the penicillin-binding proteins (PBPs) located in the cytoplasmic membrane beneath the cell walls of susceptible bacteria to inhibit the third and final stage of bacterial cell wall formation. As a result, bacterial cell membranes are unable to withstand the pressure of the hypertonic internal environment, and they rupture.

The intrinsic activity of a cephalosporin against a particular bacterial strain depends, in part, on its binding affinity to these protein receptor molecules. For example, first-generation cephalosporins usually have greater affinity for essential PBPs of staphylococci than third-generation cephalosporins. Conversely, third-generation cephalosporins usually have greater affinity for critical PBPs of the Enterobacteriaceae.

Figure 11.1
Basic structure of the penicillins and cephalosporins

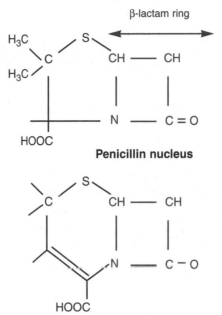

Source: Richmond MH. Beta-lactam antibiotics: the background to their use as therapeutic agents. Frankfurt: Hoeschst AG; 1981:56. Reproduced with permission.

Pharmacokinetics

Most cephalosporins are destroyed in the acid medium of the stomach and must be administered parenterally. Cephalexin (Ceporex®, Keflex®), cephradine (Anspor®, Velosef®), cefadroxil (Duricef®, Ultracef®), cefaclor (Ceclor®), cefuroxime axetil (Ceftin®), cefixime (Suprax®) and cefprozil (Cefzil®) are sufficiently stable in the stomach to be administered orally.

Once absorbed, the cephalosporins penetrate most tissues well. Effective antibiotic concentrations can be attained in synovial, pleural, peritoneal and pericardial fluids in the presence of inflammation. Because cephalosporins do not penetrate well into the eye or prostate, therapeutic levels may not be attained in these tissues. First- and second-generation cephalosporins penetrate poorly into the cerebrospinal fluid, even when the meninges are inflamed. Only third-generation cephalosporins reach therapeutic levels in the cerebrospinal fluid in the presence of inflammation.

Like the penicillins, cephalosporins are rapidly excreted by the kidneys. Probenecid can reduce their rates of excretion.

Antibacterial Spectra

Based on their antibacterial spectra, cephalosporins may be classified as first, second and third generation (Table 11.1). They may also be divided into orally and parenterally administered cephalosporins.

Injectable Cephalosporins

First-generation cephalosporins are active against most gram-positive and many gram-negative organisms. Cephalothin (Ceporacin®, Keflin®, Seffin®) is a typical first-generation injectable cephalosporin that is active against most gram-positive and many gram-negative organisms. Table 11.2 presents the antibacterial spectrum of cephalothin.

Second-generation injectable cephalosporins differ little from cephalothin with respect to their activity against gram-positive bacteria. A major difference does exist, however, in their activities against gram-negative bacteria. Second-generation cephalosporins have lower minimal inhibitory concentrations (MICs) against many gram-negative bacteria. This can be attributed to their increased affinity for penicillin-binding proteins (PBPs) of gram-negative bacteria, an increased ability to penetrate the gram-negative cell envelope, and increased resistance to beta-lactamases produced by gram-negative organisms. Cefoxitin (Mefoxin®) is noteworthy because of its activity against a range of strict anaerobes, including *Bacteroides fragilis*.

Third-generation cephalosporins are usually less active than first-generation drugs against staphylococci, but have increased potency and a wider spectrum of activity against clinically important gram-negative bacteria when compared with first- and second-generation cephalosporins. They show excellent activity against many aerobic gram-negative bacilli, including *Haemophilus influenzae* and most of the Enterobacteriaceae, including strains resistant to earlier-generation cephalosporins, penicillins and aminoglycosides. This activity is related to the agents' excellent beta-lactamase stability and high affinity for penicillin-binding proteins (PBPs). Third-generation cephalosporins offer distinct clinical advantages over earlier-generation cephalosporins against these aerobic gram-negative bacilli.

Table 11.1
Some currently available cephalosporins

First generation	Second generation	Third generation
Cephalothin	Cefamandole	Cefoperazone
Cephapirin	Cefuroxime	Cefotaxime
Cefazolin	Cefoxitin	Ceftazidime
Cephalexin*	Cefaclor*	Ceftizoxime
Cephradine*	Cefonicid	Ceftriaxone
Cefadroxil	Ceforanide	Cefixime*

* Orally active drugs

Source: Lehne RA, Moore LA, Crosby LJ, Hamilton DB (eds.), *Pharmacology for Nursing Care.* 2nd ed. Philadelphia: W.B. Saunders; 1994:944. Reproduced with permission.

Cefoperazone (Cefobid®), ceftazidime (Fortaz®, Tazicef®, Tazidime®) and ceftizoxime (Cefizox®) have antipseudomonal activity; the activity of cefotaxime (Claforan®) and ceftriaxone (Rocephin®) against *Pseudomonas aeruginosa* is variable.

Orally Effective Cephalosporins

Cephalexin (Ceporex®, Keflex®) is the standard against which all new orally effective cephalosporins must be compared. It is active against *Staphylococcus aureus,* viridans streptococci, group A streptococci, *Streptococcus pneumoniae, Neisseria meningitidis* and *N. gonorrhoeae. Salmonella, Shigella, Proteus mirabilis* and some strains of *Escherichia coli* are susceptible to cephalexin at clinically achievable concentrations. Cephalexin is inactive against *Streptococcus faecalis,* indole-positive *Proteus* species, *Pseudomonas aeruginosa, Serratia marcescens* and *Haemophilus influenzae.*

Cefaclor (Ceclor®) is a second-generation orally effective cephalosporin. It is equivalent or superior to cephalexin in activity against gram-positive cocci. It is active against *E. coli, Klebsiella pneumoniae, P. mirabilis, Shigella, Salmonella* and *H. influenzae.*

Cefuroxime axetil (Ceftin®) is an orally active prodrug of cefuroxime. After oral administration, cefuroxime axetil is hydrolyzed by nonspecific esterases to release cefuroxime into the bloodstream. As a second-generation cephalosporin, cefuroxime axetil is indicated for the treatment of patients with mild to moderately severe infections

Table 11.2
Antibacterial spectrum of cephalothin, a first-generation injectable cephalosporin

Microorganism	Sensitivity
Staphylococcus aureus (both penicillin-sensitive and penicillin-resistant)	Highly sensitive, but some resistant strains
Streptococcus pyogenes	Highly sensitive
Streptococcus pneumoniae	Highly sensitive
Streptococcus (viridans group)	Highly sensitive
Streptococcus faecalis	Some sensitivity, but many resistant strains
Clostridium perfringens	Highly sensitive
Clostridium tetani	Very highly sensitive
Corynebacterium diphtheriae	Some sensitivity
Enterobacter cloacae	Resistant
Enterobacter aerogenes	Resistant
Escherichia coli	Moderate sensitivity, but many resistant strains
Haemophilus influenzae	Moderate sensitivity, but many resistant strains
Klebsiella pneumoniae	Highly sensitive
Neisseria gonorrhoeae	Moderate sensitivity, but many resistant strains
Neisseria meningitidis	Highly sensitive, but many resistant strains
Proteus mirabilis	Some sensitivity
Proteus morganii	Resistant
Proteus rettgeri	Resistant
Proteus vulgaris	Resistant
Pseudomonas aeruginosa	Resistant
Salmonella spp.	Moderate sensitivity, but many resistant strains
Shigella spp.	Moderate sensitivity, but many resistant strains

caused by susceptible strains of a variety of gram-positive and gram-negative organisms responsible for upper and lower respiratory tract (URT, LRT) infections, urinary tract (UT) infections, skin structure infections, and gonorrhea.

Cefixime (Suprax®) is an oral third-generation cephalosporin. The drug is at least as active in vitro as other oral cephalosporins against group A streptococci and pneumococci, but staphylococci, which are susceptible to other cephalosporins, are resistant to cefixime because the drug has a low affinity for a critical beta-lactam-binding protein. Cefixime is highly active against *Neisseria gonorrhoeae, Haemophilus influenzae* and *Moraxella catarrhalis,* including beta-lactamase-producing strains usually resistant to ampicillin, amoxicillin and, occasionally, to cefaclor. *H. influenzae* and *Moraxella* are, with pneumococci, the most common bacterial pathogens in acute otitis media and sinusitis.

Cefixime is more active than other cephalosporins against many gram-negative bacilli, including *E. coli, Klebsiella, Proteus mirabilis* and *Serratia marcescens.* It has, however, no useful activity against anaerobes, *Pseudomonas,* or many strains of *Enterobacter* and *Acinetobacter.* It is less active against gram-negative bacteria than parenteral third-generation cephalosporins.

Resistance

Resistance can develop to cephalosporins by several means, including: (1) inactivation by bacterial beta-lactamases (Figure 11.2), (2) decreased permeability of the bacterial cell, which prohibits the cephalosporin from reaching the appropriate binding proteins and (3) alterations in the penicillin-binding protein(s) that prevent binding to the cephalosporin. Clinically, beta-lactamase inactivation and, to a lesser extent, altered permeability

Figure 11.2
Destruction of (a) penicillins and (b) cephalosporins by beta-lactamase

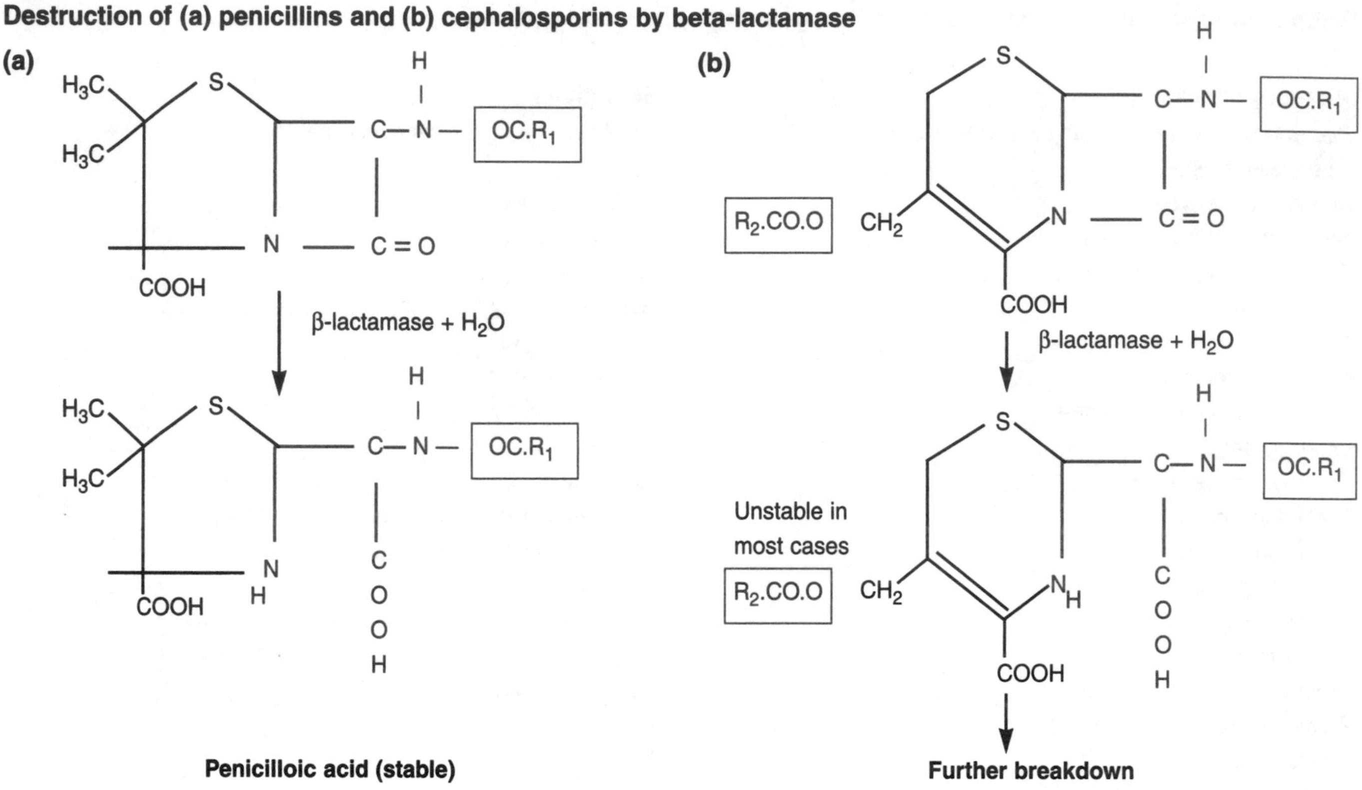

Penicilloic acid (stable)

Further breakdown

In general, the products of enzyme action on penicillins — the penicilloic acids — are stable, but the analogous products from the cephalosporins undergo further spontaneous degradation.

Source: Richmond MH. Beta-lactam antibiotics: the background to their use as therapeutic agents. Frankfurt: Hoeschst AG; 1981:58. Reproduced with permission.

are most important in gram-negative bacteria. Decreased affinity for penicillin-binding proteins occurs with some gram-positive bacteria, but it is not a common cause of clinical resistance to cephalosporins among gram-negative bacteria.

Of increasing concern is the rapid development of resistance to supposedly beta-lactamase-stable, third-generation cephalosporins, particularly by species of *Enterobacter, Serratia* and *Pseudomonas*. Therapeutic failures and relapses, as well as nosocomial spread of these organisms, have been reported. The mechanism of this resistance involves the production of large quantities of beta-lactamases that bind and inactivate third-generation cephalosporins.

Therapeutic Uses

The cephalosporins have a broad antibacterial spectrum, including penicillinase-producing *Staphylococcus aureus*. Despite this, the availabili-

ty of equally effective and less expensive alternatives has often relegated cephalosporins to the position of second-line drugs. For example, urinary tract infections caused by *Escherichia coli* may often be eradicated with cephalexin. However, ampicillin or amoxicillin are usually equally effective and cheaper. Other drugs, notably trimethoprim plus sulfamethoxazole (Bactrim®, Septra®) and trimethoprim (Proloprim®, Trimpex®) alone, cost about the same as cephalexin but are more effective in treating acute urinary tract infections. To select another example, it is uneconomical to use cephalexin to treat streptococcal pharyngitis when penicillins G or V are at least as effective and much cheaper. On the other hand, a cephalosporin may be first-line therapy when resistance has developed to the drug normally used.

Cephalosporins reduce the incidence of surgical wound infections and are very effective if used properly after a wide variety of procedures. These drugs are also often ordered before surgery.

The spectra of activity of the first- and second-generation cephalosporins are not sufficiently broad that they may be used alone in the treatment of gram-negative sepsis. They are usually administered with an aminoglycoside (Chapter 14) to treat serious infections suspected to be due to gram-negative organisms, before the results of bacteriologic tests are received.

Cefoxitin can be used to treat intra-abdominal infections resulting from a disruption of the intestinal mucosa. These infections are usually caused by gram-negative bacilli and anaerobes, in particular *Bacteroides fragilis*. Cefoxitin alone appears to be as effective as clindamycin plus an aminoglycoside for mildly to moderately ill patients with community-acquired intra-abdominal infection. It is frequently a preferred drug in such situations, provided that resistance is not a problem in the particular geographic location. For more severely ill patients and nosocomial infections, combination therapy with an anti-*B. fragilis* agent (e.g., metronidazole, clindamycin, chloramphenicol, cefoxitin, imipenem/cilastatin, ticarcillin/potassium clavulanate) plus an aminoglycoside is usually indicated.

Third-generation injectable cephalosporins have produced excellent results in gram-negative bacillary meningitis, particularly against *Escherichia coli, Klebsiella, Proteus* and *Haemophilus influenzae*. Third-generation injectable cephalosporins are also of value in the treatment of multiple resistant gram-negative infections. Other indications for these drugs include infections not responding to standard therapy, such as gram-negative pneumonia, urinary tract infections, osteomyelitis, pelvic or intra-abdominal infections and suspected sepsis in the febrile neutropenic host.

Cefixime, administered orally, is indicated for the treatment of otitis media caused by *Streptococcus pneumoniae, H. influenzae* (beta-lactamase positive and negative strains), *Moraxella catarrhalis* (beta-lactamase positive and negative strains) and *Streptococcus pyogenes*. It has been approved for acute uncomplicated cystitis and urethritis caused by *E. coli, P. mirabilis* and *Klebsiella* species. Cefixime may also be used for pharyngitis and tonsillitis caused by *S. pyogenes*. Acute bronchitis caused by *S. pneumoniae, M. catarrhalis* (beta-lactamase positive and nega-tive strains) and *H. influenzae* (beta-lactamase positive and negative strains) may also be treated with cefixime.

Adverse Effects

Cephalosporins are relatively safe drugs. In view of their structural similarities to the penicillins, it is not surprising that cephalosporins can cause hypersensitivity reactions. Allergic reactions have been reported in as many as five percent of patients receiving cephalosporins. Complaints include skin rash, urticaria, fever, serum sickness, hemolytic anemia and eosinophilia. Cephalosporins are often used to replace penicillins in patients who are allergic to the latter drugs. Although this can often be done safely, some patients are allergic to both groups of drugs.

Gastrointestinal (GI) adverse effects include nausea, vomiting and diarrhea. Pseudo-membranous colitis (as evidenced by severe diarrhea with blood, mucus or pus) can rarely occur with cephalosporin use. If this happens, the drug should be discontinued immediately and supportive measures instituted. Oral vancomycin or metronidazole can be used to eradicate the causative *Clostridium difficile*.

Other adverse effects include thrombophlebitis and pain at the site of intramuscular injection. Overgrowth of resistant organisms may occur after long-term cephalosporin administration. Patients receiving a third-generation drug should be observed for enterococcal superinfection. Finally, third-generation cephalosporins may suppress the gastrointestinal microflora, resulting in decreased vitamin K production and hypoprothrombinemia.

Table 11.3 on the next page lists the clinically significant drug interactions for the cephalosporins.

Nursing Management

Nursing management of the patient receiving any of the cephalosporins is essentially the same (Table 11.4, pages 99–100). Unique features related to each drug are included in Table 11.5 (pages 101–105).

Table 11.3
The cephalosporins: Drug interactions

Drug	Interaction
Acetylsalicylic acid (ASA)	• ASA may increase the bleeding risk with moxalactam. Avoid concurrent use
Alcohol	• Cefamandole, cefoperazone, cefotetan or moxalactam can produce a disulfiram-like effect if patients consume ethanol. Avoid alcohol and alcohol-containing medications
Aminoglycosides	• Aminoglycosides and cephalosporins may have additive nephrotoxic effects. Combined use of these drugs should be undertaken with caution. Patients with normal renal function receiving appropriate dosing and drug monitoring seldom develop nephrotoxic reactions
Antacids	• Aluminium magnesium hydroxide can decrease the absorption and reduce the effect of cefpodoxime. Give as far apart as possible
Anticoagulants, oral	• Moxalactam or cefamandole may increase the effects of oral anticoagulants. Avoid concurrent use
Diuretics	• Ethacrynic acid and furosemide increase the nephrotoxicity of cephalosporins. Monitor renal function
Colistin	• Colistin and cephalothin have been associated with increased incidence of renal toxicity. Patients should be monitored closely
Famotidine	• Famotidine, and possibly other H_2 blockers, decrease absorption and reduce effect of cefpodoxime. Monitor for decreased cefpodoxime effect
Heparin	• Possible increased bleeding risk with moxalactam. Avoid concurrent use of more than 20 000 U/day of heparin with moxalactam
Penicillins	• Possible increased cefotaxime toxicity with azlocillin or mezlocillin in patients with renal impairment due to decreased cefotaxime excretion. Decrease cefotaxime dosage if GFR < 40 mL/min
Probenecid	• Probenecid reduces the renal secretion of cephalosporins. As a result, cephalosporin levels will be higher than expected
Vancomycin	• Increased nephrotoxicity. Avoid concurrent use

Response to Clinical Challenge

Principles

The cephalosporins cause pain and irritation with IM injection. Pain is increased by the volume injected, the muscle site chosen, the skill of technique of administration, and the diluent used to reconstitute the powder (e.g., water is more painful than lidocaine or saline). The pain is also increased by the patient's fears and anxiety.

Actions

1. Discuss Marieka's experiences with the injections
2. Examine previous injection sites for inflammation
3. Explain the importance of antibiotic treatment to the patient and her family; enlist support of family
4. Discuss possibility of oral route with physician
5. Explain to Marieka that techniques can be used to reduce her pain (e.g., divide injection if volume is large and administer in 2 sites; use lidocaine as diluent — check with pharmacy; administer deep and slow; massage well following injection).

Table 11.4
Nursing management for the cephalosporins

Assessment of risk vs. benefit	Patient data	• *History:* Review for allergy — approx. 5% of pts are allergic to cephalosporins. Also, check for penicillin allergy, as some pts have cross-sensitivity • Establish baseline VS, general state of health, indicators of present infection • *Other diseases:* E.g., reduced renal function may cause toxicity, as most cephalosporins are excreted mainly by kidneys (Table 11.5 indicates exceptions that are excreted in bile) • *Age:* Infants and elderly pts may have reduced defences and increased risk for drug toxicity • *Pregnancy and lactation:* Risks to fetus and infant must be weighed against benefits of drug tx
	Drug data	• *Site and type of infection:* Drugs selected based on location of infection and causative microorganism • Culture and sensitivity results • High dose or prolonged tx may cause superinfection, resistant overgrowth or hypoprothrombinemia • Drugs cause local irritation at site of administration, e.g., GI upset, IM pain and inflammation, IV phlebitis
Implementation	Rights of administration	• Applying the "rights" helps prevent errors of administration
	Right route	• The cephalosporins are given orally and parenterally. Always ensure that the preparation is appropriate for the route
	Right time	• Most oral forms can be taken without regard to food; giving with meals may reduce GI irritation • To ensure an effective blood level, give at regularly spaced intervals ATC. The half-lives vary among drugs in this group. Note in Table 11.5 that some are given q4h while others are given q12h or od
	Right dose	• The order may specify a single dose (in mg) or state the dose by weight (mg/kg) in equally divided doses • Always refer to manufacturer's literature or label for instructions for reconstitution of powdered drugs. Use correct amount of proper diluent; mix well and allow any foam to settle before drawing up dose. Many solutions will have a yellow/amber colour and may darken with exposure to light. Do not use solutions that are cloudy or have a precipitate
	Right drug	• The generic names of this family of drugs are very similar, and confusion may occur. Always read labels carefully and check if uncertain
	Right technique	• Many of these drugs are irritating or painful by the IM and IV route. Give injections deep into a large muscle mass carefully to avoid nerves and arteries. Massage site to hasten dispersal and reduce pain

(cont'd on next page)

Table 11.4 (continued)
Nursing management for the cephalosporins

Implementation (cont'd)	Right technique (cont'd)	• Using lidocaine, a local anesthetic agent, as the diluent will reduce pain. Care must be taken not to use lidocaine that includes epinephrine, a powerful vasoconstrictor • IV administration requires knowledge of compatibility with diluents and IV solutions, correct dilution, rate of administration, and compatibility with other medications. Always refer to manufacturer's instructions for this route • Check IV sites frequently; change site every 48–72 h to minimize risk of phlebitis. When agency policy allows, the cephalosporins are given by direct IV to reduce irritation to the vein
	Nursing therapeutics	• Enhance host defences (nutrition, rest, fluids, hygiene) • *NB:* Allergy can occur at any time. Be alert for signs/symptoms and be prepared for emergency tx • Administer drugs ATC to ensure effective blood levels
	Patient/family teaching	• Educate for proper use of anti-infectives (as summarized in Chapter 9) • Review signs/symptoms of superinfection with pt and advise to report immediately • Hospitals, pharmacies, and drug companies produce leaflets for pt information. Encourage pts and families to use these resources • Advise diabetic pts not to rely on Clinitest for urine glucose monitoring: may cause false-positive results
Outcomes	Monitoring of progress	*Continually monitor:* • Clinical response indicating tx success (reduction in signs/symptoms) • For mild side effects, and treat symptomatically • For adverse effects (respond immediately to allergy, superinfection, enterocolitis, hepatotoxicity, hypoprothrombinemia) • Be aware that drugs may cause false-positive Coombs' test and Clinitest® for urine glucose

Further Reading

The choice of antibacterial drugs. *Medical Letter on Drugs and Therapeutics* 1994;36:919–925.

Handbook of antimicrobial therapy. *Medical Letter on Drugs and Therapeutics* 1992.

Mandell GL, Petri WA. Penicillins, cephalosporins, and other beta-lactam antibiotics. In: Hardman JG, Limbird LE (eds.). *Goodman and Gilman's The Pharmacological Basis of Therapeutics*. 9th ed. New York: Pergamon; 1996.

Table 11.5
The cephalosporins: Drug doses

Drug Generic name (Trade names)	Dosage	Nursing alert
A. First-Generation Cephalosporins		
cephalothin sodium (Ceporacin, Keflin)	**IV:** *Adults:* 500–2000 mg q4–6h. *Infants/children:* 80–160 mg/kg/day in divided doses. For dosage adjustment in cases of impaired renal function, consult product monograph	• Do not administer solutions that are cloudy or have a precipitate. Solution may darken at room temperature; does not affect potency. Do not administer if dark brown
cephapirin sodium (Cefadyl)	**IM/IV:** *Adults:* 500–1000 mg q4–6h. *Children:* 40–80 mg/kg/day in 4 equal doses	• Colour changes do not affect potency • Inject deep into muscle mass; massage well
cefazolin sodium (Ancef, Kefzol)	**IM/ IV:** *Adults:* For pneumococcal pneumonia, 500 mg q12h. For mild gram-pos. infections, 250–500 mg q8h. In acute uncomplicated UT Infections, 1 g q12h. In moderate or severe infections, 500–1000 mg q6–8h. In serious infections such as endocarditis, 6 g/day. *Children:* For mild to moderately severe infections, 25–50 mg/kg/day in 3–4 equal doses. For renal impairment, consult monograph	• Inject deep into large muscle mass; massage well • Monitor IV site for phlebitis • Check compatibility before adding to other medications
cephalexin (Ceporex, Keflex)	**Oral:** *Adults,* 1–4 g/day in divided doses. Usual adult dose, 250 mg q6h. *Children,* 25–50 mg/kg/day in 4 divided doses q6h	• Give with food to reduce GI irritation • Store oral suspension in refrigerator. Shake well before using
cephradine (Anspor, Velosef)	**Oral:** *Adults:* For respiratory tract infection other than lobar pneumonia, 250 mg q6h or 500 mg q12h. For pneumococcal lobar pneumonia, 500 mg q6h or 1 g q12h. For skin and soft-tissue infection, 250 mg q6h or 500 mg q12h. For UT infection, 500 mg q6h or 1 g q12h. For pts with renal impairment, consult product monograph. Children may require dosage modification proportional to their weight and the severity of infection **IM/IV:** *Adults,* 2–8 g daily in equally divided doses q4–6h. *Children > 1 year,* 50–100 mg/kg/day in equally divided doses q6h	• **PO:** Give with food to reduce GI irritation • **IM:** Give injection deep
cefadroxil (Duricef, Ultracef)	**Oral:** *Adults:* For UT infection, 1–2 g/day as single dose hs or divided into 2 daily doses. For acute pharyngitis/tonsillitis, 1 g/day in single dose or 2 divided doses for 10 days. For LRT infection, 500–1000 mg bid. For skin and soft-tissue infection, 1 g daily in single dose. *Children:* For UT and integumentary infection, acute pharyngitis or tonsillitis, and LRT infection, 30 mg/kg/day given q12h for 10 days. For pts with renal impairment, consult product monograph	• Administer without regard for food

Table 11.5 (continued)
The cephalosporins: Drug doses

Drug Generic name (Trade names)	Dosage	Nursing alert
B. Second-Generation Cephalosporins		
cefprozil (Cefzil)	**Oral:** *Adults,* 500 mg–1 g daily in 2 divided doses for up to 10 days; for infections due to *S. pyogenes,* administer for at least 10 days. Mild to moderate UT infections due to susceptible organisms may be treated with a single daily dose of 500 mg–1 g for 10 days. *Children/infants > 6 months,* 30 mg/kg/day in 2 divided doses for 10 days. Efficacy and safety in children < 6 months have not been established	• Give with food to reduce GI irritation • Refrigerate oral suspension
cefmetazole sodium (Zefazone)	**IV:** Over 3 min or by intermittent infusion over 10–60 min. *Adults,* 2 g q6–12h. For UT infections, 2 g q12h; other sites (mild to moderate infections), 2 g q8h; other sites (severe to life-threatening infections), 2 g q6h. Usual duration of tx, 5–14 days. Dosage guidelines for children have not been established. For impaired renal function, consult manufacturers' information	• Administer over 3–5 min or by intermittent infusion over 10–60 min. See manufacturer's instructions for appropriate dilution of drug, compatible diluents and IV solutions, and stability of cefmetazole in these solutions • Consult manufacturer's recommendations for pts with renal impairment
loracarbef (Lorabid)	**Oral:** For mild to moderate infections caused by susceptible bacteria. *Adults,* 200–400 mg bid. *Children/infants > 6 months,* 7.5–15 mg/kg bid. *Infants < 6 months,* efficacy and safety have not been established	• See package insert for dosages for specific indications • Dosage should be modified in pts with renal impairment; see package insert for details
cefamandole nafate (Mandol)	**IV/IM:** *Adults,* 500–1000 mg q4–8h. For life-threatening infections, up to 2 g q4h. For uncomplicated pneumonia and soft-tissue infection, 500 mg q6h. For mild UT infections, 500 mg q8h. For moderate UT infections, 1 g q8h. For severe UT infections, 1 g q4–6h. *Children,* 50–100 mg/kg/day in equal doses q4–8h. For pts with renal impairment, consult product monograph	• Solution should be light yellow or amber. Do not use if darkened or contains precipitate • Powder is difficult to reconstitute, and CO gas forms in vial. Follow manufacturer's instructions carefully. Solution stable for 24–72 h if refrigerated • May cause bleeding; monitor prothrombin time • Avoid alcohol; serious interaction

Table 11.5 (continued)
The cephalosporins: Drug doses

Drug Generic name (Trade names)	Dosage	Nursing alert
cefoxitin sodium (Mefoxin)	**IV/IM:** *Adults:* 1–2 g q6–8h. For uncomplicated pneumonia, UT or soft-tissue infection, 1 g q6–8h. For moderately severe or severe infection, 1 g IV q4h or 2 g q6–8h. For infection commonly needing antibiotics in higher dosages (e.g., gas gangrene), 2 g IV q4h or 3 g q6h. *Children:* 20–40 mg/kg q6–8h. *Infants 1 month–2 years:* 20–40 mg/kg q6–8h. *Neonates (incl. premature infants) < 1 week of age:* 20–40 mg/kg IV q12h; *1–4 weeks of age:* 20–40 mg/kg q8h	• IM injection is painful; IV administration causes irritation to vein • Each gram contains 2.3 mmol Na • Refer to manufacturer's instructions for reconstitution. May reconstitute with 0.5% lidocaine (without epinephrine) to reduce pain for IM route • Solutions containing preservatives should not be used for injections or for flushing catheters in treating neonates
cefuroxime sodium (Zinacef)	**IV/IM:** *Adults:* 2.25–9 g/day in equally divided doses q8h. For uncomplicated UT infections, skin and skin-structure infections, disseminated gonococcal infections, and uncomplicated pneumonia, 750 mg q8h. For severe or complicated infections, 1.5 g q8h. In life-threatening infections or infections due to less susceptible organisms, 1.5 g q6h may be required. In bacterial meningitis, the dose should not exceed 3 g q8h. For uncomplicated gonococcal infections, 1.5 g IM as a single dose at 2 different sites together with probenecid, 1 g orally. *Infants and children ≥ 3 months:* 50–100 mg/kg/day in equally divided doses q6–8h (not to exceed maximum adult dosage). For bacterial meningitis, 200–240 mg/kg/day in equally divided doses q6–8h	• Follow manufacturer's instructions for reconstitution • Preparation is a suspension; use 21-gauge needle • Give IM deep
cefaclor (Ceclor)	**Oral:** *Adults:* 250 mg q8–12h. Max. recomm. dose, 2 g/day. For skin and soft-tissue infections, 250 mg bid–tid. For LRT infections, 250 mg tid. *Children:* 20 mg/kg/day in divided doses q8–12h. For more serious infections, otitis media and those caused by less susceptible organisms), 40 mg/kg/day. For otitis media, administer dose q12h. For LRT infection, divide into 3 daily doses	• Store suspension in refrigerator. Stable for 14 days. Shake well before using • Administer ATC without regard to meals. May be given with food to reduce GI upset
cefonicid (Monocid)	**IM/IV:** *Adults:* 500 mg–2 g od. For uncomplicated UT infections, 500 mg od; for mild to moderate infections, 1 g od; for severe or life-threatening infections, 2 g od	• Follow manufacturer's instructions for reconstitution. Solution should be colourless to light amber • **IM:** Give deep into large muscle mass; massage well. For 2-g IM dose, divide and give in separate sites • For renal impairment, consult monograph

(cont'd on next page)

Table 11.5 (continued)
The cephalosporins: Drug doses

Drug Generic name (Trade names)	Dosage	Nursing alert
ceforanide (Precef)	**IM, IV:** *Adults,* 1–2 g/day in equally divided doses q12h. *Children,* 20–40 mg/kg/day in equally divided doses q12h	• For renal impairment dosage, consult manufacturer's product monograph
cefuroxime axetil (Ceftin)	**Oral:** *Adults/children ≥ 12 years,* 250 mg q12h; for more severe infections or those caused by less susceptible organisms, 500 mg q12h; for uncomplicated UT infections, 125–250 mg q12h. *Infants/children ≤ 12 years,* 125 mg q12h. For otitis media: *Children < 2 years,* 125 mg q12h; *children ≥ 2 years,* 250 mg q12h	• May be given without regard to meals, but absorption is enhanced when drug is administered with food • If child cannot swallow whole tablet, request alternative tx. Drug has strong, bitter taste even when crushed and mixed with food

C. Third-Generation Cephalosporins

Drug Generic name (Trade names)	Dosage	Nursing alert
cefpodoxime proxetil (Vantin)	**Oral:** For mild to moderate infections caused by susceptible bacteria. *Adults/children > 13 years:* Acute community-acquired pneumonia, 200 mg bid for 14 days; pharyngitis/tonsillitis, 100 mg bid for 10 days; skin and skin structure, 400 mg bid for 7–14 days; uncomplicated UT infections, 100 mg bid for 7 days. For uncomplicated gonorrhea (men/women) and rectal gonococcal infections (women), 200 mg in a single dose. *Children 6 months–12 years:* Acute otitis media, 5 mg/kg (max., 200 mg/dose) bid for 10 days; pharyngitis/tonsillitis, 5 mg/kg (max., 100 mg/dose) bid for 10 days	• Administer with food to enhance absorption • For pts with severe renal impairment (creatinine clearance < 30 mL/min), dosing interval should be increased to 24 h
cefixime (Suprax)	**Oral:** *Adults,* 400 mg/day. A dose of 200 mg may be given q12h prn except for UT infection, for which od dosing must be used. *Children,* 8 mg/kg/day. A dose of 4 mg/kg may be given q12h prn except for UT infection, for which od dosing must be used	• Store oral suspension at room temperature or under refrigeration. Shake well before using
cefoperazone sodium (Cefobid)	**IM/IV:** *Adults,* usually 2–4 g/day in equally divided doses q12h. In severe infections or infections caused by less sensitive organisms, dose and/or frequency may be increased. *Children,* 100–150 mg/kg/day in divided doses q8–12h. However, there is no approved labelling for use in children	• May cause hypoprothrombinemia; monitor pt • Follow maker's instructions for reconstitution • Inject deep and massage well. May use lidocaine to reduce injection pain • Monitor IV site for phlebitis. Change site q48–72h or according to agency policy • Monitor serum levels with higher doses, especially in pts with hepatic disease and/or biliary obstruction. In pts with both hepatic dysfunction and renal disease, dosage should not exceed 1–2 g/day, and serum concentrations should likewise be monitored • Avoid alcohol while on this drug

Table 11.5 (continued)
The cephalosporins: Drug doses

Drug Generic name (Trade names)	Dosage	Nursing alert
cefotaxime sodium (Claforan)	**IM/IV:** *Adults:* For uncomplicated infection, 1 g q12h. For moderately severe to severe infection, 1–2 g q8h. For very severe infection, 2 g IV q6–8h. For life threatening infection, 2 g IV q4h. For uncomplicated gonorrhea, 1 g IM as single dose. *Neonates ≤ 1 week:* 50 mg/kg IV q12h; *1–4 weeks,* 50 mg/kg IV q8h. *Infants/children < 50 kg:* 50–100 mg/kg/day IM or IV, divided into 4–6 equal doses, or up to 180 mg/kg/day for severe infection	•For renal impairment dosage, consult product monograph •Follow manufacturer's instructions for reconstitution and compatibility •Give IM deep; massage well; avoid arteries/nerves
ceftazidime pentahydrate (Fortaz, Tazicef, Tazidime)	**IM/IV:** *Adults:* For uncomplicated pneumonia or skin-structure infection, 0.5–1 g q8h. For uncomplicated UT infection, 250 mg q12h. For complicated UT infection, 500 mg q8–12h. For bone infection, 2 g IV q12h. For peritonitis, meningitis or septicemia, 2 g IV q8h. *Infants/children 1–2 months:* 25–50 mg/kg/day IV in 2 equal doses; *2 months–12 years:* 30–50 mg/kg IV q8h to a max. of 6 g/day. For pts with renal impairment, consult product monograph	•Follow manufacturer's instructions for reconstitution and stability •Lidocaine 0.5–1% may be used to reduce pain of IM injection. Give deep into muscle mass and massage well •Monitor IV site for phlebitis
ceftizoxime sodium (Cefizox)	**IM/IV:** *Adults:* For uncomplicated UT infection, 500 mg q12h. For infection at other sites, 1 g q8–12h. For severe or refractory infection, 1 g q8h to 2 g q8–12h. For life-threatening infections, 3–4 g (IV) q8h. *Infants/children 6 months–12 years,* 50 mg/kg q6–8h. For pts with renal impairment, consult product monograph	•2-g doses should be divided and given at separate sites •Consult produce monograph. Solution may be yellow/amber. Discard if cloudy •Give IM injection deep; massage well. Lidocaine 1% may be used as diluent to reduce pain •Monitor IV site for phlebitis
ceftriaxone sodium (Rocephin)	**IM/IV:** *Adults:* For moderate and severe infections, 1–2 g q24h or 0.5–1 g q12h. For uncomplicated gonorrhea, 250 mg IM as single dose. *Infants/children 1 month–12 years:* For serious miscellaneous infection, 25–37.5 mg/kg q12h. Total daily dose should not > 2 g. If body mass is > 50 kg, adult dose should be used. For meningitis, 50 mg/kg (with or without loading dose of 75 mg/kg) q12h. Total daily dose should not > 4 g	•2-g doses should be divided and given at separate sites •Consult product monograph. Solution may be yellow/amber. Discard if cloudy •Give IM deep and massage well. Lidocaine 1% may be used as diluent to reduce pain •Monitor IV site for phlebitis •Commonly used for program of home antibiotic IV tx

CHAPTER 12

The Macrolides

Topics Discussed
- Mechanism of action
- Antibacterial spectra
- Resistance
- Pharmacokinetics
- Therapeutic uses
- Adverse effects
- Nursing management

Drugs Discussed
erythromycin (eh-ree-throw-**mye**-sin)
clarithromycin (kla-ri-throw-**mye**-sin)
azithromycin (az-i-throw-**mye**-sin)

Clinical Challenge

Consider this clinical challenge as you read through this chapter. The response to the challenge appears on page 112.

Mr. J. is a 39-year-old man admitted for treatment of pneumonia due to *Streptococcus pyogenes*. He is extremely allergic to penicillin and may have cross-sensitivity to the cephalosporins.

The physician orders a regimen of IV erythromycin given by continuous infusion for 3 days, followed by 500 mg q12h given 1 h ac. After 8 h, the site is red and tender. The IV site is changed and, 48 h later, changed again. Oral dosage is commenced.

The next day when you bring the dose, Mr. J. says, "I don't want any more of this drug. It has ruined my veins, and now it's ruining my stomach."

What is your next action?

The macrolide antibiotics currently used include the prototype — erythromycin — and the recently introduced clarithromycin and azithromycin. Erythromycin, clarithromycin (Biaxin®) and azithromycin (Zithromax®) are frequently preferred alternatives to penicillin G for a number of infections in penicillin-allergic individuals. They are among the safest antibiotics in use today.

Clarithromycin and azithromycin are similar in structure to erythromycin. Their structural changes improve the stability of both clar-

ithromycin and azithromycin in acid, enhance their bioavailability and reduce gastrointestinal irritation.

Mechanism of Action

The macrolide antibiotics inhibit bacterial protein synthesis. They reversibly bind to the 50S ribosomal subunit and prevent elongation of the peptide chain, most likely by interfering with the translocation step. Macrolides do not bind to mammalian

80S ribosomes, and this accounts partly for their selective toxicity.

Macrolides may be bacteriostatic or bactericidal, depending on the concentration of the drug, organism susceptibility, growth rate and size of the inoculum. Bacterial killing is favoured by higher antibiotic concentrations, lower bacterial density and rapid growth.

Antibacterial Spectra

The antibacterial spectrum of erythromycin is similar to that of penicillin G. It includes many strains of penicillin-resistant staphylococci, *Streptococcus pyogenes*, *Streptococcus pneumoniae*, viridans streptococci, anaerobic streptococci and many strains of *Streptococcus faecalis*. Erythromycin is also effective against *Corynebacterium diphtheriae*, *Propionibacterium acnes*, *Clostridium tetani*, *Clostridium perfringens*, *Neisseria gonorrhoeae*, *Bordetella pertussis* and some species of *Brucella*. *Haemophilus influenzae* is only moderately sensitive to the drug. Oropharyngeal strains of *Bacteroides* are usually sensitive to erythromycin. The drug is also effective against *Mycoplasma pneumoniae*, *Treponema pallidum*, *Legionella pneumophila* and many species of *Rickettsia* and *Chlamydia*.

When used over short periods of time, resistance to erythromycin is not common. However, if erythromycin is used for long-term therapy or within a hospital environment, staphylococcal resistance often develops. Other bacteria that may become resistant to the drug are *Streptococcus pneumoniae*, *Streptococcus pyogenes*, the viridans streptococci and enterococci. This resistance is due to the ability of bacteria to produce an enzyme capable of destroying erythromycin.

In general, clarithromycin has an in vitro spectrum of activity that is similar to that of erythromycin, but it is two- to fourfold more active against susceptible streptococci and staphylococci; gram-positive cocci resistant to erythromycin are resistant to clarithromycin as well. The active metabolite (14-OH clarithromycin) acts in an additive or synergistic fashion against *Haemophilus influenzae*. Clarithromycin is slightly more active in vitro than erythromycin against certain pathogens responsible for atypical pneumonias (i.e., *Legionella pneumophila*, *Mycoplasma pneumoniae*, *Chlamydia pneumoniae*) and Lyme disease (*Borrellia burgdorferi*). This macrolide is somewhat more active than erythromycin against *Chlamydia trachomatis* and is considerably more active against *Ureaplasma urealyticum*. It also is active against *Toxoplasma gondii*, *Cryptosporidium* and *Mycobacterium avium* complex; it is the most active macrolide against other atypical mycobacteria.

Azithromycin, unlike erythromycin and clarithromycin, inhibits some aerobic gram-negative bacilli. The majority of these bacilli, including the Enterobacteriaceae, are intrinsically resistant to erythromycin and clarithromycin because the cell envelopes prevent passive diffusion. Organisms that are moderately susceptible to azithromycin include most *Salmonella*, *Shigella* and *Aeromonas* species, *Escherichia coli* and *Yersinia enterocolitica*. Azithromycin has excellent activity against *Vibrio cholerea* and species isolated in patients with vaginitis, such as *Gardnerella vaginalis* and *Mobiluncus*.

Resistance

Various mechanisms of acquired resistance to erythromycin have been reported. Bacteria with resistance to erythromycin are also resistant to azithromycin and clarithromycin. Decreasing binding of macrolides to their target site accounts for nearly all the resistant strains isolated from patients. This resistance is usually mediated by a plasmid (see Chapter 9 for a discussion of plasmid-mediated resistance).

Pharmacokinetics

Erythromycin is not stable in the stomach; it must be protected from gastric juices if it is to be absorbed from the intestine. This can be achieved by using enteric-coated tablets or capsules, or by applying a protective film coating to the tablets. The product ERYC® is formulated as a capsule containing enteric-coated pellets.

Erythromycin can also be protected from stomach secretions by preparing the drug as an acid-resistant ester, as in erythromycin stearate, erythromycin ethylsuccinate or erythromycin estolate. Table 12.1 on the next page lists some of the available forms of erythromycin, together with some of their more common trade names.

Table 12.1
Forms of erythromycin currently available

Orally administered	Erythromycin
	• enteric-coated tablets (E-Mycin®, Ilotycin®, Robimycin®)
	• film-coated tablets (Erythromid®)
	Erythromycin stearate
	• tablets (Erythrocin®, Bristamycin®, Erypar®, Ethril®, Pfizer-E®)
	• liquid (Erythrocin®)
	Erythromycin estolate
	• capsules (Ilosone®)
	• liquid (Ilosone®)
	Erythromycin ethylsuccinate
	• tablets (EES®, Pediamycin®)
	• liquid (EES®, Pediamycin®)
Parenterally administered	Erythromycin gluceptate (Ilotycin Gluceptate®)
	Erythromycin lactobionate (Erythrocin Lactobionate®)
Topically administered	Erythromycin (Ilotycin®)
	Erythromycin + ethyl alcohol + laureth 4 (Staticin® — used for the treatment of acne)

Despite these steps, protection against acid destruction is often not complete. Therefore, with the exception of erythromycin ethylsuccinate and erythromycin estolate, all erythromycin products should preferably be taken on an empty stomach to speed their transit into the intestine. Unfortunately, erythromycin taken on an empty stomach often causes considerable gastric distress, and food may be needed to reduce the patient's discomfort. Erythromycin ethylsuccinate and erythromycin estolate appear to be well absorbed when taken with food. In fact, maximum blood levels with erythromycin ethylsuccinate suspension or chewable tablets are obtained when the products are given immediately after meals. Both erythromycin estolate and erythromycin ethylsuccinate are hydrolyzed to erythromycin following absorption.

Once absorbed, erythromycin diffuses well throughout the body. It enters most tissue compartments, with the exception of the cerebrospinal fluid. Erythromycin is concentrated in the liver and excreted in the bile. Little erythromycin is eliminated in the urine. Its half-life ranges from one hour to more than three hours.

Clarithromycin is well absorbed from the gas-trointestinal tract, with or without food. It is metabolized in the liver, and 30% to 40% of the administered dose can be recovered in the urine. Patients with a creatinine clearance of 30 mL/min or less may require a decreased dose. Clarithromycin penetrates well into both tissues and cells, including macrophages and polymorphonuclear leukocytes. Clarithromycin is 65% to 70% bound to plasma proteins.

Food decreases the bioavailability of azithromycin. Each dose of the drug should be taken at least one hour before or two hours after a meal. Following its absorption, azithromycin concentrates inside cells, particularly macrophages and polymorphonuclear leukocytes. Azithromycin is eliminated slowly from the body. Its half-life is sixty-eight hours. Only 6% of an oral dose is excreted in the urine. Elimination in the bile, metabolism in the liver and possibly transintestinal elimination account for the clearance of azithromycin from the body.

Therapeutic Uses

Erythromycin is often used as a replacement for penicillin G or penicillin V in patients who are allergic to these drugs. Infections caused by group A streptococci, including tonsillitis, erysipelas and scarlet fever, often respond well to erythromycin. The drug can also be used as a penicillin substitute in the chemoprophylaxis of streptococcal infections. Pneumococcal infections can be treated with erythromycin. This agent can also be used as a substitute for penicillin in the treatment of the acute illness or the carrier state of diphtheria and the management of both early and late syphilis. Development of resistance has greatly restricted its value in minor staphylococcal infections.

Erythromycin is effective in the treatment of pneumonia caused by *Mycoplasma pneumoniae*. This is one of the few indications for which erythromycin is a first drug of choice. Erythromycin is effective for the treatment of Legionnaire's disease, caused by *Legionella pneumophila*. Whooping cough, produced by *Bordetella pertussis*, may also be treated with erythromycin. However, evidence for its efficacy is not overwhelming. Erythromycin is a primary treatment for *Chlamydia trachomatis* infections in infants and children, and this agent is often used in conjunction with sulfisoxazole (Pediazole®) to treat *Haemophilus influenzae*-induced otitis media in young children.

Erythromycin ophthalmic ointment is used in the treatment of superficial ocular infections involving the conjunctiva or cornea caused by organisms susceptible to erythromycin. For prophylaxis of ophthalmia neonatorum due to *N. gonorrhoeae* or *C. trachomatis*, 0.5% erythromycin ophthalmic ointment may be used.

Oral or topical erythromycin may be used in the treatment of acne vulgaris. The products are used primarily in the treatment of the inflammatory papular lesions of acne. The rationale for this use lies in the fact that erythromycin can eradicate *Propionibacterium acnes*, the anaerobic diptheroid in pilosebaceous glands that secretes a variety of enzymes, including hyaluronidase, which are capable of disrupting follicular epithelium and increasing inflammation.

Clarithromycin is indicated for the treatment of pneumonia caused by *Mycoplasma pneumoniae* or *Streptococcus pneumoniae*. It appears to be as effective as erythromycin and can be considered an alternative agent for the treatment of atypical pneumonias. Clarithromycin also is indicated for the treatment of (1) acute bacterial exacerbations

of chronic bronchitis due to *H. influenzae*, *M. catarrhalis* or *S. pneumoniae*, (2) pharyngitis/tonsillitis due to *Streptococcus pyogenes*, (3) acute maxillary sinusitis due to *S. pneumoniae* in penicillin-allergic patients and (4) uncomplicated skin and skin-structure infections due to *Staphylococcus aureus* or *S. pyogenes*.

Clarithromycin is an alternative in the treatment of infections due to *U. urealyticum*, early Lyme disease and certain opportunistic infections in AIDS or other immunocompromised patients (e.g., atypical mycobacteria, *T. gondii encephalitis*). It is considered by some to be the drug of choice for the treatment or prophylaxis of *Mycobacterium avium* complex infections.

Clarithromycin causes teratogenic effects in laboratory animals. Data in pregnant women are lacking; therefore, this drug should not be used during pregnancy, except when no alternative therapy is appropriate. Since clarithromycin is excreted in human milk, caution should be exercised when this drug is administered to nursing women.

Azithromycin is an alternative antibiotic for the treatment of mild to moderate pharyngitis/tonsillitis due to streptococcal species. It is also indicated for the treatment of (1) mild to moderate acute bacterial exacerbations of chronic bronchitis due to *H. influenzae*, *M. catarrhalis* or *Streptococcus pneumoniae*, (2) pneumonia due to *S. pneumoniae* or *H. influenzae*, (3) uncomplicated skin and skin-structure infections due to *S. aureus*, *Streptococcus pyogenes* or *Staphylococcus agalactiae* and (4) urethritis and cervicitis due to *C. trachomatis*. Azithromycin is being evaluated for the treatment of typhoid fever, Lyme disease and certain opportunistic infections in AIDS patients (e.g., *M. avium* complex, toxoplasmosis [encephalitis], cryptosporidiosis).

Penicillin is the usual drug of choice in the treatment of *S. pyogenes* pharyngitis, including the prophylaxis of rheumatic fever. Azithromycin is often effective in the eradication of susceptible strains of streptococci from the oropharynx. However, data establishing the efficacy of azithromycin in the subsequent prevention of rheumatic fever are not available at present.

Because azithromycin is mainly eliminated by the liver, it should be administered cautiously to patients with impaired hepatic function.

Table 12.2
Erythromycin: Clinically significant drug interactions

Drug	Interaction
Anticoagulants, oral	• The effects of oral anticoagulants may be increased by erythromycin lactobionate IV
Astemizole	• Astemizole metabolism may be impaired by erythromycin
Carbamazepine	• Carbamazepine blood levels may be increased by erythromycin lactobionate IV
Digoxin	• Digoxin blood levels may be increased by erythromycin lactobionate IV
Terfenadine	• Terfenadine metabolism may be impaired by erythromycin
Theophylline	• Theophylline blood levels can be increased by erythromycin
Triazolam	• Triazolam clearance may be decreased by erythromycin

Adverse Effects

With the exception of its effect on the gastro-intestinal (GI) tract, erythromycin produces a low incidence of adverse effects. The drug causes gastrointestinal upset with nausea, diarrhea and abdominal pain. Very rarely, erythromycin may cause reversible cholestatic hepatitis. This condition is characterized by clay-coloured stools, jaundice, nausea, fever, enlarged and tender liver, hyperbilirubinemia, elevated transaminase levels and dark urine. Previously believed to occur only with erythromycin estolate, cholestatic hepatitis is now known to be produced by all forms of the drug.

Both clarithromycin and azithromycin are well tolerated. Neither drug causes the high incidence of disabling nausea seen with erythromycin. Nausea, diarrhea and abdominal pain have been uncommon in clinical trials. Headache and dizziness have occurred rarely. Reversible dose-related hearing loss has been reported with high doses (e.g., ≥ 4 g/24 h) of both drugs used to treat *M. avium* infections. In general, it can be stated that clarithromycin and azithromycin are well-tolerated, albeit expensive, alternatives to erythromycin for the treatment of streptococcal pharyngitis, community-acquired respiratory infections, skin and soft-tissue infections and acute sinusitis.

In children, intravenous erythromycin may be cardiotoxic. There is growing concern that intravenous erythromycin lactobionate can cause serious cardiac adverse effects. At the time of writing this text, there were seven cases reported of a temporal association between erythromycin lactobionate and cardiac conduction disturbances. In addition, the FDA in the United States has received reports of twenty-nine cases of conduction abnormalities arising from the use of intravenous erythromycin lactobionate. These cardiac effects may be related to a quinidine-like effect of erythromycin on the heart. There may also be a connection between serum erythromycin concentrations and cardiac arrhythmias; this may explain why arrhythmias are rare complications of oral erythromycin.

Table 12.2 lists the clinically significant drug interactions for erythromycin.

Nursing Management

The nursing management of the patient receiving any of the macrolides is essentially the same (Table 12.3). Unique features related to each drug are included in Table 12.4 (pages 113–114).

Table 12.3
Nursing management for the macrolides

Assessment of risk vs. benefit	Patient data	• Establish baseline VS, general state of health, indicators of present infection • Other diseases; e.g., reduced liver or renal function may cause toxicity • *Age:* Elderly patients may have reduced defences and increased risk for drug toxicity; neonates have risk for cardiac adverse effects • *Children:* See uses and precautions in Table 12.4 • *Pregnancy and lactation:* Safety has not been established
	Drug data	• *Site and type of infection:* Select drugs based on location of infection and causative microorganism • Culture and sensitivity results • Specific drugs within group have different side effects; for erythromycin, most common are GI distress and local irritation or phlebitis with IV route; also, high dose or prolonged tx may cause hearing loss (usually reversible), superinfection or cholestatic hepatitis • Clarithromycin and azithromycin are generally well tolerated (but more expensive)
Implementation	Rights of administration	• Applying the "rights" helps prevent errors of administration
	Right route	• Macrolides are given orally and parenterally. Enteric-coated must be taken whole; chewable tablets should be chewed or crushed • Shake oral suspensions well, and use a properly calibrated device to ensure accuracy
	Right time	• Clarithromycin can be taken without regard to food; erythromycin and azithromycin are best taken on empty stomach with full glass of water. Giving erythromycin with meals may reduce GI irritation • Do not give with fruit juice
	Right dose	• Order may specify a single dose (in mg) or state the dose by weight (mg/kg/day) in equally divided doses. Calculate carefully
	Right drug	• Do not substitute one base of erythromycin for another (e.g., 250 mg of stearate base = 400 mg ethylsuccinate base)
	Right technique	• Erythromycin is irritating/painful by the IV route. IV administration requires knowledge of correct diluent and IV solution, correct dilution, and rate of administration. Always refer to manufacturer's instructions • Drug should be administered slowly (20–60 min) or by continuous infusion to reduce phlebitis. Slow rate if pain occurs; apply ice and check IV site frequently; change site q48–72 h
	Nursing therapeutics	• Enhance host defences (nutrition, rest, fluids, hygiene) • *Allergy:* Can occur at any time. Be alert for signs/symptoms, and be prepared with emergency tx • Administer drugs ATC to ensure effective blood levels

(cont'd on next page)

Table 12.3 (cont'd)
Nursing management for the macrolides

Implementation (cont'd)	Patient/family teaching	• Educate for proper use of anti-infectives (Chapter 9) • Review signs/symptoms of superinfection with pt and advise to report immediately • Instruct pt to report other signs/symptoms (e.g., jaundice or diarrhea) immediately • Discuss possibility of pregnancy; advise pt to notify physician • Emphasize importance of asking advice of pharmacist before using any macrolide with an OTC antihistamine
Outcomes	Monitoring of progress	*Continually monitor:* • Clinical response indicating tx success (reduction in signs/symptoms) • For mild side effects, and treat symptomatically • For adverse effects (respond immediately to superinfection or hepatotoxicity)

Response to Clinical Challenge

Principles

The macrolides do cause irritation; however, clarithromycin and azithromycin are less irritating, but more expensive, than erythromycin.

Patients have a right to refuse medication, but require accurate information to do so. Mr. J. needs more information about the benefits and risks of this drug and the risks of not treating the pneumonia.

Actions

1. Discuss Mr. J.'s experience of side effects (pain at IV site and GI distress); validate concerns and explain that effects are temporary and reversible
2. Explain the importance of antibiotic treatment; discuss why erythromycin was chosen (effective against organism, inexpensive, safe even with his penicillin allergy)
3. Discuss possibility of giving drug with food (which will reduce blood levels) or substituting another macrolide (more costly)
4. Ask pharmacist or physician to discuss choices with Mr. J.

Further Reading

The choice of antibacterial drugs. *Medical Letter on Drugs and Therapeutics* 1994;36:919–925.

Clarithromycin and azithromycin. *Medical Letter on Drugs and Therapeutics* 1992(May 15);34

Handbook of antimicrobial therapy. *Medical Letter on Drugs and Therapeutics* 1992.

Macrolides and lincosamides. *AMA Drug Evaluations Subscriptions;* Spring 1993.

Table 12.4
The macrolides: Drug doses

Drug Generic name (Trade names)	Dosage	Nursing alert
erythromycin (Erythromycin Base Filmtab, Erythromid, E-Mycin, Ery-Tab, Ilotycin, Robimycin, ERYC) erythromycin stearate (Erythrocin Stearate Filmtab, Bristamycin, Pfizer-E, Erypar, Ethril) erythromycin estolate (Ilosone) erythromycin ethylsuccinate (EES, Pediamycin)	**Oral:** *Adults:* 250–500 mg q6h or 333 mg q8h. Erythromycin ethylsuccinate: 400–800 mg qid. For more severe infections, up to 4 g/day. *Children:* 30–50 mg/kg/day, divided into 4 doses For prophylaxis of bacterial endocarditis in penicillin-allergic pts: Erythromycin ethylsuccinate 800 mg or erythromycin stearate 1 g 2 h before procedure, then half the dose 6 h later. *Children:* 20 mg/kg for erythromycin ethylsuccinate or erythromycin stearate	• Do not take with fruit juice. Best taken on empty stomach; if not tolerated, try coated tablets • Do not substitute tablets of one base for another (250 mg of stearate or estolate base = 400 mg of ethylsuccinate base)
erythromycin lactobionate (Erythrocin Lactobionate-IV)	**IV:** *Adults:* 250–500 mg q6h; up to 4 g/day in more severe infections. *Children:* 15–20 mg/kg/day, divided into 3–4 doses; up to 40 mg/kg/day	• Although continuous infusion is preferable, administration in divided doses not < q6h is also effective • Consult manufacturer's instructions for reconstitution • IV push is not acceptable. Do not administer with other drugs. Give slowly over 20–60 min; reduce rate if pain occurs
erythromycin gluceptate (Ilotycin Gluceptate)	**IV:** *Adults/children:* 15–20 mg/kg/day. Higher doses up to 4 g/day may be given in very severe infections	• Although continuous infusion is preferable, administration in divided doses not < q 6 h is also effective • Consult manufacturer's instructions for reconstitution • IV push is not acceptable. Do not administer with other drugs. Give slowly over 20–60 min; reduce rate if pain occurs
azithromycin (Zithromax)	**Oral:** *Adults:* For mild to moderate pharyngitis/ tonsillitis, acute bacterial exacerbations of bronchitis, pneumonia, and uncomplicated skin and skin-structure infections, 500 mg as a single dose on the first day followed by 250 mg od for 4 additional days. For non-gonococcal urethritis and cervicitis due to *C. trachomatis,* 1 g in a single dose. *Children < 16 years:* Safety and effectiveness has not been established	• Give at least 1 h ac or 2 h pc • May interfere with certain lab tests. May decrease white blood counts and platelets

Table 12.4 (continued)
The macrolides: Drug doses

Drug Generic name (Trade names)	Dosage	Nursing alert
clarithromycin (Biaxin)	**Oral:** *Adults:* For mild to moderate pharyngitis/tonsillitis due to *S. pyogenes,* 250 mg q12h for 10 days. For uncomplicated skin and skin-structure infections and acute exacerbations of chronic bronchitis due to *S. pneumoniae* or *M. catarrhalis* or pneumonia due to *S. pneumoniae* or *M. pneumoniae,* 250 mg q12h for 7–14 days. For acute exacerbations of chronic bronchitis due to *H. influenzae,* 500 mg q12h for 7–14 days. For acute maxillary sinusitis, 500 mg q12h for 14 days. Dosage reduction may be required in the elderly and in pts with renal impairment. *Children under 12 years:* Safety and effectiveness have not been established	• May be given with or without food • Avoid during pregnancy/lactation • May interfere with some lab tests. Occasionally, may decrease white blood counts

The Tetracyclines

Topics Discussed
- Mechanism of action
- Antibacterial spectra
- Resistance
- Pharmacokinetics
- Therapeutic uses
- Adverse effects
- Nursing management

Drugs Discussed
demeclocycline (dem-meh-kloe-**sye**-kleen)
doxycycline (dok-see-**sye**-kleen)
minocycline (min-oh-**sye**-kleen)
oxytetracycline (ok-see-tet-rah-**sy**-kleen)
tetracycline hydrochloride (tet-rah-**sye**-kleen hye-droe-**klor**-eyed)

Clinical Challenge
Consider this clinical challenge as you read through this chapter. The response to the challenge appears on page 120.

Mary is a 19-year-old, married university student. For 6 months, she has taken tetracycline 250 mg PO daily for treatment of acne.
    Outline a teaching plan for Mary.

The drugs tetracycline HCl (Achromycin®, Achromycin V®, Sumycin®, Tetracyn®), oxytetracycline (Terramycin®), demeclocycline (Declomycin®), doxycycline (Vibramycin®), methacycline (Rondomycin®) and minocycline (Minocin®) are collectively referred to as the tetracyclines. All tetracyclines have similar chemical structures and antibacterial spectra (Figure 13.1 on the next page). Unless otherwise stated, the term tetracycline or tetracyclines in this chapter refers to all these drugs.

Mechanism of Action

Tetracyclines are concentrated within sensitive gram-positive and gram-negative bacteria by an energy-dependent process. Once inside bacteria, tetracyclines depress protein synthesis by blocking the attachment of aminoacyl transfer RNA to the acceptor site on the messenger RNA-ribosome complex. Binding of the tetracycline antibiotic occurs primarily at the bacterial 30S ribosomal subunit.

Tetracyclines are bacteriostatic. Once bacterial cell multiplication is stopped, the host's defence mechanisms kill the pathogens. The selective toxicity of tetracyclines for sensitive bacteria, and their safety to the host, appears to depend partially on the energy-dependent uptake of the antibiotics by bacterial, but not mammalian, cells. This results in a greater accumulation of tetracyclines by bacterial cells.

Antibacterial Spectrum

The tetracyclines have a wide spectrum of activity. Although they are more effective against gram-

Figure 13.1
Structures of (a) tetracycline, (b) minocycline and (c) doxycycline

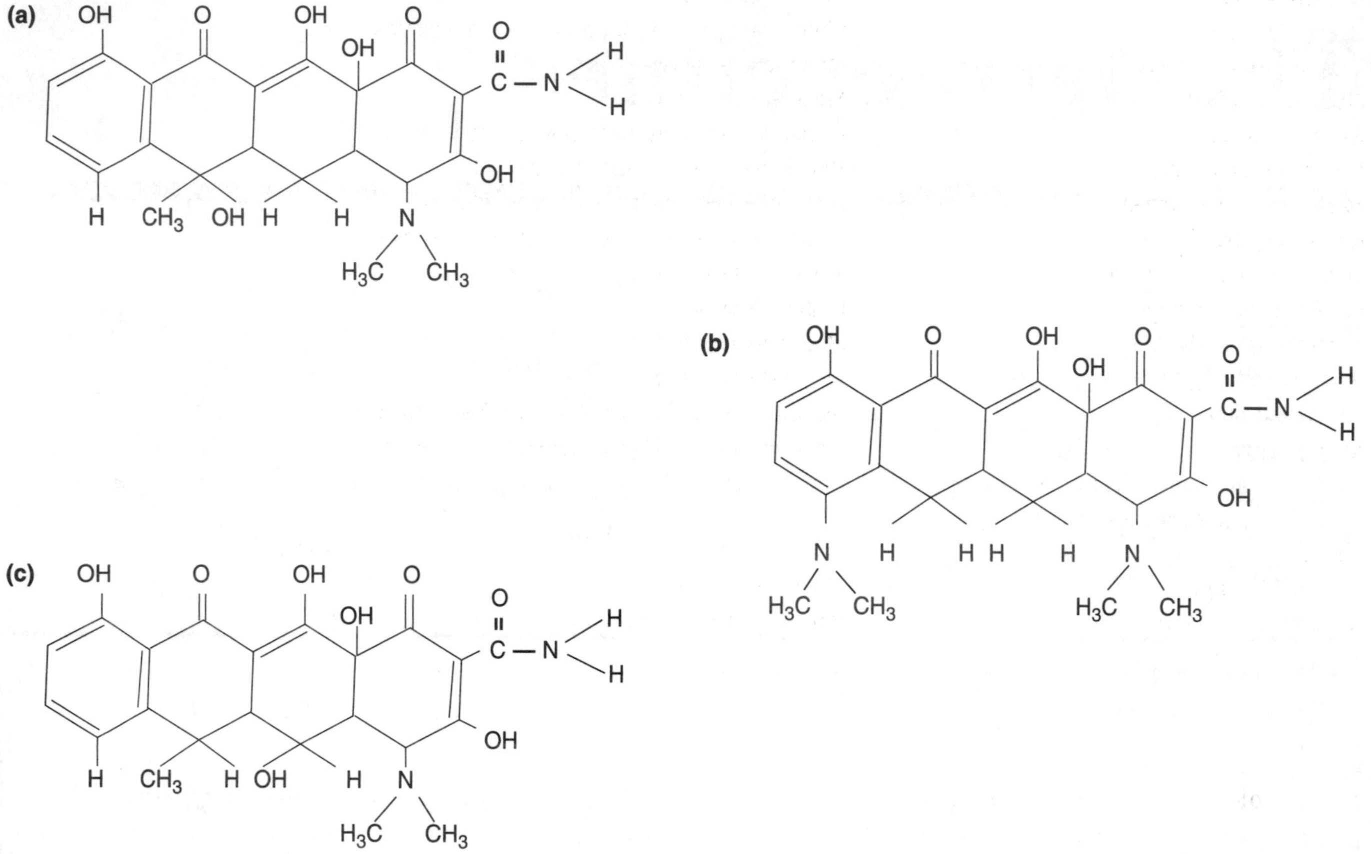

Source: Johnson GE. *PDQ Pharmacology.* Hamilton, ON: B.C. Decker; 1988:253.

positive bacteria, the drugs are also active against gram-negative bacteria, *Rickettsieae* species, *Mycoplasma* species and agents of the psittacosis–lymphogranuloma venereum group of conditions (Table 13.1). There are no major differences between the various tetracyclines. Doxycycline may be effective against some strains of *Bacteroides fragilis* that are resistant to other tetracyclines.

Resistance

Several species of bacteria have become increasingly resistant to the tetracyclines. Many Enterobacteriaceae (e.g., *Shigella, Escherichia coli*) and most *Pseudomonas aeruginosa* are resistant. Many strains of staphylococci, streptococci, pneumococci and *Bacteroides* are no longer susceptible. Emergence of high-level tetracycline-resistant *Neisseria gonorrhoeae* strains is common in areas of the world.

The primary means by which resistance develops is through alterations in bacterial cytoplasmic membrane-located proteins that result in an energy-dependent increased efflux of antibiotic from the bacterial cell. This is the explanation behind the resistance of Enterobacteriaceae. Clinical resistance can also occur as a result of the inability of tetracyclines to bind effectively to bacterial ribosomes. This is seen in various gram-positive and gram-negative bacteria, including *Neisseria*.

Pharmacokinetics

Tetracyclines are usually given orally, although formulations of tetracycline hydrochloride, tetracycline phosphate, oxytetracycline, minocycline and doxycycline are also available for parenteral administration. Absorption from the gastrointestinal tract ranges from 60% to 80% for oxytetracycline, tetracycline and demeclocycline to 95% to 100% for minocycline and doxycycline. Most

Table 13.1
Sensitivities of some organisms to the tetracyclines

Bacillus anthracis	Some sensitivity
Bacteroides spp.	Moderate sensitivity, but many resistant strains
Clostridium perfringens	Moderate sensitivity
Clostridium tetani	Moderate sensitivity
Escherichia coli	Moderate sensitivity, but many resistant strains
Haemophilus ducreyi	High sensitivity, but many resistant strains
Haemophilus influenzae	High sensitivity, but many resistant strains
Klebsiella pneumoniae	Moderate sensitivity, but many resistant strains
Listeria monocytogenese	Moderate sensitivity
Mycoplasma pneumoniae	High sensitivity
Neisseria gonorrhoeae	Moderate sensitivity
Neisseria meningitidis	Moderate sensitivity
Salmonella spp.	Moderate sensitivity, but many resistant strains
Shigella spp.	Moderate sensitivity, but many resistant strains
Staphylococcus aureus (both penicillin-sensitive and penicillin resistant)	Some sensitivity, but tetracyclines not recomm. for tx
Streptococcus pneumoniae	Moderate sensitivity, but some areas have many resistant strains
Streptococcus pyogenes	Moderate sensitivity, but many resistant strains
Treponema pallidum	Sensitive; tetracycline is recomm. in penicillin-allergic pts

tetracyclines should not be taken with milk, non-absorbable antacids or iron preparations because calcium, magnesium, aluminum and iron block tetracycline absorption. Dairy products can delay the absorption of minocycline, but food appears to have no influence on minocycline absorption. Doxycycline absorption is not significantly influenced by food or milk.

Once absorbed, tetracyclines bind in varying degrees to plasma proteins. Oxytetracycline, tetracycline and minocycline are 35%, 65% and 76% bound, respectively. Methacycline, demeclocycline and doxycycline are approximately 90% bound to plasma albumin. Tetracyclines distribute throughout the body, penetrating tissues to varying degrees. High concentrations are usually found in bile. Tetracyclines cross the placenta but have difficulty crossing the blood–brain barrier. Concentrations in the cerebrospinal fluid are only 10% to 20% of those in plasma.

Lipid solubility is a major factor in determining tetracycline diffusion. Doxycycline and minocycline are more lipophilic and penetrate tissues and secretions better than the other tetracyclines. Doxycycline diffuses well into endometrial, myometrial, prostatic and renal tissues.

Minocycline attains therapeutic concentrations in saliva and tears. The lipid solubility of minocycline can, however, be a disadvantage because it enables the drug to diffuse well into the highly lipid cells of the vestibular apparatus, leading to vestibular toxicity.

Tetracyclines bind to calcium and are retained in bones and growing teeth for long periods of time. Because they can damage developing teeth and delay the development of long bones, tetracyclines are usually contraindicated during pregnancy and in patients under eight to ten years of age.

The half-lives of the tetracyclines range from 8 h to 9 h (for tetracycline HCl and oxytetracycline) to 16 h to 18 h (for minocycline and doxycycline). The differences in half-lives are reflected in the dosage intervals for minocycline and doxycycline. Whereas most tetracyclines are recommended on a three- or four-times-daily basis, minocycline is taken twice a day and doxycycline once daily.

Renal excretion is the major route of tetracycline elimination. Minocycline has a low renal clearance, and less than 10% of a dose is recovered unchanged in urine. The drug undergoes enterohepatic circulation and may be metabolized to a considerable extent. Doxycycline elimination is independent of both renal and hepatic function. The drug is excreted in the feces, largely as an inactive chelated product. Thus, the dose of doxycycline does not require modification in patients with renal or hepatic insufficiency. Further, the inactive product has relatively less impact on the intestinal microflora, resulting in lower incidence of irritative diarrhea and candidal overgrowth.

Therapeutic Uses

Despite their broad antibacterial spectrum, tetracyclines have relatively poor activity against most pathogens and are rarely considered drugs of first choice. They are considered first-line drugs for the treatment of *Mycoplasma pneumoniae,* Rocky Mountain spotted fever, endemic typhus, *Borrelia recurrentis* (relapsing fever), chlamydial disease, nonspecific brucellosis and infections caused by *Pasteurella.*

Tetracyclines are used to treat inflammatory acne. To explain this apparently unusual use of tetracyclines, it is necessary to describe briefly the etiology of acne.

Acne vulgaris is caused by an exaggerated response of the pilosebaceous gland to the secretion of androgens. Sebum production increases, and epithelial cells lining the duct adhere to each other to form a plug that blocks the follicular channel. The resulting impaction and distention of the sebaceous glands leads to the formation of comedones and the disruption of the follicular epithelium. Discharge of the follicular contents into the dermis produces an inflammatory reaction. The presence of the anaerobic diptheroid *Propionibacterium acnes* contributes to this problem. By secreting a variety of enzymes, including hyaluridonase, it may disrupt the follicular epithelium and increase inflammation. Tetracycline antibiotics eradicate *Propionibacterium acnes* and are effective in the treatment of acne.

For most infections, tetracyclines are second- or third-line drugs, falling behind more effective agents. Conditions for which tetracyclines are backup drugs are too numerous to mention. They are listed in the *Handbook of Antimicrobial Therapy* (1992; see Further Reading at the end of the chapter).

Doxycycline and minocycline warrant special note. For most clinical conditions they offer no advantage over tetracycline HCl, and they are significantly more expensive. There are, however, a few situations in which they are superior to the other tetracyclines. Minocycline is an effective alternative to rifampicin for the eradication of meningococci, including sulfonamide-resistant bacteria from the nasopharynx.

Minocycline is most frequently prescribed for the treatment of two troublesome skin conditions. It is usually considered to be the preferred tetracycline for acne vulgaris. By eradicating the anaerobe *Propionibacterium acnes,* minocycline reduces the production of inflammatory fatty acids by the microbe and decreases inflammatory acne. Minocycline is also used to treat rosacea. Exactly why minocycline should be effective in rosacea is not known. However, its efficacy is probably unrelated to its antibacterial properties.

As mentioned previously, doxycycline is eliminated unchanged in the feces. Consequently, it does not accumulate in patients with renal or hepatic impairment and is safer than other tetracyclines in these patients. Doxycycline is the tetracycline of choice for the treatment of sinusitis and acute exacerbations of chronic bronchitis caused by pneumococci, group A streptococci and *Haemophilus influenzae*. Because it penetrates the noninflamed prostate better, doxycycline may be effective in chronic prostatitis. It is also preferred for the treatment of acute urethral syndrome because the most common causative bacteria — *Escherichia coli, Staphylococcus saprophyticus* and *Chlamydia* — are usually susceptible to the drug. Doxycycline has greater activity than the other tetracyclines against *Bacteroides fragilis*. It has been used successfully in the treatment of nongonococcal pelvic inflammatory disease produced by *E. coli,* other aerobic gram-negative coliforms and *B. fragilis.*

Tetracyclines are contraindicated in severe renal or hepatic disease. They are also normally contraindicated in pregnant or lactating women. Because of their ability to bind to calcium and affect the development of teeth and long bones, tetracyclines are contraindicated in children under eight years of age. Finally, tetracyclines should not be used in situations where bactericidal effect is essential, such as bacterial endocarditis.

Table 13.2 lists the clinically significant drug interactions for the tetracyclines.

Table 13.2
The tetracyclines: Drug interactions

Drug	Interaction
Antacids	• Antacids containing calcium, magnesium and aluminum impair the absorption of orally administered tetracyclines
Antibiotics	• Tetracyclines can block the effects of bactericidal antibiotics, such as penicillins or cephalosporins
Antiepileptics	• Carbamazepine, phenytoin or barbiturates can increase the hepatic metabolism of doxycycline and decrease its half-life
Anticoagulants	• Anticoagulants may require a reduced dosage because tetracyclines can decrease prothrombin synthesis
Oral contraceptives	• Tetracyclines can reduce the efficacy of oral contraceptives
Diuretics	• If possible, diuretics and tetracyclines should not be used together because both will increase BUN levels
Food	• Food containing calcium and magnesium can reduce tetracycline absorption. The only tetracycline that is not affected is doxycycline
Iron	• Iron blocks tetracycline absorption
Methoxyflurane	• Methoxyflurane plus a tetracycline can reduce renal function. This has occasionally led to death
Milk	• See the comments above for Food

Adverse Effects

Tetracyclines can cause nausea, vomiting, epigastric burning, stomatitis and glossitis when given orally. Administered intravenously, they can produce phlebitis. Tetracyclines can be hepatotoxic, particularly in patients with pre-existing renal or hepatic insufficiency. Hepatotoxicity does not occur frequently, but can be particularly severe during pregnancy. If given for long periods of time, tetracyclines can increase blood urea nitrogen (BUN) and occasionally cause nephrotoxicity. They should not be given with potentially nephrotoxic drugs.

As already stated, tetracyclines can stain teeth and retard bone growth if given to pregnant women after the fourth month of gestation or to children under the age of eight years.

Photosensitivity, manifested mainly as abnormal sunburn reactions, is particularly prevalent with demeclocycline therapy.

Minocycline produces vertigo in a high percentage of patients taking the drug.

Superinfection is a recognized adverse reaction to many broad-spectrum antibiotics, including tetracyclines. By suppressing the normal bacterial flora, tetracyclines enable other bacteria, such as penicillinase-producing staphylococci and *Candida,* to proliferate. Superinfections occur in the oral, anogenital and intestinal areas. The consequences of the superinfection are determined by its site. When the superinfection occurs in the oropharynx, vagina and perirectal areas, itching and discomfort may occur. If overgrowth of bowel pathogenic bacteria occurs, diarrhea is observed.

Pseudomembranous colitis, secondary to the overgrowth of *Clostridium difficile,* can also occur, particularly in elderly or debilitated patients or in those being treated with several antibiotics, immunosuppressants or corticosteroids. Symptoms include profuse, watery diarrhea, craming and fever. Strict isolation of stools and careful hand-washing are essential to prevent spread of infection. If pseudomembranous colitis develops, the tetracycline should be stopped immediately, lost electrolytes replaced and other supportive measures used as required. Oral vancomycin may be given, if necessary.

Nursing Management

The nursing management of the patient receiving any of the tetracyclines is essentially the same (Table 13.3). Unique features related to each drug are included in Table 13.4.

Response to Clinical Challenge

Principles
Mary is of childbearing age. Although she is taking a low dose of tetracycline, the long duration of her drug therapy and her lifestyle raise the question of exposure to sun.

Actions
Major points to emphasize in a teaching plan for Mary would include:
1. Store properly (airtight container; dark, cool place)
2. Dispose of any drug past expiry date
3. Take dose on empty stomach with full glass of water (and instruct which foods/other drugs to avoid)
4. Avoid exposure to sun
5. Do not take with oral contraceptives (explain risks to fetus; suggest alternative methods of birth control, or discontinuation of drug
6. Watch for signs/symptoms of superinfection (not common at this low dose)

Further Reading

The choice of antibacterial drugs. *Medical Letter on Drugs and Therapeutics* 1994;36:919–925.

Handbook of antimicrobial therapy. *Medical Letter on Drugs and Therapeutics* 1992.

Kapusnik-Unver JE, Sande MA, Chambers HF. Antimicrobial agents: tetracyclines, chloramphenicol, erythromycin, and miscellaneous agents. In: Hardman JL, Limbird LE, eds. *Goodman and Gilman's The Pharmacological Basis of Therapeutics*. 9th ed. New York: Pergamon; 1996.

Tetracyclines and chloramphenicol. *AMA Drug Evaluations Subscriptions* 1993:5.1–5.10.

Treatment of sexually transmitted diseases. *Medical Letter on Drugs and Therapeutics* 1994;36:913–918.

Table 13.3
Nursing management for the tetracyclines

Assessment of risk vs. benefit	Patient data	• Establish baseline VS, general state of health, indicators of present infection • Other diseases; e.g., reduced liver or renal function may cause toxicity, esp. in elderly pts • *Allergy:* Although not common, can occur; is more likely in pt with compromised immune system • *Neonates and children:* Risk of adverse effects to tooth and bone development • *Pregnancy and lactation:* Recommend avoiding tetracyclines
	Drug data	• *Site and type of infection:* Select drugs based on location of infection and causative microorganism • Culture and sensitivity results • Many drug reactions: Avoid with other drugs unless advised • Deteriorates into toxic product after expiry date; can cause nephrotic syndrome (nausea, vomiting, acidosis, proteinuria, hypokalomia) • Deteriorates more rapidly when exposed to heat, light, moisture • Most common side effects are GI distress and phlebitis with IV route; also, may cause superinfection, photosensitivity. • Occ. can cause serious reactions such as hepatotoxicity, nephrotoxicity, pseudomembranous colitis
Implementation	Rights of administration	• Applying the "rights" helps prevent errors of administration
	Right route	• Give orally or parenterally. IM route is very painful and should be used only when other routes are not possible
	Right time	• Best on empty stomach (1 h ac or 2 h pc) with full glass of water, but giving with meals may reduce GI irritation • Do not give with milk, dairy products, iron supplements, antacids, or laxatives containing magnesium
	Right technique	• Irritating and/or painful by IV/IM routes. IM administration should be given slowly, deep into large muscle mass, and volume not to exceed 2 mL at one site. Aspiration is essential because preparations contain local anesthetic which is harmful if injected IV • IV administration requires knowledge of correct diluent and IV solution, correct dilution and rate of administration. Always refer to manufacturer's instructions for this route • Administer drug in large volume by continuous infusion to reduce phlebitis. Check IV site frequently, and change q48–72h
	Nursing therapeutics	• Promote preventive measures (particularly hygiene) to minimize superinfections (oral, vaginal) • Administer ATC to ensure effective blood levels
	Patient/family teaching	Educate for proper use of anti-infectives, as summarized in Chapter 9. Specific points for emphasis with tetracyclines include: • *Photosensitivity:* Avoid direct exposure to sun; wear protective clothing and sunblock; effect lasts after drug tx ends

(cont'd on next page)

Table 13.3 (continued)
Nursing management for the tetracyclines

| Implementation (cont'd) | Patient/family teaching (cont'd) | • Long-term tx can cause tooth discoloration (in adults); alert pt to this effect
• *Signs/symptoms of superinfection:* Review with pt and advise to report immediately
• *Other signs/symptoms* (e.g., jaundice, severe diarrhea): Review with pt and advise to report immediately
• *Pregnancy:* Advise pt to notify physician of any possibility. Explain that drug may reduce effectiveness of oral contraceptives, and advise alternative method
• Inform diabetic pts that urine glucose testing with Clinistix®, Diastix®, or TesTape® are unreliable while taking tetracyclines |
| Outcomes | Monitoring of progress | *Continually monitor:*
• Clinical response indicating tx success (reduction in signs/symptoms)
• For mild side effects, and treat symptomatically
• For adverse effects (respond immediately to superinfection, hepatotoxicity, pseudomembranous colitis)
• *NB:* Allergy can occur at any time. Be alert for signs/symptoms; document and report to physician |

Table 13.4
The tetracyclines: Drug doses

Drug Generic name (Trade names)	Dosage	Nursing alert
tetracycline HCl (Achromycin, Achromycin V, Panmycin, Sumycin)	**Oral:** *Adults:* 250–500 mg q6h. *Children > 8 years:* 25–50 mg/kg/day in 2–4 divided doses	• Avoid exposure of drug to light or heat. Check expiry date • Give with full glass of water on empty stomach
oxytetracycline (Terramycin)	**Oral:** *Adults:* 250–500 mg qid; may be doubled in the severely ill. *Children > 8 years:* 25–50 mg/kg/ day in 4 divided doses. **IM:** Not recommended; injection can be extremely painful and, at usual dosages, serum concentrations are lower than after PO administration. No dosage recommendations given	• As for tetracycline
demeclocycline (Declomycin)	**Oral:** *Adults:* 150 mg qid or 300 mg bid. *Children > 8 years:* 6–12 mg/kg/day in 2–4 divided doses	• May be taken with food if GI irritation occurs but avoid milk, dairy products, antacids

Table 13.4
The tetracyclines: Drug doses

Drug Generic name (Trade names)	Dosage	Nursing alert
doxycycline (Doryx, Doxy-Caps, Doxychel, Doxy-Tabs, Vibramycin, Vibra-Tabs)	**Oral:** *Adults:* 200 mg on day 1, followed by maint. dose of 100 mg at same time qd. For severe infections (e.g., lung abscesses, osteomylitis) and in chronic UTI, single daily dose of 200 mg may be used throughout. For tx of acute gonococcal infections, 200 mg stat plus 100 mg hs first day, followed by 100 mg bid for 3 days. For tx of uncomplicated urethral, endocervical or vaginal infections in adults associated with *C. trachomatis* and *Ureaplasma,* 100 mg bid for at least 10 days **IV:** Only when PO tx is inadequate or not tolerated. Substitute oral tx ASAP. Duration of IV infusion may vary with dose (100–200 mg/day) but is usually 1–4 h. A recommended min. infusion time for 100 mg 0.5 mg/mL solution is 1 h. See product literature for preparation of solution for IV administration. *Adults/children > 8 years weighing ≥ 45 kg:* 200 mg on day 1, given in 1–2 infusions, followed by 100– 200 mg daily in 1–2 infusions. *Children > 8 years < 45 kg:* 4.4 mg/ kg on day 1, given in 1–2 infusions, followed by 2.2 mg/ kg–4.4 mg/kg daily in 1–2 infusions	• May be taken without regard to food • Avoid calcium, magnesium or iron supplements within 1–3 h
minocycline HCl (Minocin)	**Oral:** *Adults:* 100–200 mg initially, followed by 100 mg q12h. *Children > 13 years:* 4 mg/kg initially, then 2 mg/kg q12h. For inflammatory acne, 50–200 mg/day **IV:** Only when PO tx is inadequate or not tolerated. Substitute oral tx ASAP. Dilute drug before administration (see product literature). *Adults:* 200 mg initially, then 100 mg q12 h (max., 400 mg/day). *Children > 8 years:* 4 mg/ kg initially, then 2 mg/kg q12h	• May be taken without regard to food • **IV:** Use continuous infusion only; must be diluted in 500–1000 mL

The Aminoglycosides

Topics Discussed
- Mechanism of action
- Antibacterial spectrum
- Resistance
- Pharmacokinetics
- Therapeutic uses
- Adverse effects
- Nursing management

Drugs Discussed
amikacin sulfate (am-ih-**kay**-sin)
gentamicin sulfate (jen-tah-**mye**-sin)
kanamycin sulfate (kan-ah-**mye**-sin)
netilmicin sulfate (net-ill-**mye**-sin)
tobramycin sulfate (toe-brah-**mie**-sin)

Clinical Challenge

Consider this clinical challenge as you read through this chapter. The response to the challenge appears on page 130.

Karrie is a 23-year-old nurse who was involved in a serious car accident resulting in several injuries and a life-threatening infection. Gentamicin is ordered by the IV route. The initial serum level is drawn 15 min after the end of the infusion and indicates 4 µg/mL (8.6 µmol/L).

Two days later, Karrie complains of vertigo, stating that this occurs only when she rises from the bed, and that it slowly disappears.

A trough serum level is ordered. The resulting level is 3 µg/mL (6.5 µmol/L).

1. What action do you expect from the physician after the initial plasma level?
2. What other information would you seek?
3. Why is a trough rather than a peak level ordered?
4. When should the blood be drawn?
5. What further action do you expect from the physician?

The aminoglycoside antibiotics are a group of structurally related drugs. They derive their name from the fact that their structures contain at least one sugar attached to one or more amino groups.

The drugs discussed in this chapter are gentamicin, amikacin, kanamycin, netilmicin and tobramycin. Although streptomycin, neomycin and framycetin are also aminoglycosides, they are not presented in this chapter. Streptomycin is used primarily in the treatment of tuberculosis, and is discussed in Chapter 18. Neomycin and framycetin are used in the topical treatment of infections. Because they are not used for systemic infections, these drugs are not discussed in this chapter.

Mechanism of Action

Aminoglycosides inhibit bacterial protein synthesis and are bactericidal. They bind to the bacterial 30S ribosomal subunit of streptococci to cause a misreading of the genetic code. The proteins formed contain the wrong sequence of amino acids and have no biological value ("nonsense proteins"). Aminoglycosides block protein synthesis in other bacteria by inhibiting amino acid translocation.

Antibacterial Spectrum

Aminoglycosides are used principally to treat infections caused by sensitive strains of Enterobacteriaceae, including *Escherichia coli* and *Klebsiella, Enterobacter, Serratia* and *Proteus* species. With the exception of streptomycin and kanamycin, aminoglycosides are active against *Pseudomonas aeruginosa.* They have only limited activity against most gram-positive bacteria. They are active in vitro against certain species of streptococcus. Only minimal activity is usually found against *Streptococcus faecalis, S. pneumoniae* and streptococci of the viridans group. Although aminoglycosides inhibit staphylococci, safer drugs, such as the penicillins or cephalosporins, are usually used against these pathogens. Aminoglycosides have little activity against anaerobic microorganisms or facultative bacteria under anaerobic conditions. Facultative bacteria are not restricted to living in either aerobic or anaerobic conditions. Rather, these bacteria can live in either environment.

Gentamicin, tobramycin, amikacin and netilmicin are used extensively for the treatment of systemic infections. Although their antibacterial spectra show few qualitative differences, the various aerobic gram-negative bacilli vary in their susceptibility to the four drugs. Table 14.1 describes the differing sensitivities of six gram-negative bacilli to tobramycin and gentamicin. The purpose of this table is not to suggest that tobramycin should always be used in place of gentamicin, but rather to indicate that cultures should be performed, where practical, to determine the most appropriate aminoglycoside to treat a particular patient.

Table 14.1

In vitro activity of tobramycin and gentamicin against susceptible gram-negative organisms (percentage of isolates susceptible at 1.57 µg/mL)

	Number of strains	Tobramycin	Gentamicin
Escherichia coli	100	93%	80%
Enterobacter spp.	52	94%	81%
Proteus mirabilis	38	92%	58%
Proteus spp. (indole-positive)	26	100%	85%
Klebsiella spp.	100	100%	98%
Serratia marcescens	41	86%	88%

Resistance

Bacterial resistance can develop to aminoglycosides. The major mechanism for the development of resistance involves enzymatic inactivation of the antibiotics. Decreased uptake of the aminoglycoside by bacteria or alteration of bacterial ribosomal binding sites can also account for the development of resistance.

The aminoglycosides are inactivated by acetylation, adenylation or phosphorylation of critical binding sites. The enzymes involved in these processes are coded by genetic entities (conjugative or nonconjugative plasmids or transposable elements) that can be transferred to other gram-negative bacterial species. These transferable elements also may carry additional genes that can confer resistance to other classes of antimicrobial drugs (e.g., beta-lactams, tetracyclines) to the recipient bacterium. This may result in the simultaneous development of multiple-resistant strains.

The prevalence of individual aminoglycoside-inactivating enzymes varies widely, both with respect to geographic location and time. Thus, different patterns of aminoglycoside resistance exist among countries, among hospitals in any country, province or city, and even among wards within a hospital. As a result, physicians should rely on established tests of susceptibility to a drug to determine whether its use is appropriate in the treatment of a particular patient.

Gram-negative bacilli that are resistant to amikacin frequently are resistant to all aminoglycosides; strains of *Escherichia coli, Pseudomonas, Enterobacter,* and *Serratia* that are resistant to all aminoglycosides have been isolated. The mechanism of this resistance is thought to be decreased uptake of antibiotic by the bacterial cell.

High-level resistance to all aminoglycosides has emerged in some nosocomial strains of enterococci (*E. faecalis, E. faecium*) and has spread to other isolates of this species by transmission on plasmids and transposons that carry the genetic determinants that code these functions. In some of these isolates, concurrent resistance to other antimicrobial drugs (e.g., vancomycin, beta-lactams, erythromycin) has been observed. This represents a significant clinical challenge in that it effectively eliminates the synergy between aminoglycosides and cell wall-active agents (e.g., beta-lactams, vancomycin), which has been the mainstay of therapy for serious infections caused by these species. This may necessitate a return to single-agent treatment of these conditions and result in reduced efficacy and possibly an increase in morbidity and mortality.

Chromosomal mutations that alter the 30S ribosomal subunit binding site can result in a rapid, single-step resistance to streptomycin. This mechanism of resistance appears to be clinically important for *Mycobacterium tuberculosis* and enterococci, but not for gram-negative bacilli.

Pharmacokinetics

The aminoglycosides are very polar (water-soluble) drugs and cannot diffuse across gastrointestinal membranes. Less than one percent of an oral dose is absorbed. Aminoglycosides are absorbed rapidly from intramuscular injection sites, with peak concentrations appearing within one hour.

Aminoglycosides do not diffuse readily across body membranes. For example, concentrations of gentamicin in pleural and pericardial fluids are only one-quarter to one-half those in serum. Aminoglycoside levels in fetal serum are 20% to 40% of those in maternal serum. Aminoglycosides do not cross well into the cerebrospinal fluid, even in the presence of inflammation. If used to treat meningitis in adults, these drugs must be given intrathecally. The poorly developed blood–brain barrier of the newborn presents little impediment to drug diffusion; therefore, systemic aminoglycoside administration can produce therapeutic levels of the antibiotic in the cerebrospinal fluid of neonates. Aminoglycosides enter the perilymph of the ear, where concentrations correlate with ototoxicity.

Aminoglycosides are eliminated by renal excretion. Their half-lives of two to three hours in patients with normal kidney function are extended in patients with renal impairment. Dosages must be decreased in the neonate or adult with reduced renal function. Although formulae are provided (see Therapeutic Uses, below) to assist in dosage calculations for patients with renal impairment, they should be used as guides only when it is impossible to measure serum levels of the drug.

Therapeutic Uses

Kanamycin (Kantrex®, Klebcil®)
Kanamycin is seldom used today because of bacterial resistance. Kanamycin capsules may be given orally to sterilize the bowel preoperatively, treat intestinal infections caused by susceptible organisms or provide adjunctive treatment of neurologic manifestations associated with severe liver damage.

Gentamicin (Alcomicin®, Cidomycin®, Garamycin®)
Gentamicin is still important in the treatment of many serious gram-negative bacillary infections (e.g., caused by *E. coli, P. mirabilis,* indole-positive *Proteus, Klebsiella, Enterobacter* and *Serratia* species and *Pseudomonas aeruginosa*), although resistance to the drug is developing. In addition to the foregoing, *Salmonella* and *Shigella* species are often gentamicin-sensitive. Gentamicin can be considered for treatment of bacteremia, respiratory and urinary tract infections, infected wounds, and bone and soft-tissue infections, including peritonitis and burns complicated by sepsis. Peak serum levels should be at least 4 µg/mL (8.6 µmol/L), but should not exceed 10 µg/mL (21.6 µmol/L). Serious infections with *P. aeruginosa* may require serum levels of 6 µg/mL (12.9 µmol/L) gentamicin combined with carbenicillin (Geopen®, Pyopen®) or ticarcillin (Ticar®), piperacillin or ceftazidime. The combination produces a synergistic effect with some strains and delays the emergence of resistant organisms. For patients with impaired renal function, the half-life of gentamicin in hours can be estimated by multiplying the serum creatinine (mg/100 mL) by four. The frequency of administration (in hours) may be approximated by doubling the half-life.

Gentamicin is also applied topically for use in the treatment of primary and secondary infections caused by sensitive strains of streptococci (group A beta-hemolytic, alpha-hemolytic), *S. aureus* (coagulase-positive, coagulase-negative and some penicillinase-producing strains) and the gram-negative bacteria *P. aeruginosa, Aerobacter aerogenes, E. coli, Proteus vulgaris* and *Klebsiella pneumoniae*. Gentamicin may also be used for ocular infections caused by *S. aureus, P. aeruginosa, A. aerogenes, E. coli, P. vulgaris* or *K. pneumoniae*.

Tobramycin (Nebcin®)

Tobramycin has a similar antibacterial spectrum to that of gentamicin. It is usually active against most strains of the following organisms in vitro and in clinical infections: *P. aeruginosa; Proteus* species (indole-positive and indole-negative), including *P. mirabilis, P. morganii, P. rettgeri* and *P. vulgaris; E. coli; Klebsiella-Enterobacter-Serratia* group; *Citrobacter* species; *Providencia* species; and staphylococci, including *S. aureus* (coagulase-positive and coagulase-negative). Its minimal inhibitory concentration (MIC) against *Pseudomonas aeruginosa* is approximately one-quarter that of gentamicin. Tobramycin is considered by many to be the aminoglycoside of choice for *P. aeruginosa* infections, in which case it is combined with carbenicillin or ticarcillin, piperacillin or ceftazidime.

Tobramycin may be indicated for the treatment of the following infections when caused by susceptible organisms: septicemia, urinary tract infections, lower respiratory infections, serious skin and soft-tissue infections (including burns and peritonitis) and central nervous system infections caused by organisms resistant to antibiotics usually considered efficacious in these infections.

Effective serum concentrations of tobramycin are similar to those previously presented for gentamicin. Prolonged serum concentrations above 12 mg/L (or 12 µg/mL) should be avoided. The dosage interval in hours can be calculated for adult patients with impaired renal function by multiplying the patient's serum creatinine (mg/100 mL) by six.

Like gentamicin, tobramycin can be used for ocular infections caused by *S. aureus, P. aeruginosa, A. aerogenes, E. coli, P. vulgaris* or *K. pneumoniae*.

Amikacin (Amikin®)

Amikacin is indicated for the short-term treatment of serious infections due to amikacin-susceptible strains of *Pseudomonas aeruginosa, E. coli* and *S. aureus,* as well as *Proteus, Klebsiella-Enterobacter-Serratia, Providencia, Salmonella* and *Citrobacter* species. Among the aminoglycosides, it has the greatest resistance to bacterial aminoglycoside-inactivating enzymes. Amikacin is often considered to be the drug of choice for the initial treatment of serious gram-negative bacillary infections in hospitals, where gentamicin resistance is a problem. Amikacin's therapeutic serum concentrations range from 15–25 µg/mL (25.7–42.8 µmol/L). To obtain the dosage interval in hours for patients with impaired renal function, multiply the serum creatinine (mg/100 mL) by nine. This formula should not be used to calculate dosage for elderly patients.

Netilmicin (Netromycin®)

Netilmicin has a similar spectrum of activity to that of gentamicin and tobramycin. However, because it is less sensitive to bacterial inactivation, netilmicin is effective against some gentamicin-resistant and tobramycin-resistant strains of Enterobacteriaceae. Netilmicin is indicated for the treatment of infections caused by susceptible strains of *E. coli, Proteus* (indole-negative and some indole-positive), *Klebsiella, Enterobacter, Citrobacter* and *Staphylococcus* species. In using netilmicin, peak serum concentrations in excess of 16 mg/L (16 µg/mL) and trough levels below 4 mg/L (4 µg/mL) should be avoided. The dosage interval in hours can be calculated by multiplying the serum creatinine (mg/100 mL) by eight.

Table 14.2 on the next page lists the clinically significant drug interactions with the aminoglycosides.

Adverse Effects

Aminoglycosides accumulate in the perilymph of the inner ear, destroying both the vestibular and cochlear sensory cells. The degree of permanent damage correlates with the number of destroyed sensory hair cells in the inner ear; this in turn relates to concentration of drug and length of exposure. Patients experience tinnitus and hearing loss (usually to high-frequency tones), dizziness and

Table 14.2
The aminoglycosides: Drug interactions

Drug	Interaction
Anticoagulants, oral	• Orally administered neomycin or kanamycin may potentiate the action of coumarin anti-coagulants by reducing bacterial vitamin K production in the large intestine and/or by decreasing vitamin K absorption
Cephalothin	• An increase in nephrotoxicity has been observed in pts receiving an aminoglycoside plus cephalothin
Dimenhydrinate	• Although clinical examples are lacking, there is a possibility that the symptoms of aminoglycoside ototoxicity can be masked by dimenhydrinate
Diuretics	• Diuretics, such as ethacrynic acid and furosemide, have been associated with dysfunction of the 8th cranial nerve. Concomitant use of a potent diuretic with an aminoglycoside should be avoided. It is believed that IV diuretics may cause a rapid rise in aminoglycoside serum levels and potentiate nephrotoxicity
Muscle relaxants	• The neuromuscular blockade produced by muscle relaxants, such as succinylcholine or tubocurarine, can be potentiated by the aminoglycosides and cause respiratory paralysis. These agents should be given concomitantly only with extreme caution
Nephrotoxic drugs	• Additive or synergistic nephrotoxicity may occur when aminoglycosides are administered with certain other nephrotoxic agents. This has been documented for methoxyflurane, and aminoglycosides should not be given to pts who recently received this anesthetic unless absolutely necessary. Administration of aminoglycosides with amphotericin B, vancomycin, cisplatin, cyclosporine, or IV indomethacin also can result in increased nephrotoxicity. When nurses administer one of these combinations, they must closely monitor renal function

vertigo. Kanamycin and amikacin impair auditory functions preferentially, and gentamicin is more likely to damage vestibular function. Tobramycin causes auditory and vestibular damage with equal frequency. The diuretics ethacrynic acid (Edecrin®) and furosemide (Lasix®) potentiate aminoglycoside ototoxicity. Termination of drug treatment results in complete recovery, if hearing or balance loss, or both, are not extensive. However, if extensive damage has occurred, impairment may be permanent.

High concentrations of aminoglycosides accumulate in the renal cortex and urine. Five to seven days of therapy can cause dose-dependent damage to the proximal tubular epithelium, particularly in elderly or debilitated patients or in individuals with pre-existing renal impairment. Serum creatinine and blood urea nitrogen (BUN) increase, and severe azotemia may occur. Tobramycin and netilmicin are claimed to be less nephrotoxic than the other aminoglycosides. Concomitant therapy with furosemide, ethacrynic acid, cephalosporins or methoxyflurane (Penthrane®) increases the risk of nephrotoxicity.

Aminoglycosides can, rarely, reduce the release of acetylcholine from motor nerve terminals and cause a neuromuscular blockade, leading to flaccid paralysis and respiratory failure. The risk is greatest in patients receiving an anesthetic or a neuromuscular blocker, or those suffering from myasthenia gravis or hypokalemia. It is speculated that aminoglycosides attach to calcium binding sites on the nerves and prevent calcium from participating in the release of acetylcholine. The neuromuscular blockade is treated by administering calcium gluconate, together with an anticholinesterase drug, such as neostigmine.

Allergic reactions characterized by pruritus, rash, urticaria, and (on very rare occasions) exfoliative dermatitis have occasionally been seen following aminoglycoside administration. Drug fever, hypotension and anaphylactic shock have also been reported.

Nursing Management

The nursing management of the patient receiving any of the aminoglycosides is essentially the same (Table 14.3). Unique features related to each drug are included in Table 14.4.

Table 14.3
Nursing management for the aminoglycosides

Assessment of risk vs. benefit	Patient data	• Physician should determine any contraindications, such as allergy, and precautions, such as myasthenia gravis or renal impairment • Establish baseline VS, general state of health, indicators of present infection • Assess hearing function (audiogram may be ordered) • *Age:* E.g., elderly patient with reduced renal function may experience toxicity • *Pregnancy and lactation:* Recommended to avoid drug; may cause permanent hearing damage in fetus or infant
	Drug data	• *Site and type of infection:* Select drugs based on location of infection and causative microorganism • Culture and sensitivity results • *Many drug reactions:* Confer with pharmacist • Side effects are not common, but drug may cause superinfection and such serious reactions as ototoxicity, nephrotoxicity
Implementation	Rights of administration	• Applying the "rights" helps prevent errors of administration
	Right route	• These drugs are not given orally, except kanamycin for pre-op bowel preparation • IM route and IV infusion by small volume or direct push (depending on agency policy)
	Right time	• As with all antibiotics, give ATC to ensure effective blood levels. As shown in Table 14.4, dosage interval may be as short as q6h or as long as once daily
	Right technique	• Administer IM slowly, deep into large muscle mass; rotate sites • IV administration requires knowledge of correct diluent and IV solution, correct dilution and rate of administration. Always refer to manufacturer's instructions for this route • Administer drug in small volume by infusion over 30 min to 2 h. Flush line following infusion
	Nursing therapeutics	• Enhance host defences (nutrition, rest, fluids, hygiene) • Promote preventive measures (particularly hygiene) to minimize superinfections (oral, vaginal) • Administer drug ATC to ensure effective blood levels • Ensure that pt remains well hydrated (1500–2000 mL/day), unless fluid restriction is necessary
	Patient/family teaching	• Educate for proper use of anti-infectives, as summarized in Chapter 9. This information would apply mainly to use of topical aminoglycosides; other routes are rarely self-administered, as the pt is likely to be in hospital or on a supervised home IV program • Remind pt to notify physician if symptoms do not improve • Review signs/symptoms of adverse reactions and advise to report to physician immediately. Specifically, discuss ototoxicity: damage to 8th cranial nerve may be indicated by tinnitus (roaring, ringing, buzzing sound in either ear), or hearing loss; damage to vestibular

(cont'd on next page)

Table 14.3
Nursing management for the aminoglycosides

Implementation (cont'd)	Patient/family teaching (cont'd)	
		or cochlear sensory cells may be indicated by vertigo, dizziness, nausea or vomiting • Discuss possibility of pregnancy; advise pt to notify physician. Explain risks of lactation while on these drugs
Outcomes	Monitoring of progress	*Continually monitor:* • Clinical response indicating tx success (reduction in signs/symptoms) • For adverse effects. Respond immediately to superinfection, ototoxicity or nephrotoxicity (indicated by oliguria, proteinuria, elevated BUN and serum creatinine) • *Allergy:* Although not common, can occur at any time. Be alert for signs/symptoms; document and report to physician • Ensure that peak and trough serum levels are accurately drawn on time. Trough levels should be drawn immediately before the next dose. Peak levels vary with the drug and the route but are generally 15–30 min after IV infusion and 30–60 min after IM injection

Response to Clinical Challenge

Principles
This case study illustrates the importance of therapeutic drug monitoring (or TDM; see Chapter 5, pages 39–40; Chapter 6, pages 46–47). An understanding of pharmacokinetics and dose-response principles provides a foundation for monitoring drug therapy.

Actions
1. Peak level for IV route occurs shortly after the end of the infusion. This patient has a serious life-threatening infection, and the level is barely therapeutic. The physician will probably increase the dose
2. Inquire re: any nausea, tinnitus, or difficulty in hearing
3. Trough level indicates the lowest level in the body and can determine whether dosage interval is too short (i.e., drug is not being excreted)
4. Trough level should be drawn immediately before next dose, if possible
5. The resulting level is too high; the physician will probably reduce the dose slightly or increase the dosing interval. However, this will depend on the signs/symptoms presented by the patient, and the severity of the infection. Your observations and documentation are an essential part of this clinical situation

Further Reading

Aminoglycosides. *AMA Drug Evaluations Subscriptions* 1993:6.1–6.22.

Chambers HF, Sande MA. Antimicrobial agents: the aminoglycosides. In: Hardman JL, Limbird LE, *Goodman and Gilman's The Pharmacological Basis of Therapeutics.* 9th ed. New York: Pergamon; 1996.

The choice of antibacterial drugs. *Medical Letter on Drugs and Therapeutics* 1994;36:919–925.

Handbook of antimicrobial therapy. *Medical Letter on Drugs and Therapeutics* 1992.

Table 14.4
The aminoglycosides: Drug doses

Drug Generic name (Trade names)	Dosage	Nursing alert
gentamicin sulfate (Alcomicin, Cidomycin, Garamycin)	**IM:** For pts with normal renal function: *Adults:* For UTI, 160 mg/day or 80 mg bid for 7–10 days. For systemic infections, 3 mg/kg/day in 3 equal doses q8h for 7–10 days. For life-threatening infections, up to 5 mg/kg/day in 3–4 equal doses; reduce to 3 mg/kg/day as soon as clinically indicated. *Children:* For severe infections, 3–6 mg/kg/day in 3 equal doses q8h. If a dosage > 3 mg/kg/day is given initially, it should be reduced to 3 mg/kg/day when clinically indicated. *Premature and full-term neonates < 1 week of age,* 6 mg/kg/day in 2 equal doses q12h. *Infants > 1 week of age,* give in 3 equal doses q8h *For pts with impaired renal function:* Serum half-life can be estimated by multiplying serum creatinine level (in mg/100 mL) by 4. Frequency of administration (in h) may be approximated by doubling serum half-life **Topical:** Apply cream or ointment containing 1 mg gentamicin/g to lesion tid–qid **Ocular:** Instill 2 drops of solution containing gentamicin sulfate 5 mg/mL, or ophthalmic ointment containing gentamicin sulfate 5 mg/g, into affected eye tid–qid. Incr. dosage prn in severe infections	• Administer IM deep into large muscle mass. Rotate sites • Flush line after IV infusion • Peak levels 12 µg/mL (25.9 µmol/L) and trough levels 2 µg/mL (4.3 µmol/L) are associated with toxicity
amikacin sulfate (Amikin)	**IM:** *Adults/children/neonates,* 15 mg/kg/day, given as 7.5 mg/kg q12h. **IV:** Same dose may be given over 30–60 min *For pts with impaired renal function:* Interval between doses can be calculated by multiplying serum creatinine (in mg/100 mL) by 9 to give dosage intervals (in h). This formula should not be used to calculate dosage for elderly pts	• Administer IM deep into large muscle mass. Rotate sites • Flush line after IV infusion • Peak levels 35 µg/mL (59.5 µmol/L) and trough levels 10 µg/mL (17 µmol/L) are associated with toxicity
kanamycin sulfate (Kantrex, Klebcil)	**IM/IV:** Rarely used because of bacterial resistance. For dosage, consult product monograph **Oral:** As adjunct in extended tx of hepatic coma: *Adults,* 8–12 g/day in divided doses. As adjunct in short-term mechanical cleansings of large bowel, 1 g q1h for 4 h, followed by 1 g q6h for 36–72 h.	• Except for allergy, usually well tolerated • May be taken without regard to food

(cont'd on next page)

Table 14.4 (continued)
The aminoglycosides: Drug doses

Drug Generic name (Trade names)	Dosage	Nursing alert
netilmicin sulfate (Netromycin)	**IM/IV:** For pts with normal renal function: *Adults:* For uncomplicated UTI, 4 mg/kg/day in 2 equal doses, given q12h for 7–10 days. For systemic infections, 4–6 mg/kg/day in 2–3 equal doses q8–12h. For serious/life-threatening systemic infections, up to 7.5 mg/kg/day IV in 3 equal doses; reduce to 6 mg/kg/day as soon as indicated clinically, usually within 48 h. *Children:* 6–7.5 mg/kg/day given in 3 equal doses q8h; reduce to 6 mg/kg/day as soon as indicated clinically. *Infants/neonates > 1 week of age:* 7.5–9 mg/kg/day, given in 3 equal doses q8h. *Premature and full-term neonates < 1 week old:* 6 mg/kg/day, given in 2 equal doses q12h *For pts with impaired renal function:* Initial dose is same as that recomm. for pts with normal renal function. If serum concentrations cannot be monitored, interval between the usual single dose given at 8-h intervals can be calculated by multiplying the pt's serum creatinine level (in mg/100 mL) by 8	• Solution should be clear or pale yellow • Peak concentrations > 16 µg/mL for prolonged periods, as well as trough concentrations > 4 µg/mL, are associated with toxicity and should be avoided
tobramycin sulfate (Nebcin)	**IM/IV:** For pts with normal renal function: *Adults:* For mild to moderate infection of lower UT, 2–3 mg/kg/day od. When renal tissue is involved or in serious infections, esp. when there are signs of systemic involvement, 2–3 equally divided doses are recomm. For life-threatening infections, up to 5 mg/kg/day in 3–4 equal doses; reduce to 3 mg/kg/day as soon as indicated clinically. *Children:* 6–7.5 mg/kg/day in 3–4 equally divided doses. *Neonates ≤ 1 week old:* Up to 4 mg/kg/day in 2 equal doses q12h. *For pts with impaired renal function:* **IM:** After loading dose of 1 mg/kg, subsequent dosage must be adjusted, either with lower doses given at 8-h intervals or with normal doses at prolonged intervals. In latter situation, interval (in h) can be determined by multiplying pt's serum creatinine level by 6 **Ocular:** Instill solution containing tobramycin sulfate 5 mg/mL, as described for gentamicin sulfate	• Prolonged serum concentrations > 12 µg/mL (12 mg/L) should be avoided. Rising trough levels above 2 µg/mL (2 mg/L) may indicate tissue accumulation. Such accumulation, excessive peak concentrations, advanced age, and cumulative dose may contribute to ototoxicity and nephrotoxicity

The Sulfonamides, Trimethoprim and Trimethoprim Plus Sulfamethoxazole

Topics Discussed
- Mechanism of action
- Antibacterial spectrum
- Resistance
- Pharmacokinetics
- Therapeutic uses
- Adverse effects
- Nursing management
- Trimethoprim and trimethoprim plus sulfamethoxazole/cotrimoxazole

Drugs Discussed
sulfisoxazole (sul-fih-**sox**-ah-zole)

sulfadiazine (sul-fah-**dye**-ah-zeen)

sulfamethoxazole (sul-fah-meth-**ox**-ah-zole)

sulfacetamide (sul-fah-**see**-tah-myde)

phenazopyridine (fen-az-oh-**peer**-ih-deen)

trimethoprim (try-**meth**-oh-prim)

Clinical Challenge
Consider this clinical challenge as you read through this chapter. The response to the challenge appears on page 140.

Jack is a businessman with a history of recurring urinary tract infection (UTI). In the past, he has successfully treated such infections with a 10-day course of Azo-Gantrisin® (phenazopyridine HCl and sulfisoxazole). In this instance, Jack has been taking the drug for 5 days. He is about to embark on a business trip to Hawaii and expresses his concerns regarding continuing the medication. How will he maintain a high fluid intake on the plane? Can he discontinue the drug before his flight and resume taking it if his symptoms return?

What information do you need before you contact the physician? What actions do you expect from the doctor?

When introduced in the 1930s, the sulfonamides provided a major breakthrough in the chemotherapy of infectious disease. Unfortunately, the development of bacterial resistance has reduced the number of sulfonamides on the market to a few. These include sulfisoxazole (Gantrisin®), sulfamethoxazole (Gantanol®) and sulfadiazine. Two topical sulfonamides, mafenide acetate and silver sulfadiazine, are valuable in the treatment of burn patients. Sodium sulfacetamide is a very popular drug for ocular infections.

Mechanism of Action

Bacterial cells and mammalian cells alike require the essential vitamin folic acid. While humans absorb folic acid from their diet, bacteria cannot absorb the vitamin and must therefore synthesize it. One essential component of folic acid is para-aminobenzoic acid (PABA). Sulfonamides are structurally similar to PABA. By acting as competitive antimetabolites of PABA, sulfonamides block its incorporation into folic acid, thereby preventing folic acid synthesis and inducing bacteriostasis (Figure 15.1, page 139).This explains why sulfonamides do not reduce folic acid levels in the human host and accounts for the selective toxicity of sulfonamides in bacteria.

Antibacterial Spectrum

When first introduced, sulfonamides were effective against a wide range of gram-positive and gram-negative microorganisms, as well as *Chlamydia*. Bacteria originally sensitive included group A streptococci, pneumococci, gonococci, meningococci, *Haemophilus influenzae*, *Haemophilus ducreyi*, *Escherichia coli*, *Brucellae*, *Pasteurella pestis*, *Bacillus anthracis*, *Corynebacterium diphtheriae*, *Cholera vibrio* and *Shigellae*. However, many of these bacteria are now resistant to sulfonamides. This is particularly true for many staphylococci, enterococci, *Clostridia* and *Pseudomonas*.

Resistance

Increasing bacterial resistance has severely limited the clinical usefulness of the sulfonamides. Resistance can be chromosomally mediated or transferred by R-factor plasmids (see Chapter 9). R-factor plasmid resistance is frequently seen with Enterobacteriaceae. The mechanisms of resistance include (1) overproduction of PABA, (2) a decreased affinity of dihydropteroate synthetase (the enzyme responsible for the synthesis of folic acid) to the sulfonamide, (3) decreased permeability of the bacterium to the drug and (4) increased inactivation of the drug.

Pharmacokinetics

The sulfonamides discussed in this chapter are well absorbed from the gastrointestinal (GI) tract. They cross cell membranes freely and distribute to the brain, lung, liver, pancreas, muscle and nervous tissue. The concentrations of sulfonamides in the fetus are approximately equal to those in the mother.

Sulfonamides bind, in varying degrees, to plasma proteins. Given to a patient during the later stages of pregnancy, a sulfonamide will cross the placenta, enter the fetus and displace bilirubin from plasma albumin. In the absence of a developed blood-brain barrier, the newly freed bilirubin can enter the fetal brain to produce kernicterus. Therefore, the use of sulfonamides in pregnant women near term or in nursing mothers is inadvisable. In addition, sulfonamides should not be given to infants younger than two months old.

Some sulfonamides are extensively metabolized; others are mainly excreted unchanged by the kidneys. Only 20% of sulfisoxazole is metabolized prior to excretion. Sulfadiazine and sulfamethoxazole are 60% to 85% metabolized, respectively.

The pharmacokinetic characteristics of some commonly used sulfonamides are summarized in Table 15.1.

Therapeutic Uses

Although the value of sulfonamides has been reduced greatly by the development of bacterial resistance, these drugs have remained effective for the treatment of acute uncomplicated urinary tract infection (UTI) caused by sulfonamide-sensitive *Escherichia coli*. Sulfisoxazole (Gantrisin®) is a particularly appropriate sulfonamide because 80% of the drug is excreted unchanged in the urine. Sulfamethoxazole (Gantanol®) is less suitable because only 15% percent of a dose of this drug is excreted in an unmetabolized active form.

The combination of phenazopyridine HCl (Pyridium®) and sulfisoxazole is popular for the treatment of UTI. The two drugs can be taken as separate tablets or as the combination product Azo-Gantrisin®. Phenazopyridine is a local analgesic on the inflamed mucosa of the urinary tract. Its use reduces discomfort during the first three or four days of treatment, before sulfisoxazole has had sufficient opportunity to work. Thereafter, as bacterial counts fall, phenazopyridine is not required and treatment may be continued with sulfisoxazole alone.

Table 15.1
Characteristics of some commonly used sulfonamides

Drug	Pharmacokinetic properties	Therapeutic uses
Sulfadiazine Sulfamerazine Sulfamethazine	All are rapidly absorbed and rapidly eliminated	• Often the 3 are combined and used in products that also contain penicillin G for tx of sensitive systemic infections
Sulfisoxazole (Gantrisin®)	Rapidly absorbed; high concentration of active drug in urine	• Often used in tx of acute urinary tract infections (UTI)
Sulfamethoxazole (Gantanol®)	Rapidly absorbed; only 15% of dose found in urine unchanged	• Often combined with trimethoprim to form cotrimoxazole
Sulfamylon (Mafenide®) Silver sulfadiazine (Flamazine®)	Topical use only; can be absorbed from burned skin	• Used in tx of burn pts
Sulfacetamide sodium (Sodium Sulamyd®)	Penetrates ocular fluids and tissues in high concentrations	• Tx of conjunctivitis and corneal ulcers

Sulfadiazine may be a drug of choice in nocardiosis. It is recommended for the prophylaxis of rheumatic fever in penicillin-allergic patients. Sulfisoxazole probably is effective, but data comparing sulfadiazine and sulfisoxazole are not available.

Sulfonamides should not be used in the treatment of established streptococcal pharyngitis because they fail to eradicate the causative organism, and late sequelae (e.g., rheumatic fever, glomerulonephritis) may develop.

The use of sulfisoxazole plus erythromycin (Pediazole®) is recommended for *Haemophilus*-induced otitis media in young children.

Sulfonamides are contraindicated in patients with a history of hematologic, renal or hepatic dysfunction, allergic drug fever or skin eruptions due to sulfonamide derivatives, including antibacterial sulfonamides, oral hypoglycemics and thiazides. In addition, as mentioned earlier in this chapter, sulfonamides should not be given to premature and newborn infants, or pregnant women near parturition because of the possible occurrence of kernicterus. Other contraindications to the use of sulfonamides include uremia and a deficiency of erythrocytic glucose-6-phosphate dehydrogenase (G-6-PD). Patients with porphyria should not receive sulfonamides, because these drugs have been reported to precipitate an acute attack.

Adverse Effects

Nausea, anorexia and vomiting are seen in 5% to 10% of patients taking sulfonamides. Hypersensitivity reactions, beginning 10 to 12 days after starting therapy or within hours in a previously sensitized patient, can cause generalized skin rashes, urticaria, photodermatitis or drug fever. Patients allergic to one sulfonamide should be considered allergic to all sulfonamides.

Blood dyscrasias are rare but they can be fatal. Acute or chronic hemolytic anemia, developing within 2 to 7 days of starting therapy, or agranulocytosis, appearing between the second and sixth week of treatment in approximately 0.1% of patients, represent hypersensitivity reactions. All patients should know the symptoms of agranulocytosis and should contact their physicians immediately if they occur.

Table 15.2 on the next page lists the clinically significant drug interactions with sulfonamides.

Nursing Management

The nursing management of the patient receiving any of the sulfonamides is essentially the same (Table 15.3, pages 136–137). Unique features related to each drug are included in Table 15.4 (pages 141–142).

Table 15.2
Sulfonamides: Drug interactions

Drug	Interaction
Anesthetics; local esters	• Local anesthetic esters antagonize the antibacterial activity of sulfonamides because they are metabolized to para-aminobenzoic acid
Anticoagulants, oral	• Sulfonamides may displace oral anticoagulants from plasma proteins, thereby increasing their activity
Cyclosporine	• Sulfamethazine and sulfadiazine can decrease the effect of cyclosporine (possibly increased cyclosporine metabolism). Monitor cyclosporine concentration
Digoxin	• Sulfasalazine can possibly decrease digoxin absorption and reduce its effect. Monitor digoxin concentration
Drugs that displace sulfonamides from plasma proteins	• Sulfonamides may be displaced from plasma protein binding sites by other drugs (e.g., phenylbutazone, salicylates, probenecid), resulting in increased sulfonamide activity
Diuretics	• Diuretics, particularly thiazides, may increase the incidence of thrombocytopenia with purpura in elderly pts receiving a sulfonamide
Hypoglycemics, oral	• Sulfonamides increase the hypoglycemic effect of oral hypoglycemics. Monitor blood glucose; reaction is infrequent, but can be severe
Methotrexate	• The activity of methotrexate may be increased by a sulfonamide
Para-aminobenzoic acid (PABA)	• PABA antagonizes the antibacterial effects of sulfonamides
Phenytoin	• With the possible exception of sulfisoxazole, sulfonamides may decrease the metabolism and increase the toxicity of phenytoin. Monitor phenytoin concentration
Thiopental	• Sulfonamides have been reported to enhance the action of thiopental

---

Table 15.3
Nursing management for the sulfonamides

Assessment of risk vs. benefit	Patient data	• *History:* Physician should determine any contraindications such as allergy and precautions such as hepatic or renal impairment • Pts with allergies or asthma are at greater risk for developing hypersensitivity to these drugs • Assess to establish baseline VS, general state of health, indicators of present infection • *Pregnancy and lactation:* Avoid use of drug, which may cause kernicterus in fetus or infant
	Drug data	• *Site and type of infection:* Select drugs based on location of infection and causative microorganism • Culture and sensitivity results • Many drug reactions: confer with pharmacist • Side effects are usually mild; most common are nausea, anorexia and vomiting. Hypersensitivity and blood dyscrasias are possible

Table 15.3 (continued)
Nursing management for the sulfonamides

Implementation	Rights of administration	• Applying the "rights" helps prevent errors of administration
	Right route	• Usually, these drugs are given orally, except Bactrim®, which may be given IV if necessary
	Right time	• As with all antibiotics, give ATC to ensure effective blood levels. Dosage interval varies among drugs and depending on indication for use
	Right technique	• IV administration requires knowledge of correct diluent and IV solution, correct dilution and rate of administration. Always refer to manufacturer's instructions for this route. Drug should be administered in small volume by infusion over 60–90 min
	Nursing therapeutics	• Enhance host defences (nutrition, rest, fluids, hygiene) • Promote preventive measures (particularly hygiene) to minimize superinfections (oral, vaginal) • Administer drugs ATC to ensure effective blood levels • Ensure that pt remains well hydrated (1500–2000 mL/day), unless fluid restriction is necessary
	Patient/family teaching	• Educate for proper use of anti-infectives (see Chapter 9) • Advise pt to report to physician immediately if symptoms do not improve. Review signs/symptoms of adverse reactions and advise pt to report to physician immediately if these appear • Discuss photosensitivity; advise use of sunscreen and protective clothing • Discuss possibility of pregnancy: advise pt to notify physician. Explain risks of lactation while on these drugs
Outcomes	Monitoring of progress	*Continually monitor:* • Clinical response indicating tx success (reduction in signs/symptoms) • Note that allergy, although uncommon, can occur at any time. Be alert for signs/symptoms; document and report to physician • Respond immediately to adverse effects such as blood dyscrasias (high fever, sore throat, unusual bleeding or bruising, fatigue, jaundice; periodic blood counts may be ordered); Stevens-Johnson syndrome (fever, headache, erythematous rash, rhinitis, conjunctivitis, stomatitis). Also, sulfisoxazole can cause crystalluria and stones

Trimethoprim and Trimethoprim Plus Sulfamethoxazole (Cotrimoxazole)

Trimethoprim was combined with sulfamethoxazole in the 1960s. In Canada, as in many other countries, the combination product bears the generic name of cotrimoxazole. In other countries, such as the United States, it is referred to as trimethoprim plus sulfamethoxazole (abbreviated, in this text, TMP/SMZ). The addition of trimethoprim to sulfamethoxazole restored a credibility to the sulfonamides that had been lost after bacterial resistance to these drugs started to appear in the 1950s. Today, TMP/SMZ (cotrimoxazole) is used to treat a variety of systemic infections, many of which were handled effectively by the sulfonamides alone in their early days.

Mechanism of Action

Before folic acid can function as a vitamin it must be converted first to dihydrofolic acid, then to tetrahydrofolic acid. Trimethoprim competitively inhibits bacterial dihydrofolate reductase, the enzyme responsible for the conversion of dihydrofolic acid to tetrahydrofolic acid. In therapeutic doses it has no significant effect on the human form of the enzyme.

The TMP/SMZ (cotrimoxazole) combination contains a 1:5 ratio of trimethoprim to sulfamethoxazole. It is an effective combination, in which sulfamethoxazole reduces folic acid synthesis and trimethoprim inhibits folic acid activation (Figure 15.1).

Antibacterial Spectrum

TMP/SMZ has a broad spectrum of activity. All strains of *Staphylococcus aureus, Streptococcus pneumoniae, Streptococcus epidermidis, Streptococcus pyogenes,* viridans streptococci, *Streptococcus faecalis, Escherichia coli, Proteus mirabilis, Proteus morganii, Proteus rettgeri, Enterobacter* species, *Pseudomonas pseudomallei* and *Serratia* species are inhibited by TMP/SMZ. Although many strains of *Shigella* and *Salmonella* remain sensitive to TMP/SMZ, others have developed resistance to the antibacterial.

Resistance

Resistance can develop to trimethoprim. This may be either plasmid- or chromosome-mediated. Clinically, the most important type of acquired resistance to trimethoprim results from the production of novel trimethoprim-resistant dihydrofolate reductases. These dihydrofolate reductase enzymes are encoded on transferable plasmids or transposons and confer on the bacteria a high-level resistance to trimethoprim.

The chromosomal resistance mechanism includes (1) qualitative alteration in bacterial dihydrofolate reductase, resulting in decreased affinity for trimethoprim, (2) overproduction of the bacterial dihydrofolate reductase enzyme and (3) decreased bacterial cell wall permeability to the drug. These mechanisms usually confer a low-level resistance to trimethoprim.

Emergence of resistance to trimethoprim or cotrimoxazole varies among countries, cities and hospitals. Trimethoprim resistance, particularly high-level plasmid-mediated resistance, has been gradually increasing in the industrialized world. Three to twenty percent of *E. coli* are now resistant to trimethoprim in industrialized countries; the incidence of resistance is much higher, and can be said to be widespread, in developing nations.

Pharmacokinetics of TMP/SMZ

Both sulfamethoxazole and trimethoprim are well absorbed from the gastrointestinal tract and distribute rapidly throughout the body, including the cerebrospinal fluid. High concentrations of both drugs are found in bile. The half-life of both drugs is approximately ten hours. Although most of the trimethoprim is eliminated unchanged in the urine, approximately eighty-five percent of sulfamethoxazole is inactivated prior to renal excretion.

Therapeutic Uses of TMP/SMZ

TMP/SMZ (Bactrim®, Septra®) is used to treat a variety of systemic infections caused by gram-positive and gram-negative organisms, including infections of the upper and lower respiratory tract, urinary tract (acute, recurrent and chronic), genital tract, gastrointestinal tract, and skin and soft tissues, *Pneumocystis carinii* infections, and serious systemic infections, such as meningitis and septicemia caused by susceptible organisms.

Figure 15.1
Mechanism of action of sulfonamides and trimethoprim

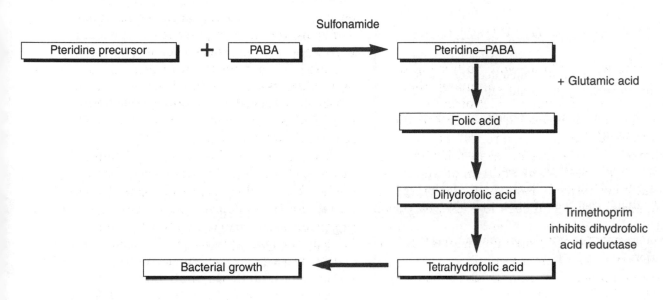

Source: Adapted from Johnson GE, *PDQ Pharmacology.* Hamilton, ON: B.C. Decker; 1988.

Some of its more common uses include acute exacerbations of chronic bronchitis caused by *Haemophilus influenzae* and *Streptococcus pneumoniae* and the treatment of acute otitis media in children and acute maxillary sinusitis in adults. Acute gonococcal urethritis can also be managed with TMP/SMZ. Gastrointestinal infections caused by *Shigellae,* including ampicillin-resistant strains, can be treated with TMP/SMZ. The combination is also effective for the treatment of typhoid fever and can be used in the management of carriers of *Salmonella typhi.* It is a treatment of choice for acute and chronic prostatitis. Trimethoprim is one of the few antibacterial agents that adequately penetrates into the uninflamed prostate.

Trimethoprim (Proloprim®, Trimpex®) is used in treating acute urinary tract infections due to susceptible strains of *E. coli* and *K. pneumoniae.* Limited clinical experience suggests the probability of therapeutic response in infections due to susceptible strains of P. mirabilis and Enterobacter. The administration of trimethoprim alone is rational, given the fact that eighty-five percent of sulfamethoxazole is inactivated before it reaches the bladder. As would be expected, trimethoprim is as effective as TMP/SMZ for the treatment of acute urinary tract infections, but has a reduced incidence of adverse effects.

Adverse Effects of TMP/SMZ

The toxicities of sulfonamides have already been described. Trimethoprim has relatively few adverse effects. They include gastric distress (nausea and vomiting), rash, itching, and very rarely leukopenia, thrombocytopenia and methemoglobinemia.

The use of high-dose TMP/SMZ to treat *Pneumocystis carinii* pneumonia (PCP) in HIV-infected patients can significantly increase serum potassium concentrations. Because this can lead to life-threatening hyperkalemia, HIV patients should have their electrolyte levels closely monitored, particularly during days 7 to 10 of treatment.

Response to Clinical Challenge

Principles

Review the concepts related to drug compliance in Chapters 1 and 3. Jack should be provided sufficient information to make an informed decision. Before calling the physician you should ask:

• Which symptoms have improved (e.g., urinary frequency? burning?)
• How long is the plane flight? Can Jack organize his dosage schedule around this time?
• In previous episodes of UTI, how long did he take the medication? Was the infection cured?

When you contact the physician, you can report this information.

Actions

The physician may consider a stat urine for C&S; if it is sterile, Jack can discontinue the medication. The physician may consider changing the prescription to another medication that does not require similar attention to fluid intake.

To meet Jack's current needs, the physician may also suggest that Jack skip one dose just before flight time and resume taking the drug when he arrives at his destination. Though not ideal, this may be the best compromise.

If Jack continues the drug, remind him about photosensitivity: advise him to use a sunscreen and wear protective clothing (though he likely won't appreciate this in Hawaii!).

Further Reading

The choice of antibacterial drugs. *Medical Letter on Drugs and Therapeutics* 1994;36:919–925.

Greenberg S, et al. Trimethoprim-sulfamethoxazole induces reversible hyperkalemia. *Ann Int Med* 1993;119(August 15):291–295.

Gregor J, et al. Acute psychosis associated with oral trimethoprim-sulfamethoxazole therapy. *Can J Psychiatry* 1993;38(2):56–58.

Handbook of antimicrobial therapy. *Medical Letter on Drugs and Therapeutics* 1992.

Leiner S. Recurrent urinary tract infections in otherwise healthy adult women. *Nurse Practitioner* 1995;20(2):48, 51–52, 54–56.

Mandel GL, Petri WA. Antimicrobial agents: sulfonamides, trimethoprim-sulfaxethoxazole, quinolone, and agents for urinary tract infections. In: Hardman JL, Limbird LE, eds. *Goodman and Gilman's The Pharmacological Basis of Therapeutics.* 9th ed. New York: Pergamon; 1996:1057–1072.

Sulfonamides and trimethoprim. In: *AMA Drug Evaluation Subscriptions* 1993:7.1–7.20.

Table 15.4
The sulfonamides, trimethoprim and trimethoprim plus sulfamethoxazole: Drug doses

Drug Generic Name (Trade Names)	Dosage	Nursing Alert
sulfadiazine	**Oral:** *Adults:* Initially, 2–4 g; then 1 g q4–6h. *Children and infants > 2 months old:* Initially, 75 mg/kg, then 150 mg/kg/day in 4–6 divided doses. Should not exceed 6 g/day. Duration of tx for nocardiosis is 4–6 months or more. For prophylaxis of rheumatic fever, *pts < 27 kg:* 500 mg/day; *pts > 27 kg:* 1 g/day. For prophylaxis of meningococcal disease (only if *N. meningitidis* isolate is known to be susceptible): *Adults:* 1 g bid for 2 days. *Children 1–12 years:* 500 mg bid for 2 days. *Infants 2 months to 1 year:* 500 mg od for 2 days	• Take with full glass of water on empty stomach
sulfisoxazole	**Oral:** *Adults:* 2–4 g stat; then 4–8 g/24 h in 4–6 divided doses. *Children > 2 months old:* 75 mg/kg stat; then 150 mg/kg/day in divided doses q4–6h, max. 6 g/day	• Administer at evenly spaced intervals ATC with full glass of water • Tablets may be crushed if difficult to swallow • Maintain fluid balance of 1500 mL output (may require 3–4 L daily intake)
sulfamethoxazole (Gantanol)	**Oral:** *Adults:* 2 g stat; then 1 g q12h. For severe infection, 1 g tid. *Children > 2 months old:* 50–60 mg/kg stat; then 50% of this amount q12h (max., 75 mg/kg/24 h)	• Take with full glass of water (tablets and oral suspension)
trimethoprim (Proloprim, Trimpex)	**Oral:** *Adults/children > 12 years:* 100 mg q12h for 10 days	• Stress that full course of tx must be completed
trimethoprim + sulfamethoxazole; cotrimoxazole; TMP/SMZ (Bactrim, Septra)	**Oral:** *Adults/children > 12 years:* 2 adult tabs or 1 DS tab bid. For severe infections: Increase dosage to 3 adult or 1.5 DS tabs bid. *Children < 12 years:* 3 mg trimethoprim/kg + 15 mg sulfamethoxazole/kg bid for at least 5 days. For prophylaxis and for *Salmonella* carriers: 1 adult tab or 0.5 DS tab bid. For acute salmonellosis: Tx should be continued for at least 7 days after defervescence. Carriers should continue tx until repeated stool cultures are negative. For uncomplicated gonorrhea *(adults/children):* 2 adult or 1 DS tab qid for 2 days. For *Pneumocystis carinii* pneumonitis *(adults/children):* 5 mg trimethoprim/kg + 25 mg sulfamethoxazole/kg qid for at least 14 days	• Do not confuse adult tablets with DS tablets: dose differs • IV route used only when necessary; generally does not cause irritation

Table 15.4 (continued)
The sulfonamides, trimethoprim and trimethoprim plus sulfamethoxazole: Drug doses

Drug Generic name (Trade names)	Dosage	Nursing alert
trimethoprim + sulfamethoxazole; cotrimoxazole; TMP/SMZ (Bactrim, Septra) (cont'd)	**IV:** *Adults/children over 2 months with normal renal function:* For severe UTI and shigellosis, 8–10 mg/kg daily (based on the trimethoprim component) in 2–4 equally divided doses at intervals of 6, 8, or 12 h for up to 14 days for severe UTI or 5 days for shigellosis For *P. carinii pneumonia:* 15 to 20 mg/kg daily (based on the trimethoprim component) in 3 or 4 equally divided doses at 6- or 8-h intervals for up to 14 days. A longer course of tx, usually 21 days, is required in AIDS pts. Monitoring serum trimethoprim concentrations to maintain levels of 5–8 µg/mL may decrease the incidence of serious adverse reactions in AIDS pts and allow successful completion of tx IV preparation is contraindicated in infants < 2 months	

The Fluoroquinolones

Topics Discussed
- Mechanism of action
- Pharmacokinetics
- Antibacterial spectrum
- Resistance
- Therapeutic uses
- Adverse effects
- Nursing management

Drugs Discussed
ciprofloxacin (sip-roe-**flox**-ah-sin)
enoxacin (ee-**nox**-ah-sin)
lomefloxacin (loe-mee-**flox**-ah-sin)
nalidixic acid (nal-ih-**dik**-sik)
norfloxacin (nor-**flox**-ah-sin)
ofloxacin (oh-**flox**-ah-sin)

Clinical Challenge
Consider this clinical challenge as you read through this chapter. The response to the challenge appears on page 149.

Mrs. S. is a 73-year-old woman who fell and broke her hip. Following surgery, she developed severe osteomyelitis evidenced by swollen hip and thigh, difficulty with any motion or weightbearing, pain and fever.

Surgical drainage of the infection has been completed. She has returned home and will receive wound care and Cipro IV® through the hospital's home care program. She and her family have been taught care of the central line, and an RN visits twice daily to administer medications and monitor Mrs. S.'s condition.

1. State the desired outcomes for Mrs. S., including expected progress and warning signs/symptoms of side effects or adverse reactions.
2. State your response for 1 week, 4 weeks and 7 weeks of therapy.
3. What actions can Mrs. S. take to prevent risk for superinfection?

The fluoroquinolones are the latest group of antibiotics to be introduced. They were preceded by nalidixic acid (NegGram®), a quinolone that has been used for decades solely for the treatment of urinary tract infections. Because nalidixic acid is structurally similar to the fluoroquinolones and has essentially the same mechanism of action, it is discussed in the same chapter as these new antibacterials.

The currently available fluoroquinolones include ciprofloxacin (Cipro®), enoxacin (Penetrex®), lomefloxacin (Maxaquin®), norfloxacin (Noroxin®) and ofloxacin (Floxin®). All five drugs can be taken orally. Ciprofloxacin and ofloxacin are also available in parenteral formulations. Figure 16.1 on the next page provides the chemical structures of the fluoroquinolones.

Figure 16.1
Chemical structures of fluoroquinolones

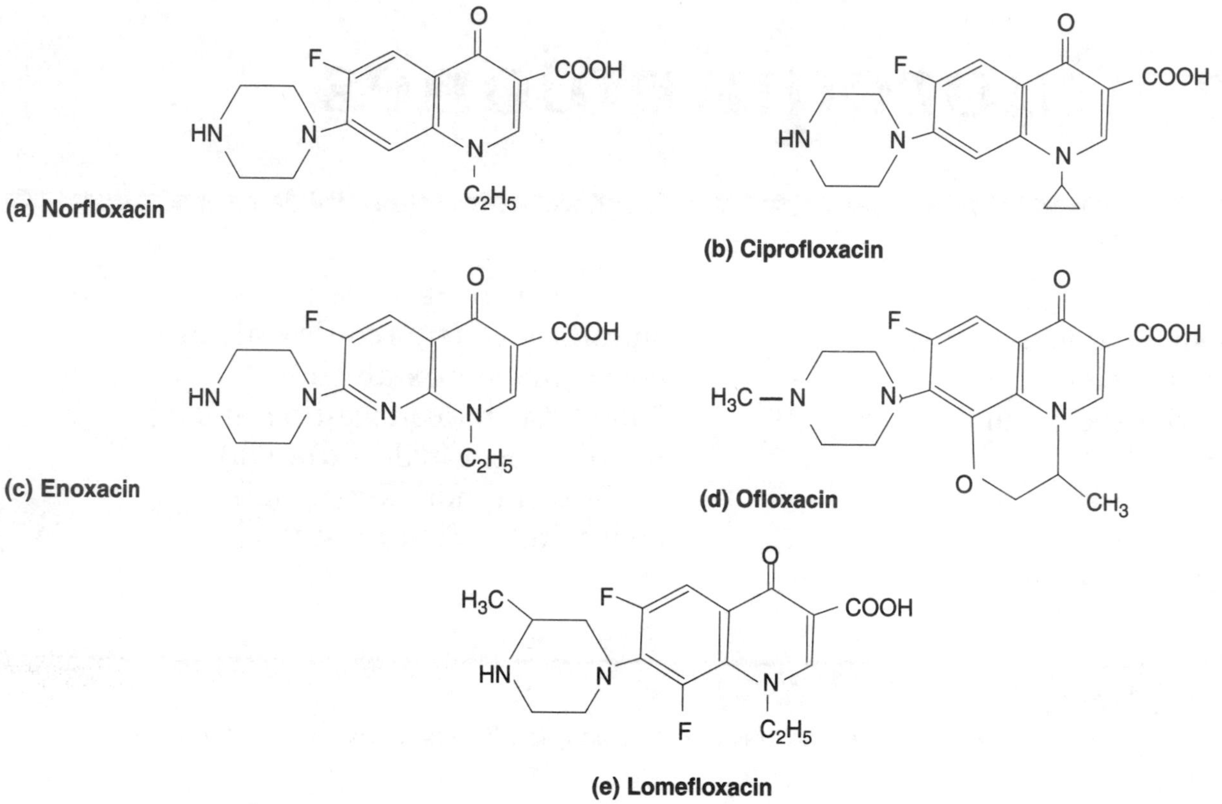

(a) Norfloxacin

(b) Ciprofloxacin

(c) Enoxacin

(d) Ofloxacin

(e) Lomefloxacin

Source: AMA Drug Evaluations Subscriptions; 1993. Reproduced with permission.

Mechanism of Action

Fluoroquinolones inhibit DNA synthesis by a specific action on DNA gyrase, the enzyme responsible for the unwinding and supercoiling of bacterial DNA within the bacterium before its replication.

Pharmacokinetics

Nalidixic acid is rapidly and almost completely absorbed from the intestinal tract. Once absorbed, it is converted to an active metabolite, hydroxynalidixic acid, and an inactive glucuronide in the liver. Nalidixic acid and its metabolites are eliminated through the kidney, and urine concentrations are severalfold greater than those of serum. About 80% of administered nalidixic acid is eliminated as the active hydroxynalidixic acid.

The fluoroquinolones are rapidly, but variably, absorbed following oral administration. Oral bioavailability is approximately 40% to 50% for norfloxacin, 60% to 70% for ciprofloxacin and 90% to 100% for enoxacin, lomefloxacin and ofloxacin.

All the fluoroquinolones appear to distribute widely in body fluids and tissues: they penetrate into blister fluid, bile, saliva, sputum, peritoneal fluid, macrophages, polymorphonuclear neutrophils, lung, liver, kidney, gall bladder, skeletal muscle, uterus, cervix, vagina and bone. In the urine, all the fluoroquinolones reach concentrations that exceed the minimum inhibitory concentrations (MICs) of most urinary tract pathogens for at least twelve hours.

In patients with inflamed meninges, ciprofloxacin and ofloxacin may reach concentrations in the cerebrospinal fluid that exceed the MIC90 for most gram-negative pathogens that cause bacterial meningitis, including *Pseudomonas aeruginosa, Salmonella* species, and other Enterobacteriaceae. However, concentrations of these drugs achieved in the cerebrospinal fluid are not adequate to treat meningitis caused by staphylococci, *Streptococcus pneumoniae,* group B streptococci, and *Listeria monocytogenes.*

Fluoroquinolones are eliminated by the liver,

gastrointestinal tract and kidney. All fluoro-quinolones can be recovered in urine, and the drugs appear to be cleared by both glomerular filtration and tubular secretion.

Antibacterial Spectrum

Nalidixic acid is active against many gram-negative bacteria commonly found in urinary tract infections (UTIs). These include indole-positive *Proteus* strains, *Escherichia coli*, *Proteus mirabilis* and *Klebsiella. Pseudomonas aeruginosa* are not sensitive to nalidixic acid.

Fluoroquinolones are effective against most aerobic gram-negative and some gram-positive bacteria. Ciprofloxacin generally is the most active fluoroquinolone in vitro, especially against susceptible gram-negative bacteria (e.g., *Pseudomonas* species). It is less active against gram-positive organisms. Specific differences in potency among the fluoroquinolones exist for some organisms; however, the clinical significance of these differences depends on such factors as the pharmacokinetic properties and relative toxicities of the various drugs.

The fluoroquinolones are highly active against most Enterobacteriaceae, including *Escherichia coli*, *Klebsiella*, *Enterobacter*, *Proteus mirabilis*, *P. vulgaris*, *Morganella morganii*, *Providencia*, *Citrobacter* and *Serratia*. These drugs are active against *Pseudomonas aeruginosa*, including strains that are resistant to other antibacterials.

The gram-negative coccobacilli, *Haemophilus influenzae* and *H. ducreyi*, and the gram-negative cocci, *Neisseria meningitidis*, *N. gonorrhoeae* and *Moraxella catarrhalis*, are highly susceptible to the fluoroquinolones. The beta-lactamase-producing strains of organisms are also susceptible.

The fluoroquinolones are active against some gram-positive bacteria, although inhibitory concentrations generally are higher than for gram-negative bacteria. All of the fluoroquinolones are active against staphylococci (*S. aureus*, *S. epidermidis*), including methicillin-resistant strains. Ciprofloxacin and ofloxacin are the most active. Some centres report a substantial increase in the percentage of isolates of methicillin-resistant *S. aureus* that are resistant to the fluoro-quinolones.

Streptococci, including *S. pyogenes* (group A),

S. agalctiae (group B), *S. pneumoniae* and viridans streptococci, are usually highly susceptible. Enterococci (*E. faecalis*) are only moderately susceptible to ciprofloxacin and ofloxacin. Norfloxacin, enoxacin and lomefloxacin are less active, although concentrations achieved in urine are usually adequate for urinary tract infections caused by *E. faecalis*.

The fluoroquinolones are active in vitro against *Legionella pneumophila*. Ciprofloxacin and ofloxacin are active against *Mycobacterium tuberculosis* and certain atypical mycobacteria.

Resistance

Bacterial resistance to nalidixic acid is a problem when the drug is used chronically, and this has limited its long-term use. Plasmid-mediated, transferable resistance to the fluoroquinolones has not been reported. However, resistance can be caused by chromosomal mutations. These involve alterations in DNA gyrase or changes in outer membrane proteins that affect bacterial membrane permeability. At this point, it is not known whether acquired resistance to the fluoroquinolones will become a major clinical problem.

Therapeutic Uses

Nalidixic acid is indicated for the treatment of acute or chronic urinary tract infections due to one or more species of nalidixic acid-sensitive gram-negative pathogenic organisms, in particular *E. coli*, *Proteus*, *Aerobacter* and *Klebsiella* species. It is useful in mixed urinary tract infection when the nalidixic acid-sensitive gram-negative rods predominate. As previously mentioned, bacterial resistance may develop when nalidixic acid is used chronically. Thus, the drug is not recommended for long-term prophylaxis of urinary tract infections.

Because fluoroquinolones are well absorbed, distribute well throughout the body and have a broad spectrum of bactericidal activity, they are used to treat a wide range of infections.

Ciprofloxacin may be used for the treatment of patients with acute bronchitis and acute pneumonia, urinary tract infections, skin and soft-tissue infections, bone and joint infections, and infectious diarrhea, caused by a wide range susceptible organisms.

Ofloxacin is indicated for the treatment of adults with lower respiratory tract infections, including pneumonia, and acute exacerbations of chronic bronchitis due to *H. influenzae* or *S. pneumoniae*. It is also used to treat uncomplicated cystitis or complicated urinary tract infections due to *E. coli, K. pneumoniae* or *P. mirabilis*. Ofloxacin is used to treat prostatitis due to *E. coli*. Sexually transmitted diseases due to *N. gonorrhoeae* and nongonococcal urethritis and cervicitis due to *Chlamydia trachomatis* can also be treated with ofloxacin. Finally, ofloxacin can be used in mild to moderate skin and skin-structure infections due to *S. aureus* and *S. pyogenes*.

Lomefloxacin is used in acute exacerbations of chronic bronchitis of mixed etiology that does not involve *Streptococcus pneumoniae*. It is also used in uncomplicated and complicated infections of the upper and lower urinary tract. Lomefloxacin appears, on the basis of limited data, to be effective in the treatment of acute and chronic bacterial prostatitis, infectious diarrhea, bone and joint infections, infections of the skin and skin structures and sexually transmitted diseases (e.g., chancroid due to *Haemophilus ducreyi*).

Norfloxacin is indicated for the treatment of upper and lower urinary tract infections, specifically complicated and uncomplicated cystitis, pyelitis and pyelonephritis caused by susceptible strains of *E. coli, K. pneumoniae,* unspecified *Klebsiella,* unspecified *Citrobacter, P. mirabilis, S. aureus, S. faecalis* and *P. aeruginosa*.

Enoxacin appears to be effective for complicated urinary tract infections. Single doses have been beneficial in uncomplicated urethral and endocervical gonorrhea. Additional clinical trials are required before determining enoxacin's spectrum of indications, dosage range and usefulness, relative to the other fluoroquinolones.

Adverse Effects

Nausea, vomiting, diarrhea and abdominal pain are the most commonly reported adverse effects of nalidixic acid. Other adverse effects include allergic reactions (rashes, urticaria, eosinophilia), photosensitivity and visual disturbances (blurring of vision, photophobia, changes in colour vision). Its central nervous system adverse effects are drowsiness, weakness, dizziness, headaches and, on very rare occasions, convulsions.

The fluoroquinolones are well tolerated and rarely require discontinuation because of adverse effects. The most frequent adverse effects involve the gastrointestinal tract and the central nervous system. Nausea, headache and dizziness occur most commonly. Abdominal pain, dyspepsia, flatulence, vomiting, diarrhea and stomatitis are also encountered. The adverse effects involving the central nervous system include malaise, drowsiness, weakness, insomnia, restlessness and agitation. Depression, hallucinations, visual disturbances, psychosis and convulsive seizures are rare.

Anaphylactic reactions, including cardiovascular collapse, have occurred rarely in patients receiving therapy with a fluoroquinolone.

Superinfection can occur in patients receiving long-term treatment with a fluoroquinolone.

The fluoroquinolones are contraindicated in children because of potential adverse effects on developing bone and cartilage. In recent studies, however, these drugs have shown efficacy and lack of arthropathy when administered to pediatric patients for prophylaxis of bacterial infections and other indications. Additional data are required to confirm these findings before these drugs can be recommended in children under 18 years of age.

Table 16.1 lists the clinically significant drug interactions with nalidixic acid and the fluoroquinolones.

Nursing Management

The nursing management of the patient receiving any of the fluoroquinolones is essentially the same (Table 16.2). Unique features related to each drug are included in Table 16.3 (pages 150–152).

Table 16.1
Nalidixic acid and the fluoroquinolones: Drug interactions

Drug	Interaction
Aluminum, magnesium and calcium, iron and zinc	• The divalent and trivalent cations in antacid and mineral products appear to reduce the gastrointestinal absorption of fluoroquinolones
Anticoagulants, oral	• Nalidixic acid and the fluoroquinolones have been reported to increase the effects of warfarin and its derivatives. During concomitant administration of these drugs, the prothrombin time or other appropriate coagulation tests should be closely monitored
Caffeine	• Ciprofloxacin and enoxacin reduce the clearance of caffeine. Excessive caffeine intake should be avoided
Cyclosporine	• Possible cyclosporine toxicity with ciprofloxacin or norfloxacin. Monitor renal status: concentrations of both drugs may remain within normal range; adjustment of cyclosporine dosage may avoid nephrotoxicity. Effectiveness of decreased cyclosporine dosage in avoiding rejection has not been established. Ofloxacin or enoxacin may not interact
Didanosine	• Decreased ciprofloxacin effect due to decreased absorption. Avoid concurrent use, or take in separate doses no less than 2 h apart
Pentoxifylline	• Headache may be due to pentoxifylline toxicity with ciprofloxacin. Avoid concurrent use
Probenecid	• Probenecid blocks the renal tubular secretion of ciprofloxacin and norfloxacin
Ranitidine	• May decrease absorption and effect of enoxacin. Avoid concurrent use
Sucralfate	• Sucralfate before ciprofloxacin produces a 30% decrease in ciprofloxacin absorption. Avoid concurrent use
Theophylline	• Nalidixic acid and some fluoroquinolones (e.g., ciprofloxacin, enoxacin, norfloxacin) increase plasma theophylline concentrations. Pts may experience theophylline toxicities (nausea, vomiting, CNS stimulation, cardiovascular instability and convulsions). These effects are seen most frequently with enoxacin and, to a much lesser extent, with ciprofloxacin

Table 16.2
Nursing management for the fluoroquinolones

Assessment of risk vs. benefit	Patient data	• *History:* Physician should determine any contraindications such as allergy and precautions such as hepatic or renal impairment. Pts with allergies or asthma are at greater risk for developing hypersensitivity to these drugs. Administer with extreme caution for pts with hx of CNS disorders, as there is increased risk for seizures • Assess to establish baseline VS, general state of health, indicators of present infection • *Pregnancy and lactation:* Recommend avoidance, as drugs may cause arthropathy in the fetus or infant
	Drug data	• *Site and type of infection:* Select drugs based on location of infection and causative microorganism • Culture and sensitivity results • *Some serious drug interactions:* Confer with pharmacist • Note drug-food interactions with this class (Table 16.1) • Side effects are usually mild; most common are nausea, headache and dizziness. Phototoxicity is possible, esp. with lomefloxacin. With long-term tx, superinfections can occur. Serious adverse reactions such as hypersensitivity and nephrotoxicity are possible though rare. Crystalluria has occurred if urine is alkaline

(cont'd on next page)

Table 16.2 (continued)
Nursing management for the fluoroquinolones

Implementation	Rights of administration	• Using the "rights" helps prevent errors of administration
	Right route	• Usually, these drugs are given PO, except Cipro IV® and ofloxacin
	Right time	• As with all antibiotics, give ATC to ensure effective blood levels. Dosage interval varies among drugs and depending on indication for use
	Right technique	• IV administration requires knowledge of correct diluent and IV solution, correct dilution and rate of administration. Always refer to manufacturer's instructions for this route. Drug should be administered in small volume by infusion over 60 min. Rapid infusion causes phlebitis
	Nursing therapeutics	• Enhance host defences (nutrition, rest, fluids, hygiene) • Promote preventive measures (particularly hygiene) to minimize superinfections (oral, vaginal). Intestinal superinfections caused by depletion of normal GI flora can be minimized by dietary measures (e.g., eating yoghurt, buttermilk) • Administer ATC to ensure effective blood levels • Ensure that pt remains well hydrated (1500–2000 mL/day), unless fluid restriction is necessary
	Patient/family teaching	• Educate for proper use of anti-infectives (Chapter 9) • *Review drug-food interactions:* Advise limiting or eliminating caffeine and separating administration of any antacids, calcium or iron supplements by at least 2 h • Remind pt to notify physician if symptoms do not improve. Review signs/symptoms of adverse reactions and advise to report to physician immediately. Discuss likelihood of dizziness and advise safety precautions (e.g., avoid driving until effects of drug are known; change position slowly) • *Discuss photosensitivity:* Advise use of sunscreen, protective clothing • *Discuss possibility of pregnancy:* Advise patient to notify physician. Explain risks of lactation while on these drugs
Outcomes	Monitoring of progress	*Continually monitor:* • Clinical response, indicating tx success (reduction in signs/symptoms) • Note that allergy, although uncommon, can occur at any time: be alert for signs and symptoms; document and report to physician • With long-term therapy, observe for superinfections • Respond immediately to adverse effects (e.g., CNS effects such as hallucinations, depression or seizures)

Response to Clinical Challenge

Principles

The most essential desired outcome for Mrs. S. is to cure the osteomyelitis. This will have other outcomes such as increased mobility, function and comfort and decreased pain. The expected rate of progress is slow; therefore, Mrs. S. will require encouragement during the first weeks of therapy. There should be some continual improvement in her clinical signs/symptoms.

Regarding drug monitoring, the major concept is an understanding of the relationship of dose and duration of therapy to the onset of side effects and adverse reactions. In the early course of therapy, Mrs. S. will probably experience the common side effects; these may abate with continued use. As therapy is prolonged, Mrs. S. is at increased risk for superinfection. As well, the site must be monitored for signs of infection/inflammation. Allergic responses can occur at any time during the course of treatment.

Actions

A plan of care for Mrs. S. would include the following goals:

• Week 1: Minor clinical improvement with minor nausea, periods of dizziness and headaches.
• Week 4: Mrs. S. should be afebrile, with improved joint mobility, decreased swelling and pain. She should also tolerate the drug better, maintain her fluid intake, and consume yoghurt and buttermilk to prevent intestinal overgrowth. (Observe her for signs of allergic response and superinfection.)
• Week 7: Mrs. S. should be weightbearing with some discomfort, but visible external swelling. Lab work should indicate reduced infection and normal renal function. The IV site should appear healthy; there should be no superinfection.

Further Reading

Bailey J, et al. Ciprofloxacin-induced acute interstitial nephritis. *Am J Nephrol* 1992;12:271–273.

The choice of antibacterial drugs. *Medical Letter on Drugs and Therapeutics* 1994;36:919–925.

Fluoroquinolone antimicrobial drugs. *AMA Drug Evaluation Subscriptions* 1993; 2. Systemic anti-infectives:8.1–8.14.

Handbook of antimicrobial therapy. *Medical Letter on Drugs and Therapeutics* 1992.

Mandel GL, Petri WA. Antimicrobial agents: sulfonamides, trimethoprim-sulfamethoxazole, quinolones, and agents for urinary tract infections. In: Hardman JL, Limbird LE. *Gilman and Gibson's The Pharmacological Basis of Therapeutics*. 9th ed. New York: Pergamon; 1996:1057–1072.

Table 16.3
The fluoroquinolones: Drug doses

Drug Generic name (Trade names)	Dosage	Nursing alert
nalidixic acid (NegGram)	**Oral:** *Adults:* Initially, 1 g qid for 1–2 weeks. Max. 4 g/day. For prolonged tx, total dose/day may be reduced to 2 g after initial tx. *Children < 12 years:* Initially, 55 mg/kg/day, given in 4 divided doses. For prolonged tx, total daily dose may be reduced to 33 mg/kg/day	• May be taken with or without food. Liberal fluid intake. Avoid antacids within 2 h. Take with food to help reduce GI side effects
ciprofloxacin (Cipro IV)	**IV:** *Adults:* For moderate/severe/complicated UTI: 200–400 mg q12h. For moderate/severe respiratory tract infections: 400 mg q8–12h. Skin or skin-structure, blood or bone infections: 400 mg q12h. As with oral ciprofloxacin, the duration of tx depends on the severity of infection; in general, the drug should be continued for at least \2 days after s/s of infection have disappeared. The usual duration of tx is 7–14 days but may be 6 weeks or longer for some infections (e.g., bone and joint, prostatitis) *Adults with CrCl ≥ 30 mL/min,* usual dose; *CrCl < 30 mL/min and pts on hemodialysis or peritoneal dialysis:* Use recommended dose od or half usual dose bid	• Follow manufacturer's instruction for dilution and infuse over 60 min; causes phlebitis if rate too fast • Use large vein, if possible
ciprofloxacin HCl (Cipro)	**Oral:** *Adults:* For mild to moderate UTI: 250 mg q12h. For severe or complicated UTI, bacterial prostatitis, mild to moderate respiratory tract, bone and joint, skin and skin-structure infections, and infectious diarrhea: 500 mg q12h. Also for pts with typhoid fever. For severe or complicated respiratory tract, bone and joint, and skin and skin-structure infections: 750 mg q12h. Usual tx is 7–14 days, but more prolonged tx may be required for severe or complicated infections. Bone and joint infections may require tx for 4–6 weeks or longer; infectious diarrhea for 5–7 days. For acute cystitis in women, 3 days' tx may be adequate For uncomplicated urethral, endocervical, rectal and pharyngeal gonorrhea (including PPNG infections): 500 mg as a single dose For chancroid: 500 mg q12h for 3 days	• Oral ciprofloxacin can be taken with or without meals. The preferred time of dosing is 2 h pc, with a glass of water. Concurrent use of antacids or sucralfate should be avoided. Remind pt to limit caffeine intake. Maintain fluid intake to reduce risk of crystalluria, unless fluids restricted

Table 16.3 (continued)
The fluoroquinolones: Drug doses

Drug Generic name (Trade names)	Dosage	Nursing alert
ciprofloxacin HCl (Cipro) (cont'd)	For prevention of gram-negative bacillary infection in neutropenic adults with acute leukemia: 500 mg q12h *Creatinine clearance > 30 mL/min:* No dose adjustment. *CrCl < 30 mL/min and pts or hemodialysis or peritoneal dialysis:* Use recommended dose od or half-dose bid For severe infections and severe renal impairment, a unit dose of 750 mg may be administered at the intervals noted above. However, pts should be monitored carefully, and serum concentrations should be measured periodically. Peak concentrations (1–2 h after dosing) > 5 µg/mL should be avoided. For pts with changing renal function or those with renal impairment and hepatic insufficiency, measurement of serum concentrations may provide additional guidance for adjusting dosage	
enoxacin (Penetrex)	**Oral:** *Adults:* For mild to moderate acute UTI: 200 mg q12h for 7 days. For complicated or severe UTI: 400 mg q12h for 14 days. For uncomplicated gonococcal urethritis or cervicitis: 400 mg in a single dose for 1 day. Manufacturer recommends reducing dose by 50% in pts with creatinine clearances < 30 mL/min	•Concurrent use of antacids, calcium or iron supplements or sucralfate should be avoided; separate by 2 h. Preferred time is 2 h pc. Liberal fluid intake, unless contraindicated
lomefloxacin HCl (Maxaquin)	**Oral:** *Adults:* For mild to moderate acute exacerbation of chronic bronchitis or cystitis: 400 mg od for 10 days. For complicated UTI: 400 mg od for 14 days. For prophylaxis for transurethral surgical procedures: 400 mg 2–6 h prior to surgery *Adults with renal impairment (CrCl 10–40 mL/min):* An initial loading dose of 400 mg followed by maintenance doses of 200 mg od for duration of tx. Hemodialysis pts should receive same regimen as those with impaired renal function. Serial determination of lomefloxacin serum concentrations is recommended to guide dosage adjustments	•Lomefloxacin may be taken with or without meals. Concurrent use of antacids, calcium and iron supplements or sucralfate should be avoided. Photosensitivity is more common with this drug. Liberal fluid intake, if allowed

(cont'd on next page)

Table 16.3 (continued)
The fluoroquinolones: Drug doses

Drug Generic name (Trade names)	Dosage	Nursing alert
norfloxacin (Noroxin)	**Oral:** *Adults:* For uncomplicated UTI: 400 mg bid for 7–10 days. For complicated UTI: 400 mg bid for 10–21 days (max., 800 mg/day). Adults with renal impairment, 400 mg od when CrCl is ≤ 30 mL/min/1.73 m² but > 6.6 mL/min/1.73m². When CrCl is > 30 mL/min/ 1.73 m², dosage modification is unnecessary For acute bacterial prostatitis: 400 mg bid for at least 10 days; 4–6 weeks of tx is usually required for chronic prostatitis For uncomplicated urethral or endocervical gonorrhea: 800 mg as a single dose For bacterial gastroenteritis: 400 mg bid for 3–5 days. For prevention of gram-negative bacillary infections in neutropenic adults with acute leukemia: 400 mg bid	• Norfloxacin is taken 1 h ac or 2 h pc with a glass of water. Pts should be well hydrated. Concurrent use of antacids, calcium or iron supplements or sucralfate should be avoided
ofloxacin (Floxin)	**Oral:** *Adults:* For LRT, uncomplicated and complicated skin and skin-structure infections: 400 mg q12h for 10 days. For acute pelvic inflammatory disease: 400 mg q12h for 10–14 days. For acute uncomplicated gonorrhea: 400 mg single dose. For cervicitis/urethritis due to *C. trachomatis* or mixed infections due to *C. trachomatis* and *N. gonorrhea:* 300 mg q12h for 7 days. For acute cystitis: 200 mg q12h for 3 days. For uncomplicated UTIs: 200 mg q12h for 7 days. For complicated UTIs: 200 mg q12h for 10 days. For prostatitis: 300 mg q12h for 6 weeks **IV:** *Adults:* Same doses as oral, administered over 60 min. For pts with CrCl < 20 mL/min: half recommended dose q24h	• **PO:** Do not take antacids, zinc or iron preparations within 2 h of ofloxacin • **IV:** Premixed ofloxacin in dextrose injection in bottles and flexible containers requires no further dilution prior to administration (see manufacturer's labelling for instructions). Since these injections contain no preservatives or bacteriostatic agents, they should be used promptly after opening; unused portions should be discarded

CHAPTER 17

Miscellaneous Antibiotics and Antibacterials

Topics Discussed
- Mechanisms of action
- Pharmacokinetics
- Antibacterial spectra
- Resistance
- Therapeutic uses
- Adverse effects
- Nursing management

Drugs Discussed
chloramphenicol (klor-am-**fen**-ih-kole)
vancomycin (van-koe-**mye**-sin)
nitrofurantoin (nye-troe-fyoor-**an**-toe-in)
imipenem (ih-mee-**pen**-em)
cilastatin (sil-a-**stat**-in)

Clinical Challenge
Consider this clinical challenge as you read through this chapter. The response to the challenge appears on page 161.

J.K. is a 37-year-old man with rheumatic heart disease who is scheduled for surgery. One dose of vancomycin IV is ordered pre-op.

1. Determine the rate of infusion.
2. Determine the time of administration in relation to the surgery.
3. State administration precautions.

Chloramphenicol (Chloromycetin®)

Mechanism of Action
Chloramphenicol penetrates readily into bacteria. It blocks protein synthesis by binding to the 50S subunit of the bacterial 70S ribosome and inhibiting the formation of peptide bonds among amino acids. Bacterial and mammalian ribosomes differ, and the ability of chloramphenicol to affect primarily the bacterial ribosomes accounts for its selective effect on protein synthesis in microorganisms.

Pharmacokinetics
Chloramphenicol is well absorbed from the gastrointestinal tract. The drug is lipid soluble, and once absorbed penetrates most tissues and body fluids readily. This includes the cerebrospinal fluid. Concentrations in brain are higher than those in plasma. Therapeutic concentrations are achieved in synovial, pleural and ascitic fluid. Chloramphenicol penetrates intracellularly, which facilitates its efficacy against phagocytosed organisms.

Chloramphenicol is primarily eliminated by hepatic metabolism. In patients with normal liver function, approximately ninety percent of the drug is conjugated to its inactive glucuronide. The mean elimination half-life in adults and children is approximately four hours.

Patients with hepatic dysfunction (e.g., cirrhosis) conjugate chloramphenicol at a slower rate. In these individuals, the dose of chloramphenicol must be reduced to prevent toxic levels from occurring. Likewise, neonates and premature infants cannot metabolize chloramphenicol well, and its elimination in them is significantly slower. These patients must also receive lower doses of the antibiotic to prevent it from accumulating to toxic levels in the body.

Antibacterial Spectrum

Chloramphenicol has a broad spectrum of activity. It is bacteriostatic against many gram-positive and gram-negative microorganisms as well as *Chlamydia* and *Rickettsia*. In Canada and the United States, *Salmonella* species, including *S. typhi,* generally are susceptible to chloramphenicol. Enterobacteriaceae are variable in their response to chloramphenicol. Most strains of *Escherichia coli, Klebsiella pneumoniae* and *Proteus mirabilis* are inhibited by chloramphenicol, but the majority of strains of *Serratia, Providencia, Proteus rettgeri* and *Pseudomonas aeruginosa* are resistant.

Resistance

Resistance has developed in some gram-positive and gram-negative bacteria to chloramphenicol. In most cases, this appears to be due to the ability of the bacteria to chemically inactivate chloramphenicol. *Pseudomonas aeruginosa* and some strains of *Proteus* and *Klebsiella* have become resistant as a result of a change in permeability that prevents chloramphenicol from entering the bacterial cells.

Therapeutic Uses

Chloramphenicol has severe toxicities (see later discussion) and it should not be used to treat minor infections. However, it penetrates the cerebrospinal fluid and brain tissue well and is active against a number of important microbial pathogens, including some for which alternative drug therapies are limited. Therefore, chloramphenicol is recommended for well-defined indications in seriously ill patients, when the location of the infection, the susceptibility of the causative organism, or individual patient characteristics limit or prevent the use of less toxic agents.

Chloramphenicol's indications include (1) acute infections cause by *Salmonella typhi* (chloramphenicol is not recommended for routine treatment of the typhoid carrier state), (2) serious infections caused by susceptible strains of (a) *Salmonella* species with systemic involvement, (b) *H. influenzae,* specifically, meningeal infections, (c) *Rickettsia;* psittacosis in children, (d) various gram-negative bacteria causing bacteremia, meningitis or other serious gram-negative infections, (e) other susceptible organisms that have demonstrated resistance to other appropriate antimicrobial agents, and (3) cystic fibrosis regimens.

Chloramphenicol is prepared in ocular formulations for use in the treatment of superficial conjunctival and/or corneal infections. It is also used topically in the ear because it is effective against a wide range of pathogens causing external otitis. These include *Staphylococcus aureus, Escherichia coli,* strains of *Pseudomonas* and *Proteus* species. If signs of drug-induced local irritation appear, chloramphenicol should be discontinued. Blood dyscrasias have been reported following topical use in the ear.

Table 17.1 lists the clinically significant drug interactions of chloramphenicol; Table 17.2 gives the nursing management for patients taking this drug.

Adverse Effects

Chloramphenicol can cause a dose-dependent depression of bone marrow. Its therapeutic concentration in plasma ranges from 5–20 µg/mL (approximately 15–62 µmol/L). When its plasma concentration exceeds 25 µg/mL (77.3 µmol/L), anemia — sometimes with leukopenia or thrombocytopenia — can occur. This effect is reversible if the drug is discontinued. It should not be confused with choramphenicol-induced aplastic anemia, which is almost invariably fatal. Reported in one in 25 000 to one in 40 000 patients, aplastic anemia can occur after only one dose of chloramphenicol or several weeks or months after the drug is stopped.

Newborns, particularly premature infants, metabolize chloramphenicol slowly. The half-life of the drug is increased from four hours in the adult to twenty-six hours in babies less than two weeks of age. This fact must be taken into account in calculating dosage. Otherwise, toxic levels of the drug can accumulate, leading to the grey-baby syndrome, a condition characterized by abdominal distention, vomiting, cyanosis, irregular respiration, a fall in body temperature and cardiovascular collapse.

Table 17.1
Cloramphenicol: Drug interactions

Drug	Interaction
Anticoagulants, oral	• Chloramphenicol can inhibit the metabolism of dicoumarol. It may also decrease vitamin K production by gut bacteria and the production of prothrombin by liver cells. Therefore, concomitant use of chloramphenicol and dicoumarol should be avoided. If chloramphenicol must be used, warfarin might be preferable to dicoumarol. Test prothrombin times at more frequent intervals
Barbiturates	• Chloramphenicol may decrease the metabolism and increase the toxicity of barbiturates; barbiturates can increase the metabolism and decrease the effect of chloramphenicol. Monitor barbiturate and chloramphenicol concentrations in epileptics. Avoid concurrent use in others
Bone marrow depressants	• Bone marrow depressants (e.g., antineoplastics) have additive effects with chloramphenicol and should not be used concomitantly
Cephalosporins	• The bacteriostatic effects of chloramphenicol may interfere with the bactericidal effects of cephalosporins. If both drugs are essential, give the cephalosporin a few hours or longer before chloramphenicol
Cyclophosphamide	• Cylcophosphamide metabolism may be inhibited by chloramphenicol, resulting in an increase in cyclosphosphamide's effects
Hypoglycemics, oral	• Chloramphenicol may increase the hypoglycemic effects of these drugs. Monitor blood glucose
Penicillins	• As for cephalosporins
Phenytoin	• Phenytoin metabolism may be inhibited by chloramphenicol, increasing the effect of phenytoin. If necessary, decrease phenytoin dose
Rifampin	• Rifampin can increase chloramphenicol metabolism and decrease its effects. Avoid concurrent use

Table 17.2
Nursing management for chloramphenicol

Assessment of risk vs. benefit	Patient data	• *History:* Physician should determine any contraindications such as allergy or blood dyscrasias and precautions such as hepatic impairment • Assess to establish baseline VS, general state of health, indicators of present infection • *Pregnancy and lactation:* Recommend avoidance while taking drug: may cause grey-baby syndrome • *Geriatric pts:* monitor more closely if liver function is reduced
	Drug data	• *Site and type of infection:* Select drugs based on location of infection and causative microorganism • Culture and sensitivity results • *Some serious drug interactions:* Confer with pharmacist • Most serious adverse reaction is bone marrow depression: monitor CBC and clinical symptoms
Implementation	Rights of administration	• Using the "rights" helps prevent errors of administration
	Right route	• Give PO or IV
	Right time	• As with all antibiotics, give ATC to ensure effective blood levels

(cont'd on next page)

Table 17.2 (continued)
Nursing management for chloramphenicol

Implementation (cont'd)	Rights of administration (cont'd)	
	Right technique	• IV administration requires knowledge of correct diluent and IV solution, correct dilution and rate of administration. Always refer to manufacturer's instructions for this route. Drug should be administered in small volume by infusion over 30–60 min. May be given by direct IV (if policy allows)
	Nursing therapeutics	• Enhance host defences (nutrition, rest, fluids, hygiene)
		• Instruct pt that bitter taste lasts only 2–3 min during administration
		• *Emotional support:* Most pts have serious illnesses
	Patient/family teaching	• Educate for proper use of anti-infectives (Chapter 9)
		• Pt's need for information may be limited by serious illness
		• Discuss possibility of pregnancy: Advise pt to notify physician. Explain risks of lactation while on this drug
Outcomes	Monitoring of progress	*Continually monitor:*
		• Clinical response, indicating tx success (reduction in signs/symptoms)
		• Be alert for signs/symptoms of bone marrow depression. Monitor CBC and platelet count; weekly (or more frequent) serum levels; document and report changes immediately to physician

Vancomycin (Vancocin®, Vancoled®)

Mechanism of Action

Vancomycin inhibits cell wall synthesis in susceptible bacteria. However, it is structurally and pharmacodynamically very different from the penicillins and cephalosporin beta-lactam antibiotics that also inhibit cell wall synthesis. It does not depend on binding to penicillin-binding proteins (PCPs) for its action, but instead binds to a different component of the cell wall to interfere with the elongation of the peptidoglycan backbone of the wall. This specificity of action partly explains the minimal resistance shown to vancomycin to date.

Pharmacokinetics

Vancomycin is not absorbed if given orally, and it irritates if given intramuscularly. Therefore, it should be administered only intravenously, except when it is given orally for treatment of *Clostridium difficile* toxic colitis. In this situation, the intent is not to have the drug absorbed.

Vancomycin is eliminated by glomerular filtration. It is not metabolized. Its dosage must be reduced, based on creatinine clearance, in patients with reduced renal function.

Antibacterial Spectrum

Vancomycin is active only against gram-positive bacteria. The antibiotic cannot penetrate the outer membrane that surrounds gram-negative species and, as result, is ineffective in treating gram-negative infections. Vancomycin is one of the most potent antibiotics against *Staphylococcus aureus* and *S. epidermidis,* including methicillin- and cephalothin-resistant strains.

Streptococcus pyogenes and *S. pneumoniae* (including penicillin-G-resistant strains) are highly susceptible to vancomycin. The drug usually inhibits the growth of viridans streptococci, *S. bovis, S. agalactiae* (group B), and enterococci (e.g., *E. faecalis*). However, vancomycin may not be bactericidal against some strains of these species, particularly the enterococci. Antibacterial synergism against enterococci is usually obtained when

Table 17.3
Vancomycin: Drug interactions

Drug	Interaction
Cephalosporins	• Vancomycin and some cephalosporins may show additive nephrotoxicity. Avoid concurrent use
Cholestyramine	• May bind and inactivate oral vancomycin; should not be given concurrently to treat pseudomembranous colitis
Digoxin	• Absorption may be decreased. Monitor digoxin concentration
Ototoxic or nephro- toxic drugs	• Other ototoxic or nephrotoxic drugs (e.g., aminoglycosides, loop diuretics) should be given cautiously when vancomycin is administered because of potential for additive effects
IV solutions of incompatible drugs	• Vancomycin has been reported to incompatible with IV solutions of many drugs, including heparin, chloramphenicol, methicillin, adrenal corticosteroids, aminophylline, barbiturates, chlorothiazide, phenytoin, sodium bicarbonate, sulfisoxazole and warfarin

vancomycin is combined with an aminoglycoside, particularly gentamicin or streptomycin.

Gram-positive bacilli that are susceptible to vancomycin include *Clostridia* (including *C. difficile*), *Corynebacteria*, *Bacillus anthracis*, *Listeria monocytogenes*, *Actinomyces* species and lactobacilli.

Resistance

During the first thirty years of its use, the development of resistance to vancomycin was not a serious clinical problem. In the last ten years, however, vancomycin-resistant gram-positive bacteria have been isolated from patients who were treated with this antibiotic. In most cases, resistance to vancomycin is attributable to the production of a new cell wall component that prevents the drug from binding to the wall. Resistance to vancomycin is reported from *Enterococcus faecalis* from a plasmid-mediated effect that results in the production of a protein that blocks vancomycin from binding to its normal receptor.

Therapeutic Uses

Vancomycin should be used only in serious gram-positive infections that are not treatable with other antibiotics. It is recommended for serious methicillin-sensitive staphylococcal infections in patients who cannot take a penicillin or cephalosporin (e.g., immediate-type hypersensitivity) or who have not responded to these drugs.

Vancomycin is the drug of choice for serious infections caused by methicillin-resistant *S. aureus* (MRSA) and coagulase-negative staphylococci,

including methicillin-resistant *S. epidermidis* (MRSE). Often the addition of other drugs (e.g., rifampin, gentamicin) to a vancomycin regimen increases the rate of response.

MRSE has become an important cause of infections associated with indwelling devices, including prosthetic heart valves. Vancomycin is the drug of choice for treating these infections.

The combination of vancomycin with gentamicin or streptomycin (for susceptible strains) is the regimen of choice for enterococcal endocarditis in penicillin-allergic patients. Intravenous vancomycin is useful for prophylaxis of infective endocarditis in high-risk patients who are allergic to penicillins and are undergoing dental or certain other surgical procedures.

Oral vancomycin is the drug of choice for the treatment of confirmed antibiotic-associated pseudomembranous colitis caused by *Clostridium difficile.*

Table 17.3 lists the clinically significant drug interactions with vancomycin; Table 17.4 gives the nursing management of patients taking this drug.

Adverse Effects

Vancomycin's most common adverse effect is called "red-neck" or the "red-man" syndrome. This is a nonimmunologic, dose-dependent, glycopeptide-induced anaphylactoid reaction, characterized by one or more of the following signs and symptoms: erythematous macular rash involving the face, neck, upper torso, back and arms; flushing; pruritus; pain and muscle spasms in the chest; tachycardia; hypotension. The exact mechanism of this reaction is unknown. It occurs coincident with

Table 17.4
Nursing management for vancomycin

Assessment of risk vs. benefit	Patient data	• *History:* Physician should determine any contraindications such as allergy and precautions such as renal impairment • Assess to establish baseline VS, general state of health, indicators of present infection • *Pregnancy and lactation:* Safety not established • *Geriatric pts:* Monitor more closely if renal function is reduced; may be more prone to ototoxicity
	Drug data	• Drug is used only for serious gram-positive infections • Culture and sensitivity results • *Some serious drug interactions:* Confer with pharmacist • If given with anesthetics, increases reactions including hypotension, flushing and urticaria (administer 1 h pre-op)
Implementation	Rights of administration	• Using the "rights" helps prevent errors of administration
	Right route	• Not absorbed PO; causes tissue damage IM. Used only IV, except for tx of colitis
	Right time	• As with all antibiotics, give ATC to ensure effective blood levels
	Right technique	• IV administration requires knowledge of correct diluent and IV solution, correct dilution and rate of administration. Always refer to manufacturer's instructions for this route. Drug should be administered in small volume by infusion over 60 min. Not given by direct IV
	Nursing therapeutics	• Enhance host defences (nutrition, rest, fluids, hygiene) • Monitor site carefully; can cause extravasation and necrosis • Monitor BP • *Emotional support:* Most pts have serious illnesses
	Patient/family teaching	• Educate for proper use of anti-infectives (Chapter 9) • Pt's need for information may be limited by serious illness • *Discuss possibility of pregnancy:* Advise pt to notify physician. Explain risks of lactation while on this drug
Outcomes	Monitoring of progress	*Continually monitor:* • Clinical response indicating tx success (reduction in signs/symptoms) • Be alert for signs/symptoms of red-neck syndrome or ototoxicity; document and report immediately to physician • Weekly (or more frequent) serum levels • Audiogram or general hearing assessment (esp. in geriatric pts)

an increase in plasma histamine levels. Pre-treatment with antihistamines, such as hydroxyzine or diphenhydramine, is effective in preventing this reaction.

Ototoxicity has been associated with the use of vancomycin; however, this association has not been definitely correlated. On the basis of the current information, it is reasonable to conclude that, in certain patients (e.g., those with impaired renal function, the elderly, those receiving other potentially ototoxic drugs and those with pre-existing hearing loss), vancomycin could reduce hearing ability, ranging from tinnitus and loss of high-frequency acuity to loss of conversational-frequency range.

Dose-dependent nephrotoxicity was a problem with earlier preparations of vancomycin. With the newer products, this reaction occurs infrequently and is reversible.

Nitrofurantoin (Macrodantin®, Macrobid®)

Mechanism of Action, Antibacterial Spectrum and Pharmacokinetics

The mechanism of action of nitrofurantoin is unclear. The drug inhibits a variety of enzyme systems in bacteria and is active against common urinary pathogens. Most strains of *Escherichia coli* are susceptible. About two-thirds of the strains of other coliforms are also susceptible. *Staphylococcus aureus, S. saprophyticus* and enterococci (*Enterococcus faecalis*) are also susceptible to nitrofurantoin.

Susceptible bacteria do not readily develop resistance to nitrofurantoin during therapy.

Nitrofurantoin is well absorbed from the upper small intestine. Once absorbed, it is concentrated in the urine. Bacteria in the lower urinary tract are exposed to high concentrations of the drug, and this fact accounts for the clinical efficacy of nitrofurantoin in the treatment of lower urinary tract infections.

A major limitation to the use nitrofurantoin in the past has been high incidence of gastrointestinal irritation produced by the drug (see Adverse Effects, below). Fortunately, it has been possible to reduce this effect by changing the crystal size of the drug. Nitrofurantoin was originally formulated as a microcrystal that dissolved quickly in the gastrointestinal tract. This was later replaced by macrocrystalline nitrofurantoin (Macrodantin®). This product is as effective as the discontinued microcrystalline nitrofurantoin, but because it dissolves more slowly it produces less gastrointestinal intolerance.

More recently a product called Macrobid® has been introduced. This product provides a two-component drug delivery system, with one part providing for the relatively rapid dissolution and absorption of nitrofurantoin, and the second allowing for prolonged drug absorption. The advantages of this combination include reduced gastrointestinal distress plus decreased dosage frequency (from four times daily to twice daily).

Therapeutic Uses

Nitrofurantoin is indicated for the treatment of urinary tract infections (e.g., pyelonephritis, pyelitis, cystitis) that are due to susceptible strains of *E. coli*, enterococci, *S. aureus* and certain susceptible strains of *Klebsiella, Enterobacter* and *Proteus* species. It is not indicated for the treatment of associated renal cortical or perinephric abscesses.

Anuria, oliguria or significant impairment of renal function (creatinine clearance < 60 mL/min) are contraindications to the use of nitrofurantoin, for two reasons. First, patients with renal impairment have difficulty eliminating the drug, and second, the drug may fail to achieve therapeutic concentrations in the bladder.

Adverse Effects

Gastrointestinal irritation is the most common adverse effect of nitrofurantoin. Symptoms include anorexia, nausea and vomiting; diarrhea and abdominal pain occur less frequently. These effects have been partially overcome by changing the crystal size of the drug (see discussion above).

Nitrofurantoin can cause allergic reactions including rashes, urticaria, angioneurotic edema, eosinophilia and fever. An acute pulmonary reaction, characterized by fever, myalgia, dyspnea, pulmonary infiltration and pleural effusion can also result from nitrofurantoin administration. A second type of pulmonary reaction involving pneumonic complications can be produced by nitrofurantoin, involving shortness of breath on exertion and cough. Both types of pulmonary reactions usually disappear when the drug is stopped.

A sensorimotor peripheral neuropathy has been associated with nitrofurantoin use, and is seen most often in patients with impaired renal function. Nitrofurantoin has also been reported to produce megaloblastic anemia and cholestasis. In patients deficient in glucose-6-phosphate dehydrogenase, the drug can produce hemolysis.

Table 17.5 on the next page lists the clinically significant drug interactions with nitrofurantoin; Table 17.6 gives the nursing management of patients receiving this drug.

Table 17.5
Nitrofurantoin: Drug interactions

Drug	Interaction
Antacids	• Antacids containing magnesium trisilicate, when administered concomitantly with nitrofurantoin, reduce both the rate and extent of absorption. The mechanism for this interaction probably is adsorption of nitrofurantoin onto the surface of the magnesium trisilicate
Drugs that reduce renal function	• Nitrofurantoin should not be given with drugs that produce impaired renal function
Uricosuric drugs	• Uricosuric drugs, such as probenecid and sulfinpyrazone, may inhibit the renal tubular secretion of nitrofurantoin. The resulting increase in serum levels may increase toxicity, and the decreased urinary levels could lessen its efficacy as a UT antibacterial

Table 17.6
Nursing management for nitrofurantoin

Assessment of risk vs. benefit	Patient data	• *History:* Physician should determine any contraindications such as allergy or G-6-PD deficiency and precautions such as renal impairment or diabetes (neuropathy more common in diabetics) • Assess to establish baseline VS, general state of health, indicators of present infection • *Pregnancy and lactation:* Safety not established • *Geriatric pts:* Monitor more closely if renal function is reduced
	Drug data	• Drug is used in UTI (acute or chronic prophylaxis) • Culture and sensitivity results • *Some drug interactions:* Confer with pharmacist • GI irritation is most common side effect • Most serious adverse reactions are allergic responses (respiratory reaction) and peripheral neuropathy
Implementation	Rights of administration	• Using the "rights" helps prevent errors of administration
	Right route	• Give PO
	Right time	• As with all antibiotics, give ATC to ensure effective blood levels
	Right technique	• Store in light-resistant container. Do not crush tablets or open capsules
	Nursing therapeutics	• Enhance host defences (nutrition, rest, fluids, hygiene) • Promote liberal fluid intake. Monitor fluid balance
	Patient/family teaching	• Educate for proper use of anti-infectives (Chapter 9) • Advise pt that urine may become dark brown (no significance) • *Discuss possibility of pregnancy:* Advise patient to notify physician. Explain risks of lactation while on this drug
Outcomes	Monitoring of progress	*Continually monitor:* • Clinical response indicating tx success (reduction in signs/symptoms) • Be alert for signs/symptoms of allergic reactions or neuropathy

Imipenem Plus Cilastatin Sodium (Primaxin®)

Mechanism of Action

Imipenem is a beta-lactam bactericidal antibiotic that inhibits cell wall synthesis in aerobic and anaerobic gram-positive and gram-negative bacteria. It is metabolized to inactive, potentially nephrotoxic derivatives by a dihydropeptidase enzyme located in the brush border of the proximal renal tubules. Because of this, only very low concentrations of imipenem can be found in the urine.

Cilastatin blocks the metabolism and inactivation of imipenem in the kidney. By combining cilastatin with imipenem, it is possible to attain antibacterial concentrations of imipenem in the urine.

Antibacterial Spectrum

Imipenem has a wide spectrum of activity. Most aerobic and anaerobic gram-positive and gram-negative species are susceptible. Imipenem owes its activity to three major factors: (1) it readily penetrates the cell wall of gram-positive and gram-negative bacteria, (2) it is highly resistant to the activity of most beta-lactamases, whether they are of plasmid or chromosomal origin and (3) it preferentially binds to a critical penicillin-binding protein, PBP-2.

Therapeutic Uses

Neither imipenem nor cilastatin is appreciably absorbed from the gastrointestinal tract; therefore, these drugs must be injected. The combination of imipenem plus cilastatin is indicated in the treatment of serious infections when caused by sensitive bacteria. Lower respiratory tract infections, urinary tract infections, intra-abdominal and gynecological infections and septicemia caused by susceptible bacteria may be treated with imipenem plus cilastatin. Endocarditis caused by *Staphylococcus aureus* also may be treated with the combination, as can bone, joint and skin-structure infections produced by susceptible bacteria.

Adverse Effects

The combination of imipenem and cilastatin is generally well tolerated. The most common adverse effects include nausea, diarrhea and vomiting. However, this combination product can produce severe allergic reactions. As a result, imipenem plus cilastatin should be administered with caution to any patient who has demonstrated some form of allergy, particularly to structurally related drugs (e.g., penicillins, cephalosporins). If an allergic reaction to Primaxin® occurs, discontinue the drug. Serious hypersensitivity reactions may require epinephrine and other emergency measures.

Table 17.7 lists the clinically significant drug interactions with imipenem plus cilastatin.

Table 17.8 on the next two pages gives the dosages for all the drugs discussed in this chapter.

Response to Clinical Challenge

Principles

The manufacturer's instructions should be followed for the IV administration of any drug. The powdered drug is reconstituted with sterile water for injection, mixed well and then added to 100–200 mL of IV solution (0.9% NaCl, D5W, D10W, Ringer's lactate).

Actions

1. Rate of administration: give over 60 min.
2. Give 1 h pre-op to avoid interaction with anesthetics.
3. Precautions include using a pump device to control the rate of flow (rapid administration can cause hypotension or red-neck syndrome). Monitor frequently for extravasation; this drug can cause necrosis. Never give IM.

Table 17.7
Imipenem plus cilastatin: Drug interactions

Drug	Interaction
Cyclosporine	• Acute CNS disturbances (e.g., agitation, confusion, severe tremor) occurred in renal transplant pts receiving cyclosporine and imipenem/cilastatin concomitantly. Avoid concurrent use in pts with decreased renal function

Table 17.8
Miscellaneous antibiotics and antibacterials: Drug doses

Drug Generic name (Trade names)	Dosage	Nursing alert
chloramphenicol (Chloromycetin)	**Oral, IV:** *Adults,* 50 mg/kg/day in divided doses q6h for most indications (e.g., typhoid fever, rickettsial infections); 100 mg/kg/day in divided doses q6h for meningitis and brain abscess. *Children,* 50–75 mg/kg daily in divided doses q6h for most indications; 75–100 mg/kg daily in divided doses q6h for meningitis *Neonates: > 7 days weighing > 2 kg,* 50 mg/kg/day in divided doses q12 h; *< 7 days weighing > 2 kg,* 25 mg/kg od; *1.2–2 kg,* 25 mg/kg od; *< 1.2 kg,* 22 mg/kg od In pts with impaired hepatic function, dosage reductions may be necessary. Clear guidelines are not available and, ideally, serum concentrations should be monitored. In adults, an initial loading dose of 1 g followed by 500 mg q6h has been suggested	• If agency policy allows, may be given by direct IV over 1 min. May be given intermittently over 30–60 min. Consult manufacturer's instructions for preparation; do not use cloudy solutions. Check site for phlebitis. Give oral dose with full glass of water without food. May cause false-positive Clinitest®; use alternative to test urine glucose. Serum concentrations of chloramphenicol should be monitored periodically for patients of all ages
vancomycin HCl (Vancocin, Vancoled)	**IV:** *Adults of average size with normal renal function:* 1 g (15 mg/kg) q12h (preferred) or 500 mg (6.5–8 mg/kg) q6h. Monitor serum concentrations in the elderly. In severely ill patients, 1 g may be given q8h for 2–3 days until the infection is under control. Intrathecal administration also may be necessary in CNS infections. Morbidly obese patients may require higher doses, which should be based on total body weight, creatinine clearance and measurement of serum concentrations *Children/infants > than 1 month with normal renal function:* 40 mg/kg daily given in 4 divided doses. Larger doses (e.g., 60 mg/kg daily in 4 divided doses) may be required in patients with CNS infections; intrathecal administration also may be necessary (see below) *Infants 8 days to 1 month with normal renal function:* Initially, 15 mg/kg followed by 10 mg/kg q8h. *Infants 0–7 days with normal renal function:* Initially, 15 mg/kg followed by 10 mg/kg q12h. Monitor serum vancomycin concentrations in neonates	• Follow manufacturer's instructions to prepare; administer IV infusion over 60 min. Monitor carefully for extravasation, as severe necrosis can result. Do not give IM. To give by N/G tube, dilute IV dosage form

Table 17.8 (continued)
Miscellaneous antibiotics and antibacterials: Drug doses

Drug Generic name (Trade names)	Dosage	Nursing alert
vancomycin (Vancocin, Vancoled) (cont'd)	Pts with impaired renal function must receive reduced dosages; monitor peak and trough vancomycin serum concentrations to achieve peak concentrations of 30–40 µg/mL and trough concentrations between 5–10 µg/mL **Intrathecal:** *Adults:* 20 mg/day. *Neonates/ children:* 5–20 mg/day. If intraventricular instillation is employed, initial dose should not exceed 5 mg. Monitor CSF vancomycin concentrations to ensure levels are adequate but not excessive. See product insert for instructions on preparing vancomycin solutions for intrathecal use **Oral:** *Adults:* 125–500 mg q6h. The lower dose is effective for most cases of confirmed pseudomembranous colitis caused by *C. difficile. Children:* 50 mg/kg/day in divided doses q6h (max., 2 g/day)	
nitrofurantoin monohydrate (Macrobid)	**Oral:** *Adults/children > 12 years:* 100 mg q12h for 7 days. Tx for acute UTI should be continued for 7 days or for at least 3 days after sterility of the urine is observed	• Give with food or milk q12h. May cause false-positive glucose with Clinitest®
nitrofurantoin macrocrystals (Macrodantin)	**Oral:** *Adults:* 50–100 mg qid. *Children:* 5–7 mg/kg/24 h, given in divided doses qid. Tx should be continued for at least 1 week or for at least 3 days after sterility of the urine is obtained	• Give with food or milk to minimize GI upset
imipenem plus cilastatin sodium (Primaxin)	**IV:** *Adults:* Mild infections, 250 mg q6h. Moderate infections, 500 mg q8h. Severe (fully susceptible) infections, 500 mg q6h. Severe infections due to less-susceptible organisms, 1000 mg q8h. Life-threatening conditions, 1000 mg q6h	• Consult manufacturer's instructions for reconstitution. Doses < 500 mg may be given over 20–30 min; doses of 1 g should be given over 40–60 min. Do not give direct IV. Give by IV infusion only

Further Reading

The choice of antibacterial drugs. *Medical Letter on Drugs and Therapeutics* 1994;36:919–925.

Handbook of antimicrobial therapy. *Medical Letter on Drugs and Therapeutics* 1992.

Miscellaneous antibacterial drugs. *AMA Drug Evaluation Subscriptions* 1993; 2. Systemic anti-infectives:9.1–9.23.

Other beta-lactam antimicrobial agents. *AMA Drug Evaluation Subscriptions* 1992; 2. Systemic anti-infectives:3.8–3.12.

Tetracyclines and chloramphenicol. *AMA Drug Evaluation Subscriptions* 1993; 2. Systemic anti-infectives:5:11–5.18.

Antitubercular Drugs

Topics Discussed
- Treatment of tuberculosis
- Drugs of first choice
- Alternative drugs
- Mechanisms of action
- Pharmacokinetics
- Antibacterial spectra
- Therapeutic uses
- Adverse effects
- Nursing management

Drugs Discussed
aminosalicylic acid (a-meen-oh-sal-i-**sill**-ik)
capreomycin (kap-ree-oh-**mye**-sin)
cycloserine (sye-kloe-**seer**-een)
ethambutol (e-**tham**-byoo-tole)
isoniazid (eye-soe-**nye**-a-zid)
pyrazinamide (peer-a-**zin**-a-mide)
rifampin (rif-**am**-pin)
streptomycin (strep-toe-**mye**-sin)

Clinical Challenge

Consider this clinical challenge as you read through this chapter. The response to the challenge appears on page 176.

Jerry is a 21-year-old college student who has just returned from an extensive trip across Canada and some European countries. He travelled by bus, train and plane and stayed in many hostels. A travelling companion has just been diagnosed with TB, and Jerry is given a skin test with PPD which reads positive after 72 h.

A definitive diagnosis is made by chest X-ray and sputum for culture and sensitivity. Jerry has a nonresistant form of *Mycobacterium tuberculosis* and is placed on a 6-month course of therapy. For the initial phase (2 months) he must take isoniazid, rifampin and pyrazinamide daily. The physician also orders pyridoxine. Jerry undergoes several other tests prior to beginning drug therapy and asks many questions about the tests and the drugs.

1. How is a skin test with PPD done, and what does it indicate?
2. What is the rationale for each drug?
3. What tests will be done prior to initiating drug therapy, and why?
4. Two weeks after therapy begins, Jerry visits the TB clinic. What tests and observations will be made at this time to determine his response to drug therapy?

Tuberculosis (TB) is caused by *Mycobacterium tuberculosis*. This bacillus can remain dormant in the human host for years. Tuberculosis has been a major public health problem since the industrial revolution, when poor living and working conditions favoured its spread. Beginning in the late 1940s and early 1950s, effective drug treatment appeared to have defeated tuberculosis. However, the last ten years have seen a major resurgence in the disease, and today TB is the most common cause of death from a single infectious agent in the world. Approximately ten million people in the United States are asymptomatically infected with tubercle bacilli. Since 1990, approximately 25 000 new cases of tuberculosis and 2000 deaths annually have been reported in the United States.

Two major reasons explain the return of tuberculosis: the epidemic of human immunodeficiency virus (HIV) and the transmission of multiple-drug resistant (MDR) strains of tuberculosis. HIV infection is the most important risk factor to reactivation of latent tuberculosis and progression to active disease. Tuberculosis is one of the most common opportunistic infections affecting AIDS patients worldwide. Nearly fifty percent of HIV-seropositive individuals in Africa are infected with the tubercle bacillus.

The appearance of multiple-drug resistance compounds the problem of treating tuberculosis. At a time when we have more immunocompromised patients susceptible to the disease, we find that the drugs that worked well in the past are often not effective now. Outbreaks of multiple-drug resistant tuberculosis were reported before AIDS appeared on the scene, but these were isolated events. However, in the 1980s reports were received from various parts of the world about outbreaks of multiple-drug resistant TB in non-HIV-infected, immunocompetent individuals. These reports are ominous, for they predict the future difficulties we may face in treating tuberculosis. The problem of multiple-drug resistant TB, together with the increasing number of HIV-infected individuals who are at particular risk for infection with *M. tuberculosis,* must be faced in the immediate future if we are to treat a disease we previously considered to be well controlled.

Treatment of Tuberculosis

Two main principles govern the treatment of tuberculosis. First, patients must be treated with two or more drugs to prevent the emergence of resistant strains, which occur naturally. Second, treatment must be continued for long enough to sterilize the lesions and prevent relapse. Because of the slow growth rate of *M. tuberculosis* and its intracellular location, drug administration must be used for a longer period of time than is usual in other infectious disease.

Antituberculous drugs are classed into first-line agents and alternative drugs on the basis of their efficacy, activity and risk for adverse reactions. First-line drugs include isoniazid, rifampin, ethambutol and pyrazinamide. Their pharmacologic properties and therapeutic uses are discussed in this chapter, together with those of the alternative drugs streptomycin, aminosalicylic acid, cycloserine and capreomycin. Alternative drugs are indicated only when the *M. tuberculosis* is resistant to the first-line agents.

The current recommended treatment for pulmonary tuberculosis is a six-month regimen of isoniazid, rifampin and pyrazinamide for two months, followed by isoniazid and rifampin for four months. When isoniazid resistance is suspected, ethambutol should be added. A nine-month regimen of isoniazid and rifampin, following an initial two-week period of added ethambutol, is also effective.

Drugs of First Choice

Isoniazid (INH®, Nydrazid®)

Mechanism of action. The mechanism of action of isoniazid is not known. It is speculated that the drug blocks the synthesis of mycolic acids by *Mycobacterium tuberculosis*. These acids are normal constituents of the bacterial cell wall. In their absence, the integrity of the cell wall is reduced, and cell death occurs. Lower concentrations of isoniazid are bacteriostatic; higher levels are bactericidal.

Pharmacokinetics. Isoniazid is rapidly absorbed from the gastrointestinal tract and distributed throughout the body. Antacids reduce

Figure 18.1
Distribution of the isoniazid (INH) half-lives in 336 experimental subjects

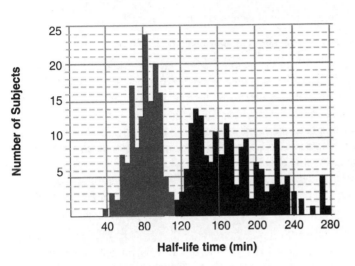

Figure 18.2
Serum isoniazid (INH) levels of 341 subjects at 180 min after IV injection of 5 mg/kg of INH

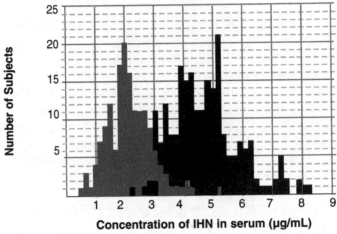

Source for both figures: Tiitinen H. Isoniazid and ethionamide serum levels and inactivation in Finnish subjects. *Scand J Resp Dis* 1969;50:110–124. Reproduced with permission.

Colour columns refer to 143 rapid inactivators grouped according to their INH half-lives; black columns refer to 198 slow inactivators.

peak serum levels of the drug. Substantial concentrations of isoniazid are found in pleural effusions and the cerebrospinal fluid. Isoniazid crosses the placenta and can also be found in breast milk in concentrations equivalent to those in plasma.

Isoniazid is inactivated by acetylation. Patients can be characterized as either slow or rapid metabolizers of the drug. Approximately sixty percent of North Americans are slow acetylators and should receive lower doses of isoniazid. Rapid acetylators require more frequent dosing. (Approximately eighty percent of Chinese, Japanese and Inuit are fast acetylators.) Figures 18.1 and 18.2 present the bimodal distribution in isoniazid metabolism and its effects on drug concentration in human serum.

Antibacterial spectrum. The clinical usefulness of isoniazid is limited to the eradication of *Mycobacterium tuberculosis* and some atypical mycobacterial infections. Organisms of other generae and fungi are not affected unless extremely high concentrations of isoniazid are present. Unfortunately, *M. tuberculosis* can become resistant to this drug.

Therapeutic uses. Isoniazid is one of the safest and most effective drugs for the treatment

of tuberculosis. Its ability to reach high concentrations in all body fluids, including the cerebrospinal fluid, combined with its antibacterial activity, makes it appropriate for the treatment of all types of TB infections. Isoniazid is included in first-line drug combinations. It is also considered a drug of choice when single-agent treatment is used prophylactically in patients who show positive skin reactions, but who are otherwise radiographically or clinically negative.

Table 18.1 on the next page lists the clinically significant drug interactions with isoniazid.

Adverse effects. In spite of its wide acceptance, isoniazid can adversely affect both the central and peripheral nervous systems. Its most frequent adverse effect is a dose-related peripheral neuritis, characterized by numbness and tingling in the lower extremities. This is seen most often in undernourished or alcoholic patients or in slow acetylators. If the drug is withdrawn soon after the onset of the symptoms, the adverse effects usually reverse rapidly. However, if therapy is continued in the face of patient complaints, residual problems may persist for up to one year following cessation of treatment. The routine use of 15 to 50 mg/day of pyridoxine has been recommended to prevent

Table 18.1
Isoniazid: Drug interactions

Drug	Interaction
Acetaminophen	• Concurrent use of acetaminophen may increase the potential for hepatotoxicity and nephrotoxicity
Antacids	• Antacids containing aluminum may inhibit the absorption of isoniazid from the GI tract
Disulfiram	• Disulfiram plus isoniazid can produce behavioural changes (e.g., psychotic reactions)
Drugs interacting strongly with cytochrome P450	• Isoniazid modifies the actions of cytochrome P450, and drugs that affect or are affected by this cytochrome may have their effects modified by isoniazid. Isoniazid inhibits the metabolism of phenytoin, increasing phenytoin plasma levels. The concomitant use of isoniazid with oral anticoagulants (i.e., coumarin and indandione derivatives) may result in enhanced anticoagulant effect due to the inhibition of the enzymatic metabolism of anticoagulants. Isoniazid may decrease the hepatic metabolism of benzodiazepines. It may also decrease the metabolism and increase the plasma concentrations of theophylline. Inducers of cytochrome P450 (e.g., carbamazepine, rifampin, phenobarbital, primidone, alcohol) may increase the formation of hepatotoxic metabolites of isoniazid and the subsequent risk for hepatitis and/or hepatic necrosis. The concurrent use of prednisolone and possibly other adrenal corticosteroids may increase the hepatic metabolism and/or excretion of isoniazid, decreasing its plasma concentrations and effectiveness, especially in fast acetylators
Food	• Isoniazid is closely related chemically to the monoamine oxidase inhibitors (MAOIs). Ingestion of certain fish (e.g., smoked or pickled fish, skipjack tuna, sardines) or cheese (e.g., Parmesan) may induce a typical tyramine syndrome of palpitations, severe general flushing, conjunctival injection, headache, dyspnea, tightness of the chest, tachypnea and sweating. The reaction is thought to be due to the inhibition of plasma MAO and diamine oxidase by isoniazid, thus interfering with the metabolism of tyramine and histamine found in fish and cheese
Ketokonazole and miconazole	• Use of ketoconazole and miconazole may increase the potential for isoniazid hepatotoxicity

---

peripheral neuritis, increased to 100 to 300 mg daily in patients with pre-existing neuritis.

The central nervous system adverse effects include symptoms of excitability, extending from irritability and restlessness to seizures. Hyperglycemia, metabolic acidosis and seizures can occur following isoniazid overdosage, and death or prolonged coma has occurred from persistent seizures, even when conventional doses have been given. The drug should be used with caution in patients with a known history of seizures.

Allergic reactions to isoniazid include fever and skin rashes. It can also cause a syndrome similar to systemic lupus erythematosus.

Isoniazid causes subclinical hepatic injury, with abnormal serum transaminase (AST) and bilirubin values, in ten to twenty percent of patients. Although most patients can continue to take the drug and apparently recover, a few progress to clinically overt hepatitis. There does not appear to be a correlation between plasma isoniazid concentrations and drug-induced hepatotoxicity. Its incidence increases with age, being uncommon in patients under thirty-five.

Rifampin (Rifadin®, Rimactane®)

Mechanism of action and antibacterial spectrum. Rifampin forms a stable complex with DNA-dependent RNA polymerase to inhibit RNA synthesis. It is effective against most gram-positive bacteria, as well as many gram-negative microbes, such as *Escherichia coli, Pseudomonas,* indole-positive and indole-negative *Proteus* and *Klebsiella.* It is particularly effective and bactericidal against *Mycobacterium tuberculosis.* Rifampin also increases the in vitro activity of streptomycin and isoniazid against *M. tuberculosis.*

Pharmacokinetics. Rifampin is well absorbed when taken orally. Maximum serum

Table 18.2
Rifampin: Drug interactions

Drug	Interaction
Aminosalicylic acid (PAS)	• Aminosalicylic acid can reduce rifampin absorption
Anticoagulants, antidiabetics, contraceptives, corticosteroids, digitalis, narcotics	• Rifampin increases the metabolism of many drugs that are metabolized by cytochrome P450. The metabolism of oral anticoagulants, oral antidiabetic drugs, beta blockers, chloramphenicol, ciprofloxacin, clofibrate, oral contraceptives, corticosteroids, cyclosporine, diazepam, digoxin, digitoxin, diltiazem, disopyramide, glucocorticoids, haloperidol, narcotics, mexiletine, nifedipine, phenytoin and other anticonvulsants, progestins, quinidine, theophylline and verapamil can be increased by rifampin
Fluconazole	• The plasma concentrations of fluconazole may be lowered when this drug is used with rifampin. The dose may need to be increased
Halothane	• Halothane plus rifampin can result in increased risk for hepatotoxicity
Isoniazid	• Isoniazid plus rifampin increases the risk for hepatotoxicity
Ketoconazole	• When rifampin and ketoconazole are used together, the serum concentrations of both drugs may be lower
Probenecid	• Probenecid can increase the blood levels of rifampin
Trimethoprim	• Use of trimethoprim with rifampin may significantly increase the elimination of trimethoprim and shorten its elimination half-life

concentrations are seen within two to three hours. Its absorption is reduced if the drug is taken immediately following a meal or together with aminosalicylic acid. Once absorbed, rifampin distributes widely in body tissue and fluids, reaching therapeutic levels in the cerebrospinal and pleural fluids. Rifampin is metabolized in the liver and excreted in the bile. Its metabolite is biologically active. Some unaltered drug is reabsorbed from the gastrointestinal tract following biliary excretion.

Therapeutic uses. Resistance develops readily if rifampin is used alone. Thus, it is always used together with other agents for the treatment of tuberculosis. In combination with isoniazid or isoniazid and ethambutol, rifampin is effective in the initial treatment of moderate and advanced pulmonary tuberculosis. Rifampin should also be included in retreatment protocols for patients who have not received the drug during their initial therapy. It is also useful in treating extrapulmonary TB, including miliary tuberculosis and tuberculosis meningitis. Rifampin alone is used for preventive therapy as an alternative to isoniazid in patients who cannot tolerate the latter drug or

who have a high probability of contact with an isoniazid-resistant strain.

Rifampin can be included in the treatment of *Mycobacterium leprae*. Its efficacy is increased by concomitant use of dapsone (Avlosulfon®). Rifampin can also be used for short-term treatment of meningococcal carriers, but resistance can develop quickly, even when treatment is only two to three weeks. Because of this, rifampin is not usually used to treat clinical infections.

Table 18.2 lists the clinically significant drug interactions with rifampin.

Adverse effects. The most common adverse effects of rifampin are gastrointestinal disturbances and nervous system complaints characterized by drowsiness, ataxia, dizziness, headache and fatigue. Liver damage is the most serious adverse effect.

The dosage interval is important with rifampin. If used once or twice weekly, as opposed to daily, it is more likely to produce fever, chills, aches, nausea and vomiting. Immune thrombocytopenia and hemolytic anemia, as well as acute renal failure, have also been reported in patients receiving intermittent therapy.

Table 18.3
Ethambutol: Drug interactions

Drug	Interaction
Rifampin	• Rifampin may increase the rate of elimination of ethambutol

Rifampin causes a reddish discoloration to all body secretions and excretions (e.g., saliva, tears, perspiration, sputum, feces and urine).

Rifampin is a potent inducer of hepatic cytochrome P450 enzymes and has produced clinically important interactions with many drugs (Table 18.2).

Ethambutol (Myambutol®)

Mechanism of action, pharmacokinetics and therapeutic uses. Ethambutol interferes with protein metabolism in *Mycobacterium tuberculosis*. The drug is rapidly absorbed from the gastrointestinal tract. In patients with tuberculous meningitis, it enters the cerebrospinal fluid in therapeutic levels. Ethambutol is eliminated primarily by renal excretion and has a half-life of three hours in patients with normal kidney function. Its dose should be reduced in patients with renal impairment.

Resistance builds quickly if ethambutol is used alone. Therefore, it is used as an adjunct to isoniazid and rifampin. Ethambutol is used in short-course chemotherapy when resistance to isoniazid or rifampin is suspected. In retreatment and cases of primary resistance, ethambutol is of great value when combined with other effective antitubercular drugs.

Adverse effects. Generally, ethambutol is well tolerated. Its major adverse effect is unilateral or bilateral retrobulbar neuritis. Occurring after two or more months of treatment, this most commonly involves the central fibres of the optic nerve and is characterized by a loss of central vision and disturbances in colour discrimination. Less often, the peripheral fibres of the optic nerve are affected, in which case there may be a constriction of the peripheral fields of vision with no loss of visual acuity. These effects are usually reversible if the drug is withdrawn. Nevertheless, patients should have a complete ophthalmologic examination before therapy is instituted to establish an accu-rate baseline for future reference. Because of difficulty in evaluating visual function in children, ethambutol is recommended only for adults.

Ethambutol can produce occasional mild gastrointestinal upset and allergic reactions, which include dermatitis, pruritus and, very rarely, anaphylaxis. The drug can also produce dizziness, mental confusion, fever, malaise and headache. Ethambutol can interfere with uric acid excretion. The precipitation of acute gout has been reported following its administration. Peripheral neuritis has been rarely reported.

Table 18.3 lists the clinically significant drug interactions with ethambutol.

Pyrazinamide

Pharmacokinetics. Pyrazinamide is an analogue of nicotinamide. Its mechanism of action is not known. It is absorbed from the gastrointestinal tract and distributed widely in body tissues. The drug also penetrates macrophages and tuberculous cavities. Pyrazinamide is metabolized in the body to pyrazinoic acid, and this metabolite appears to be responsible for the hyperurecemic effect of pyrazinamide. Renal glomerular filtration serves as the major excretory pathway for pyrazinamide and its metabolites. The half-life of pyrazinamide is nine to ten hours.

Therapeutic uses. When given with isoniazid, pyrazinamide is effective against resistant strains of *M. tuberculosis*. In the past, pyrazinamide has been only sparingly used in Western Europe and North America. Despite its clinical efficacy, concern over its hepatic toxicity (see Adverse Effects) relegated it to alternative drug status. However, its potent tuberculocidal activity has resulted in a reassessment of its value as shorter regimens for the treatment of TB have become recommended. In addition, reducing pyrazinamide's dose decreased its toxicity. As a result, pyrazinamide is now considered a first-line drug in the treatment of tuberculous. One definite advantage to this drug is that it is relatively inexpensive.

Pyrazinamide is now used in combination with drugs such as isoniazid, rifampin and ethambutol for the abbreviated (i.e., six to nine months) treatment of tuberculosis. Pyrazinamide can also be given on an intermittent basis, once or twice a week, and still produce acceptable cure rates.

Adverse effects. Pyrazinamide can be hepatotoxic; this effect appears to be dose related. When the drug was originally studied, it became apparent that 3 g/day was effective when given with isoniazid in the initial treatment of tuberculosis. However, this dose produced a fourteen percent incidence of hepatotoxicity and at least one death. This led to the abandonment of pyrazinamide as a first-line drug for the treatment of tuberculosis. Reducing the daily dose from 40 to 70 mg/kg to 15 to 30 mg/kg decreased the risk for hepatotoxicity, while maintaining its clinical efficacy.

Hyperuricemia has been reported in all patients receiving pyrazinamide, and clinical gout has occurred in some. Pyrazinamide-induced gout does not respond to uricosuric treatment with probenecid. Acetylsalicylic acid (ASA), in doses of 2.3 g/day, reverses the hyperuricemic effect of pyrazinamide.

Alternative Drugs

Streptomycin

Mechanism of action and therapeutic uses. Streptomycin is an aminoglycoside antibiotic (see Chapter 14). It is bactericidal, principally for extracellular (including cavitary) tubercle bacilli. This action is likely due to a direct action of the drug on the bacterial ribosome to inhibit protein synthesis. Streptomycin is not absorbed from the gastrointestinal tract and therefore must be injected intramuscularly.

The greatest value of streptomycin is in the early weeks or months of therapy when it appears to enhance the effects of the oral agents. The combination of intramuscular streptomycin and isoniazid has an immediate, marked, suppressive effect on susceptible organisms that has often been life-saving in critical situations. Streptomycin is also useful in intermittent therapy. It should be discontinued when the sputum becomes negative.

Adverse effects. The adverse effects of streptomycin include ototoxicity and nephrotoxicity. (The adverse effects of the aminoglycoside antibiotics, together with their drug interactions, are presented in Chapter 14. Although streptomycin is not specifically included there, the discussion in Chapter 14 is general for this group of antibiotics and applies also for streptomycin.)

Aminosalicylic Acid, PAS (Parasal Sodium®, Teebacin Acid®)

Mechanism of action and therapeutic uses. Aminosalicylic acid (or PAS, as it is often called) is structurally similar to para-aminobenzoic acid (PABA). By acting as an antimetabolite of the latter compound, PAS prevents the utilization of PABA in the synthesis of folic acid by *Mycobacterium tuberculosis*.

PAS is indicated for the treatment of active pulmonary and extrapulmonary tuberculosis when the infecting organisms are known or strongly suspected to be susceptible to the drug and resistant to the first-line drugs. PAS is much less effective than other antituberculous drugs. When used alone, its antimycobacterial effect is scarcely discernible, and bacterial resistance develops rapidly. When included in a regimen with isoniazid and rifampin, PAS may delay the development of resistance to these drugs.

Table 18.4 on the next page lists the clinically significant drug interactions with aminosalicylic acid (PAS).

Adverse effects. Gastrointestinal irritation, sometimes leading to bleeding, is the most common adverse effect of aminosalicylic acid. The drug is used with caution when treating ulcer patients. Aminosalicylic acid can produce allergic reactions, including fever, rash, pruritus and hepatotoxicity. PAS should be used with caution in patients with renal or cardiac failure because larger doses of the sodium salt can cause sodium overload and fluid retention.

Capreomycin (Capastat®)

Capreomycin is a polypeptide antibiotic isolated from a species of Streptomyces. It is only rarely used in the treatment of tuberculosis.

Table 18.4
Aminosalicylic acid (PAS): Drug interactions

Drug	Interaction
Anticoagulants, oral	• Oral anticoagulants may require dosage adjustment in the presence of PAS
Diphenhydramine	• Diphenhydramine may impair the absorption of PAS
Para-aminobenzoic acid (PABA)	• PABA may reduce or block the effects of PAS
Probenecid	• Probenecid inhibits the renal excretion of PAS
Rifampin	• PAS can reduce the absorption of rifampin

Capreomycin is indicated in pulmonary infections caused by susceptible strains when the primary drugs (isoniazid, streptomycin, ethambutol, pyrazinamide and rifampin) cannot be used because of toxicity or the presence of resistant bacilli. If capreomycin is used alone, resistance develops rapidly. Capreomycin is usually reserved for retreatment programs when parenteral therapy is indicated.

Capreomycin is both ototoxic and nephrotoxic. It should not be used with other antibiotics with similar properties.

Table 18.5 lists the clinically significant drug interactions with capreomycin.

Cycloserine (Seromycin®)

Mechanism of action and therapeutic uses. Cycloserine is structurally similar to alanine, and competes with alanine to prevent cell wall formation by *Mycobacterium tuberculosis*. Cylcoserine is a broad-spectrum antibiotic. It is effective against *M. tuberculosis,* as well as both gram-positive and gram-negative bacteria. Cycloserine, administered orally, is an effective antimycobacterial drug if patients can tolerate it. It is indicated for the treatment of active pulmonary and extrapulmonary tuberculosis caused by susceptible strains, but is used only when treatment with the primary antituberculous drugs (isoniazid, ethambutol, rifampin, pyrazinamide, streptomycin) has proven inadequate.

Adverse effects. The limiting factor in the use of cycloserine is its central nervous system toxicity. Appearing within a few weeks of starting the drug, the effects include headache, tremor, dysarthria, vertigo, confusion, somnolence, nervousness, irritability and psychotic states. Patients may also demonstrate catatonic and depressed reactions, hyperreflexia, visual disturbances and grand mal seizures or absence attacks. These usually disappear if the drug is stopped.

Table 18.6 lists the clinically significant drug interactions with cycloserine.

Nursing Management

Table 18.7 gives the nursing management of the patient receiving antitubercular drugs. Table 18.8 (page 174) summarizes the monitoring of adverse reactions to antitubercular drugs and Table 18.9 (pages 175–176) lists the dosages of all drugs discussed in this chapter.

Table 18.5
Capreomycin: Drug interactions

Drug	Interaction
Polymyxin B, colistin, aminoglycosides, vancomycin	• These drugs plus capreomycin may have additive toxicities on the eight cranial nerves or on peripheral neuromuscular function

Table 18.6
Cycloserine: Drug interactions

Drug	Interaction
Alcohol	• Alcohol increases the risk of epileptic seizures occurring with cycloserine
Ethionamide	• Ethionamide and cycloserine have additive CNS toxicity
Isoniazid	• Isoniazid and cycloserine have additive CNS toxicity

Table 18.7
Nursing management for the antitubercular drugs

Assessment of risk vs. benefit	Patient data	• *History:* Physician should determine any contraindications such as acute liver disease or active gout and precautions such as alcohol abuse, malnutrition, diabetes or renal impairment that may affect half-life. Baseline lab tests of liver function (e.g., AST, ALT and serum bilirubin) • Assess to establish baseline VS, general state of health, clinical indicators of present infection • Pregnancy: Risk category C (animal studies show adverse effects to fetus but human data are unknown or insufficient); benefits may be acceptable despite the risks • Geriatric pts: At greater risk for hepatotoxicity, peripheral neuritis
	Drug data	• Select drugs based on culture and sensitivity results. Combinations are used to reduce incidence of resistance • Some serious drug interactions: Confer with pharmacist Most serious adverse reactions are outlined in Table 18.8 with monitoring parameters
Implementation	Rights of administration	• Using the "rights" helps prevent errors of administration
	Right route	• Usually given PO, but isoniazid can be given IM and rifampin IV
	Right time	• Dosage schedule varies with drug and with reason and phase of treatment; may be daily or biweekly
	Right technique	• IV administration requires knowledge of correct diluent and IV solution, correct dilution and rate of administration. Always refer to manufacturer's instructions for this route
	Nursing therapeutics	• Assess individuals having immediate contact with patient (family, other patients, caregivers). May include tuberculin skin test with purified protein derivative (PPD). (Refer to agency procedure for correct technique and interpretation of test.) • Enhance host defences (nutrition, rest, fluids, hygiene) • Emotional support: Long-term tx can be discouraging; some pts may also have HIV • Universal precautions to prevent spread of infection (including self-care for caregivers)

(cont'd on next page)

Table 18.7 (continued)
Nursing management for the antitubercular drugs

Implementation (cont'd)	Patient/family teaching	• Educate for proper use of anti-infectives (Chapter 9) • Pt's need for information may be influenced by length of time required for tx or limited by serious illness • Compliance and follow-up are essential factors in successful tx: review principles of patient education (Chapter 3) • Pts/families should know warning signs/symptoms of the possible toxicities of drugs (see Table 18.8) • Warn pts to avoid alcohol (increases risk for hepatotoxicity) • Discuss possibility of pregnancy: Advise pt to notify physician and discuss birth control methods; oral contraceptives may not be effective if taking rifampin *Specific points related to drugs:* • Rifampin causes a reddish discoloration to all body secretions and excretions (saliva, tears, perspiration, sputum, feces and urine); may permanently stain soft contact lenses
Outcomes	Monitoring of progress	*Continually monitor:* • Clinical response indicating tx success (reduction in signs/symptoms) • Be alert for signs/symptoms of adverse reactions; document and report immediately to physician

Table 18.8
Monitoring adverse reactions to antitubercular drugs

Adverse reaction	Drug	Observations
Hepatotoxicity	isoniazid rifampin pyrazinamide	• Baseline liver function tests (e.g., ALT, AST, bilirubin) • Frequent monitoring of liver enzymes (every 2–4 weeks). Minor elevations may be acceptable; significant elevations require discontinuation of drug • Clinical symptoms (nausea, anorexia, fatigue, malaise, jaundice, dark urine)
Peripheral neuritis	isoniazid	• Tingling, numbness, burning pain in hands or feet
Optic neuritis	ethambutol	• Baseline ophthalmic exam • Clinical symptoms: blurred vision, reduced visual field, reduced colour discrimination (esp, red and green)
Ototoxicity **Nephrotoxicity**	streptomycin capreomycin	• Review in Chapter 14
CNS toxicity	cycloserine	• Headache, tremor, vertigo, confusion, irritability, psychotic states

Table 18.9
The antituberculars: Drug doses

Drug Generic name (Trade names)	Dosage	Nursing alert
A. First-Line Drugs		
ethambutol HCl (Myambutol)	**Oral:** *Adults/children ≥ 13 years:* Initially, in pts who have not received previous anti-TB tx, 15 mg/kg as single oral dose q24h. Retreatment in patients who have received previous anti-TB treatment, 25 mg/kg as single oral dose q24h. Concurrently administer at least one other anti-TB drug. After 60 days of ethambutol administration, decrease dose to 15 mg/kg and give as single oral dose q24h	• Give at same time each day with food or milk to reduce GI irritation
isoniazid (INH, Nydrazid)	**Oral/IM:** *Adults:* For prophylaxis, 300 mg/day in a single dose. For tx of active TB, 5 mg/kg od (max., 300 mg). For disseminated TB and pulmonary disease caused by atypical mycobacteria, 10–20 mg/kg/day. *Infants /children:* For active TB, 10–20 mg/kg/day. For preventative tx, 10 mg/kg/day (max. 300 mg/day) in 1 dose	• Best absorbed on empty stomach but may be taken with food to reduce GI upset, increase compliance • **IM:** Give deep into large muscle mass, massage well and rotate sites. Solutions crystallize at cool temperature; store at room temperature
pyrazinamide	**Oral:** *Adults/children:* 15–30 mg/kg daily in one or more doses (max., 2 g/day)	• Calculate doses carefully. Do not exceed maximum dose
rifampin (Rifadin, Rimactane)	**Oral:** *Adults:* 10 mg/kg/day or biweekly (max., 600 mg/day). *Children:* 10–20 mg/kg daily or biweekly (max., 600 mg/day). **IV:** *Adults:* Dosage is same as for oral preparation and should be reserved for pts who cannot take this drug PO	• The drug should be given in a single dose 1 h ac (usually breakfast) or 2 h pc • Important to give daily, not intermittently, to reduce adverse effects • Food may reduce GI irritation • Follow manufacturer's instructions for IV reconstitution. Administer 100 mL over 30 min and 500 mL over 3 h
B. Alternative Drugs		
aminosalicylic acid, PAS (Parasal Sodium)	**Oral:** *Adults:* Administer (with INH and/or streptomycin) 10–12 g/day in 2–3 divided doses. *Children:* 150–300 mg/kg/day in 3–4 divided doses, not to exceed adult dosage	• May be taken with food or pc to reduce GI disturbances or with aluminum hydroxide antacid gel. Deteriorates rapidly when exposed to moisture, heat and light • Store tabs in a light-proof and moisture-resistant container. Discard if brownish or purplish discoloration occurs

(cont'd on next page)

Table 18.9 (continued)
The antituberculars: Drug doses

Drug Generic name (Trade names)	Dosage	Nursing alert
capreomycin sulfate (Capastat)	**IM:** *Adults:* 15 mg/kg (approx. 1 g/day) for 2–4 months, followed by 1 g 2–3x/week for 6–12 months or longer prn. Most pts tolerate 1 g/day for 2–4 months and occasionally for as long as 6 months. Daily dose should not > 20 mg/kg	• Refer to manufacturer's instructions to reconstitute powder. Solution may change colour without loss of potency. Do not use if precipitate forms. • Administer deep into large muscle mass; aspirate to avoid inadvertent IV injection (can cause neuromuscular blockade). Rotate sites
cycloserine (Seromycin)	**Oral:** *Adults:* Initially, 250 mg bid q12h for the first 2 weeks. Can increase by 250 mg every few days (if tolerated) until tx serum levels are obtained. Usual dosage: 500 mg to 1 g (max.) daily in divided doses	• Monitor blood levels. Best results occur with peak serum concentrations of 25–30 µg/mL. Serum levels in excess of 30 µg/mL have been associated with toxicity and should be avoided. Blood used to determine serum drug concentrations should be drawn before pt's first dose of the day
streptomycin	**IM only:** *Adults:* 15 mg/kg/day (max. 1 g). *Children:* 20–30 mg/kg/day (max. 1 g). Total dose, not > 120 g	• Inject deeply into large muscle mass; rotate site. Draw blood for serum levels 30–60 min after IM infection. Peak levels: 5–25 µg/mL (5–25 mg/L). Trough: not > 5 µg/mL (5 mg/L)

Response to Clinical Challenge

Principles

Patient/family education is an essential component of successful treatment of TB. Regular follow-up visits for monitoring and compliance to dosage schedule can be promoted by effective education strategies. To achieve this goal, the nurse must have a thorough understanding of TB, the diagnostic tests used for the disease and for drug monitoring as well as competence in patient education. Brief answers are provided for each question posed in this clinical challenge; details are found in the chapter.

Actions

1. A skin test with PPD (purified protein derivative of the tubercle bacillus) is done by injection. It is interpreted in 48–72 h; an area of induration (hardness), not merely erythema (redness), indicates exposure to the bacillus.

2. Isoniazid, rifampin and pyrazinamide are ordered to eradicate the *Mycobacterium tuberculosis* and are given together to prevent development of resistance. Pyridoxine (vitamin B6) is given to prevent peripheral neuropathy from isoniazid. With his travelling, Jerry may presently be deficient in this vitamin, depending on his diet.

3. Skin test, chest X-ray, sputum specimen will be done for diagnosis. Liver function tests, general physical exam and VS are conducted for baseline. Discussion regarding alcohol use is important to determine risk.

4. Based on the known toxicities of these drugs, liver enzymes will be taken to determine hepatic effects, and Jerry will be asked for any new signs/symptoms that may indicate drug adverse reactions. He will also be asked questions regarding his compliance to the drug schedule and any difficulties he encounters in following this regime.

Further Reading

Antimycobacterial drugs. *AMA Drug Evaluations* 1994; 3. Miscellaneous anti-infectives:1.1–1.4.

Drugs for tuberculosis. *Medical Letter on Drugs and Therapeutics* 1993;35:906–912.

Handbook of antimicrobial therapy. *Medical Letter on Drugs and Therapeutics* 1992.

Mandel GL, Petri WA. Antimicrobial agents: drugs used in the chemotherapy of tuberculosis and leprosy. In: Hardman JL, Limbird LE, eds. *Goodman and Gilman's The Pharmacological Basis of Therapeutics*. 9th ed. New York: Pergamon; 1996:1155–1174.

CHAPTER 19

Drugs Used for Systemic Fungal Infections

Topics Discussed
- Pharmacotherapy of Fungal Diseases
- Mechanisms of action
- Pharmacokinetics
- Antifungal spectra
- Therapeutic uses
- Adverse effects
- Nursing management

Drugs Discussed
amphotericin B (am-foe-**ter**-ih-sin)
fluconazole (flew-**kon**-ah-zole)
flucytosine (flew-**sye**-toe-seen)
itraconazole (it-trah-**kon**-ah-zole)
ketoconazole (kee-toe-**kon**-ah-zole)

Clinical Challenge

Consider this clinical challenge as you read through this chapter. The response to the challenge appears on page 186.

A 31-year-old woman is admitted to hospital and diagnosed with a fungal infection. Treatment with ketoconazole is initiated. Her history indicates that she has been healthy except for a chronic sinus infection. She states that she uses oral contraceptives, occasional acetaminophen for headaches and terfenadine for the sinus problem. The following day she faints, without injury. Her BP is normal but her pulse is irregular. The physician is notified.

1. What is a possible explanation for the patient's fainting?
2. What actions on the part of the physician do you predict?
3. How could this episode have been prevented?

Pharmacotherapy of Fungal Diseases

Fungal diseases can be either superficial or systemic. Systemic infections constitute a major therapeutic problem and can have a significant fatality rate. Systemic "opportunistic infections" occur commonly in debilitated and immunosuppressed patients. They include candidiasis, aspergillosis, cryptococcosis and phycomycosis. Other systemic infections, including blastomycosis, coccidioidomycosis, histoplasmosis and sporotrichosis, occur less frequently.

This chapter discusses drugs used to treat systemic fungal infections. The treatment of fungal infections of the skin, hair, nails, gastrointestinal tract and vagina is discussed in Chapter 24.

The treatment of systemic fungal infections is unsatisfactory. At the present time only a limited number of drugs are available, and their use is often associated with severe adverse effects. In addition, patients with systemic mycotic infections may be very ill with other diseases. Antibiotics or antibacterials are used on occasion to treat systemic mycotic infections. Penicillin G, for example, can be given intravenously for the treatment of actinomycosis. Patients allergic to penicillin can be given erythromycin, a cephalosporin, a tetracycline or clindamycin. Sulfonamides are the drugs of choice for nocardiosis. If they cannot be used, ampicillin, erythromycin or a tetracycline may be given. The pharmacology of these drugs is presented elsewhere in this text and will not be repeated here.

Amphotericin B (Fungizone®)

Mechanism of Action
Amphotericin B is a fungistatic drug. It works by interacting with ergosterol, a fungal membrane sterol, to increase the membrane permeability of sensitive fungi. The result of this action is that small molecules leak from the cells and amino acid uptake is impaired.

Amphotericin B does not affect bacteria because, with the exception of *Mycoplasma,* sterols are not found in bacterial cell membranes. However, mammalian cell membranes contain sterols, and this partly explains amphotericin B's toxicity in humans.

Pharmacokinetics
Amphotericin B is poorly absorbed from the intestinal tract and must be administered intravenously to produce a systemic effect. After intravenous injection, the drug is rapidly concentrated in body tissues. Its initial half-life is twenty-four hours. However, because of its extensive storage in body tissues, amphotericin B has a second half-life of fifteen days as the drug is eliminated very slowly from its storage sites. Amphotericin B crosses the blood–brain barrier, but its concentration in the cerebral spinal fluid is lower than that found in blood.

The major route of excretion for amphotericin B is extrarenal; thus, a dosage adjustment is not needed for patients with impaired kidney function. About five percent of an amphotericin B dose is excreted daily as active drug. Amphotericin B can be found in urine for at least seven weeks after treatment is stopped.

Antifungal Spectrum
Amphotericin B is used to treat systemic infections caused by *Cryptococcus neoformans, Histoplasma capsulatum, Coccidioides immitis, Blastomyces dermatitidis* and *Sporothrix schenckii.*

Therapeutic Uses
Amphotericin B is a broad-spectrum antifungal drug used for the treatment of patients with progressive, potentially fatal disseminated mycotic infections. It can also be used to treat opportunistic infections in immunosuppressed patients caused by *Candida, Cryptococcus* and *Torulpsis.* Because the drug does not diffuse well into the cerebrospinal fluid, intrathecal administration may be required for central nervous system infections.

Adverse Effects
Amphotericin B must be used with considerable care. The most common early adverse effect is an acute febrile reaction beginning about two hours after starting the infusion and peaking approximately one hour later. An antipyretic, such as ASA, may reduce the fever.

A dose-dependent azotemia can also result from amphotericin B use. Although this is usually temporary, ceasing when the drug is stopped, permanent damage may be evident, particularly in patients with pre-existing renal impairment. More severe nephrotoxicity is manifested by hyponatremia, hypokalemia and renal tubular acidosis. If this occurs, the dose should be reduced, the patient hydrated, and serum electrolytes adjusted. Other nephrotoxic drugs should be discontinued. Renal function and serum electrolytes should be monitored twice weekly.

Reversible normocytic, normochromic anemia is common with prolonged therapy. Blood transfusion may be required.

Hypersensitivity reactions are not usual. However, amphotericin B can produce generalized pain, seizures and anaphylactic shock. The drug can also cause headache, fever, chills, anorexia and vomiting.

Table 19.1 on the next page lists the clinically significant drug interactions with amphotericin B.

Table 19.1
Amphotericin B: Drug interactions

Drug	Interaction
Aminoglycoside antibiotics	• Aminoglycoside antibiotics are nephrotoxic and should not be given with amphotericin B
Antibiotic and anti-neoplastic drugs	• Antibiotics and antineoplastics should be avoided if possible in pts receiving amphotericin B, because their use may result in deep fungal infections. Antineoplastics may also increase the risk of renal damage
Corticosteroids	• Corticosteroids may predispose pts to systemic fungal infections. Furthermore, they may enhance the potassium depletion produced by amphotericin B
Cyclosporine	• Cyclosporine and amphotericin B produce increased renal toxicity. Avoid concurrent use, if possible
Digitalis	• Digitalis toxicity is increased by hypokalemia. Amphotericin B may produce hypokalemia. Monitor potassium concentration
Skeletal muscle relaxants	• Skeletal muscle relaxants produce increased neuromuscular blockade because of hypokalemia. Monitor potassium concentration and neuromuscular status

Flucytosine (Ancotil®, Ancobon®)

Mechanism of Action

Flucytosine is fungistatic. It is a structural analogue of cytosine, an essential component in body functions. Flucytosine is taken up into fungal cells via cytosine permease. Once in the fungal cell, flucytosine is deaminated by fungal cytosine deaminase to form fluorouracil (5-FU) and fluorodeoxyuridine monophosphate. Fluorouracil is incorporated into fungal RNA and inhibits protein synthesis. It is probably the metabolite responsible for bone marrow depression. Fluorodeoxyuridine monophosphate inhibits DNA synthesis.

Pharmacokinetics

Flucytosine is well absorbed from the intestinal tract. The drug can be found in the serum thirty minutes after oral administration. Flucytosine is widely distributed in body fluids and readily crosses the blood–brain barrier to enter the cerebrospinal fluid. The drug is excreted primarily by the kidneys, and most of it can be found unchanged in the urine. Its dosage schedule must be modified in patients with impaired renal function. Flucytosine has a half-life of three to five hours.

Antifungal Spectrum

Flucytosine inhibits the growth of *Cryptococcus neoformas, Candida albicans, Torulopsis glabrata, Sporothrix schenckii, Cladosporium* species and *Phialophora* species, the fungi responsible for chromomycosis. Resistance has been reported to flucytosine. This may reflect a deficiency in the enzymes involved in the transport of the drug into the cytoplasm, or it may be due to a compensatory ability of the organism to increase its rate of pyrimidine synthesis.

Therapeutic Uses

Administered orally, flucytosine is given for the treatment of serious infections caused by susceptible strains of *Candida* or *Cryptococcus,* or both. Flucytosine passes easily into the cerebrospinal fluid and enters the aqueous humor and bronchial secretions in concentrations adequate to inhibit sensitive fungi. Septicemia, endocarditis and urinary tract infections caused by *Candida* have been treated effectively. Meningitis and pulmonary infections caused by *Cryptococcus* have also responded to flucytosine. Limited trials in patients with *Candida* pulmonary infections, *Cryptococcus septicemias* or cryptococcal urinary tract infections support the use of flucytosine in these conditions. Flucytosine also has been used in the treatment of chromomycosis caused by *Fonsecaea pedrosoi, Cladosporium carrioni* and *Philaphora verrucosa.*

Table 19.2
Flucytosine: Drug interactions

Drug	Interaction
Drugs that depress bone marrow	• Drugs that depress bone marrow may predispose patients to the bone marrow depressing effects of flucytosine
Drugs that reduce renal function	• Drugs known to reduce renal function (e.g., diuretics, aminoglycoside antibiotics, amphotericin B) should be used carefully because flucytosine is excreted primarily by the kidneys

Because resistance may develop to flucytosine during therapy, it is usually combined with amphotericin B. The administration of flucytosine often allows the use of lower doses of amphotericin B.

Adverse Effects

Reversible neutropenia, together with occasional thrombocytopenia, are the principal adverse effects of flucytosine. The drug can also cause nausea, eosinophilia and skin rashes. Flucytosine is capable of producing reversible hepatic dysfunction. Patients sometimes experience confusion, hallucinations, headache and vertigo. A few cases of irreversible bone marrow failure have been reported. Patients with a limited bone marrow reserve, such as individuals receiving cytotoxic drug treatment, may be prone to develop hematological adverse effects when treated with flucytosine.

Table 19.2 lists the clinically significant drug interactions with flucytosine.

Azole Antifungal Drugs

The azoles are an expanding group of antifungal drugs. They include the topical products clotrimazole, econazole, miconazole and terconazole, which are discussed in Chapter 24.

The current chapter discusses the azoles that are used systemically. These are ketoconazole (Nizoral®), fluconazole (Diflucan®) and itraconazole (Sporanox®). Ketoconazole is an imidazole because it has two nitrogens in the azole ring. Fluconazole and itraconazole have three nitrogens and are called triazoles. These structural differences may account for the differences in the adverse effects between ketoconazole and fluconazole or itraconazole.

Mechanism of Action

All azoles have the same mechanism of action: they bind to the heme iron of cytochrome P450 and inhibit the demethylation of 14-alpha-methylsterols to ergosterol. Ergosterol is the main sterol in the fungal cell membrane. The effect of this action is to alter the permeability of the fungal cell membrane. Both fluconazole and itraconazole have greater specificity for fungal cytochrome P450 than for the mammalian cytochrome. This may account for the relatively low toxicity of triazoles in clinical trials compared with the imidazoles.

Pharmacokinetics

Ketoconazole is well absorbed from the gastrointestinal tract. It is best absorbed in conditions of low pH. Histamine$_2$ (H$_2$) antagonists (e.g., cimetidine, famotidine, nizatidine and ranitidine) and antacids reduce ketoconazole absorption. Ketoconazole is distributed widely through the tissues and tissue fluids but does not reach therapeutic concentrations in the central nervous system unless high doses are given. The drug is inactivated in the liver and excreted in the bile and urine. Its half-life in plasma is eight hours.

Fluconazole is well absorbed and can be given orally or intravenously. Its oral bioavailability is over ninety percent. Fluconazole penetrates into all body tissues and fluids, and its apparent volume of distribution approximates that of the total body water. Its terminal plasma elimination half-life is approximately thirty hours. The long plasma elimination half-life provides the basis for once-daily dosing.

The pharmacokinetics of fluconazole do not appear to be affected by age alone, but are markedly affected by a reduction in renal function. There is an inverse relationship between the elimination half-life and creatinine clearance. Thus, the dose of fluconazole should be reduced in patients with impaired renal function.

Itraconazole, like ketoconazole, requires a low

gastric pH to be absorbed. The absorption of itraconazole is variable, with peak concentrations of 0.02 to 0.18 mg/L being measured following a 100-mg dose. Food enhances itraconazole absorption. Itraconazole's concentration is two to twenty times higher in lipophilic tissues than in plasma. The plasma half-life of itraconazole following a single dose is 15 h to 20 h, and 30 h to 35 h after multiple doses. Itraconazole is metabolized by the liver and excreted through the bile. A metabolite, hydroxyitraconazole, is active as an antifungal.

Antifungal Spectrum

Ketoconazole is effective against a variety of fungi and yeasts, including *Blastomyces dermatitidis, Candida, Coccidioides immitis, Histoplasma capsulatum* and dermatophytes.

Fluconazole has broad-spectrum activity. Animal models have shown it to be effective in the treatment of aspergillosis, blastomycosis, candidiasis, cryptococcosis and histoplasmosis.

Itraconazole has an antifungal spectrum similar to that of ketoconazole, except that it is also active against *Aspergillus* species and *Sporothrix schenckii*.

Therapeutic Uses

Ketoconazole is indicated for the treatment of serious life-threatening systemic fungal infections in normal, predisposed or immunocompromised patients for whom alternative therapy is considered inappropriate or has been unsuccessful. This includes systemic candidiasis, chronic mucocutaneous candidiasis, coccidioiodomycosis and paracoccidioiodomycosis, histoplasmosis and chromomycosis. Ketoconazole is not indicated in the treatment of fungal infections in CNS infections because it penetrates poorly into the central nervous system.

Fluconazole is approved for the treatment of oropharyngeal and esophageal candidiasis. It is also effective for the treatment of serious systemic candidal infections, including urinary tract infections (UTI), peritonitis and pneumonitis. Fluconazole is also indicated for the treatment of cryptococcal meningitis. The drug is used for the prevention of the recurrence of cryptococcal meningitis in patients with acquired immunodeficiency syndrome (AIDS). Oral fluconazole has also been approved for the treatment vaginal candidiasis. A single oral dose of fluconazole is at least as effective as intravaginal treatment of vulvovaginal candidiasis and is often preferred.

Itraconazole is indicated for the treatment of the following fungal infections in normal, predisposed or immunocompromised patients: invasive and noninvasive pulmonary aspergillosis; oral and oral/esophageal candidiasis; chronic pulmonary histoplasmosis; cutaneous and lymphatic sporotrichosis; paracoccidioidomycosis; chromomycosis; blastomycosis.

Adverse Effects

Ketoconazole's most common adverse effects are nausea and pruritus. Patients may also experience headache, dizziness, abdominal pain, constipation, diarrhea, somnolence and nervousness. Concern is greatest over the possible hepatotoxic effects of ketoconazole. Cases of fatal, massive hepatic necrosis have been reported. As previously stated, liver function should be monitored periodically and the drug stopped if signs of hepatocellular dysfunction appear. Ketoconazole can block adrenal steroid synthesis. Approximately ten percent of men on the drug experience gynecomastia.

Table 19.3 lists the clinically significant drug interactions with the azoles.

Cases of idosyncratic hepatocellular dysfunction have been reported during ketoconazole treatment. It is important to recognize that liver disorders can occur during therapy. These can be fatal unless properly recognized and managed. Liver function tests such as SGT, alkaline phosphatase, AST (SGOT), ALT (SGPT) and bilirubin should be performed before treatment and at periodic intervals during treatment (monthly or more often), particularly in patients who are expected to be on prolonged therapy or who have a history of significant alcohol consumption. Likewise, the concurrent use of ketoconazole with hepatotoxic drugs should be most carefully monitored, especially in these patients.

For fluconazole, the two most serious adverse effects noted during clinical trials were exfoliative skin disorders and hepatic necrosis. Because most patients had serious underlying diseases (AIDS or malignancy) and were receiving multiple concomitant medications, including many known to be hepatotoxic or associated with exfoliative skin disorders, the causal association of these reactions with fluconazole is uncertain.

Table 19.3
The azoles: Drug interactions

Drug	Interaction
Astemizole	• Ketoconazole inhibits the metabolism of astemizole, resulting in an increase in the plasma level of astemizole and its active metabolite. This can prolong QT intervals
Antacids, anticholinergics, H2 blockers, omeprazole	• Drugs that reduce gastric acid secretion or neutralize stomach acid may reduce the absorption of ketoconazole or itraconazole because their bioavailability depends on gastric acidity
Anticoagulants, oral	• Ketoconazole, itraconazole and fluconazole enhance the anticoagulant effect of warfarin. Monitor pts carefully
Cyclosporine	• Cyclosporine plasma concentrations may be increased by ketoconazole, fluconazole or itraconazole
Digoxin	• Digoxin plasma concentrations may be increased by itraconazole
Hydrochlorothiazide	• Hydrochorothiazide may increase fluconazole plasma levels
Isoniazid	• Plasma concentrations of azole antifungal drugs are reduced when given concurrently with isoniazid
Phenytoin	• Fluconazole can increase the AUC of phenytoin by up to 75%. Phenytoin can decrease the plasma concentrations of itraconazole
Rifampin	• Rifampin has been reported to decrease the plasma concentrations of ketoconazole, fluconazole and itraconazole
Sulfonylurea oral hypoglycemics	• Severe hypoglycemia has been reported in patients concomitantly receiving azole antifungal agents and oral hypoglycemic drugs
Terfenadine	• Ketoconazole inhibits the metabolism of terfenadine, resulting in increased plasma concentrations of terfenadine and a delay in the elimination of its acid metabolite. These effects may result in prolonged QT intervals
Theophylline	• The plasma clearance of theophylline may be decreased by fluconazole

Patients with baseline abnormal liver function tests and those who develop abnormal liver function tests during fluconazole therapy should be monitored for the development of more severe hepatic injury. Immunocompromised patients, (especially those with AIDS) who develop rashes during treatment with fluconazole should be monitored carefully. If lesions progress, fluconazole should be discontinued.

Other adverse effects of fluconazole include nausea, headache, skin rash, vomiting, abdominal pain and diarrhea.

The incidence of adverse effects with itraconazole was 6.8% in short-term and 20.6% in long-term trials. Gastrointestinal adverse effects were most frequently reported, followed by dermatological reactions (rash and pruritus), headache and effects involving the respiratory system.

The liver and biliary system was also implicated in adverse events, with an incidence rate 2.7% of patients on long-term treatment. For therapy longer than thirty days with itraconazole, liver function should be monitored by appropriate tests. Patients who develop abnormal liver function tests during itraconazole therapy should be monitored for the development of more severe hepatic injury.

Nursing Management

The nursing management of the patient receiving antifungal drugs is presented in Table 19.4 on the next page. Unique features related to individual drugs are given in Table 19.5 (pages 185–186).

Table 19.4
Nursing management for the antifungal drugs

Assessment of risk vs. benefit	Patient data	• *History:* Physician should determine whether severity of infection warrants use of drug. Baseline lab tests of liver function (e.g., AST, ALT, serum bilirubin) and renal function • Assess to establish baseline VS, general state of health, clinical indicators of present infection • *Pregnancy:* Risk category C (animal studies show adverse effects to fetus but human data are unknown or insufficient). Benefits may be acceptable despite the risks
	Drug data	• Select drugs based on culture and sensitivity results • *Some serious drug interactions:* Confer with pharmacist • Most serious adverse effects are renal and hepatic toxicity and hematologic effects of bone marrow depression. Amphotericin is most toxic of this class
Implementation	Rights of administration	• Using the "rights" helps prevent errors of administration
	Right route	• Give IV and PO
	Right time	• See Table 19.5. Dosage schedules vary among drugs in this class
	Right technique	• IV administration requires knowledge of correct diluent and IV solution, correct dilution and rate of administration. Always refer to manufacturer's instructions for this route. Specific precautions with this group because bacteriostatic agent is not added; therefore, very strict aseptic technique is required. Rate must be carefully controlled
	Nursing therapeutics	• Enhance host defences (nutrition, rest, fluids, hygiene) • *Emotional support:* Long-term tx can be discouraging; some pts may also have HIV • Universal precautions to prevent spread of infection (including self-care for caregivers)
	Patient/family teaching	• Educate for proper use of anti-infectives (Chapter 9) • Pt's need for information may be influenced by length of time required for tx or limited by serious illness • Compliance and follow-up are essential factors in successful tx: review principles of pt education in Chapter 3 • Explain that successful tx may require weeks or months • Pts/families should know warning signs/symptoms of possible toxicities of drugs. Report immediately: rash, fever, sore throat, diarrhea, nausea, vomiting, unusual bleeding or bruising, weakness, dark urine or jaundice • Warn pts to avoid alcohol (increases risk of hepatotoxicity) • Discuss possibility of pregnancy: Advise pt to notify physician; discuss birth control methods
Outcomes	Monitoring of progress	*Continually monitor:* • Clinical response indicating tx success (reduction in signs/symptoms) • Be alert for signs/symptoms of adverse reactions; document and report immediately to physician • Blood tests to monitor renal, hepatic and bone marrow function may be ordered (weekly or periodically)

Table 19.5
The antifungals: Drug doses

Drug Generic name (Trade names)	Dosage	Nursing alert
amphotericin B (Fungizone IV)	**Slow IV infusion:** Usually 250 µg/kg/day initially; increase gradually as tolerance permits. Optimal dose unknown. Total daily dose may range up to 1 mg/kg, or alternate-day dosages to 1.5 mg/kg. Under no circumstances should total daily dose exceed 1.5 mg/kg. Several months of tx may be necessary	• Follow manufacturer's instructions for reconstitution. Do not use if precipitate forms. Use infusion pump, in-line filter and distal vein site. Infuse slowly; monitor vasomotor status. Stable in room light for 8 h. Use very strict aseptic technique; no bacteriostatic agent in the solution. Heparin may be added to reduce phlebitis
fluconazole (Diflucan)	**Oral/IV:** PO and IV dosages are equivalent. *Adults:* Administering loading dose on day 1 of tx (2x usual daily dose) results in plasma concentrations close to steady state by day 2. For acute infections, give loading dose equal to 2x the daily dose, not to exceed a max. single dose of 400 mg on day 1. Oropharyngeal candidiasis: 200 mg on day 1, followed by 100 mg/day. Continue for at least 2 weeks. Esophageal candidiasis: 100–200 mg/day. Continue for a min. of 3 weeks and for at least 2 weeks following resolution of symptoms. Systemic candidiasis: 200–400 mg/day. Continue for a min. of 4 weeks and for at least 2 weeks after resolution of symptoms. Cryptococcal meningitis: 200–400 mg/day. Although the duration of tx is unknown, initial tx should last a min. of 10 weeks. Prevention of recurrence of cryptococcal meningitis in AIDS: 200 mg/day. Vaginal candidiasis: Single dose of 150 mg PO. *For children's dosages, consult product information*	• May be given without regard to food. • **IV:** Use infusion pump; rate not to exceed 200 mg/h. Remove protective overwrap just before use and check inner bag for leaks. Solution may have slight opacity which diminishes over time; do not use if cloudy or has precipitate. Do not connect in series with other infusions. For pts with impaired renal function, consult product monograph
flucytosine (Ancotil, Ancobon)	**Oral:** *Adults/children with normal renal function:* Usually, 37.5 mg/kg at 6-h intervals. Reduce dose in pts with renal impairment according to manufacturer's instructions	• Drug may be written as 5-FC. This is part of the drug name, not the dose. Nausea and vomiting may be avoided if drug is given over 15-min interval at each dosing period. Tx plasma level is 30–60 µg/mL
itraconazole (Sporanox)	**Oral:** Oral/esophageal candidiasis: 100 mg daily for 2 weeks. Increase to 200 mg/day in pts with AIDS or neutropenia. Tx should last 4 weeks. Blastomycosis and chronic pulmonary histoplasmosis: 200 mg od. If necessary, increase in 100-mg increments to max. 400 mg/day. Continue tx for a min. of 3 months and until clinical parameters and lab tests indicate active fungal infection has subsided	• Capsules must be swallowed whole. For max. absorption, it is essential to administer itraconazole immediately after a full meal. Doses > 200 mg/day should be given in 2 divided doses and taken at same time qd

(cont'd on next page)

Table 19.5 (continued)
The antifungals: Drug doses

Drug Generic name (Trade names)	Dosage	Nursing alert
itraconazole (Sporanox) (cont'd)	Pulmonary aspergillosis: 200 mg/day for 3–4 months. Invasive pulmonary aspergillosis: 200 mg bid for 3–4 months. Sporotrichosis: 100 mg od for 3 months. Paracoccidio-idomycosis: 100 mg od for 6 months. Chromomycosis due to *Fonsecaea pedrosoi:* 200 mg/day for 6 months. Chromomycosis due to *Cladosporium carrionii:* 100 mg/day for 3 months	
ketoconazole (Nizoral)	**Oral:** *Adults:* 200 mg od. Pts who fail to respond and have inadequate blood levels (< 1 µg/mL) may receive 400 mg. *Children ≤ 20 kg:* 50 mg od; *20–40 kg:* 100 mg od; *> 40 kg:* 200 mg od	• Daily dose may be divided and given with food to reduce GI distress. If pt has hypochlorhydria, dissolve drug in 4 mL of 0.2 N HCl, sip through glass or plastic straw to protect teeth and follow with a glass of water. Avoid administration with antacids, H$_2$ blockers

Response to Clinical Challenge

Principles
Serious drug interactions can occur with this group of drugs. The interdisciplinary team needs to be vigilant to prevent such interactions.

1. The patient may be experiencing serious cardiac effects due to the combination of the terfenadine and the ketoconazole.
2. The physician should order an ECG and VS monitoring. The nurse should ensure that the patient is not continuing to take the OTC terfenadine.
3. Admission history should clearly identify all medications the patient is presently taking. The nurse should ensure that the information is obtained and documented; the pharmacist should advise regarding potential drug interactions; and the physician should use precautions when prescribing drugs that may interact.

Further Reading

Bennet JE. Antimicrobial agents: antifungal drugs. In: Hardman JE, Limbird LE, eds. *Goodman and Gilman's The Pharmacological Basis of Therapeutics.* 9th ed. New York: Pergamon; 1996:1175–1190.

Drugs for AIDS and associated infections. *Medical Letter on Drugs and Infections* 1993;35:900–905.

Drugs used for systemic mycoses. *AMA Drug Evaluations* 1991; 3. Miscellaneous anti-infectives:2.1–2.23.

Itraconazole. *Medical Letter on Drugs and Therapeutics* 1993;35:887–892.

Oral fluconazole for vaginal candidiasis. *Medical Letter on Drugs and Therapeutics* 1994;36:926–932.

Systemic antifungal drugs. *Medical Letter on Drugs and Therapeutics* 1994;36:913–918.

CHAPTER 20

Antiviral Drugs

Topics Discussed
- Definition of serotype, virion, genome, retrovirus, transcription, opportunistic infection
- Drugs for the treatment of AIDS
- Supportive therapy for AIDS patients
- Mechanism of action and pharmacologic effects
- Nursing management for AIDS
- Drugs for the treatment of other viral infections

Drugs Discussed
acyclovir (ay-**sye**-kloe-veer)
amantadine (ah-**man**-tah-deen)
didanosine (dye-**dan**-oh-seen)
foscarnet sodium (foss-**kar**-net)
ganciclovir (gan-**sye**-kloe-veer)
idoxuridine (eye-doks-**yoor**-ih-deen)
pentamidine (pen-**tam**-ih-deen)
ribavirin (rye-bah-**vye**-rin)
trifluridine (try-**flyoor**-ih-deen)
vidarabine (vye-**dar**-ah-been)
zalcitabine (zal-**syte**-ah-been)
zidovudine (zye-**dov**-yoo-deen)

Clinical Challenge
Consider this clinical challenge as you read through this chapter. The response to the challenge appears on page 201.

Miss Kent, a 73-year-old woman, visits the community clinic with a red, sore left eye. Herpes simplex is diagnosed and she is given a prescription for trifluridine (Viroptic®) solution 1%. She is told to instill one drop q2h during waking hours (maximum, 9 drops/day) and to return in 3 days.

Outline a teaching plan and approaches you would employ to ensure that Miss Kent uses this drug effectively.

With the development of an increasing number of antibiotics capable of eradicating many bacterial diseases, attention is switching to antiviral drugs. The general public is increasingly alarmed about viral diseases, particularly as they relate to the sexually transmitted infections herpes genitalis and acquired immunodeficiency syndrome (AIDS). Publicity given to these problems has overshadowed the fact that the great majority of viral infections occur without any accompanying illness. If this were not the case, respiratory viruses belonging to hundreds of *serotypes* (the categories into which bacteria, fungi or viruses are placed, based on the antigens each contains or the antibodies it produces) would immobilize humankind. When a viral infection does produce sickness, the illness is usually self-limited and of short duration, and results in long-term immunity to the virus involved.

However, new antiviral drugs must be developed. At present the treatment of viral disorders is almost entirely of a preventative nature. Because of effective programs, humans have been immunized against many viral disorders, including poliomyelitis, measles, rubella, mumps and yellow fever. Immunization procedures have also been developed against influenza and rabies.

Immunization, however, has two major shortcomings. It is of prophylactic value only and has no benefit once the individual has contracted the disease. Furthermore, scientists have been unable to develop specific immunization procedures for many viral disorders. Therefore, it is important to develop drugs capable of eradicating viral infections after they have been contracted.

Viruses are among the simplest living organisms. They are composed of one or more strands of a linear or helical nucleic acid core, consisting of either DNA or RNA. Viruses must enter living cells to maintain their growth and to reproduce. Thus, they are essentially intracellular parasites that utilize many of the biochemical mechanisms and products of the host cell to sustain their viability. This makes it difficult to find a drug that is selective for the virus and that does not interfere with host cell function.

A mature virus is called a *virion*. It can exist outside a host cell and still retain its infective properties. However, to reproduce, the virus must enter the host cell, take over the host cell's mechanisms for nucleic acid and protein synthesis, and direct the host cell to make new viral particles.

Viruses are divided into two classes, depending on whether their nucleic acid is deoxyribonucleic acid (DNA) or ribonucleic acid (RNA). The nucleic acid core, referred to as the *genome,* is surrounded by a protein-containing shell.

Viruses reproduce only inside living cells. The larger and more complex the virus, the greater the likelihood that a drug can interrupt its activity. Most viruses causing human disease are very small RNA viruses. Up to the present time they have remained largely refractive to drug treatment.

Prior to discussing individual drugs used to treat viral disorders, we will spend a short time describing the multiplication cycle of viruses so that the reader will be better prepared to understand the means by which drugs can interfere with a virus's life cycle.

Antiviral drugs may (1) inhibit the penetration of a virus into the host cell, (2) impair the uncoating of the viral nucleic acid molecule or (3) prevent viral replication.

This chapter will be divided into two parts: drugs for the treatment of AIDS and drugs for the treatment of other viral diseases. The importance given to the treatment of AIDS, together with the rapid expansion of research into anti-AIDS drugs, makes a separate section in this chapter mandatory.

Drugs for the Treatment of AIDS

Retroviruses form a subgroup of RNA viruses which, in order to replicate, must first "reverse transcribe" the RNA of the genome into DNA (*transcription* describes the synthesis of RNA from DNA). Once in the form of DNA, the viral genome is incorporated into the host cell genome, allowing it to take full advantage of the host cell's transcription/translation machinery for the purpose of replication. Once incorporated, the viral DNA is virtually indistinguishable from the host's DNA and, in this state, the virus may persist for as long as the cell lives. As it is virtually invulnerable to attack in this form, any treatment must be directed at another state of the life cycle and must necessarily continue until all virus-carrying cells have died.

Acquired immunodeficiency syndrome (AIDS) is caused by the human immunodeficiency virus (HIV), a retrovirus. It is important to understand this relationship, as the expressions HIV and AIDS are often used synonymously. Treatment directed against HIV should reduce the progression of AIDS.

Drugs are currently used (1) to combat the virus or (2) to treat infections that have arisen as result of the host's reduced immune response. These two groups of agents will be discussed separately.

Anti-HIV Drugs

Therapeutic advances against HIV have been unprecedented, compared with those against other viral diseases. Because of the rapidly expanding nature of this field of research, comments made in this text may well be outdated by the time of publication.

Zidovudine, AZT, Azidothymidine (Retrovir®)

Mechanism of action and pharmacologic effects. Zidovudine is a thymidine analogue that is converted into zidovudine triphosphate, which then competes with host thymidine triphosphate and is incorporated into the growing viral DNA during reverse transcription of the viral RNA. Since this compound is missing a crucial hydroxyl group, no additional nucleosides can be added to the DNA strand, and this results in early termination of viral DNA chain elongation.

It is generally assumed that the value of zidovudine lies in its selective capacity to be incorporated by the retroviral reverse transcriptase, rather than by the host cell polymerase. There appears to be little doubt the zidovudine delays the fall in T4 cells in patients infected with HIV.

Therapeutic uses. Zidovudine is indicated for the management of adult patients with HIV infection who have evidence of impaired immunity (CD4 cell count of approximately 500/mm³ or less) before therapy is begun. The drug is also indicated for HIV-infected children over three months of age who have advanced symptomatic HIV diseases.

Adverse effects. Most patients develop nausea and headache over the first couple of weeks of treatment with zidovudine, but these effects are usually transient. Some develop insomnia, myalgia, fever, asthenia, diarrhea and abdominal pain. Although these symptoms are common, they rarely cause withdrawal of the drug.

Bone marrow depression is a far more worrying consideration. In all the placebo-controlled studies, but most frequently in patients with advanced symptomatic HIV disease, anemia and granulocytopenia were the most significant adverse events observed. Significant anemia most commonly occurs after four to six weeks of therapy, but may occur as early as two weeks. In many cases, dose adjustment, discontinuation of zidovudine and/or blood transfusions were required. Frequent blood counts are strongly recommended in patients with advanced HIV disease receiving this drug.

Table 20.1 lists the clinically significant drug interactions with zidovudine.

Didanosine, ddI (Videx®)

Mechanism of action and pharmacologic effects. Didanosine (ddI) is a synthetic, purine nucleoside analogue active against HIV. In the cell, ddI is converted to dideoxyadenosine, which is then phosphorylated to dideoxyadenosine triphosphate (ddATP). ddATP is the compound that inhibits viral reverse transcriptase and acts as a chain terminator in a manner similar to that of AZT.

Therapeutic uses. Didanosine is indicated for the treatment of adults and children over six months of age who have advanced HIV disease and who are intolerant of zidovudine therapy, or who have demonstrated significant clinical or immunologic deterioration during zidovudine therapy.

Adverse effects. The major toxicities of didanosine are pancreatitis and peripheral neuropathy. Pancreatitis can occur in patients receiving didanosine at or below the recommended dose; this condition can be fatal. Peripheral neuropathy is usually characterized by symmetrical distal numbness, tingling and pain in the feet or hands.

Additional adverse effects include headache, diarrhea, asthenia, insomnia, nausea and vomiting, rash or pruritus, abdominal pain, CNS depression, constipation, stomatitis, myalgia, arthritis, taste loss or perversion, pain, dry mouth, alopecia and dizziness.

Table 20.1
Zidovudine: Drug interactions

Drug	Interaction
Ganciclovir	• Ganciclovir may increase the potential for hematologic toxicity with zidovudine
Nephrotoxic or cytotoxic drugs	• Nephrotoxic or cytotoxic drugs or other drugs that cause bone marrow depression (e.g., antineoplastic drugs) plus zidovudine may have increased risk for toxicity

Table 20.2
Didanosine (ddI): Drug interactions

Drug	Interaction
Ketoconazole	• Ketoconazole absorption may be reduced by didanosine
Quinolone antibiotics	• Didanosine may reduce the plasma concentrations of quinolone antibiotics

Table 20.2 lists the clinically significant drug interactions with didanosine.

Zalcitabine; Dideoxycytidine, ddC (Hivid®)

Mechanism of action and pharmacologic effects. Zalcitabine is also known as dideoxycytidine (ddC), a synthetic nucleoside analogue. This compound is converted to its active metabolite dideoxycytidine triphosphate (ddTP) within cells. ddTP inhibits viral reverse transcriptase and terminates the DNA chain. Thus, in the presence of ddTP, HIV cannot synthesize DNA from its RNA.

Therapeutic uses. Zalcitabine is used in combination with zidovudine for the treatment of adult patients with advanced HIV infection (CD4 cell counts < 300 cells/mm^3) who have demonstrated significant clinical or immunologic deterioration.

Table 20.3 lists the clinically significant drug interactions with zalcitabine.

Adverse effects. The major clinical toxicity of zalcitabine, possibly or probably related to drug treatment, is peripheral neuropathy, which occurred in 25% to 34% of subjects treated in phase 2 and phase 3 monotherapy studies. Zalcitabine-related peripheral neuropathy is a sensorimotor neuropathy, characterized initially by numbness and burning dysasthesia involving the distal extremities.

Fatal pancreatitis has been documented with the administration of zalcitabine alone or in combination with zidovudine. Other serious toxicities of the drug include esophageal ulcers, cardiomyopathy/congestive heart failure and anaphylactoid reactions.

Ribavirin (Virazole®)

Ribavirin is marketed as an aerosol treatment for infants with respiratory viral infections (see Drugs for the Treatment of Other Antiviral Agents, page 192). The drug has also been tested for its anti-HIV effects. Its mechanism of action is thought to involve alterations of the intracellular guanosine pool and the guanylation step required for 51-capping of viral messenger RNA. Ribavirin has caused suppression of HIV replication in continuous cell lines and human peripheral blood leukocytes.

Supportive Therapy for AIDS Patients

People living with AIDS are susceptible to *opportunistic infections* (i.e., infections that would not normally be found in patients with normal host defence mechanisms). The appropriate use of antibiotics, antifungals and antivirals can significantly prolong life in the HIV-infected individual. Many of the drugs used in these conditions have previously been described in earlier chapters. At this point, it is appropriate to review only those drugs that have not yet been discussed.

Foscarnet Sodium (Foscavir®)

Mechanism of action and pharmacologic effects. Foscarnet inhibits the DNA polymerase of

Table 20.3
Zalcitabine (ddC): Drug interactions

Drug	Interaction
Drugs associated with peripheral neuropathy	• These drugs should be avoided when possible because their concomitant use with zalcitabine has the potential to cause peripheral neuropathy

Table 20.4
Foscarnet: Drug interactions

Drug	Interaction
Pentamidine	• Pentamidine and foscarnet produce additive hypocalcemia. Fatal hypocalcemia has been reported when foscarnet was given with parenteral pentamidine. Monitor calcium concentrations

human herpes viruses and the reverse transcriptase of HIV at a different site from nucleoside analogues such as ganciclovir, acyclovir or zidovudine. In vitro foscarnet inhibits replication of cytomegalovirus (CMV), herpes simplex (HSV) 1 and 2, varicella zoster (VZV) and HIV at concentrations easily achieved with parenteral therapy. Clinical isolates of CMV resistant to ganciclovir and of HSV and VZV resistant to acyclovir have generally been susceptible to foscarnet.

Therapeutic uses. Foscarnet has been approved for intravenous treatment of CMV retinitis in patients with AIDS. This condition occurs in up to 30% of patients with AIDS and often causes blindness. The drug has been as effective as ganciclovir for treatment of sight-threatening CMV retinitis in AIDS patients and can be used to treat ganciclovir-resistant CMV infections. However, foscarnet is much more expensive than ganciclovir. There is no consensus on which of the two should be used for initial treatment of CMV retinitis. However, foscarnet appears to be the drug of choice for the treatment of acyclovir-resistant HSV and VZV infections.

Adverse effects. Foscarnet is less well tolerated than ganciclovir, except that ganciclovir is myelosuppressive, while foscarnet generally is not. The most common dose-limiting adverse effect of foscarnet is nephrotoxicity; prehydration with IV saline decreased the risk in one uncontrolled trial.

Foscarnet binds divalent metal ions, such as calcium. Metabolic abnormalities (e.g., hypocalcemia, hypomagnesemia, hypophosphatemia, hypokalemia), which are all apparently related to this effect, occur commonly. High maintenance doses of foscarnet cause a decrease in ionized calcium (with normal total serum calcium concentrations) that may cause neurological and cardiac toxicity. Other adverse effects have included nausea, seizures, neutropenia, neuropathy, arrhythmia, nephrogenic diabetes insipidus and penile ulcers.

Table 20.4 lists the clinically significant drug interactions with foscarnet.

Ganciclovir Sodium (Cytovene®)

Ganciclovir is a synthetic nucleoside analogue that inhibits the replication of herpes viruses both in vitro and in vivo. The drug is indicated for the treatment of cytomegalovirus (CMV) retinitis in immunocompromised individuals, such as patients with AIDS, those with iatrogenic immunosuppression secondary to organ transplantation or those undergoing chemotherapy for neoplasia. The emergence of clinically significant viral resistance to ganciclovir has been reported.

During clinical trials, ganciclovir treatment was withdrawn or interrupted in approximately 32% of the patients because of adverse effects. The most frequent adverse events involved the hematopoietic system. Neutropenia occurred in 38% and thrombocytopenia in 19% of patients.

Table 20.5 lists the clinically significant drug interactions with ganciclovir.

Pentamidine Isethionate (Pentacarinat®, NebuPent®, Pneumopent®)

Pneumocystis carinii pneumonia (PCP) occurs in approximately 80% of AIDS patients and is an

Table 20.5
Ganciclovir: Drug interactions

Drug	Interaction
Imipenem + cilastatin	• Imipenem plus cilastatin (Primaxin®) taken with ganciclovir produce generalized seizures
Zidovudine	• Zidovudine taken with ganciclovir produces neutropenia

important cause of death. Most initial episodes of PCP in HIV-positive patients occur when the blood CD4+ lymphocyte count is less than 200 cells/mm^3, or less than 20% of total lymphocytes. A recurrence rate has been reported of up to 60% within one year after the initial episode of PCP.

Current therapies for PCP use cotrimoxazole (trimethoprim plus sulfamethoxazole) and parenteral pentamidine. Either therapy is effective but adverse effects limit their effectiveness. Pentamidine should be given parenterally only in a hospital setting with facilities to monitor blood glucose, blood counts, and renal and hepatic functions. Fatalities due to severe hypotension, hypoglycemia and cardiac arrhythmias have been reported in patients treated with parenteral pentamidine. Profound severe hypotension may result after a single dose.

Aerosolized pentamidine isethionate (NebuPent®, Pneumopent®) once a month is effective in preventing recurrence of PCP in AIDS patients and is probably effective in preventing first episodes. Pentamidine isethionate powder (Pentacarinat®), approved for intravenous or intramuscular injection, can also be aerosolized and inhaled by patients with AIDS.

Nursing Management

Table 20.6 describes the nursing management of the patient receiving antiviral drugs for the treatment of AIDS. Dosage details of specific drugs are given in Table 20.11 (pages 198–201).

Drugs for the Treatment of Other Viral Infections

Acyclovir (Zovirax®)

Mechanism of action and therapeutic uses. Acyclovir is metabolized to acyclovir triphosphate, which inhibits DNA polymerase and viral multiplication in herpes simplex types 1 and 2, varicella zoster, herpes simiae (B virus) and Epstein-Barr virus.

Acyclovir is available in parenteral, oral and topical formulation. When injected, it is indicated for the treatment of initial and recurrent mucosal and cutaneous herpes simplex infections in immunocompromised adults and children. The parenteral form is also approved for severe initial episodes of herpes simplex infections in patients who may not be immunocompromised. Oral acyclovir may be indicated in the treatment of initial episodes of herpes genitalis and the suppression of unusually frequent recurrences of herpes genitalis.

Acyclovir is applied topically for management of initial episodes of genital herpes simplex infections. It is also indicated in the management of non–life-threatening cutaneous herpes simplex virus infections in immunocompromised patients.

Adverse effects. Acyclovir appears to be a relatively safe drug, but a few patients have experienced delirium. Although it cannot be established that this was a result of acyclovir treatment, it must be borne in mind. Other reported adverse effects include inflammation and/or phlebitis (13.8%) at the injection site, and diaphoresis, hematuria, hypotension, headache and nausea, each of which occurred in 1.6% of patients treated. Hives have been reported in 4.7% of patients on parenteral acyclovir. Nausea and vomiting may be encountered with oral acyclovir. Other adverse effects include headache, diarrhea, skin rash, vertigo and arthralgia. Topical acyclovir may produce discomfort when applied.

Table 20.7 on page 194 lists the clinically significant drug interactions with acyclovir.

Table 20.6
Nursing management for antiviral drugs in the treatment of AIDS

Assessment of risk vs. benefit	Patient data	• Physician should determine whether severity of present or future infection warrants use of drug. Baseline blood tests • Assess to establish baseline VS, general state of health, clinical indicators of present infection • *Pregnancy:* Risk category C (animal studies show adverse effects to fetus but human data are unknown or insufficient). Benefits may be acceptable despite the risks
	Drug data	• Each drug in this category has some serious adverse reactions
Implementation	Rights of administration	• Using the "rights" helps prevent errors of administration
	Right route	• Give IV and PO
	Right time	• See Table 20.11. Dosage schedules vary among drugs of this class. Ideally administered ATC
	Right technique	• IV administration requires knowledge of correct diluent and IV solution, correct dilution and rate of administration. Always refer to manufacturer's instructions for this route. Specific precautions with this group because rapid administration causes greater toxicity. Rate must be carefully controlled. An infusion pump is advised
	Nursing therapeutics	• Enhance host defences (nutrition, rest, fluids, hygiene) • *Emotional support:* Long-term tx required, with side effects and risks for adverse reactions. Drugs do not promise a cure • Universal precautions to prevent spread of infection (including self-care for caregivers)
	Patient/family teaching	• Pt's need for information may be influenced by length of time required for tx or limited by serious illness • Compliance and follow-up are essential factors in successful tx. Review principles of pt education in Chapter 3 • Remind pt that HIV can still be transmitted to others • Pts/families should know warning signs/symptoms of possible toxicities of drugs. Report immediately: rash, fever, sore throat, diarrhea, nausea, vomiting, unusual bleeding or bruising, weakness, numbness, pain or tingling in hands or feet • *Discuss possibility of pregnancy:* Advise pt to notify physician and discuss birth control methods
Outcomes	Monitoring of progress	*Continually monitor:* • Clinical response: Reduced incidence of opportunistic infections indicate tx success (but not cure) • Be alert for signs/symptoms of adverse reactions (e.g., bone marrow depression, pancreatitis, peripheral neuropathy, severe hypotension); document and report immediately to physician • Blood tests to monitor bone marrow function may be ordered (weekly or periodically)

Table 20.7
Acyclovir: Drug interactions

Drug	Interaction
Narcotics (meperidine and congeners)	• Acyclovir may decrease the renal excretion of meperidine and increase its toxicity. This interaction might also occur with other narcotics
Probenecid	• Probenecid may decrease the renal excretion of acyclovir and increase its toxicity

Amantadine (Symmetrel®)

Mechanism of action and therapeutic uses. Amantadine may inhibit penetration of influenza A viruses into the host cell or reduce the uncoating of those viruses that do penetrate the cell. The drug is therefore indicated in the prevention and treatment of respiratory infections caused by influenza A virus strains. Amantadine may have its greatest value in patients at high risk for developing influenza because of underlying disease, such as the elderly in hospitals or nursing homes. The drug does not interfere with immunization, and patients may receive amantadine while waiting for the effects of immunization to appear. If used to treat an influenza A virus infection, amantadine must be started within forty-eight hours of the onset of symptoms.

Adverse effects. Amantadine is generally well tolerated; high doses are more likely to produce adverse effects. The drug is excreted unchanged by the kidneys, and patients with compromised renal function may experience drug-related toxicities with normal doses. The more important adverse effects of amantadine are orthostatic hypotensive episodes, congestive heart failure, depression, psychosis and urinary retention. Other adverse effects include acute neurotoxicity consisting of tremors, hallucinations and abnormal behaviour. Some patients experience depression, confusion, detachment, lethargy, nervousness and dizziness. Occasionally, physical manifestations of central nervous system toxicity occur, including nausea, vomiting, ataxia and slurred speech.

Table 20.8 lists the clinically significant drug interactions with amantadine.

Idoxuridine (Herplex®)

Mechanism of action and therapeutic uses. Idoxuridine is incorporated into viral DNA, destabilizing the nucleic acid and altering viral protein synthesis. Ophthalmic idoxuridine is used topically in the treatment of herpes simplex keratitis only. Epithelial infections, especially initial attacks, characterized by the presence of a dendritic figure, are highly responsive to idoxuridine. Infections located in the stroma have shown a less favourable response. In recurrent cases, idoxuridine will often control the current episode of the viral infections, but scarring that resulted from previous attacks will not be corrected.

Adverse effects. Idoxuridine can cause clouding of the cornea and small defects in the corneal epithelium. It may also cause local irritation, itching, mild edema and photophobia.

Ribavirin (Virazole®)

Mechanism of action and therapeutic uses. Ribavirin is active against respiratory syncytial (RS) virus. Its mechanism of action is not known. Ribavirin is indicated only for lower respiratory tract infections due to RS virus. Ribavirin aerosol treatment must be accompanied by (and does not replace) standard supportive respiratory and fluid management for infants and children with severe respiratory tract infections.

Table 20.8
Amantadine: Drug interactions

Drug	Interaction
Anticholinergics	• Amantadine taken with anticholinergics can cause hallucinations, confusion and nightmares. Decrease the anticholinergic dosage before starting amantadine

Table 20.9
Vidarabine: Drug interactions

Drug	Interaction
Corticosteroids	• Corticosteroids are usually contraindicated in the tx of keratoconjunctivitis. If vidarabine tx is combined with topical corticosteroid tx for associated conditions, the hazards of customary corticosteroid-induced ocular abnormalities must be considered. These include corticosteroid-induced glaucoma or cataract formation and progression of bacterial infections

Adverse effects. Serious adverse events that have occurred during ribavirin therapy have included worsening of respiratory status, bacterial pneumonia and pneumothorax. It is not clear whether these effects are related to the use of ribavirin.

Trifluridine (Viroptic®)

Mechanism of action and therapeutic uses. Trifluridine is phosphorylated by a cellular thymidine kinase to its nucleotide monophosphate. Trifluridine monophosphate and its metabolites inhibit the following DNA viruses: herpes simplex types 1 and 2, varicella zoster, adenovirus and vaccinia virus. Trifluridine is indicated for the treatment of primary keratoconjunctivitis and recurrent epithelial keratitis due to herpes simplex viruses types 1 and 2.

Adverse effects. The most common adverse effect is burning upon instillation and superficial punctate keratitis.

Vidarabine (Vira-A®)

Mechanism of action and therapeutic uses. Vidarabine is adenine arabinoside. The drug probably impairs the initial steps in the synthesis of viral DNA. Intravenous vidarabine is infused for the treatment of herpes simplex virus encephalitis. It appears to slow the process of neurologic deterioration but cannot reverse existing damage. Maximum benefits, involving alterations in morbidity and the prevention of serious neurologic sequelae, depend on early diagnosis and treatment. Controlled studies indicate that vidarabine therapy reduces the mortality rate from 70% to 28%.

Intravenous vidarabine may also be effective in decreasing both the mortality and morbidity of neonatal herpes simplex infections, particularly milder forms of the disease. It has prevented severe ocular and neurologic sequelae in neonates with only localized skin, eye or mouth infections. In neonates with central nervous system and disseminated disease, the drug has reduced both morbidity and mortality.

Intravenous vidarabine has proven beneficial in the treatment of immunocompromised adults and children with localized zoster and chicken pox infections, respectively.

Vidarabine may also be applied in the eye for the treatment of herpes keratoconjunctivitis manifested by dendritic keratitis or geographic corneal ulcers. It may also be indicated in patients who have developed toxic or allergic manifestations to idoxuridine.

Adverse effects. Intravenous vidarabine produces nausea, vomiting, diarrhea and anorexia. Its effects on the central nervous system can also include dizziness, hallucinations, ataxia and psychosis. When applied topically in the form of an ophthalmic preparation, the most common adverse effects are burning, irritation, lacrimation, pain and photophobia.

Table 20.9 lists the clinically significant interactions with vidarabine.

Nursing Management

Table 20.10 on the next page describes the nursing management of patients receiving general antiviral therapy. Dosage details of specific drugs are given in Table 20.11 (pages 198–201).

Table 20.10
Nursing management of antiviral drugs

Assessment of risk vs. benefit	Patient data	• Physician should determine whether severity of infection warrants use of drug • Assess to establish baseline VS, general state of health, clinical indicators of present infection • *Pregnancy:* Risk category C (animal studies show adverse effects to fetus but human data are unknown or insufficient). Benefits may be acceptable despite the risks
	Drug data	• Each drug in this category has some serious adverse reactions
Implementation	Rights of administration	• Using the "rights" helps prevent errors of administration
	Right route	• Give by IV, oral, topical or ophthalmic routes
	Right time	• See Table 20.11. Dosage schedules vary among drugs of this class. Ideally administered ATC
	Right technique	• *Ophthalmic administration:* Ensure correct technique (including asepsis, cleansing eyes correctly, hand washing, proper placement of eye dropper for instillation) • IV administration requires knowledge of correct diluent and IV solution, correct dilution and rate of administration. Always refer to manufacturer's instructions for this route. Specific precautions with this group because rapid administration causes greater toxicity. Rate must be carefully controlled. An infusion pump is advised
	Nursing therapeutics	• IV route may require large-volume infusions; monitor fluid intake and output. Maintain hydration to prevent renal damage • Avoid cross-contamination of infected sites through hygiene and clean, loose dressings, if necessary • Drugs do not promise a cure for all herpes viruses; pt can still spread infection to others during tx • Universal precautions to prevent spread of infection (including self-care for caregivers)
	Patient/family teaching	• Teach correct technique for instillation of eye drops. Remind to avoid use of eye makeup, eye cleansing products and to use separate face cloth or towel. Provide a patient teaching aid such as that illustrated in Figure 20.1. • Instruct patient how to apply topical ointment using a finger cot or glove and avoiding contamination to clean sites. Keep infected area clean and dry • Although these drugs are generally well tolerated, pts/families should know warning signs/symptoms of possible toxicities. Report immediately: rash, severe CNS symptoms (e.g., confusion), cardiac effects (fainting, irregular heartbeat) • *Discuss possibility of pregnancy:* Advise pt to notify physician and discuss birth control methods

Table 20.10 (continued)
Nursing management of antiviral drugs

Outcomes	Monitoring of progress	*Continually monitor:*
		• *Clinical response:* Reduced incidence of opportunistic infections indicate tx success (but not cure)
		• Be alert for signs/symptoms of ADRs (e.g., bone marrow depression, pancreatitis, peripheral neuropathy, severe hypotension); document and report immediately to physician
		• Blood tests to monitor bone marrow function may be ordered (weekly or periodically)

Figure 20.1
Patient teaching tool

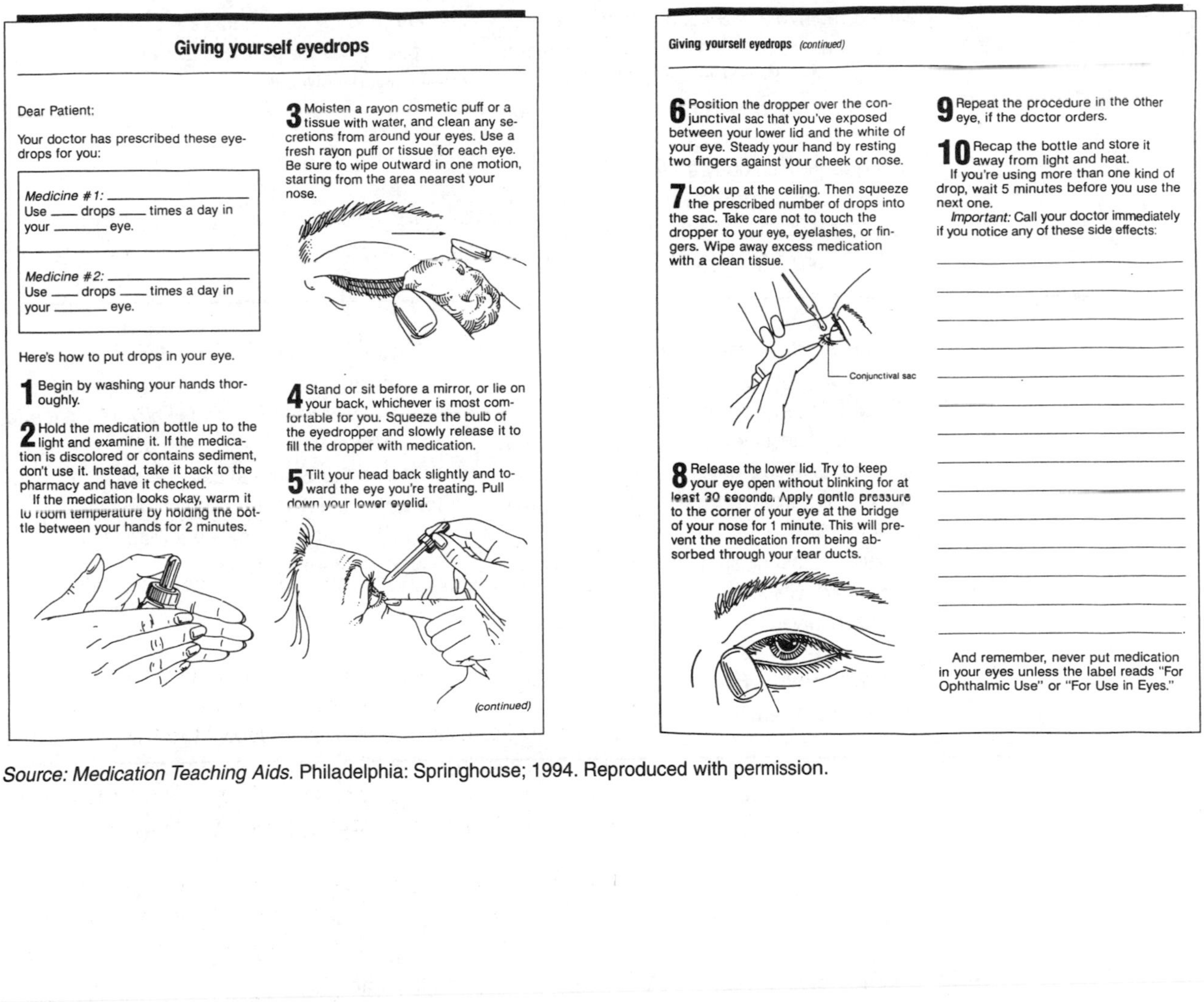

Giving yourself eyedrops

Dear Patient:

Your doctor has prescribed these eyedrops for you:

Medicine #1: _____
Use ____ drops ____ times a day in your _____ eye.

Medicine #2: _____
Use ____ drops ____ times a day in your _____ eye.

Here's how to put drops in your eye.

1 Begin by washing your hands thoroughly.

2 Hold the medication bottle up to the light and examine it. If the medication is discolored or contains sediment, don't use it. Instead, take it back to the pharmacy and have it checked.
   If the medication looks okay, warm it to room temperature by holding the bottle between your hands for 2 minutes.

3 Moisten a rayon cosmetic puff or a tissue with water, and clean any secretions from around your eyes. Use a fresh rayon puff or tissue for each eye. Be sure to wipe outward in one motion, starting from the area nearest your nose.

4 Stand or sit before a mirror, or lie on your back, whichever is most comfortable for you. Squeeze the bulb of the eyedropper and slowly release it to fill the dropper with medication.

5 Tilt your head back slightly and toward the eye you're treating. Pull down your lower eyelid.

(continued)

Giving yourself eyedrops *(continued)*

6 Position the dropper over the conjunctival sac that you've exposed between your lower lid and the white of your eye. Steady your hand by resting two fingers against your cheek or nose.

7 Look up at the ceiling. Then squeeze the prescribed number of drops into the sac. Take care not to touch the dropper to your eye, eyelashes, or fingers. Wipe away excess medication with a clean tissue.

— Conjunctival sac

8 Release the lower lid. Try to keep your eye open without blinking for at least 30 seconds. Apply gentle pressure to the corner of your eye at the bridge of your nose for 1 minute. This will prevent the medication from being absorbed through your tear ducts.

9 Repeat the procedure in the other eye, if the doctor orders.

10 Recap the bottle and store it away from light and heat.
   If you're using more than one kind of drop, wait 5 minutes before you use the next one.
   Important: Call your doctor immediately if you notice any of these side effects:

_____
_____
_____
_____
_____
_____
_____
_____
_____

And remember, never put medication in your eyes unless the label reads "For Ophthalmic Use" or "For Use in Eyes."

Source: Medication Teaching Aids. Philadelphia: Springhouse; 1994. Reproduced with permission.

Table 20.11
The antivirals: Drug doses

Drug Generic name (Trade names)	Dosage	Nursing alert
A. Drugs for the Treatment of AIDS		
didanosine, ddl (Videx)	**Oral:** *Adults:* Dosing q12h. Adult patients should take 2 tablets at each dose so that adequate buffering is provided to prevent gastric degradation. Dose dependent on weight: ≥ 60 *kg:* tablets 200 mg bid, powder 250 mg bid; < 60 *kg:* tablets 125 mg bid, powder 167 mg bid. *Children:* Dosing q8h. To prevent gastric degradation, children > 1 year of age should receive a 2-tablet dose; children < 1 year should receive a 1-tablet dose. Limited data suggest an oral dose of 200–300 mg/m^2/day, up to a max. of 250 mg/ day for tablet formulation. Recommended dose in children depends on body surface areas: ≥ 0.9 *m^2,* 75 mg tid (powder, 90 mg tid); *0.6–0.8 m^2,* 50 mg tid (powder, 60 mg tid); ≤ 0.5 *m^2,* 25 mg tid (powder, 30 mg tid)	• Give on empty stomach. Food reduces absorption by 50% • Tabs should be chewed thoroughly or crushed. May be given as a dispersion (add tabs to 25 mL water and stir thoroughly); take immediately. Pharmacy-prepared admixture should be shaken thoroughly prior to administration • Drug contains sodium (2 tabs = 529 mg, 1 packet = 1.38 g). Use care to avoid dispersal of powder into air
foscarnet sodium (Foscavir)	**IV:** *Adults with normal renal function:* Induction tx, 60 mg/kg at a constant rate over a min. of 1 h, q8h for 2–3 weeks, depending on response. Adequate hydration is recommended to establish diuresis both prior to and during tx. Maintenance tx for adults with normal renal function, 90–120 mg/kg/day over 2 h; because higher plasma concentrations may be associated with increased toxicity, most pts should be given the 90 mg/kg/day regimen initially. All doses must be individualized on the basis of the pt's renal function (see manufacturer's recommended dosage)	• Cautious use in pts with reduced renal function, decreased calcium levels before tx and in those receiving other drugs known to influence serum calcium levels. Ensure adequate hydration (add 2.5 L normal saline over 24 h when foscarnet is given as a continuous infusion; add 0.5–1 L normal saline to each infusion while on intermittent tx)
ganciclovir sodium (Cytovene)	**IV:** Initially, 5 mg/kg q12h for 14–21 days, given as constant infusion over 1 h. After induction tx, recommended dose is 5 mg/kg given as IV infusion over 1 h daily for 7 days/ week, or 6 mg/kg daily for 5 days/week **Oral:** For pts with stable CMV following at least 3 weeks of tx with IV solution, the maintenance-dose capsule os 100 mg tid with food; alternatively, 500 mg 6x/day with food	• Use infusion pump to control rate of infusion over 1 h. Never give IM or SC. Maintain hydration • IV solution prepared in biologic cabinet; gown, gloves and mask required • Stable at room temperature for 12 h. Do not refrigerate

Table 20.11 (continued)
The antivirals: Drug doses

Drug Generic name (Trade names)	Dosage	Nursing alert
pentamidine isethionate (Pentacarinat, NebuPent, Pneumopent)	**Inhalation:** Dose specific to device for delivery. For prophylaxis against PCP in pts at high risk for the disease: *Adults:* 300 mg od q4weeks; administered by Respirgard II® nebulizer. **IM/IV:** *Adults:* 4 mg/kg daily for 14–21 days. Pts with renal failure (CrCl < 35 mL/min): For life-threatening infections, 4 mg/kg daily for 7–10 days; then 4 mg/kg on alternate days to complete course of 14 doses. For less severe infections, 4 mg/ kg on alternate days for 14 doses	• Follow instructions with inhaler device • **IV:** Reconstitute according to manufacturer's instructions and infuse over 1 h
zalcitabine; dideoxycytidine, ddC (Hivid)	**Oral:** Daily recommended combination regimen: One 0.75-mg tablet, administered concomitantly with 200 mg zidovudine q8h (total daily dose, 2.25 mg zalcitabine and 600 mg zidovudine)	• Administer ATC on empty stomach
zidovudine; azidothymidine, AZT (Retrovir)	**Oral:** *Adults:* For asymptomatic HIV infection, 100 mg q4h while awake for a total daily dose of 500 mg. For symptomatic HIV disease, 100 mg q4h ATC for total daily dose of 600 mg. *Children:* 3 months to 12 years, 180 mg/m^2 q6h (750 mg/m^2/day). Do not exceed 200 mg for any individual dose **IV:** 1–2 mg/kg administered as 1-h infusion q4h ATC (6x daily). Pts should receive IV zidovudine only until PO tx can be administered	• Store capsules in a cool place, protect from light. Should be swallowed whole • **IV:** Infuse over 1 h. Follow manufacturer's instructions for dilution

B. Drugs for the Treatment of Other Viral Infections

acyclovir sodium (Zovirax)	**IV:** *Adults,* 5 mg/kg infused at constant rate over 1 h q8h (15 mg/kg/day) in pts with normal renal function for 7 days. *Children < 12 years,* 250 mg/m^2 infused at constant rate over 1 h q8h (750 mg/m^2/day) for 7 days	• For pts with renal failure: Consult product monograph • **IV:** Follow manufacturer's instructions for reconstitution and give over 1 h. Rotate site to prevent phlebitis. Maintain hydration to prevent renal damage • **PO:** Give with or without food • **Topical:** Apply with finger cot or glove

(cont'd on next page)

Table 20.11 (continued)
The antivirals: Drug doses

Drug Generic name (Trade names)	Dosage	Nursing alert
B. Drugs for the Treatment of Other Viral Infections (cont'd)		
acyclovir (Zovirax) (cont'd)	**Oral:** Initial infection, 200 mg q4h while awake, for total of 1 g/day for 10 days. Suppressive tx for recurrent disease, 200 mg tid; increase if breakthrough occurs to 200 mg 5x/day. If necessary, consider 400 mg bid. May be continued for up to 12 months. Pts with CrCl < 10 mL/min/1.73 m² , 200 mg q12h **Topical:** Apply 5% ointment liberally to affected area 4–6x/day for 10 days	
amantadine HCl (Symmetrel)	**Oral:** *Adults,* 200 mg/day. Geriatrics, 100 mg/day. *Children: 9–12 years,* 100 mg bid; *1–9 years,* 4.5–9 mg/kg/day (not > 150 mg/day) in 2–3 equal doses	• If CNS effects develop on od dosage, give in doses of 100 mg bid • For older pts or those who experience CNS side effects, divide daily dose and give bid; avoid hs (may cause insomnia) • If pt has difficulty swallowing, contents of capsule may be mixed with food
idoxuridine (Herplex)	**Ophthalmic:** One drop 0.1% solution q1h during the day and q2h at night until definite improvement occurs as demonstrated by lack of staining with fluorescein; dosage is then reduced to 1 drop q2h during the day and q4h at night. Tx should be continued for 3–5 days after healing appears complete but not for more than 14–21 days	• Wash hands before and after procedure. Cleanse eyes before instillation. Do not contaminate dropper by touching eye or lids
ribavirin (Virazole)	Read Viratek Small Particle Aerosol Generator (SPAG) operator's manual. Start tx ASAP, within 3 days of infection. Tx is carried out continuously, apart from time required for ancillary care, for not less than 3 and no more than 7 days	• Discard and replace solution q24h. Reconstitute according to instructions. Do not use in ventilator equipment; may precipitate and cause malfunction
trifluridine (Viroptic)	**Ophthalmic:** *Adults:* Initially, 1 drop 1% solution onto cornea of affected eye q2h while awake (max., 9 drops/day). Continue until healing starts. Then, 1 drop q4h for max. 5 drops/day. Continue for 7 days post re-epithelialization. If no improvement after 7 days of	• Wash hands before and after procedure. Cleanse eyes. Do not contaminate dropper by touching eyes or lids

Table 20.11 (continued)
The antivirals: Drug doses

Drug Generic name (Trade names)	Dosage	Nursing alert
trifluridine (Viroptic) (cont'd)	full tx, or complete re-epithelialization has not occurred after 14 days, other forms of tx should be considered. Avoid administration of full dosage for more than 21 days	
vidarabine (Vira-A)	**IV:** *Adults/children:* For herpes simplex encephalitis, 15 mg/kg/day for 10 days. For herpes simplex infection in neonates, 15 mg/kg/day for 10 days. For varicella zoster in immunocompromised patients, 10 mg/kg/day for 5 days	•**IV:** Reconstitute according to manufacturer's instructions. Give daily dose in large volume over 12–24 h. Infusion pump recommended. Monitor fluid intake
	Ophthalmic: 1.5 cm ointment in conjunctival sac 5x/day at 3-h intervals until corneal re-epithelialization has occurred. Continue tx for 7 days more at reduced dosage (e.g., bid) to prevent recurrence	•**Ophthalmic:** Wash hands before and after procedure. Cleanse eyes. Do not contaminate dropper by touching eyes or lids

Response to Clinical Challenge

Principles
Miss Kent is a "young-older adult"; assess her hearing and visual ability before any teaching occurs.

Actions
Determine Miss Kent's previous experience with eye drops. Use a patient teaching aid demonstrating the correct technique (see Figure 20.1, page 197). Instruct her and ask her to instill one drop while you observe.

The teaching plan should include:
- wash hands prior to instilling eye drops
- cleanse eye
- instill without touching dropper to eye or to lid
- apply gentle pressure to lacrimal sac to prevent systemic absorption of the drug
- do not use any other eye drops at the same time
- if dose missed, instill drop as soon as remembered, unless next dosage time is close; do not double dose
- common side effects include mild, transient burning or irritation to the eye
- contact physician if eye pain is more severe or if healing does not occur
- if vision is blurred, avoid dangerous activities and wear sunglasses to avoid photophobia

Further Reading

Bennet JE. Antimicrobial agents: antiviral drugs. In: Hardman JL, Limbird LE, *Goodman and Gilman's The Pharmacological Basis of Therapeutics.* 9th ed. New York: Pergamon; 1996:1191–1224.

Drugs for AIDS and associated infections. *Medical Letter on Drugs and Therapeutics* 1993;35:900–905.

Drugs for non-HIV viral infections. *Medical Letter on Drugs and Therapeutics* 1994;36:27–32.

Drugs for sexually transmitted diseases. *Medical Letter on Drugs and Therapeutics* 1994;36:1–6.

Drugs for viral infections. *Medical Letter on Drugs and Therapeutics* 1992;34:867–873.

Handbook of antimicrobial therapy. *Medical Letter on Drugs and Therapeutics* 1992.

CHAPTER 21

Antimalarial Drugs

Topics Discussed
- Life cycle of the malarial parasite
- Rationale of drug treatment of malaria
- Drugs effective against the erythrocytic form of the plasmodium
- Drugs effective against the exoerythrocytic form of the plasmodium
- Drugs effective against both forms of the plasmodium
- Nursing management

Drugs Discussed
chloroquine (**klor**-oh-kwin)
quinine (kwin-**een**)
quinidine (**kwin**-ih-deen)
mefloquine (**meff**-loe-kwin)
primaquine (**prim**-ah-kween)
pyrimethamine (pirr-ih-**meth**-ah-meen)
sulfadoxine (sul-fah-**dok**-seen)

Clinical Challenge

Consider this clinical challenge as you proceed through this chapter. The response to the challenge appears on page 210.

H.K. is a 36-year-old businessman. Of Jamaican descent, he lives in Canada but frequently travels. His next trip will take him to an area with endemic malaria.

What baseline information will be needed before a drug is ordered? Of the drugs available, which might be avoided?

Outline a teaching plan for Mr. K. What community resources might supply more information prior to his trip?

Malaria remains one of the major health problems of the world. Because of this disease, as many as three million lives may be lost annually in Africa, India, Southeast Asia and Central and South America. Malaria is a result of infection with protozoa of the genus *Plasmodium*. Spread by the bite of the female *Anopheles* mosquito, it has largely been eradicated in the United States by insecticide-spraying programs.

Malaria produces paroxysms of severe chills, fever and profuse sweating that vary in severity depending on the species of *Plasmodium* involved. Of the more than forty species of this genus, only

four — *Plasmodium falciparum, Plasmodium vivax, Plasmodium malariae* and *Plasmodium ovale* — affect humans, and all are transmitted in the saliva of the *Anopheles* mosquito.

P. falciparum causes malignant tertian malaria, the most dangerous form of human malaria. Because of its potential to invade erythrocytes of any age, this species can produce an overwhelming parasitemia and fulminating infection in the nonimmune patient that, if untreated, may rapidly cause death. Delay in treatment until after demonstration of parasitemia may lead to an irreversible state of shock, and death may ensue even after the peripheral blood is free of parasites. If treated early, the infection usually responds readily to appropriate antimalarial drugs and relapses will not occur.

P. vivax infection has a low mortality rate in untreated adults and is characterized by relapses that occur as long as two years after primary infection.

P. malariae induced malaria is generally characterized by fever spikes every seventy-two hours. Clinical attacks may occur years after infection, but are much rarer than after infections with *P. vivax.*

P. ovale causes a rare malarial infection with a periodicity and relapses similar to those of *P. vivax,* but it is milder and more readily cured.

Life Cycle of the Malarial Parasite

The life cycle of the malarial parasite is illustrated in Figure 21.1. The female *Anopheles* mosquito is the vector for malaria. By taking its pound of flesh, and a little blood as well, from a human carrying the male and female sexual forms of the parasite, it becomes the carrier of the plasmodium. Once in the stomach of the mosquito, the male gametocyte fertilizes the female to form a zygote, which then penetrates the stomach wall, forming a cyst on its outer surface. Numerous cell divisions take place to produce an oocyst containing thousands of sporozoites. Rupture of the cysts results in the release of sporozoites, which are carried to the mosquito's salivary glands. When the mosquito subsequently goes on a hunting foray, she may bite an unfortunate human, injecting sporozoites into the blood of the new host.

Once injected into the host's blood, the sporozoites accumulate within liver parenchymal cells, where they divide to form a hepatic schizont containing numerous merozoites. This is referred to as the *exoerythrocytic* phase of malaria. Merozoites require six to twelve days to develop, after which time they leave the liver and invade the host's erythrocytes to produce the *erythrocytic* phase of

Figure 21.1
Life cycle of the malarial parasite

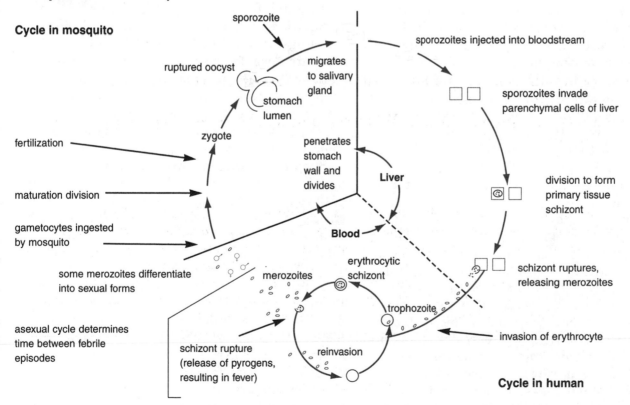

Source: Pratt WB. *Chemotherapy of Infection.* New York: Oxford Press; 1977. Reproduced with permission.

malaria or erythrocytic schizogony. Schizonts formed in the red blood cells grow and eventually rupture the erythrocytes, releasing merozoites, lytic materials and parasitic toxins into the blood. The recurrent chills and fever experienced by patients are due to the release of the latter two materials.

Merozoites released from the red blood cells may either reinvade erythrocytes, producing the same series of events just described, or undergo sexual division in blood to form male and female gametocytes. It is these promiscuous little rogues that are ingested by the passing mosquito — all of which brings us back to the point where we started this trip through the stomach, stinger and saliva of the mosquito, and liver and erythrocytes of the human.

Rationale of Drug Treatment of Malaria

Ideally, it would be best to treat the mosquito rather than the human. By adopting this approach only the purveyors of the plasmodium would be exposed to the adverse effects of pharmacotherapy. Alas, however, this is not possible with the current state of knowledge. There is no drug for the bug. Our only approach is to spray copious amounts of insecticides in its general vicinity.

True, in Canada and the northern United States, we can always claim smugly that we could freeze the mosquito's stinger for at least nine months of the year. However, this approach is more academic than practical because the little *Anopheles* is more prudent than humans and refuses to take up residence in such inhospitable surroundings.

Returning to spraying, no one would question the success of the program. However, mosquito resistance to insecticides is a constant problem and explains, in part, the continued presence of malaria. It is therefore necessary to administer drugs capable of treating the disease in humans.

Transferring our attention from mosquitoes to humans, it would obviously be best if we could prevent viable plasmodia from reaching the liver. However, here again we fail. At present there are no drugs that stand between the bite of the mosquito and the liver of the human. As a result, we are left with treating the infection within the liver or the erythrocyte.

Because the fever and chills of malaria result from the release of lytic materials and parasitic toxins from the ruptured erythrocyte, drugs that prevent plasmodia from prospering in red blood cells may make the patient asymptomatic. However, they do not eradicate *P. vivax* and *P. ovale* because when therapy is stopped, merozoites harboured in the liver return to the blood and reinfect erythrocytes. *P. vivax* and *P. ovale* can be eliminated only by drugs that attack the hepatic forms of plasmodia. This approach is reasonable in areas such as Canada and the United States, where malaria is not endemic. In endemic areas, however, continual reinfection is likely, and drug therapy is usually aimed only at suppressing the symptoms of malaria by treating the erythrocytic stage.

The preceding comments pertain only to the treatment of *P. vivax* and *P. ovale*. When the liver schizont containing *P. falciparum* ruptures, spilling merozoites into the blood, these latter organisms do not reinfect the liver. As a result, the successful treatment of the initial malarial attack usually results in complete eradication of the plasmodium from the body. It is also likely that *P. malariae* does not have exoerythrocytic forms.

Drugs work within the liver or erythrocytes. They are given for the purpose of (1) suppressive therapy, (2) treating an acute attack (clinical cure), (3) producing a radical cure or (4) preventing infection with malaria (chemoprophylaxis).

Suppressive therapy is exactly as the name indicates: it suppresses malaria but does not cure it. Suppressive therapy involves the use of drugs to prevent or restrict the erythrocytic asexual stage of the disease. Chloroquine is usually the drug of choice. Chloroquine-resistant *P. falciparum* can be treated with pyrimethamine plus sulfadoxine (Fansidar®). Mefloquine (Lariam®) may also be given. This drug is used both to suppress and to treat malaria. It is considered alternative therapy to chloroquine or hydroxychloroquine in the suppressive therapy of malaria. The principal use of mefloquine is malaria chemoprophylaxis in travellers to areas where chloroquine-resistant and/or pyrimethamine/sulfadoxine-resistant strains of *P. falciparum* are most likely to be present.

Suppressive therapy may be curative if used

for years, such that the life of the patient exceeds (it is hoped) the life of the parasite. Usually, however, malarial attacks can recur if suppressive therapy is stopped. Suppressive therapy is recommended during periods of exposure to the mosquito and for several weeks after leaving a malarious zone of the world. Short-term suppressive treatment may also be of value in patients with a history of malaria who are undergoing severely stressful situations.

Acute attacks of malaria likewise are treated with drugs that are effective against the erythrocytic stage of the plasmodium. Cure of an acute attack of malaria caused by *P. vivax, P. ovale, P. malariae* or chloroquine-sensitive strains of *P. falciparum* is readily accomplished with a three-day course of chloroquine phosphate. If oral administration is not feasible, chloroquine hydrochloride may be administered intravenously until an oral preparation can be used. Alternatively, oral quinine sulfate can be given or, in severe attacks, quinidine gluconate can be administered by slow intravenous infusion if parenteral chloroquine hydrochloride is not available.

Malaria caused by *P. falciparum* from an area in which multiple-drug resistance is known to occur should be assumed to be resistant to chloroquine and treated as such. Treatment should be initiated with oral quinine sulfate, if possible. In severe life-threatening attacks, when parenteral administration is necessary, the administration of quinidine gluconate by slow intravenous infusion is the treatment of choice.

When oral medication can be tolerated, sulfadiazine and pyrimethamine or the combination of pyrimethamine/sulfadoxine (Fansidar®) can be given with quinine sulfate. Alternatively, tetracycline plus quinine or quinidine may be substituted for the sulfonamide/pyrimethamine combination. Oral mefloquine may also be used to treat mild to moderate acute malaria caused by mefloquine-sensitive strains of *P. falciparum* (both chloroquine-sensitive and chloroquine-resistant strains) or by *P. vivax.*

Radical cure implies the elimination of the hepatic forms of *P. vivax* and *P. ovale.* This is usually attempted after the initial acute attack is treated. Primaquine is often employed for this purpose.

Chemoprophylactic therapy can significantly reduce the morbidity and mortality of malaria. Chloroquine phosphate remains first-line therapy for chloroquine-sensitive *P. falciparum, P. malariae, P. ovale* and *P. vivax.* Mefloquine is recommended for malaria chemoprophylaxis in areas where chloroquine-resistant *P. falciparum* malaria is endemic.

Drugs Effective against the Erythrocytic Forms of the Plasmodium

Chloroquine (Aralen®) and Hydroxychloroquine (Plaquenil®)

Mechanism of action and therapeutic uses. Chloroquine and hydroxychloroquine are concentrated within the parasitized erythrocyte, where they may act by inhibiting nucleic acid synthesis by the plasmodium. Both drugs are effective against all four types of malaria, with the exception of chloroquine-resistant *P. falciparum.* They destroy the erythrocytic stages of the infection and are used both to prevent and to treat attacks. Chloroquine is the drug of choice for treatment of acute attacks. Neither chloroquine nor hydroxychloroquine will eradicate plasmodia from the liver. If this is desired, these drugs should be followed by primaquine therapy. Chloroquine resistance should be considered if a good response is not noted in two to three days.

Adverse effects. Adverse reactions to chloroquine include dizziness, headache, itching, skin rash, vomiting and blurring of vision. In low suppressive doses, these effects are minor. They are seen more frequently, and with greater intensity, if higher doses are given. Nausea and vomiting can occur with either drug. This can be reduced by taking the drugs with food. Chloroquine and hydroxychloroquine concentrate in melanin-containing areas of the body. Prolonged administration of high doses can produce corneal deposits, leading to blindness. Neither drug should be used in patients with retinal or visual field defects.

Table 21.1 on the next page lists the clinically significant drug interactions with chloroquine and hydroxycholoquine.

Table 21.1
Chloroquine and hydroxychloroquine: Drug interactions

Drug	Interaction
Chlorpromazine	• Chloroquine may increase chlorpromazine toxicity. Monitor chlorpromazine concentration
Cimetidine	• Cimetidine may decrease the metabolism and increase the toxicity of chloroquine. Monitor for symptoms of toxicity
Digoxin	• Hydroxychloroquine may increase digoxin toxicity. Monitor digoxin concentration
Penicillamine	• Chloroquine may increase penicillamine toxicity. Monitor penicillamine concentration or for clinical signs of toxicity
Promethazine	• Promethazine may increase chloroquine toxicity. Monitor for symptoms of toxicity

Quinine

Mechanism of action and therapeutic uses. Quinine's mechanism of action in the treatment of malaria is not known. It may reduce the ability of the parasite to feed within the erythrocyte. Although quinine is effective in both suppressing and treating malarial attacks, its use in malaria would probably be of historical interest only, had resistance not developed in *P. falciparum* to chloroquine and hydroxychloroquine. When used against *P. falciparum,* quinine is usually combined with pyrimethamine and a sulfonamide, such as sulfadiazine. Alternatively, uncomplicated attacks can be treated with quinine, plus tetracycline or clindamycin.

Adverse effects. Quinine often causes cinchonism. This term is derived from the fact that quinine is obtained from the bark of the cinchona tree. Cinchonism symptoms are similar to those produced by high doses of ASA (salicylism) and include nausea, vomiting, diarrhea, sweating, blurred vision, ringing in the ears and impaired hearing. In addition, patients may rarely experience leukopenia and agranulocytosis. High concentrations of quinine can cause hypotension and depress myocardial function.

Table 21.2 lists the clinically significant drug interactions with quinine.

Mefloquine Hydrochloride (Lariam®)

Mechanism of action and therapeutic uses. Mefloquine's exact mechanism of action is not known. The drug is an effective blood schizon-

Table 21.2
Quinine: Drug interactions

Drug	Interaction
Antacids	• Antacids may increase quinine toxicity. Avoid concurrent use
Anticoagulants	• Quinine may increase the effects of anticoagulants because it can depress the formation of prothrombin
Barbiturates	• Quinine may decrease phenobarbital metabolism and increase its toxicity. Monitor phenobarbital concentration
Carbamazepine	• Quinine may decrease carbamazepine metabolism and increase its toxicity. Monitor carbamazepine concentration
Cimetidine	• Cimetidine may decrease quinine metabolism and increase its toxicity
Digoxin	• Quinine may increase digoxin toxicity. Monitor digoxin concentration
Neuromuscular blockers	• Quinine may potentiate effects of neuromuscular blockers (especially pancuronium, succinylcholine and tubocurarine)

Table 21.3
Mefloquine: Drug interactions

Drug	Interaction
Beta blockers	• Mefloquine plus a beta blocker can produce ECG abnormalities or cardiac arrest
Chloroquine	• Mefloquine plus chloroquine may increase the risk for convulsions
Quinidine	• Mefloquine plus quinidine may produce ECG abnormalities or cardiac arrest
Quinine	• Mefloquine plus quinine may increase the risk for convulsions or ECG abnormalities or cardiac arrest
Valproic acid	• Mefloquine has lowered valproic acid levels and resulted in a loss of seizure control. Monitor the valproic acid blood levels of pts given mefloquine and adjust dose of valproic acid appropriately

ticide. That is to say, it acts against the mature form of the parasite. Mefloquine has no activity against exoerythrocytic forms of *P. vivax,* but does kill the asexual erythrocytic forms of *P. falciparum* and *P. vivax.*

Mefloquine is indicated for the treatment of mild to moderate acute malaria cause by mefloquine-susceptible strains of *P. falciparum* or *P. vivax.* Administration of primaquine is necessary to eliminate exoerythrocytic (hepatic phase) *P. vivax.* The primary use of mefloquine is in the chemoprophylaxis of malaria in travellers to areas where there is risk of chloroquine-resistant *P. falciparum* infection or where *P. falciparum* infection is resistant to both chloroquine and pyrimethamine/sulfadoxine (Fansidar®).

Adverse effects. Mefloquine is well tolerated in doses used for chemoprophylaxis or treatment of malaria. Its most common adverse effects are nausea, vomiting, myalgia, abdominal pain, anorexia, diarrhea, dizziness, tinnitus, headache and rashes.

Table 21.3 lists the clinically significant drug interactions with mefloquine.

Drug Treatment of the Exoerythrocytic Forms of the Plasmodium

Primaquine

Mechanism of action and therapeutic uses. The mechanism of action of primaquine may be related to the fact that it causes the mitochondria of the exoerythrocytic (hepatic) forms of plasmodia to swell and become vacuolated.

Primaquine is effective only against the exoerythrocytic stage of the plasmodium. Primaquine is important because it is the only agent effective against the liver forms of the plasmodium. It is used to provide a radical cure of malaria caused by *P. vivax* and *P. ovale.* Primaquine is similarly taken to prevent an attack after departure from areas where *P. vivax* and *P. ovale* are endemic. Because primaquine will also kill the sexual forms in the blood, it can be given to eradicate gametocytes in patients recovering from *P. falciparum* malaria.

Adverse effects. Primaquine is a relatively safe drug. It can produce occasional gastrointestinal distress, nausea, headache, pruritus and leukopenia. Agranulocytosis may occur very rarely. Five to ten percent of black males, dark-skinned Caucasians (such as Native Americans), Asians and people from Mediterranean areas demonstrate a primaquine sensitivity that can result in acute hemolytic anemia. Extensive investigations into primaquine sensitivity has determined that these subjects have a genetically determined deficiency in the erythrocytic enzyme glucose-6-phosphate dehydrogenase (G-6-PD). Without pursuing the biochemical aberrations that occur in these patients, it is enough to say that the deficiency in the enzyme enables primaquine to produce hemolysis. In addition to hemolysis, patients who are deficient in G-6-PD may also develop methemoglobinemia when treated with primaquine.

Table 21.4 on the next page lists the clinically significant drug interactions with primaquine.

Table 21.4
Primaquine: Drug interactions

Drug	Interaction
Quinacrine	• Quinacrine appears to potentiate the actions of primaquine. Therefore, the concomitant use of quinacrine and primaquine is contraindicated. Primaquine should not be administered to pts who have received quinacrine recently

Drugs That Inhibit Both Forms of the Plasmodium

Pyrimethamine (Daraprim®)

Mechanism of action and therapeutic uses. Pyrimethamine inhibits the enzyme dihydrofolic acid reductase, preventing the activation of folic acid. The reduction of folic acid by dihydrofolic acid reductase is essential to humans as well as plasmodia. Pyrimethamine has selective toxicity for the parasite because it binds very strongly to the dihydrofolic acid reductase from plasmodia and very weakly to the human enzyme.

Pyrimethamine is used prophylactically against all susceptible strains of plasmodia. Because of the widespread existence and rapid development of resistance to pyrimethamine by *P. falciparum,* it should never be used alone in the treatment of malaria. It has, however, been used successfully in combination with other agents. The drug is often used in combination with sulfadoxine to treat chloroquine-resistant *P. falciparum.* The combination product containing both pyrimethamine and sulfadoxine carries the trade name Fansidar®. Sulfadoxine reduces the formation of folic acid by plasmodia, and pyrimethamine inhibits the activation of any folic acid that is formed by the malarial parasite. The combination increases the activities of both drugs many times, decreases the number of resistant strains, and delays the development of resistance. The addition of quinine to pyrimethamine and a sulfonamide assists in controlling symptoms during the initial stages of an acute attack by chloroquine-resistant *P. falciparum.*

Pyrimethamine is also combined with mefloquine and sulfadoxine. Mefloquine is an effective blood schizonticide against *P. falciparum, P. vivax* and *P. malariae.* It destroys the early asexual blood stages and therefore acts earlier than pyrimethamine/sulfadoxine. It is not an effective tissue schizonticide.

Adverse effects. Pyrimethamine is a relatively safe drug, and few adverse effects are associated with normal doses. Signs of toxicity at higher doses, such as those used in the treatment of toxoplasmosis, include anorexia, vomiting, anemia, leukopenia and thrombocytopenia. In addition, atrophic glossitis has been reported. These effects reflect the inhibition of human dihydrofolate reductase. An acute dose of pyrimethamine can produce central nervous system stimulation, including convulsions.

Multiple-dose regimens of pyrimethamine/sulfadoxine (Fansidar®) are associated with severe cutaneous adverse reactions. Toxic epidermal necrolysis, Stevens-Johnson syndrome or erythema multiforme can occur. Other adverse effects attributed to the combination of pyrimethamine plus sulfadoxine include agranulocytosis, aplastic anemia, thrombocytopenia, leukopenia, neutropenia, hemolytic anemia, purpura, hypoprothrombinemia, methemoglobinemia and eosinophilia. Gastrointestinal adverse effects include glossitis, stomatitis, gastritis, dyspepsia, dry mouth, black tongue, gastroenteritis, anorexia, nausea, vomiting, abdominal pains, diarrhea, pancreatitis and pseudomembranous enterocolitis. Abnormal liver function tests have also been observed (elevated SGPT, SGOT, alkaline phosphatase and bilirubin).

Table 21.5 lists the clinically significant drug interactions with pryimethamine.

Nursing Management

Table 21.6 describes the nursing management of the patient receiving antimalarial drugs. Dosage details of specific drugs are given in Table 21.7 (pages 211–213).

Table 21.5
Pyrimethamine: Drug interactions

Drug	Interaction
Antacids	• Antacids may decrease pyrimethamine's effects. Give at least 4 h apart
Dapsone	• Pyrimethamine plus dapsone can produce agranulocytosis. Avoid concurrent use
Lorazepam	• Lorazepam, administered concurrently with pyrimethamine, may induce hepatotoxicity
Myelosuppressive agents	• Myelosuppressive agents interact with pyrimethamine, which may cause an exacerbation of the myelosuppressive effects of cytostatic agents, especially those of the antifolate drug methotrexate. Convulsions have occurred after the concurrent administration of methotrexate and pyrimethamine to children with CNS leukemia. Cases of bone marrow aplasia have been associated with the administration of daunorubicin, cytosine arabinoside and pyrimethamine to pts with acute myeloid leukemia
Phenothiazines	• Pyrimethamine may increase chlorpromazine toxicity. Monitor chlorpromazine concentration

Table 21.6
Nursing management of antimalarial drugs

Assessment of risk vs. benefit	Patient data	• Physician should order baseline blood tests • Assess for baseline VS, general state of health (incl. cardiac, renal and liver function), genetic risks such as G-6-PD deficiency, hx of allergic reactions, eye exam (if applicable) • For tx of present infection, assess current clinical indicators • *Pregnancy:* Most drugs in the group are risk category C (animal studies show adverse effects to fetus but human data are unknown or insufficient). Benefits may be acceptable despite the risks
	Drug data	• Each drug in this category has some serious adverse reactions, as discussed in text • Drug–food interactions are important; e.g., chloroquine and alcohol can cause liver toxicity (some tonic water products contain quinine which can be additive to drug tx!)
Implementation	Rights of administration	• Using the "rights" helps prevent errors of administration
	Right route	• Give PO — preferred route except for chloroquine hydrochloride (IM/SC) and quinidine gluconate (IV)
	Right time	• Drugs should be taken with food/meals; all cause gastric irritation. Ideally administered at regular intervals to ensure blood levels
	Right technique	• IV administration requires knowledge of correct diluent and IV solution, correct dilution and rate of administration. Always refer to manufacturer's instructions for this route. Specific precautions because rapid administration causes greater toxicity. Rate must be carefully controlled. An infusion pump is advised

(cont'd on next page)

Table 21.6 (continued)
Nursing management of antimalarial drugs

Implementation (cont'd)	Nursing therapeutics	• Emphasis differs if drug is used to treat malarial infection or for prophylaxis • If current infection, enhance host defences (nutrition, rest, fluids, hygiene) • For prophylaxis, pt teaching becomes of prime importance
	Patient/family teaching	• Compliance and follow-up are essential factors in successful tx. Review principles of pt education in Chapter 3 • Some drugs cause dizziness; pt should exercise caution until response to drug is known • Pt should take drug and return for follow-up as instructed (for blood tests and eye exams, if required). Use of sunglasses and avoiding exposure to sun can reduce risks of eye and skin reactions • Pts/families should know warning signs/symptoms of possible toxicities of drugs. Report immediately: rash, fever, sore throat, unusual bleeding or bruising, weakness, visual changes or ringing in ears. Other troublesome side effects should also be reported • Encourage discussion on risks of drug tx (side effects/adverse reactions) versus risk of contracting malaria • Discuss possibility of pregnancy; advise patient to notify physician and discuss birth control methods
Outcomes	Monitoring of progress	*Continually monitor:* • Clinical response • Be alert for signs and symptoms of adverse reactions (e.g., skin rash, blood dyscrasias, retinal damage); document and report immediately to physician • Blood tests to monitor bone marrow function may be ordered periodically

Response to Clinical Challenge

Principles

Before a drug is selected, risk can be assessed by a general examination and history. The physician and nurse will determine present renal, hepatic, cardiac and retinal health and inquire regarding previous drug allergies.

Because of his Jamaican heritage, H.K. may have G-6-PD deficiency, which can be determined by a blood test. If positive, primaquine will be avoided.

Actions

A general teaching plan should include a specific discussion of common side effects and recognition of adverse reactions. Teaching should also include a discussion of the risks of drug therapy versus the risks of contracting malaria.

Providing H.K. with written materials may increase compliance and understanding. Local community resources may include: public health clinic, travel bureau, library, infection control department.

Table 21.7
The antimalarials: Drug doses

Drug Generic name (Trade names)	Dosage	Nursing alert
chloroquine phosphate (Aralen Tablets)	**Oral:** For clinical attack of malaria: *Adults,* 600 mg base (1 g salt), followed by 300 mg base (500 mg salt) in 6 h and daily for next 2 days. *Children,* 10 mg base/kg initially (max., 600 mg base), followed by 5 mg base/kg in 6 h and daily for the next 2 days For prophylaxis of malaria: *Adults,* 300 mg base (500 mg salt). *Children,* 5 mg base/kg. The dose is given once weekly on the same day of the week beginning 1–2 weeks before the individual enters the malarious area, during, and tor 4–8 weeks after leaving the area. Primaquine should be added to regimen immediately after the individual has left an area endemic for *P. vivax* or *P. ovale,* particularly if exposure has been heavy and prolonged and if the person is not G-6-PD deficient	•Take same time daily with a meal. Check dose; e.g., 500 mg tab contains 300 mg base (active drug) and 200 mg phosphate
chloroquine hydrochloride (Aralen Injection Solution)	**IM/SC:** For tx of clinical attack of malaria: *Adults,* 2.5 mg base/kg q4h or 3.5 mg base/kg q6h, repeated prn (max., 25 mg/kg/day). Usual dose, 200–250 mg base q6h for 3 days. Oral preparation should be substituted ASAP **IV:** For tx of clinical attack of malaria: *Adults,* 10 mg base/kg, preferably infused over 4 h, while monitoring CV status to detect hypotension or arrhythmias; 5 mg base/kg is then given q12h, preferably infused over 2 h (max., 25 mg/kg/day) until pt is alert. *Children,* Initially, 1.25 mg base/kg/h is infused continuously for 8 h, immediately followed by 0.62 mg base/kg for 24 h	•Close monitoring of blood glucose, BP, HR, ECG is advisable. Carefully map site and aspirate to avoid inadvertent injection into vein. Severe reactions can occur with this route. Check dose carefully; e.g., 50 mg/mL solution contains 40 mg base (active drug)
quinine sulfate	**Oral:** For tx of chloroquine-sensitive malaria when chloroquine is contraindicated or not tolerated. *Adults,* 650 mg quinine sulfate (or 10 mg/kg) q8h for 3 days. *Children,* 25 mg/kg/day in divided doses q8h for 3 days. *P. falciparum* infections acquired in SE Asia, particularly Thailand, should be treated for 7 days	•Give with food to reduce GI irritation and reduce bitter taste. Do not crush tablets •Read label carefully. Do not confuse with quinidine

(cont'd on next page)

Table 21.7 (continued)
The antimalarials: Drug doses

Drug Generic name (Trade names)	Dosage	Nursing alert
quinine sulfate (cont'd)	For tx of chloroquine-resistant *P. falciparum* malaria: *Adults,* give the above dose. To prevent recrudescences (a fresh outbreak), pyrimethamine 25 mg bid is added for first 3 days and sulfadiazine 500 mg qid for 5 days, or the fixed-dose combination of pyrimethamine/sulfadoxine (Fansidar®) (3 tabs as a single dose) can be added to the regimen	
quinidine gluconate	**IV:** For tx of severe malaria: *Adults/children/ infants:* a loading dose of 10 mg salt/kg (equivalent to 6.2 mg of quinidine base) is infused over 1–2 h while monitoring for hypotension and widening of the QRS interval; if either occurs, rate should be decreased or infusion discontinued. A constant infusion of 0.02 mg salt/kg/min is given after loading dose	• Read manufacturer's instructions for reconstitution. Use only clear, colourless solution. Use infusion pump to control rate. Do not exceed 1 mL/min
mefloquine HCl (Lariam)	**Oral:** Begin 1 week prior to entering the area and continue for 4 weeks after leaving the area. For prophylaxis of malaria: *Adults,* 250 mg of base weekly. *Children (> 15 kg),* 4 mg/kg (max., 250 mg) weekly. For tx of malaria: *Adults,* 1.25 g base given as a single oral dose. *Children,* 25 mg/kg in a single dose	• Establish schedule to ensure drug is taken weekly. Take with food and a full glass (250 mL) of water
primaquine phosphate	**Oral:** For tx of malaria (radical cure) due to *P. vivax* and *P. ovale* or to prevent relapses in travellers after their return from malarious areas when exposure to *P. vivax* and *P. ovale* was prolonged. *Adults,* 15 mg daily for 14 days, preferably consecutively with chloroquine or other tx, which is given on the first 3 days of an acute attack. *Children,* 0.3 mg/kg, with the same regimen as for adults	• For pts with G-6-PD deficiency, consult manufacturer's information for dosage • Drug should be taken with food, same time each day
pyrimethamine (Daraprim)	**Oral:** For prophylaxis of malaria, the following doses are given once weekly on the same day of the week: *Adults/children > 10 years,* 25 mg; *children ≤ 2 years,* 6.25–12.5 mg; *3–10 years,* 12.5–25 mg. Start 1 day before entering endemic area and continue for 4 weeks after return or 6–10 weeks after exposure	• Drug should be taken with food • Establish schedule to ensure drug is taken weekly

Table 21.7 (continued)
The antimalarials: Drug doses

Drug Generic name (Trade names)	Dosage	Nursing alert
pyrimethamine + sulfadoxine (Fansidar) Tablets containing pyrimethamine 25 mg + 500 mg sulfadoxine	**Oral:** For self-tx of acute attack of chloro-quine-resistant *P. falciparum* malaria. Give as single dose. *Adults,* 3 tablets. *Children 9–14 years,* 2 tablets; *4–8 years,* 1 tablet; *1–3 years,* 1/2 tablet; *< 1 year,* 1/4 tablet	• Drug should be taken with food

Further Reading

Handbook of antimicrobial therapy. *Medical Letter on Drugs and Therapeutics* 1992.

Advice for the travelers. *Medical Letter on Drugs and Therapeutics* 1994;36:919–925.

Antiprotozoal drugs. *AMA Drug Evaluations* 1991; 3. Miscellaneous anti-infectives:3.1–3.41.

Tracey JW, Webster LT Jr. Drugs used in the chemotherapy of protozoal infections: Malaria. In: Hardman JL, Limbird LE, eds. *Goodman and Gilman's The Pharmacological Basis of Therapeutics.* 9th ed. New York: Pergamon; 1996.

CHAPTER 22

Antiprotozoal Drugs

Topics Discussed
- Trichomoniasis
- Amebiasis
- Giardiasis
- Pneumocystosis
- Toxoplasmosis
- Drugs used to treat the above conditions
- Nursing management

Drugs Discussed
emetine (**em**-a-teen)
furazolidone (fyoor-a-**zole**-i-done)
iodoquinol (eye-oh-doe-**kwin**-ol)
metronidazole (me-troe-**nie**-da-zole)
paromomycin (par-oh-moe-**my**-sin)
pyrimethamine (pirr-i-**meth**-a-meen)

Clinical Challenge

Consider this clinical challenge as you read through this chapter. The response to the challenge appears on page 220.

Lois is a 27-year-old woman who works as a receptionist in the clinic. She has vaginitis and the physician has ordered metronidazole. She is going on a weekend trip and will be driving for 3 h to attend her brother's birthday party. While you are reviewing the possible side effects with her, she asks the following questions:

- Could I delay starting the drug until Monday?
- Could I take the drug today but skip the weekend?
- Does my husband also have to be treated?

Identify the principles on which to base your responses. Outline a teaching plan.

The preceding chapter dealt with the treatment of malaria, a protozoal disease caused by the genus *Plasmodium*. Strictly speaking, malaria should be discussed together with all other protozoal diseases. However, we did not take this approach because of the serious nature of malaria and its prevalence in the world.

The present chapter continues our discussion of the treatment of protozoal diseases and concentrates on trichomoniasis, amebiasis, giardiasis, pneumocystosis and toxoplasmosis — conditions that also present health hazards.

Trichomoniasis

Vaginal infections caused by *Trichomonas vaginalis* are common and occur most frequently during the reproductive years when estrogen levels are high. The disease presents in females as vaginitis: symptomatic women typically have a diffuse, malodorous, yellow-green discharge with vulvar irritation. Diagnosis usually is made by direct microscopic visualization (wet preparation) or by culture. Male partners are usually asymptomatic but can act as reservoirs for reinfection.

Table 22.1
Metronidazole: Drug interactions

Drug	Interaction
Alcohol	•Metronidazole has a disulfiram (Antabuse®)-like effect when consumed with ethanol. Signs/symptoms include nausea, vomiting and headache. Pts should be warned to abstain from alcohol during tx
Anticoagulants	•Oral anticoagulants, such as warfarin, may have increased effects if given with metronidazole
Disulfiram	•Disulfiram and metronidazole have been reported to produce psychotic episodes and confusion in some pts
Lithium	•Concomitant use of lithium and metronidazole may result in lithium intoxication due to decreased renal clearance of lithium. Persistent renal damage may develop. When metronidazole must be administered to patients receiving lithium, it may be prudent to consider tapering or discontinuing lithium temporarily, when feasible. Otherwise, levels of lithium, creatinine and electrolytes, along with urine osmolality, should be frequently monitored
Phenobarbital	•Metabolism of metronidazole has been reported to increase with the concurrent administration of phenobarbital. Increased doses of metronidazole should be considered
Phenytoin	•Pts maintained on phenytoin were found to have toxic levels after oral metronidazole administration. Phenytoin concentrations returned to therapeutic blood levels after stopping metronidazole

Thus, both partners should be treated. Infections often recur.

Trichomonal vaginitis, urethritis and prostatovesiculitis are classified as sexually transmitted diseases (STDs). Although in theory, infections may be acquired from contaminated items (e.g., towels, toilet seats), no well-documented cases of nonvenereal transmission have been reported.

Metronidazole is the sole drug of choice for the treatment of trichomoniasis.

Metronidazole (Flagyl®, Protostat®)

Mechanism of action and therapeutic uses. Metronidazole is rapidly and completely absorbed after oral administration. The drug is well distributed to various tissues, reaching therapeutic concentrations in vaginal secretions, semen, saliva, breast milk and cerebrospinal fluid. It is mainly cleared by oxidative metabolism in the liver. Both the parent drug and its metabolites are excreted in the urine, which may become reddish-brown during treatment.

Adverse effects. The adverse effects of metronidazole are usually mild. These include nausea, anorexia, diarrhea, epigastric pain,

cramping and an unpleasant metallic taste. More serious adverse effects, such as numbness in extremities and neurotoxicity, have been rarely reported. Because the drug causes an adverse reaction when ethanol is consumed (Antabuse®-like effects), patients should be cautioned to avoid consuming alcohol during treatment.

Table 22.1 lists the clinically significant drug interactions with metronidazole.

Amebiasis

Amebiasis is caused by infection with the protozoan *Entamœba histolytica,* which occurs in all parts of North America and throughout the world. Patients become infected when they ingest mature cysts (Figure 22.1 on the next page). Once in the small bowel the cysts disintegrate, releasing four amebae, which in turn divide to form eight trophozoites. The trophozoites are carried into the large intestine, where they may live and multiply for a time in the crypts of the bowel. Some trophozoites invade the intestinal epithelium, where they form new cysts and produce ulceration. Although diarrhea often occurs at this point, ulceration does not usually result in prolonged diarrhea or abdominal pain.

Figure 22.1
Life cycle of *Entamœba histolytica*

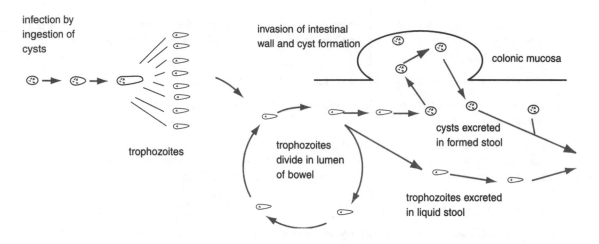

infection by ingestion of cysts

trophozoites

invasion of intestinal wall and cyst formation

colonic mucosa

trophozoites divide in lumen of bowel

cysts excreted in formed stool

trophozoites excreted in liquid stool

Source: Pratt WB. *Chemotherapy of Infection.* New York: Oxford Press; 1977. Reproduced with permission.

Interestingly, patients with diarrhea do not spread the disease because the trophozoites are not allowed sufficient time in the bowel to mature into active cysts before they are eliminated. However, cysts formed from the trophozoites on the colonic surface and subsequently passed in formed feces can lead to spread of the disease.

Amebiasis is not always limited to the bowel. If trophozoites are absorbed through the ulcerated intestinal mucosa, they can locate in the liver. Amebicides can be divided into drugs that are effective against either the intestinal or the extraintestinal form of the disease.

Treatment of Amebiasis

The choice of drug(s) to treat amebiasis depends principally on the severity of the disease and site of involvement (luminal or extraintestinal). These are summarized in Table 22.2. (For dosages of each drug, consult Table 22.5, pages 221–222.)

Within endemic areas, asymptomatic carriers generally are not treated. Elsewhere, the asymptomatic cystic carrier is treated with a luminal amebicide (i.e., a drug that kills amebae within the lumen of the gastrointestinal tract).

The pharmacology of each drug used to treat amebiasis is described in the paragraphs that follow.

Iodoquinol (Diodoquin®, Yodoxin®)

Mechanism of action and therapeutic uses. Iodoquinol blocks several important parasitic enzymes. It is the drug of choice for the treatment of asymptomatic amebiasis. Metronidazole plus iodoquinol is first-choice therapy for mild to moderate or severe intestinal disease and for hepatic abscess therapy. Iodoquinol plus either emetine or dehydroemetine represents second-line treatment for severe intestinal disease. Emetine, or dehydroemetine, combined with iodoquinol plus chloroquine is considered alternative therapy to metronidazole plus iodoquinol for hepatic amebic abscesses.

Adverse effects. Headaches, diarrhea, nausea, vomiting, anal pruritus and skin rashes are seen occasionally following use of iodoquinol. Because it contains iodine, iodoquinol can cause occasional enlargement of the thyroid and should thus not be given to patients with known iodine sensitivity or to those with hepatic damage. Further, iodoquinol has caused subacute myeloptic neuropathy when used in high doses. Patients so afflicted experience weakness, dysesthesia, peripheral neuropathy and sometimes blindness. The drug is therefore contraindicated in patients with pre-existing optic neuropathy.

Table 22.2
Recommended therapy for amebiasis

Type of infection	Therapy of choice	Alternative therapy
Asymptomatic (cyst-carrier state)	Iodoquinol	Paromomycin sulfate or diloxanide furoate
Mild to moderate intestinal disease	Metronidazole followed by iodoquinol	Metronidazole followed by paromomycin
Severe intestinal disease	Metronidazole followed by iodoquinol	Dehydroemetine or emetine followed by iodoquinol
Tissue abscess (usually hepatic)	Metronidazole followed by iodoquinol	Dehydroemetine or emetine plus iodoquinol with or without chloroquine phosphate

Source: Antiprotozoal drugs. *AMA Drug Evaluations* 1991; 3. Miscellaneous anti-infectives:3.1–3.41. Reproduced with permission.

Metronidazole (Flagyl®, Protostat®)

The actions, adverse effects and drug interactions of metronidazole have been described under the treatment of trichomoniasis earlier in this chapter. With respect to its use for the treatment of amebiasis, metronidazole becomes concentrated within *E. histolytica,* where it inhibits hydrogen production, thereby blocking the ability of the parasite to synthesize chemicals vital to its survival. The drug has little activity on the metabolic processes of humans because it is not retained in high concentrations in mammalian cells. Because most of an oral dose of metronidazole is absorbed, it is given with another luminal amebicide (usually iodoquinol) to eradicate organisms in the intestine and avoid relapse.

Emetine and Dehydroemetine

Mechanism of action and therapeutic uses. Emetine and dehydroemetine are injected intramuscularly to circumvent the nausea and vomiting produced by oral administration and the severe cardiotoxicities of intravenous treatment. The drugs block protein synthesis in both parasitic and mammalian cells but are more toxic to the protozoa. Both agents are amebicidal in the intestinal lumen against trophozoites of *E. histolytica* but are not active against cysts.

Emetine or dehydroemetine may be combined with iodoquinol as alternative therapy to metronidazole plus iodoquinol in the treatment of severe intestinal disease. These drugs are now only rarely used.

Adverse effects. Emetine and dehydroemetine can produce serious local and systemic reactions. The drugs cause pain, tenderness and muscular weakness at the injection site. Stimulation of intestinal smooth muscle is common. Patients may complain of diarrhea, cramps and vomiting.

Severe cardiovascular adverse reactions, including hypotension, tachycardia, chest pain, shortness of breath and changes in the electrocardiogram (prolongation in the P-R and Q-T intervals, as well as a flattening of the T waves) can occur. Careful monitoring of the patient is essential. Patients should be hospitalized and kept in bed during treatment. It is essential to follow the patient closely, including frequent electrocardiograms, to prevent lasting heart damage.

Paromomycin Sulfate (Humatin®)

Paromomycin is an aminoglycoside antibiotic (see Chapter 14). It is an alternative to iodoquinol for asymptomatic amebiasis, and may also be used as second-line therapy to metronidazole plus iodoquinol for mild to moderate amebic intestinal disease.

The nursing management related to the use of paromomycin sulfate is the same as that discussed in Chapter 14 for the other aminoglycoside antibiotics (see Table 14.3, pages 129–130).

Giardiasis

Giardiasis is an intestinal infection by *Giardia lamblia*. The disease may be transmitted by beavers (hence, "beaver fever") who contaminate waters in mountainous watersheds. Once ingested, the motile trophozoite of *G. lamblia* attaches to the intestinal mucosa, where it can cause a foul diarrhea and/or flatulence, abdominal distention, pain and vomiting. Giardiasis may also be associated with other parasitic or bacterial infections of the intestine.

Treatment of Giardiasis

Metronidazole has become the drug of choice in giardiasis because it has good activity and usually is well tolerated in both children and adults. Quinacrine (Atabrine®) can be given to severely affected adults who can tolerate it; however, its toxic effects (e.g., nausea and vomiting, skin disorders, psychosis) may necessitate discontinuing the drug. Because children, in particular, do not tolerate quinacrine well, metronidazole or furazolidone (Furoxone®) are more commonly prescribed for them.

The pharmacology of metronidazole is presented earlier in this chapter.

Furazolidone (Furoxone®)

Furazolidone's mechanism of antigiardial action is unclear. However, the drug does interfere with several bacterial enzymes, and this may account for its activity. Furazolidone is claimed to be effective in more than ninety percent of cases.

The most common adverse effects of furazolidone are nausea, vomiting and a vesicular or morbilliform pruritic rash. Furazolidone can also cause agranulocytosis. Patients with glucose-6-phosphate dehydrogenase (G-6-PD) deficiency can experience acute hemolysis.

Table 22.3 lists the clinically significant drug interactions with furazolidone.

Pneumocystosis

Pneumocystosis is caused by *Pneumocystis carinii*, an opportunistic parasite that infects mainly children and patients receiving immunosuppressive drugs. *P. carinii* pneumonia is also prevalent in patients with acquired immunodeficiency syndrome (AIDS; see Chapter 20). Patients often appear pale and experience a dry cough, dyspnea, tachypnea and chest discomfort. Infants have difficulty feeding, fail to gain weight, and sometimes have foamy saliva.

The treatment of pneumocystosis with pentamidine is presented in Chapter 20. Trimethoprim plus sulfamethoxazole (Bactrim®, Septra®) is an alternative agent; the pharmacology of this combination, together with its dose for the treatment of *P. carinii* infections, is presented in Chapter 15.

Toxoplasmosis

Toxoplasmosis is caused by the nonfacultative intracellular protozoan *Toxoplasma gondii*. Cats are hosts for both the enteric sexual and extraintestinal asexual forms. Humans contract toxoplasmosis by ingesting cysts, often from poorly cooked or raw meat, or oocysts from cat feces. The symptoms of toxoplasmosis range from none to encephalitis and death. The most common include retinochoroiditis, lymphadenopathy, fever and, on occasion, a rash on the palms and soles.

Toxoplasmosis is treated with pyrimethamine (Daraprim®) plus trisulfapyrimidines. The pharmacology of pyrimethamine is presented in Chapter 21.

Table 22.3
Furazolidone: Drug interactions

Drug	Interaction
Adrenergic drugs, tricyclic antidepressants, foods containing tyramine	• Furazolidone inhibits monoamine oxidase. A hypertensive reaction may occur if furazolidone is given with adrenergic drugs, TCAs or foods containing significant amounts of tyramine (e.g., cheese, red wine)
Alcohol	• Furazolidone produces a disulfiram-like reaction in some pts, if taken with alcohol

Nursing Management

The nursing management of the patient receiving antiprotozoal drugs is described in Table 22.4. Dosage details are given in Table 22.5 (pages 221–222).

Table 22.4
Nursing management of antiprotozoal drugs

Assessment of risk vs. benefit	Patient data	• *History:* Physician should establish liver function, hx allergic reactions (e.g., to iodine) • Assess for baseline VS, general state of health, learning ability for self-medication • For tx of present infection, assess current clinical indicators • *Pregnancy:* Most drugs in this group are risk category B (human data unknown or insufficient). Not recommended in first trimester; benefits must outweigh risks
	Drug data	• Most common side effects are r/t GI distress. Others are caused by CNS effects (e.g., headache, dizziness) • Each drug in this category has some serious adverse reactions: iodoquinol — optic neuropathy; metronidazole — CNS toxicity, leukopenia; emetine and dehydroemetine — cardiac toxicity; furazolidone — agranulocytosis, hemolysis with G-6-PD deficiency. • *Drug interactions:* Several summarized in text. NB reaction with alcohol, which can be severe
Implementation	Rights of administration	• Using the "rights" helps prevent errors of administration
	Right route	• PO most common, but parenteral route can be used for severe infections. Vaginal route also common for metronidazole
	Right time	• Drugs should be taken with food/meals; all cause gastric irritation. Ideally administered at regular intervals to ensure blood levels
	Right technique	• IV administration of metronidazole and pentamidine requires knowledge of correct diluent and IV solution, correct dilution and rate of administration. Always refer to manufacturer's instructions for this route. Should be infused slowly. An infusion pump is advised • **IM:** Inject emetine deeply and slowly
	Nursing therapeutics	• Emphasis depends on indication for use, e.g., treating trichomoniasis vaginalis versus amebiasis. For any infection, enhance host defences (nutrition, rest, fluids, hygiene) • With emetine and dehydroemetine, bedrest is advised • Implement infection control methods relevant for intestinal disease
	Patient/family teaching	• Pts/families should understand transmission of intestinal and/or vaginal infections and daily hygiene to prevent infecting others.

(cont'd on next page)

Table 22.4 (continued)
Nursing management of antiprotozoal drugs

Implementation (cont'd)	Patient/family teaching (cont'd)	• With vaginal infection, partner may also be treated. Management of common side effects should be discussed (e.g., for dry mouth, review Chapter 28; for dizziness or headache, avoid driving or activities that require alertness until response to medication is known). Encourage pt to tolerate some side effects, e.g., unpleasant metallic taste with metronidazole • Stress importance of avoiding alcohol while taking metronidazole or furazolidone; may cause severe reaction • Pts/families should know warning signs/symptoms of possible toxicities of drugs. Report immediately: rash, fever, sore throat, unusual bleeding or bruising, excessive weakness, vertigo • *Discuss possibility of pregnancy:* Advise pt to notify physician; discuss birth control methods
Outcomes	Monitoring of progress	*Continually monitor:* • Clinical response. With intestinal infections, stool examinations will be conducted during and after tx • Be alert for signs/symptoms of adverse reactions, e.g., skin rash, blood dyscrasias, retinal damage. Document and report immediately to physician • With long-term tx, blood tests may be ordered periodically

Response to Clinical Challenge

Principles
All anti-infectives have greater success with the maintenance of an effective blood level. This is achieved by dosing at regular intervals, based on the half-life of the specific drug.

Vaginal infections may be transmitted to a sexual partner and cause reinfection following drug therapy.

Actions
Metronidazole has a half-life of 8–9 h. Treatment of vaginal infection caused by *Trichomonas vaginalis* can be achieved by three options:

• 2-g single dose (PO)
• 250 mg tid x 10 days (PO)
• 500 mg daily x 10–20 days (vaginal).

Lois should not start and then stop drug therapy. She should discuss dosage options with the physician, together with necessity of treating her husband.

A general teaching plan should include the following points:

• avoid alcohol (severe reaction)
• avoid driving until response to drug is known
• expect side effects (GI distress, which can be reduced by taking drug with food; dry mouth and unpleasant metallic taste, which can sometimes be moderately reduced by good oral hygiene, sugarless gum/candy; discolored urine (no action required)
• report other reactions and any signs/symptoms of superinfection.

Table 22.5
The antiprotozoals: Drug doses

Drug Generic name (Trade names)	Dosage	Nursing alert
dehydroemetine	**IM:** For amebiasis: *Adults:* 1–1.5 mg/kg/day for 5 days. Max. dose, 90 mg/day, followed by 650 mg of iodoquinol PO tid for 20 days. Max., 2 g/day. *Children:* Not > 1–1.5 mg/kg/day in 2 doses for 5 days, followed by 30–40 mg/kg/day of iodoquinol PO in 3 doses for 20 days. Max., 2 g/day	• Inject slowly and deeply. Aspirate to avoid inadvertent injection into blood vessel. Instruct pt to refrain from exercise and exertion during tx (drug very irritating to tissue)
emetine	**IM:** For amebiasis: *Adults:* 1 mg/kg/day (max., 60 mg/day) for 5 days, followed by 650 mg iodoquinol PO tid for 20 days. *Children:* Not > 0.5 mg/kg bid for 5 days, followed by 30–40 mg/kg/day of iodoquinol PO in 2–3 doses for 20 days. Max., 2 g/day	• As for dehydroemetine
furazolidone (Furoxone)	**Oral:** For giardiasis: *Adults:* 100 mg qid for 7–10 days. *Children:* 6 mg/kg/day divided into 4 equal doses, with meals for 7–10 days. Do not give to children < 1 month of age	
iodoquinol (Diodoquin, Yodoxin)	**Oral:** For asymptomatic amebiasis (cyst-carrier state): *Adults:* 650 mg tid for 20 days. Max. dose, 2 g/day. *Children:* 30–40 mg/kg/day in 2–3 doses for 20 days. Max. dose, 2 g/day. Refer also to dosage instructions for adults and children under metronidazole	• Tablets may be crushed and mixed with food
metronidazole (Flagyl, Protostat)	**Oral:** For amebiasis (intestinal disease or tissue abscess): *Adults:* 750 mg tid for 10 days, followed by 650 mg of iodoquinol tid for 20 days. Max. dose, 2 g/day. *Children:* 35–50 mg/kg/day in 3 divided doses for 10 days, followed by iodoquinol 30–40 mg/kg/day in 3 doses for 20 days. Max dose, 2 g/day For giardiasis: *Adults:* 250–500 mg tid for 5–7 days or 2 g/day as single dose for 3 days. *Children:* 5 mg/kg tid for 5–7 days	• Warn pts not to consume alcohol. Vaginal inserts or cream should be inserted deep into the vagina. To facilitate disintegration of insert, it may be immersed in water for a few seconds just before introduction into vagina. Keep applicator clean

(cont'd on next page)

Table 22.5 (continued)
The antiprotozoals: Drug doses

Drug Generic name (Trade names)	Dosage	Nursing alert
metronidazole (Flagyl, Protostat) (cont'd)	For trichomoniasis: *Single dose* (for both women and men), 2 g as a single dose after a meal. *Standard 10-day tx: Women:* 250 mg bid, morning and night for 10 days. *Men:* 250 mg bid for 10 days. For both men and women, it may occasionally be necessary to give a second day 10-course after 4–6 weeks. *Vaginal insert:* One 500-mg insert every night for 10–20 days, even during menstruation. *Vaginal cream:* One applicatorful 1x or 2x daily into the vagina for 10–20 days, even during menstruation	
paramomycin sulfate (Humatin)	**Oral:** *Adults/children:* 25–35 mg/kg/day in 3 divided doses with meals for 7–10 days. This course of tx may be repeated after a 2-week interval	• Give with food
pyrimethamine (Daraprim)	**Oral:** For toxoplasmosis: *Adults:* Initially, 100–150 mg in 2 equal doses daily for 3 days, followed by 25–50 mg/day for 3–4 weeks plus trisulfapyrimidines 2–6 g daily in 4–6 divided doses for 3–4 weeks. *Children:* 2 mg/kg/day (max., 25 mg/day) for 3 days, then 1 mg/kg/day (max., 25 mg/day) for 4 weeks. This should be given with 100–200 mg/kg/day of trisulfapyrimidines in 4–6 divided doses for 3–4 weeks. *Infants:* 2 mg/kg/day for 3 days, then 1 mg/kg/day every 2–3 days for 4 weeks	• Give with milk or food to reduce GI distress
quinacrine HCl (Atabrine Hydrochloride)	**Oral:** For giardiasis: *Adults:* 100 mg tid pc for 5 days. Although not commonly used in children, a recommended dose is 2 mg/kg tid pc for 5 days (max., 300 mg/day)	• Give pc

Further Reading

Antiprotozoal drugs. *AMA Drug Evaluations* 1991; 3. Miscellaneous anti-infectives:3.1–3.41.

Drugs for parasitic infections. *Medical Letter on Drugs and Therapeutics* 1993(December 10):35.

Handbook of antimicrobial therapy. *Medical Letter on Drugs and Therapeutics* 1992.

Tracey JW, Webster LT, Jr. Drugs used in the chemotherapy of protozoal infections. In: Hardman JL, Limbird LE, eds. *Goodman and Gilman's The Pharmacological Basis of Therapeutics.* 9th ed. New York: Pergamon; 1996:987–1008.

CHAPTER 23

Drugs Used to Treat Worm Infections (Anthelmintics)

Topics Discussed
- Cestodes (tapeworms)
- Nematodes (roundworms)
- Trematodes (flukes)
- Drugs used to treat worm infections: mechanisms of action, therapeutic uses, adverse effects
- Nursing management

Drugs Discussed
mebendazole (meh-**ben**-dah-zole)
niclosamide (nik-**loe**-sah-myde)
piperazine (**pie**-per-ah-zeen)
praziquantel (praz-zee-**kwahn**-tel)
pyrantel (pirr-**ran**-tel)
pyrvinium (peer-**vin**-ee-um)
thiabendazole (thye-ah-**ben**-dah-zole)

Clinical Challenge

Consider this clinical challenge as you read through this chapter. The response to the challenge appears on page 228.

Barry J. is 7 years old. His father brings him to the clinic with his 5-year-old sister. A stool specimen has been sent for examination, and the report states, "Enterobius vermicularis."

Explain to the family:

- the diagnosis
- the treatment
- the actions the family should take.

What are the drugs of choice and the advantages of each?

Worms, or *helminths*, have plagued humankind since the beginning of time. Despite recent developments in drug therapy, they continue to extract a tremendous cost in human suffering. Even today, approximately fifty percent of humans are infected with worms. It has been estimated that the number of worm infections harboured by humans exceeds the world's population; meaning that, at this moment, millions of people are providing nice, warm hostels for more than one type of worm.

Helminths can be divided into cestodes (flatworms), nematodes (roundworms) and trematodes (flukes) (Table 23.1 on the next page). Worms can also be classified according to the parts of the body they infect. Some infect only the gastrointestinal tract; others live in body tissues.

Table 23.1
Classification of human helminths

Biological Classification	Examples
Cestodes (flatworms or tapeworms)	*Tænia saginata* *Tænia solium*
Nematodes (roundworms)	*Ascaris lumbricoides* (roundworm) *Enterobius vermicularis* (pinworm) *Necator americanus, Ancylostoma duodenale* (hookworms)
Trematodes (flukes)	*Schistosoma* spp.

Table 23.2
Drugs used to treat worm infections

Helminths	Drugs
Cestodes	Niclosamide Praziquantel
Nematodes	
Ascaris lumbricoides	Pyrantel Mebendazole Piperazine
Enterobius vermicularis	Mebendazole Pyrantel pamoate Piperazine Pyrvinium pamoate
Strongyloides stercoralis	Thiabendazole Pyrvinium pamoate
Trichuris trichiura	Mebendazole Thiabendazole
Necator americanus and *Ancylostoma duodenale*	Mebendazole Pyrantel pamoate Thiabendazole Bephenium Hydroxynaphthoate
Trematodes	
Schistosoma hæmotobium and *Schistosoma mansoni*	Niridazole Stibophen

Anthelmintic drugs can act locally on worms in the gastrointestinal tract or systemically on worms that have migrated into various tissues. Most common intestinal parasites can be eliminated easily and safely with an appropriate anthelmintic that works inside the intestinal lumen. Tissue infections (e.g., muscle, liver, lung) may be more difficult to treat, are often of longer duration (subchronic to chronic) and occasionally require additional supportive procedures, including surgery, for cure. Table 23.2 summarizes the drugs currently used to treat the various types of worm infections.

Cestodes (Tapeworms)

Tapeworm infections occur when humans eat uncooked meat or fish containing encysted larvae. The tapeworm is segmented and flat, with a small sucker on its head (called the *scolex*). Once larvae are ingested, the sucker attaches to the host's small intestine, and the worm grows by producing one segment after another. The extent to which the worm can grow is illustrated by the fact that the fish tapeworm (*Diphyllobothrium latum*) can reach a length of ten metres and may contain three to four thousand segments.

It is not surprising that patients with tapeworms encased within the lumen of their intestinal tracts may experience symptoms. What is remarkable is that many individuals show few effects. The symptoms of tapeworm infection may include vague abdominal discomfort and pain, weakness, weight loss, epigastric fullness and anemia.

Taenia saginata and *Taenia solium* are the two chief tapeworms infecting humans. Improperly cooked beef is the source of *T. saginata* (beef tapeworm). Although the tapeworm can grow to ten metres in humans, it cannot propagate in the intestines. The fertilized eggs of *T. saginata* can form larvae only in the gastrointestinal tract of cattle. *T. solium* differs from the beef tapeworm in two respects. First, it is obtained from uncooked pork (pork tapeworm), and second, it can propagate in the gastrointestinal tract of humans. If this happens, larvae hatched in the gastrointestinal tract are carried into the blood and spread throughout the body, developing into space-occupying masses in the orbit of the eye, brain, muscle, liver and other organs.

Niclosamide (Niclocide®)

Mechanism of action, therapeutic uses and adverse effects. Tapeworms derive most of their energy in the intestine from anaerobic metabolism, and niclosamide inhibits anaerobic metabolism in the helminth. As a result, the scolex releases its hold on the intestinal wall and the worm is passed in the feces.

Niclosamide is administered orally to treat both beef and pork tapeworms. Because the drug is not absorbed from the gastrointestinal tract, tapeworms are exposed to high concentrations of it. In the case of *T. solium,* viable eggs may be released when segments of the worm are destroyed. Therefore, a laxative is usually administered one or two hours after the drug to prevent cysticercosis (a disease caused by the presence of tapeworm larvae). The drug is also given to eradicate fish tapeworm (*Diphyllobothrium latum*) and dwarf tapeworm (*Hymenolepis nana*).

Niclosamide produces few adverse effects. Some patients complain of abdominal pain, and others may experience diarrhea.

Praziquantel (Biltricide®)

Mechanism of action, therapeutic uses and adverse effects. Praziquantel causes an efflux of intracellular calcium, resulting in tetanic paralysis of worms and their subsequent removal from their sites of attachment. The drug has a broad spectrum of activity against trematodes (flukes) and cestodes (tapeworms). Praziquantel is as effective as niclosamide and appears quite safe in treating intestinal tapeworm infections caused by *T. saginata* (beef tapeworm), *T. solium* (pork tapeworm) and *D. latum* (fish tapeworm). When given daily for two weeks, praziquantel is also effective in the treatment of cysticercosis caused by pork tapeworm (*T. solium*).

Large doses of praziquantel have commonly been associated with dizziness, headache, malaise, abdominal pain and nausea. However, these effects are generally mild and transient. Praziquantel frequently causes drowsiness, and patients should be advised to use caution while driving or performing activities that require mental alertness until one day after the last dose is taken. The drug can also cause a syndrome consisting of headache, hyperthermia, seizures, intracranial hypertension and/or arachnoiditis (inflammation of the arachnoid membrane) in patients treated for neurocysticerosis (the presence of tapeworm larvae in nervous tissue), especially those with multiple brain cysts. It is presumed that these effects result from an inflammatory response to dead and dying organisms in the central nervous system and cerebrospinal fluid. They may be prevented by prior or concurrent corticosteroid therapy, or both. Praziquantel is contraindicated in the treatment of ocular cysticerosis because the destruction of parasites within the eye may cause irreparable lesions.

Table 23.3 lists the clinically significant drug interactions with praziquantel.

Nematodes (Roundworms)

Nematodes, or roundworms, are the most common helminths bothering humans. Depending on the particular worm involved, they may be found within the gastrointestinal tract or in the tissues of the body. The next few pages will discuss the main characteristics of the more common roundworm infections and the drugs used to treat them.

Ascaris lumbricoides (Roundworm)

Ascaris lumbricoides is the most common human parasite. It is found in about one-third of the world's population — about one billion people. Commonly call a roundworm, it should not be confused with the general classification of round-

Table 23.3
Praziquantel: Drug interactions

Drug	Interaction
Carbamazepine	• Carbamazepine increases metabolism of praziquantel and decreases its effect. Monitor for decreased response to praziquantel
Phenytoin	• Phenytoin increases metabolism of praziquantel and decreases its effect. Monitor for decreased response to praziquantel

worms (nematodes), of which it is only one member. Infection with *A. lumbricoides* is more prevalent in warmer areas of the world, but is also seen in colder climates.

Humans become infected with roundworms when they ingest embryonated eggs. Children playing in sandboxes provide an excellent example of how this can happen. The larvae hatch in the duodenum and are absorbed into the blood. Carried to the alveoli, they ascend the airways to reach the epiglottis and are swallowed. Upon their return to the small intestines, the larvae develop into male and female roundworms. At this stage patients may be asymptomatic or may experience abdominal distress (epigastric pain, nausea, vomiting and anorexia). More serious problems are created if the worms migrate into the pancreatic and bile ducts, gall bladder or liver, or if they completely obstruct the appendix or intestinal lumen.

Because of the possibility of serious complications, ascariasis (the disease caused by the roundworm) should always be treated. Pyrantel pamoate and mebendazole are the drugs of choice. Piperazine citrate is an alternative.

Pyrantel pamoate (Antiminth®, Combantrin®).

Pyrantel pamoate is poorly absorbed from the gastrointestinal tract. Administered orally, it paralyzes roundworms. A single oral dose of pyrantel pamoate is the drug of choice for the treatment of *A. lumbricoides*. The drug is also indicated for the treatment of pinworms (enterobiasis) and hookworms (*Ancylostoma duodenale, Necator americanus*). It is not recommended for pregnant patients or for children under one year of age. Sufficient drug may be absorbed to produce headache, irritability, insomnia, dizziness and drowsiness. Abdominal cramps have also been reported.

Mebendazole (Vermox®).

Mebendazole is also poorly absorbed from the gastrointestinal tract. It inhibits glucose uptake by *A. lumbricoides,* depletes the worm's supply of glycogen and lowers adenosine triphosphate (ATP) synthesis. In addition to *A. lumbricoides,* mebendazole is used to eradicate *Enterobius vermicularis* (pinworm) and *Trichuris trichiura* (whipworm). Hookworm infections caused by *A. duodenale* or *N. americanus* may also be treated with mebendazole. As well, it has been used to treat infections caused by *T. solium* (pork tapeworm).

Patients treated with mebendazole may suffer diarrhea, vomiting and/or abdominal pain. Other adverse effects reported include drowsiness, itching, headache and dizziness. Special attention should be given to patients with intestinal pathology (e.g., Crohn's ileitis, ulcerative colitis).

Table 23.4 lists the clinically significant drug interactions with mebendazole.

Piperazine citrate (Vermizine®) and piperazine adipate (Entacyl®).

Piperazine produces a flaccid paralysis in the worm, which is eliminated in the feces. Piperazine is well absorbed from the gastrointestinal tract, and most of the drug is eliminated in urine within twenty-four hours. Piperazine is effective against *A. lumbricoides* (roundworm) and *E. vermicularis* (pinworm). Given as either the citrate, phosphate or adipate salts, it cures more than eighty percent of roundworm infections when given for two days.

Piperazine is generally well tolerated. Its adverse reactions include gastrointestinal upset,

---

Table 23. 4
Mebendazole: Drug interactions

Drug	Interaction
Insulin and oral hypoglycemics	• Mebendazole may increase insulin secretion. This would potentiate exogenous insulin and oral hypoglycemic drugs
Carbamazepine and phenytoin	• Carbamazepine and phenytoin decrease the plasma concentration of mebendazole when mebendazole is used in large doses
Cimetidine	• Cimetidine inhibits mebendazole metabolism and increases mebendazole serum concentration. Determination of plasma concentrations of mebendazole is recommended to allow dosage adjustment.

Table 23.5
Piperazine: Drug interactions

Drug	Interaction
Phenothiazines	• Phenothiazines and piperazine should be taken concomitantly with caution because piperazine can exaggerate phenothiazine-induced extrapyramidal effects

urticaria and dizziness. It can also cause neurologic symptoms that include hypotonia and ataxia — the so-called worm-wobble effect. Visual disturbances and exacerbations of epilepsy can also occur. Piperazine is contraindicated in patients with impaired renal or hepatic function, convulsive disorders or a history of hypersensitivity reactions to piperazine or its salts.

Table 23.5 lists the clinically significant drug interactions with piperazine.

Enterobius vermicularis (Pinworm)

Enterobius vermicularis, also called oxyuris, is the infamous pinworm, the most common human helminth in Canada and the United States. As any parent with young children will readily attest, this little fellow can make life very difficult around the house. Not content to torment children, it can also weigh heavily on the minds of men and women of all walks of life. Its ability to tickle the seats of the mighty has led to the development of many drugs, all capable of giving this parasite a well-deserved shellacking.

Pruritus in the perianal and perineal regions is the most common consequence of pinworm infections. Scratching may lead to infection. In female patients the worms may migrate to the genital tract. Because pinworm infections are often found in several members of the same family, it is appropriate to treat the entire family and close friends of an infected child.

Pinworms are treated with mebendazole, pyrantel pamoate, piperazine and pyrvinium. All but the last drug were discussed previously in this chapter.

Pyrvinium pamoate (Povan®, Vanquin®). The mechanism of action of pyrvinium is not known. Given orally, it is not well absorbed. Pyrvinium pamoate is considered an alternative drug to pyrantel pamoate or mebendazole for the treatment of *E. vermicularis.* Pyrvinium is given in a single dose, but the treatment is repeated in two weeks to clear any worms that have matured from the remaining eggs. The drug has few adverse effects. Patients should be warned that feces will be stained a bright red, and that this effect is harmless. Pyrvinium may occasionally cause a photosensitive skin rash.

Strongyloides stercoralis (Threadworm)

Strongyloides stercoralis (threadworm) is encountered frequently in the tropics. It can also be common in the southern United States. Threadworm infections are often found in conjunction with other worm infestations. Thiabendazole is the drug of choice; pyrvinium pamoate is a back-up agent.

Thiabendazole (Mintezol®). Thiabendazole is rapidly absorbed from the gastrointestinal tract and metabolized in the liver. Its mechanism of action is not known. Nematodes sensitive to this drug include *A. lumbricoides* (roundworm), *E. vermicularis* (pinworm), *T. trichiura* (whipworm), *N. americanus* and *A. duodenale* (hookworm). The adverse effects of thiabendazole limit it as a drug of first choice to the treatment of *S. stercoralis.* About one-third of patients taking the drug experience anorexia, nausea, vomiting, drowsiness or vertigo. Pruritus, rash, diarrhea, hallucinations, crystalluria and leukopenia occur less frequently.

Trichuris trichiura (Whipworm)

Whipworm infections are found throughout the world. They are more prevalent in warm, humid climates. *Trichuris trichiura* is often found in patients suffering from roundworm and hookworm infections. Usually whipworm infections do not cause major problems, except in severely infected children.

Mebendazole is the drug of first choice for the treatment of whipworms. Thiabendazole is the back-up drug. Both agents were discussed earlier in this chapter.

Necator americanus and *Ancylostoma duodenale* (Hookworm)

Hookworms burrow through the skin of humans and are transported via blood to the alveoli. After ascending the respiratory tree to the epiglottis they are swallowed, after which they reach the intestinal lumen. Within the intestine, hookworms attach to the mucosa and cause ulcerations, abdominal fullness and epigastric pain. Because hookworms can suck blood from the intestinal mucosa, patients may demonstrate progressive hypochromic, microcytic anemia of the nutritional-deficiency type. Other problems created by hookworms are localized erythema and severe itching at the point where larvae penetrate the skin. The passage of large numbers of larvae through the lungs can cause pneumonitis.

Mebendazole and pyrantel pamoate are recommended for the treatment of hookworms. Both of these drugs have been discussed previously.

Trematodes (Flukes)

Trematodes are nonsegmented flattened worms. Usually, they have two suckers — one at the mouth and the other located on the ventral surface. Trematode larvae are acquired by humans through food (aquatic vegetation, fish, crayfish) and by direct penetration of the skin. Most trematodes mature in the intestinal tract (intestinal flukes); others migrate and mature in the liver and bile duct (liver flukes), whereas still others penetrate the intestinal wall and are carried to the lung (lung flukes).

The symptoms vary, depending on the location of the flukes. Diarrhea, abdominal pain and anorexia are often seen, regardless of the infection site. Lung flukes cause coughs, chest pain and hemoptysis. Liver flukes can block the bile duct, enlarge the liver and produce right-quadrant pain and diarrhea.

As schistosomiasis (also called bilharziasis) is rarely seen in North America, it is beyond the scope of this book to discuss the use of niridazole (Ambilhar®) to treat infections of *Schistosoma haematobium* and *Schistosoma mansoni,* or the use of stibophen for infections caused by *Schistosoma mansoni.* By the same token, space limitations prevent a discussion of the use of antimony potassium tartrate for the treatment of *Schistosoma japonicum* infections, biothionol as the drug of first choice in the treatment of infections caused by *Paragonimus westermani* (lung fluke) and *Fasciola hepatica* (sheep liver fluke), or chloroquine phosphate as the drug of first choice in the treatment of *Clonorchis sinensis* (liver fluke) infections. Nurses requiring the use of these drugs should consult reference texts, such those cited under the section headed Further Reading at the end of this chapter.

Nursing Management

The nursing management of the patient receiving anthelmintic drugs is described in Table 23.6. Dosage details are given in Table 23.7 (pages 230–231).

Response to Clinical Challenge

Principles

Barry has the most common helminth infestation — pinworms. Several drugs can be chosen for treatment. The entire family will be treated because it is likely that others are infected. Each family member should be taught good personal hygiene, particularly after bowel movements. This includes good hand washing and cleaning of fingernails.

Actions

Two drugs of choice are mebendazole and pyrantel. Mebendazole has the advantage that it can be swallowed whole, chewed, or crushed and mixed with food (likely more appealing to the 5- and 7-year-olds in this family). Pyrantel has the advantage of a single-dose treatment which is repeated after 2 weeks. Both drugs have few side effects, are generally well tolerated and do not require laxatives administered for successful treatment.

Table 23.6
Nursing management for the anthelmintics

Assessment of risk vs. benefit	Patient data	• *History:* Physician should establish liver function, hx allergic reactions • Assess for baseline VS, general state of health, learning ability for self-medication • For tx of present infection, assess current clinical indicators • *Pregnancy:* Most drugs in this group are risk category B or C (benefits must outweigh risks)
	Drug data	• Generally well tolerated with few adverse risks. • Most common side effects are r/t GI distress. Some drugs cause CNS effects, e.g., headache, dizziness • *Drug interactions:* Several summarized in text
Implementation	Rights of administration	• Using the "rights" helps prevent errors of administration
	Right route	• Give PO
	Right time	• All drugs are given orally; dosage regime varies with drug and indication for use
	Right technique	• Check before crushing tablets; some should be taken whole
	Nursing therapeutics	• Implement infection control methods relevant for intestinal disease
	Patient/family teaching	• Most drugs will be self-administered. Ensure pt is taught how/when to take drug and that doses for adults and children differ. Stress hygiene to prevent reinfestation of self or others, including cleaning clothing and bedding. Advise pt to avoid preparation of food for others while infected • Advise pt that some drugs in this class cause dizziness • *Discuss possibility of pregnancy:* Advise pt to notify physician; discuss birth control methods
Outcomes	Monitoring of progress	*Continually monitor:* • Clinical response • With intestinal infections, stool examinations will be conducted during and after tx

Table 23.7
The anthelmintics: Drug doses

Drug Generic Name (Trade Names)	Dosage	Nursing Alert
mebendazole (Vermox)	**Oral:** *Children > 2 years/adults:* For whipworm (trichuriasis), roundworm (ascariasis), hookworm (ancylostomiasis), threadworm (strongyloidiasis), tapeworm (taeniasis) and mixed infections, 1 tablet (100 mg) a.m. and hs for 3 days. For enterobiasis, 1 tablet (100 mg) only. If not cured after 3 weeks, give second course	• Tablets may be chewed, crushed and mixed with food or swallowed whole. Do not give to pregnant women, particularly in first trimester. Caution should be used when administering to nursing women
niclosamide (Niclocide)	**Oral:** For intestinal tapeworm infections except *H. nana* (e.g., diphyllobothriasis, dipylidiasis, taeniasis): *Adults,* 2 g (4 tablets) as a single dose. *Children > 34 kg (75 lb),* 1.5 g (3 tablets) as a single dose; *11–34 kg (25–75 lb),* 1 g (2 tablets) as a single dose *For H. nana* (dwarf tapeworm): *Adults,* 2 g (4 tablets) on day 1, followed by 1 g (2 tablets) daily for 6 days. *Children > 34 kg (75 lb),* 1.5 g (3 tablets) on day 1, then 1 g (2 tablets) daily for 6 days; *11–34 kg (25–75 lb),* 1 g (2 tablets) on day 1, then 0.5 g (1 tablet) for 6 days	• Pt should omit breakfast but may eat 2 h after last dose. Take entire daily dose at one time. Tablets should be chewed thoroughly and swallowed with a little water • Physician may order a laxative to expel worms
piperazine adipate (Entacyl)	**Oral:** For roundworms and pinworms (ascariasis or enterobiasis); one-day tx. **Granules:** *Children 2–8 years,* 1 packet (2 g); *8–14 years,* 1 packet (2 g) 2x in 1 day (total, 4 g). *Children > 14 years/adults,* 1 packet (2 g) 3x in 1 day (total, 6 g). **Suspension:** *Children < 2 years,* 5 mL (1 tsp) 3x in 1 day; *2–8 years,* 10 mL (2 tsp) 2x in 1 day; *8–14 years,* 10 mL (2 tsp) 3x in 1 day; *> 14 years/adults,* 15 mL (3 tsp) 3x times in 1 day. Repeat in 2 weeks	• Dissolve 1 packet in 60 mL (2 oz) water, milk or fruit juice. Best absorbed on empty stomach. Do not substitute piperazine citrate; dosage differs
piperazine citrate (Vermizine)	**Oral:** For roundworms (ascariasis): *Adults/children,* 75 mg/kg (max., 3.5 g) od for 2 days. For pinworms (enterobiasis): *Adults/children,* 65 mg/kg (max., 2.5 g) od for 7 days. Repeat after 1 week	• Do not substitute piperazine adipate; dosage differs. Best absorbed on empty stomach
praziquantel (Biltricide)	**Oral:** For tapeworms (taeniasis, diphyllobothriasis and dipylidiasis): *Adults/children > 4 years,* 10–20 mg/kg in a single dose. For hymenolepiasis: *Adults/children > 4 years,* 25 mg/kg in a single dose.	• Swallow quickly; has very bitter taste. Do not crush or chew tablets

Table 23.7 (continued)
The anthelmintics: Drug doses

Drug Generic Name (Trade Names)	Dosage	Nursing Alert
praziquantel (Biltricide) (cont'd)	For cysticercosis: *Adults/children > 4 years,* 50 mg/kg/day in 3 equal doses q4–6h for 14 days. Concomitant corticosteroid tx (e.g., dexamethasone 6–16 mg/day, prednisone 30–40 mg/day) is recommended in selected pts with cerebral involvement and elevated intracranial pressure. May repeat in 3–6 months	
pyrantel pamoate (Antiminth, Combantrin)	**Oral:** For pinworms/roundworms: *Adults/ children* (1 single daily dose): ≤ *11 kg,* 1 tablet or 2.5 mL; *12–23 kg,* 2 tablets or 5 mL, *24–45 kg,* 4 tablets or 10 mL; *46–68 kg,* 6 tablets or 15 mL; *> 68 kg,* 8 tablets or 20 mL. For hookworms: Same dosage as above, given od for 3 days. One tablet contains 125 mg pyrantel base; 1 mL contains 50 mg pyrantel base	• Do not exceed recommended dose. Shake liquid well and take at one time, with food, milk or juice • Advise rigorous cleaning of living quarters and clothing; strict attention to personal hygiene • Should not be taken if pregnant, unless essential for pt's welfare
pyrvinium pamoate (Povan, Vanquin)	**Oral:** For pinworms: Single dose of 50 mg/ 10 kg. Repeat in 2 weeks	• Take immediately pc
thiabendazole (Mintezol)	**Oral:** For threadworm (strongyloidiasis): 25 mg/kg bid (max., 3 g/day) for 2 days. Continue tx for at least 5 days in pts with disseminated infections (hyperinfection syndrome). Immunocompromised pts may require more prolonged tx	• Tablet should be chewed and taken with food. Shake suspension well • A significant number of pts may require more than 2 days' tx to achieve negative stool samples; follow-up stool samples should be obtained

Further Reading

Anthelmintics. *AMA Drug Evaluations* 1992; 3. Miscellaneous anti-infectives:4.1–4.32.

Drugs for parasitic infections. *Medical Letter on Drugs and Therapeutics* 1993(December 10); 35.

Handbook of antimicrobial therapy. *Medical Letter on Drugs and Therapeutics* 1992.

Tracy JW, Webster LT Jr. Drugs used in the chemotherapy of helminthiasis. In: Hardman JL, Limbird LE, eds. *Goodman and Gilman's The Pharmacological Basis of Therapeutics.* 9th ed. New York: Pergamon; 1996:1009–1026.

CHAPTER 24

Drugs for the Treatment of Topical Infections

Topics Discussed
- Antibacterial drugs
- Antifungal drugs
- Mechanisms of action and pharmacologic effects
- Therapeutic uses
- Adverse effects
- Drug interactions
- Nursing management

Drugs Discussed
amphotericin (am-foe-**ter**-ih-sin)
bacitracin (bass-ih-**tray**-sin)
clotrimazole (kloe-**trye**-mah-zole)
econazole (ee-**kon**-ah-zole)
framycetin (frah-mye-**see**-tin)
fusidic acid (few-**sid**-ik)
gentamicin (jen-tah-**mye**-sin)
griseofulvin (gris-ee-oh-**ful**-vin)
haloprogin (hal-oh-**proe**-jin)
ketoconazole (kee-toe-**kon**-ah-zole)
mafenide acetate (mah-**fen**-eyed **ass**-eh-tayt)
miconazole (mye-**kon**-ah-zole)
mupirocin (myoo-**peer**-oh-sin)
neomycin (nee-oh-**mye**-sin)
nystatin (nye-**stat**-in)
silver sulfadiazine (sul-fah-**dye**-ah-zeen)
terbinafine (ter-**bin**-ah-feen)
tioconazole (tye-oh-**kon**-a-zole)
tolnaftate (tole-**naff**-tayt)

Clinical Challenge

Consider this clinical challenge as you read through this chapter. The response to the challenge appears on page 237.

Jock is a 19-year-old hockey player who visits the team doctor for a check-up. Tinea pedis (athlete's foot) is diagnosed, and tioconazole 1% cream bid is ordered.

1. How should the cream be applied?
2. What side effects may occur?
3. How long will treatment be required?
4. What actions would you recommend to this young athlete?

Previous chapters in Unit 3 have concentrated on specific groups of anti-infective agents and their use in the treatment of infections within various body systems. This chapter addresses topical infections and describes the pharmacologic properties, therapeutic uses, adverse effects and interactions of drugs designed specifically for their treatment. Nurses will find this material most useful because of the prevalence of these infections in the general population.

Antibacterial Drugs

Streptococcus pyogenes and *Staphylococcus aureus* are the most common causative bacteria in primary skin infections. Other common pathogens are *Escherichia coli* and *Pseudomonas aeruginosa*, together with *Klebsiella, Enterobacter, Pasteurella* and *Proteus* species.

Aminoglycoside Antibiotics: Gentamicin (Garamycin®), Framycetin (Soframycin®), Neomycin (Myciguent®)

Therapeutic uses. The mechanism of action and antibacterial spectra of aminoglycoside antibiotics are presented in Chapter 14. Used topically, these drugs are effective in the treatment of primary and secondary skin infections caused by sensitive strains of streptococci, *Staphylococcus aureus, Pseudomonas aeruginosa, Enterobacter aerogenes, Escherichia coli, Proteus vulgaris* and *Klebsiella pneumoniae.*

Gentamicin, framycetin and neomycin are often applied for the treatment of skin infections. Neomycin is often combined with polymyxin B, and either bacitracin or gramicidin. Framycetin is available alone or combined with dexamethasone; it is also impregnated into a light-weight paraffin gauze dressing. Gentamicin is applied topically for infected severe burns when the causative bacteria is *Pseudomonas aeruginosa.*

Adverse effects. Hypersensitivity reactions, usually of the delayed type, are the most common adverse effects of the aminoglycosides. If gentamicin is applied to a large denuded surface, it may be absorbed in sufficient quantity to produce systemic toxicity (see Chapter 14).

Mafenide (Sulfamylon®) and Silver Sulfadiazine (Flamazine®, Silvadene®)

Mechanism of action, therapeutic uses and adverse effects. Mafenide is a sulfonamide that is used in conjunction with debridement for the prevention and treatment of infection, particularly by *Pseudomonas aeruginosa,* in second- or third-degree burns. In addition to typical sulfonamide-type allergic reactions, mafenide can produce pain or a burning sensation.

Silver sulfadiazine is effective in vitro against various strains of the following pathogens isolated from infected burn wounds: *Pseudomonas aeruginosa, Enterobacter aerogenes, Escherichia coli, Proteus mirabilis, Proteus vulgaris, Staphylococcus aureus, Klebsiella, Aerobacter niger* and *Candida albicans.* The drug owes its activity to the formation of silver chloride, silver protein complexes and sodium sulfadiazine. Both sulfadiazine and silver exert bacteriostatic effects.

Silver sulfadiazine is indicated for the treatment of leg ulcers, burns, skin grafts, incisions and other clean lesions, abrasions, minor cuts and wounds. It is particularly valuable in the treatment and prophylaxis of infections in victims of serious burns. Silver sulfadiazine does not penetrate so well as mafenide, but systemic effects have been reported following the application of the drug to large surface areas. However, it also does not produce the pain on application that characterizes mafenide. As well, the incidence of allergic reactions is lower.

Bacitracin (Baciguent®)

Bacitracin is an excellent topical antibiotic that is active against staphylococci and streptococci. Although severe allergic disorders have been seen when bacitracin is applied locally, these are very rare.

Fusidic Acid, Sodium Fusidate (Fucidin Topical®)

Mechanism of action and pharmacologic effects. Fusidic acid inhibits bacterial protein synthesis by interfering with amino acid transfer from aminoacyl-sRNA to protein on the ribosomes. Fusidic acid may be bacteriostatic or bactericidal, depending on the inoculum size. Fusidic acid is virtually inactive against gram-negative bacteria.

Therapeutic uses and adverse effects. Fusidic acid is indicated for the treatment of primary and secondary skin infections caused by sensitive strains of *S. aureus,* streptococcus species and *C. minutissimum.* Primary skin infections that may be expected to respond to treatment with fusidic acid topical include impetigo contagiosa and erythrasma. Fusidic acid is also used in secondary skin infections such as infected wounds and infected burns. Resistance to fusidic acid has readily been induced in vitro. The development of resistance has also been shown to occur in the clinical setting. Mild irritation has occasionally been reported in patients with dermatoses treated with fusidic acid.

Mupirocin (Bactroban®)

Mechanism of action, therapeutic uses and adverse effects. Mupirocin exerts a bactericidal action against sensitive organisms by inhibiting bacterial protein synthesis. It reversibly and specifically binds to bacterial isoleucyl transfer-RNA synthetase. Mupirocin is indicated for the topical treatment of impetigo caused by sensitive strains of staphylococcus and streptococcus species as well as for other superficially infected dermatoses and lesions that are moist and weeping. For abrasions, minor cuts and wounds, the use of mupirocin may prevent development of infection by sensitive gram-positive organisms. No cross-resistance has been shown between mupirocin and other commonly used antibiotics.

Topical mupirocin compares well with fusidic acid for skin infections. Although both appear equally effective in the topical treatment of acute bacterial skin infections, mupirocin has been reported to be particularly effective against primary skin infections, impetigo, and staphylococcal and streptococcal infections. In addition, fusidic acid is used systemically for severe staphylococcal infections; induction of resistant bacteria is therefore a concern. Mupirocin is unsuitable for systemic administration, and its topical use cannot influence subsequent systemic treatment of severe infections.

Local adverse reactions have been reported with mupirocin. These include itching, burning, erythema, stinging and dryness.

Miscellaneous Drugs

Gramicidin is effective against many gram-positive bacteria. It is often incorporated into creams, together with polymyxin B (Polysporin®), neomycin (Spectrocin®) and polymyxin B plus neomycin (Neosporin®) for the treatment of superficial bacterial skin infections.

Iodochlorhydroxyquin, or clioquinol (Vioform®), has both antibacterial and antifungal activities. It is applied topically to treat dermatoses and infections in which a mild antibacterial and antifungal effect is desired. Unfortunately, the drug may stain fabrics and hair.

Polymyxin B has bactericidal action against most gram-negative bacilli except *Proteus* species. It is particularly effective against *Pseudomonas aeruginosa, E. coli, Enterobacter* and *Klebsiella* species. Polymyxin B is not active against gram-positive bacteria or fungi.

Betadine contains 10% povidone-iodine USP (1% available iodine). It is available as a solution, ointment, shampoo and skin cleanser, and is also impregnated into gauze pads. Povidone-iodine is bactericidal and fungicidal. Unlike iodine, it does not stain natural fabrics.

Antifungal Drugs

Dermatophytosis (fungal infections) may involve the skin, hair and nails. Dermatophytes show specificity for the type of keratin they invade. *Microsporum* species usually attack hair; *Trichophyton,* the skin, hair and nails; and *Epidermophyton,* the skin.

Topically Applied Antifungal Drugs

Amphotericin B (Fungizone®)
Amphotericin B is active against *Candida* species and can be used to treat cutaneous and mucocutaneous infections. Topical applications can cause local irritation, pruritus and skin rash.

Clotrimazole (Canesten®, Lotrimin®, Gyne-Lotrim®, Mycelex®, Myclo®)

Therapeutic uses and adverse effects. Clotrimazole is effective against a wide range of fungi, including *Microsporum* and *Trichophyton* species. Topical creams and solutions are used to treat tinea pedis, tinea cruris and tinea corporis caused by *Trichophyton rubrum, Trichophyton mentagrophytes* and *Epidermophyton floccosum,* as well as candidiasis caused by *Candida albicans,* and tinea versicolor produced by *Microsporum furfur.* Vaginal creams and tablets are used in the treatment of vaginal candidiasis and trichomoniasis. Although skin reactions have been reported, clotrimazole is generally well tolerated.

Econazole (Ecostatin®, Spectazole®)

Therapeutic uses and adverse effects. Econazole exhibits a broad spectrum of fungistatic activity in vitro against species of the genus *Candida*. Vaginal ovules are used to treat vulvovaginal candidiasis (moniliasis). Topical creams are employed in the treatment of tinea pedis, tinea cruris, tinea corporis, tinea versicolor and cutaneous candidiasis. Econazole may occasionally cause itching, burning or other local irritations.

Haloprogin (Halotex®)

Therapeutic uses and adverse effects. Haloprogin is used in the topical treatment of superficial fungal infections of the skin, such as tinea pedis, tinea cruris, tinea corporis and tinea manuum due to infection by *Trichophyton rubrum*, *T. tonsurans*, *T. mentagrophytes*, *Microsporum canus* and *Epidermophyton floccosum*. The drug is also useful in the treatment of tinea versicolor due to *Microsporum furfur* and for monilial infections of the skin caused by *Candida albicans*. Topical application occasionally causes irritation, burning, vesicle formation and pruritus.

Miconazole (Micatin®, Monistat-Derm®, Monistat®)

Therapeutic uses and adverse effects. Miconazole is applied topically to inhibit *Epidermophyton*, *Microsporum* and *Trichophyton* species, as well as *Candida*. Infections often treated with miconazole include tinea pedis, tinea cruris, tinea corporis, tinea unguium and tinea versicolor. Rarely, mild pruritus, irritation and burning at the site of application have been reported.

Terconazole (Terazol®)

Therapeutic uses and adverse effects. Terconazole exhibits fungicidal activity in vitro against the genus *Candida*. Both the yeast and mycelial form of *C. albicans* are sensitive to terconazole. Terconazole vaginal ovules and cream are indicated for the local treatment of vulvovaginal candidiasis (moniliasis). Both dosage forms of terconazole have been associated with a higher incidence of headache. However, the overall degree of safety of terconazole appears to be high.

Tioconazole (Gyno-Trosyd®, Trosyd®)

Therapeutic uses and adverse effects. Tioconazole is indicated for the topical treatment of patients with tinea pedis, tinea cruris and tinea corporis caused by *T. rubrum*, *T. mentagrophytes*, and *E. floccosum;* cutaneous candidiasis due to *C. albicans;* tinea (pityriasis) versicolor caused by *M. furfur*. One percent tioconazole dermal cream is well tolerated. Some patients (7.2%) have reported symptoms of local irritation; the most commonly observed symptoms include burning sensation (3.2%), itching (2.8%), erythema (1.5%), rash (0.8%) and edema (0.2%).

Tolnaftate (Tinactin®)

Therapeutic uses and adverse effects. Tolnaftate is used for the topical treatment of tinea pedis, tinea cruris, tinea corporis and tinea manuum due to infection with *T. rubrum*, *T. mentagrophytes*, *T. tonsurans*, *M. audouini*, *E. floccosum* and for tinea versicolor due to *M. furfur*. Good results can be anticipated in patients with recent, mild fungus infection of the scalp (tinea capitis) treated with tolnaftate solution. Tolnaftate preparations are essentially nonsensitizing and do not ordinarily sting or irritate intact or broken skin in either exposed or intertriginous areas.

Orally Administered Antifungal Drugs

Griseofulvin (Fulvicin-U/F®, Fulvicin-P/G®, Grifulvin V®, Grisactin®, Grisactin Ultra®, Gris-PEG®, Grisovin-FP®)

Therapeutic uses and adverse effects. Griseofulvin is effective orally against superficial infections caused by fungi responsible for dermatomycoses. It is useful in the treatment of fungal infections of the scalp and glabrous skin.

Griseofulvin is less effective in chronic infections of the feet, palms and nails. Because these

Table 24.1
Griseofulvin: Drug interactions

Drug	Interaction
Alcohol	• Alcohol should be forbidden during tx with griseofulvin as griseofulvin may augment or potentiate the effects of alcohol, leading to tachycardia, flushing, and more serious consequences
Anticoagulants, oral	• The activity of oral anticoagulants may be reduced by griseofulvin because griseofulvin can increase their metabolism
Barbiturates	• Griseofulvin can increase the metabolism and decrease the activity of barbiturates
Contraceptives, oral	• Oral contraceptives may have decreased contraceptive effects if griseofulvin is taken

chronic infections tend to cause hyperkeratosis, concomitant topical keratolytic therapy is almost always necessary.

Griseofulvin is absorbed over a prolonged period of time from the gastrointestinal tract. Its absorption is greatly increased by reducing the particle size of the drug. Once absorbed, griseofulvin is deposited in the stratum corneum of the skin, the keratin of the nails and the hair, thus preventing fungal invasion of newly formed cells.

Its adverse effects include headache, skin rashes, dryness of the mouth and gastrointestinal disturbances. Photosensitivity reactions may be associated with griseofulvin, and patients should be warned to avoid exposure to intense, natural or artificial sunlight. Should a photosensitivity reaction occur, lupus erythematosus may be aggravated. Griseofulvin can cause hepatotoxicity. It is contraindicated in patients with acute intermittent porphyria, a history of porphyria, or hepatocellular failure. The drug is also contraindicated in patients who are hypersensitive to it.

Table 24.1 lists the clinically significant drug interactions with griseofulvin.

Orally and Topically Administered Antifungal Drugs

Ketoconazole (Nizoral®)

Therapeutic uses and adverse effects. The use of oral ketoconazole to treat systemic fungal infections is described in Chapter 19. Ketoconazole has a broad spectrum of antifungal activity. It may be considered for treatment of severe, recalcitrant dermatophytoses unresponsive to other forms of therapy.

Cases of idiosyncratic hepatocellular dysfunction have been reported during oral ketoconazole treatment. Liver disorders can occur during therapy; these can be fatal unless properly recognized and managed. Liver function tests such as SGGT, alkaline phosphatase, SGPT, SGOT and bilirubin should be performed before treatment and at periodic intervals during it (monthly or more frequently), particularly in patients who are expected to receive prolonged therapy or who have a history of significant alcohol consumption. Likewise, the concurrent use of ketoconazole with potentially hepatotoxic drugs should be most carefully monitored, especially during prolonged therapy or in patients whose history includes significant alcohol consumption.

The other adverse effects of orally administered ketoconazole include nausea and/or vomiting (3%), gastrointestinal hemorrhage (<1%), abdominal pain (1.2%) and diarrhea (<1%).

Ketoconazole inhibits certain hepatic oxidase systems. Thus, it may decrease the elimination of coadministered drugs whose metabolism depends on the enzymes (see Table 19.3, page 183).

Ketoconazole cream (2%) is applied topically for the treatment of tinea pedis, tinea corporis and tinea cruris by *Trichophyton rubrum, Trichophyton mentagrophytes* and *Epidermophyton floccusum;* in the treatment of tinea versicolor (pityriasis) caused by *Malassazeia furfur (Pityrosporum orbiculare);* and in the treatment of seborrhoeic dermatitis caused by *Pityrosporum ovale.* Ketoconazole cream appears to be well tolerated by the skin.

Ketoconazole shampoo is indicated for the topical treatment and prophylaxis of pityriasis capitis infections (dandruff) in which the yeast *Pityrosporum* is involved.

Nystatin (Candex®, Mycostatin®, Nilstat®)

Therapeutic uses and adverse effects. Nystatin is effective against *Candida* species. Topical creams, ointments, powders and vaginal tablets are available for the treatment of mycotic infections caused by *Candida albicans*. Vaginal preparations may also be used during pregnancy to prevent thrush in the newborn. Because nystatin is not absorbed from the gastrointestinal tract, it is taken orally to prevent or treat candidal infections of the oral cavity or esophagus, for intestinal candidiasis and for protection against candidal overgrowth during antimicrobial or corticosteroid therapy. Large oral doses occasionally cause gastrointestinal distress, diarrhea, nausea and vomiting.

Terbinafine (Lamisil®)

Therapeutic uses and adverse effects. Terbinafine is an allylamine that has a broad spectrum of antifungal activity. At low concentrations, terbinafine is fungicidal against dermatophytes, moulds and certain dimorphic fungi.

Terbinafine interferes specifically with fungal sterol biosynthesis at an early step. This leads to a deficiency in ergosterol and to an intracellular accumulation of squalene, resulting in fungal cell death.

Oral terbinafine is indicated in the treatment of onychomycosis (fungal infection of the nail) caused by dermatophyte fungi. Terbinafine appears to be more effective than griseofulvin in the treatment of onychomycosis. Whereas griseofulvin is required for five to six months for fingernails and eight to eighteen months for toenail infections, terbinafine is usually given for six weeks to three months. Terbinafine also has a lower relapse rate than griseofulvin.

Terbinafine tablets are also approved for the treatment of ringworm (tinea corporis, tinea cruris and tinea pedis) and yeast infections of the skin caused by genus *Candida* (e.g., *C. albicans*) where oral therapy is considered appropriate owing to the site, severity or extent of the infection.

Compared with other oral antifungals, terbinafine appears to be safer; its side effects are mild and transient. The most common are gastrointestinal symptoms or skin reactions.

One percent terbinafine cream is indicated in the treatment of fungal infections of the skin caused by dermatophytes, such as *Trichophyton,* as well as yeast infections of the skin, principally those caused by genus *Candida* (e.g., *C. albicans*). It is effective and requires shorter periods of therapy than other topical imidazoles, such as clotrimazole, ketoconazole and tioconazole.

Nursing Management

The nursing management of the patient receiving drugs for the treatment of topical infections is described in Table 24.2 on the next page. Dosage details for individual drugs are given in Table 24.3 (pages 239–242).

Response to Clinical Challenge

1. *Application:* Wash area thoroughly and dry; gently massage cream into affected and surrounding area every morning and evening.
2. *Side effects:* This drug is usually well tolerated, but Jock may experience local irritation (burning, itching, redness).
3. *Duration of treatment:* Will vary with extent of infection, but may be as long as 6 weeks.
4. *Patient teaching:* Keep feet clean and dry; wear well-ventilated shoes and change them daily; change socks frequently; do not miss any doses; do not use any other creams/lotions on infected area; return for follow-up exam as instructed.

Further Reading

Balfour JA, Faulds D. Terbinafine. A review of its pharmacodynamic and pharmacokinetic properties, and therapeutic potential in superficial mycoses. *Drugs* 1992;43:259–284.

Handbook of antimicrobial therapy. *Medical Letter on Drugs and Therapeutics* 1992.

Table 24.2
Nursing management of topical anti-infectives

Assessment of risk vs. benefit	Patient data	• *History:* Physician should establish liver function, hx allergic reactions • Assess for baseline VS, general state of health, learning ability for self-medication • For tx of present infection, assess current clinical indicators (e.g., appearance and size of infected area) • *Pregnancy:* Most drugs in the group are risk category B or C (i.e., benefits must outweigh risks)
	Drug data	• Topical application is generally well tolerated with few adverse risks. Application to large areas may cause systemic absorption. • Oral route is associated with higher incidence of side effects or adverse reactions • Most common side effects are related to local irritation (i.e., itching, burning, redness). This must be distinguished from allergic reaction. Some drugs do cause CNS effects, e.g., headache, dizziness with ketoconazole • *Drug interactions:* Most significant occur with griseofulvin (see Table 24.1). Other lotions/creams should not be used concurrently without advice from physician/pharmacist
Implementation	Rights of administration	• Using the "rights" helps prevent errors of administration
	Right route	• Topical route for most of these agents; griseofulvin, ketoconazole, nystatin and terbinafine also given PO
	Right time	• Schedule varies with drug and indications for use. Generally, the schedule for topical application can vary with pt's lifestyle. Vaginal applications should be inserted hs to facilitate remaining at site
	Right technique	• Application of topical medications requires asepsis, protection of self from medication, knowledge of whether to massage into site and whether a dressing should be applied • In general, application should be made with gloved hand or spatula. Area should be cleansed thoroughly and dried prior to new application. Infected and surrounding area should be covered. For intertriginous areas (areas of the body where two skin surfaces may rub together such as axilla, underneath large breasts, inner thighs), lotions or powders are preferred over creams. Apply sparingly and smoothly
	Nursing therapeutics	• Implement infection control methods to prevent spread or reinfection. Maintain asepsis (e.g., use spatula to remove cream from container)
	Patient/family teaching	• Most drugs will be self-administered. Ensure pt is taught how/when to apply/take drug

Table 24.2 (continued)
Nursing management of topical anti-infectives

Implementation (cont'd)	Patient/family teaching (cont'd)	• Stress hygiene to prevent reinfection of self or others, e.g., separate towels, clean clothing and bedding; clean, well-ventilated shoes and frequent changing of socks for athlete's foot • Explain possible local reactions and how to observe for improvement • Even if condition has improved, drug should be continued to prescribed duration to prevent recurrence. Advise pt to contact physician if no improvement in condition • Oral route has more side effects and pts should be so advised. For griseofulvin, pts should avoid exposure to ultraviolet light (photosensitivity) and alcohol (serious reaction) • Advise pt that some drugs in this class cause dizziness • *Discuss possibility of pregnancy:* Advise pt to notify physician; discuss birth control methods
Outcomes	Monitoring of progress	*Continually monitor:* • Clinical response. Drug tx will continue even after apparent improvement

Table 24.3
Topical anti-infectives: Drug doses

Drug Generic name (Trade names)	Dosage	Nursing alert
A. Aminoglycoside Antibiotics		
framycetin sulfate–gramicidin (Soframycin Ointment)	**Topical:** Apply locally 2–4x/day as prescribed	• Observe for sensitivity
framycetin sulfate gauze dressing (Sofra-Tulle)	**Topical:** Apply single layer directly to wound and cover with appropriate dressing. If wound is exudative, dressings should be changed at least daily. In case of leg ulcers, cut dressing accurately to size of ulcer to decrease risk of sensitization and to avoid contact with surrounding healthy skin	• Store dressing flat, at cool temperature
gentamicin sulfate (Garamycin)	**Topical:** Cream or ointment should be applied gently to lesions tid–qid	• Cleanse area; cover with gauze dressing if desired
neomycin sulfate (Myciguent)	**Topical:** Apply to affected areas 2–5x/day.	• Cleanse area and pat dry. Apply thin film of ointment • Discontinue use if sensitization occurs. Observe for superinfection

(cont'd on next page)

Table 24.3 (continued)
Topical anti-infectives: Drug doses

Drug Generic name (Trade names)	Dosage	Nursing alert
B. Sulfonamides		
mafenide acetate (Sulfamylon)	**Topical:** Apply thin layer 1–2x/day	• Clean and debride wounds before applying cream with sterile glove • Monitor for local pain or irritation
silver sulfadiazine (Flamazine, Silvadene)	**Topical:** Apply 3–5 mm of cream. Reapply at least q24h	• Cleanse area; apply with sterile glove or non-metallic spatula. Reapply if cream has been removed by pt activity. Wound may be dressed or left open
C. Miscellaneous Antibiotics		
bacitracin compound (Baciguent)	**Topical:** Apply liberally 1 or more times/day	• Cleanse area; apply liberally and cover with dry, sterile dressing • Observe for sensitivity reactions
fusidic acid, sodium fusidate (Fucidin Topical)	**Topical:** Apply small amount of ointment or cream tid–qid until favourable results are achieved. Apply single layer of intertulle directly to wound and cover with dressing	• Cleanse area. If wound is exudative, dressings should be changed at least 1x/day • Observe for sensitivity to fusidic acid and its salts, or to lanolin
mupirocin (Bactroban)	**Topical:** Apply small amount to affected area tid for up to 10 days	• Avoid contact with eyes. Ointment is not suitable for ophthalmic or intranasal use • Dressing may be used
D. Topically Applied Antifungal Drugs		
amphotericin B (Fungizone)	**Topical:** Apply 3% cream, ointment or lotion bid–tid prn **Instill (in eye):** Drops containing 0.5–1.5 mg/mL; 1 drop q30min, then q1h	• Wear gloves to apply liberally and rub in well • Avoid occlusive dressings. May stain clothing (usually comes out when washed)
clotrimazole (Canesten, Lotrimin, Gyne-Lotrimin, Mycelex, Myclo-Derm)	**Topical:** *Skin infections:* Apply cream or solution to selected and surrounding areas bid, a.m. and p.m. *Vaginal trichomoniasis:* 1 (100-mg) tablet intravaginally for 6 days, preferably hs. *Vaginal candidiasis:* 1 (200-mg) tablet intravaginally for 3 days, preferably hs; or 1 (100-mg) tablet intravaginally for 6 days, preferably hs. *Vaginal cream:* 1 full applicator 1% cream intravaginally for 6 days preferably hs; or 1 full applicator 2% cream for 3 days, preferably hs	• Cleanse area and dry well. Apply thin coat and massage gently • **Vaginal:** Insert deep into vagina using applicator (except if pregnant). Cleanse equipment well after use

Table 24.3 (continued)
Topical anti-infectives: Drug doses

Drug Generic name (Trade names)	Dosage	Nursing alert
D. Topically Applied Antifungal Drugs (cont'd)		
econazole nitrate (Ecostatin, Spectazole)	**Cream:** Apply bid (a.m. and hs) **Vaginal:** 1 ovule for 3 nights	•Cleanse area, then apply cream and massage gently into affected and surrounding areas. Cleanse vaginal applicator well after use
haloprogin (Halotex)	**Topical:** Apply cream or solution (10 mg/g or 10 mg/mL) bid	•Avoid contact with eyes
miconazole nitrate (Micatin, Monistat-Derm, Monistat 7)	**Cream:** Apply thin layer to affected area bid for 1–2 weeks **Vaginal cream:** 1 applicatorful od hs for 7 nights **Vaginal suppositories:** 1 suppository od for 7 nights	•Massage gently until cream disappears. Read manufacturer's instructions •Cleanse applicator after each use
tioconazole (Gyno-Trosyd, Trosyd)	**Topical** (Trosyd): For tinea versicolor, treat for 7–28 days. For tinea pedis, up to 6 weeks may be required in severe cases. For dermatophyte infections and cutaneous candidiasis at other sites, treat for 2–4 weeks **Intravaginal** (Gyno-Trosyd): 1 applicatorful, preferably hs	•Massage gently into affected and surrounding areas bid, a.m. and hs. Apply sparingly under breasts or inner thighs and smooth in well to avoid macerating effects •Observe for local transient reaction
tolnaftate (Tinactin)	**Topical:** Provided as solution, powder, cream or aerosol powder. All should be applied according to directions bid. Usually, 2–3 weeks' tx is adequate, but 4–6 weeks may be required	•**Powder:** Apply small amount and rub in gently. **Cream:** Massage gently until it disappears. **Solution:** 1 drop to each lesion, then massage. **Spray:** Spray liberally on affected area
E. Orally Administered Antifungal Drug		
griseofulvin (Fulvicin-U/F, Fulvicin-P/G, Grifulvin V, Grisactin, Grisactin Ultra, Gris-PEG, Grisovin FP)	**Oral:** Microcrystalline form: *Adults:* For less serious infections, 500 mg daily (125 mg qid or 250 mg bid); for severe infections, 750 mg–1 g daily in divided doses. *Children:* Approx. 10 mg/kg/day in single or divided doses with meals	•Give with meal to reduce GI irritation. Fatty foods promote absorption

(cont'd on next page)

Table 24.3 (continued)
Topical anti-infectives: Drug doses

Drug Generic name (Trade names)	Dosage	Nursing alert

E. Orally Administered Antifungal Drug (cont'd)

griseofulvin (Fulvicin-U/F, Fulvicin-P/G, Grifulvin V, Grisactin, Grisactin Ultra, Gris-PEG, Grisovin-FP) (cont'd)	Ultramicrocyrstalline form: *Adults:* For tinea corporis, tinea cruris and tinea capitis, 330 mg daily in single or divided doses. For more difficult fungal infections (e.g., tinea pedis and tinea unguium), 660 mg in divided doses. *Children:* Approximately 5.5 mg/kg/day	

F. Orally and Topically Administered Antifungal Drugs

ketoconazole (Nizoral)	**Oral:** *Adults,* 200 mg od, not to exceed 400 mg. *Children > 40 kg,* 200 mg od; *20–40 kg,* 100 mg od; *≤ 20 kg,* 50 mg od, not to exceed 100–400 mg. **Topical cream:** Apply od for tinea pedis (4–6 weeks), tinea corporis (3–4 weeks), tinea cruris (2–4 weeks), tinea versicolor and cutaneous candidiasis (2–3 weeks) **Topical shampoo:** Apply to wet scalp, work into lather and leave on for 3–5 min before rinsing with water. For pityriasis capitis infections (dandruff) involving *Pityrosporum:* 2x weekly for 4 weeks. Prophylaxis 1x every 1–2 weeks	• **Oral:** Best absorbed in acid medium with citrus juice, coffee or tea. Do not give with antacids • **Topical:** Cover affected and surrounding areas and rub in gently. **Shampoo:** Keep out of eyes and off eyelids
nystatin (Candex, Mycostatin, Nadostine, Nilstat)	**Oral:** (Tablets) *Adults,* 500 000–1 000 000 U tid. (Suspension) *Adults/children,* 400 000–600 000 U qid. *Infants,* 200 000 U qid. *Premature and low birthweight infants,* 100 000 U qid. **Vaginal:** 100 000–200 000 U/day for 2 weeks. **Topical:** Apply cream or ointment (100 000 U/g) to lesions bid. Use powder for moist lesions bid–tid	• **Suspension:** Shake well before use. Hold half of each dose for some time in either side of mouth before swallowing. • **Topical:** Apply liberally
terbinafine HCl (Lamisil)	**Oral:** *Adults,* 125 mg bid or 250 mg daily. For onychomycosis of fingers and toes, 6 weeks–3 months. Infection of the big toenail may require 6 months or more. For tinea pedis, 2–6 weeks; for tinea corporis and tinea cruris, 2–4 weeks **Topical:** Apply cream od–bid. For tinea corporis/cruris, 1–2 weeks; tinea pedis, 1 week; cutaneous candidiasis, 2 weeks; pityriasis versicolor, 2 weeks	• Tx varies according to indication and severity of infection. Complete resolution of signs/symptoms may not occur until several weeks after mycological cure • Avoid contact with eyes. Do not use occlusive dressing

Drugs Used in the Treatment of Cancer

Millions of human cells divide and differentiate every day. Under normal circumstances, cell division, differentiation and growth are controlled by the cell's own genes, by contacts with surrounding cells and by various growth and inhibitory substances. When this control is lost, cancer develops.

The past twenty-five years have seen a massive push in the fight against cancer. While this effort has brought about an improved understanding of the nature of the illness and some spectacular advances in treatment, still the incidence of cancer has not decreased, nor has overall mortality from the disease been affected.

Unit 4 presents an overview of the chemotherapy of cancer. It describes the basic mechanisms by which drugs may decrease cancer growth, their effect on tumour size and the cell cycle and — most importantly for nurses — the adverse effects that are common to most anticancer drugs.

Because of the complexity of cancer chemotherapy, Unit 4 does not attempt to detail the treatment of particular types of cancer or the approved uses for each anticancer drug. This information cannot be provided in a text of this size and should be obtained from books dedicated solely to the treatment of cancer.

CHAPTER 25

Antineoplastic Drugs

Topics Discussed
- Definition of neoplasia, persistant proliferation, invasive growth, metastasis, selective toxicity, growth fraction
- Relationship of growth fraction to choice of anticancer drugs and success of chemotherapy
- Classification of antineoplastic drugs
- Adverse effects
- Nursing management

Drugs Discussed
actinomycin D (ak-tin-oh-**mye**-sin)

aminoglutethimide (ah-meen-oh-glew-**teth**-ih-myde)

asparaginase (as-**par**-ah-jin-ase)

bleomycin (blee-oh-**mye**-sin)

buserelin (byoo-seh-**ree**-lin)

busulphan (byoo-**sul**-fan)

carboplatin (kar-boe-**plat**-in)

carmustine; BCNU, BiCNU (kar-**muss**-teen)

chlorambucil (klor-**am**-byoo-sill)

cisplatin (sis-**plat**-in)

cladribine (**klad**-rib-een)

cyclophosphamide (sye-kloe-**foss**-fah-myde)

cytarabine (sye-**tare**-ah-been)

dacarbazine (dah-**kar**-ba-zeen)

dactinomycin (dak-tin-oh-**mye**-sin)

daunorubicin (dawn-oh-**roo**-bih-sin)

docetaxel (doe-see-**tak**-sil)

doxorubicin (dox-oh-**roo**-bih-sin)

etoposide (ee-**toe**-poe-side)

floxuridine (flox-**yoor**-ih-deen)

fludarabine (floo-**dar**-ah-been)

fluorouracil (flyoor-oh-**yoor**-ah-sill)

flutamide (**flew**-tah-myde)

goserelin (**goe**-seh-rell-in)

hydroxyurea (hye-drox-ee-yoo-**ree**-ah)

idarubicin (eye-dah-**roo**-bih-sin)

ifosfamide (eye-**foss**-fah-myde)

leuprolide (lew-**proe**-lyde)

lomustine; CCNU, CeeNU (loe-**muss**-teen)

mechlorethamine; nitrogen mustard (mek-klor-**eth**-ah-meen)

megestrol (meh-**jess**-trole)

melphalan (**mel**-fah-lan)

mercaptopurine; 6-MP (mer-kap-toe-**pyoor**-een)

methotrexate (meth-oh-**trex**-ate)

methyl lomustine; methyl CCNU (**meth**-ill loe-**muss**-teen)

mitotane (**mye**-toe-tane)

mitomycin C (mye-toe-**mye**-sin)

paclitaxel (pack-lih-**tak**-sill)

pentostatin; DCF (pen-toe-**stat**-in)

plicamycin; mithramycin (plye-kah-**mye**-sin)

pipobroman (pye-poh-**broe**-man)

procarbazine (proe-**kar**-bah-zeen)

streptozocin (strep-toe-**zoss**-in)

tamoxifen (tah-**mock**-see-fen)

teniposide; VM-26 (ten-**ip**-oh-syde)

testolactone (tes-toe-**lack**-tone)

thioguanine (thye-oh-**gwan**-een)

thiotepa (thye-oh-**tepp**-ah)

vinblastine (vin-**blass**-teen)

vincristine (vin-**kriss**-teen)

vindesine (**vin**-dah-seen)

vinorelbine (vin-or-**ell**-been)

Clinical Challenge

Consider this clinical challenge as you read through this chapter. The response to the challenge appears on page 252.

You are working in a women's health clinic. As part of the breast health program, the clinic is participating in a large, multicentre study of prevention of breast cancer using tamoxifen. A double-blind, randomized trial using tamoxifen 20 mg/day versus placebo has begun, and you are recruiting volunteer subjects. To fulfill your role in this research you need to understand the use of placebos in a double-blind trial and answer subjects' questions about the drug tamoxifen (e.g., What is the action of the drug? What side effects may occur? What are the indications for notifying the clinic?).

Mrs. E.H. is a 53-year-old client who is participating in the study. She asks, "Are there other benefits — not just prevention of breast cancer? What side effects may I expect?"

What answers would you provide?

This chapter reviews drugs used in the treatment of cancer, which are variously called anticancer or *antineoplastic* drugs. Because of the complexity of the subject, we will not discuss in detail these drugs' mechanisms of action nor their precise therapeutic applications. Instead, we will concentrate on the general principles that guide the use of antineoplastic agents and the adverse effects common to most of them.

Although we discuss the treatment of cancers in general, nurses will recognize that the term cancer refers to many different disorders and not to a single disease entity. Perhaps no word strikes fear into the human heart so much as cancer. This is understandable, because as mortality from infectious disease has declined (largely as a result of the new antibacterials), cancer has emerged as a leading cause of death. The number of deaths due to cancer in North America is second only to those caused by heart failure. In women between the ages of thirty and fifty-four and in children aged three to fourteen, cancer leads all other causes of mortality.

Yet, cancer is predominantly a disease of the elderly: more than half of all reported cases occur in people over the age of 65. Thus, the aging of the population in the industrialized world is the major factor in the disease's increased incidence. Gender is the second most important determinant, with males accounting for the majority of newly diagnosed cases. When mortality is broken down into tumour types, lung cancer is clearly responsible for the heightened incidence of cancer in men.

Cancer, or *neoplasia,* arises from transformed cells. It is characterized by an uncontrolled cellular proliferation that takes place at the expense of the host. Neoplastic cells have three common characteristics: persistent proliferation, invasive growth and the formation of metastases.

Persistent proliferation refers to the ability of cancer cells to undergo unrestrained growth and division, and is the most distinguishing aspect of malignant cells. This is in marked contrast to normal cells, whose proliferation is carefully controlled. Persistent proliferation in cancer is due to the fact that malignant cells are unresponsive to the feedback mechanisms that regulate cellular proliferation in healthy tissue. Thus, cancer cells are able to continue multiplying under conditions that would suppress further growth and division of normal cells. As a result of persistent proliferation, cancerous tissues continue to grow, unless intervention is instituted, until they cause the host's death.

Invasive growth refers to the ability of cancer cells to move into territory normally belonging to cells of a different type. Under normal conditions, the various types of cells that compose a tissue remain segregated from one another. That is to say, cells of one type do not invade areas in the body that are the normal habitat of cells of a different type. Malignant cells are not fettered by these constraints and, as a result, cells of a solid tumour can penetrate adjacent tissues.

Cancer cells can also form *metastases,* or secondary tumours that appear at other locations in the body. They result from malignant cells breaking away from the original tumour and migrating via the lymphatic or circulatory systems to other parts of the body, where they produce a new tumour.

Cancer may be treated by surgery, irradiation and drug therapy (chemotherapy). For most solid tumours, surgery or radiation therapy, or both, are preferred. These forms of treatment can often cure or control tumours locally. However, because of the ability of tumours to metastasize, many patients eventually die because of metastases in distant sites. Therefore, effective systemic therapy with drugs is needed to cure most cancers.

The goal of cancer chemotherapy is to kill malignant tumour cells and spare normal host cells. This is called *selective toxicity.* Selective toxicity is not a new concept in this text. In Unit 3, we saw how it forms the basis of all antibiotic, antifungal, antiviral, antiprotozoal and anthelmintic therapy. However, selective toxicity is easier to achieve in anti-infective therapy because mammalian and bacterial cells, for example, differ markedly in their structure and metabolic processes. This is not case in cancer. Normal and malignant cells do not show such major differences, and this fact is most significant for cancer treatment. It is virtually impossible to kill large numbers of cancer cells without destroying at least some normal cells.

Anticancer drugs suppress all proliferating cells, both normal and neoplastic. This effect accounts for their major toxicities on such rapidly dividing normal cells as bone marrow, gastrointestinal and germinal epithelia, hair follicles and lymphoid organs. Thus, successful anticancer therapy is defined differently than successful anti-infective treatment. Successful antineoplastic treatment depends on killing malignant tumour cells with doses of anticancer drugs that allow recovery of normal proliferating cells. To understand how this can be achieved, it is important to review the relationship of cellular growth fraction to cancer chemotherapy.

Relationship of Growth Fraction to Choice of Anticancer Drugs and Success of Chemotherapy

Figure 25.1 presents the cell cycle. Every cell that divides passes through specific phases before undergoing mitosis. During the synthesis (S) phase, lasting from six to fifty hours, DNA synthesis increases and chromosomal material doubles. Thereafter the cell proceeds through the G_2 phase, lasting about six hours, during which time a series of biochemical events occur that prepare the cell for mitosis. After mitosis (the M-phase), new cells enter the G_1 phase. Depending on the cells involved, G_1 may last minutes or years. Cells progressing through G_1, S, G_2 and mitosis are said to be "in cycle." Cells not actively dividing are said to be in the G_0 (or gap) phase.

Every tissue, whether normal or neoplastic, has a portion of its cells that are not actively dividing. They can be found side by side with dividing cells. The number of cells in cycle divided by the total number of cells in the tissue is the *growth fraction.* The growth fraction does not remain constant. Larger tumours have smaller growth fractions. If the size of the tumour is reduced, either by surgery, radiotherapy or antineoplastic drugs, more resting cells begin to cycle.

Figure 25.1
The cell cycle

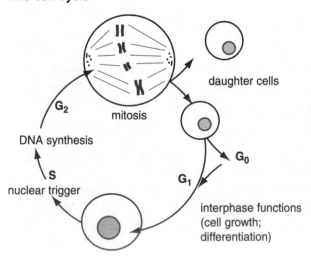

Cells in cycle ⇄ Resting cells

Anticancer drugs are more effective against proliferating cells than cells in G_0 because antineoplastic agents usually kill cells by disrupting either DNA synthesis or mitosis, functions that occur only in proliferating cells. Thus, as a general rule, antineoplastic drugs are much more toxic to tissues that have a high growth fraction than to tissues whose growth fraction is low. Solid tumours (e.g., those of the lung, breast, stomach, colon and rectum) have a low growth fraction and often respond poorly to anticancer drugs. Disseminated tumours (e.g., leukemias and lymphomas) have a high growth fraction and generally respond well to antineoplastic drugs.

Chemotherapy against cancer that employs a combination of drugs is considerably more effective than therapy with just one drug. The benefits of combination therapy are (a) suppression of drug resistance, (b) enhancement of therapeutic effects and (c) reduced injury to normal cells. If several drugs are selected, with different mechanisms of action, drug resistance occurs less frequently and more malignant cells are killed. Furthermore, so long as drugs are selected that do not have overlapping toxicities, oncologists can extend anticancer action beyond what might be safely achieved using any one of these chemicals alone.

Drug Resistance

Many patients treated with cancer chemotherapy fail to respond from the outset. For these patients, their cancers are resistant to drug therapy. Other patients respond initially, and subsequently relapse. For these individuals, their cancers have developed resistance to chemotherapy. The presence of drug-resistant tumour cells is an important factor in the success or failure of cancer chemotherapy.

Several explanations can be offered for the apparent development of drug resistance. Cancers are not composed of homogeneous cells. Rather, human tumours contain various subpopulations of cells that differ genetically and structurally from one another: some are sensitive to a particular drug, others are not. Given the number of cells present within most tumours at the time of diagnosis — 1×10^8 to 1×10^9 — it seems likely that at least one resistant subpopulation will be

Figure 25.2
Cellular resistance to anticancer drugs

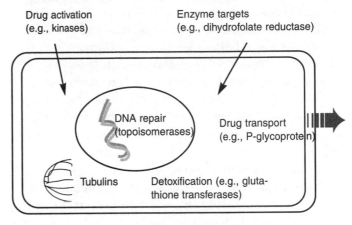

Source: Sikic BI. The rational basis for cancer chemotherapy. In: Craig CR, Stitzel RE. *Modern Pharmacology.* 4th ed. Boston: Little, Brown; 1994:663–672.

present for each individual antineoplastic drug. Killing of the sensitive cells leads to the proliferation of the resistant. The use of combination chemotherapy, whereby all cells in a tumour may respond to at least one of the drugs, reduces the chance that this form of drug resistance will develop.

Drug resistance can also develop in cell lines that were originally sensitive. This form of drug resistance has been extensively studied, and many mechanisms of cellular resistance to anticancer drugs have been elucidated. Figure 25.2 depicts the major mechanisms of cellular resistance to anticancer drugs.

Resistance to an anticancer drug can develop at its molecular site of action. In the case of methotrexate, resistance develops, in part, because of an alteration in the structure of the target enzyme, dihydrofolate reductase, resulting in reduced drug affinity. In addition, some cancer cells increase their dihydrofolate reductase content and this, too, contributes to the development of methotrexate resistance.

Tumour cells may become generally resistant to a variety of anticancer drugs because they either fail to take up or to retain sufficient drug. This type of resistance is called multidrug resistance. It is the major form of resistance shown to anthracyclines, vinca alkaloids, etoposide, paclitaxel and dactinomycin. Multidrug resistance results from the production of a high-molecular-weight membrane protein called the P-glycoprotein, which acts to increase the efflux of antineoplastic drugs out of cancer and normal cells.

Resistance can develop to alkylating agents (see discussion, below) because of changes in cell DNA repair capabilities, increases in thiol content (which subsequently serves as alternative and benign targets of alkylation), decreases in cell permeability and increases in glutathion transferase activity. The last-named phenomenon increases the cellular detoxification of alkylating agents.

Some drugs must be metabolically activated to function as anticancer agents. These include the antimetabolites 6-fluorouracil and 6-mercaptopurine. These drugs may be ineffective if a tumour is lacking the enzymes required for their activation. The reverse is also true. Some drugs, such as cytarabine and bleomycin, can be metabolically inactivated by resistant tumours.

Classification of Antineoplastic Drugs

Classification Based on Cell Cycle

Antineoplastics are characterized as *cell-cycle independent* if they affect cells during any phase of the cycle, including resting or G_0 cells, or *cell-cycle dependent*, if they affect only cells that are actively cycling at the time of exposure to drugs. Anticancer drugs may also be phase dependent if one specific phase of the cycle is the principal site of drug action. For example, the vinca alkaloids vinblastine, vincristine, vindesine and vinorelbine block mitosis and are considered phase-dependent drugs.

Classification Based on Mechanism of Action or Source

Although it is useful to classify drugs in relation to the cell cycle, it is more practical to categorize them in terms of their mechanisms of action or source. This system of classification is described below.

Table 25.1 provides a listing of antineoplastic drugs according to their mechanisms of action or source.

Alkylating agents. As shown in Table 25.1, alkylating agents are a heterogeneous group of drugs and form the largest class of anticancer drugs. By definition, alkylating agents are drugs that can introduce alkyl groups into nucleophilic sites on other molecules. Their most important targets are the pyrimidine and purine bases in DNA. These drugs interfere with RNA transcription, thereby inhibiting cell growth and causing death. The degree to which each drug can alkylate DNA correlates well with its cytotoxicity. This interaction also accounts for the mutagenic and carcinogenic properties of the alkylating agents. By attaching to components of DNA molecules, alkylating agents inhibit DNA replication and transcription, leading to cell death.

Because alkylation reactions can take place at any time during the cell cycle, alkylating agents are considered nonspecific to cell cycle. However, most of these drugs are more toxic to proliferating cells than to cells in G_0. This is because alkylation of DNA produces its most detrimental effects when cells attempt to replicate DNA. Resting cells are often able to repair damage to DNA before that damage can affect cell function.

Antimetabolites. The antimetabolites listed in Table 25.1 are structurally similar to important chemicals in the body. These structural similarities allow antimetabolites to compete with normal body metabolites for vital enzymes. If an antimetabolite replaces the normal metabolite on a vital enzyme, it blocks reactions that are essential to cell function and life.

The means by which an antimetabolite works can be illustrated by describing the mechanism of action of methotrexate. Methotrexate is similar in structure to dihydrofolate, a metabolite of folic acid, and it competes with dihydrofolate for binding to the enzyme dihydrofolate reductase. The reduction of dihydrofolate by dihydrofolate reductase plays a pivotal role in the transfer of single-carbon units that are necessary in DNA and purine biosynthesis. When methotrexate competes successfully with dihydrofolate for binding sites on dihydrofolate reductase, it inhibits DNA and purine synthesis.

Cytosine, thymine and uracil are pyrimidines. They are employed in the biosynthesis of nucleic acids (DNA and RNA). Cytosine arabinoside, also known as cytarabine, and 5-fluorouracil, also known as 5-FU, are two antimetabolites of pyrim-

Table 25.1
Antineoplastic drugs according to mechanism of action or source

Classification	Drug	Trade name(s)
Alkylating agents	busulphan	Myleran
	carboplatin	Paraplatin, Paraplatin-AQ
	carmustine (BCNU)	BCNU, BiCNU
	chlorambucil	Leukeran
	cisplatin	Platinol, Platinol-AQ
	cyclophosphamide	Cytoxan, Procytox
	dacarbazine	DTIC
	ifosfamide	Ifex
	lomustine (CCNU)	CeeNU
	mechlorethamine HCl (nitrogen mustard)	Mustargen
	melphalan	Alkeran
	streptozocin	Zanosar
	thiotepa	
Antimetabolites	cladribine	Leustatin
	cytarabine	Cytosar, Tarabine
	floxuridine	FUDR
	fludarabine	Fludara
	fluorouracil (5-FU)	Adrucil, Efudex, Fluoroplex
	hydroxyurea	Hydrea
	mercaptopurine (6-MP)	Purinethol
	methotrexate (amethopterin)	Folex
	thioguanine	Lanvis
Antibiotics	bleomycin	Blenoxane
	dactinomycin (actinomycin D)	Cosmegen
	daunorubicin (daunomycin)	Cerubidine
	doxorubicin	Adriamycin PFS, Adriamycin RDF, Rubex
	idarubicin	Idamycin
	mitomycin	Mutamycin
	pentostatin (DCF)	Nipent
	plicamycin (mithramycin)	Mithracin
Plant-derived products	docetaxel	Taxotere
	etoposide	VePesid
	paclitaxel	Taxol
	teniposide (VM-26)	Vumon
	vinblastine	Alkaban AQ, Velbe, Velben, Velsar
	vincristine	Oncovin, Vincasar PFS
	vindesine	Eldesine
	vinorelbine	Navelbine
Hormones and drugs that affect hormone balance	aminoglutethimide	Cytadren
	buserelin	Suprefact
	flutamide	Euflex, Eulexin
	goserelin	Zoladex
	leuprolide	Leupron, Lupron
	megestrol	Megace
	mitotane	Lysodren
	tamoxifen	Nolvadex, Tamofen
	testolactone	Teslac
Miscellaneous antineoplastics	asparaginase	Elspar, Kidrolase
	procarbazine	Matulane, Natulan

idines. Like all pyrimidine antimetabolites, these drugs are metabolized into compounds that are structurally very similar to pyrimidines. Because of this structural similarity, the drugs can replace pyrimidines in key metabolic reactions and thus bring about cell death.

Adenine, guanine and hypoxanthine are purines. Purines, like pyrimidines, are used in the synthesis of DNA and RNA. Administering a purine analogue, such as thioguanine, 6-mercaptopurine (6-MP) or fludarabine, blocks vital metabolic functions and kills cells.

Antitumour antibiotics. Bleomycin, dactinomycin, daunorubicin, doxorubicin, idarubicin, mitomycin, pentostatin, and plicamycin are cytotoxic compounds produced by microorganisms. In all cases, the antitumour antibiotics produce their cytotoxic effects through direct interaction with DNA.

Plant-derived products. Vinblastine, vincristine, vindesine and vinorelbine are either naturally occurring or semisynthetic products derived from the *Vinca rosea* plant (periwinkle). They are often called the vinca alkaloids. These have been used in the treatment of cancer since the introduction of vinblastine and vincristine in the early 1960s.

Vinca alkaloids strongly bind to tubulin, a class of proteins that form the mitotic spindle during cell division. These drugs disrupt mitotic spindle formation during mitosis at the metaphase of the cell cycle. Cell death results from an inability to segregate chromosomes properly. Vinca alkaloids are usually regarded as M-phase specific in the cell cycle.

Paclitaxel (Taxol®) is a naturally occurring chemical that is obtained from the yew tree (genus Taxus). It binds specifically and reversibly to tubulin and stabilizes microtubules in the polymerized form. The stabilization of microfilaments disrupts mitosis and kills cells.

Docetaxel (Taxotere®) is a semisynthetic anticancer drug that belongs to the taxoid family. Docetaxel is a mitotic spindle poison that increases the rate of microtubule assembly and inhibits the depolymerization of microtubules. Docetaxel is approved for the treatment of patients with locally advanced or metastatic breast cancer in whom pre-

vious therapy has failed. It is also indicated for the treatment of patients with locally advanced or metastatic non–small-cell lung cancer after failure of platinum-based chemotherapy.

Etoposide (VePesid®) is a semisynthetic derivative of podophyllotoxin that is produced in the roots of the American mandrake, or May apple. Its mechanism of action is not well understood. It does not bind to microtubules but does form a complex with an enzyme in the body that results in a single-strand breakage of DNA. Etoposide is most lethal to cells in the S and G_2 phases of the cell cycle.

Hormones and drugs that alter hormone balance. Estrogens, progestins, androgens and corticosteroids are used in the treatment of various cancers. Estrogens are employed in the treatment of prostatic cancer and in the management of five-year postmenopausal breast tumours. Androgens are sometimes given to premenopausal patients with mammary cancer. Progestins are used on occasion to treat kidney and endometrial carcinomas. Corticosteroids, particularly prednisone, are administered in high doses to patients with lymphomas and some other cancers.

The rationale behind the use of these drugs is the belief that some cancers are hormone dependent. For example, if a prostatic cancer is androgen dependent, treatment with estrogens, together with castration, is reasonable. The converse is also true. If breast cancer in premenopausal patients is estrogen dependent, the use of androgens makes sense. Corticosteroids induce a regression of lymphoid tissue by causing a breakdown of existing lymphocytes and inhibiting the production of new lymphocytes. The biochemical mechanism behind these actions is not clear.

Tamoxifen competitively blocks estrogen receptors. Certain forms of cancer, notably breast cancer in premenopausal women, often depend on endogenous estrogens for growth. When given in high doses, tamoxifen prevents endogenous estrogens from stimulating their receptors and significantly reduces cancer growth.

Tamoxifen may also have some benefits with long-term use. It may reduce LDL-cholesterol, with a potential reduction in coronary disease. Long-term use appears to have no adverse effects on bone density; however, there may be a possible association with endometrial cancer. The most frequent side effects are hot flashes, irregular menses, vaginal depression and nausea. Psychological depression also can occur, but generally the drug is well tolerated.

Flutamide is a potent nonsteroidal antiandrogen. It inhibits androgen uptake and/or inhibits nuclear binding of androgen in target tissues. Flutamide is well absorbed from the gastrointestinal tract. It is rapidly and completely metabolized, but its major metabolite has comparable antiandrogenic activity to flutamide. Flutamide is approved for use in combination with LHRH agonistic analogues (such as leuprolide acetate) for the treatment of metastatic prostatic carcinoma (Stage D_2). Flutamide prevents stimulation of tumour growth that may occur as a result of the transient increase in testosterone secretion after the initiation of leuprolide therapy.

Leuprolide and buserelin are synthetic derivatives of gonadotropin-releasing hormone (GnRH/LHRH). Chronic exposure of the pituitary to these agents abolishes gonadotropin release and results in markedly decreased estrogen and testosterone production by the gonads. These drugs are indicated for palliative treatment of patients with hormone-dependent advanced carcinoma of the prostate gland. They are also useful in breast cancers.

Goserelin acetate is also a synthetic analogue of GnRH. Administered chronically, goserelin inhibits gonadotropin production, resulting in gonadal and accessory sex organ regression. Goserelin is indicated for the palliative treatment of patients with hormone-dependent advanced carcinoma of the prostate.

Miscellaneous antineoplastics.
Asparaginase (Elspar®, Kidrolase®) is an enzyme extracted from cultures of *Escherichia coli*. It converts asparagine to aspartic acid. Certain cancers are unable to make asparagine and are dependent on the blood to bring them adequate amounts. In the absence of asparagine, because of its hydrolysis to aspartic acid, they cannot proliferate. Asparaginase is not toxic to normal cells, which have the ability to synthesize asparagine. Asparaginase appears to act selectively during the G_1 phase of the cell cycle.

Procarbazine (Matulane®, Natulan®) is converted to its active metabolite in the liver of the patient. Following activation, it can cause chromosomal damage and suppress DNA, RNA and protein synthesis.

Adverse Effects of Antineoplastic Drugs

Antineoplastic drugs are cellular poisons that kill both malignant and normal cells. The selective toxicity seen with antibiotics, antifungals, antivirals and anthelmintics — in which the drug attacks preferentially the microbe, fungus, virus or worm, leaving the host cells largely unaffected — is not seen with antineoplastics. For example, a drug that blocks DNA or RNA synthesis and/or function will damage both normal and malignant cells. This is particularly true for cell-cycle independent drugs. Cell-cycle dependent drugs will also damage both normal and neoplastic tissue, but these agents show a selectivity for tissues with the highest percentage of cells "in cycle." This means that they can rapidly kill both cancer cells and normal cells with a rapid turnover (e.g., bone marrow, gastrointestinal tract, hair). They also damage the immune system, resulting in a fall in production of both T- and B-lymphocytes.

The hematopoietic system is particularly at risk when antineoplastic drugs are administered. Patients often show pancytopenia as the production of red cells, white cells and platelets falls. The decrease in platelets predisposes patients to hemorrhage. A decrease in neutrophils, together with the fall in B- and T-lymphocytes, places patients at risk with respect to infections.

The mucosal cells of hollow organs normally have a rapid rate of turnover. By inhibiting cell duplication, antineoplastics damage the gastrointestinal and genitourinary tracts. This can lead to ulceration and bleeding.

Antineoplastic treatment is perhaps most obvious when one looks at the hair and nails of patients receiving therapy. Alopecia and baldness are common adverse effects.

Antineoplastics increase tissue breakdown, raising both the purine load and the production of uric acid. If the uric acid concentration increases above 12 mg/100 mL (750 µmol/L) of blood, kidney damage can occur. Allopurinol (Zyloprim®) blocks xanthine oxidase, thereby decreasing uric acid production. It is often administered to patients receiving antineoplastics to decrease uric acid formation. Care must be taken when it is used together with 6-mercaptopurine, because this latter drug is metabolized by xanthine oxidase. Lower doses of 6-mercaptopurine must be used to compensate for the reduced rate of inactivation.

Vinca alkaloids interfere with the microtubular structures important to nerve cell function. As a result, they can produce significant nerve damage. Some drugs, notably busulphan, can cause pulmonary fibrosis.

Nausea and vomiting are often experienced by patients receiving anticancer drugs. These effects are particularly pronounced with cisplatin (Platinol®). A combination of antiemetics, with different mechanisms of action, is usually more effective than giving a single agent. Drugs of choice include diphenhydramine, droperidol, ondansetron (Zofran®) and prochlorperazine. Metoclopramide (Maxeran®, Reglan®) increases gastric emptying and is often helpful in reducing nausea and vomiting due to anticancer drugs.

Doxorubicin (Adriamycin®) and daunomycin (Cerubidine®) can cause dose-dependent cardiac arrhythmias and, eventually, heart failure. This danger is minimized by reducing the dosages of these drugs. Both drugs are red dyes and can produce red urine. Patients should be informed of this fact to prevent unnecessary alarm.

Procarbazine (Natulan®) is metabolized to a monoamine oxidase inhibitor. It can produce a variety of central nervous system effects. Patients should be warned to refrain from eating or drinking foods containing tyramine (e.g., cheese, red wine). The toxicities of monoamine oxidase inhibitors are explained in Chapter 46.

Caution should be taken in the intravenous administration of dactinomycin (Cosmegen®), cytosine arabinoside (Cytosar®), nitrogen mustards and vinca alkaloids. Extravasation of these drugs can cause tissue damage.

Nursing Management

It is beyond the scope of this text to discuss in detail the complete nursing care for cancer patients. Readers are referred to a medical-surgical or oncological nursing text for a comprehensive discussion of other aspects of oncological nursing care.

Table 25.2 summarizes the general nursing management of patients receiving antineoplastic drugs. Table 25.3 on page 254 specifies nursing management of common adverse drug reactions.

Response to Clinical Challenge

First, explain the purposes of the trial, discuss informed consent with E.H. and ensure that she meets the eligibility criteria for the study. (Recall the nursing responsibilities in research discussed in Chapter 1.) Ensure that she understands that she may receive either the placebo or the actual drug, and that neither she nor you will know whether she is placed in the experimental or the control group.

Explain the mechanism of action, potential benefits and possible side effects of the drug (as described in this chapter).

Further Reading

Camp-Sorrell D. Controlling the adverse effects of chemotherapy. *Nursing* 1991;21(4):34–41.

Crawley MM. Recent advances in chemotherapy: administration and nursing implications. *Nurs Clin North Am* 1990;25(2):377–391.

Creaton E, Leonard FE, Day AL. A hospital-based chemotherapy education and training program. *Cancer Nurs* 1991;14(2):79–90.

Drugs of choice for cancer chemotherapy. *Medical Letter on Drugs and Therapeutics* 1991;33:21–28.

Erlichman C. The pharmacology of anticancer drugs. In: Tarnock IF, Hill RP, eds. *The Basic Science of Oncology.* Toronto: Pergamon Press; 1987:292–307.

Graydon J, Blubela N. Fatigue reducing strategies used by patients receiving treatment for cancer. *Cancer Nurs* 1995;18(1):23–28.

Mayer D. What are patients asking about tamoxifen use? *Can Oncol Nurs J* 1994;4(4):196.

McDaniel R, Nelson R. Sensory perceptions of women receiving tamoxifen for breast cancer. *Cancer Nurs* 1995;18(3):215–221.

Miaskowski C. Chemotherapy update. *Nurs Clin North Am* 1991;26(2):331–340.

Table 25.2
Nursing management of the antineoplastic drugs

Assessment of risk vs. benefit	Patient data	• Physician should determine baseline lab tests of liver, hematologic and renal function • Lifespan and developmental considerations: Because these drugs are used for life-threatening illnesses, they may be used across the lifespan in spite of risks to specific age groups • *Pregnancy:* Risk category D (animal studies show adverse effects to fetus but benefits may be acceptable despite risks)
	Drug data	• Select drugs based on type and location of cancer • *Some serious drug interactions:* Confer with pharmacist • *Some serious adverse effects:* See Table 25.3.
Implementation	Rights of administration	• Using the "rights" helps prevent errors of administration
	Right route	• Give IV and PO
	Right time	• Protocols have been developed for the scheduling of these drugs based on body weight, type and location of cancer. Schedules vary: may be given several times daily or once weekly
	Right technique	• These drugs are toxic; thus, agency policies and procedures must be followed carefully • In many institutions, only certified nurses or physicians administer these drugs IV. Preparation of solutions is conducted using a laminar flow hood. IV administration requires knowledge of correct diluent and IV solution, correct dilution and rate of administration. Always refer to manufacturer's instructions for this route • Rate must be carefully controlled and site frequently monitored: extravasation can cause tissue sloughing • Specific precautions with this group because these drugs can also produce adverse effects in people handling them
	Nursing therapeutics	• Enhance host defences and general state of health through good nutrition, rest, fluids and hygiene measures • Encourage daily fluid intake of 2–3 L to prevent dehydration due to vomiting, promote urinary excretion of drug and minimize adverse renal effects • Scheduling of meals and antiemetic administration is also important. Provide small, bland meal prior to drug and prophylactic or routine schedule of the antiemetic • Avoid vaccinations while on tx • To prevent bleeding, avoid IM injections and other invasive tx, if platelet count is reduced • Emotional support: Adverse effects of tx can be discouraging
	Patient/family teaching	• Pt's need for information may be influenced by the length of time required for tx or limited by serious illness • Compliance and follow-up are essential factors in successful treatment; review principles of pt education in Chapter 3

(cont'd on next page)

Table 25.2 (continued)
Nursing management of the antineoplastic drugs

Implementation (cont'd)	Patient/Family teaching (cont'd)	• Explain that successful tx of cancer may require weeks or months • Pts/families should know warning signs/symptoms of possible toxicities of drugs (see Table 25.3) • *Discuss possibility of pregnancy:* Advise pt to notify physician; discuss birth control methods
Outcomes	Monitoring of progress	*Continually monitor:* • Signs/symptoms of adverse reactions; document and report immediately to physician • Blood tests for renal, hepatic and bone marrow function may be ordered (weekly or periodically)

Table 25.3
Nursing management of adverse reactions to antineoplastic drugs

Reaction	Signs/symptoms	Nursing management and teaching
Nausea and vomiting May be caused by: • direct irritation of oral drugs on gastric mucosa • stimulation of the chemo-receptor trigger zone • psychogenic, r/t anticipatory reaction	Nausea may occur prior to, during or following drug administration. It may be mild to severe, constant or intermittent. Vomiting may lead to fluid or electrolyte imbalances	• Determine probable cause • Bland food prior to drug may reduce direct irritating effects • Schedule antiemetic drug appropriately • Minimize psychological reaction through reassurance, relaxation, meditation • Adapt drug schedule to lifestyle, when possible • Promote nutrition and fluid intake
Stomatitis • Because drugs do not have selective toxicity but affect all proliferating cells, oral mucosa may be damaged • Temporary condition, but may be severe and debilitating	Soreness, burning in mouth and tongue; open sores may occur	• Frequent mouth care • Soft foods and fluids • Maintain nutrition (problem exacerbated with poor nutritional status) • Topical analgesic may be required
Alopecia • May affect all body hair (eyebrows, eyelashes, body hair as well as scalp) • May be very distressing to pt	Reversible hair loss usually occurs gradually and unevenly	• Provide emotional reassurance • Discuss use of makeup, hairpieces, head covers
Bone marrow suppression Common and most serious reaction; includes: • anemia	Fatigue, pallor, shortness of breath with reduced red blood cell count	• Monitor lab values (RBC, Hgb, hematocrit) • Blood transfusion administration, if ordered • Promote iron-rich foods • Iron supplement may be given
• leukopenia	Infection (fever, cough, sore throat, dysuria)	• Monitor temperature • Report signs of infection immediately • Avoid crowds and others with known infections
• thrombocytopenia	Easy bruising, petechiae or bleeding (gums, bowel, bladder, hypermenorrhea)	• Reduce risk of bleeding by using soft toothbrush, electric razor, stool softener to reduce straining • Avoid IM injections • Apply firm pressure after venipuncture for 5 min • Avoid ASA, anticoagulants

Autonomic Nervous System Pharmacology and Neuromuscular Blocking Drugs

The pharmacology of the autonomic nervous system is presented in this text before discussion of drugs that affect particular body systems. The reason for this order is that drugs affecting the autonomic nervous system (ANS) influence many areas of the body. Autonomic pharmacology thus forms the basis for understanding the effects of drugs on many systems. For example, it would be most difficult to discuss cardiovascular pharmacology or gastrointestinal pharmacology without first understanding the importance of ANS innervation to these systems and the manner in which drugs may tamper with it.

Somatic nerves are not part of the autonomic nervous system. The means by which drugs may influence the transmission of impulses from somatic nerves to skeletal muscles is discussed in Unit 5 because of the similarities between autonomic pharmacology and the pharmacology of drugs affecting motor end-plate function.

CHAPTER 26

Introduction to the Transmission of Autonomic and Somatic Nerves

Topics Discussed
● Definition of neurotransmitter, cholinergic, adrenergic, nicotinic, muscarinic
● Divisions and functions of the autonomic nervous system
● Interactions between sympathetic and parasympathetic divisions of the autonomic nervous system
● Neurotransmitters — their synthesis, actions and inactivation
● Autonomic receptors

Divisions of the Autonomic Nervous System

The autonomic nervous system (ANS) innervates smooth muscles, cardiac muscle and glands. It has also been called the involuntary or visceral nervous system. Its functions include the control of heart rate, blood pressure, secretions (e.g., sweat, salivation, stomach), pupil diameter, accommodation of the eye, gastrointestinal motility and bronchodilatation.

The autonomic nervous system consists of two divisions, called sympathetic and parasympathetic. These divisions have certain common anatomical characteristics:

• They originate within the central nervous system.
• Their activities and integration are controlled from within the brain.

• Each sympathetic and parasympathetic nerve contains a preganglionic neuron, whose cell of origin lies within the central nervous system, and a postganglionic neuron, whose cell of origin lies within one of the ganglia outside the central nervous system. The two neurons synapse at a ganglion. Ganglia are collections of neurons located outside the central nervous system.

The Sympathetic Division of the Autonomic Nervous System
The preganglionic sympathetic nerves leave the spinal cord from the first thoracic to the second lumbar segments. Once outside the spinal cord, the preganglionic fibres synapse with their postganglionic nerves at ganglia located in three major areas of the body:

• Most preganglionic sympathetic nerves travel to ganglia that lie in two chains, one on each side of the vertebral column. These are called the *vertebral* or *paravertebral ganglia.*

• Some preganglionic sympathetic nerves travel to the abdominal cavity where they meet their postganglionic counterparts at *prevertebral ganglia.* The prevertebral ganglia are the celiac, superior mesenteric, inferior mesenteric, and aorticorenal ganglia.

• Finally, a few prevertebral sympathetic nerves run to the urinary bladder and rectum where they synapse with the postganglionic fibres. The ganglia that provide the meeting place for these pre- and postganglionic fibres and which lie near the organs innervated are called *terminal ganglia.*

Functionally, paravertebral, prevertebral and terminal ganglia are identical. They have the same neurotransmitter (acetylcholine) and the same receptors, and they are all affected in the same way by drugs.

Stimulation of the sympathetic division of the autonomic nervous system, usually referred to simply as the sympathetic nervous system (SNS), prepares the body to meet situations of mild to severe stress. Standing can be considered a very mild stress. In this position blood must be returned to the heart against the pull of gravity. To meet this situation the sympathetic nerves to veins are stimulated and the blood vessels constrict, returning blood to the heart. During conditions of more acute stress, such as a final examination, stimulation of the sympathetic nervous system increases heart rate, cardiac output and intermediary metabolism, dilates the bronchioles and redistributes blood from the gastrointestinal tract to the skeletal muscles. Obviously, defecation is not desired at such a moment. Therefore, sympathetic nervous system stimulation reduces peristalsis.

Drugs that either increase or decrease sympathetic nervous system activity have profound effects. For example, fatigue is common in patients receiving sympathetic blocking drugs, particularly if they are stressed and cannot generate the increase in cardiac output and intermediary metabolism required to meet the needs of the body.

The Parasympathetic Division of the Autonomic Nervous System

Most parasympathetic preganglionic fibres originate in the midbrain or medulla oblongata. After leaving the central nervous system, they travel directly to the organs innervated, where they meet their postganglionic nerves at ganglia that are found close to or within the organs. A few preganglionic parasympathetic nerves leave the central nervous system from the sacral portion of the spinal cord. They too synapse with the postganglionic nerves in ganglia that are close to or within the innervated organs. All parasympathetic ganglia are identical with respect to the neurotransmitter released, receptors stimulated and reaction to drugs.

If it may be said that sympathetic stimulation prepares the body to meet stress, the parasympathetic division carries on many of the mundane day-to-day activities. Parasympathetic stimulation increases the flow of saliva and promotes peristalsis. The use of a parasympathomimetic drug can make patients feel they are drowning in their own saliva and unwilling to venture more than a few paces from the nearest washroom. Parasympathetic stimulation also constricts the pupil in the presence of bright light and allows the ciliary body to accommodate the lens for near vision. Stimulation of the parasympathetic vagus nerve slows heart rate.

Interaction Between the Sympathetic and Parasympathetic Divisions of the Autonomic Nervous System

The autonomic nervous system innervates blood vessels, the heart, glands and smooth muscle. Many organs receive nervous supply from both the sympathetic and parasympathetic divisions. These include the heart, bronchi, gastrointestinal tract, sex organs and bladder. Some organs are innervated by only one division. These include sweat glands, piloerector muscles and arterioles, which receive only sympathetic innervation.

In general, if an organ is innervated by both the sympathetic and parasympathetic divisions, their actions are antagonistic. For example, sympathetic stimulation increases heart rate and force of contraction while parasympathetic stimulation produces bradycardia. Sympathetic activation dilates the pupil; parasympathetic activation constricts it.

In a few organs the two divisions do not behave antagonistically. Both sympathetic and parasympathetic stimulation produce saliva. Parasympathetic activation of the salivary glands, such as occurs at the smell of appetizing food, causes the secretion of a copious amount of thin, watery saliva. Students exposed to the rigors of oral examinations know only too well the consequences of the sympathetic stimulation of the salivary glands. A thick, mucilaginous saliva is produced, making it difficult for candidates to unstick their tongues from the roofs of their mouths.

Special attention must be paid to the innervation of the arterioles and veins. These vessels are innervated mainly by the sympathetic nervous system (SNS). As a result, the contractile state is determined by the extent of the sympathetic stimulation at any moment. Increased sympathetic activity produces both a rise in peripheral resistance, due to constriction of the arterioles, and an increase in venous return to the heart, as a result of vasoconstriction in the veins. Any condition, disease or drug that blocks SNS innervation of these vessels produces both a decrease in peripheral resistance, due to a dilatation of the arterioles, and postural hypotension, as a result of vasodilatation in the veins. When the patient stands, blood cannot be returned to the heart because the veins cannot constrict. With the sudden decrease in venous return to the heart, the amount of blood pumped to the brain is reduced dramatically, and the patient may faint.

Neurotransmitters

Chemical Transmission of Impulses

The ability of the autonomic nervous system to produce a physiologic response is dependent on the transmission of impulses to effector cells. *Conduction,* an electrical phenomenon, is the very rapid passage of impulses along a nerve fibre. The process of passing this impulse across a synapse from one neuron to another or to an effector cell is called *transmission.* This is a chemical rather than an electrical process and is dependent on neurotransmitters — chemicals produced and stored in the axon terminal of the neuron. *Neurotransmitters* are the messengers by which nerve cells communicate (Figure 26.1).

The neurotransmitter in the ganglia of both parasympathetic and sympathetic nerves is acetylcholine (Figure 26.2). When an impulse reaches the end of a preganglionic nerve, acetylcholine is released and crosses the ganglionic synapse to stimulate the postganglionic neuron.

Acetylcholine is also the neurotransmitter released by all postganglionic parasympathetic nerves. In this case it is responsible for the stimulation of innervated tissue. A few postganglionic sympathetic nerves also release acetylcholine. The most notable example of this is the sympathetic innervation of sweat glands.

Somatic nerves release acetylcholine, which stimulates the motor end-plates of skeletal muscles. Somatic and autonomic nerves that release acetylcholine are called *cholinergic.*

Figure 26.1
The synapse

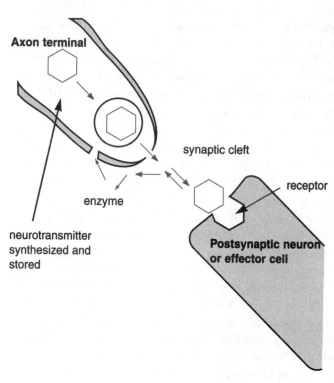

Figure 26.2
Chemical transmission of impulses

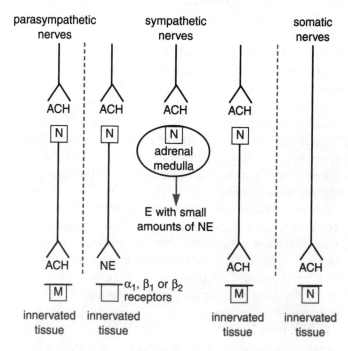

ACH = acetylcholine; NE = norepinephrine; E = epinephrine;
N = nicontinic receptors; M = muscarinic receptors

Sympathetic stimulation is mediated by the chemicals *epinephrine* and *norepinephrine*. (In many parts of the world, these are called adrenaline and noradrenaline, respectively.) Functions mediated by either or both are called *adrenergic*.

It is important to recognize the physiological functions of each chemical. Epinephrine is an emergency hormone and is released by adrenal medullae in response to stress. It increases heart rate and force of contraction, shunts blood from the gastrointestinal tract, where it is not needed during stress, to the skeletal muscles, where it is required. Epinephrine also dilates the bronchioles and increases intermediary metabolism. In other words it prepares individuals for either fight or flight, depending on their particular preference (flight is safer; if caught, you can always fight).

Norepinephrine is not usually considered a hormone, although small amounts may be secreted by the adrenal medullae. Instead, norepinephrine should be considered a neurotransmitter, released by the very great majority of postganglionic sympathetic nerves. Its physiological function is to assist in routine cardiovascular control. It is responsible for control of vascular tone. Increased norepinephrine release by the appropriate nerves constricts arterioles and increases peripheral resistance. As suggested above, the simple act of standing up increases norepinephrine release from nerves innervating veins. This causes vasoconstriction and promotes adequate venous return to the heart. Norepinephrine released by the cardiac sympathetic accelerator nerves increases heart rate.

In addition to their peripheral actions, norepinephrine and acetylcholine produce central nervous system (CNS) effects. Norepinephrine is involved with mood, arousal level and positive reinforcement. Acetylcholine may excite or inhibit CNS activity. It is found in several regions, including the reticular system and the cerebellum, and is implicated in parkinsonism. Blocking acetylcholine activity in the central nervous system produces memory impairment, confusion, disorientation and slurred speech. This is important to remember when studying ANS pharmacology, because drugs that act peripherally may also have CNS side effects.

Figure 26.3
Synthesis of acetylcholine

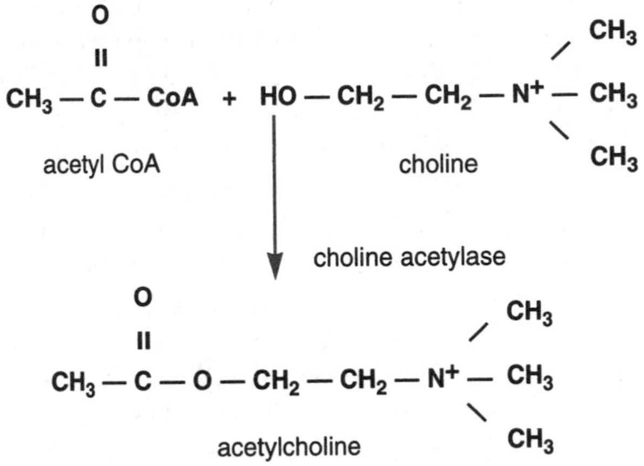

$$CH_3 - \overset{\overset{\displaystyle O}{\|}}{C} - CoA \; + \; HO - CH_2 - CH_2 - \overset{\diagup CH_3}{\underset{\diagdown CH_3}{N^+}} - CH_3$$

acetyl CoA   choline

↓ choline acetylase

$$CH_3 - \overset{\overset{\displaystyle O}{\|}}{C} - O - CH_2 - CH_2 - \overset{\diagup CH_3}{\underset{\diagdown CH_3}{N^+}} - CH_3$$

acetylcholine

Figure 26.4
Inactivation of acetylcholine

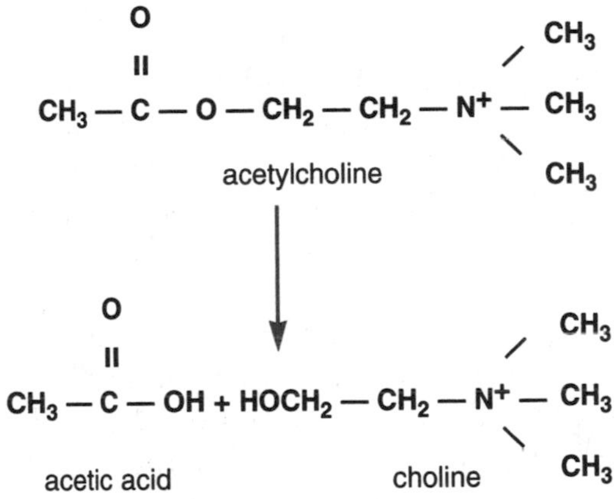

$$CH_3 - \overset{\overset{\displaystyle O}{\|}}{C} - O - CH_2 - CH_2 - \overset{\diagup CH_3}{\underset{\diagdown CH_3}{N^+}} - CH_3$$

acetylcholine

↓

$$CH_3 - \overset{\overset{\displaystyle O}{\|}}{C} - OH + HOCH_2 - CH_2 - \overset{\diagup CH_3}{\underset{\diagdown CH_3}{N^+}} - CH_3$$

acetic acid   choline

Synthesis and Inactivation of the Neurotransmitters

Acetylcholine is synthesized within nerves from choline and acetylcoenzyme A by the enzyme choline acetylase (Figure 26.3). It is stored intraneuronally within vesicles until such time as a wave of depolarization releases it. The enzyme *acetylcholinesterase,* also formed within cholinergic nerves, rapidly inactivates acetylcholine, once it has been released, by hydrolyzing it to acetic acid and choline (Figure 26.4).

Acetylcholinesterase, or true cholinesterase as it is sometimes called, should not be confused with pseudocholinesterase. The latter enzyme is found in the serum and is therefore also called *serum cholinesterase.* Whereas it can also hydrolyze acetylcholine, its specificity is not limited to this chemical. Serum cholinesterase can inactivate a number of drugs containing ester groups, including procaine and succinylcholine.

The synthesis of norepinephrine and epinephrine is more complex (Figure 26.5). The precursor of these chemicals is the amino acid tyrosine. Tyrosine is first converted to dopa (dihydroxyphenylalanine) and then to dopamine (dihydroxyphenylethylamine). Dopamine is subsequently metabolized to norepinephrine, within sympathetic nerves, or norepinephrine and epinephrine, within chromaffin tissue and the brain. The rate-limiting step in the formation of epinephrine and norepinephrine involves the conversion of tyrosine to dopa. Once formed, both epinephrine and norepinephrine are stored in small particles called granules. Their release occurs when the adrenal medullae or sympathetic nerves are stimulated.

Epinephrine, norepinephrine and dopamine are often called the catecholamines. When doctors order a catecholamine analysis of blood or urine, they are attempting to determine the extent of sympathetic nervous system activity as a prelude to diagnosing the cause of a disease. For example, in a very small number of people hypertension (high blood pressure) may be caused by a tumour of chromaffin tissue. The adrenal medullae are the major sites of chromaffin tissue in the body. A tumour of chromaffin tissue is called a pheochromocytoma. Patients so afflicted will have very high concentrations of epinephrine, and possibly also norepinephrine, in their blood and urine.

The inactivation of epinephrine and norepinephrine once they have been released has been the subject of considerable research. It is now known that norepinephrine, released by sympathetic postganglionic fibres, is removed from innervated tissue by neuronal reuptake and diffusion away in the blood. These are the main means by which the effects of released norepinephrine are terminated. Small amounts of the released neurotransmitters are inactivated by the enzymes catechol O-methyltransferase and monoamine oxidase.

Epinephrine is secreted into the blood and carried throughout the body. Its effects on any particular tissue may be terminated by diffusion away in the blood or uptake into sympathetic nerves innervating the organ concerned. Similar to norepinephrine, epinephrine may, in part, be inactivated by monoamine oxidase and catechol O-methyltrans-

Figure 26.5
Synthesis of norepinephrine and epinephrine

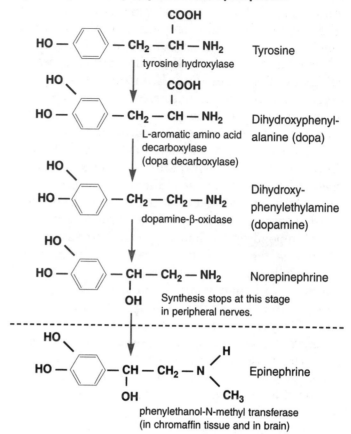

ferase. Enzymatic inactivation may be a more important means of terminating epinephrine's effects because it is carried in blood throughout the body and will have a greater opportunity to encounter the inactivating enzymes.

Autonomic Receptors

Cholinergic Receptors

Following their release, acetylcholine, epinephrine and norepinephrine stimulate autonomic receptors on or in the tissues affected (see Figure 26.2, page 258). In the case of acetylcholine the cholinergic receptors are classified as *nicotinic* or *muscarinic*. This distinction goes back many decades to the time when it was demonstrated that small doses of nicotine stimulated cholinergic receptors in both sympathetic and parasympathetic ganglia. It was also determined at that time that nicotine did not stimulate the organs innervated by parasympathetic nerves. The cholinergic receptors in these tissues were called muscarinic because they were stimulated by small amounts of the chemical muscarine, obtained from mushrooms. Muscarine did not stimulate autonomic ganglia. This was the first evidence that the cholinergic receptors in ganglia are not identical to those found in innervated tissues.

Skeletal muscles have cholinergic receptors which are stimulated by acetylcholine released from somatic nerves. These receptors also are stimulated by low doses of nicotine and are classified as nicotinic. It would be convenient, at this point, if we could state that cholinergic receptors in the ganglia and on skeletal muscle are identical because they both are stimulated by nicotine. However, Nature is never that kind to the suffering student. On the contrary, there is evidence that the nicotinic receptors in ganglia are not identical to the nicotinic receptors on skeletal muscle.

Evidence to support this statement can be found in the abilities of drugs to block selectively either ganglia or neuromuscular junctions. *Ganglionic blockers* are drugs that competitively prevent acetylcholine from uniting with ganglionic nicotinic receptors. These drugs, in usual therapeutic doses, do not stop acetylcholine, released by somatic nerves, from stimulating the nicotinic receptors on skeletal muscle. *Neuromuscular blockers,* such as tubocurarine, block competitively nicotinic receptors at the motor end-plate. In normal therapeutic doses they do not block the ganglia. If the nicotinic receptors on skeletal muscle were identical to those in the ganglia, tubocurarine should block both. By the same token, ganglionic blockers should also paralyze skeletal muscles. The fact that ganglionic blockers affect only ganglia and tubocurarine only skeletal muscles indicates that the two groups of nicotinic receptors are not identical.

Adrenergic Receptors

Epinephrine and norepinephrine stimulate adrenergic receptors. It has been known for many years that epinephrine can cause either an excitation or inhibition of smooth muscle contraction. For example, it constricts the blood vessels in the peritoneal area and dilates those in skeletal muscle. To explain these disparate actions, the existence of two types of adrenergic receptors, called alpha (α) and beta (β), were proposed. Stimulation of the alpha receptors on blood vessels produces vasoconstriction. Beta-receptor stimulation causes vasodilatation.

To fulfill its function as an emergency hormone, epinephrine must stimulate both types of receptors at the same time. This is essential if it is to redistribute blood in the body, moving it from areas not involved in the body's response to stress and shifting it to tissues responsible for meeting emergency situations. Epinephrine accomplishes this by constricting blood vessels (alpha stimulation) supplying the gastrointestinal tract and dilating (beta stimulation) those perfusing skeletal muscles. The bronchodilatation produced by epinephrine is also a beta-receptor mediated response.

The general rule may be stated that alpha-receptor stimulation produces excitation and beta-receptor stimulation causes inhibition. The exception to this rule can be found in the heart. In this tissue the chronotropic and inotropic effects of epinephrine are mediated by the beta receptors. Drugs that are only beta stimulants increase heart rate and force of contraction, and drugs that block beta receptors decrease heart rate. Alpha stimulants usually slow the heart beat.

Norepinephrine can also stimulate both alpha and beta receptors. It is, however, a far more effective alpha stimulant. This is consistent with its physiological role to maintain normal vascular tone. The degree of vasoconstriction under resting conditions is determined by the quantity of norepinephrine released by sympathetic nerves. When relatively large amounts are secreted, alpha receptors are stimulated and the blood vessels involved constrict. A decrease in norepinephrine release allows the vessels to relax.

Norepinephrine, released by the cardiac accelerator nerves, stimulates the beta receptors to increase heart rate and force of contraction. This is one of the few areas of the body where the beta-receptor stimulant effects of norepinephrine can be seen.

Not all beta receptors are identical. The beta receptors in the heart differ from those elsewhere in the body. Accordingly, the receptors in the heart are designated beta$_1$ (β_1); those in other parts of the body are beta$_2$ (β_2). Drugs have been synthesized that are capable of stimulating beta$_2$ receptors more selectively. Used to treat bronchial asthma, their advantage over previous agents (which stimulate both beta$_1$ and beta$_2$ receptors) is that the newer drugs dilate the bronchioles without producing marked tachycardia.

Finally, a new form of the alpha receptor has been found. It has been known for some time that the secretion of large amounts of norepinephrine reduces the subsequent release of this neurotransmitter. Recent work has suggested the presence of a receptor on the nerve ending. When norepinephrine, which has been released by the nerve, stimulates this presynaptic receptor on the outside of the nerve membrane it reduces the subsequent secretion of the neurotransmitter. The new receptor has been designated alpha$_2$ (α_2). It differs from the alpha receptor previously described (now called alpha$_1$) in two ways. Alpha$_1$ receptors are located in the tissue innervated. Alpha$_2$ receptors are found on the nerve membrane itself. Stimulation of alpha$_1$ receptors causes smooth muscle excitation. Stimulation of alpha$_2$ receptors reduces the subsequent secretion of norepinephrine.

Figure 26.6 summarizes the classes of autonomic nervous system drugs.

A moment of quiet contemplation reviewing Figure 26.2 (page 258) and Table 26.1 will indicate the possibility of tampering selectively with one or another aspect of autonomic function. Subsequent chapters in Unit 5 will discuss the pharmacology and nursing process related to drugs that influence one or more of these sites.

Further Reading

Hoffman BB, Lefkowitz RJ, Taylor, P. Neurohumoral transmission: the autonomic and somatic motor nervous systems. In: Hardman JG, Limbird LE, *Goodman and Gilman's The Pharmacological Basis of Therapeutics*. 9th ed. New York: Pergamon Press; 1996:105–140.

Fleming WW. Introduction to the autonomic nervous system. In: Craig CR, Stitzel RE, eds. *Modern Pharmacology*. 4th ed. Boston: Little, Brown; 1994:101–114.

Table 26.1
Location of autonomic receptors

Organ	Sympathetic receptor	Sympathetic response	Parasympathetic response
CNS		alertness/arousal excitement nervousness/anxiety	
CVS			
Heart			
• SA node	β_1	rate ↑	rate ↓
• AV node	β_1	conduction ↑	conduction ↓
• His-Purkinje	β_1	↑automaticity	little effect
• ventricles	β_1	↑force of contraction	no innervation
Blood vessels			
• skin, mucosa	α_1	constrict	no innervation
• skeletal muscle	β_2	dilate	no innervation
	α_2	constrict	
• abdominal (viscera)	α_1	constrict	no innervation
	β_2	dilate	
• renal	dopaminergic	dilate	no innervation
EYE			
• iris (radial muscle)	α_1	contract (mydriasis)	no innervation
• iris (circular muscle)		no innervation	constrict (miosis)
• ciliary body sphincter		no innervation	constrict ; accommodation for near vision

Figure 26.6
Classes of autonomic nervous system drugs

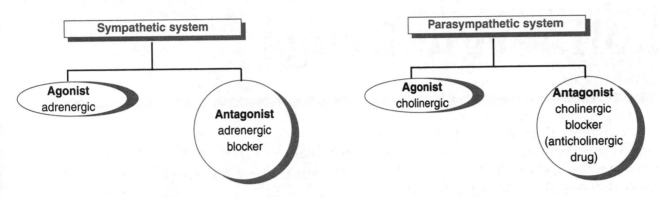

Table 26.1 (continued)
Location of autonomic receptors

Organ	Sympathetic receptor	Sympathetic response	Parasympathetic response
LUNGS			
• bronchial muscle	β_2	relax (dilate)	constrict
• bronchial gland secretion	α_1, β_2	inhibit	stimulate
GI TRACT			
• motility	α_1, β_2	decrease	increase
• sphincters	α_1	contract	relax
• secretions			increase
• salivary glands	α_1	thick, mucous secretion	thin, watery secretion
• gallbladder and ducts	β_2	relax	contract
LIVER	α_1, β_2	release of glucose glycogenolysis	storage of glucose glycogen synthesis
SPLEEN	α	contracts: discharges stored blood into circulation	no innervation
GLANDS			
• sweat	cholinergic	increased	no innervation
• lachrymal		no innervation	tear secretion
• nasal/pharyngeal		no innervation	copious secretions
PANCREAS	α_2	inhibits insulin secretion	
	β_2	stimulates insulin release	
KIDNEY	β_1	increases renin secretion vasoconstriction: reduced urine	no innervation
BLADDER			
• sphincter	α_1	contract	relax
• detrusor	β_2	relax	contract
SEX ORGANS			
• male	α_1	ejaculation	erection
• female			
• uterus: pregnant	α_1	contraction	
	β_2	relaxation	
nonpregnant	β_2	relaxation	

Cholinergic Drugs

Topics Discussed

Direct-Acting Cholinergics:
- Mechanism of action and pharmacologic effects
- Therapeutic uses
- Adverse effects
- Nursing management

Indirect-Acting Cholinergics (Cholinesterase Inhibitors):
- Mechanism of action and pharmacologic effects
- Therapeutic uses
- Adverse effects
- Nursing management

Drugs Discussed

Direct-Acting Cholinergics:
bethanechol (beh-**than**-eh-kole)
carbamylcholine (car-ba-mill-**coal**-een)
pilocarpine (pye-loe-**kar**-peen)

Indirect-Acting Cholinergics:
ambenonium (am-bin-**noh**-nee-yum)
demecarium (dem-ah-**care**-ee-yum)
echothiophate (ek-oh-**thye**-oh-fate)
edrophonium (ed-roe-**fone**-ee-yum)
isoflurophate (eye-soh-**flyoor**-oh-fate)
neostigmine (nee-oh-**stig**-meen)
physostigmine (fye-zoe-**stig**-meen)

Clinical Challenge

Consider this clinical challenge as you read through this chapter. The response to the challenge appears on page 270.

J. is a 3-year-old boy, brought into emergency by his mother, who reports that he has suddenly become very ill. J. lives on a farm and recently his father has been spraying with insecticides. The physician contacts the nearest poison control centre and is informed that this insecticide contains an anticholinesterase chemical.

1. What symptoms will this boy display?
2. What drugs could be used to treat this child?

Cholinergic drugs mimic the effects of acetylcholine. They may act directly, by stimulating muscarinic or nicotinic receptors, or indirectly, by inhibiting the enzyme acetylcholinesterase, thereby allowing acetylcholine to accumulate around the receptors.

Acetylcholine itself is not suitable for use as a drug. It cannot be given orally; it is rapidly destroyed by both acetylcholinesterase and pseudocholinesterase; and its action is nonspecific, affecting both nicotinic and muscarinic receptors.

Ideally, cholinergic drugs should rectify these obvious sins of acetylcholine, and to a degree, they do. Some cholinergic drugs can be given orally.

Cholinergic drugs all have longer durations of action than acetylcholine and some specificity for either the nicotinic or muscarinic receptors. They may be divided into (1) direct-acting and (2) indirect-acting cholinergic drugs. Direct-acting cholinergics interact directly with muscarinic and/or nicotinic receptors. Indirect-acting cholinergics do not directly stimulate cholinergic receptors. Rather, they inhibit cholinesterase, the enzyme responsible for the inactivation of acetylcholine. The increased concentrations of acetylcholine that accumulate around both nicotinic and muscarinic receptors account for the cholinergic effects seen in patients.

Direct-Acting Cholinergic Drugs

Mechanism of Action and Pharmacologic Effects

The direct-acting cholinergics stimulate muscarinic receptors. In some cases they also stimulate nicotinic receptors. Their pharmacologic effects include salivation, secretion of sweat, vasodilatation, bronchiolar constriction, increased gastrointestinal activity, gastric acid secretion and increased urinary bladder tone.

The effects of these drugs on the cardiovascular system are complex. They stimulate the muscarinic receptors in the heart to produce bradycardia. This action may be offset by a reflex increase in sympathetic stimulation to the heart caused by the peripheral vasodilatation produced by these drugs.

The most commonly used direct-acting cholinergics are carbamylcholine (Carbachol®), bethanechol (Urecholine®) and pilocarpine (Isopto Carpine®).

Therapeutic Uses

Carbamylcholine and bethanechol stimulate muscarinic, and to some extent nicotinic, receptors. They are given orally or parenterally for the treatment of postoperative intestinal atony or urinary retention.

Pilocarpine and carbamylcholine are instilled in the eye to produce miosis by stimulating the muscarinic receptors on the circular muscle of the iris (Figure 27.1). The resulting increase in the

Figure 27.1
Autonomic innervation of the iris and ciliary body

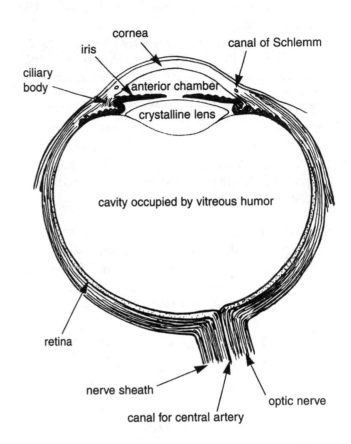

drainage of aqueous humor through the canals of Schlemm lowers the intraocular pressure, thereby aiding in the treatment of glaucoma. Glaucoma is a condition in which intraocular pressure increases, potentially causing damage to the retina and/or optic nerve. Both drugs can also be used to produce miosis during ocular surgery.

Adverse Effects

When given systemically, these drugs stimulate muscarinic receptors throughout the body. As a result, their adverse effects include sweating, abdominal cramps, salivation, flushing of the skin, asthmatic attacks, headache and a fall in blood pressure.

Bethanechol and carbamylcholine are contraindicated in patients with bronchial asthma, peptic ulcers, pronounced bradycardia or hypotension, vasomotor instability, coronary artery disease, epilepsy and parkinsonism. Many of these contraindications require little comment. For obvious reasons, a drug that constricts bronchioles, increases gastric acid secretion, slows the heart and dilates blood vessels is contraindicated in the above conditions.

It is perhaps less obvious why these drugs are contraindicated in parkinsonism. Patients with parkinsonism have a relatively large amount of acetylcholine in the brain, compared with the levels of dopamine. It is this imbalance of acetylcholine relative to dopamine in brain basal ganglia that is responsible for the problems in muscle movement. Administering a cholinergic drug to a parkinsonian patient accentuates the imbalance and worsens the disease.

Nursing Management

Table 27.1 describes the nursing management of the patient receiving direct-acting cholinergic agonists. Dosage details for all drugs discussed in this chapter are given in Table 27.4 (pages 271–272).

Indirect-Acting Cholinergic Drugs (Cholinesterase Inhibitors)

Mechanism of Action and Pharmacologic Effects

The indirect-acting cholinergic drugs inhibit acetylcholinesterase. They are thus called cholinesterase inhibitors or anticholinesterases. By inhibiting the inactivation of acetylcholine they increase cholinergic stimulation. Cholinesterase inhibitors may be divided into the reversibly and irreversibly acting drugs. The effects of the former last a few hours, the latter several days or weeks.

The reversibly acting cholinesterase inhibitors include physostigmine (Eserine®, Antilirium®), demecarium (Humorsol®), neostigmine (Prostigmin®), pyridostigmine (Mestinon®), ambenonium (Mytelase®) and edrophonium (Tensilon®). Isoflurophate (DFP®, Floropryl®) and echothiophate (Echodide®, Phospholine Iodide®) are two of the more commonly used irreversibly acting cholinesterase inhibitors. A spin-off from the war-gas industry, irreversibly acting cholinesterase inhibitors were developed to poison people. Long after the war buffs lost interest in them, these agents remain as valuable drugs in the treatment of disease.

The pharmacologic effects of the cholinesterase inhibitors are similar to those listed for the direct-acting cholinergics. They include a generalized parasympathomimetic action, including salivation, increased gastrointestinal activity and urinary bladder tone, as well as vasodilatation and increased sweating.

Therapeutic Uses

Cholinesterase inhibitors are used for their effects on the eye, the skeletal muscles and the gastrointestinal and urinary tracts. When instilled in the eye, the drug's the inhibition of acetylcholinesterase in the iris increases parasympathetic stimulation of the circular muscle, producing miosis. The resulting increase in the drainage of aqueous humor through the canals of Schlemm lowers intraocular pressure and is of value in the treatment of glaucoma. As previously explained, glaucoma is a condition in which the intraocular pressure increases, potentially causing damage to the retina and the optic nerve. The drugs used most frequently to treat glaucoma are demecarium, isoflurophate and echothiophate.

The systemic administration of a cholinesterase inhibitor can have a dramatic effect on skeletal muscle function. The inhibition of acetylcholinesterase increases acetylcholine stimulation of nicotinic receptors on the motor end-plates of skeletal muscle.

Pyridostigmine, neostigmine and ambenonium have been used to great advantage in the treatment of myasthenia gravis, a disease characterized by decreased neuromuscular transmission, together with weakness and fatiguability of skeletal muscles. Myasthenia gravis is caused by an autoimmune response to the nicotinic receptors on motor end-plates. Antibodies are formed that reduce the number of receptors. Cholinesterase inhibitors increase acetylcholine concentration around nicotinic receptors on skeletal muscle. They are used to increase skeletal muscle strength in patients with myasthenia gravis.

In addition to their ability to increase acetylcholine concentration, both neostigmine and pyridostigmine directly stimulate skeletal muscle nicotinic receptors. Experiments performed with denervated tissue, in which there is neither acetylcholine nor acetylcholinesterase, have shown that the drugs can stimulate skeletal muscle.

Table 27.1
Nursing management of direct-acting cholingergics

Assessment of risk vs. benefit	Patient data	• Physician should determine any contraindications (see Adverse Effects in text). Rule out intestinal obstruction • Assess to establish baseline VS, general state of health • *Pregnancy and lactation:* Safety not established
	Drug data	• Relatively short-acting; poor oral absorption
Implementation	Rights of administration	• Using the "rights" helps prevent errors of administration
	Right route	• Give PO, SC or instill into eye
	Right dose	• Do not substitute oral and SC doses; higher dose required PO
	Right time	• Give oral dose on empty stomach to prevent nausea. Do not instill drops concurrently with other drops
	Right technique	• Never give IM or IV; may cause immediate, severe cholinergic crisis (see Outcomes, below)
	Nursing therapeutics	• **PO/SC:** Observe pt closely for 30–60 min after administration. Have bedpan/commode or bathroom easily accessible. Ensure safety; drug may cause hypotension/dizziness. Remind pt to call for assistance prn • Post-void residual may be ordered
	Patient/Family teaching	• General education for drug tx • For ophthalmic use, ensure that pt can correctly instill in eye and apply light lacrimal pressure to prevent systemic absorption. Emphasize importance of washing hands prior to instillation. Reassure that blurred vision will improve with continued use; if blurring persists, consult physician. Avoid dangerous activity until response to drug is known • *Discuss possibility of pregnancy:* Advise pt to notify physician. Explain risks of lactation while on these drugs
Outcomes	Monitoring of progress	*Continually monitor:* • For tx of postoperative or postpartum urinary retention. Frequently monitor response and output; if voiding does not occur within 1 h, notify physician • For glaucoma, evaluate changes in vision or eye irritation. Encourage pt to have follow-up eye exam to determine ocular pressure • Be alert for signs/symptoms of cholinergic crisis (excessive stimulation of cholinergic receptors causing salivation, diaphoresis, hiccuping, nausea, vomiting or abdominal cramps and bronchoconstriction; may also result in CNS effects of slurred speech, respiratory arrest and seizure). Have respiratory support and atropine on hand; report immediately to physician

Obviously, this direct action complements their anticholinesterase effects in the treatment of the myasthenic patient.

Neostigmine is also used after surgery to reverse the skeletal muscle paralysis produced by tubocurarine and other drugs with similar actions. Tubocurarine is a competitive blocker of nicotinic receptors on skeletal muscle. Its effects can be reversed by increasing acetylcholine concentration in the vicinity of the receptors.

Neostigmine can be employed for the treatment of postoperative intestinal atony or urinary retention. The rationale for its use is the same as presented for the direct-acting cholinergics.

One additional use of an anticholinesterase drug deserves attention. Parenteral physostigmine (Antilirium®) can be used to treat patients poisoned with anticholinergics or tricyclic antidepressants. The latter group has extensive anticholinergic properties. Physostigmine is used in preference to neostigmine or pyridostigmine because it will cross the blood-brain barrier and can, therefore, antagonize both the central and peripheral toxicities of the anticholinergics and antidepressants. Neostigmine or pyridostigmine do not cross the blood-brain barrier and are ineffective in combatting the action of anticholinergics or antidepressants within the brain.

Adverse Effects

The adverse effects of cholinesterase inhibitors result from an accumulation of acetylcholine throughout the body, producing a generalized stimulation of all cholinergic receptors. These include peripheral muscarinic and nicotinic receptors, as well as cholinergic receptors in the central nervous system. Obviously, these effects are much more intense when the drugs are administered systemically than when they are instilled in the eye. In spite of this comment, many patients have experienced systemic adverse effects when irreversibly acting agents have been applied to the eye.

It is beyond the scope of this book to list all the effects of a cholinergic crisis. However, *muscarinic stimulation* produces miosis, ocular pain, bronchoconstriction, increased bronchial secretion, salivation, abdominal cramps and diarrhea.

The consequences of excessive *nicotinic stimulation* include skeletal muscle paralysis. If large doses are used, sufficient acetylcholine may accumulate around skeletal muscle receptors to produce a depolarizing block of the motor end-plates. This effect requires an explanation. In the normal course of neuromuscular transmission acetylcholine is released. It stimulates nicotinic receptors and depolarizes motor end-plates. The beginning of muscle contraction occurs. However, the contraction of muscles requires many waves of depolarization. For this to happen, acetylcholine must first be destroyed to allow motor end-plates to repolarize so that they can accept the next impulse. If large doses of a cholinesterase inhibitor are used, acetylcholine is not metabolized and repolarization does not take place. Successive waves of depolarization can not occur and muscular paralysis ensues.

High doses of cholinesterase inhibitors can also affect the *central nervous system* to produce slurred speech, ataxia, confusion, convulsions and paralysis of the respiratory centre. If untreated, the patient will die from respiratory failure.

The treatment of a cholinergic crisis involves the use of large doses of atropine, a competitive blocker of muscarinic receptors. However, atropine does not affect nicotinic receptors on skeletal muscle. If these are paralyzed, it may be necessary to ventilate the patient. If the patient has absorbed an irreversibly acting cholinesterase inhibitor it may be possible to "reactivate" the enzyme by administering the drug pralidoxime (PAM). This chemical may remove the irreversible inhibitor from the cholinesterase enzyme.

Although we have concentrated on the toxicities of the cholinesterase inhibitors that are used as drugs, nurses should be aware that many individuals are poisoned by anticholinesterases used as insecticides. Two popular insecticides that are irreversibly acting cholinesterase inhibitors are malathion and parathion. They may be swallowed or accidentally absorbed through the skin or lungs.

Table 27.2 lists the clinically significant drug interactions with indirect-acting cholinergic drugs.

Nursing Management

Table 27.3 describes the nursing management of the patient receiving indirect-acting cholinergics (cholinesterase inhibitors). Dosage details for all drugs discussed in this chapter are given in Table 27.4 (pages 271–272).

Table 27.2
The indirect-acting cholinergics: Drug interactions

Drug	Interaction
Beta blockers	• Prolonged bradycardia and hypotension have been reported with the beta blockers atenolol or nadolol and neostigmine. This interaction may also occur with physostigmine. Because of multiple case reports, the concurrent use of a beta blocker and neostigmine or physostigmine should be avoided, if possible. Shorter-acting beta blockers, such as propranolol and especially esmolol, may cause a less severe reaction
Sympathomimetic amines	• Sympathomimetic amines increase myopia with pilocarpine. The mechanism of this interaction has not been established. Monitor pts for change in refraction

Table 27.3
Nursing management of indirect-acting cholinergics

Assessment of risk vs. benefit	Patient data	• Physician should determine any contraindications (see Adverse Effects in text) • Assess to establish baseline VS, general state of health • *Pregnancy and lactation:* Safety not established
	Drug data	• For tx of chronic glaucoma, myasthenia gravis and to reverse effects of neuromuscular blockade agents used during surgery. Duration of action varies from a few hours to several days/weeks
Implementation	Rights of administration	• Using the "rights" helps prevent errors of administration
	Right route	• Give PO, SC, IV, IM or instill into eye
	Right dose	• Do not substitute oral and SC doses; higher dose required PO
	Right time	• Give oral dose with food or milk to prevent nausea. Do not instill drops concurrently with other drops. Drug schedule for tx of myasthenia gravis must be individualized
	Right technique	• Give IV doses slowly using infusion pump. Check agency policy regarding direct-push administration
	Nursing therapeutics	• For tx of myasthenia gravis, establish a careful dosage schedule and observe drug effects (e.g., improvement in ability to swallow or raise eyelids and reduced fatigue). Differentiate myasthenia crisis (extreme muscle weakness due to insufficient drug) from cholinergic crisis (may also have extreme muscle weakness but accompanied by other signs of cholinergic stimulation, as outlined)
	Patient/family teaching	• General education for drug tx • For myasthenia gravis, pt/family need information and reassurance to manage drug tx. The constant challenge is to provide sufficient drug to enhance muscle strength; excessive drug dose also causes muscle weakness. Help pt to develop a systematic approach to assessing muscle strength and keep track of each drug dose and its effects

(cont'd on next page)

Table 27.3 (continued)
Nursing management of indirect-acting cholinergics

| Implementation (cont'd) | Patient/Family teaching (cont'd) | • For ophthalmic use, ensure that pt can correctly instill in eye and apply light lacrimal pressure to prevent systemic absorption. Emphasize importance of washing hands prior to instillation. Reassure that blurred vision will improve with continued use; if blurring persists, consult physician. Avoid dangerous activity until response to drug is known
• For tx of myasthenia gravis, monitor muscle strength and daily function. For glaucoma, evaluate changes in vision or eye irritation. Encourage pt to have follow-up eye exam to determine ocular pressure.
• *Discuss possibility of pregnancy:* Advise pt to notify physician. Explain risks of lactation while on these drugs |
| Outcomes | Monitoring of progress | *Continually monitor:*
• For tx of postoperative or postpartum urinary retention. Frequently monitor response and output: if voiding does not occur within 1 h, notify physician
• For glaucoma, evaluate changes in vision or eye irritation. Encourage pt to have follow-up eye exam to determine ocular pressure
• Be alert for signs/symptoms of cholinergic crisis (excessive stimulation of cholinergic receptors causing salivation, diaphoresis, hiccuping, nausea, vomiting or abdominal cramps and broncho-constriction; may also result in CNS effects of slurred speech, respiratory arrest and seizure). Have respiratory support and atropine on hand; report immediately to physician |

Response to Clinical Challenge

Principles

J. has been poisoned with an insecticide containing a cholinesterase inhibitor (anticholinesterase agent). By blocking the enzyme cholinesterase, the action of the neurotransmitter acetylcholine is prolonged at cholinergic receptors. This causes increased response of the parasympathetic system (see Table 26.1, pages 262–263).

1. This would cause the following symptoms:
CNS: Ataxia, slurred speech, confusion, seizures, respiratory arrest
Eye: Miosis

Respiratory: Bronchoconstriction (wheezing, dyspnea)
CVS: Bradycardia
GI: Increased tone (cramps, nausea, vomiting), salivation
GU: Urination

2. Treatment is based on blocking the action of acetylcholine at the muscarinic and nicotinic receptors. The muscarinic actions of acetylcholine can be blocked by administering atropine (see Chapter 28). Atropine will not block the nicotinic effects of the cholinesterase inhibitor on skeletal muscles. With respiratory paralysis, mechanical ventilation may be required. Timely administration of pralidoxime may remove the cholinesterase inhibitor from the enzyme.

Table 27.4
The cholinergics: Drug doses

Drug Generic name (Trade names)	Dosage	Nursing alert
A. Direct-Acting Cholinergics		
bethanechol chloride (Urecholine)	**Oral:** 10–50 mg tid or qid. **SC:** Usual dose, 5 mg	•Never give IM or IV. Give on empty stomach. Note variation in PO and SC doses; they are not interchangeable. Monitor VS x 1h after SC administration. Test dose may be ordered
carbamylcholine chloride (Carbachol)	*For systemic use:* **Oral:** 1–4 mg. **SC:** 0.25–0.5 mg *For ophthalmic use:* 0.01%: Instill 0.5 mL into the anterior chamber. 0.75, 1.5, and 3%: 1–2 drops instilled into the eye 2–3x daily	•Do not give IV or IM
pilocarpine (Miocarpine, Pilopine AS)	*Chronic glaucoma:* **Topical,** to the conjunctiva, 1 drop 0.5%–4% solution up to 4x/day *Acute angle-closure glaucoma:* **Topical,** to the conjunctiva, 1 drop 1%–2% solution q5–10 min for 3–6 doses, then 1 drop q1–3h until intraocular pressure is reduced	•Monitor for local reaction (discontinue) and for systemic toxicity, if drug used frequently. Check label. Available as 1%, 2%, 4% or 6% solution. Also available as a gel
B. Indirect-Acting Cholinergics (Reversibly Acting Anticholinesterases)		
neostigmine (Prostigmin)	**Oral:** For myasthenia gravis. *Adults:* Initially, 15 mg q3–4h; adjust in accordance with the pt's requirements. *Children:* 2 mg/kg/day in divided doses prn **IM/SC:** For exacerbations of myasthenia gravis when oral therapy is impractical. *Adults,* 0.5 mg. Adjust subsequent dosage according to response. *Infants and children,* 0.01–0.04 mg/kg q2–3h Atropine (0.01 mg/kg IM or SC) should not be used routinely but should be available to control adverse effects	•Give oral dose with food or milk to reduce GI effects

(cont'd on next page)

Table 27.4 (continued)
The cholinergics: Drug doses

Drug Generic name (Trade names)	Dosage	Nursing alert
B. Indirect-Acting Cholinergics (Reversibly Acting Anticholinesterases) (cont'd)		
neostigmine (Prostigmin) (cont'd)	**IV:** For tx of exacerbations of myasthenia gravis or when pt cannot take anticholinesterase agents orally. Infusion rate by IV pump should parallel the rate at which oral medication is given. For example, if pt normally takes 60 mg pyridostigmine qid, neostigmine 4 mg should be infused over the 24-h period (neostigmine 1 mg IV is equivalent to pyridostigmine 60 mg PO)	• Give IV slowly; do not exceed 1 mg/min. Use infusion pump. Have atropine and respiratory support available
physostigmine (Antilirium)	To help control CNS reactions and some arrhythmias in pts poisoned with TCAs or anticholinergics. **IV:** *Adults,* 0.5–1 mg slowly (1 mg/min). May repeat dose if life-threatening signs/symptoms recur. *Children,* 0.5 mg given slowly. If toxic effects persist and no cholinergic effects are produced, repeat dose at 5-min intervals to max. dose of 2 mg. Lowest total effective dose should be repeated if life-threatening signs/symptoms recur	• Give slowly; do not exceed 1 mg/min. Use infusion pump • Use only clear solution; darkening indicates loss of potency
C. Indirect-Acting Cholinergics (Irreversibly Acting Anticholinesterases)		
demecarium bromide (Humorsol)	*For glaucoma:* **Instill:** 1 drop 0.125%–0.25% solution in conjunctival sac q12–48h	• Use aseptic technique and correct procedure for instillation into eye
echothiophate iodide (Phospholine Iodide)	*For glaucoma:* **Instill:** 1 drop 0.03%–0.125% solution in conjunctival sac q12–48h (0.25% may be required in highly pigmented eyes)	• Use aseptic technique and correct procedure for instillation into eye. If possible, instill hs; causes transient blurred vision
isoflurophate (Floropryl)	*For glaucoma.* **Instill:** Initially, 1/4" strip 0.025% ointment q8–72h.	• Use aseptic technique and correct procedure for instillation into eye

Further Reading

Brown JH, Taylor Palmer. Muscarinic receptor agonists and antagonists. In: Hardman JG, Limbird LE, eds. *Goodman and Gilman's The Pharmacological Basis of Therapeutics.* 9th ed. New York: Pergamon; 1996: 141–160.

Colasanti BK. Directly acting cholinomimetics. In: Craig CR, Stitzel RE, eds. *Modern Pharmacology.* 4th ed. Boston: Little, Brown; 1994:145–150.

Hoover DB. Cholinesterases and cholinesterase inhibitors. In: Craig CR, Stitzel RE, eds. *Modern Pharmacology.* 4th ed. Boston: Little, Brown; 1994: 161–168.

Taylor P. Anticholinesterase agents. In: Hardman JG, Limbird LE, eds. *Goodman and Gilman's The Pharmacological Basis of Therapeutics.* 9th ed. New York: Pergamon; 1996:161–176.

CHAPTER 28

Anticholinergic Drugs

Topics Discussed

- Atropine
- Atropine-like mydriatics and cycloplegics
- Atropine-like antispasmodics
- Atropine-like antiasthmatics
- Anticholinergic properties of other categories of drugs
- Risks of anticholinergics for older adults
- Nursing management

Drugs Discussed

atropine (**at**-troe-peen)
cyclopentolate (sye-kloe-**pen**-toe-late)
glycopyrrolate (glye-koe-**pye**-roe-late)
homatropine (home-at-**troe**-peen)
hyoscine (**hye**-oh-seen)
hyoscyamine (hye-oh-**sye**-ah-meen)
ipratropium (ip-rah-**troe**-pee-um)
isopropamide (eye-soe-**proe**-pah-myde)
methantheline (meh-**than**-the-leen)
oxybutynin (ox-ee-**byoo**-tin-in)
oxyphenonium (ox-ee-fen-**oh**-nee-yum)
pirenzepine (peer-**en**-zeh-peen)
propantheline (proe-**pan**-the-leen)
scopolamine (scoe-**pole**-ah-meen)

Clinical Challenge

Consider this clinical challenge as you read through this chapter. The response to the challenge appears on page 277.

Mr. D.T. has recently experienced an exacerbation of irritable bowel syndrome. An anticholinergic agent, isopropamide, is useful to treat the symptoms. The dosage range is 5–10 mg q12h PO. The physician orders 10 mg bid, which Mr. T. takes regularly for 5 days.

On a home visit, you are discussing his recent problems and drug therapy. He states that he feels worse than before. Now he has trouble focussing to watch TV and difficulty voiding; his mouth is so dry he has lost his appetite. His wife reports that last night he seemed vague and forgetful.

What is the most likely cause of Mr. T.'s present sign/symptoms? What actions do you recommend?

Anticholinergic drugs block stimulation of cholinergic receptors by acetylcholine. They are also referred to as *cholinergic blocking drugs*. Since acetylcholine is the neurotransmitter at autonomic ganglia, postganglionic cholinergic neuromuscular junctions and somatic motor end-plates, it would be logical to assume on the basis of their name that anticholinergic drugs block all types of cholinergic receptors. However, in its usual context the expression means only the competitive blockade of muscarinic receptors. In this text anticholinergic drugs can be taken to mean *antimuscarinic agents*.

Anticholinergics are best studied by discussing atropine first. It is the standard drug in this category and the chemical against which all other agents should be compared. If nurses understand the actions of atropine, they will have little difficulty incorporating newer anticholinergics into their therapeutic armamentarium.

Atropine

Mechanism of Action and Pharmacologic Effects

Atropine is obtained from the belladonna plant. It combines reversibly with muscarinic receptors, preventing stimulation by acetylcholine. Atropine blocks muscarinic receptors throughout the body. This includes all receptors innervated by parasympathetic postganglionic nerves and those few muscarinic receptors that receive innervation from cholinergic sympathetic nerves. Because atropine is a competitive blocker of muscarinic receptors, its effects can be overcome if large amounts of acetylcholine accumulate around the receptors. It is possible, therefore, to reverse the effects of atropine by administering a cholinesterase inhibitor.

If nurses understand the actions of parasympathetic nerves, they will have no difficulty remembering atropine's effects. Parasympathetic stimulation decreases heart rate; increases respiratory tract, salivary gland and gastric secretion; stimulates motor activity in the stomach, duodenum, jejunum, ileum and colon; constricts the pupil; and enables the eye to accommodate for near vision. Sympathetic cholinergic stimulation increases the secretion of sweat. (See Table 26.1, pages 262–263.)

The cholinergic block induced by atropine produces exactly the opposite effects. It increases heart rate, decreases the secretions of the respiratory tract, salivary and sweat glands, reduces gastric secretion and motor activity of the stomach, duodenum, jejunum, ileum and colon, dilates the pupil and produces a paralysis of accommodation for near vision (cycloplegia).

Not all cholinergic functions are equally susceptible to the blocking actions of atropine. Secretions of the sweat, salivary and respiratory tract glands are most easily depressed. Larger systemic doses are required to produce dilatation of the pupil (mydriasis), cycloplegia and inhibition of vagal tone to the heart. Still higher doses of atropine are needed to inhibit parasympathetic activity to the gastrointestinal tract, ureter and urinary bladder. A reduction in gastric secretion requires the highest doses of atropine, and there is some suggestion that it is impossible to obtain this effect with normal therapeutic quantities.

Therapeutic Uses

One of the major uses of atropine has been to modify gastrointestinal function. Prior to the introduction of the histamine$_2$ blocker cimetidine (Tagamet®), atropine and atropine-like drugs were widely used in the management of peptic ulcers. They were used alone and in combination with antacids and CNS depressants. Many of these products had only minimal effect. As suggested above, very high doses of atropine, and most atropine-like drugs, must be used to inhibit gastric acid secretion and reduce gastrointestinal motility.

Atropine is well established as a component of preanesthetic medications. It is used because of its ability to inhibit the secretions of the salivary glands and the respiratory tract. Scopolamine (or hyoscine) is also derived from belladonna. It mimics the peripheral effects of atropine but has a greater effect on the brain, producing considerable drowsiness, euphoria and amnesia. Scopolamine can cause fatigue and sleep and is used as one component of preanesthetic medication.

Atropine can be used to treat bradycardia and syncope caused by a hyperactive carotid sinus reflex. In this condition even a small increase in blood pressure stimulates the carotid sinus pressor receptors to slow the heart reflexly by increasing vagal stimulation. As a result of the abrupt fall in heart rate, patients may faint. Atropine blocks muscarinic receptors on the heart and prevents the action of the vagus nerve. It can also assist in the treatment of A-V conduction disturbances caused by increased vagal activity.

The use of atropine to treat the toxicities of the cholinesterase inhibitors is mentioned in Chapter 27. Patients treated with neostigmine, pyridostigmine or ambenonium for myasthenia gravis may also receive atropine, or an atropine-like drug, to minimize the consequence of acetylcholine accumulation around muscarinic receptors. However, neither atropine nor any other anticholinergic drug should be routinely incorporated into the patient's therapeutic regimen. Masking the signs of increased muscarinic stimulation may lead to cholinergic crisis.

Atropine and scopolamine are effective in preventing motion sickness, although the mechanism of this effect is not clear. The scopolamine-impregnated disc, known either as Transderm-Scop or Transderm-V, can be stuck behind the ear, and scopolamine will be absorbed through the skin over a period of thirty-six to forty-eight hours. There is little doubt that travellers will spend considerably less time in the washroom on ocean cruises if they premedicate with atropine or scopolamine. However, the drug is not advised for drivers of automobiles because it causes drowsiness and blurred vision.

Adverse Effects

The adverse effects of atropine result from its ability to diminish or block most cholinergic functions in the body. These have been listed above (Mechanism of Action and Pharmacological Effects). However, a desired effect for one patient may be an adverse effect for another. For example, if atropine is used to decrease the flow of saliva, its

---

Box 28.1

Signs and symptoms of atropine toxicity (anticholinergic crisis)

✔ Hot as a Hare	Fever, tachycardia, weakness
✔ Dry as a Bone	Dry mouth, difficulty swallowing, thirst
✔ Red as a Beet	Skin is hot, flushed and dry
✔ Blind as a Bat	Blurred vision, photophobia
✔ Mad as a Hatter	Confusion, disorientation, incoherence

---

adverse effects include cycloplegia, mydriasis, tachycardia, decreased gastrointestinal and urinary bladder activity and reduced sweat production. On the other hand, if the drug is given to reduce vagal effects on the heart, an increase in heart rate is the desired and not an adverse effect. In that case, the dry mouth joins the other actions of atropine as an adverse effect. The major difference between atropine and scopolamine is the ability of the latter agent to produce a marked CNS depression.

Box 28.1 summarizes the symptoms of atropine toxicity (anticholinergic crisis). The treatment of anticholinergic toxicity involves removing the drug from the body by the use of activated charcoal or the induction of emesis. The cholinesterase inhibitor (see Chapter 27) physostigmine is used as the antidote for anticholinergic poisoning.

Table 28.1 lists the clinically significant drug interactions with the anticholinergics.

Table 28.1
The anticholinergics: Drug interactions

Drug	Interaction
Amantadine	•Amantadine and anticholinergics can produce hallucinations, confusion and nightmares. Decrease dosage of anticholinergic before starting amantadine
Cimetidine	•High doses of propantheline decrease the effects of cimetidine. Avoid concurrent high doses of anticholinergics with cimetidine
Haloperidol	•Anticholinergics can decrease the effects of haloperidol. Monitor haloperidol effects and, if necessary, its serum concentration
Levodopa	•Anticholinergics can decrease levodopa absorption and its effects. Monitor clinical status of pt

Atropine-Like Mydriatics and Cycloplegics

Atropine is an effective mydriatic and cycloplegic. It does, however, have a long duration of action. Patients would obviously not wish to walk around for a day or more unable to accommodate for near vision and with one or both pupils the size of small bowling balls just because a physician needed to produce mydriasis for a short period of time.

Synthetic or semisynthetic anticholinergics, such as cyclopentolate (Cyclogyl®) and homatropine, may be substituted for atropine when a shorter duration of action is desired. The drugs are used to produce mydriasis in order to allow for a thorough retinal examination. They are also used to treat iritis, iridocyclitis, keratitis and choroiditis. The cycloplegic effects are desirable for accurate measurement of refractive errors.

Atropine-Like Antispasmodics

Many synthetic and semisynthetic anticholinergics have been placed on the market for the adjunctive treatment of peptic ulcers, intestinal spasms and irritable bowel syndrome. The drugs are claimed to be more effective than atropine and produce a lower incidence of systemic adverse effects. To a degree these claims may be justified. Most of the drugs are less readily absorbed from the intestinal tract than atropine and do not cross the blood-brain barrier as readily as atropine. This should reduce their systemic and CNS adverse effects.

It is beyond the scope of this book to discuss all atropine substitutes. Some of the more popular ones include the semisynthetic drug homatropine methyl bromide and the synthetic compounds glycopyrrolate (Robinul®), isopropamide (Darbid®), methantheline (Banthine®), oxyphenonium (Antrenyl®) and propantheline (Probanthine®).

Attention should be drawn to pirenzepine (Gastrozepin®). This anticholinergic effectively inhibits gastric acid secretion. It is effective as adjunctive therapy in disorders where the inhibition of gastric acid secretion is likely to be beneficial, specifically: duodenal ulcer and nonmalignant gastric ulcer. However, modern treatment of peptic ulcers no longer relies solely on reducing gastric acid secretion. The role of drugs that decrease gastric acid secretion in the treatment of peptic ulcers is discussed in detail in Chapter 59.

Oxybutynin chloride (Ditropan®) is an anticholinergic that has both antimuscarinic and direct antispasmodic actions on smooth muscle. The drug is indicated for the relief of symptoms associated with voiding in patients with uninhibited neurogenic and reflex neurogenic bladder.

Atropine-Like Antiasthmatics

Ipratropium bromide (Atrovent Inhaler®) is an anticholinergic drug that is administered by inhalation. It blocks the action of the vagus nerve by competitively blocking the effects of acetylcholine at parasympathetic (cholinergic) receptors. This results in reduced bronchomotor tone. Ipratropium is poorly absorbed and causes few systemic effects. In the treatment of asthma, it is a less effective bronchodilator than inhaled beta$_2$ stimulant, but has additive effects when used in conjunction with a beta$_2$ agonist. (See Chapter 69 for detailed information on the treatment of asthma.)

Ipratropium is an equally or more effective bronchodilator than beta$_2$ agonists in the treatment of chronic obstructive pulmonary disease (COPD), such as chronic bronchitis or emphysema.

Ipratropium is also available as a nasal spray that is effective in the treatment of watery rhinorrhea associated with vasomotor rhinitis.

Anticholinergic Properties of Other Categories of Drugs

Many commonly used drugs not normally classified as anticholinergics have significant anticholinergic actions. These are usually considered adverse effects. For example, many antidepressant and most antipsychotic medications block cholinergic receptors, and this causes such adverse effects as dry mouth, blurred vision, urinary retention and constipation. These effects may cause the patient to discontinue the drugs. The anticholinergic effects of these drugs are discussed in more detail in the chapters devoted to each group of agents.

Risks of Anticholinergics for Older Adults

Drugs that block cholinergic receptors present special risks to the older adult, as age-related changes in body function may be exacerbated by anticholinergic therapy. For example, older men are more likely to have prostatic hypertrophy, which causes difficulty voiding. Adding anticholinergic drugs to the situation may increase the problem and lead to urinary retention. Similarly, older people have slower intestinal peristalsis and are more prone to constipation, particularly if anticholinergic therapy is associated with inactivity in a hospital. Giving an anticholinergic may have positive results from the surgeon's point of view but it also increases the likelihood of postoperative abdominal distention. Further, older people often notice a decrease in production of saliva (dry mouth); this effect will be even more noticeable following administration of an anticholinergic drug. Finally, glaucoma, hypertension and coronary artery disease are contraindications to the use of anticholinergic drugs, and these conditions are more prevalent in the aging population.

These risks can be addressed by thorough assessment prior to administration to detect precautions or contraindications. It is essential that nurses ensure careful dosing of anticholinergics and monitor closely patient response to these drugs.

Nursing Management

Table 28.2 on the next page describes the nursing management of the patient receiving anticholinergic drugs. Drug dosage details for individual drugs are given in Table 28.3 (pages 279–280).

Further Reading

Brown JH, Taylor P. Muscarinic receptor agonists and antagonists. In: Hardman JG, Limbird LE, eds. *Goodman and Gilman's The Pharmacological Basis of Therapeutics.* 9th ed. New York: Pergamon; 1996: 141–160.

Hoover DB. Muscarinic blocking drugs. In: Craig CR, Stitzel RE, eds. *Modern Pharmacology.* 4th ed. Boston: Little, Brown; 1994:151–160.

Response to Clinical Challenge

Principles

Anticholinergic drugs block parasympathetic receptors in the eye, salivary glands and bladder. As well, the drug can cross the blood-brain barrier and cause confusion. These effects are dose related. Older adults should receive lower doses of these drugs.

Actions

The most likely cause of the signs/symptoms is excessive dosage of the isopropamide. The appropriate action is to notify the physician, discuss the findings and discuss dosage reduction. If the symptoms do not abate, the drug should be discontinued and another substituted.

Table 28.2
Nursing management of the anticholingergics

Assessment of risk vs. benefit	Patient data	• Physician should determine any contraindications such as those described in text (see Adverse Effects). Particularly, assess for CV disease or glaucoma • Assess to establish baseline VS, general state of health • *Pregnancy and lactation:* Safety not established
	Drug data	• Response is dose related; greater doses generally cause more side effects
Implementation	Rights of administration	• Using the "rights" helps prevent errors of administration
	Right route	• Most commonly given PO. Drops are instilled into eye. Injectable forms are available; check carefully which route (IM, IV or SC) is allowed. Scopolamine is available in patch formulation
	Right dose	• Do not substitute oral and SC doses; a higher dose is required PO
	Right time	• Give oral dose 30–60 min ac and avoid administration with antacids. Preoperative medications must be given at a specified time before surgery; check orders
	Right technique	• Check injectable form carefully; some drugs can be given IV, others IM or SC. Do not instill eyedrops concurrently with other drops
	Nursing therapeutics	• Some side effects can be minimized through simple actions, e.g.: *dry mouth (xerostomia)* — use sugarless gum/candy, rinse mouth frequently, drink low-calorie beverages; *constipation* — increase fluid and fibre intake and maintain activity if possible; *blurred vision/photophobia* — reduce light or advise use of dark glasses; *urinary retention* — advise pt to void prior to administration; *hyperthermia due to suppression of sweating* — advise pt to limit exposure to heat and to minimize strenuous exercise
	Patient/family teaching	• Educate for drug tx. The use of the ipratropium inhaler is described in Chapter 69. For ophthalmic use, instruct pt re: hygiene and correct technique of administration • Remind pt to avoid hazardous activities until response to drug is known • *Discuss possibility of pregnancy:* Advise pt to notify physician. Explain risks of lactation while on these drugs
Outcomes	Monitoring of progress	*Continually monitor:* • For tx of GI disorders, monitor response and improvement in symptoms. Monitor urinary output • For mydriatic or cycloplegic action, evaluate changes in vision or eye irritation. Be alert for signs/symptoms of adverse reactions, esp. tachycardia

Table 28.3
The anticholinergics: Drug doses

Drug Generic name (Trade names)	Dosage	Nursing alert
atropine	*Preoperative:* To inhibit salivary and respiratory secretions, **IM:** 0.4–0.6 mg approx. 0.5 h preop. To block the cardiac vagal nerves, **IM/IV:** 1.5–2 mg To treat bradyarrhythmias, **IV:** *Adults:* Initially, 0.4–1 mg every 1–2h prn (max., 2 mg). *Children:* 0.01–0.03 mg/kg Reversal of adverse muscarinic effects of anticholinesterases, **IV:** *Adults:* 0.6–1.2 mg for each 0.5–2.5 mg of neostigmine methylsulfate or 10–20 mg of pyridostigmine bromide concurrently with antichollnesterase Organophosphate poisoning, **IM/IV:** *Adults:* 1–2 mg initially, then 1–2 mg q20–30min prn. In severe cases, 2–6 mg may be used initially and repeated q5–60min prn. May be followed by oral tx. *Children:* 0.05 mg/kg q10–30min prn **Ophthalmologic:** For anterior uveitis or postoperative mydriasis, *Adults:* 1 drop 1%–2% solution instilled od; more frequent use (max., tid) may be required for severe inflammation. *Children,* 0.5% solution or ointment od–tid To break posterior synechiae: 1 drop 2% solution (alternately with phenylephrine 10%) q5–10min for 5 applications of each For malignant (ciliary block) glaucoma: Initially, 1 drop 1%–2% solution and 1 drop phenylephrine 10% tid or qid. For maintenance, 1 drop 1% or 2% solution/day or every other day	• Drug supplied in light-resistant container. Read labels carefully; available in many strengths • **IV:** Administer by direct push over 1–2 min. Check agency policy for this procedure • **Ophthalmic:** Ensure asepsis and correct technique of administration
ipratropium bromide (Atrovent)	**Inhalation:** Adjust to meet needs of pt. Recommended dosage is 2 metered doses (actuations; 40 µg, total) tid or qid. Some pts may need up to 4 metered doses (actuations; 80 µg, total) at a time to obtain max. benefit during early tx	• Assess respiratory status (rate, breath sounds, degree of dyspnea, pulse) before administration and at peak of medication. Confer with physician about alternative medication if severe bronchospasm is present, because onset of action is too slow for pts in acute distress. If paradoxical bronchospasm (wheezing) occurs, withhold medication and notify physician immediately • Assess for allergy to atropine and belladonna alkaloids; pts with these allergies may also be sensitive to ipratropium

(cont'd on next page)

Table 28.3 (continued)
The anticholinergics: Drug doses

Drug Generic name (Trade names)	Dosage	Nursing alert
pirenzepine (Gastrozepin)	**Oral:** 50 mg bid, a.m. and p.m. In pts with more pronounced symptoms, dosage may be 50 mg tid	• Tablets should be taken 30 min or more ac with a little liquid
scopolamine, hyoscine (Transderm-Scop, Transderm–V)	Prevention of s/s of motion sickness, such as nausea and vomiting. **Topical:** *Adults,* 1 disk 12 h before antiemetic protection is required. Not suitable for use in children and may not be suitable for elderly pts	• Apply to clean, dry area behind ear; use even pressure to ensure good contact with skin. Wash hands thoroughly before and after application. Patch is effective for 3 days; is waterproof
scopolamine, hyoscine	*Preoperative:* To induce drowsiness, fatigue, sleep, euphoria, amnesia and to decrease respiratory and salivary secretions. **Oral:** *Adults,* 1 mg. **IM/IV:** *Adults,* 0.4–0.6 mg. *Infants 4–7 months,* 0.1 mg; *7 months–3 years,* 0.15 mg. *Children 3–8 years,* 0.2 mg; *8–12 years,* 0.3 mg	• **IV:** Dilute with sterile water and inject slowly by direct push. Check agency policy. Pre-op medications must be given at specified time prior to surgery; check orders

Adrenergic Drugs

Topics Discussed
● For each drug: Mechanisms of action, pharmacologic effects, therapeutic uses, adverse effects
● Newer adrenergic bronchodilators
● Stimulation of adrenergic receptors: Summary of effects
● Special considerations for the older adult
● Nursing management

Drugs Discussed
albuterol (al-**byoo**-ter-ole)
dobutamine (doe-**byoo**-tah-meen)
dopamine (**dope**-ah-meen)
ephedrine (ef-**fed**-drin)
epinephrine (ep-ee-**nef**-rin)
fenoterol (fen-oh-**ter**-ole)
isoproterenol (eye-soh-proe-**ter**-eh-nole)
metaproterenol (met-ah-pro-**ter**-eh-nole)
metaraminol (met-ah-**ram**-in-ole)
norepinephrine (nor-ep-ee-**nef**-rin)
orciprenaline (or-sih-**pren**-ah-leen)
phenylephrine (fen-ill-**eff**-rin)
procaterol (proe-**kat**-er-ole)
pseudoephedrine (syoo-doe-eh-**fed**-rin)
salbutamol (sal-**byoo**-tah-moel)
salmeterol (sal-**met**-er-ole)
terbutaline (ter-**byoo**-tah-leen)

Clinical Challenge
Consider this clinical challenge as you read through this chapter. The response to the challenge appears on page 289.

You are one of the nurses at a summer camp for children aged 10 to 13. A 12-year-old girl, Mona, has a known allergic response to some foods and to bee sting. She carries an anaphylaxis kit with her including a tourniquet, two auto injectors with 0.5 mg/mL of epinephrine, and anti-histamine tablets.

During a hike, she is stung by a bee on her right calf.

1. Upon Mona's arrival, what would you check in her kit?
2. What signs/symptoms might she experience after being stung?
3. What are the therapeutic actions of epinephrine, and why is it indicated in this situation?
4. What is the self-administration technique for the injection?
5. What observations would you make following the injection?
6. What other actions would be appropriate?

Drugs can activate adrenergic receptors, either directly or indirectly, by four basic mechanisms (see Table 29.1 on the next page):

• direct receptor binding
• promotion of norepinephrine release from sympathetic nerve endings
• blockade of norepinephrine reuptake by sympathetic nerve endings
• inhibition of the enzymatic inactivation of norepinephrine.

Table 29.1
Mechanisms of adrenergic receptor activation

Mechanism of stimulation	Examples
1. Direct mechanism	
•Binding to receptor to cause activation	Epinephrine
	Isoproterenol
	Ephedrine*
2. Indirect mechanisms	
•Promotion of NE release	Ephedrine*
	Amphetamines
•Inhibition of NE reuptake	Cocaine
	Tricyclic antidepressants
•Inhibition of MAO	MAO inhibitors

NE = Norepinephrine, MAO = monamine oxidase

*Ephedrine is a mixed-acting drug that activates adrenergic receptors directly and also promotes release of norepinephrine.

Source: Lehne RA. Adrenergic agonists. In: *Pharmacology for Nursing Care.* Philadelphia: W.B. Saunders; 1994:166. Reproduced with permission.

Note that only the first mechanism is direct. With the other three mechanisms, receptor activation occurs by an indirect process.

Drugs that release norepinephrine from sympathetic nerve endings work within the nerve to trigger the secretion of norepinephrine. The norepinephrine that is released from the nerve is then free to stimulate sympathetic receptors.

Compounds that block the reuptake of norepinephrine by sympathetic nerve endings act on the neuronal membrane. Because neuronal reuptake is the main means by which norepinephrine is removed from the area around receptors, drugs that block neuronal reuptake increase the concentration of norepinephrine in contact with sympathetic receptors.

Inhibition of the enzymatic inactivation of norepinephrine plays a minor role in terminating the effects of this chemical because, as just stated, neuronal reuptake, not enzymatic inactivation, is the main means by which norepinephrine's actions are terminated. Thus, drugs that inhibit norepinephrine inactivation do not significantly increase sympathetic nervous system activity.

A quick review of the mechanisms by which norepinephrine is inactivated in the body, as presented in Chapter 26, will help nurses understand the relative importance of drugs that block norepinephrine reuptake and the compounds that inhibit norepinephrine's enzymatic inactivation.

Direct-acting adrenergic drugs (mechanism 1, above) stimulate alpha$_1$, beta$_1$ or beta$_2$ receptors, or all three. Table 29.2 summarizes the types of adrenergic receptors stimulated by various categories of adrenergic drugs. These drugs mimic, at least in part, the effects of sympathetic nervous system stimulation.

Adrenergic drugs are best studied by reviewing first the actions of epinephrine, norepinephrine (levarterenol) and isoproterenol, because all newer compounds have been designed to reproduce some of the actions of these three chemicals.

Epinephrine, Adrenaline (Adrenalin®)

Mechanism of Action and Pharmacologic Effects

Epinephrine is an emergency hormone released by the adrenal medullae in times of stress. The chem-

Table 29.2
Receptor specificity of representative adrenergic agonists

Catecholamines		Noncatecholamines	
Drug	**Receptors activated**	**Drug**	**Receptors activated**
Epinephrine	$\alpha_1, \alpha_2, \beta_1, \beta_2$	Ephedrine*	$\alpha_1, \alpha_2, \beta_1, \beta_2$
Norepinephrine	$\alpha_1, \alpha_2, \beta_1$	Phenylephrine	α_1
Isoproterenol	β_1, β_2	Terbutaline	β_2
Dopamine†	α_1, β_1, dopamine		

α = alpha β = beta

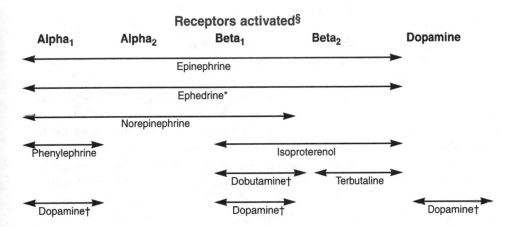

Receptors activated§

*Ephedrine is a mixed-acting agent that causes NE release and also activates alpha and beta receptors directly.

†Receptor activation by dopamine and dobutamine is dose dependent.

§This chart presents the same information on receptor specificity given above in tabular form. Arrows indicate the range of receptors that the drugs can stimulate (at usual therapeutic doses).

Source: Lehne RA. Adrenergic agonists. In: *Pharmacology for Nursing Care.* Philadelphia: W.B. Saunders; 1994:169. Reproduced with permission.

ical is known as adrenaline in many parts of the world. (Adrenalin® — without the e on the end — is a trade name.) Epinephrine stimulates alpha$_1$, beta$_1$ and beta$_2$ receptors. When epinephrine is secreted by the adrenals, it increases heart rate and force of contraction (beta$_1$), dilates bronchioles (beta$_2$) and redistributes blood in the body by constricting the blood vessels in the peritoneal cavity (alpha$_1$) and dilating those in skeletal muscle, myocardium and liver (beta$_2$). Other effects of epinephrine include contraction of the radial muscles in the iris (alpha$_1$) and constriction of the blood vessels in the skin (also alpha$_1$).

Nurses often see the last-named effects — dilatation of the pupils and constriction of the blood vessels in the skin. Patients about to receive a needle or undergo some other stressful procedure are "all eyes" and have a complexion that closely resembles stripped whitefish. This is simply a manifestation of the patient's fight-or-flight mechanism and should not overly concern the nurse.

Epinephrine also increases the respiratory rate and tidal volume, thereby reducing alveolar carbon dioxide. This effect, together with the increase in cardiac output, improves tissue oxygenation. At the same time, epinephrine increases the concentrations of glucose, lactate and free fatty acids in the blood. All are necessary if the stimulated tissues are to receive the metabolic materials to meet their increased needs.

The effects of injected epinephrine may differ from those observed when the chemical is released from the adrenals. This difference is due to the fact that the quantities injected may exceed the amounts normally secreted by the adrenals. If epinephrine is infused at a rate that approximates the physiological release (10–30 µg/min), heart rate and cardiac output increase and blood is shunted according to the route outlined above.

If, however, epinephrine is infused in supraphysiological amounts, it produces a generalized alpha$_1$-mediated effect on blood vessels. All blood vessels in the body will constrict. Although heart rate may increase initially, it will later decrease, and bradycardia will ensue in response to the increase in blood pressure.

To understand why heart rate falls when blood pressure increases, nurses should recognize that the body has two pressor receptors that prevent extreme episodes of hypertension that could cause stroke or myocardial infarction. These receptors, found in the aortic arch and the carotid sinus, return blood pressure to a safe level by decreasing cardiac output. When any drug, such as epinephrine, produces a major increase peripheral resistance, it alerts the pressor receptors to impending danger. They, in turn, stimulate the vagus nerves to slow the heart and decrease the cardiac output. The resulting fall in cardiac output returns blood pressure towards normal, thereby protecting the body.

Therapeutic Uses

Epinephrine cannot be given orally because it is inactivated in the gastrointestinal tract. It is usually administered intramuscularly or subcutaneously. Occasionally epinephrine is given by inhalation to produce bronchodilatation.

The therapeutic uses of epinephrine are based on its actions on the cardiovascular system and bronchioles. By stimulating beta$_2$ receptors, epinephrine dilates bronchioles. Because of its potency and rapid onset of action, it can be used to treat status asthmaticus, an emergency situation. It has also been used in the past on a chronic basis to treat bronchial asthma. However, more selective beta$_2$ stimulant drugs are available, and these have largely replaced inhalation epinephrine for this indication.

Epinephrine may be injected to treat acute hypersensitivity or anaphylactic reactions. The release of histamine in these conditions constricts bronchioles and dilates blood vessels. Epinephrine is the drug of choice because its pharmacologic

effects are opposite to those of histamine. It dilates the bronchioles constricted by histamine and constricts the blood vessels dilated by histamine.

Anyone who has enjoyed a visit to the dentist may remember the cardiac palpitations experienced shortly after the local anesthetic was injected. These effects are due to the absorption of epinephrine from the local anesthetic-epinephrine mixture. Epinephrine is routinely added to solutions of local anesthetics as a vasoconstrictor to keep the local anesthetic local for as long as possible.

Epinephrine is used in attempts to restore cardiac rhythm in patients following cardiac arrest.

Adverse Effects

The adverse effects of epinephrine resemble a very acute case of stage fright. These include fear, anxiety, tension, restlessness and throbbing headache — effects often experienced by performers before going on stage. Once in front of the audience, tremor, weakness, pallor, respiratory difficulties and palpitations take over. This may seem a cavalier way to view the adverse effects or toxicities of epinephrine, but thinking of them in this way facilitates recall by association.

The inadvertent intravenous injection of a large dose of epinephrine can cause cerebral hemorrhage and cardiac arrhythmias. The cerebral hemorrhage results from the abrupt increase in blood pressure.

Norepinephrine, Noradrenaline, Levarterenol (Levophed®)

Mechanism of Action and Pharmacologic Effects

Norepinephrine (also known as noradrenaline and levarterenol) must feel much like a younger child at school who is always compared to an older sibling. Although sharing some characteristics with epinephrine, norepinephrine is not able to do everything epinephrine can. This only stands to reason: norepinephrine is not an emergency hormone. It should, therefore, not be expected to shunt blood from one part of the body to another, increase respiration or stimulate intermediary metabolism. Rather, it is a neurotransmitter, primarily responsible for cardiovascular control.

Norepinephrine is a potent alpha$_1$ stimulant, affecting both arterioles and veins. It has little activity on beta$_2$ receptors. The release of norepinephrine throughout the body constricts arterioles and increases peripheral resistance. One manifestation of norepinephrine-induced arteriolar constriction is a reduction in blood flow through skeletal muscles. This is in contrast to the increase in skeletal muscle blood flow produced by the beta$_2$-stimulating actions of epinephrine.

As mentioned above, norepinephrine constricts veins. The simple act of standing releases norepinephrine from nerves innervating these vessels. The ensuing vasoconstriction prevents blood from accumulating in the lower extremities of the body and ensures adequate venous return to the heart.

Like epinephrine, norepinephrine stimulates beta$_1$ receptors in the heart. The release of norepinephrine by the sympathetic cardiac accelerator nerves increases heart rate. On the other hand, the infusion of norepinephrine slows the heart. In this situation, the alpha$_1$-mediated increase in peripheral resistance alerts the carotid sinus and aortic arch pressure receptors to the presence of possible danger. They, in turn, stimulate the parasympathetic vagus nerves to the heart. The bradycardiac effect of vagal stimulation is greater than the direct beta$_1$-stimulant effect of norepinephrine. As a result, the heart rate falls.

Therapeutic Uses
Similar to epinephrine, norepinephrine cannot be given orally. It is injected intravenously for the maintenance of blood pressure in acute hypotensive states, surgical and nonsurgical trauma, central vasomotor depression and hemorrhage.

Adverse Effects
Norepinephrine can produce bradycardia, as a result of the increase in peripheral resistance (see Mechanism of Action and Pharmacologic Effects). The consequences of an overdosage are similar to those of epinephrine. They include hypertension, headache and severely decreased blood flow producing renal or hepatic failure. Local tissue necrosis may occur at the injection site.

Isoproterenol (Isuprel®)

Mechanism of Action and Pharmacologic Effects
Isoproterenol is a potent stimulant of beta$_1$ and beta$_2$ receptors. It increases both heart rate and force of contraction, a beta$_1$-mediated effect, while decreasing peripheral resistance and blood pressure, a beta$_2$ response. Isoproterenol also dilates the bronchioles as a result of its ability to stimulate beta$_2$ receptors.

Therapeutic Uses
Isoproterenol can be used to treat bronchial asthma but has three major drawbacks. First, it cannot be given orally. Although oral and sublingual products are on the market, their effects are unpredictable. Therefore, isoproterenol is usually given by inhalation for the treatment of asthma. Second, it stimulates both beta$_1$ and beta$_2$ receptors. As a result, it usually produces both bronchodilatation along with annoying tachycardia. Finally, isoproterenol has a short duration of action of two to three hours. Newer adrenergic bronchodilators, such as albuterol/salbutamol, terbutaline and fenoterol, circumvent these problems. They have a more selective action on beta$_2$ receptors, may be administered both orally and by inhalation, and have a longer duration of action than isoproterenol.

Isoproterenol is also available in a parenteral formulation. Given by injection, the drug is used for the prevention or treatment of (1) Adams-Stokes syndrome and other episodes of heart block, except when caused by ventricular tachycardia or fibrillation, (2) cardiac arrest, (3) carotid sinus hypersensitivity, (4) ventricular arrhythmias, especially certain types of ventricular tachycardia and fibrillation, (5) laryngobronchospasm during anesthesia and (6) as adjunctive therapy in shock. The cardiac effects are due to the beta$_1$ stimulation produced by isoproterenol. The use of the drug to modify cardiac function has decreased over the past two decades.

Adverse Effects
The adverse effects of isoproterenol are predictable. Excessive sympathetic beta-receptor stimulation leads to tachycardia, palpitation, nervousness, nausea and vomiting. Other adverse effects

are headache, flushing of the skin, tremor, dizziness, weakness, precordial distress or anginal-type pain. Again, these effects can be accounted for by the vasodilatation and cardiac stimulation produced by the drug.

Ephedrine

Ephedrine is not a new adrenergic drug. Prior to its introduction in North America in 1924, it had been used for about 2000 years in China. It is an $alpha_1$, $beta_1$ and $beta_2$ stimulant and can also produce CNS excitation.

Oral ephedrine is used alone and in combination with theophylline as a bronchodilator. Because it is a less effective bronchodilator and also increases heart rate, ephedrine has largely been replaced by $beta_2$ stimulants, such as albuterol/salbutamol, fenoterol and terbutaline. In addition, ephedrine produces unwanted vasoconstriction and CNS stimulation.

Use is made of the $alpha_1$ stimulant properties of ephedrine in various cold remedies to constrict blood vessels in the nose and reduce tissue swelling. It may be given orally or instilled locally when its nasal vasoconstrictor action is desired.

Table 29.3 lists the clinically significant drug interactions with adrenergic drugs.

Dopamine (Dopastat®, Intropin®, Revimine®)

Mechanism of Action and Pharmacologic Effects

Dopamine is the precursor of norepinephrine, as well as a transmitter in its own right within the brain. When injected as a drug, dopamine stimulates the $beta_1$ receptors in the heart to increase both heart rate and stroke volume. It produces a smaller increase in heart rate than isoproterenol.

Low to intermediate therapeutic doses of dopamine have no effect on peripheral resistance. Dopamine stimulates specific dopamine receptors on the kidney blood vessels to increase the glomerular filtration rate, renal blood flow and sodium excretion.

Therapeutic Uses

Dopamine is used in the treatment of shock patients (see Chapter 37) who are experiencing decreased renal function and normal, or low, peripheral resistance. Dopamine is also used to treat chronic refractory heart failure (see Chapters 32 and 37).

Adverse Effects

Dopamine produces tachycardia, anginal pain, arrhythmias, headache and hypertension. Nausea and vomiting may also be seen. As mentioned before, low to medium therapeutic doses of dopamine increase renal blood flow. High doses of the drug constrict renal blood vessels.

(For the clinically significant drug interactions with dopamine, refer to Table 32.10 on page 337.)

Dobutamine (Dobutrex®)

Mechanism of Action and Pharmacologic Effects

Dobutamine stimulates $beta_1$ receptors in the heart. It produces a greater increase in contractile force than in heart rate. Dobutamine does not dilate renal blood vessels, or increase either glomerular filtration rate or sodium excretion. The major advantage of dobutamine over the other adrenergics is its apparent ability to increase cardiac output with minimal effects on heart rate.

Therapeutic Use

Dobutamine is used in the treatment of acute congestive heart failure (CHF). Patients with acute CHF benefit from the increase in cardiac output provided by dobutamine and a decrease in pulmonary wedge pressure (see Chapter 32).

Pulmonary wedge pressure is a reflection of the capacity of the left ventricle to accept blood coming back from the lungs. In CHF the pulmonary wedge pressure increases because the heart cannot pump all the blood that should be returned in the pulmonary vessels. By increasing cardiac output, dobutamine reduces pulmonary wedge pressure.

Patients who have just undergone cardiopulmonary bypass operations will also benefit from dobutamine.

Adverse Effects

The adverse effects of dobutamine are similar to those previously described for dopamine.

(For the clinically significant drug interactions with dobutamine, refer to Table 32.10 on page 337.)

Table 29.3
The adrenergics: Drug interactions

Drug	Interaction
Antidepressants, tricyclic	•TCAs may increase severalfold the pressor responses to epinephrine and norepinephrine
Antidiabetics	•Adrenergics may decrease the effects of antidiabetic drugs. Monitor blood glucose
Antihistamines	•The effects of epinephrine can be potentiated by some antihistamines
Beta blockers	•Pts receiving nonselective beta blockers show an exaggerated alpha$_1$ (vasoconstrictor) response to epinephrine. This can produce hypertension and reflex vagal-induced bradycardia. Beta blockers can decrease the antianaphylactic effect of epinephrine. The effects of beta agonists are blocked by beta blockers
Enflurane	•Enflurane plus sympathomimetic amines have resulted in cardiac arrhythmias. Monitor cardiac rhythm
Furosemide	•Furosemide and sympathomimetics can produce hypokalemia
Guanethidine, guanadrel	•Guanethidine and guanadrel will have decreased antihypertensive effects in the presence of a sympathomimetic amine. Guanethidine increases the response to norepinephrine
Halothane	•Halothane and epinephrine have been implicated in possible fatal arrhythmias
Insulin	•Adrenergics can decrease the effect of insulin. Monitor blood glucose
Isoflurane	•Isoflurane plus adrenergics have resulted in cardiac arrhythmias. Monitor cardiac rhythm
Monoamine oxidase inhibitors	•MAOIs and adrenergics, except isoproterenol, can produce severe hypertension and possible crisis. This effect may occur with OTC products. Avoid concurrent use
Thiazide diuretics	•Thiazide diuretics and sympathomimetics can produce hypokalemia.
I-Thyroxin	•The effects of epinephrine are potentiated by I-thyroxin

Phenylephrine (Neosynephrine®)

Phenylephrine is an adrenergic drug with major cardiovascular effects. It stimulates alpha$_1$ receptors. When given orally, subcutaneously or intravenously it raises both systolic and diastolic blood pressure. As might be expected, the increase in peripheral resistance produces reflex bradycardia by stimulating the vagus nerves. Phenylephrine can be used systemically to increase blood pressure in hypotensive conditions. It is also used to dilate the pupils. Its greatest use is as a nasal vasoconstrictor in cold preparations. In this situation it is taken orally, together with an antihistamine and an analgesic, or instilled locally in the nose as drops or mist.

Newer Adrenergic Bronchodilators

Metaproterenol/Orciprenaline (Alupent®), Albuterol/Salbutamol (Proventil®, Ventolin®), Terbutaline (Brethine®, Bricanyl®), Fenoterol (Berotec®), Procaterol (Pro-Air®), Salmeterol (Serevent®)

These newer bronchodilators were discussed earlier in this chapter (see Isoproterenol/Therapeutic Uses). They have the following advantages over isoproterenol:

• They preferentially stimulate beta$_2$ receptors.
• They may be given orally or by inhalation.
• They have a longer duration of action than isoproterenol.

The availability of the beta$_2$ stimulants has drastically reduced the use of isoproterenol and ephedrine.

Despite their relative selectivity for beta$_2$ receptors, these drugs can produce palpitations, tachycardia, nervousness and tremor. The tachycardia reflects the fact that, in higher doses, the drugs stimulate beta$_1$ receptors. Other side effects, which can also be attributed to their sympathomimetic actions, are nausea and vomiting.

Salmeterol (Serevent®) is the most recent beta$_2$ stimulant to be introduced for the treatment of asthma. Its properties and recommended clinical use separate it from the older beta$_2$ agonists. Compared to the older beta$_2$ stimulants, salmeterol has a slower onset of action (10–20 min) and is longer-acting (12 h) and offers more effective protection against histamine-induced bronchoconstriction. Salmeterol is recommended in patients with reversible obstructive airway disease who are using optimum anti-inflammatory treatment and experiencing breakthrough symptoms requiring a regular inhaled short-acting bronchodilator more than twice daily. In short, salmeterol appears to be preferred in patients who have first been prescribed fenoterol, salbutamol or terbutaline, plus an inhaled corticosteroid, and still require effective treatment. Salmeterol would appear to fill an important void between the use of beta$_2$ stimulants, plus inhaled corticosteroids, and systemic corticosteroid therapy. Chapter 69 details the use of these drugs in the treatment of asthma.

(For the clinically significant drug interactions with beta$_2$ bronchodilators, refer to Table 69.1 on page 821.)

Stimulation of Adrenergic Receptors: Summary of Effects

From the preceding discussion, it is clear that the effects of adrenergic drugs depend on the particular receptors stimulated. Drugs that stimulate alpha$_1$ receptors, for example, produce different effects and are used for different therapeutic purposes than compounds that are beta agonists.

Table 29.4 summarizes the therapeutic and adverse effects of drugs that stimulate alpha$_1$, beta$_1$ or beta$_2$ receptors.

Special Considerations for the Older Adult

Adrenergic drugs present special risks to the older adult for two main reasons. First, the older patient is "brittle," with changes in cardiovascular, renal and ocular function (among others) modifying the response to drugs. For example, visual changes in the aging eye result in slower response to alterations in light, with yellowing opacities of the lens requiring more light. In addition, the lens responds slower to changes from near to far vision. If these patients are treated with drugs that either dilate or constrict the pupil, the result could be blurred vision, resulting in falls, social isolation and sensory deprivation.

Older patients are also more likely to have

Table 29.4
Therapeutic and adverse effects of adrenergic drugs (with respect to receptors stimulated)

Receptor	Therapeutic effect	Adverse effect
Alpha$_1$	Adjunct to local anesthesia	• Bradycardia
	Hemostasis	• Hypertension
	Mydriasis (for surgery)	• Tissue necrosis
	Nasal decongestion	
	Vasoconstriction (elevate blood pressure, treat shock)	
Beta$_1$	Reverse cardiac arrest	• Arrhythmias
	Positive inotropic action: increase force of contraction (tx heart failure and shock)	• Angina (increase cardiac O_2 demand)
Beta$_2$	Bronchodilation (tx asthma, allergic reactions)	• Hyperglycemia

advanced atherosclerosis. In this case, drugs that normally constrict or dilate blood vessels are less likely to produce significant changes in the elderly.

Older patients may also have reduced density of adrenergic receptors. This can account for the decreased efficacy of beta$_2$ adrenergic bronchodilators.

In treating older patients, nurses should keep in mind that the elderly have a reduced capacity to respond to many drugs and also a decreased ability to adjust to those drug responses that are produced. In this situation, the adage of drug dosing for the elderly, "start low and go slow," is most important.

Nursing Management

Table 29.5 describes the nursing management of the patient receiving adrenergic drugs. Dosage details for individual drugs are given in Table 29.6 (pages 291–292).

Response to Clinical Challenge

1. Check expiry date of all drugs, colour of solution in auto injector. Ask Mona if she has used the auto injector and review steps of self-administration with her.
2. Mona may experience edema and redness at site, generalized edema, hypotension evidenced by dizziness, weakness or pallor, wheezing or dyspnea.
3. Epinephrine is a general adrenergic stimulant which will increase heart rate and force of contraction, dilate bronchioles and redistribute blood circulation. It will, therefore, reduce the edema, raise the blood pressure and alleviate the respiratory distress that Mona is experiencing due to her allergic reaction.
4. Mona should remove the safety cap from the auto injector, place the injector at a right angle against her thigh, press hard and hold in place until the injector functions, remove and massage area.
5. The onset of drug action should occur in 5–10 minutes and the above symptoms should reduce.
6. Remove the stinger if possible, apply tourniquet to leg for 10 min above site, apply ice pack, have Mona lie quietly, seek medical treatment.

Table 29.5
Nursing management of the adrenergics

Assessment of risk vs. benefit	Patient data	• *History:* Physician should determine any contraindications such as those described in text (see Adverse Effects). Particularly, assess for CV disease, diabetes, hyperthyroidism, glaucoma • Assess to establish baseline VS, general state of health • *Pregnancy and lactation:* Safety not established. Should be used only if benefits outweigh risks
	Drug data	• Response depends on specificity of action on adrenergic receptors, e.g.: *epinephrine, ephedrine* — $\alpha_1, \beta_1, \beta_2$; *norepinephrine* — α_1 (when infused as a drug); *isoproterenol* — β_1, β_2; *dopamine, dobutamine* — β_1 • Actions and side effects are dose related; increasing dose may cause increased response at other receptors • All drugs in this class are potent

(cont'd on next page)

Table 29.5 (continued)
Nursing management of the adrenergics

Implementation	Rights of administration	• Using the "rights" helps prevent errors of administration
	Right route	• Give PO, SC, IM, IV, by ophthalmic drops or inhaler. Check form carefully (e.g., suspension may be given SC but not IM or IV)
	Right dose	• All drugs are potent. Check doses very carefully; e.g., may be ordered as µg/kg and available supply may state mg/mL. Epinephrine is supplied as 1% (1:100), 0.1% (1:1000) and 0.01% (1:10 000) solutions
	Right time	• Many of these drugs are used in emergency situations and titrated to pt's response • For IV route, use infusion pump to control rate • Drug interactions can be serious (causing hypertension, hypotension, cardiac arrhythmias, hyperglycemia). Check complete drug regimen with physician or pharmacist
	Right technique	• For infusion, follow manufacturer's instructions for reconstitution and compatability. Always check solution — do not use if discolored or if there is a precipitate • IV should be given in central line or large vein; powerful vasoconstricting action may cause venous damage. If drug extravasates into surrounding tissue, can cause ischemia and necrosis. Observe site frequently; if extravasation occurs, affected area should be infiltrated with 10–15 mL saline solution containing 5–10 mg phentolamine (see Chapter 30) • For use of inhalers, see Chapter 69
	Nursing therapeutics	• Some side effects can be minimized; e.g., *hypotension* — pt to remain supine during and following administration; *local irritation* — for SC/IM, massage injection site well; for IV, use large vein and change site regularly; *emotional support* — drug is often used for serious or life-threatening illness such as shock and CHF. Pts/families require information and reassurance
	Patient/family teaching	• Educate for general drug tx (see Chapter 3) • For ophthalmic use, instruct pt re: hygiene and correct technique for administration • For auto injector, ensure that pt/family know technique of self-administration • For IV, instruct pt to inform nurse immediately of any pain at site • *Discuss possibility of pregnancy:* Advise pt to notify physician. Explain risks of lactation while on these drugs
Outcomes	Monitoring of progress	*Note:* Because of the serious nature of the indications for use of these drugs, constant monitoring and titration of the dose is required. • *Monitoring includes:* BP, HR, ECG rhythm, respirations, CNS status, peripheral perfusion, renal output and hemodynamic parameters (measurements of CO, preload, afterload). Blood gases and electrolytes may also be monitored frequently

Table 29.6
The adrenergics: Drug doses

Drug Generic name (Trade names)	Dosage	Nursing alert
dobutamine HCl (Dobutrex)	**IV:** *Adults:* Usually, 2.5–10 µg/kg/min. Rarely, up to 40 mg/kg/min	• Solution should be further diluted before administration to at least 50 mL (see manufacturer's literature for recommended diluents) and should be used within 24 h. Discard any solution that is discolored, cloudy or has precipitate. Drug is incompatible with alkaline solutions and should not be mixed with sodium bicarbonate injection • Use infusion pump. Rate is titrated according to pt response • IV site should be large vein or central line. Observe site frequently for extravasation • Monitor urine output and ECG closely during infusion
dopamine HCl (Dopastat, Intropin, Revimine)	**IV:** *Adults:* 0.5–5 µg/kg/min initially; increase at 10- to 30-min intervals up to 50 µg/kg/min	• Discard unused solution within 24 h. Discard if solution is discolored, cloudy or has precipitate • Use infusion pump. Rate is titrated according to pt response (see Table 29.5) • IV site should be large vein or central line. Observe site frequently for extravasation • Monitor urine output and ECG closely during infusion
epinephrine, adrenaline (Adrenalin)	Anaphylactic shock: **SC/IM:** *Adults:* 0.5 mg. May repeat in 5 min; may be followed by IV administration. **IV:** *Adults:* 0.1–0.25 mg (max., 0.5 mg). May repeat q5–15min or follow with infusion at 1 µg/min; may increase to a max. of 4 µg/min. *Children:* **IM/IV/SC:** 10 µg/kg (up to 0.3 mg); may repeat q5–15min Asthma: **SC:** *Adults:* 0.2–0.5 mg q20 min – 4 h (max., 1 mg/dose)	• Read label carefully; drug is supplied as 1:100, 1:1000 and 1:10 000 solutions. (*Example:* A 1:100 solution contains 1 g/ 100 mL, or 1000 mg/100 mL, or 10 mg/mL) • Use tuberculin syringe for accuracy • Shake well prior to use. Do not use if discolored or contains a precipitate • Massage injection site well; causes irritation and local vasoconstriction • Suspension for SC only; do not use IV or IM
isoproterenol (Isuprel)	**IV:** *Adults:* 2 mg (10 mL) diluted in 500 mL D5W is infused at a rate of 0.25–1 mL/min (1–4 µg/min) with continuous monitoring of ECG. Rate of infusion is determined by chronotropic response. *Children:* 0.1–0.25 µg/kg/min	• Supplied as 1:5000 solution (1 mL = 200 µg). Calculate doses carefully • Prepare IV solution according to manufacturer's instructions or agency protocol • Use infusion pump for accuracy. Rate is continuously adjusted according to pt's response. Continuous cardiac and BP monitoring required

Table 29.6 (continued)
The adrenergics: Drug doses

Drug Generic Name (Trade Names)	Dosage	Nursing Alert
norepinephrine, noradrenaline, levarterenol bitartrate (Levophed)	**IV:** *Adults,* 8–12 µg/min initially, then 2–4 µg/min maintenance infusion rate, titrated by BP response	•Use infusion pump to control rate; continuous cardiac and BP monitoring required •Monitor IV site frequently to prevent extravasation. (If occurs, site should be injected with phentolamine.) Do not stop infusion suddenly; discontinue gradually with continuous monitoring

Further Reading

Hoffman BB, Lefkowitz RJ. Catecholamines, sympathomimetic drugs and adrenergic receptor antagonists. In: Hardman JG, Limbird LE, eds. *Goodman and Gilman's The Pharmacological Basis of Therapeutics.* 9th ed. New York: Pergamon; 1996: 199–248.

Lee TJF, Stitzel RE. Adrenomimetic drugs. In: Craig CR, Stitzel RS, eds. *Modern Pharmacology.* 4th ed. Boston: Little, Brown; 1994:115–128.

Antiadrenergic Drugs

Topics Discussed
- Alpha$_1$ receptor blockers
- Beta blockers
- Labetalol: Alpha and beta blocker
- Mechanism of action, pharmacologic effects, therapeutic uses and adverse effects for each drug discussed
- Adrenergic neuron blockers
- Special considerations for the older adult
- Nursing management

Drugs Discussed
acebutolol (ass-seh-**byoo**-toe-lole)
atenolol (at-**ten**-oh-lole)
clonidine (**klon**-ih-deen)
doxazosin (dok-**say**-zoe-sin)
guanethidine (gwahn-**eth**-ih-deen)
labetalol (lah-**bet**-ah-lole)
methyldopa (meth-il-**doe**-pah)
metoprolol (meh-**troe**-proe-lole)
nadolol (**nay**-doe-lole)
oxprenolol (ox-**pren**-oh-lole)
pindolol (**pin**-doe-lole)
prazosin (**pra**-zoe-sin)
propranolol (proe-**pran**-oh-lole)
reserpine (reh-**ser**-peen)
sotalol (**soe**-tah-lole)
terazosin (ter-**az**-oh-sin)
timolol (**tim**-oh-lole)

Clinical Challenge

Consider this clinical challenge as you read through this chapter. The response to the challenge appears on page 310.

Alan is a young actor with diabetes controlled by insulin and a history of allergies. As a young child, he had asthma but has not had any recent episodes.

During a clinic visit, he discusses the stage fright he experiences prior to a performance and mentions that another actor recommended he try propranolol. Alan asks your advice.

1. Why would propranolol be suggested?
2. What consequences might occur if Alan were to take this drug?
3. What would you tell Alan?

Antiadrenergic drugs are used to block, in whole or in part, the sympathetic nervous system. The effects they produce are due to the degree to which they decrease adrenergic functions. They are used in the treatment of hypertension, cardiac arrhythmias, angina pectoris and migraine headaches, to mention but four disorders.

This chapter describes the pharmacology and nursing actions related to the use of antiadrenergic drugs. Their clinical value in the treatment of specific conditions is discussed in greater detail in other chapters of this book.

Antiadrenergic drugs are classified either as *adrenergic receptor blockers,* which block either alpha$_1$ or beta receptors, or *adrenergic neuron blockers,* which inhibit the release of norepinephrine from peripheral sympathetic nerves or sympathetic neurons within the central nervous system (Figure 30.1).

These two classifications differ significantly in their pharmacologic effects. Adrenergic neuron blockers reduce most sympathetically mediated functions. Alpha and beta blockers, on the other hand, prevent only those activities mediated by their respective receptors.

Alpha$_1$ Receptor Blockers

Doxazosin (Cardura®), Prazosin (Minipress®), Terazosin (Hytrin®)

Mechanism of action and pharmacologic effects. Alpha$_1$ receptor blockers prevent norepinephrine from stimulating alpha$_1$ receptors. Their effects depend on the degree of sympathetic tone existing prior to the administration of the blocker.

For example, an alpha$_1$ receptor blocker has minimal effect on the blood pressure of a recumbent subject because, in a reclining position, sympathetic nerves release little norepinephrine. However, the situation is very different when someone is standing. In this position, the person depends on an increased release of norepinephrine in the veins to constrict these vessels and maintain venous return. If the veins cannot constrict (e.g., after administration of an alpha$_1$ blocker), blood return to the heart is compromised and cardiac output falls. This, in turn, dramatically lowers blood pressure. (Recall that blood pressure is determined by cardiac output together with peripheral resistance.)

An abrupt fall in blood pressure seen when a patient stands is called *orthostatic hypotension* or *postural hypotension.* Alpha$_1$ blockers can produce severe orthostatic hypotension if care is not taken to titrate their dose gradually according to the needs of the individual patient.

Alpha$_1$ blockers also decrease peripheral resistance. Because this function is controlled by the diameter of the arterioles, and the calibre of these vessels is partially controlled by the release of norepinephrine, alpha$_1$ blockers, which block the effects of norepinephrine, dilate arterioles and thus decrease peripheral resistance. This action, together with the fall in cardiac output secondary to a reduction in venous return, accounts for the ability of alpha$_1$ blockers to decrease blood pressure.

One additional consequence of the decrease in

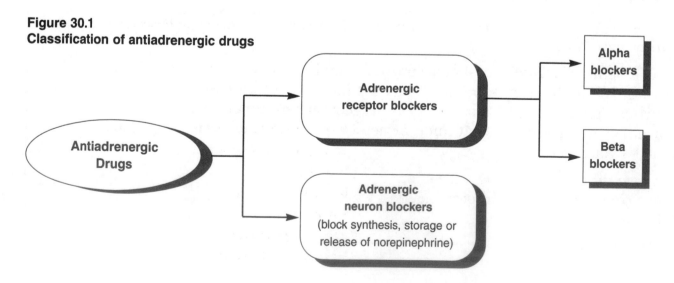

Figure 30.1
Classification of antiadrenergic drugs

Table 30.1
Alpha₁ receptor blockers: Drug interactions

Drug	Interaction
Alcohol	• Additive hypotension with acute ingestion of alcohol
Antihypertensive drugs	• Antihypertensive drugs add to the hypotensive effects of alpha₁ blockers
Diuretics	• Diuretics increase the antihypertensive effects of alpha₁ blockers

peripheral resistance by alpha₁ blockers is a reflex increase in heart rate. This results from the actions of the carotid sinus and aortic arch pressor receptors. When these receptors sense a fall in blood pressure, they reflexly increase heart rate by decreasing vagal stimulation to the heart in an attempt to restore blood pressure to its previous level. This is, of course, to no avail because there just is not enough blood returning to the heart to allow cardiac output to increase. The only effect of this playback mechanism is to produce an often disturbing increase in heart rate (tachycardia). The whole process in not unlike the actions of governments: despite the good intentions, the ultimate effect only increases inconvenience.

Table 30.1 lists the clinically significant drug interactions with alpha₁ receptor blockers.

Therapeutic uses. Doxazosin, prazosin and terazosin are useful in treating high blood pressure (see Chapter 36). They are often used in a general treatment program in conjunction with a diuretic and/or other antihypertensive drug as needed for proper patient response.

Adverse effects. The adverse effects of blocking alpha₁ receptors include postural hypotension and reflex tachycardia. Nasal stuffiness is another consequence of vasodilatation. Blocking alpha₁ receptors in the iris produces parasympathetic predominance and constriction of the pupil (miosis).

Beta Blockers

Nonselective Beta Receptor Blockers

Propranolol (Inderal®)

Mechanism of action and pharmacologic effects. The introduction of beta blockers in the 1960s represented a major therapeutic advance. Propranolol was the first beta blocker accepted in most countries of the world. It blocks the ability of epinephrine and norepinephrine to stimulate the beta₁ and beta₂ receptors (Table 30.2).

Propranolol produces major effects on the cardiovascular system. Similar to alpha₁ receptor blockers, the consequences of propranolol treatment are determined by the degree of sympathetic stimulation that existed prior to drug treatment.

Table 30.2
Distribution of beta receptors

Organ	Receptor type	Effects of stimulation
Heart	β_1	• Increase in heart rate
	β_1	• Increase in cardiac contractility
	β_1	• Acceleration of A-V conduction
Bronchi	β_2	• Dilatation
Arterioles	β_2	• Dilatation
Kidney	β_1	• Release of renin
Metabolism	β_2	• Increase in blood sugar
	β_1	• Increase in free fatty acids

For example, in the resting individual with low sympathetic drive, propranolol has little effect on the heart. However, in the stressed or exercising human, whose myocardial function depends heavily on sympathetic stimulation, propranolol reduces or prevents the usual increase in heart rate, A-V conduction, force of contraction and cardiac output.

Propranolol lowers blood pressure. Part of this action is due to a decrease in cardiac output. The drug also reduces sympathetic nervous system activity in the brain, and this may play a role in its antihypertensive effects. In addition, propranolol decreases renin release by the kidney, and this may also be a factor in the fall in blood pressure.

Beta$_2$ receptors mediate adrenergic bronchodilatation. Propranolol blocks this effect and should not be given to asthmatic patients. If propranolol is given to an asthmatic, bronchiolar constriction occurs, the forced expiratory volume in one second (FEV_1) falls, and the patient is placed in jeopardy.

Propranolol can have marked effects on intermediary metabolism. Sympathetic stimulation increases plasma free fatty acid levels. Propranolol blocks this effect. The drug also has major effects on carbohydrate metabolism, and should thus be used with caution in insulin-dependent diabetics. Following the injection of insulin, the blood sugar falls. This triggers the release of epinephrine, whose hyperglycemic effects offset, in part, the action of insulin. The resulting blood sugar is a balance between the hypoglycemic action of insulin and the hyperglycemic effects of the released epinephrine. If a diabetic patient is treated with propranolol, the effects of insulin are greater because the beta blocker decreases the effects of the released epinephrine.

Pharmacokinetics. Propranolol is usually administered orally. It is completely absorbed but subject to extensive first-pass metabolism. Only twenty to thirty percent of the oral dose survives hepatic metabolism to reach the systemic circulation. In addition, there is considerable person-to-person variability in the extent of first-pass metabolism. This is one factor that accounts for the wide range of doses required to treat patients. Patients who require larger doses may inactivate a higher percentage of the absorbed drug during first pass

through the liver. It is not uncommon to find patients managed adequately for angina pectoris on as little as 80 mg daily, whereas others may need 320 mg/day of the drug for the same condition.

Therapeutic uses. Propranolol is used to prevent angina pectoris attacks (see Chapter 34). By reducing sympathetic stimulation to the heart, the drug decreases the oxygen requirements of the myocardium, protecting the patient with chronic stable angina.

Propranolol is also used to treat essential hypertension (see Chapter 36). Its mechanism of action in reducing blood pressure has been described above.

Because propranolol reduces sympathetic stimulation of the atria and A-V node, it is a valuable drug in the treatment of adrenergically induced supraventricular arrhythmias (see Chapter 33). It is also of value in reducing mortality in patients who have suffered a myocardial infarct.

Propranolol is also used to prevent migraine headaches (see Chapter 56). Although its mechanism of action in this condition is still not clear, chronic propranolol use reduces the incidence of vascular headaches.

Obviously, propranolol is an ideal drug for the patient with a pheochromocytoma, a condition characterized by very high concentrations of epinephrine (and sometimes also norepinephrine) in the blood and urine. However, this condition is very rare, and most nurses may never encounter it.

Adverse effects. Bradycardia and congestive heart failure are the most obvious adverse effects of propranolol. Nature did not provide humans with sympathetic innervation of the heart just so that pharmacologists could block it with propranolol (or any other beta blocker, for that matter). A complete block of sympathetic impulses to the heart runs the risk of reducing heart rate and cardiac output to the point where heart failure ensues.

A block of beta$_2$ receptors in the bronchioles can produce bronchoconstriction in an asthmatic patient.

The other adverse effects of propranolol are not so easily explained. They include nausea, vomiting, constipation or diarrhea. Central nervous system effects include depression, disturbed sleep and nightmares. These effects, more often than any of the others, are the reasons given by patients for stopping (or wanting to stop taking) propranolol. Allergic reactions to propranolol include rash, fever and purpura.

Nadolol (Corgard®), Sotalol (Sotacor®) and Timolol (Blocadren®)

Nadolol, sotalol and timolol are three additional nonselective beta blockers. Nadolol is more water-soluble than propranolol and is less likely to enter the brain to produce CNS effects (see Chapter 36). Nadolol has a half-life of approximately twenty-four hours, considerably longer than the half-lives of four to six hours for propranolol and timolol. As a result, nadolol can be administered once daily. Nadolol is approved for the prophylaxis of angina pectoris and the treatment of hypertension.

Sotalol has a half-life of seventeen hours after oral administration. It is considered primarily to be an antiarrhythmic drug that prolongs repolarization (Class III) and also has beta-adrenergic blocking activity (Class II; see Chapter 33). Sotalol has been approved for oral treatment of life-threatening ventricular arrhythmias. Although it can also be used to treat hypertension or prevent attacks of angina pectoris, it proarrhythmic effects limit sotalol's use in these conditions to patients who require the drug for the treatment of ventricular arrhythmias.

Timolol is similar to propranolol. It has a half-life of three to four hours. It is used to prevent attacks of angina pectoris and to treat hypertension, and has been shown to reduce the likelihood of death if administered to patients after a myocardial infarct.

Cardioselective Beta Blockers

Acebutolol (Monitan®, Sectral®), Atenolol (Tenormin®), Metoprolol (Betaloc®, Lopresor®, Lopressor®) and Esmolol (Brevibloc®)

Acebutolol, atenolol, esmolol and metoprolol are called cardioselective, suggesting that the only receptors blocked are those in the heart. This is not true. Although they do block more easily the receptors in the heart, these drugs can diminish beta$_2$ receptor effects in the bronchioles and blood vessels if sufficiently high doses are used. Table 30.3 on the next page lists the differences between nonselective and cardioselective beta blockers.

Acebutolol differs pharmacodynamically from atenolol, esmolol and metoprolol. The latter three are competitive inhibitors of beta$_1$ receptors. Acebutolol, on the other hand, is a partial agonist, affecting beta$_1$ receptors. The mechanism of action of partial-agonist beta blockers is explained below.

Attention has been focussed on the reduced ability of the cardioselective drugs to block beta receptors in bronchioles. None of these drugs should be used in the asthmatic patient. These patients depend greatly on sympathetic activity to maintain their airways, and any degree of bronchoconstriction places them at risk.

There are a few situations in which the cardioselective beta blockers are preferred over propranolol. They are better drugs in the diabetic patient receiving insulin because they do not reduce the epinephrine-induced effects on blood glucose as much as propranolol.

Acebutolol, atenolol and metoprolol may also be better than the nonselective beta blockers in their effects on peripheral circulation. During periods of stress, propranolol, timolol and nadolol may increase peripheral resistance. This occurs because of the release of epinephrine which, in the face of a beta$_2$ block, produces a generalized alpha$_1$ vascular stimulation. For example, a patient, after waiting anxiously in the doctor's office, may show an abnormally elevated diastolic pressure because of the effects of released epinephrine on the alpha$_1$ receptors ("white-coat hypertension"). Theoretically at least, this effect should not be seen in patients who receive a cardioselective beta blocker because the epinephrine released is free to stimulate both alpha$_1$ and beta$_2$ receptors, with the effects of one offsetting those of the other.

Atenolol and acebutolol are water-soluble beta blockers. They are eliminated by renal excretion and have longer half-lives than other beta blockers, with the exception of nadolol. As a result, atenolol can be administered once a day, and acebutolol twice daily. Their water solubility also reduces entry into the brain, and this may be accompanied by fewer CNS adverse effects.

Acebutolol, atenolol and metoprolol have the

Table 30.3
Effects resulting from administration of different beta blockers

	Nonselective	Cardioselective	Partial agonist
Heart rate and force of contraction (β_1)	Decrease (both rate and force of contraction)	Decrease (both rate and force of contraction)	Decrease (both rate and force of contraction). Fall in resting heart rate is less with this group of β-blockers because of their partial-agonist activity
Peripheral resistance (β_2)	Increases, owing to the fact that α_1 receptors can act unopposed because β_2 receptors are blocked	Little effect because β_2 receptors are not blocked by cardioselective β-blockers	Possible slight decrease because of the β_2-agonist properties
Renin release (β_1)	Decreases	Decreases	Decreases
Bronchioles (β_2)	Bronchoconstriction in asthmatics	Less bronchoconstriction in asthmatics but cardioselective β-blockers are not recommended for these pts	Asthmatics have reduced capacity to dilate bronchioles if a partial-agonist β-blocker is used
Glucose metabolism (β_2)	Reduced hyperglycemic response to epinephrine. Use caution in diabetics because insulin can produce increased hypoglycemia if it is given to a pt on a nonselective β-blocker	Little effect	Reduced response to epinephrine because partial-agonist β-blockers are not as potent β_2 stimulants as endogenously released epinephrine

same basic clinical indications and adverse effects as propranolol. Esmolol has a unique therapeutic use. With a very short elimination half-life of nine minutes, esmolol is used to control the ventricular response in atrial flutter or fibrillation, particularly after cardiac surgery. Both its therapeutic and adverse effects usually disappear within thirty minutes.

Beta Blockers with Intrinsic Sympathetic Activity (ISA): Partial-Agonist Beta Blockers

Acebutolol (Monitan®, Sectral®), Oxprenolol (Trasicor®) and Pindolol (Visken®)

Acebutolol, oxprenolol and pindolol are not true beta blockers. In contrast to the drugs previously mentioned in this section, which attach to beta receptors and block them, acebutolol, oxprenolol and pindolol have affinity for the receptors and, once attached, stimulate them. However, because they have much less intrinsic sympathetic activity

(ISA) than either epinephrine or norepinephrine, the degree of beta stimulation is less when acebutolol, oxprenolol or pindolol occupies the receptor in place of the normal mediators epinephrine and norepinephrine. These drugs are sometimes called *partial agonists,* a term that reflects their limited ability to stimulate adrenergic receptors.

Acebutolol differs from oxprenolol and pindolol because it is a cardioselective partial agonist, affecting only beta$_1$ receptors. It is for this reason that it was also presented above under the topic of cardioselective beta blockers. Oxprenolol and pindolol act on both beta$_1$ and beta$_2$ receptors.

Partial agonists do not reduce the resting heart rate as much as other beta blockers because their intrinsic sympathetic activity ensures some degree of sympathetic stimulation. During times of stress, however, when an increase in heart rate and cardiac output are required to meet the needs of the body, patients given a partial agonist still have diminished myocardial function when compared with untreated subjects.

It is also claimed that beta blockers with ISA can stimulate beta$_2$ receptors to produce bronchodilatation and vasodilatation in the resting patient. The clinical significance of this fact is not obvious. Partial agonists may also dilate peripheral blood vessels, and this can reduce coldness and intermittent claudication. Most beta blockers can increase serum cholesterol. The clinical significance of this is not clear. However, beta blockers with ISA or partial-agonist activity may be preferred in patients with high serum cholesterol because they usually do not increase blood lipids.

Acebutolol and pindolol are effective in the treatment of angina pectoris and hypertension. Oxprenolol is approved only for the treatment of hypertension.

The pharmacologic properties, adverse effects of acebutalol, oxprenolol and pindolol are similar to those for the other beta blockers.

Table 30.4 lists the clinically significant drug interactions with beta receptor blockers.

Table 30.4
Beta blockers: Drug interactions

Drug	Interaction
Alcohol	• Additive hypotension may occur with acute ingestion of alcohol
Antiarrhythmic drugs (disopyramide, lidocaine, tocainide, perhaps other Class I antiarrhythmics)	• These drugs, plus a beta blocker, can result in exaggeration of unwanted effects of antiarrhythmic agents (e.g., enhanced myocardial depression, hypotension, bradycardia, A-V blockade, asystole)
Antiasthmatics	• The bronchodilator actions of selective beta$_2$ stimulants (e.g., fenoterol, procaterol, salbutamol, terbutaline) are blocked by nonselective beta blockers, including those with partial-agonist activity. Cardioselective beta blockers are less likely to affect the actions of beta$_2$ stimulants
Antidiabetic agents	• Nonselective beta blockers reduce glycogen breakdown and delay the rise in blood glucose after insulin- or oral hypoglycemic-induced hypoglycemia. Furthermore, nonselective beta blockers modify the normal physiologic reactions to hypoglycemia. In the presence of a nonselective beta blocker, the hypoglycemic reaction is accompanied by bradycardia rather than tachycardia, and a rise in diastolic BP
Atropine	• Atropine and other anticholinergics may prevent bradycardia produced by beta blockers
Clonidine	• Clonidine plus a nonselective beta blocker can lead to potentiation of the hypertensive response during clonidine withdrawal
Digoxin	• Digoxin may demonstrate reduced inotropic effects in the presence of a beta blocker. Beta blockers and digoxin are additive in depressing A-V conduction. Use beta blockers with caution in pts receiving digoxin who develop bradycardia
Doxazosin, prazosin, terazosin	• An alpha$_1$ receptor blocker, together with a beta blocker, can produce increased postural (orthostatic) hypotension after the first dose of the alpha$_1$ blocker
Epinephrine	• Epinephrine can increase blood pressure in pts taking nonselective beta blockers
Nifedipine	• Nifedipine plus a beta blocker can occasionally provoke severe hypotension and overt heart failure in a susceptible pt with poor myocardial reserve
Sympathomimetics	• Large doses of sympathomimetics plus a nonselective beta blocker can result in hypertension
Verapamil	• Verapamil plus a beta blocker can result in enhanced myocardial depression, hypotension, bradycardia, A-V blockade and asystole

Labetalol (Trandate®): Alpha and Beta Blocker

Mechanism of Action and Pharmacologic Effects

Labetalol blocks both alpha and beta receptors. Although it is more potent as a beta blocker, its antihypertensive effects are due primarily to alpha$_1$ receptor antagonism, resulting in decreased peripheral resistance. The reflex tachycardia normally seen with arteriolar dilatation is prevented by the partial beta blockade. Heart rate usually does not slow when labetalol is administered. Presumably the increase in sympathetic stimulation, secondary to vasodilatation, compensates partially for the beta blockade.

Therapeutic Uses

Labetalol is used in the treatment of essential hypertension (see also Chapter 36). Although some authorities may recommend the drug for initial therapy, most physicians prefer to add it to existing therapeutic regimens if the need arises.

Adverse Effects

The most serious reported adverse effects of labetalol are severe postural hypotension, jaundice and bronchospasm. Nausea and vomiting may also be experienced with the drug.

Table 30.5 lists the clinically significant drug interactions with labetalol.

Adrenergic Neuron Blockers

Peripherally Acting Drugs

These drugs derive their name from their ability to inhibit the formation, storage or release of norepinephrine from postganglionic sympathetic nerve endings. They do not block adrenergic receptors. The consequences of administering an adrenergic neuron blocker are more devastating than either alpha$_1$ or beta blockers because it abolishes all sympathetic function, not merely those activities mediated by one receptor or another.

Adrenergic neuron blockers lower blood pressure by reducing peripheral resistance and decreasing cardiac output. Peripheral resistance decreases because the drugs inhibit sympathetic function in the arterioles. Cardiac output falls as a result of dilatation of the veins and reduction in venous return. The consequences of venodilatation are not limited solely to a decrease in cardiac output. The inability of the veins to constrict when an individual stands allows blood to pool in the lower extremities of the body, producing postural or orthostatic hypotension.

The decrease in cardiac output and blood pressure reduces renal blood flow. This causes a retention of body fluids as less blood is filtered and a higher percentage of the glomerular filtrate is reabsorbed. The resulting increase in blood and extracellular fluid volume diminishes the hypotensive effects of the drugs.

The sympathetic nervous system is antagonistic to the actions of the parasympathetic nervous system in the gastrointestinal tract. Under normal

Table 30.5
Labetalol: Drug interactions

Drug	Interaction
Antidiabetic drugs	• Antidiabetic drugs may have increased hypoglycemic effect when labetalol is used concomitantly
Antihypertensive drugs and diuretics	• Antihypertensives and diuretics increase the hypotensive effects of labetalol
Cimetidine	• Cimetidine increases the bioavailability of labetalol. Use special care in establishing dose in these pts
Halothane	• Halothane increases the hypotensive effects of labetalol. High doses of halothane (3%) with labetalol predispose pts to the myocardial depressant effects of halothane and an undesirable reduction in myocardial performance
Nitroglycerin	• Nitroglycerin adds to the hypotensive effects of labetalol

conditions the stimulant effects of the latter are offset, in part, by the inhibitory actions of the former. A reduction in sympathetic outpourings, as produced by adrenergic neuron blockers, leads to parasympathetic dominance. This causes increased gastrointestinal motility and diarrhea.

The patient treated with one of these drugs may be a sad sight. If forced to stand up quickly (e.g., in response to a peristaltic urge), he or she may suffer an acute attack of postural hypotension and faint. In male patients, adrenergic neuron blockers inhibit erection and ejaculation. This situation can be stressful for both the patient and his sexual partner. It may be most difficult to convince either of them that the patient is in better shape than he has been in years because his diastolic pressure has been reduced!

In view of this catastrophic picture, it seems a little mundane to mention that patients receiving adrenergic neuron blockers often complain of a stuffy nose. This effect is due to vasodilatation of the blood vessels perfusing the mucous membranes of the nasopharynx.

Reserpine (Serpasil®)

Mechanism of action and pharmacologic effects. Reserpine was originally obtained from the plant *Rauwolfia serpentina* (hence the trade name Serpasil®). It is now chemically synthesized. Reserpine depletes sympathetic nerve endings of their supply of norepinephrine and as a result depresses sympathetic functions both within the brain and in peripheral tissues. It produces seda-

tion and depression as well as reduction in cardiac output and increased postural hypotension. Reserpine also depletes dopamine stores in the brain and produces extrapyramidal, or parkinsonian, effects.

Therapeutic uses. Reserpine was the first adrenergic neuron blocker introduced into patient care. Initially, it was marketed as a tranquilizer and then later as an antihypertensive. It has been largely replaced for both indications by newer drugs. The majority of patients receiving reserpine are older and have been taking the drug for many years for treatment of hypertension. There appears to be no justification for starting patients on reserpine today.

Adverse effects. The adverse effects of reserpine are directly attributable to the depletion of norepinephrine and inhibition of sympathetic nervous system activity. The drug can produce a marked depression in the patient's mood. It often causes bradycardia and postural hypotension. Nasal congestion is common. The inhibition of sympathetic activity in the gastrointestinal tract allows the parasympathetic nervous system to act unopposed. As a result, reserpine treatment produces increased gastric secretion, nausea, vomiting, anorexia, aggravation of peptic ulcer or ulcerative colitis, increased intestinal motility and diarrhea. Impotence or decreased libido are also consequences of use.

Table 30.6 lists the clinically significant drug interactions with reserpine.

Table 30.6
Reserpine: Drug interactions

Drug	Interaction
Barbiturates	•Reserpine can cause hypotension during thiopental anesthesia. Discontinue reserpine 2 weeks before giving anesthesia
Diazoxide	•Reserpine and diazoxide can cause severe additive hypotension. Avoid concurrent use
Enflurane, halothane, isoflurane, nitrous oxide	•Reserpine, together with these anesthetics, can cause additive hypotension. Monitor BP
Monoamine oxidase inhibitors	•Reserpine plus a MAOI can precipitate mania due to the release of accumulated 5-hydroxytryptamine (5-HT). Avoid concurrent use

Guanethidine (Ismelin®)

Mechanism of action and therapeutic use. Guanethidine has been used for more than thirty years for the treatment of hypertension. It reduces the levels of norepinephrine in sympathetic nerve endings. As a result, guanethidine reduces venous return and decreases both heart rate and cardiac output. Consistent with these effects, guanethidine reduces kidney perfusion, with the result that salt and water are retained.

Adverse effects. The major adverse effects of guanethidine are those described for adrenergic blockers in general. Guanethidine does not cross the blood-brain barrier; thus, the CNS effects reported for reserpine are not encountered with guanethidine. Patients treated with guanethidine should not be given a tricyclic or tetracyclic antidepressant because these drugs prevent the effect of guanethidine on sympathetic nerve endings.

Table 30.7 lists the clinically significant drug interactions with guanethidine.

Centrally Acting Drugs

Central sympathetic inhibitors act within the brain to impair sympathetic centres. They are used primarily to lower blood pressure. The use of clonidine and methyldopa in the treatment of hypertension is described in more detail in Chapter 36.

Clonidine (Catapres®)

Clonidine is a potent antihypertensive drug. It is claimed to lower blood pressure by stimulating the alpha$_2$ receptors in the brain. Stated simply, this means that by stimulating these receptors on the sympathetic nerves in the brain, clonidine prevents the neurons from releasing norepinephrine. This inhibits sympathetic centres in the brain, with the result that peripheral sympathetic nerves, which depend on stimulation from the central sympathetic centres, are also blocked.

Clonidine can produce postural hypotension, but its effects are not pronounced. It often produces dry mouth and sedation. These effects can be severe. Impotence occurs occasionally. Treatment with clonidine leads to the retention of sodium, chloride and water. Similar to guanethidine, patients receiving clonidine should not be given tricyclic or tetracyclic antidepressants, as these can diminish or abolish the actions of the drug.

Table 30.8 lists the clinically significant drug interactions with clonidine.

Methyldopa (Aldomet®)

Methyldopa inhibits sympathetic centres in the brain, thereby reducing peripheral sympathetic nervous system function. Methyldopa decreases peripheral resistance and this accounts, at least in part, for the fall in blood pressure. Its effects on

---

Table 30.7
Guanethidine: Drug interactions

Drug	Interaction
Alcohol	• Acute ingestion of alcohol may lead to additive hypotension
Antidepressants, tricyclic	• TCAs decrease the antihypertensive effect of guanethidine. Use alternative antihypertensive
Contraceptives, oral	• Oral contraceptives decrease the effects of guanethidine. Avoid concurrent use
Enflurane, halothane, isoflurane, nitrous oxide	• Guanethidine, together with these anesthetics, can cause additive hypotension. Monitor BP
Minoxidil	• Minoxidil and guanethidine can produce severe hypotension. Avoid concurrent use
Phenothiazines	• Phenothiazines decrease the antihypertensive effect of guanethidine. Avoid concurrent use, if possible
Sympathomimetic amines	• Sympathomimetic amines decrease the antihypertensive effect of guanethidine. Avoid concurrent use

Table 30.8
Clonidine: Drug interactions

Drug	Interaction
Alcohol	• Additive sedation can occur with the use of alcohol
Antidepressants, tricyclic	• TCAs decrease the antihypertensive effect of clonidine. Beta blockers, diuretics or, in some pts, methyldopa can be used as alternatives
Beta blockers, nonselective	• Nonselective beta blockers may exaggerate the vasoconstrictor response when clonidine is withdrawn. Withdraw beta blocker before stopping clonidine
Levodopa	• Clonidine can decrease the effect of levodopa. Use an alternative antihypertensive drug
Naloxone	• Naloxone can decrease the effect of clonidine. Monitor BP and clinical status
Tolazoline	• Tolazoline can decrease the antihypertensive effect of clonidine. Avoid concurrent use

cardiac output are still disputed. Some studies report a fall in cardiac output that correlates with the decrease in blood pressure, while other investigations report no effect on cardiac output.

The adverse effects of methyldopa include sedation, postural hypotension, edema and impotence. These can be attributed to sympathetic blockade. Other adverse reactions are not so easily explained. They include drug fever, hepatic dysfunction, hemolytic anemia and lactation (in either sex). These occur only rarely. A problem for the clinical chemist is the fact that up to twenty-five percent of patients taking 1000 mg of methyldopa daily for six months or more develop a positive direct Coombs' test. This has no clinical significance, but it makes cross-matching blood difficult.

Table 30.9 lists the clinically significant drug interactions with methyldopa.

Table 30.9
Methyldopa: Drug interactions

Drug	Interaction
Alcohol	• Acute ingestion of alcohol can lead to additive hypotension
Beta blockers	• Methyldopa and beta blockers can produce a hypertensive reaction if patient releases catecholamine due to unopposed alpha-adrenergic stimulation. Avoid concurrent use
Contraceptives, oral	• Oral contraceptives can decrease the antihypertensive effect of methyldopa. Avoid concurrent use
Diazoxide	• Diazoxide and methyldopa can produce severe additive hypotension. Avoid concurrent use within 6 h
Digoxin	• Digoxin and methyldopa can produce sinus bradycardia. Monitor heart rate
Haloperidol	• Haloperidol plus methyldopa can produce dementia. Monitor, and discontinue both drugs if dementia occurs
Hypoglycemics, sulfonylureas	• Methyldopa can increase tolbutamide's hypoglycemia. Monitor blood glucose
Iron, oral	• Oral iron may decrease the hypotensive effect of methyldopa by reducing its absorption. Monitor BP
Lithium	• Methyldopa can increase lithium toxicity. Monitor lithium concentration and clinical status. Lithium concentrations may remain near upper normal limit
Monoamine oxidase inhibitors	• MAOIs may produce hallucinations in pts receiving methyldopa. Avoid concurrent use

Special Considerations for the Older Adult

The aging process causes a reduced compensatory response to changes in body position. The alpha adrenergic blockers produce a "first-dose" effect of marked orthostatic hypotension with dizziness or syncope. The combination of aging plus drug action may have serious consequences, such as falls, fractures, hospitalization and surgery. With aging, changes in renal and hepatic function may occur. The older individual will metabolize many drugs more slowly, increasing the risk for accumulation and toxicity.

Beta blockers should also be used cautiously in older patients, meaning lower doses and smaller increases. Many people over seventy have type II diabetes, which is often controlled by diet and exercise or may require the use of oral hypoglycemic agents (discussed in Chapter 65). Beta blockers may interfere with this control or may mask the symptoms of hypoglycemia, leading to dizziness and falls.

A final note of caution relates to the diagnosis of hypertension in the aging population. The blood pressure should be carefully and accurately measured on two occasions before the diagnosis is made, and monitoring should continue after drug treatment is initiated. (Chapter 36 discusses the treatment of hypertension in greater detail.)

Nursing Management

Table 30.10 summarizes the nursing management of patients receiving antiadrenergic drugs. Drug doses of individual drugs are given in Table 30.11 (pages 306–310).

Table 30.10
Nursing management of the antiadrenergics

Assessment of risk vs. benefit	Patient data	• *History:* Physician should determine any contraindications such as those described in text (see Adverse Effects). Particularly, assess for CV disease, diabetes, asthma, COPD or myasthenia gravis • Assess to establish baseline VS, general state of health. Baseline BP in both arms should be taken lying, sitting and standing. Liver or kidney disease may affect rate of drug metabolism • *Pregnancy and lactation:* Safety not established. Should be used only if benefits outweigh risks • *Age:* Older adults usually more sensitive to drug action and slower to metabolize; doses should be lower
	Drug data	• Response depends on specificity of action on adrenergic receptors, e.g.: *propranolol* is a nonselective β-blocker; *doxazosin, prazosin, terazosin* block α_1 receptors; *atenolol, metoprolol, esmolol* block β_1 receptors; *acebutolol, oxprenolol, pindolol* are partial agonists as well as β-blockers; *labetalol* blocks both α and β receptors; *reserpine, guanethidine, methyldopa* block adrenergic neurons • Actions and side effects are dose related; increasing dose may cause increased response at other receptors • Some drugs undergo significant first-pass metabolism (see pharmacokinetics of propranolol), which accounts for much larger oral than parenteral doses. The absorption of some drugs in this class is enhanced with food; others may be given without regard to meals • Drug class has many clinically significant drug interactions; verify total drug regimen with pharmacist or physician

Table 30.10 (continued)
Nursing management of the antiadrenergics

Implementation	Rights of administration	• Using the "rights" helps prevent errors of administration
	Right route	• Give PO, SC, IM, IV, via dermal patch. Check available form carefully; e.g., regular tablet may be crushed, but long-acting form should not be crushed or chewed
	Right dose	• Drug doses in this class vary significantly • Oral and parenteral doses may differ considerably
	Right time	• Many of these drugs are used to control hypertension or angina; regular administration to maintain effective blood levels is essential. Missed doses should be given as soon as remembered • Do not discontinue beta blockers suddenly; may cause angina and precipitate myocardial infarction
	Right technique	• **Oral:** Tablets should be stored in airtight, light-resistant container • **IV:** follow manufacturer's instructions for reconstitution and compatibility. Check agency policy regarding direct IV administration. Continuous cardiac monitoring is required for this route
	Nursing therapeutics	• Some side effects can be minimized; e.g., *hypotension* — pt to remain supine during and following IV administration; *dizziness* — pt should change positions slowly, avoid dangerous activities until response to drug is known; *dry mouth* — good oral hygiene, sugarless gum/candy
	Patient/family teaching	• Educate for drug tx (see Chapter 3) • Emphasize first-dose effect of α-blockers and orthostatic hypotension with all drugs in this class. Because of long-term use of these drugs for control of hypertension and angina, education should be an important part of the nursing plan (see Chapter 36) • *Discuss possibility of pregnancy:* Advise pt to notify physician. Explain risks of lactation while on these drugs
Outcomes	Monitoring of progress	*Continually monitor:* • Pulse; consult physician for dosage change if P < 50 • BP (lying/sitting and standing) • Blood glucose levels, if pt is diabetic • Observe for adverse reactions, esp. in CV, respiratory functions • Some drugs cross blood-brain barrier; observe for insomnia, nightmares, depression

Table 30. 11
The antiadrenergics: Drug doses

Drug Generic name (Trade names)	Dosage	Nursing alert
A. Alpha₁ Receptor Blockers		
doxazosin mesylate (Cardura)	**Oral:** *Adults:* 1 mg, given od. To minimize postural hypotension, do not exceed this dose. Max. reduction in BP normally occurs 2–6 h after dose. Dose may be slowly increased prn. Usual dose range, 1–8 mg od. Max. recommended dose, 16 mg od	•Give hs to minimize adverse effects. Warn pt of postural hypotension; teach to rise slowly
prazosin HCl (Minipress)	**Oral:** *Adults:* Give starting dose of 0.5 mg with food, preferably with evening meal, at least 2–3 h before retiring. Increase dose gradually, with 0.5 mg being given bid or tid for at least 3 days. Unless adverse effects occur, increase dose to 1 mg bid or tid, prn, for at least a further 3 days. Increase subsequent doses gradually prn. Max., 20 mg/day	•Warn pt of first-dose orthostatic hypotension, which may occur 30 min to 2 h after dose. Monitor BP. Do not give initial dose > 0.5 mg to older adult. Check fluid and electrolyte status; hypotension is more severe in volume-depleted or sodium-restricted pt
terazosin HCl (Hytrin)	**Oral:** *Adults:* Initially, 1 mg hs for all pts. Usual dose range, 1–5 mg od. Max. dose, 20 mg/day	•Give hs to minimize adverse effects. Warn pt of postural hypotension; teach to rise slowly
B. Nonselective Beta Blockers		
nadolol (Corgard)	Angina pectoris: **Oral:** *Adults:* Initially, 80 mg/day. Increase prn by 80-mg increments weekly to obtain satisfactory response. Max. recommended daily dose, 240 mg Hypertension: **Oral:** *Adults:* Initially, 80 mg/day. Increase prn by 80-mg increments weekly to obtain satisfactory response. Max. recommended daily dose, 320 mg	•May be given with food or on empty stomach •Monitor pulse; notify physician if P < 50
propranolol HCl (Inderal)	Angina pectoris: **Oral:** *Adults:* Initially, 20–40 mg bid ac. If satisfactory response is not obtained after 1 week, increase to 80 mg bid. Average optimum dose appears to be 160 mg/day Arrhythmias: **Oral:** *Adults:* 10–30 mg tid or qid, ac and hs. **IV:** Reserved for life-threatening arrhythmias or those occurring under anesthesia. Usual dose is 1–3 mg, administered under careful monitoring (ECG, CVP). Rate of administration should not exceed 1 mg/min Hypertension: **Oral:** *Adults:* Initially, 40 mg bid; increase prn in 1 week to 80–160 mg bid. For most pts, dosage is within the range of 160–320 mg/day	•Oral and IV doses not interchangeable •Give with food. Regular tablets may be crushed and mixed with food if pt has difficulty swallowing. Do not crush or chew long-acting form

Table 30. 11 (continued)
The antiadrenergics: Drug doses

Drug Generic name (Trade names)	Dosage	Nursing alert
B. Nonselective Beta Blockers (cont'd)		
sotalol HCl (Betapace, Sotacor)	Ventricular arrhythmias: **Oral:** *Adults:* Adjust dosage gradually, allowing 2–3 days between dosing increments. Initially, 80 mg bid. Increase prn to 240–320 mg/day. In most pts, tx response is obtained at a total daily dose of 160–320 mg/day given in 2 divided doses. Max., 640 mg/day	• Food reduces absorption; administer on empty stomach • Notify physician if P < 50
timolol maleate (Blocadren)	Angina pectoris: **Oral:** *Adults:* Initially, 5 mg bid or tid. Increases may be made prn at intervals of not less than 3 days. First increase should not exceed 10 mg/day. Subsequent increases should not exceed 15 mg/day. Max. total daily dose, 45 mg Hypertension: **Oral:** *Adults:* Initially, 5–10 mg bid. Dosage may be increased prn at intervals of 2 weeks by 5 mg bid. Max. total daily dose, 60 mg Preventive use in ischemic heart disease: **Oral:** *Adults:* Initially, 5 mg bid. If no adverse reactions occur, increase dose to 10 mg bid after 2 days Migraine prophylaxis: **Oral:** *Adults:* Initially, 10 mg bid, up to 30 mg/day	• If migraine tx is not effective after 6–8 weeks, discontinue. May be given without regard to food. May be crushed if necessary • Confer with physician if P < 50
C. Cardioselective Beta Blockers		
acebutolol HCl (Monitan, Sectral)	Angina pectoris: **Oral:** *Adults:* Initially, 200 mg bid. Increase after 2 weeks, prn, to a max. of 300 mg bid. Usual maintenance dose is in the range of 200–600 mg/day, given in 2 divided doses Hypertension: **Oral:** *Adults:* Initially, 100 mg bid. Increase after 1 week, prn, to 200 mg bid. Some pts may require further increments of 100 mg bid at intervals of not less than 2 weeks, to a max. of 400 mg bid	• Do not discontinue suddenly; may cause MI or angina • May be given without regard to food • Confer with physician if P < 50 • Lower doses should be used for geriatric pts

(cont'd on next page)

Table 30. 11 (continued)
The antiadrenergics: Drug doses

Drug Generic name (Trade names)	Dosage	Nursing alert
C. Cardioselective Beta Blockers (cont'd)		
atenolol (Tenormin)	Angina pectoris: **Oral:** *Adults:* Initially, 50 mg od. If optimum response is not achieved within 1 week, increase to 100 mg od. Some pts may require 200 mg/day Hypertension: **Oral:** *Adults:* 50 mg od. If adequate response is not achieved within 1–2 weeks, increase to 100 mg od	• May give without regard to food. May be crushed • Confer with physician if pulse <50
metoprolol tartrate (Betaloc, Lopresor, Lopressor)	Angina pectoris: **Oral:** *Adults:* Initially, 50 mg bid for first week. Increase by 100 mg/day for the next week, prn. Usual maint. dose, 200 mg/day Hypertension: **Oral:** *Adults:* Initially, 50 mg bid. Increase prn after 1 week to 100 mg bid. In some cases, daily dosage may need to be increased by further 100-mg increments at intervals of not less than 2 weeks up to a max. of 200 mg bid Acute tx for myocardial infarction prophylaxis: **IV:** *Adults:* 5 mg q2min for 3 doses; 15 min after last IV dose, start PO 50 mg q6h for 48 h, then 100 mg bid	• Oral dose should be given with food. Do not crush or chew extended-release tablets • **Direct IV:** Check agency policy. Continuous cardiac monitoring required

D. Beta Blockers with Intrinsic Sympathetic Activity (ISA): Partial-Agonist Beta Blockers

Note: For acebutolol, which is a cardioselective beta blocker with ISA, consult information provided under Cardioselective Beta Blockers (page 307)

oxprenolol HCl (Trasicor)	Hypertension: **Oral:** *Adults:* Initially, 20 mg tid, followed by upward titration of dose tid, with increases of 60 mg/day at 1–2 week intervals, prn. Once optimal dose has been established, total daily dose may be given bid	• Do not crush or chew slow-release tabs

Table 30. 11 (continued)
The antiadrenergics: Drug doses

Drug Generic name (Trade names)	Dosage	Nursing alert
D. Beta Blockers with Intrinsic Sympathetic Activity (ISA): Partial-Agonist Beta Blockers (cont'd)		
pindolol (Visken)	Angina pectoris: **Oral:** *Adults:* Give tid or qid. Initially, 5 mg tid with meals. Increase after 1–2 weeks, prn. Usual maint. dose, 15 mg up to 40 mg/day Hypertension: **Oral:** *Adults:* Initially, 5 mg bid, with breakfast and evening meal. Increase prn after 1–2 weeks to 10 mg bid. If further increases are needed after 1–2 weeks, give 15 mg bid. Doses > 30 mg daily must be given tid. Pts treated satisfactorily on 10–20 mg/day may take total dose in a.m. with breakfast	• Give with meals. May crush if necessary
E. Alpha and Beta Blocker		
labetalol HCl (Normodyne, Trandate)	Hypertension: **Oral:** *Adults:* Initially, 100 mg bid. Adjust dose thereafter, prn. Usual maint. dose, 200–400 mg bid. Pts may require up to 1200 mg/day. **IV:** *Adults:* Initially, 20 mg by slow injection over 2 min. Additional injections of 40 mg can be given at 10-min intervals until a desired supine BP is achieved or total 300 mg has been injected	• **Oral:** Give with food to enhance absorption • **IV:** Check manufacturer's instructions for reconstitution and agency policy on direct injection. May be given at 2 mg/min; use infusion pump for accuracy
F. Adrenergic Neuron Blockers		
reserpine (Serpasil)	Hypertension: **Oral:** *Adults* (not receiving other antihypertensive drugs): Initially, 0.5 mg daily for 1–2 weeks. Maint. dose, 0.125–0.25 mg/day	• Take with food or milk to reduce GI irritation • Store in airtight, light-resistant container
guanethidine (Ismelin)	Hypertension: **Oral:** *Adults:* Initially, 10 mg od in single dose, preferably in a.m. If necessary, increase daily dosage by 1 10-mg tablet at intervals of not less than 1 week until desired BP is achieved. Usual daily dose, 25–50 mg	• May crush tabs and mix with food, if necessary

(cont'd on next page)

Table 30. 11 (continued)
The antiadrenergics: Drug doses

Drug Generic name (Trade names)	Dosage	Nursing alert
F. Adrenergic Neuron Blockers (cont'd)		
clonidine HCl (Catapres)	**Hypertension: Oral:** *Adults,* 0.1 mg bid, a.m. and hs. Maint. dose: After 2–4 weeks, further increments of 0.1 mg/day may be necessary. Maintenance: 0.2–0.6 mg/day in divided doses	• Last dose of day should be given hs to ensure BP control during sleep
methyldopa (Aldomet)	**Hypertension: Oral:** *Adults:* Usual starting dose, 250 mg bid or tid in the first 48 h. Daily dosage can then be increased or decreased, preferably at intervals of not less than 2 days, until adequate response is achieved. Usual daily maint. dose, 500 mg to 2 g in 2–4 doses. Max. recommended dose, 3 g **IV** (methyldopate): *Adults:* 250–1000 mg q6h	• To minimize sedation, start dosage increases in evening • Shake suspension well before using • **IV:** Follow manufacturer's instructions for reconstitution; infuse over 30–60 min

Response to Clinical Challenge

Principles

1. Anxiety is a generalized response that produces emotional and physical reactions. The physical component is mediated primarily by the sympathetic nervous system (increased heart rate, dry mouth, sweaty palms, GI distress, to name but a few common signs/symptoms). A nonselective beta blocker, such as propranolol, reduces the sympathetic response. However, this is not a recommended use for this drug.

2. Because Alan has other chronic conditions, he is at greater risk for adverse reactions. Beta blockers can disrupt diabetic control by affecting release of glycogen from the liver and reducing the usual warning signs of hypoglycemia. Although his asthma has not been a recent problem, Alan could experience problems due to bronchoconstriction (an adverse effect of beta blockers).

Actions

3. Advise Alan to take medications only after consultation with his physician. Suggest that alternative methods (both pharmacological and nonpharmacological) can be used to control anxiety, and discuss these with him.

Further Reading

Hoffman BB, Lefkowitz RJ. Catecholamines, sympathomimetic drugs, and adrenergic receptor antagonists. In: Hardman JG, Limbird LE, eds. *Goodman and Gilman's The Pharmacological Basis of Therapeutics.* 9th ed. New York: Pergamon; 1996: 199–248.

Westfall DP. Adrenoceptor antagonists. In: Craig CR, Stitzel RE, eds. *Modern Pharmacology.* 4th ed. Boston: Little, Brown; 1994:129–143.

Neuromuscular Blocking Drugs

Topics Discussed
- Competitive (nondepolarizing) blockers
- Noncompetitive (polarizing) blockers
- For each drug discussed: Mechanism of action, pharmacologic effects, therapeutic uses, adverse effects
- Nursing management

Drugs Discussed
atracurium besylate (at-trah-**cure**-ee-um)

doxacurium (dox-ah-**cure**-ee-yum)

gallamine triethiodide (**gal**-ah-meen try-eth-**eye**-oh-dyde)

metocurine (met-oh-**cure**-een)

mivacurium chloride (mye-vah-**cure**-ee-um)

pancuronium bromide (pan-cure-**oh**-nee-yum)

pipecuronium (pip-eh-kyoor-**oh**-nee-um)

rocuronium (roe-cure-**oh**-nee-yum)

succinylcholine chloride (suk-sin-ill-**koe**-leen)

tubocurarine chloride (tyoo-boh-**cure**-ar-reen)

vecuronium bromide (vee-cure-**oh**-nee-yum)

Clinical Challenge

Consider this clinical challenge as you read through this chapter. The response to the challenge appears on page 319.

C.J. is a 76-year-old man who has just had surgery for a total right hip replacement for treatment of severe osteoarthritis. At the time of entering the Post Anesthetic Recovery Room (PARR), his blood pressure is 140/80; pulse 60 and regular; respiration 18, spontaneous and shallow. He is responding to verbal commands, can swallow and speak, but his eyelids remain closed.

For his surgery, Mr. J. received succinylcholine, propofol, fentanyl, vecuronium and morphine. Immediately after surgery, he was given neostigmine and atropine. Ten minutes after admission to PARR, Mr. J. still has not opened his eyes; he does not speak or swallow with verbal instruction, shows jerky movements of the limbs and seems very restless.

What is the probable cause of his response? What is the appropriate action?

Acetylcholine released from somatic nerves stimulates nicotinic receptors on motor end-plates to contract skeletal muscles. Because nicotinic receptors on skeletal muscle are not identical to nicotinic receptors in autonomic ganglia, it is possible to block skeletal muscle function without altering autonomic activities.

The drugs discussed in this chapter are used to block skeletal neuromuscular transmission. They can be classified, on the basis of their mechanisms of action, into competitive (nondepolarizing) and noncompetitive (or depolarizing) blockers.

Competitive (Nondepolarizing) Blockers

Tubocurarine

Mechanism of action and pharmacologic effects. Tubocurarine is the best-known competitive blocker of the actions of acetylcholine on skeletal muscle nicotinic receptors. South American Indians recognized the ability of tubocurarine to paralyze skeletal muscles hundreds of years ago and utilized the drug, a naturally occurring chemical obtained from the curare plant, as their drug of choice for dispatching adversaries. Delivered with considerable velocity on the end of an arrow, tubocurarine served these people well. The unlucky foe on the receiving end of the arrow found it most difficult to flee, as his legs soon became paralyzed. Shortly thereafter respiration failed, as both the intercostal and diaphragmatic muscles succumbed to the effects of the drug.

Anesthetists make use of the same property of the drug to relax skeletal muscles during surgery. However, in contradistinction to the natives of South America, anesthetists do not stand around the curarized individual while respiration becomes ever more feeble. In the clinical situation, patients receiving tubocurarine are artificially ventilated until the drug's effects subside.

Tubocurarine also releases histamine from mast cells. This may account for the bronchospasm, hypotension and excessive bronchial and salivary secretion that can accompany use of the drug. Heparin, also stored in mast cells, is released by tubocurarine, causing decreased blood coagulability.

Therapeutic uses. The primary indication for neuromuscular blockers such as tubocurarine is as adjuvant drugs in surgical anesthesia. They are also administered to facilitate intubation and provide skeletal muscle relaxation during surgery. Neuromuscular blockers relax skeletal muscles and reduce the concentration of anesthetic required, thereby decreasing the risk of cardiovascular and respiratory depression. Muscular relaxation can be used to assist in the alignment of a fracture or the relocation of a dislocated joint.

The actions of tubocurarine can be terminated by administering a cholinesterase inhibitor, such as neostigmine. The increase in acetylcholine concentration around nicotinic receptors overcomes the effects of competitive blockers. However, acetylcholine also accumulates around muscarinic receptors. To prevent muscarinic stimulation, an anticholinergic, such as atropine, can also be given.

Other Drugs

Atracurium Besylate (Tracrium®), Gallamine Triethiodide (Flaxedil®), Pancuronium (Pavulon®), Vecuronium Bromide (Norcuron®)

These drugs are also competitive blockers of acetylcholine on nicotinic skeletal muscle receptors. Pancuronium is used extensively. It is about five times more potent than tubocurarine and has little histamine-releasing action.

Recently, several newer competitive neuromuscular blockers have arrived on the market. Their properties are summarized below.

Metocurine (Metubine®). This drug is a methyl analogue of tubocurarine that produces nondepolarizing (competitive) neuromuscular blockade at the myoneural junction. Recent clinical findings suggest that metocurine reaches the neuromuscular junction more rapidly than does tubocurarine. After intravenous injection, there is rapid onset (1–4 min) of muscle relaxation, with maximum twitch inhibition (96%) in 1.5–10 min. The maximum effect lasts 35–60 min. The time for recovery to 50% of control twitch response is in excess of 3 h. Metocurine is indicated as an adjunct to anesthesia to induce skeletal muscle relaxation. It may be employed to reduce the intensity of muscle contractions in pharmacologically or electrically induced convulsions. It may also be employed to facilitate the management of patients undergoing mechanical ventilation.

Mivacurium chloride (Mivacron®). This recently introduced neuromuscular blocker has a faster onset and shorter duration of action than the other competitive neuromuscular blockers, and it does not demonstrate cumulative effects during prolonged treatment. Mivacurium's effects last approximately 13–24 min. Because mivacurium is metabolized by plasma cholinesterase, the same enzyme that destroys succinylcholine, its duration of action is prolonged in patients with low plasma cholinesterase activity. With its shorter duration of action, mivacurium would appear to offer advantages for routine nonemergency intubations and for short procedures. Furthermore, because cumulative effects do not accrue during prolonged treatment with mivacurium, therapy can be continued without affecting the recovery time.

Pipecuronium (Arduan®). This long-acting, nondepolarizing neuromuscular blocking agent has minimal adverse cardiovascular effects. It is used as a skeletal muscle relaxant during general anesthesia and for endotracheal intubation. The drug is not recommended for procedures that last fewer than 90 min or for patients requiring prolonged mechanical ventilation in intensive care units.

Doxacurium (Nuromax®). This is a long-acting, nondepolarizing neuromuscular blocking agent similar to pipecuronium. It is used as a skeletal muscle relaxant during general anesthesia and for endotracheal intubation. Although small decreases in heart rate and mean arterial pressure occur in some patients who receive doxacurium, clinical studies have found no adverse cardiovascular effects in patients with heart disease receiving up to three times the usual effective dose. As with pipecuronium, which it closely resembles in activity, the duration of block is prolonged in patients with renal failure.

Rocuronium bromide (Zemuron®). This is a new short-onset, intermediate-acting, nondepolarizing neuromuscular blocking drug that is being promoted particularly for use in rapid endotracheal intubation. Rocuronium has the fastest onset of action of any nondepolarizing neuromuscular blocking agent to become available in North America, but in the doses required for rapid onset, it also has a long duration of action. Whether it could sometimes replace succinylcholine for emergency endotracheal intubation remains to be determined.

Noncompetitive (Depolarizing) Blockers

Succinylcholine Chloride (Anectine®, Quelicin®, Sucostrin®, Sux-Cert®)

Mechanism of action and pharmacologic effects. Succinylcholine depolarizes nicotinic receptors on motor end-plates, producing muscle fasciculations. In this regard it is similar to the initial actions of acetylcholine. In the case of acetylcholine, however, the neurotransmitter is metabolized, allowing the end-plate to repolarize before it is subsequently depolarized by the next series of acetylcholine molecules. It is a series of depolarization-repolarization cycles that is responsible for purposeful muscle movement. If the motor end-plate cannot repolarize, the cycle is broken and purposeful muscle action is prevented.

This is what happens when succinylcholine is administered. Although it is metabolized rapidly by pseudocholinesterase to succinic acid and choline, its rate of inactivation is considerably slower than acetylcholine's. Because of this, it remains attached to nicotinic receptors, preventing motor end-plate repolarization and paralyzing muscles. However, as stated above, succinylcholine is inactivated rapidly. Therefore, it must be given by continuous intravenous drip if prolonged muscular relaxation is required. Some individuals have an atypical pseudocholinesterase, incapable of metabolizing succinylcholine. If the drug is given to these patients, it will have a prolonged duration of action.

Table 31.1 on the next page lists the clinically significant drug interactions with neuromuscular blocking drugs.

Table 31.1
Neuromuscular blockers: Drug interactions

Drug	Interaction
Aminoglycoside antibiotics	• Aminoglycoside antibiotics potentiate the actions of neuromuscular blocking drugs
Beta blockers	• Beta blockers have been reported both to prolong and to reverse neuromuscular blockade with tubocurarine. Monitor neuromuscular status
Benzodiazepines	• Diazepam can prolong the effects of succinylcholine
Cyclophosphamide	• Cyclophosphamide inhibits cholinesterase and prolongs succinylcholine's effects. Measure plasma cholinesterase and decrease succinylcholine dosage accordingly
Digoxin	• Neuromuscular blockers increase the incidence of digoxin arrhythmias
Diuretics	• Furosemide and thiazides increase the effects of neuromuscular blockers. Monitor neuromuscular status
Lithium	• Lithium prolongs neuromuscular blockade. Monitor neuromuscular status
Metaclopramide	• Metaclopramide prolongs effect of succinylcholine. Give with caution
Monoamine oxidase inhibitors	• Phenelzine inhibits cholinesterase and prolongs effect of succinylcholine. Measure plasma cholinesterase and reduce succinylcholine dosage accordingly
Narcotics	• Narcotics increase central respiratory depression and respiratory muscle paralysis with tubocurarine. Use with caution
Quinidine	• Quinidine increases neuromuscular blockade. Use with caution
Tamoxifen	• Tamoxifen prolongs atracurium's effects. Monitor closely
Theophylline	• Theophylline can produce arrhythmias with pancuronium. Theophylline also decreases neuromuscular blockade. Avoid concurrent use

Therapeutic uses. Succinylcholine chloride is used in surgery as a skeletal muscle relaxant. Its effects cannot be reversed by the injection of an anticholinesterase. As explained in Chapter 27, the accumulation of large amounts of acetylcholine can, in itself, lead to a depolarizing block. Bearing in mind that succinylcholine is inactivated by pseudocholinesterase, the injection of an anti-cholinesterase, such as neostigmine, that inhibits both acetylcholinesterase and pseudo-cholinesterase, will not only allow acetylcholine to accumulate but will also reduce the rate at which succinylcholine is metabolized. These effects combine to increase the duration of the depolarization block.

Nursing Management

Table 31.2 summarizes the nursing management of the patient receiving a neuromuscular drug. Dosage details of individual drugs are given in Table 31.3 (pages 316–318).

Table 31.2
Nursing management of the neuromuscular blocking drugs

Assessment of risk vs. benefit	Patient data	• *History:* Physician should determine contraindications (e.g., allergy) and precautions (e.g., cardiac disease, electrolyte disorders, hepatic impairment) • Assess for baseline data (particularly BP, P, R, T). • *Age:* These drugs are used across the lifespan but should be given cautiously to older adults. Children may require higher doses of some drugs in this class and may be more sensitive to the effects of others. • *Pregnancy:* Risk category C (animal studies show adverse effects to fetus but human data are unknown or insufficient); benefits may be acceptable despite risks
	Drug data	• Select drugs based on duration of action and pt profile • Duration of action varies: may be ultra-short (succinylcholine, 4–6 min), short-acting (mivacurium, 13–245 min), intermediate-acting (pancuronium, 35–45 min) or long-acting (pipecuronium, 90–120 min) • Intensity and duration of paralysis may be prolonged by some drugs; confer with pharmacist • Most serious adverse effects are respiratory depression and CV effects (bradycardia, hypotension)
Implementation	Rights of administration	• Using the "rights" helps prevent errors of administration
	Right route	• Give IV, except succinylcholine and tubocurarine, which may be given IM if necessary
	Right dose	• See Table 31.3. Calculate dilution in IV fluid and infusion rates carefully; usually ordered as dose/kg. High individual variability in response to these drugs; dose is determined by response as well as age and weight
	Right time	• May be given by rapid bolus, intermittent or continuous infusion. Check local policies for approved procedures and recommended administration
	Right technique	• IV administration requires knowledge of correct diluent and IV solution, correct dilution and rate of administration. Always refer to manufacturer's instructions for this route. Pump device recommended to control rate of infusion. Equipment for intubation, mechanical ventilation and O_2 tx must be readily available
	Nursing therapeutics	• Neuromuscular blockers do not produce analgesia; carefully monitor for pain and administer analgesics concurrently when required. Drugs also do not produce unconsciousness; be aware of communications and explain all procedures to pt • Maintain fluid and electrolyte balance; more serious adverse reactions can occur • Frequently check function of mechanical ventilator • Position pt; provide frequent skin care

(cont'd on next page)

Table 31.2 (continued)
Nursing management of the neuromuscular blocking drugs

Implementation (cont'd)	Patient/family teaching	• *Preoperative:* Explain drug action and that residual effects such as muscle weakness disappear soon after medication is stopped
Outcomes	Monitoring of progress	*Continually monitor:* • Clinical response indicating tx success (paralysis, skeletal muscle relaxation) • Respiratory status during and following tx until pt is fully recovered. Paralysis occurs progressively in the muscles of the eyelids, mouth and jaw, limbs, abdomen, glottis, intercostals and, finally, the diaphragm. Recovery occurs in the reverse order. Full recovery is evidenced by ability to cough/swallow, lift head voluntarily, grip hand (muscle strength). Use peripheral nerve stimulation to monitor response for prolonged drug tx • Use of reversing agents, such as edrophonium or neostigmine, may be useful for the competitive blockers but cannot be used for the noncompetitive blocker succinylcholine • Be alert for signs/symptoms of adverse reactions, particularly CV and respiratory; document and report immediately to physician

Table 31.3
The neuromuscular blockers: Drug doses

Drug Generic name (Trade names)	Dosage	Nursing alert
A. Competitive Neuromuscular Blockers		
atracurium besylate (Tracrium)	**IV:** *Adults/children ≥ 2 years:* Initially, 0.4–0.5 mg/kg; subsequent doses, 0.08–0.1 mg/kg. If given after succinylcholine-assisted intubation, 0.3–0.4 mg/kg is recommended initially	• Follow manufacturer's instruction for reconstitution. Do not mix with acidic or alkaline solutions. Never give IM • Initial dose by bolus over 1 min. Subsequent doses may be give by infusion. Check agency policy • Intermediate-acting duration, 20–30 min. Cardiac and respiratory monitoring required
doxacurium chloride (Nuromax)	**IV:** *Adults:* 50 µg/kg (may need up to 80 µg/kg prolonged effect; 25 µg/kg for succinylcholine-assisted intubation) initially, followed 60–100 min later by 5–10 µg/kg, repeated prn. *Children 2–12 years:* 30–50 µg/kg initially; maint. dose may be required more frequently than in adults	• Follow manufacturer's instructions for reconstitution. Diluted solutions should be discarded after 8 h

Table 31.3 (continued)
The neuromuscular blockers: Drug doses

Drug Generic name (Trade names)	Dosage	Nursing alert
A. Competitive Neuromuscular Blockers (cont'd)		
gallamine triethiodide (Flaxedil)	**IV:** *Adults/children:* 1 mg/kg initially (not to exceed 100 mg/dose), followed by 0.3–0.5 mg/kg. *Infants up to 1 month:* Initially, 1 mg/kg, followed by doses of 0.5 mg/kg	• Give only as bolus over 30–60 s. Intermediate-acting duration, 15–30 min. Cardiac and respiratory monitoring required
metocurine iodide (Metubine Iodide)	For endotracheal intubation: **IV:** 0.2–0.4 mg/kg, initially. Supplemental doses average 0.5–1 mg Electroshock tx: **IV:** 1.75–5.5 mg. Average dose, 2–3 mg	• Not recommended for IM administration. Should be administered IV as sustained injection over 30–60 s. Care must be taken to avoid overdosage
mivacurium chloride (Mivacron)	**IV:** *Adults:* Initial bolus dose, 0.15 mg/kg. Maint. dosing of 0.1 mg/kg generally is required approximately 15 min following initial dose. *Children 2–12 years:* 0.2 mg/kg	• Initial dose given by bolus over 5–15 s. Short-acting duration, 10–15 min. Maint. doses may be given by continuous infusion • Follow manufacturer's instructions for reconstitution. Check local policies. Dose is highly individualized; must be adapted for pts with renal or hepatic disease or obesity
pancuronium bromide (Pavulon)	**IV:** *Adults/children:* Initially, 0.04–0.1 mg/kg; for intubation, 0.1 mg/kg; subsequently, 0.01–0.02 mg/kg, repeated prn (usually, q20–40min).	• Usually given by bolus. May be given, but not stored, in plastic syringe. Intermediate action, 35–45 min
pipecuronium bromide (Arduan)	**IV:** *Adults:* 70–85 μg/kg (dosage adjustments required for obesity or renal impairment). If given following recovery from succinylcholine during intubation, decrease dose to 50 μg/kg (70–85 μg/kg, if longer paralysis desired). Additional doses of 10–15 μg/kg may be required as maintenance (dosage reduction recommended if using concurrent inhalation anesthetics). *Children 1–14 years,* 57 μg/kg. *Infants 3 months to 1 year,* 40 μg/kg	• Store at room temperature. Read manufacturer's instructions for reconstitution Refrigerate reconstituted solution and use within 24 h • Do not dilute into, or administer from, large-volume IV solutions
rocuronium bromide (Zemuron)	Refer to detailed manufacturer's information for recommended dosages	

(cont'd on next page)

Table 31.3 (continued)
The neuromuscular blockers: Drug doses

Drug Generic name (Trade names)	Dosage	Nursing alert
A. Competitive Neuromuscular Blockers (cont'd)		
tubocurarine chloride	**IV:** *Adults/children:* 0.2–0.5 mg/kg initially, followed by 0.04–0.1 mg/kg. *Infants ≤ 1 month:* 0.3 mg/kg initially, followed by 0.1 mg/kg. For detailed instructions on dosages for use as (a) adjunct to general anesthesia, (b) adjunct to electroconvulsive therapy, (c) aid to mechanical ventilation or (d) diagnosis of myasthenia gravis, refer to manufacturer's information	• Usual route is IV bolus, but can be given IM if no venous access. Long-acting duration, 35–60 min
vecuronium bromide (Norcuron)	**IV:** *Adults* (for intubation): 0.08–0.1 mg/kg; subsequent intraoperative doses, 0.01–0.015 mg/kg, repeated prn or a maint. infusion of approximately 1 µg/kg/min. If vecuronium is given after succinylcholine-assisted intubation, 0.04–0.06 mg/kg is recommended as initial dose. *Children 1–10 years:* May require slightly larger initial dose and more frequent supplemental doses than adults. *Infants < 1 year:* Are more sensitive to vecuronium than adults; recovery time may be more prolonged	• May be given by bolus or infusion. Follow manufacturer's instructions for reconstitution. Do not mix with alkaline solutions. Intermediate duration, 25–30 min
B. Noncompetitive Neuromuscular Blockers (cont'd)		
succinylcholine chloride (Anectine, Quelicin, Sucostrin, Sux-Cert)	**IV:** *Adults:* Initially, 0.3–1.5 mg/kg; subsequent doses, 0.01–0.05 mg/kg. For continuous infusion, a 0.1% (1 mg/mL) or 0.2% (2 mg/mL) solution is administered at an average rate of 2.5–7.5 mg/min. Dose necessary to maintain paralysis is reduced in pregnant women. *Infants:* 2 mg/kg. *Children:* 1 mg/kg. **IM** (when a suitable vein is not accessible): *Adults/infants/older children:* Up to 3–4 mg/kg (not to exceed total dose of 150 mg)	• Usual route is IV, but can be given IM. Continuous infusion not recommended for neonates and infants, since tachyphylaxis occurs with a cumulative dose of 4 mg/kg and phase II block at about 6 mg/kg • When IM injection is warranted, give deep into muscle mass • Ultrashort-acting duration, 4–6 min. No specific antidote; repeated doses or prolonged use not advised

Response to Clinical Challenge

Principles
It is probable that Mr. J. is experiencing incomplete reversal of the neuromuscular blocking agent (vecuronium) used during surgery. The short-acting succinylcholine is used for intubation but repeated or prolonged use is not recommended. Vecuronium would be given for skeletal muscle relaxation during the procedure. Its duration is 25–30 min and could be repeated if necessary.

Actions
The immediate action is to notify the physician and administer antidotes such as neostigmine and atropine. The neostigmine is a cholinergic agonist which will provide an antidote to the vecuronium at the neuromuscular receptors. (Note that this reversing agent should not be used for succinylcholine overdose, but the duration of this drug, given at intubation, is long past.) Atropine, an anticholinergic, will prevent excessive stimulation of the vagal nerve to the heart, thus preventing bradycardia.

Refer to Chapters 27 and 28 for more information on cholinergic and anticholinergic drugs.

Further Reading

Ellis M, Klein D. Implementing neuromuscular blockade monitoring in a surgical intensive care unit. *Clin Nurse Spec* 1995;9(3):134–139.

Embree P. Long-acting nondepolarizing neuromuscular blocking agents. *AANA Journal* 1993;61(4):83–87.

Levy L, et al. Neuromuscular blockage: nursing interventions and case studies from infancy to adulthood. *Crit Care Nurs Q* 1993;15(4):53–57.

Susla G. Neuromuscular blocking agents in critical care. *Nurs Clin North Am* 1993;5(2):296–311.

Taylor Palmer. Agents acting at the neuromuscular and autonomic ganglia. In: Hardman JG, Limbird LE, eds. *Goodman and Gilman's The Pharmacological Basis of Therapeutics*. 9th ed. New York: Pergamon; 1996:161–176.

Volle RL, Miyamoto MD. Drugs that affect neuromuscular transmission. In: Craig CR, Stitzel RE, eds. *Modern Pharmacology*. 4th ed. Boston: Little, Brown;1994: 177–184.

Cardiovascular Pharmacology

Unit 6 deals with cardiovascular pharmacology. Beginning with a discussion of drugs used for the treatment of congestive heart failure, it proceeds through antiarrhythmic drugs, antianginal drugs, drugs for the treatment of peripheral and cerebral vascular disorders, antihypertensive drugs and antihypotensive drugs.

The importance of these drugs cannot be overstated. Without them, countless millions would either die or have their lifestyle severely hampered by such conditions as congestive heart failure (CHF), supraventricular and ventricular arrhythmias, angina pectoris, hypertension, hypotension or shock.

The importance of the material presented in Unit 5 will now become apparent. To understand cardiovascular pharmacology and its attendant nursing process, nurses require a good knowledge of autonomic physiology and pharmacology and the nursing measures pertinent to it. If the material in the following chapters seems difficult, readers are encouraged to refer back to the relevant chapters in Unit 5.

CHAPTER 32

Drugs for the Treatment of Congestive Heart Failure

Topics Discussed
- Hemodynamics
- Definition of cardiac output, preload, afterload, vasodilator
- Congestive heart failure (CHF)
- Drug treatment of CHF: Drugs that decrease preload or afterload; inotropic drugs
- For each drug discussed: Mechanism of action, pharmacological effects, therapeutic use, adverse effects
- Nursing management
- Approach to the treatment of CHF

Drugs Discussed

Diuretics:
bumetanide (byoo-**met**-ah-nyde)
chlorthalidone (klor-**thal**-ih-doan)
ethacrynic acid (eth-ah-**krin**-ic)
furosemide (fur-**oh**-seh-mide)
hydrochlorothiazide (hye-droe-klor-oh-**thye**-ah-zide)
metolazone (meh-**tole**-ah-zone)

Nitrates:
isosorbide dinitrate (eye-soe-**sor**-byde dye-**nye**-trate)

ACE Inhibitors:
captopril (**kap**-toe-pril)
enalapril (en-**al**-ah-pril)
lisinopril (lye-**sin**-oh-pril)

Inotropic Drugs:
amrinone (**am** rin-none)
digoxin (dye-**jox**-in)
dobutamine (doe-**byoo**-tah-meen)
dopamine (**dope**-ah-meen)

Clinical Challenge

Consider this clinical challenge as you read through this chapter. The response to the challenge appears on page 339.

Mrs. Gupta is 83 years old. She was admitted to your medical cardiac unit after a short stay in CCU for treatment of heart failure. She has been stable for the past 24 h. This morning her ECG rhythm shows atrial fibrillation at a rate of 49 beats per minute with frequent PVCs. She tells you she feels weak and has no appetite. Her serum digoxin level is 2.3 mmol/L. She is due for her regular dose of digoxin 0.25 mg PO.

What are your concerns? What actions will you take? What is your rationale? What nursing monitoring do you recommend?

Hemodynamics

Hemodynamics is the study of the blood flow through the heart and blood vessels. Nurses perform hemodynamic assessments each time they take a blood pressure or palpate for peripheral pulses. It is important for us now to review the major factors that control hemodynamics in the healthy human and compare these with the situation seen in congestive heart failure (CHF) before we proceed to a discussion of the treatment of heart failure.

Throughout our discussions of CHF, we will be discussing cardiac output (CO). *Cardiac output* is the amount of blood ejected by the heart each minute. Depending on age, physical conditioning and body size, normal CO values range from 4–8 L/min. Cardiac output is controlled by heart rate (HR) and stroke volume (SV):

$$CO = HR \times SV$$

An increase in either heart rate or stroke volume produces a commensurate increase in cardiac output.

Both the sympathetic and parasympathetic nervous systems affect heart rate. Parasympathetic stimulation releases acetylcholine and slows heart rate. Sympathetic stimulation releases norepinephrine and increases both heart rate and stroke volume. For example, when a person is forced to run across the street, the sympathetic nerves innervating the heart release more norepinephrine. This stimulates the heart to increase heart rate and cardiac output. Once our pedestrian reaches the other side of the road and is safely out of the way of traffic, sympathetic stimulation decreases and parasympathetic predominance returns. At this time, the heart slows and cardiac output falls.

Nurses may also be aware of the terms preload and afterload.

Preload is defined as the amount of blood in the ventricles at the end of diastole, as represented by the pressure that the volume exerts on the ventricular wall. Stated simply, it is the volume in the ventricular "tank" just before systolic ejection. The pressure measurement taken is termed the end-diastolic pressure (EDP), and it is a direct reflection of the end-diastolic volume (EDV). If more blood is returned to the heart, preload increases. If

the heart cannot pump the increase in venous return, end-diastolic pressure also increases.

In a normal heart, the organ is able to handle an increase in venous return. As more blood is returned to the heart, stroke volume increases and cardiac output goes up. Thus, an increase in preload does not result in venous congestion because all the extra blood returned to the heart is quickly pumped back into the arterial circulation.

This is not the case in patients with heart failure. In these people, the heart is damaged and cannot handle the venous return. As a result, if the right side of the heart is damaged, blood accumulates in the systemic veins. If the damage is primarily to the left side of the heart, the accumulation of blood occurs in the pulmonary veins. In either case, venous congestion occurs.

Afterload is the resistance to systolic contraction and ejection. It is determined mainly by the systemic vascular resistance in the arterioles of the body. The greater the pressure within the arterioles, the higher the afterload. When the afterload is increased, the heart must work harder to pump blood throughout the body.

Systemic vascular resistance can be altered by drugs. Drugs that constrict the arterioles increase systemic vascular resistance and afterload. These drugs make it more difficult for the heart to pump blood. The reverse is also true. Drugs that dilate arterioles (e.g., ACE inhibitors or nitroglycerin) lower the systemic vascular resistance and afterload. As a result, they make it easier for the heart to pump blood and increase cardiac output.

Congestive Heart Failure

Congestive heart failure (CHF) is a condition in which the ability of the heart to pump blood is impaired, causing fluid to back up in the lungs and other tissues.

CHF can also be divided into left-sided and right-sided heart failure. Reference has been made to the consequences of right-sided or left-sided heart damage. If the difficulty is left-sided failure, the heart is unable to pump blood returned from the lungs. As a result, pulmonary congestion occurs, bringing with it dyspnea (difficult or painful breathing) and orthopnea (difficult breathing except in an upright position). If the difficulty is right-sided failure, the heart is unable to accommodate blood returned to it via the systemic veins. Orthopnea and paroxysmal nocturnal dyspnea are less common but systemic venous congestion occurs, leading to ankle edema, congestive hepatomegaly and systemic venous distention.

The differentiation between left-sided and right-sided heart failure is somewhat fallacious because their symptoms often overlap. For example, subjects with left-sided failure may experience edema and patients with right-sided failure often suffer from exertional dyspnea.

The contractility of the heart is reduced in low-output CHF. Contractility is defined as the force with which the heart contracts for any given fibre length. Initially, decreased contractility of the heart may not be evident because of two compensatory mechanisms. These are an increase in both heart size and sympathetic nervous system activity. They are depicted in Figure 32.1.

The increase in heart size can be understood when it is recognized that a decrease in myocardial contractility, stroke volume and cardiac output produces an increase in end-systolic and diastolic volumes (an increase in preload). To compensate for these phenomena the heart dilates. The larger heart allows for an increase in force of contraction, offsetting for a time the initial defect in myocardial contractility.

Sympathetic stimulation increases heart rate and improves myocardial contractility, thereby helping to maintain cardiac output. Unfortunately, increased sympathetic stimulation produces a generalized vasoconstriction. Although this assists in maintaining blood pressure, it also increases afterload and reduces tissue perfusion.

Sympathetic stimulation also releases renin from the kidney. Renin, in turn, is converted first to angiotensin I and then to angiotensin II.

Figure 32.1
Effects of a decrease in myocardial contractility with the development of CHF

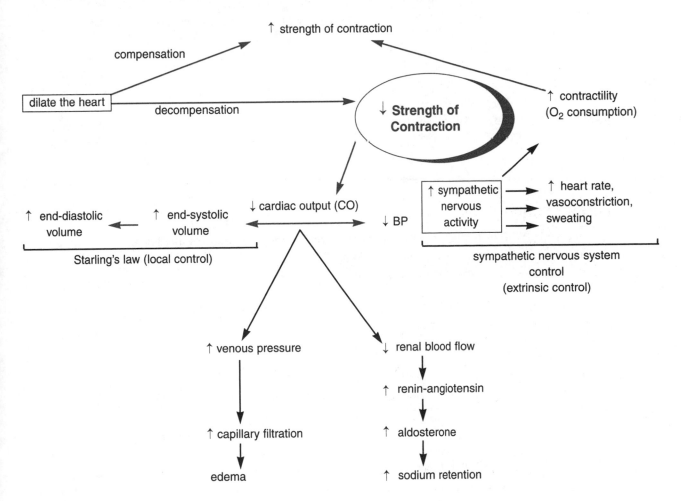

Angiotensin II is a potent vasoconstrictor that increases peripheral resistance and afterload. It also stimulates the secretion of the mineralocorticoid aldosterone from the adrenal cortex, leading to the retention of salt and water by the body and the formation of edema and an increase in preload.

Eventually, as myocardial contractility continues to deteriorate, the compensatory mechanisms are insufficient to maintain cardiac output. At this point CHF occurs. Figures 32.2 and 32.3 describe the compensating mechanisms in heart failure and the reasons for the formation of edema. Box 32.1 summarizes the causes and effects of CHF.

Drug Treatment of CHF

CHF may be treated by drugs that (1) decrease preload (diuretics and nitrates), (2) reduce afterload (angiotensin-converting enzyme inhibitors) or (3) increase myocardial contractility (inotropic drugs).

As previously explained, preload refers to the cardiac filling pressure or venous return to the right side of the heart. Afterload is the systemic vascular resistance against which the heart must pump to circulate blood throughout the body. The use of diuretics (to decrease preload), vasodilators (to reduce afterload), and inotropic agents (to increase myocardial contractility) is depicted in Figure 32.4 on page 326.

Figure 32.2
Compensating mechanism in heart failure

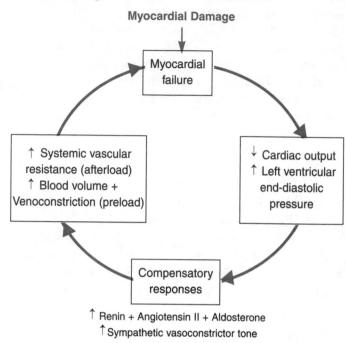

Source: Bristol-Myers Squibb. Reproduced with permission.

Box 32.1
Causes and effects of CHF

➤ Heart failure occurs when the heart does not pump enough blood to meet the needs of the tissues
➤ Low cardiac output leads to congestion, dyspnea and edema
➤ The compensating mechanisms in heart failure are:
  • enlarged heart
  • increased release of renin, resulting in increased angiotensin II and aldosterone secretion
    — angiotensin II constricts renal vessels
    — aldosterone promotes salt and water retention
  • increased sympathetic stimulation
    — stimulation of beta$_1$ receptors in the heart increases heart rate
    — stimulation of alpha$_1$ receptors on blood vessels increases peripheral resistance and venous return
➤ The consequences of the compensating mechanisms include increased:
  • blood volume
  • venoconstriction (preload)
  • systemic vascular resistance (afterload)

Figure 32.3
Renal causes of edema in CFH

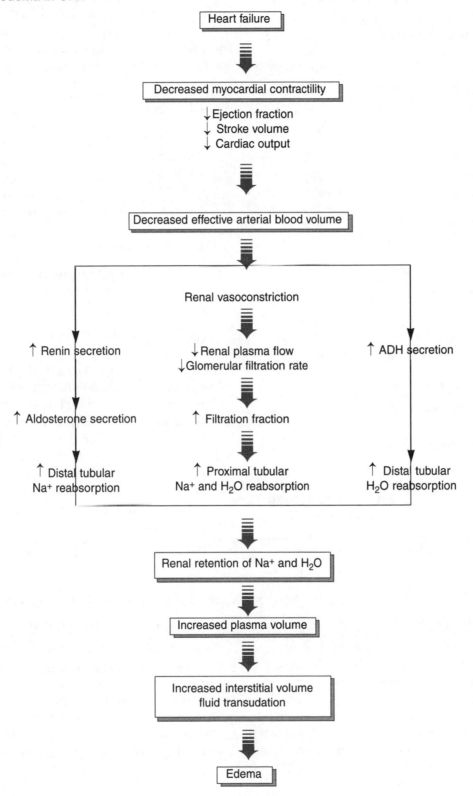

Source: Young JB, Roberts R. Heart failure. In: Dirks JH, Sutton RAL, eds. *Diuretics, Physiology, Pharmacology and Clinical Use.* Philadelphia: W.B. Saunders; 1986:156. Reproduced with permission.

Figure 32.4
Use of diuretics, vasodilators and inotropic drugs to treat CHF

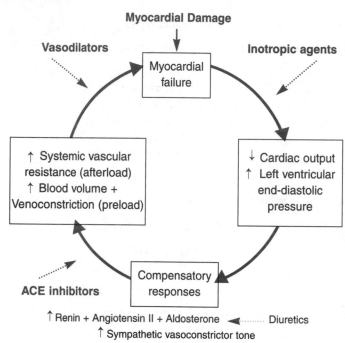

ACE = Angiotensin-converting enzyme

Source: Bristol-Myers Squibb. Reproduced with permission.

Drugs That Decrease Preload

Diuretics

Mechanism of action and pharmacologic effects. The pharmacologic actions of these drugs is presented in detail in Chapter 39. These drugs, which include the thiazides, chlorthalidone and loop diuretics, increase sodium, chloride and water excretion. They decrease blood volume and lower cardiac filling pressure, thereby reducing both pulmonary congestion and peripheral edema.

Therapeutic uses. Diuretics are first-line agents for all grades of cardiac failure when sinus rhythm is present. They are usually sufficient alone in mild CHF. When the patient is afflicted with more severe heart failure, diuretics are usually given with other drugs, such as a vasodilator and/or digoxin. When symptoms are mild, the less potent thiazides and chlorthalidone may suffice. In more severe cases, a loop diuretic, such as furosemide, may be required.

Potassium loss is a common problem encountered with thiazides, chlorthalidone and loop

diuretics. This effect can be reduced by combining these drugs with a potassium-sparing diuretic, such as triamterene, amiloride or spironolactone, or by adding a potassium chloride preparation to the therapeutic regimen. In all cases, careful monitoring of fluid and electrolyte levels is necessary.

Adverse effects. Diuretics, particularly loop diuretics, frequently produce adverse effects, including hypovolemia, reduced renal perfusion, increased blood urea, hyponatremia and hypokalemia. (Elderly patients are especially at risk.) Mild to moderate hypokalemia can potentiate digoxin toxicity. Other adverse effects of diuretics, which include hyperglycemia, hypercalcemia, magnesium depletion and hyperlipidemia, are discussed in Chapter 39.

Nursing management. The nursing management of patients receiving diuretics is described in Table 39.4 (page 439).

Nitrates

Mechanism of action and pharmacologic effects. Nitrates dilate veins, thereby decreasing venous return (preload). These drugs also dilate arterioles and reduce afterload, but their major beneficial effect in CHF can be attributed to venodilatation. Isosorbide dinitrate is the nitrate product used most frequently. It is orally effective for four to six hours.

Table 32.1 lists the clinically significant drug interactions with diuretics.

Therapeutic uses. Isosorbide dinitrate produces a significant, but small, improvement in exercise tolerance. When administered together with hydralazine, isosorbide dinitrate improved two-year survival in one multicentre trial.

Adverse effects. Headache and hypotension are the most common adverse effects of isosorbide dinitrate. The chronic use of any nitrate can lead to the development of tolerance. If the drug is then withdrawn, rebound vasoconstriction can occur.

Table 32.2 lists the clinically significant drug interactions with isosorbide dinitrate.

Nursing management. The nursing management of patients receiving nitrates is described in Table 34.2 (page 374).

Table 32.1
Diuretics: Drug interactions

Drug	Interaction
Allopurinol	• Hydrochlorothiazide has increased allopurinol toxicity. Monitor renal and hepatic function
Aminoglycoside antibiotics	• Furosemide and aminoglycoside antibiotics have increased ototoxicity and nephrotoxicity. Avoid concurrent use, if possible
ACE inhibitors	• Giving an ACEI plus a diuretic to a CHF pt can produce a powerful hypotensive effect, possibly leading to postural hypotension. This can best be avoided by stopping the diuretic a few days before starting with low doses of the ACEI. Thereafter, it may be possible to reintroduce the diuretic and increase the dose of the ACEI slowly. Monitor BP. There is also increased risk for renal failure with an ACEI, especially in pts with renal artery stenosis. Monitor BP, renal function
Cholestyramine	• Cholestyramine can decrease diuretic absorption and effects. Give at least 6 h apart
Corticosteroids	• Corticosteroids' potassium-lowering effects are increased by diuretics
Cyclosporine	• Cyclosporine plus a diuretic can produce gout or renal toxicity. Avoid concurrent use, if possible
Digoxin	• Diuretics increase digoxin toxicity. Monitor potassium and magnesium concentrations
Insulin and oral hypoglycemics	• Insulin and oral hypoglycemics may have their hypoglycemic effects reduced by diuretics
Lithium	• Lithium plasma levels and toxicity can be increased by diuretics. Monitor lithium concentration
Neuromuscular blocking agents	• Diuretics increase neuromuscular blockade. Monitor neuromuscular status and potassium concentration and discontinue diuretic, if time allows
Nonsteroidal anti-inflammatory drugs	• NSAIDs may inhibit the diuretic and antihypertensive response to diuretics. Monitor BP, diuretic effect and sodium concentration
Phenytoin	• Phenytoin can decrease furosemide absorption and effect. Monitor diuretic effect
Probenecid	• Probenecid can decrease the effect of furosemide; avoid concurrent use, if possible. While diuresis is decreased by 1 g of probenecid daily, it may be increased by 2 g daily

Table 32.2
Isosorbide dinitrate: Drug interactions

Drug	Interaction
Diazoxide	• Diazoxide and isosorbide dinitrate can produce severe additive hypotension. Avoid concurrent use within 6 h

Drugs That Decrease Afterload

Angiotensin-Converting Enzyme Inhibitors (ACEIs) — Captopril (Capoten®), Enalapril (Vasotec®), Lisinopril (Prinivil®, Zestril®)

Mechanism of action and pharmacologic effects. Drugs that dilate precapillary resistance vessels (arterioles) are called vasodilators. By dilating precapillary resistance vessels, vasodilators decrease peripheral resistance (afterload) and increase cardiac output (see Figure 32.5).

Myocardial failure increases renin secretion by the kidneys. Renin is converted to angiotensin I which, in turn, is changed into angiotensin II by the angiotensin-converting enzyme (ACE). Angiotensin II has two major effects: it constricts

Figure 32.5
Consequences of reducing the systemic vascular resistance (SVR) on the cardiac output (CO) of the normal heart and the heart in failure

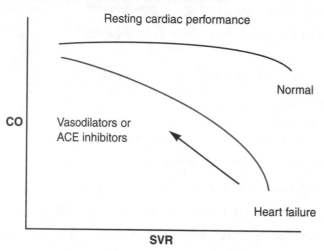

Source: Bristol-Myers Squibb. Reproduced with permission.

blood vessels and increases aldosterone secretion (Figure 32.6).

ACEIs block the conversion of angiotensin I to angiotensin II. By inhibiting the enzymatic conversion of angiotensin I to angiotensin II, ACEIs dilate arterioles and veins, reducing, respectively, afterload and preload. In addition, as presented in Figure 32.7, by decreasing aldosterone secretion, ACEIs reduce blood volume, further contributing to their ability to decrease preload.

Therapeutic uses. The therapeutic value of ACEIs can be attributed to their actions on both veins and arterioles. Venodilatation leads to a decrease in both right- and left-sided filling pressures. Arteriolar dilatation decreases peripheral resistance, leading to a reduction in afterload on the heart. The consequences of these effects include an improvement in cardiac output. ACEIs are effective in chronic CHF. Blood pressure often falls initially, but usually returns to a value not significantly below the pretreatment level, if the patient was not hypertensive.

The effects of ACEIs depend on the patient's salt balance. Sodium depletion activates the renin-angiotensin system and increases ACEI activity. Patients on high-dose diuretic therapy are most likely to experience a severe fall in blood pressure following the first dose(s) of the drugs. As a result, it is often recommended that diuretic therapy be

Figure 32.6
Contribution of the renin-angiotensin system to CHF

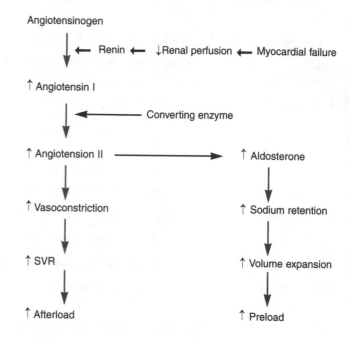

Figure 32.7
Effect of captopril on the renin-angiotensin-aldosterone system in CHF

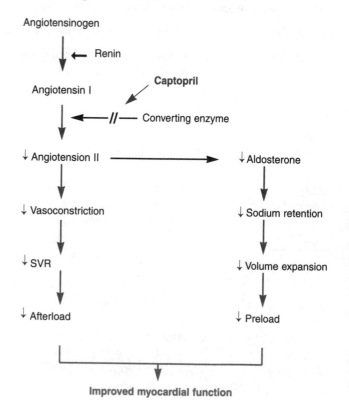

stopped a few days before starting an ACEI to minimize the initial hypotensive effects of the drugs.

Adverse effects. ACEIs are usually safe in normal doses, but they can produce hypotension. These drugs can also cause reversible deterioration of renal function in patients with pre-existing chronic renal disease or renal artery stenosis.

Captopril's adverse effects include loss of taste, proteinuria, dermatologic reactions and neutropenia. However, the likelihood of these effects' occurring is markedly reduced if the dose of the drug is kept at (or below) 150 mg/day. The presence of pre-existing renal disease also increases the risk for adverse effects.

Angioedema (0.2%) has been reported in patients treated with enalapril. Enalapril can cause pruritus or a rash, in addition to the hypotension referred to before.

Angioedema has also been reported in patients on lisinopril. In some patients with CHF who have normal or low blood pressure, additional lowering of blood pressure may occur with lisinopril. If hypotension occurs, a reduction of the dose or discontinuation of therapy should be considered. As previously suggested, agranulocytosis and bone marrow depression have been caused by ACEIs. Several cases of agranulocytosis and neutropenia have been reported in which a causal relationship to lisinopril cannot be excluded.

Table 32.3 lists the clinically significant drug interactions with ACEIs.

Nursing management. The nursing management of patients receiving ACEIs is described in Table 32.4 on the next page. Dosage details for individual drugs are given in Table 32.12 (pages 340–343).

Inotropic Drugs

Digoxin (Lanoxin®)

Mechanism of action and pharmacologic effects. Inotropic drugs increase myocardial contractility. Digoxin accomplishes this by increasing intracellular concentrations of calcium ions (Ca^{++}). Secondary to this ability, digoxin also decreases both heart rate and heart size in patients with CHF. Increased heart rate and size arise only as compensatory mechanisms to assist the organ to meet the blood flow needs of the tissues. Once

---

Table 32.3
Angiotensin-converting enzyme inhibitors (ACEIs): Drug interactions

Drug	Interaction
Allopurinol	• Possible increased susceptibility to Stevens-Johnson syndrome and hypersensitivity reactions with captopril. Avoid concurrent use, if possible, esp. in pts with renal failure
Azathioprine	• Azathioprine and an ACEI may cause anemia in renal transplant pts. Avoid concurrent use
Cimetidine	• Severe neuropathies with captopril. Monitor neurological function in pts with renal impairment
Diuretics	• Diuretics plus an ACEI can produce a powerful hypotensive effect in CHF pts. This can best be avoided by stopping the diuretic a few days before starting with low doses of the ACEI. Thereafter, it may be possible to reintroduce the diuretic and increase the dose of the ACEI. Diuretics plus ACEIs increase the risk for renal failure, especially in pts with bilateral renal artery stenosis. Monitor BP, renal function
Hypoglycemics, oral	• Increased hypoglycemic effect with captopril and enalapril. Monitor blood glucose
NSAIDs	• NSAIDs reduce the ability of ACEIs to dilate blood vessels
Potassium-sparing diuretics and potassium supplements	• Potassium-sparing diuretics (amiloride, triamterene, spironolactone) or potassium supplements can produce hyperkalemia when used with ACEIs, because ACEIs decrease aldosterone secretion and retain potassium

Table 32.4
Nursing management of the angiotensin-converting enzyme inhibitors (ACEIs)

Assessment of risk vs. benefit	Patient data	• Physician should determine drug dosage and indication. Safety not established in children. Baseline assessment of BP, pulse, electrolytes and CBC • *Pregnancy:* Risk category C (first trimester) and D (second and third trimesters). Human fetal risk has been demonstrated. In certain clinical situations, benefits may outweigh the risks
	Drug data	• May cause hypotension; use cautiously with other drugs that lower BP (e.g., diuretics) and during surgery. In sodium-depleted pts, a single dose of enalapril can substantially lower BP
Implementation	Rights of administration	• Using the "rights" helps prevent errors of administration
	Right route	• Most commonly given PO but may be given IV for acute situations
	Right time	• See Table 32.12. Dosage schedules among drugs in this class vary
	Nursing therapeutics	• Plan care to accommodate pt's level of energy. Encourage pt to maintain highest level of function by balancing activity and rest
	Patient/family teaching	• Pt's need for information may be influenced by length of time required for tx or limited by serious illness. Compliance and follow-up are essential factors in successful tx; review principles of pt education in Chapter 3 • For captopril, advise pt that changes in taste generally reverse within 8–12 weeks of tx • Teach precautions r/t hypotension (see Chapter 36) and instruct how to monitor own BP, if pt desires • Pts/families should know warning signs/symptoms of possible toxicities of drugs. Report immediately: rash, fever, sore throat, chest pain, irregular heartbeat, or swelling of face, eyes, lips, or tongue, especially difficulty breathing • Discuss dietary precautions regarding sodium and potassium • *Discuss possibility of pregnancy:* Advise pt to notify physician; discuss birth control methods
Outcomes	Monitoring of progress	*Continually monitor:* • *BP, P:* Sometimes dramatic drop in BP occurs with first dose; tx can continue with caution • Observe progress of CHF (i.e., edema, dyspnea, rales). Monitor white cell count and any signs/symptoms of neutropenia or agranulocytosis

digoxin improves contractility, and end-systolic and end-diastolic volumes decrease, the stimulus to heart enlargement disappears and it returns to a more normal size.

Similarly, the improved cardiac output of the digitalized heart removes the need for increased sympathetic stimulation. Vagal (parasympathetic) tone increases and the heart slows. Tissue perfusion is also improved because the reduction in sympathetic stimulation to the arterioles (precapillary resistance vessels) allows these vessels to dilate. Edema is reduced or eliminated because the improved cardiac output increases kidney perfusion and/or reduces pre-existing venous congestion.

Digoxin also influences the electrical activities of the heart, decreasing sympathetic stimulation to the organ and return normal vagal activity to the sinoatrial (S-A) and atrioventricular (A-V) nodes. This reduces impulse formation in the S-A node and decreases the conduction of electrical activity between the atria and ventricles. In higher therapeutic doses, digoxin also has a direct depressant effect on A-V conduction.

The delay in A-V conduction benefits the patient with atrial flutter or fibrillation. By reducing the speed at which impulses are transmitted to the ventricles, the ventricular rate of contraction is reduced. This allows more time for these chambers to fill, and cardiac efficiency is improved.

Not all electrical changes produced in the heart by digoxin benefit the patient. The drug can also produce an increase in conductivity and a decrease in the refractory period in the atria. As a result, atrial flutter can be converted to atrial fibrillation.

Greater toxic significance is attached to the actions of digoxin on the electrical activity of the ventricles. The drug reduces the resting potential of Purkinje cells and increases their automaticity while decreasing their refractory periods. When these actions are combined with a decrease in A-V conduction so that normal impulses from the atria have difficulty reaching the ventricles, the stage is set for one or more Purkinje cells to serve as ectopic pacemakers. This is seen with toxic doses of the drug.

Pharmacokinetics. Digoxin can be given intravenously or orally. Its action is relatively rapid, beginning within five to thirty minutes after intravenous injection and one to two hours after ingestion. Digoxin is excreted unchanged in the urine and has a half-life of about 1.5 days in patients with normal renal function. Digoxin's clearance varies directly with creatinine clearance, and its dosage must be reduced in proportion to a decrease in creatinine clearance. Elderly patients should be given reduced maintenance dosages of digoxin.

The toxic levels of digoxin are only two to three times higher than its therapeutically effective concentrations. In view of this, methods have been developed to measure the concentrations of the cardiac glycosides in the serum of patients. Most hospital laboratories have a rapid radioimmunoassay method for the measurement of serum digoxin. The therapeutic window usually falls between 0.5–2.0 nanograms/mL (1.0–2.6 nmol/L). This has been a great help in managing patients. As serum levels of digoxin approach 2.0 nanograms/mL (2.6 nmol/L), the physician is alerted to possible toxicities. Concentrations below 0.5 nanograms of digoxin per millilitre (1.0 nmol/L) of serum are usually ineffective. However, nurses should be aware that these values are only aids in the clinical management of the individual, and must be taken in context with the condition of the patient. Several clinical conditions, such as hypokalemia, hypothyroidism, age and myocardial infarction, can increase the actions of digoxin on the heart. In the final analysis, the physician's clinical judgment must serve as the basis for patient management.

Therapeutic uses. CHF is the major indication for the use of digoxin. The increased myocardial contractility improves cardiac output and tissue perfusion and reduces venous congestion. Patients with CHF due to coronary heart disease, hypertensive heart disease, aortic stenosis, aortic insufficiency, mitral insufficiency or congenital heart disease with left-to-right shunts respond better to digoxin than those with CHF due to cardiomyopathy or cor pulmonale.

Diuretics complement digoxin because they reduce blood volume and venous congestion. However, care must be taken to prevent hypokalemia. It is usually necessary to use a potassium-sparing diuretic with the thiazide, chlorthalidone, metolazone or loop diuretic, or to supplement the patient's diet with potassium.

Digoxin's place in the treatment of patients

with cardiac failure and atrial fibrillation is accepted. By slowing the ventricular rate, digoxin allows more time for filling. This action, combined with its inotropic effects, improves cardiac output and gives patients significant clinical benefits.

Digoxin's role in treating congestive heart failure patients with sinus rhythm is controversial. There is no evidence that the drug improves long-term survival in patients with cardiac failure. Because of its toxicities and the recent introduction of ACEIs in the treatment of heart failure, the use of digoxin in patients with CHF and normal sinus rhythm may well fall to third-line therapy, behind diuretics and ACEIs.

Because of its ability to increase A-V conduction time, digoxin is widely used in the treatment of supraventricular tachyarrhythmias. The most common use for the drug is the treatment of atrial fibrillation with a rapid ventricular response. By the same token, atrial flutter can also be managed by digoxin to produce a ventricular rate of 70–100 beats per minute.

Paroxysmal supraventricular tachycardia can also be treated with digoxin, provided that it can be established that digoxin is not the cause of the arrhythmia. Digoxin can often be successful in interrupting the re-entrant circuit in the Wolff-Parkinson-White syndrome. However, it is contraindicated in patients in whom the syndrome is associated with atrial fibrillation.

Adverse effects. The adverse effects of digoxin may be divided into those involving the heart and those occurring in other tissues. The toxic effects on the heart are due to alterations in electrical activity.

Digoxin can affect the atria, the A-V conduction system or the ventricles. Within the atria digoxin can cause a marked sinus bradycardia, due to withdrawal of sympathetic stimulation and reinsertion of parasympathetic (vagal) activity. In addition, digoxin can affect atrial rhythm. As a result of an increase in automaticity, premature beats or paroxysmal or nonparoxysmal atrial tachycardia may be seen. Mention has already been made of the fact that digoxin may convert atrial flutter to atrial fibrillation.

The effects of digoxin on A-V conduction have also been discussed. The impediment to the conduction of impulses from the atria to the ventricles may be either a beneficial or a toxic effect, depending on the condition of the patient. Obviously, patients with atrial flutter or fibrillation will benefit from some degree of A-V block. However, a complete heart block is a sign of impending digitalis intoxication. At this point, accelerated A-V junctional rhythms may be produced because of the ability of high levels of digoxin to increase the automaticity of this tissue. A-V junctional tachycardia can occur.

The most common ventricular rhythm disturbance caused by digitalis is premature ventricular depolarizations. These appear as coupled beats (bigeminy), with an ectopic beat following immediately upon the normal beat. The word ectopic can be defined as pertaining to a structure out of place. An ectopic beat, therefore, relates to a beat that emanates from an unusual site in the heart. Coupled beats can lead to trigeminy (i.e., the occurrence of three beats in rapid succession), ventricular tachycardia and ventricular fibrillation.

The toxic effects of digoxin on the heart are seen more often when high concentrations of the drug are present. However, they can also occur with normal, or even low levels of the drug, depending on the clinical condition of the patient.

Tolerance to digoxin is reduced in old age, renal insufficiency or hypothyroidism and following acute myocardial infarction, among other conditions. Patients who fall into one or more of these categories may experience toxic reactions to digoxin with relatively low doses of the drug.

In addition, hyperkalemia (high plasma potassium concentration) can increase the A-V block produced by digoxin, and hypokalemia (low plasma potassium concentration) can enhance the increase in automaticity of an ectopic pacemaker.

It is apparent from the discussion that digoxin can produce just about any kind of arrhythmia imaginable. Table 32.5 summarizes the frequency of various kinds of arrhythmias in patients bothered with digitalis-induced cardiac arrhythmias.

Physicians treat digoxin-induced tachyarrhythmias by first withdrawing the drug. Depending on the degree of intoxication, this may be all the treatment required. If potassium levels are low, potassium chloride may be given in divided doses totalling 50–80 mEq for adults (5–8 mEq/h), provided renal function is adequate. When correction of the arrhythmia is urgent, and the serum

Table 32.5
Frequency of cardiac arrhythmias in patients with digitalis intoxication

	% arrhythmias
Ventricular premature beats	33%
Ventricular tachycardia	8%
Nonparoxysmal A-V junctional tachycardia	17%
A-V junctional escape rhythms	12%
Atrial tachycardia with block	10%
Second- and third-degree A-V block	18%
S-A block with sinus arrest	2%

Source: Huffman DH. Clinical use of digitalis glycosides. *Am J Hosp Pharm* 1976;33:179–185. Reproduced with permission.

potassium concentration is low or normal, potassium is administered intravenously in 5% dextrose in water. A total of 40–100 mEq (30 mEq/500 mL) at a rate of 20 mEq/h may be given unless limited by pain due to local irritation. Additional amounts may be given if the arrhythmia is uncontrolled and the potassium well tolerated. Electrocardiographic monitoring is indicated to avoid potassium toxicity (e.g., peak of T-waves). Children must be given reduced doses of potassium chloride. Nurses are referred to detailed information on specific products for pediatric doses of potassium.

Potassium should not be used (and may be dangerous) for severe or complete heart block due to digoxin and unrelated to tachycardia. The electrocardiogram should be observed continuously so that the infusion may be stopped promptly when the desired effect is achieved.

Other agents that have been used in the treatment of digoxin intoxication include lidocaine, phenytoin, quinidine, procainamide and beta blockers. The three last-mentioned agents should be used with caution when A-V block is a component of digoxin intoxication because they may exaggerate this arrhythmic property.

Purified digoxin-specific antibody fragments (Fab fragments) bind with digoxin, and the resulting complex is excreted by the kidney. This approach to treating digoxin toxicity appears to be highly effective. For example, consider the case of a 20-month-old child who ingested about 40 digoxin tablets (0.25-mg strength) and had a serum digoxin of 13.6 ng/mL. This child was treated with IV digoxin-specific Fab fragments, after skin testing for allergy. Twelve hours later no digoxin was detectable. After two more days, the child was discharged.

The adverse effects of digoxin on tissues other than the heart involve primarily the gastrointestinal tract. Anorexia, nausea and vomiting represent some of the earliest signs of digitalis poisoning. Abdominal discomfort and diarrhea may also be seen. Neurological effects, including headache, fatigue, malaise and drowsiness, may be produced by digitalis. In addition, vision may also be blurred in some patients.

Table 32.6 on the next page lists the clinically significant drug interactions with digoxin.

Nursing management. The nursing management of patients receiving digoxin is described in Table 32.7 on page 335. Dosage details of individual drugs are given in Table 32.12 (pages 340–343).

Amrinone (Inocor®)

Mechanism of action and pharmacologic effects. Amrinone is a potent inotropic vasodilator. It inhibits the enzyme phosphodiesterase, thereby increasing the uptake of calcium by myocardial cells. This action likely accounts for its ability to increase myocardial contractility. It may also be the explanation for amrinone's ability to dilate vascular smooth muscle. Amrinone decreases both preload and afterload. It improves resting and exercise hemodynamics, increases left ventricular ejection fraction and improves ventricular capacity.

Therapeutic uses. Amrinone has been used in patients with severe chronic CHF not adequately controlled by digoxin, diuretics, antiarrhythmic drugs and vasodilators. The drug has also been used in patients with refractory acute heart failure due to myocardial infarction. If amrinone is used with hydralazine, patients experience greater improvement in resting hemodynamics and exercise tolerance than if either drug is used alone.

Adverse effects. Administration of amrinone has reduced platelet counts to 100×10^9 platelets/L (100 000 platelets/mm^3) in 2.4% of patients. Blood platelet counts should be

Table 32.6
Digoxin: Drug interactions

Drug	Interaction
Amiodarone	• Amiodarone increases digoxin serum concentrations
Antacids	• Antacids decrease digoxin absorption and reduce its effect. Give as far apart as possible; monitor digoxin levels
Calcium	• Calcium and digoxin have similar effects on the myocardium. Parenteral calcium has been reported to precipitate cardiac arrhythmias in pts receiving digoxin
Cholestyramine and colestipol	• These drugs bind digoxin in the intestine, decrease its absorption and reduce its effects. Give digoxin 30 min before either drug and monitor digoxin concentration
Cyclosporine	• Cyclosporine decreases renal clearance of digoxin and increases its toxicity. Monitor digoxin concentration
Diuretics	• With the exception of potassium-sparing diuretics, diuretics can cause hypokalemia and increase digoxin toxicity
Itraconazole	• Itraconazole can increase digoxin toxicity (mechanism not established). Monitor digoxin concentration
Methyldopa	• Methyldopa and digoxin can cause sinus bradycardia. Monitor heart rate
Metoclopramide	• Metoclopramide may decrease digoxin absorption
Penicillinamine	• Penicillinamine can decrease digoxin's effect (mechanism not established). Monitor digoxin concentration
Phenytoin	• Phenytoin can increase the metabolism and decrease the effect of digoxin. Monitor digoxin concentration
Propafenone	• Propafenone increases serum digoxin concentrations
Quinidine	• Quinidine can increase serum digoxin levels by reducing the renal and nonrenal clearance of the drug. GI disturbances and ventricular arrhythmias have occurred. Reduce digoxin dose by 50% before starting quinidine. Monitor pts carefully, esp. during first 5 days of combined tx. If quinidine is stopped, monitor pts for underdigitalization
Rifampin	• Rifampin can decrease serum digoxin concentration
Verapamil	• Verapamil can increase digoxin toxicity. Monitor digoxin concentration. Quinidine and verapamil may be synergistic in their effect on digoxin

determined before and during amrinone therapy. Clinically significant lowering of platelet counts to $\leq 50 \times 10^9$ platelets/L ($\leq 50\ 000$ platelets/mm^3) warrants discontinuation of amrinone therapy. Amrinone has been reported to produce fever and nephrogenic diabetes insipidus. Hepatotoxicity has occurred rarely.

Table 32.8 (page 336) lists the clinically significant drug interactions with amrinone.

Nursing management. The nursing management of the patient receiving amrinone is described in Table 32.9 (page 337). Dosage details of individual drugs are found in Table 32.12 (pages 340–343).

Dobutamine (Dobutrex®)

Dobutamine stimulates beta$_1$ receptors in the heart. In contrast to other sympathomimetics, it increases cardiac output with minimal effects on heart rate, thereby reducing myocardial oxygen requirements. Dobutamine does not produce renal vasodilatation, or increase glomerular filtration or sodium excretion.

Intravenous dobutamine is used for short-term therapy to increase cardiac output in patients with severe chronic cardiac failure.

Dobutamine's diverse effects include tachycardia, anginal pain, arrhythmias, headache and hypertension. Nausea and vomiting may also be seen.

Table 32.7
Nursing management of digoxin

Assessment of risk vs. benefit	Patient data	• Physician should determine drug dosage and indication. Obtain baseline assessment of weight, BP, P (apical and radial rate, rhythm and quality), electrolytes • *Pregnancy:* Risk category C (first trimester). Adverse effects have been demonstrated in animals; insufficient human data. In some clinical situations, benefits may outweigh risks
	Drug data	• Narrow tx range; doses must be calculated carefully and serum monitoring may be appropriate • Should not be used in A-V block • Dosage adjustment required in renal impairment and with elderly pts. Cautious use following MI
Implementation	Rights of administration	• Using the "rights" helps prevent errors of administration
	Right route	• Give IV, PO. Follow agency and manufacturer's instructions for direct IV administration
	Right time	• See Table 32.12
	Right technique	• Check agency policy and medical orders; may require monitoring apical pulse for 1 min prior to administration (see Monitoring of Progress, below)
	Nursing therapeutics	• Plan care to accommodate pt's level of energy. Encourage pt to maintain highest level of function by balancing activity and rest
	Patient/Family teaching	• Compliance and follow-up are essential factors in successful tx. Review principles of pt education in Chapter 3 • Discuss dietary precautions regarding sodium and potassium. Instruct pt to monitor pulse. Review both cardiac and noncardiac signs/symptoms of toxicity with pt/family. Remind pts not to use OTCs without advice of pharmacist or physician
Outcomes	Monitoring of progress	*Continually monitor:* • BP and P (rate, rhythm, quality). Monitor pulse for bigeminy and other dysrhythmias, including PVCs and A-V block. (*Note:* withholding drug for bradycardia alone, without other dysrhythmias or signs of toxicity, is often inappropriate and may only lead to inadequate blood levels.) • For progress of CHF (i.e., edema, dyspnea, rales, energy level) • For evidence of toxicity (incidence is reported as 11%–23% and mortality is as high as 39%). Watch for: anorexia, lethargy, visual disturbances, disorientation, blurred or yellow vision, dizziness, difficulty swallowing • *Serum blood levels:* Tx levels are reported as 1–2.6 nmol/L. Blood should be drawn at least 8 h after last dose or just prior to next dose

Table 32.8
Amrinone: Drug interactions

Drug	Interaction
Disopyramide	• Disopyramide and amrinone should be administered cautiously together until additional clinical experience is available

Dopamine (Dopastat®, Intropin®, Revimine®)

Dopamine exerts an inotropic effect on the myocardium, resulting in increased cardiac output through stimulation of beta cardiac receptors. Dopamine's use is usually not associated with a tachyarrhythmia. At low and intermediate therapeutic doses, dopamine usually increases systolic and pulse pressure with either no effect or a slight increase in diastolic pressure. Total peripheral resistance is usually unchanged. At higher doses dopamine causes alpha adrenergic stimulation.

Blood flow to peripheral vascular beds may decrease while mesenteric flow increases. As previously mentioned in Chapter 30, dopamine has been reported to dilate the renal vasculature by stimulating dopamine receptors. This action is accompanied by increases in glomerular filtration rate, renal blood flow and sodium excretion.

Table 32.10 lists the clinically significant drug interactions with dobutamine and dopamine.

Nursing management. The nursing management of the patient receiving dobutamine or dopamine is described in Table 32.11 (page 338). Dosage details for individual drugs are given in Table 32.12 (pages 340–343).

Approach to the Treatment of Congestive Heart Failure

A diuretic, to reduce preload, should be the first form of drug therapy in patients with CHF. Usually, the drug selected is hydrochlorothiazide, given in the morning or twice daily. If a stronger drug is required for more severe disease or in patients with renal insufficiency, furosemide is the agent of choice. The potassium-sparing diuretics spironolactone, triamterene or amiloride may be combined with the primary diuretic to reduce the risk of hypokalemia. If another drug is required to reduce preload further, isosorbide dinitrate may be given (40 mg four times daily).

If the symptoms of heart failure are not controlled adequately with diuretic therapy, either digoxin or an ACE inhibitor may be added. There appears to be little doubt as to the efficacy of digoxin in patients with atrial fibrillation. However, the role of the drug in patients with normal sinus rhythm is being questioned.

Angiotensin-converting enzyme inhibitors are particularly useful additions to diuretic therapy because they reduce both hyponatremia and urinary potassium loss. If an ACEI is used, however, the patient should not receive a potassium-sparing diuretic or potassium supplements. Failure to heed this advice can lead to significant hyperkalemia. Care should also be taken in starting an ACEI in patients previously receiving diuretic therapy. The physician may wish to reduce the dose of the diuretic or stop it two to three days before beginning ACEI treatment. In addition, it is recommended that the patient receive low doses of the ACEI initially. After the patient has demonstrated the ability to tolerate these doses, the physician can gradually increase the dose of the ACEI to meet the individual needs of the patient.

The treatment of CHF due to outflow obstruction is more complicated, because small reductions in ventricular filling pressures and aortic impedance can cause a major decrease in cardiac output. As a result, diuretics should be used with greater caution and afterload reduction is generally contraindicated. Furthermore, digoxin can worsen outflow obstruction in hypertrophic cardiomyopathy. Despite the lack of good data to support its efficacy, propranolol is generally used to reduce the number of anginal attacks and decrease syncope. Calcium channel blockers (nifedipine and verapamil) may offer another alternative. Nifedipine and propranolol reduce left ventricular outflow gradient.

Table 32.9
Nursing management of amrinone

Assessment of risk vs. benefit	Patient data	• Physician should determine drug dosage and indication. Assess for baseline readings of BP, P, body mass • *Pregnancy:* Risk category C (adverse effects have been demonstrated in animals; insufficient human data). In some clinical situations, benefits may outweigh risks
	Drug data	• May cause hypotension; use cautiously with other drugs that lower BP (e.g., diuretics) and during surgery • Known to cause allergic reactions; check hx for allergy to drug or bisulfites
Implementation	Rights of administration	• Using the "rights" helps prevent errors of administration
	Right route	• Give IV only. Follow agency policy for direct IV administration. Follow manufacturer's instructions for reconstitution for continuous infusion. Drug is compatible only with sodium chloride. Solution should be clear yellow; stable for 24 h. Use infusion pump to ensure accurate dosage
	Right time	• See Table 32.12
	Nursing therapeutics	• Plan care to accommodate pt's level of energy. Encourage pt to maintain highest level of function by balancing activity and rest
	Patient/family teaching	• Pt's need for information may be influenced by length of time required for tx or limited by serious illness • Pts/families should know warning signs/symptoms of possible toxicities of drug. Report immediately: dyspnea, chest pain, allergic reactions, easy bruising • Advise pt to change position slowly (dizziness may occur due to hypotensive effects)
Outcomes	Monitoring of progress	*Continually monitor:* • BP, P; fluid I/O, body mass, platelet count • Observe progress of CHF (i.e., edema, dyspnea, rales, activity tolerance)

Table 32.10
Dobutamine and dopamine: Drug interactions

Drug	Interaction
Antidepressants, tricyclic	• TCAs may potentiate the pressor responses to dobutamine and dopamine
Halogenated anesthetics	• Halogenated anesthetics increase cardiac autonomic irritability and sensitize the myocardium to the actions of dobutamine and dopamine
Monoamine oxidase inhibitors	• MAOIs reduce the rate of dobutamine and dopamine inactivation
Sympathomimetics	• Use dobutamine or dopamine cautiously in pts receiving sympathomimetics concomitantly

Table 32.11
Nursing management of dobutamine and dopamine

Assessment of risk vs. benefit	Patient data	• Physician should determine drug dosage and indication. Assess for baseline figures of BP, P, body mass
		• *Pregnancy:* Risk category C (adverse effects have been demonstrated in animals; insufficient human data). In some clinical situations, benefits may outweigh risks.
	Drug data	• May cause hypotension; use cautiously with other drugs that lower BP and during surgery
		• Known to cause allergic reactions; check hx for allergy to drug or bisulfites
Implementation	Rights of administration	• Using the "rights" helps prevent errors of administration
	Right route	• Give by IV only. Dopamine should be given in a large central line because of the dangers of tissue necrosis with extravasation. Follow manufacturer's instructions for reconstitution for continuous infusion. Solution is stable for 24 h. Use infusion pump to ensure accurate dosage
	Right dose	• See Table 32.12. A titration protocol chart is recommended for accurate dosage calculation
	Nursing therapeutics	• Plan care to accommodate pt's level of energy. Encourage pt to maintain highest level of function by balancing activity and rest
	Patient/family teaching	• Pt's need for information may be influenced by length of time required for tx or limited by serious illness
		• Pts/families should know warning signs/symptoms of possible toxicities of drug. Report immediately: dyspnea, chest pain, signs of allergic reactions, numbing, tingling or burning of extremities
Outcomes	Monitoring of progress	*Continually monitor:* • Cardiac function • BP, peripheral circulation (palpate peripheral pulses) • Fluid I/O; body mass

Acute heart failure is a medical emergency and is treated by drugs that decrease preload, reduce afterload and increase myocardial contractility. Parenteral furosemide is used to reduce preload in the treatment of acute heart failure associated with increased left ventricular end-diastolic pressure. Nitroprusside can be used to decrease afterload. Nitroprusside has been successful in the treatment of acute left ventricular failure due to hypertension. It decreases both peripheral resistance and pulmonary congestion.

As suggested earlier, the efficacy of digoxin to treat patients with acute heart failure and normal sinus rhythm is questionable. Dopamine and dobutamine are adrenergic drugs widely used for the patient with low cardiac output when left ventricular end-diastolic pressure is normal or increased. Low doses of dopamine (5 µg/kg/min) increase cardiac output and preserve renal blood flow, while producing only a small increase in peripheral resistance. Dobutamine is particularly valuable in treating heart failure without hypotension. If hypotension is present, dopamine may be preferred.

The place of amrinone must still be established. Although this drug is an effective inotrope, it can cause serious adverse effects (see earlier discussion).

Response to Clinical Challenge

Principles

Because of her age, Mrs. Gupta may excrete digoxin more slowly through her kidneys. She may be experiencing toxicity evidenced by atrial fibrillation, weakness, anorexia and bradycardia. Although her serum level is within norms, it is at the high end.

Digoxin has a narrow therapeutic margin and many patients experience serious side effects. The atrial fibrillation is a potentially serious dysrhythmia. The detection of toxicity depends on clinical observation as well as the serum drug level. The dose (0.25 mg) may be too high given her age.

Actions

• Monitor apical-radial rate.

• Check serum potassium level (both hypokalemia and hyperkalemia increase toxic effects of digoxin).

• Discuss observations and concerns with physician.

• Continue to monitor pulse (rate, rhythm, quality); inquire whether she is experiencing other signs/symptoms of toxicity.

Further Reading

Armstrong P, Moe G. Medical advances in the treatment of congestive heart failure. *Circulation* 1993;88(6): 2941–2951.

Drugs for chronic heart failure. *Medical Letter on Drugs and Therapeutics* 1993;35:40–42.

Drugs used for heart failure. *AMA Drug Evaluations Subscriptions* 1993 (Summer);1:7.1–7.18.

Gawlinski A, Jensen G. The complications of cardiovascular aging. *Am J Nurs* 1991;91(11):26–30.

McDonnell D. The use of central nervous system manisfestations in the early detection of digitalis toxicity. *Heart Lung* 1993;22:477–481.

Murphy T. Digoxin toxicity: ventricular dysrhythmias to watch for. *Am J Nurs* 1993;93(12):37–41.

Nagelhout JI. Pharmacologic treatment of heart failure. *Nurs Clin North Am* 1991;26:401–416.

Noll M. Advances in cardiovascular pharmacology. *J Cardiovasc Nurs* 1993;8(1):vi–vii.

Pahor M et al. The impact of age on risk of adverse drug reactions to digoxin. *J Clin Epidemiol* 1993;46(11):1805–1814.

Walthal S et al. Routine withholding of digitalis for heart rate below 60 beats per minute: widespread nursing misconceptions. *Heart Lung* 1993;22: 472–476.

Table 32.12
Treatment of congestive heart failure (CHF): Drug doses

Drug Generic name (Trade names)	Dosage	Nursing alert
A. Thiazide and Thiazide-Like Diuretics That Decrease Preload		
hydrochlorothiazide (Esidrix, HydroDIURIL)	**Oral:** *Adults:* 25–200 mg/day initially; mainte-nance, 25–100 mg/day. *Children:* 2 mg/kg/day in 2 divided doses	• May give with food or milk to reduce GI irritation • Usually given in a.m. to prevent nocturia. May crush tablets and mix with food/fluid • May interfere with some lab tests
chlorthalidone (Hygroton)	**Oral:** *Adults:* 50–100 mg/day	• Same as for hydrochlorothiazide
metolazone (Zaroxolyn)	**Oral:** *Adults:* 2.5–10 mg/day	• May give with food or milk to reduce GI irritation • Usually given in a.m. to prevent nocturia, but intermittent dose schedule may be required to control edema • Do not substitute or crush extended-release tablet
B. Loop Diuretics That Decrease Preload		
furosemide (Lasix)	**IV:** *Adults: 20–40 mg.* **Oral:** *Adults:* 40–80 mg; max., 200 mg/day	• May be given with food to reduce GI irrita-tion. May crush tablets and mix with food/fluid • Do not use discoloured solutions or tabs. Follow agency policy for intermittent infusion or direct IV administration. Use solution within 24 h
ethacrynic acid (Edecrin)	**IV:** *Adults:* 50 mg (0.5–1 mg/kg). **Oral:** *Adults:* Begin with 50 mg od pc and increase gradual-ly by 50 mg/day prn to 150–200 mg/day over 4 days. *Children:* Initially, 25 mg; increase by 25-mg increments until satisfactory response is obtained	• Same as for furosemide
bumetanide (Burinex, Bumex)	**Oral:** *Adults:* Usual total daily dosage is 0.5–2.0 mg, given as single dose. If neces-sary, a second or third dose may be given at 4- or 5-h intervals. Max. recommended daily dose, 10 mg. In pts with hepatic failure, keep dosage to a minimum — a maint. dose as low as 0.5 mg/day should be considered, and total daily dosage should not exceed 5 mg **IV:** *Adults* (for pulmonary edema): Initially, 0.5–1 mg. A second or third dose may be given at intervals of 2–3 h, but daily dose should not exceed 10 mg	• *Note potency:* 1 mg bumetanide equals 40 mg furosemide • May give with food. Follow agency policy for intermittent infusion or direct IV administration

Table 32.12 (continued)
Treatment of congestive heart failure (CHF): Drug doses

Drug Generic name (Trade names)	Dosage	Nursing alert
C. Vasodilators That Decrease Preload		
isosorbide dinitrate (Isordil, Sorbitrate)	**Oral:** Up to 40 mg qid	• Administer 1 h ac or 2 h pc with glass of water to enhance absorption. Do not crush extended-release tabs. *Chewable:* Should be chewed and held in mouth for 2 min before swallowing. *Sublingual:* Hold under tongue until dissolved
D. Vasodilators That Decrease Afterload (ACE Inhibitors)		
captopril (Capoten)	**Oral:** *Adults:* Initially, 6.25–12.5 mg tid. The dosage may be increased to a max. of 150 mg/day	• Food reduces absorption. Give 1 h ac or 2 h pc. Tabs may be crushed. Tabs may have a sulfur-like odour
enalapril (Vasotec)	**Oral:** *Adults:* Initially, 2.5 mg/day in 1 or 2 doses. Dosage can be increased gradually to a max. of 20 mg/day	• Diuretic tx should be discontinued (2–3 days) to avoid precipitous fall in BP
lisinopril (Prinivil, Zestril)	**Oral:** *Adults:* Initially, 2.5 mg/day. If required, increase gradually. Usual effective dosage range is 5–20 mg/day given od. Dosage titration should be performed over a 2- to 4-week period, or more rapidly if indicated by the presence of residual signs/symptoms of heart failure	• Monitor BP after first dose. May drop sharply, especially if a diuretic is also used
E. Inotropic Drugs digoxin (Lanoxin)	The following dosages are given to pts who have not received digitalis for at least 2 weeks. Smaller loading and maintenance doses should be used in small or elderly pts and in those with impaired renal function, electrolyte disturbances (particularly hypokalemia) or metabolic abnormalities (particularly hypothyroidism) **Oral:** *Adults:* Average digitalizing dose, 0.75–1.5 mg. For rapid digitalization: Initially, 0.5–0.75 mg, followed by 0.25–0.5 mg q6–8h until full digitalization is achieved. For slow digitalization and maintenance: 0.125–0.5 mg/day (0.125–0.25 mg in the elderly), depending on lean body mass and renal function as determined by creatinine clearance. Dose should be reduced as renal function decreases. Institution of maintenance tx without a loading dose is suitable for many pts with CHF	• **PO:** Give without regard to food. Separate from antacids by 2 h. May crush tabs • Narrow tx range: calculate doses carefully. Digoxin 0.25 mg tab = 0.2 mg liquid-filled cap • Monitor apical pulse for dysrhythmias, including bradycardia. Follow agency policy or medical orders for withholding dose if pulse is too low

(cont'd on next page)

Table 32.12 (continued)
Treatment of congestive heart failure (CHF): Drug doses

Drug Generic name (Trade names)	Dosage	Nursing alert
E. Inotropic Drugs (cont'd) digoxin (Lanoxin) (cont'd)	Tx serum levels are achieved after 6–7 days of maintenance tx in pts with normal renal function. Single daily doses are usually satisfactory for maintenance; however, it may be necessary to give 2 divided doses to some pts with recurrent supraventricular tachyarrhythmias *For infants and children,* the following digitalizing doses are given in divided amounts at 6-h intervals (to ensure adequate absorption, it may be desirable to initiate tx by the IV route and then substitute oral tx, with lower dose given first): *Premature infants,* 0.02–0.03 mg/kg; *full-term newborn infants,* 0.025–0.035 mg/kg; *1 month to 2 years,* 0.035–0.06 mg/kg; *2–5 years,* 0.03–0.04 mg/kg; *5–10 years,* 0.02–0.035 mg/kg; *> 10 years,* 0.01–0.015 mg/kg. Daily oral maint. dose is 20%–30% of the oral loading dose in premature infants and 25%–35% of the oral loading dose in full-term infants and children. More gradual digitalization can be accomplished by initiating tx with the appropriate maintenance dose **IV:** *Adults* (average digitalizing dose): 0.5–1 mg. Initially, 0.25–0.5 mg, followed by 0.25 mg, is given at 4- to 6-h intervals prn to a total dose of 1 mg. For maintenance, 0.125–0.5 mg daily *For infants and children,* the following digitalizing doses of the pediatric solution are given in divided amounts at 6-h intervals: *Premature infants,* 0.015–0.025 mg/kg; *full-term newborn infants,* 0.02–0.03 mg/kg; *1 month to 2 years,* 0.03–0.05 mg/kg; *2–5 years,* 0.025–0.035 mg/kg; *5–10 years,* 0.015–0.03 mg/kg. Daily IV maint. dose is 20%–30% of the oral loading dose in premature infants and 25%–30% of the oral loading dose in full-term infants and children	• **IV:** Follow agency policy for IV administration. Observe site carefully for extravasation; can damage tissues. Use pump to ensure accuracy. Monitor plasma levels. Administer diluted solution immediately. Do not use if solution has precipitate or is discoloured

Table 32.12 (continued)
Treatment of congestive heart failure (CHF): Drug doses

Drug Generic Name (Trade Names)	Dosage	Nursing Alert
E. Inotropic Drugs (cont'd)		
amrinone (Inocor)	**IV:** *Adults:* Initially, 0.75 mg/kg, given as bolus injection over 2–3 min. If needed, an additional bolus injection of 0.75 mg/kg may be given 30 min after initiation of tx. For maintenance, drug is infused at a rate of 5–10 µg/kg/min. Total daily dose should not exceed 10 mg/kg	• Monitor BP, HR, CVP (if available) during tx with amrinone • Follow agency policy for direct IV administration or continuous infusion. Use infusion pump to ensure accurate rate. Solution should be clear yellow
dobutamine HCl (Dobutrex)	Solution should be further diluted before administration to at least 50 mL (see manufacturer's literature for recommended diluents) and should be used within 24 h. Dobutamine is incompatible with alkaline solutions and should not be mixed with sodium bicarbonate injection **IV:** *Adults:* Rate of infusion required to increase cardiac output usually ranges from 2.5–10 µg/kg/min. Rarely, infusion rates up to 40 µg/kg/min may be required	• Solution may slightly pink. Follow agency policy for continuous infusion; use infusion pump to ensure accuracy. Administration protocols should be available for quick, accurate dosage calculations. Rate is titrated according to pt's response • Continuously monitor HR, BP
dopamine HCl (Dopastat, Intropin, Revimine)	Dopamine should be administered through a central venous line. Peripheral IV administration, even with a large-bore needle, should be avoided **IV:** *Adults:* A solution containing 400 µg/mL is prepared by diluting the contents of an ampule, vial or additive syringe with sterile sodium chloride injection or 5% dextrose injection. (This is a more dilute solution than that recommended by the manufacturer.) Initially, the dilute solution is infused at a rate of 2–5 µg/kg/min. In more seriously ill patients, an initial infusion rate of 5 µg/kg/min may be increased gradually to 5–10 µg/kg/min and, rarely, to 20–50 µg/kg/min. The urine output and electrocardiogram should be monitored closely during the infusion	• Same as for dobutamine • Discard yellow, brown or cloudy solutions

Drugs for the Treatment of Cardiac Arrhythmias

Topics Discussed
- Etiology of cardiac arrhythmias
- Pharmacologic approaches to treating tachyarrhythmias
- For each drug discussed: Mechanism of action, pharmacological effects, therapeutic uses, adverse effects
- Classification of antiarrhythmic drugs
- Nursing management

Drugs Discussed
adenosine (ad-**en**-oh-seen)
amiodarone (am-ee-**oh**-dah-rone)
bretylium (bree-**till**-ee-yum)
digoxin (dye-**jox**-in)
disopyramide (dye-soe-**peer**-ah-myde)
esmolol (**ez**-moe-lole)
flecainide (**flek**-ah-nyde)
lidocaine (**lye**-doe-kane)
mexiletine (mex-**ill**-eh-teen)
moricizine (more-**iss**-siz-een)
phenytoin (fen-ih-**toe**-in)
procainamide (proe-**kane**-ah-myde)
propafenone (proe-pah-**feen**-own)
propranolol (proe-**pran**-oh-lole)
quinidine (**kwin**-ih-deen)
sotalol (**soe**-tah-lole)
tocainide (toe-**kay**-nyde)
verapamil (ver-**ap**-ah-mil)

Clinical Challenge

Consider this clinical challenge as you read through this chapter. The response to the challenge appears on page 366.

Mr. W., aged 78, is admitted to the CCU for emergency treatment of ventricular dysrhythmia. Lidocaine is ordered. A loading dose is to be administered over 2–3 min, followed by an infusion of 1 mg/min.

1. Given Mr. W.'s age, what do you predict should be the loading dose?
2. Is the infusion dose within the recommended range?
3. Calculate the infusion rate to administer this dose.
4. What is the therapeutic plasma range? What signs/symptoms would indicate toxicity?

Etiology of Cardiac Arrhythmias

Cardiac arrhythmias — more appropriately called cardiac dysrythmias — are caused by disorders of rate, rhythm, origin or conduction within the heart. They may be produced by drugs, such as digoxin, or by cardiac disease. It has been estimated that between eighty and ninety percent of patients with myocardial infarcts have cardiac arrhythmias at some time during their hospital management. The significance of this becomes apparent when it is recognized that death following an infarct usually results from ventricular arrhythmias.

Cardiac tachyarrhythmias are the result of disorders of impulse formation, impulse conduction or both.

Disorders of Impulse Formation

The heart has many cells that have the potential to act as pacemakers. These cells, found in specialized conducting systems, such as the A-V node, the A-V bundle and the Purkinje network in the ventricles, depolarize spontaneously. This is the property of *automaticity*.

Although possessing the potential to act as ectopic pacemakers, these "latent pacemakers" do not usually trigger heartbeats. The S-A node is the most rapidly depolarizing tissue in the heart. Under normal circumstances it serves as the site for impulse formation. Once the S-A node reaches its threshold it sends an electrical wave throughout the heart, depolarizing all "latent pacemakers" before they have a chance to act as sites of impulse formation. If, however, the normal S-A pacemaker node is damaged, or the rate at which its impulses are conducted throughout the heart is reduced, a formerly latent pacemaker may reach its threshold potential and fire before a depolarization wave sweeps over it from the S-A node. If this happens, it becomes an ectopic site for impulse formation.

Disorders of Impulse Conduction

Disorders of impulse conduction are more often the cause of cardiac arrhythmias. A-V blocks or bundle branch blocks are obvious causes of abnormal heart rhythms and need little explanation. It is more difficult to explain the etiology of paroxysmal atrial tachycardia, A-V nodal tachycardias and ventricular tachycardias because they depend on the complex condition known as re-entry (Figure 33.1).

If a localized area of the heart is damaged by a myocardial infarct, the transmission of impulses along a portion of a normal conducting system may be blocked in one direction. In Figure 33.1, impulse

Figure 33.1
The phenomenon of re-entry

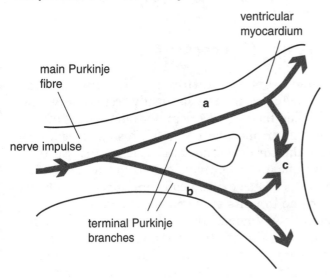

A. Impulse conduction with healthy myocardium

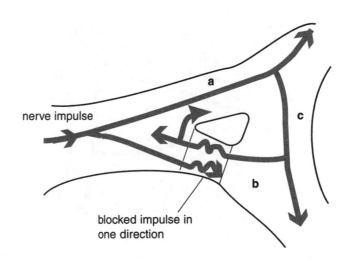

B. Impulse conduction impaired by myocardial infarct

transmission is blocked unidirectionally along pathway (b). As a result, the impulse that travels along (a) and (c) is allowed to come up (b) in a retrograde manner and re-enter (a) in the manner shown. This results in an extra heartbeat. If it happens at several sites, it can produce severe tachyarrhythmia leading to fibrillation.

Pharmacologic Approaches to Treating Tachyarrhythmias

Cardiac tachyarrhythmias can be treated by either (1) reducing the rate at which ectopic pacemakers depolarize or (2) modifying the conduction defects that lead to re-entry arrhythmias. Quinidine, procainamide, propranolol and phenytoin act by the first mechanism. These drugs decrease the rate of firing of ectopic pacemakers. As explained below, these drugs also modify impulse conduction.

Re-entry-mediated ectopic rhythms can be altered either by increasing conductivity in the damaged tissue, in effect overcoming the block, or by decreasing further the conduction velocity, thereby converting a unidirectional block to a bidirectional one. Lidocaine and phenytoin are claimed to increase conductivity through damaged tissue. Quinidine, procainamide and propranolol have the opposite effect. By decreasing conductivity, they convert a unidirectional block into a bidirectional

**Figure 33.2
Bidirectional block**

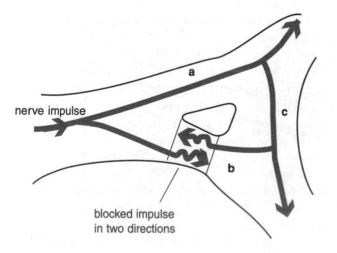

nerve impulse

blocked impulse
in two directions

one. A bidirectional block is depicted in Figure 33.2.

With the exception of digoxin and adenosine, antiarrhythmic drugs can be placed into one of four categories (see next section). Because the inotropic properties of digoxin were described in Chapter 32, only its antiarrhythmic effects will be described here. Because adenosine does not fit conveniently into one of the four major categories of antiarrhythmic drugs, it will also be discussed separately.

Digoxin (Lanoxin®)

Mechanism of action, pharmacologic effects and therapeutic uses. The complex actions of digoxin and the other cardiac glycosides have been explained in Chapter 32. As an antiarrhythmic drug, digoxin lengthens A-V nodal conduction time and functional refractory period. Many cardiologists consider digoxin the drug of choice to slow the ventricular response in patients with atrial fibrillation or flutter. Patients with stable, chronic atrial fibrillation usually respond better to digoxin than patients with unstable, acute atrial fibrillation. If digoxin proves unsatisfactory alone, it may be combined with propranolol or verapamil.

Generally, digoxin is contraindicated or given very cautiously in the presence of type I A-V block. Digoxin should also not be used as the only drug in Wolff-Parkinson-White patients because it can increase the ventricular response to atrial fibrillation or flutter.

Adenosine (Adenocard®)

Mechanism of action and pharmacologic effects. Adenosine is a naturally occurring purine nucleoside formed as a degradation product of adenosine triphosphate (ATP). This agent is a potent dilator of coronary arteries, and its antiadrenergic and negative chronotropic actions can decrease cardiac oxygen consumption. In the heart, adenosine inhibits sinus node automaticity and depresses A-V nodal conduction and refractoriness. Thus, adenosine is effective in terminating paroxysmal supraventricular tachycardic arrhythmias involving the A-V node in the re-entrant circuit. A-V re-entry, in which an accessory conduction

Table 33.1
Adenosine: Drug interactions

Drug	Interaction
Carbamazepine	• The effects of adenosine are prolonged in pts receiving carbamazepine
Dipyridamole	• Dipyridamole blocks adenosine uptake and potentiates its effects; a lower dose (25%) should be used in these pts
Theophylline	• Theophylline blocks the receptor responsible for adenosine actions and therefore, a larger dose of adenosine may be required to obtain the desired effect

pathway is present (e.g., Wolff-Parkinson-White syndrome), may also be involved. Adenosine will terminate the arrhythmia only if the arrhythmia is due to re-entry. The drug should not be used in atrial flutter, atrial fibrillation or atrial or ventricular tachycardias, as it may produce transient A-V or ventriculoatrial block.

Therapeutic uses. Adenosine is used as first-line therapy for acute termination of A-V nodal re-entrant tachycardia and other supraventricular tachycardias in which the re-entry loop involves the A-V node.

Adverse effects. Symptomatic adverse effects are common and include transient nausea, metallic taste, dyspnea, chest pain, ventricular ectopy, headache and flushing. The chest pain may resemble the pain of cardiac ischemia in patients with chronic stable angina or mimic that of duodenal ulcer.

Table 33.1 lists the clinically significant drug interactions with adenosine.

Classification of Antiarrhythmic Drugs

Antiarrhythmic drugs can be classified into one of four categories. These are summarized in Table 33.2 on the next page.

• Class I antiarrhythmic drugs act on receptors in the cardiac sodium channel to reduce sodium entry at the time the cell membrane rapidly depolarizes. As a result, these drugs decrease the rate of depolarization. In their presence, cells require a greater (more negative) potential before they can propagate an impulse to adjacent cells (i.e., they increase the threshold to impulse propagation).

Class I antiarrhythmic drugs also increase the repolarization time, decrease conduction velocity, prolong the effective refractory period and decrease automaticity.

• Class II antiarrhythmic drugs are beta blockers (see Chapter 30). Because these agents competitively block beta adrenergic receptors, they inhibit sympathetic stimulation of cardiac beta receptors.

• Class III antiarrhythmic drugs prolong the duration of cardiac action potential without changing the rate at which fibres depolarize.

• Class IV antiarrhythmic drugs block the slow inward calcium current occurring in rapid depolarization and the early stages of repolarization (phase 2).

Class IA: Quinidine, Procainamide, Disopyramide

Mechanism of action and pharmacologic effects. Quinidine, procainamide and disopyramide reduce the maximal rate of depolarization. They increase the threshold for excitation, depress conduction velocity and prolong the effective refractory period in the atrial, His-bundle, and ventricular conducting systems. These drugs also exert a direct anticholinergic (atropine-like) effect on the muscarinic receptors of the heart (see Chapter 28).

Therapeutic uses and adverse effects. Quinidine is used to treat both atrial and ventricular arrhythmias. It has been used to maintain sinus rhythm after cardioversion in supraventricular arrhythmias. The drug is also often used with digoxin to treat atrial fibrillation. Because quinidine has an atropinic action, it increases A-V con-

Table 33.2
Classification of the antiarrhythmics (antidysrhythmics)

Class/Action	Drugs	Use
IA • Reduce rate of depolarization • Increase threshold to stimulation • Depress conduction rate • Prolong refractory period in the atrial, His-bundle, and ventricular systems	Quinidine Procainamide (Pronestyl®) Disopyramide (Norpace®, Rhythmodan®)	• Decrease ectopic impulse formation • Treat atrial and ventricular arrhythmias
IB • Lengthen effective refractory period only in the ventricular conduction system	Lidocaine (Xylocaine®) Mexiletine (Mexitil®) Phenytoin (Dilantin®) Tocainide (Tonocard®)	• Treat ventricular arrhythmias
IC • Reduce membrane responsiveness	Flecainide (Tambocor®) Moricizine (Ethmozine®) Propafenone (Rythmol®)	• Treat ventricular tachyarrythmias
Class II • Block beta receptors	Propranolol (Inderal®)	• Treat catecholamine-induced arrhythmias, digitalis arrhythmias, atrial fibrillation and paroxysmal atrial tachycardia
Class III • Increase refractory period in atrial, A-V nodal, His-Purkinje and ventricles	Amiodarone (Cordarone®)	• Treat ventricular arrhythmias not responsive to first-line agents
Class IV • Block calcium channels • Depress A-V conduction	Verapamil (Calan®, Isoptin®)	• Treat supraventricular tachyarrhythmias and A-V re-entrant tachycardia

duction. Digoxin, on the other hand, decreases A-V conduction. By combining the two drugs, the physician can slow the atria with quinidine and reduce A-V conduction with digoxin.

Quinidine's toxicities are usually dose related. At plasma concentrations above 8 µg/mL the direct depressant effects on A-V conduction appear and the QRS complex widens. As the concentration rises, S-A block or arrest, high-grade A-V block, ventricular arrhythmias or asystole may occur. These effects can also be produced by small amounts of quinidine in individuals allergic to the drug, or in patients with congestive heart failure or renal impairment. The other adverse effects of quinidine include diarrhea, nausea and vomiting, headache, vertigo, palpitations, tinnitus and visual disturbances.

Gastrointestinal symptoms are the most common adverse reactions. They occur even when drug concentrations in the plasma are low. This type of adverse reaction is apparent almost immediately after quinidine is started, and in some cases forces early discontinuation of the drug. The central and peripheral nervous systems are rarely affected.

Table 33.3 lists the clinically significant drug interactions with quinidine.

Procainamide (Pronestyl®, Procan®) has essentially the same therapeutic effects and clinical indications as quinidine. In contrast to quinidine, procainamide has little atropinic action. It is used mainly for the treatment of ventricular arrhythmias. Procainamide is also employed in the treatment of atrial fibrillation and paroxysmal supraventricular tachycardias. Effective

Table 33.3
Quinidine: Drug interactions

Drug	Interaction
Acetylsalicylic acid	• ASA can produce bleeding in pts receiving quinidine. Avoid concurrent use
Amiodarone	• Amiodarone can increase quinidine toxicity. Monitor quinidine concentration
Antacids	• Antacids may decrease the renal excretion of quinidine and increase its toxicity. Monitor quinidine concentration
Anticholinergics	• Anticholinergics have additive anticholinergic effects with quinidine
Anticoagulants, oral	• Oral anticoagulants may show increased activity, because quinidine depresses the formation of prothrombin and inhibits the synthesis of vitamin K-sensitive clotting factors
Beta blockers	• Ophthalmic timolol can increase bradycardia. Use a cardioselective ophthalmic beta blocker. Metoprolol can decrease quinidine metabolism. Monitor metoprolol concentration or cardiac status
Cimetidine	• Cimetidine can increase quinidine toxicity. Monitor quinidine concentration
Dextromethorphan	• Quinidine can decrease the metabolism of dextromethorphan and increase its toxicity. Avoid concurrent use
Digoxin	• Quinidine can reduce the excretion and tissue binding of digoxin, leading to possible digoxin toxicity. Digoxin concentration may not correlate with cardiac effects. Reduce digoxin dose by 50% before starting quinidine. Monitor pts carefully, particularly during the initial 5 days of combined tx. If quinidine is discontinued, pts should be monitored for underdigitalization
Flecainide	• Quinidine may decrease the metabolism of flecainide, leading to flecainide toxicity. Monitor flecainide concentration or ECG
Haloperidol	• Quinidine may increase the effects of haloperidol. Monitor clinical status or haloperidol concentration
Metoclopramide	• Metoclopramide may decrease the effect of sustained-release quinidine preparations. Monitor quinidine concentrations
Neuromuscular blocking drugs	• Quinidine can additively increase the activity of neuromuscular blocking drugs. Use with caution
Phenytoin	• Phenytoin can increase the metabolism and decrease the effect of quinidine. Monitor quinidine concentration
Potassium	• Quinidine's activity is increased by hyperkalemia and decreased by hypokalemia
Primidone	• Primidone can increase the metabolism and decrease the effect of quinidine. Monitor quinidine concentrations
Rifampin	• Rifampin increases the metabolism and decreases the effect of quinidine. Monitor quinidine concentrations
Verapamil	• IV verapamil can produce hypotension with quinidine. Avoid concurrent use

therapeutic blood levels of procainamide lie between 4–8 µg/mL. Hypersensitivity to procainamide is an absolute contraindication to its use; thus, cross-sensitivity to procaine and related drugs must be borne in mind. Procainamide should not be administered to patients with complete A-V heart block. It is also contraindicated in cases of second-degree and third-degree A-V block unless an electric pacemaker is operative. Procainamide may also be contraindicated in patients with myasthenia gravis.

Procainamide may cause less anorexia, nausea and vomiting than quinidine. A reversible lupus erythematosus-like syndrome may result from its use. Both procainamide and its active metabolite N-acetylprocainamide are eliminated by the

Table 33.4
Procainamide: Drug interactions

Drug	Interaction
Amiodarone	• Amiodarone can increase procainamide toxicity. Monitor procainamide concentration
Beta blockers	• The cardiac depressant action of beta blockers is potentiated in pts with acute MI by the prior administration of procainamide
Cholinergic drugs	• Cholinergics may antagonize the anticholinergic activity of procainamide
Cimetidine	• Cimetidine decreases the renal excretion and increases the toxicity of procainamide. Monitor procainamide concentration
Ranitidine	• Ranitidine decreases both the absorption and renal excretion of procainamide. This can result in either an increase in procainamide toxicity or a decrease in its effects. Monitor procainamide concentration
Trimethoprim	• Trimethoprim may decrease the renal clearance of procainamide and increase its toxicity. Monitor procainamide concentration

kidneys and will accumulate in patients with renal impairment unless lower doses are given. Unless the serum concentrations of procainamide can be measured, it is better not to use the drug in end-stage renal failure. Granulocytopenia may follow the use of procainamide.

Table 33.4 lists the clinically significant drug interactions with procainamide.

Disopyramide (Norpace®, Rythmodan®) has actions similar to those of quinidine. Some clinicians believe this drug should be reserved for patients who are not in heart failure and who cannot tolerate quinidine or procainamide.

Disopyramide is eliminated by both hepatic metabolism and renal excretion. Its dosage should be reduced in patients with liver or kidney impairment. The drug is contraindicated in the presence of shock, renal failure, severe intraventricular conduction defects, pre-existing second- and third-degree A-V block (if no pacemaker is present) or known hypersensitivity to the drug. It should not be used in the presence of uncompensated or inadequately compensated congestive heart failure because it can worsen CHF. Severe hypotension occurring after disopyramide administration has been observed, usually in patients with primary myocardial disease (cardiomyopathy) and in patients with inadequately compensated CHF or advanced myocardial disease with low output state.

Other adverse effects of disopyramide include heart block, ventricular fibrillation, and tachy-arrhythmias. Its pronounced anticholinergic effects are often marked, and the drug is contraindicated in most patients with glaucoma or in those with urinary retention (treatment must often be stopped because of this latter effect).

Table 33.5 lists the clinically significant drug interactions with disopyramide.

Class IB: Lidocaine, Mexiletine, Phenytoin, Tocainide

Mechanism of action and pharmacologic effects. Similar to the drugs in Class IA, lidocaine, mexiletine, phenytoin and tocainide decrease conduction. However, in contrast to the Class IA drugs — which lengthen the effective refractory period in the atrial, His-bundle and ventricular conducting systems — Class IB agents lengthen the effective refractory period only in the ventricular conducting system. As a result, Class IB drugs cannot be used to treat atrial arrhythmias.

Therapeutic uses and adverse effects. Lidocaine (Xylocaine®) depresses automaticity in the ventricles. It has little effect on the atria and, in usual doses, does not depress myocardial contractility. It is used for the immediate control of ventricular premature extrasystoles and ventricular tachycardia. Ventricular arrhythmias secondary to cardiac surgery, cardiac catheterization, acute myocardial infarction and electrical conversion are treated with lidocaine. Although phenytoin is preferred, lidocaine can be used to treat digitalis-induced arrhythmias.

Table 33.5
Disopyramide: Drug interactions

Drug	Interaction
Anticoagulants, oral	• Conflicting reports suggest that disopyramide decreases the metabolism and increases the effects of oral anticoagulants. Avoid concurrent use, if possible
Beta blockers	• Disopyramide and beta blockers have additive effects on myocardial contractility. This can lead to cardiac failure. Monitor cardiac status
Erythromycin	• Erythromycin can increase disopyramide toxicity, probably as a result of decreased disopyramide metabolism. Avoid concurrent use
Phenytoin	• Phenytoin increases the concentration of a toxic metabolite of disopyramide, thereby both decreasing disopyramide's effect and increasing its toxicity. Avoid concurrent use, if possible
Rifampin	• Rifampin decreases disopyramide's effect, probably due to increased metabolism. Avoid concurrent use, if possible

The serum therapeutic window for lidocaine is 1–5 µg/mL (4.3–21.3 µmol/L). Serum levels below 1 µg/mL (4.3 µmol/L) are usually ineffective. Lidocaine concentrations in serum above 5 µg/mL (21.3 µmol/L) usually herald the start of central nervous system depression, stimulation or seizures.

Lidocaine's major toxicities involve the central nervous and cardiovascular systems. Patients may experience drowsiness, paresthesias, muscle twitching, convulsions, coma, respiratory depression and depressed myocardial contractility. Lidocaine is rapidly metabolized. Patients with hepatic insufficiency and those over the age of seventy should, as a rule, receive half to two-thirds the usual loading dose, and lower than normal maintenance doses.

Lidocaine is contraindicated in patients with known hypersensitivity to local anesthetics of the amide type; Adams-Stokes syndrome; or severe degrees of S-A, A-V or intraventricular block. It should be used with caution in patients with bradycardia or severe digoxin intoxication. Constant ECG monitoring is essential for the proper administration of lidocaine. Signs of excess depression of cardiac contractility (e.g., prolongation of P-R interval, QRS complex, aggravation of arrhythmias) should signal prompt cessation of the intravenous injection.

Table 33.6 lists the clinically significant drug interactions with lidocaine.

Mexiletine (Mexitil®) is similar in structure and activity to lidocaine. Given orally, mexiletine is used to treat or prevent ventricular ectopy and tachycardia. The drug is also used to suppress ventricular arrhythmias in survivors of acute myocardial infarction following therapy with lidocaine. Mexiletine may be as effective as procainamide and better tolerated. It appears to be less effective in patients with long-standing refractory ventricular arrhythmias. The concomitant use of propranolol may allow for a lower dose of mexiletine and better arrhythmia control.

Mexiletine's cardiovascular toxicities include sinus bradycardia or tachycardia, atrial fibrillation, hypotension, dyspnea and ventricular tachyarrhythmias, including torsade de pointes.

Table 33.6
Lidocaine: Drug interactions

Drug	Interaction
Beta blockers	• Beta blockers decrease the metabolism and increase the toxicity of lidocaine. Monitor lidocaine concentrations
Cimetidine	• Cimetidine may decrease lidocaine clearance
Propafenone	• Propafenone may have additive CNS toxicity with lidocaine. Monitor clinical status

Table 33.7
Mexiletine: Drug interactions

Drug	Interaction
Metoclopramide	• Metoclopramide may increase the rate of absorption of mexiletine
Narcotics	• Narcotics can slow the rate of absorption of mexiletine
Phenytoin	• Phenytoin increases the metabolism and decreases the effect of mexiletine. Monitor mexiletine concentration
Rifampin	• Rifampin increases the metabolism and decreases the effect of mexiletine. Monitor mexiletine concentration
Tobacco (smoking)	• Tobacco smoking may increase the metabolism and decrease the effect of mexiletine. Monitor mexiletine concentration

Mexiletine is contraindicated in the presence of second- or third-degree A-V block in the absence of a pacemaker. It is also contraindicated in cardiogenic shock. The drug should be used with caution in patients with hypotension or CHF because of its potential for depression of myocardial contractility. Caution should also be exercised when mexiletine is used in patients with severe first-degree A-V block or intraventricular conduction abnormalities. If the drug is given to a patient with the sick sinus syndrome, severe bradycardia and prolongation of sinus node recovery time may occur. Patients with severe bradyarrhythmias should not be given mexiletine. The extracardiac adverse reactions attributed to mexiletine include nausea, vomiting, malaise, dizziness, tremor, diplopia, paresthesias, confusion and ataxia.

Table 33.7 lists the clinically significant drug interactions with mexiletine.

Phenytoin (Dilantin®) depresses spontaneous atrial and ventricular automaticity without altering intraventricular conduction. It may also increase conduction through damaged Purkinje fibres. The drug is used mainly to reverse digitalis-induced arrhythmias.

The adverse effects of phenytoin include fatigue, dizziness, ataxia, nausea, vomiting, pruritus and rashes. If the drug is given rapidly intravenously, it can cause a slowing of the heart rate, myocardial depression, hypotension, reduction in A-V conduction and, very occasionally, cardiac arrest. Phenytoin is contraindicated in sinus bradycardia, S-A block, second- and third-degree A-V block and Adams-Stokes syndrome.

Phenytoin interacts with many drugs. These interactions are given in Table 49.2 (page 575).

Tocainide (Tonocard®) is structurally related to lidocaine and has similar electrophysiologic properties. In therapeutic doses, tocainide decreases the effective refractory period of the atrium, A-V node and right ventricle without affecting A-V conduction. Tocainide does not alter heart rate. Peripheral and pulmonary vascular resistance may increase slightly.

Tocainide is indicated only for the treatment of symptomatic ventricular arrhythmias in patients not responding to other therapy, or when other therapy was not tolerated. Tocainide should be used with caution in patients with heart failure or with minimal cardiac reserve because of the potential for aggravating the degree of heart failure. It should also be used with caution in patients who are receiving beta blockers or other antiarrhythmics, or both.

Nausea and tremor are the most common adverse effects of tocainide. It can also cause anorexia, vomiting, abdominal pain and constipation. Tocainide's other adverse effects include dizziness, lightheadedness, confusion, anxiety and paresthesias. The drug can also cause hypotension, bradycardia, palpitations, chest pain, conduction disturbances and left ventricular failure. Reports of hematological disorders, including leukopenia, agranulocytosis, bone marrow depression, hypoplastic anemia and thrombocytopenia, have caused concern with its use.

Table 33.8 lists the clinically significant drug interactions with tocainide.

Table 33.8
Tocainide: Drug interactions

Drug	Interaction
Cimetidine	• Cimetidine can possibly decrease tocainide absorption and decrease its effect. Monitor tocainide concentration. Ranitidine does not appear to interact
Rifampin	• Rifampin can increase the metabolism and decrease the effect of tocainide. Monitor tocainide concentration

Class IC: Flecainide, Moricizine, Propafenone

Mechanism of action and pharmacologic effects. Drugs in Class IC depress the rate of rise of the membrane action potential. They have minimal effects on the duration of the membrane action potential and on the effective refractory period of ventricular myocardial cells.

Therapeutic uses and adverse effects. Flecainide acetate (Tambocor®) depresses sinus node automaticity, prolongs conduction (particularly in the His-Purkinje system and ventricles) and increases ventricular refractoriness. Flecainide is rapidly absorbed from the gastrointestinal tract: peak plasma levels are attained in three hours. Its bioavailability is not affected by food. When given in multiple doses, the drug has a half-life of twenty hours. Its half-life is increased in patients with CHF or renal failure. Flecainide is indicated for the treatment of documented ventricular arrhythmias, such as sustained ventricular tachycardia, that are judged life-threatening. Because of the proarrhythmic effects of flecainide, the drug should be reserved for patients in whom the benefits of treatment are believed to outweigh the risks.

In postmyocardial infarction patients, flecainide was found to be associated with a 5.1% mortality rate and nonfatal cardiac arrest. The most serious adverse reactions reported with flecainide were new or exacerbated ventricular arrhythmias, which occurred in 6.8% of patients, and new or worsened CHF, which occurred in 3.9% of patients. The adverse effects of flecainide include blurred vision and dizziness. Flecainide may also cause headache, nausea, fatigue, nervousness, tremor and paresthesias.

Table 33.9 lists the clinically significant drug interactions with flecainide.

Moricizine (Ethmozine®), like other Class I antiarrhythmic drugs, reduces the fast inward sodium current of the action potential. It does not readily fit into any of the subclasses of sodium channel blocking drugs and has proven difficult to subclassify within the Class I antiarrhythmic agents.

Table 33.9
Flecainide: Drug interactions

Drug	Interaction
Amiodarone	• Amiodarone can possibly increase the toxicity of flecainide (mechanism not established). Monitor flecainide concentration
Beta blockers	• Beta blockers produce an additive decrease in cardiac contractility with flecainide. Monitor CV status
Digoxin	• Flecainide can increase the serum levels of digoxin
Quinidine	• Quinidine may decrease the metabolism and possibly increase the toxicity of flecainide. Monitor flecainide concentration and ECG
Verapamil	• Verapamil and flecainide have additive effects on conduction and contractility. Their use together can lead to asystole and cardiogenic shock. Monitor ECG and CV status

Table 33.10
Moricizine: Drug interactions

Drug	Interaction
Cimetidine	• Cimetidine may decrease the metabolism and increase the toxicity of moricizine. Monitor moricizine concentrations
Theophylline	• Moricizine may increase the metabolism and decrease the effect of theophylline. Monitor theophylline concentration

In patients with impaired left ventricular function, moricizine has minimal effects on measurements of cardiac performance such as cardiac index, stroke volume index, pulmonary capillary wedge pressure, and systemic or pulmonary vascular resistance or ejection fraction, either at rest or during exercise. A small but consistent increase occurs in resting blood pressure and heart rate. Exercise tolerance in patients with ventricular arrhythmias is not affected. In those with a history of heart failure or angina pectoris, exercise duration and rate-pressure product with maximal exercise are unchanged during administration. Nevertheless, worsened heart failure has been attributed to use of moricizine in some patients with severe underlying disease.

Moricizine is used to suppress life-threatening ventricular arrhythmias; it has been reported to be more effective than disopyramide or low doses of propranolol, but less effective than flecainide, in suppressing premature ventricular complexes. In one study, moricizine did not improve the survival rate and increased the incidence of adverse events in patients following myocardial infarction. Moricizine is more effective in preventing recurrences of nonsustained than sustained ventricular tachycardia. However, the drug has limited efficacy and carries considerable risk of inducing life-threatening proarrhythmias in patients with serious ventricular arrhythmias and inducible sustained tachycardia.

The cardiovascular adverse effects of moricizine include worsening of arrhythmias, conduction disturbances and heart failure. Nausea and dizziness sufficient to discontinue the drug have been reported. In a few patients drug-related fever, elevation of serum aminotransferase or bilirubin, or thrombocytopenia have been detected. The discontinuation of the moricizine phase of the cardiac arrhythmic suppression trial (CAST) study due to a lack of benefit emphasizes that physicians should use moricizine only after a careful evaluation of the potential benefits and risks.

Table 33.10 lists the clinically significant interactions with moricizine.

Propafenone (Rythmol®) slows atrial, ventricular, A-V node, His-Purkinje and accessory pathway conduction. The drug can be used orally for the suppression of the following ventricular arrhythmias when they occur singly or in combination: episodes of ventricular tachycardia; premature (ectopic) ventricular contractions, such as premature ventricular beats of unifocal or multifocal origin; couplets; R on T phenomenon, when of sufficient severity to require treatment.

Propafenone's adverse effects include worsening of congestive heart failure, A-V and intraventricular conduction disturbances and ventricular arrhythmias. The drug can also cause nausea, diarrhea, constipation, paresthesias and taste disturbances.

Table 33.11 lists the clinically significant drug interactions with propafenone.

Class II: Beta Blockers

Mechanism of action and pharmacologic effects. By blocking $beta_1$ receptors in the heart, beta blockers reduce cardiac output, diminish myocardial oxygen requirements and prevent cardiac arrhythmias, particularly those caused by increased sympathetic activity. The cardiac effects of beta blockade include bradycardia, decreased contractility, increased A-V conduction time and reduced automaticity.

Therapeutic uses. Propranolol (Inderal®) and acebutolol (Monitan®, Sectral®) are indicated for

Table 33.11
Propafenone: Drug interactions

Drug	Interaction
Anticoagulants, oral	• Propafenone can increase the effect of warfarin, probably by reducing its metabolism. Monitor prothrombin time
Beta blockers	• Propafenone can decrease the elimination and increase the plasma levels of propranolol and metoprolol. A reduction in beta blocker dosage may be necessary. Monitor clinical status
Cimetidine	• Cimetidine can increase propafenone plasma levels. Monitor plasma concentrations of propafenone and clinical status
Digoxin	• Propafenone may increase the serum levels and toxicity of digoxin (mechanism not established). Monitor digoxin concentration
Lidocaine	• Propafenone can increase the CNS toxicity of lidocaine. Monitor clinical status

the treatment of arrhythmias. Beta blocker treatment is best suited for catecholamine-induced arrhythmias. Propranolol is also used for atrial flutter and fibrillation, paroxysmal atrial tachycardia and digitalis-induced arrhythmias.

Esmolol (Brevibloc®) is a beta$_1$ cardioselective beta blocker. Higher doses will block beta$_2$ receptors. Esmolol is administered only intravenously. It has a rapid onset and a short duration of action. This drug is indicated in the perioperative management of tachycardia and hypertension in patients in whom there is a concern for compromised myocardial oxygen balance and who, in the judgment of the physician, are clearly at risk for developing hemodynamically induced myocardial ischemia. Esmolol is also indicated for the rapid control of ventricular rate in patients with atrial fibrillation or atrial flutter in acute situations when the use of a short-acting agent is desirable.

Metoprolol, propranolol and timolol are used prophylactically after myocardial infarction to reduce the incidence of sudden death.

Adverse effects. The major adverse effects of these drugs are bradycardia, CHF, cardiac arrest (in patients with A-V block) and bronchospasm. Beta blockers can precipitate heart failure in patients with heart disease. They are contraindicated in bronchospasm, including bronchial asthma, and allergic rhinitis during the pollen season; sinus bradycardia and greater than first-degree block; cardiogenic shock; right ventricular failure secondary to pulmonary hypertension; and congestive heart failure unless the failure is secondary to

a tachyarrhythmia treatable with a beta blocker. Chronic occlusive peripheral vascular disease is a relative contraindication to the use of nonselective beta blockers.

Sudden withdrawal of a beta blocker in patients with angina pectoris can precipitate worsening of angina, cardiac arrhythmias and acute myocardial infarction.

The drug interactions for beta blockers are presented in Table 30.4 (page 299).

Class III: Amiodarone, Bretylium, Sotalol

Mechanism of action and pharmacologic effects. The drugs in Class III possess diverse pharmacologic properties. However, they all share the capacity to prolong the duration of action potentials and refractoriness in the Purkinje and ventricular muscle fibres. All these drugs have significant interactions with the autonomic nervous system.

Therapeutic uses and adverse effects. Amiodarone (Cordarone®) possesses the basic pharmacologic properties of Class III antiarrhythmic drugs as presented above. It also depresses sinus node automaticity and slows conduction in the atria, A-V node, His-Purkinje system and ventricles. The prominent effect seen after acute intravenous administration of amiodarone is slow conduction and prolonged refractoriness of the A-V node. The drug may also have a marked negative inotropic effect following acute intravenous administration.

Amiodarone has the potential for serious toxicity. Because of this, and the substantial management difficulties associated with its use, the drug is indicated for treatment of patients with life-threatening cardiac arrhythmias (e.g., ventricular tachycardia, ventricular fibrillation) that are refractory to other treatment.

Amiodarone is contraindicated in severe sinus node dysfunctions, sinus bradycardia, and second- and third-degree A-V block. It is also contraindicated in patients with episodes of bradycardia sufficient to cause syncope, unless used in conjunction with a pacemaker.

Amiodarone can be a most toxic drug. The most serious and potentially life-threatening adverse effects associated with its use are pulmonary fibrosis, aggravation of arrhythmias and cirrhotic hepatitis. It can also cause anorexia, nausea, vomiting, abdominal pain and constipation. Other effects include headache, weakness, myalgia, tremor, ataxia, paresthesias, depression, insomnia, nightmares and hallucinations. Peripheral neuropathy, accompanied by histologic changes in nerve fibres, can also occur. Amiodarone can cause photosensitivity reactions.

Its effects on the cardiovascular system include myocardial depression, hypotension, sinoatrial block, A-V block, ventricular arrhythmias, fatal CHF, cardiogenic shock and cardiac arrest. Hypersensitivity pneumonia and pulmonary fibrosis have developed in some patients taking amiodarone. Elevated serum creatinine levels have been reported in patients receiving this drug.

Table 33.12 lists the clinically significant drug interactions with amiodarone.

Bretylium (Bretylol®) was originally marketed as an adrenergic neuron blocker (see Chapter 30) to be used in the treatment of hypertension. However, tolerance develops to its antihypertensive effects, and the drug is absorbed poorly from the gastrointestinal tract. Bretylium is currently used only intravenously as an antiarrhythmic drug.

Bretylium has two actions: it directly modifies the electrical properties of the myocardium, and it depresses the adrenergic neuronal transmission following a brief period of increased norepinephrine release. With respect to its primary antiarrhythmic actions, bretylium suppresses ventricular fibrillation and ventricular arrhythmias. As a result of these actions, bretylium may be of value as the last resort in life-threatening ventricular arrhythmias, principally ventricular tachycardia and fibrillation, which are resistant to conventional antiarrhythmic drug therapy.

There is no evidence that prophylactic bretylium confers clinical benefit in patients with recent but uncomplicated myocardial infarction. In such patients, bretylium injection may lead to unpredictable cardiovascular effects. Therefore, the drug should not be used to prevent the development of arrhythmias in patients with recent myocardial infarction.

The major adverse effects of bretylium relate to its modification of adrenergic function. The catecholamines released shortly after its injection increase blood pressure and heart rate. They may also cause anxiety, excitement, flushing, substernal pressure sensation, headache and angina pectoris.

The intravenous use of bretylium to treat acute arrhythmias is associated with a profound, long-lasting hypotension resulting from the peripheral vasodilatation; more than ten percent of patients will require discontinuation of bretylium because of hypotension. Rapid intravenous administration may initiate nausea and vomiting.

Table 33.13 lists the clinically significant drug interactions with bretylium.

Sotalol (Betapace®, Sotacor®) possesses both beta blocking effects (Class II) and cardiac action potential duration prolongation properties (Class III). As a beta blocker, sotalol is non-cardioselective (see Chapter 30). Whereas significant beta blockade may occur at oral doses as low as 25 mg, Class III effects are seen at daily doses of 160 mg and above. The antiarrhythmic activity of sotalol appears to be primarily due to the drug's Class III property.

Sotalol is approved for the treatment of documented life-threatening ventricular arrhythmias such as sustained ventricular tachycardia. It may also be used for the treatment of patients with documented symptomatic ventricular arrhythmias when the symptoms are of sufficient severity to require treatment. Because of its proarrhythmic effects, sotalol should be reserved for patients in whom, in the opinion of the physician, the benefits of treatment clearly outweighs the risks.

For patients with sustained ventricular tachycardia, sotalol therapy should be initiated in the hospital. Hospitalization may also be required for

Table 33.12
Amiodarone: Drug interactions

Drug	Interaction
Anticoagulants, oral	• Amiodarone decreases the metabolism and increases the effect of oral anticoagulants. Monitor prothrombin time. This effect may persist for several months after stopping amiodarone
Benzodiazepines	• Benzodiazepines may increase the cardiovascular toxicity of amiodarone (mechanism not established). Monitor CV status closely
Beta blockers	• Beta blockers can produce symptomatic bradycardia or sinus arrest if given to a pt receiving amiodarone
Cholestyramine	• Cholestyramine decreases the absorption and effect of amiodarone. Avoid concurrent use
Dextromethorphan	• Amiodarone may decrease the metabolism of dextromethorphan in extensive metabolizers and increase its toxicity. Monitor clinical status
Digoxin	• Amiodarone may increase digoxin toxicity (mechanism not established). Monitor digoxin concentration. Digoxin can also produce symptomatic bradycardia or sinus arrest if given with amiodarone
Fentanyl	• Amiodarone has increased cardiovascular toxicity with fentanyl (mechanism not established). Monitor CV status
Flecainide	• Amiodarone may increase flecainide toxicity (mechanism not established). Monitor flecainide concentration
Halogenated anesthetics (enflurane, halothane, isoflurane)	• These drugs increase the cardiovascular toxicity of amiodarone (mechanism not established). Monitor CV status
Phenytoin	• Amiodarone decreases phenytoin metabolism and increases its toxicity. Monitor phenytoin concentration
Procainamide	• Amiodarone increases procainamide toxicity (mechanism not established). Monitor procainamide concentration
Quinidine	• Amiodarone increases quinidine toxicity (mechanism not established). Monitor quinidine concentration
Thyroid hormones	• Amiodarone decreases the effect of thyroxin because it decreases the conversion of thyroxin (T4) to triiodothyronine (T3). Switch to triiodothyronine
Verapamil	• Verapamil can produce symptomatic bradycardia or sinus arrest if given to a pt receiving amiodarone

---

Table 33.13
Bretylium: Drug interactions

Drug	Interaction
Quinidine, procainamide, propranolol	• Adding bretylium to any of these drugs may significantly prolong A-V transmission time and could aggravate pre-existing block. Observe pts carefully

---

certain other patients, depending on cardiac status and underlying cardiac disease.

Sotalol is contraindicated in patients with bronchial asthma, allergic rhinitis, severe sinus node dysfunction, sinus bradycardia, second- and third-degree A-V block (unless a functioning pacemaker is present) and congenital or acquired long Q-T syndrome. The drug is also contraindicated in cardiogenic shock, severe or uncontrolled CHF, hypokalemia and anesthesia with agents that produce myocardial depression.

Like other antiarrhythmics, sotalol may initiate arrhythmias. There is a suggestion that it may cause early sudden death in a postinfarction patient population. The most commonly observed effects leading to its discontinuation include fatigue, bradycardia, dyspnea, proarrythmia, asthenia (weakness or loss of strength) and dizziness. Sotalol's drug interactions are the same as those listed for beta blockers in general in Table 30.4 (page 299).

Class IV — Calcium Channel Blockers: Verapamil

Mechanism of action and pharmacologic effects. Calcium channel blockers, such as verapamil (Calan®, Isoptin®) selectively inhibit the slow-channel calcium ion transport into cardiac tissue. This slow inward current links myocardial excitation to contraction and control of energy storage and utilization. The pacemaker cells of the S-A node and cells in the proximal region of the A-V node are depolarized primarily by the calcium current. Blocking the calcium channel has the effect of depressing A-V conduction.

Therapeutic uses and adverse effects. Administered intravenously, verapamil can be used to treat paroxysmal supraventricular tachycardia (e.g., atrial fibrillation or atrial flutter of recent onset with rapid ventricular response). Oral verapamil is indicated for the treatment of atrial fibrillation or flutter with rapid ventricular response not otherwise controllable with digitalis preparations. Oral verapamil is also indicated as follow-up treatment to the use of injectable verapamil in paroxysmal supraventricular tachycardia.

Because of its potent A-V nodal depressant activity, verapamil should be used with caution, or not at all, in patients with A-V nodal dysfunction, including those taking digitalis. Contraindications to the use of verapamil also include acute myocardial infarction, severe congestive heart failure (unless secondary to a supraventricular tachycardia amenable to verapamil therapy), cardiogenic shock or sever hypotension, second- or third-degree A-V block, sick sinus syndrome (except in patients with a functioning artificial ventricular pacemaker) and marked bradycardia. The concomitant use of verapamil with beta blockers or cardiac depressant drugs is contraindicated.

The incidence of adverse effects from verapamil is nine percent, lower than for most other antiarrhythmic drugs. The most common adverse effect following intravenous administration is a transient and mild fall in arterial blood pressure. There have been reports of serious adverse effects, including hypotension, bradycardia and, on rare occasions, ventricular asystole.

Oral verapamil almost invariably causes constipation. Nausea, vomiting, lightheadedness, headache, flushing, nervousness, rashes and pruritus also may occur following oral treatment.

The drug interactions for verapamil are listed in Table 36.3 (page 394).

Nursing Management

The nursing management of patients receiving antidysrhythmic drugs is described in Table 33.14. Dosages for individual drugs are given in Table 33.15 (pages 361–366).

Box 33.1 and Figure 33.3 illustrate a sample patient/family teaching for an antidysrhthmic drug.

Table 33.14
Nursing management for antidysrhythmic drugs

Assessment of risk vs. benefit	Patient data	• Physician should determine whether any underlying causes of the dysrhythmia can be corrected, particularly electrolyte imbalances. The drugs in this category have specific contraindications; these should be determined before tx begins • *Assess:* Baseline data on VS must be determined prior to first dose • *Pregnancy:* Most drugs in this class are in risk category C (animal studies show adverse effects to fetus but human data are unknown or insufficient); benefits may be acceptable despite risks. Exceptions include lidocaine, moricizine and sotalol, which are in risk category B (studies in animals may or may not have shown risk; if risk is shown in animal studies, no risk has been shown in human studies)
	Drug data	• Some serious drug interactions; confer with pharmacist • Most serious adverse effects occur in CNS and CV system
Implementation	Rights of administration	• Using the "rights" helps prevent errors of administration
	Right route	• Give IV, PO
	Right dose	• Some drugs in this class are prepared in various salts, e.g., quinidine. Do not substitute various preparations, as the dose of the active drug may vary. Do not substitute long-acting forms
	Right time	• See Table 33.15. Note variation in dosage schedules between drugs in this class
	Right technique	• IV administration requires knowledge of correct diluent and IV solution, correct dilution and rate of administration. Always refer to manufacturer's instructions for this route. Rate must be carefully controlled using an infusion pump. Follow agency policy regarding direct push or loading doses
	Nursing therapeutics	• Some drugs in this class cause GI irritation (nausea, diarrhea) which can often be minimized by administration with food • Allergy to quinidine can be prevented by giving a test dose. Generally, the CNS and CVS adverse effects can be minimized by maintaining tx serum levels • Infusions must be discontinued when cardiac dysrhythmia is corrected or adverse effects appear. CPR equipment and emergency drug supply must be kept immediately available during IV administration
	Patient/family teaching	• Review principles of pt education in Chapter 3 • Pt's need for information may be influenced by length of time required for tx or limited by serious illness • Compliance and follow-up are essential factors in successful tx • For a sample teaching plan, see product insert for amiodarone (Figure 33.3 on next page; also see Box 33.1)

(cont'd on next page)

Table 33.14 (continued)
Nursing management for antidysrhythmic drugs

Implementation (cont'd)	Patient/Family teaching (cont'd)	• Patients/families should know warning signs/symptoms of possible toxicities of drugs. Report immediately • *Discuss possibility of pregnancy:* Advise pt to notify physician; discuss birth control methods
Outcomes	Monitoring of progress	*Note:* For most agents in this class, initial doses and all IV therapy require continuous ECG monitoring • Be alert for signs/symptoms of adverse reactions; document and report immediately to physician

---

Box 33.1
General patient/family teaching for proper use of an antidysrhythmic drug

✔ Instruct patient to take pulse.
✔ Take medication as ordered; never double a dose to make up for a missed one.
✔ Remind patient to change positions slowly and to avoid dangerous activities if drowsiness or dizziness occur.
✔ Instruct patient not to take OTCs without advice and to limit use of alcohol
✔ Patients/families should know warning signs/symptoms of possible toxicities of drug.

Figure 33.3
Sample teaching plan for amiodarone

AMIODARONE
(a mee' oh da rone)

OTHER NAME: Cordarone

WHY is this drug prescribed?
Amiodarone is used to treat and prevent the recurrence of irregular heartbeat. It slows down nerve activity in the heart and relaxes an overactive heart.

WHEN should it be used?
Amiodarone is usually taken once or twice a day. Follow the instructions on your prescription label carefully, and ask your pharmacist or doctor to explain any part that you do not understand. It is important that you take this medication exactly as your doctor has prescribed it. Do not stop taking amiodarone without consulting your doctor. This medication must be taken regularly for one to three weeks before a response is seen and for several months before the full effect is felt.

HOW should it be used?
Amiodarone comes in tablets. Your prescription label tells you how much to take at each dose. Ask your pharmacist any questions you have about refilling your prescription.

What SPECIAL INSTRUCTIONS should I follow while using this drug?
Keep all appointments with your doctor and the laboratory so that your response to this medication can be evaluated. Blood tests, EKGs (electrocardiograms), and chest X-rays may be performed periodically. Your dosage may need to be adjusted (or the drug may be stopped temporarily), depending on your response.
Follow your doctor's advice on smoking and diet, including beverages containing alcohol and caffeine. Cigarettes and caffeine-containing beverages may increase the irritability of your heart and interfere with the action of amiodarone.

What should I do IF I FORGET to take a dose?
Omit the missed dose and take only the next regularly scheduled dose. Do not take a double dose to make up for the missed one.

What SIDE EFFECTS can this drug cause? What can I do about them?
Nausea, vomiting, constipation, loss of appetite, abdominal pain. Take amiodarone with meals. Tremors; lack of coordination or difficulty walking; dizziness, weakness, or fatigue; difficulty sleeping or sleep disturbances; headache; sexual disturbances; weight loss; abnormal taste or smell; vision disturbances such as blurred vision, halos around objects, sensitivity to light, and dry eyes; flushing; swelling of feet, ankles, or lower legs; blue-gray discoloration of skin (especially face and hands) and sensitivity of skin exposed to sunlight. Contact your doctor, especially if these effects are severe or persist.
Cough, shortness of breath or painful breathing, swelling of abdomen (accumulation of fluid), irregular or rapid heartbeat. Contact your doctor immediately (these effects can occur even after you stop taking this medication).

What OTHER PRECAUTIONS should I follow while using this drug?
Before taking amiodarone, tell your doctor if you have a history of lung, liver, heart, or thyroid disease.
Before taking amiodarone, tell your doctor what prescription and nonprescription drugs you are taking, especially phenytoin, warfarin or other anticoagulants ("blood thinners"), digoxin, flecainide, procainamide, quinidine, and other heart medications (including those for irregular heartbeat). Women who are pregnant or breast-feeding or who plan to become pregnant should inform their doctors.
This medication can make your skin more sensitive to sunlight (and sunlamps) than usual. This effect may continue for weeks or months after you stop taking amiodarone. If you will be outside for long periods, wear protective clothing and use a sunscreen preparation. Sun exposure may make you more likely to develop a blue-gray skin discoloration, which may not go away completely after discontinuation of amiodarone.
Before having surgery, tell the doctor or dentist in charge that you are taking amiodarone (or if you have taken the drug within the past two months).

What STORAGE CONDITIONS are necessary for this drug?
Keep this medication in the container it came in, tightly closed, and out of the reach of children. Store it at room temperature and protect it from light.

Source: American Society of Hospital Pharmacists, 1991.

Table 33.15
The antiarrhythmics: Drug doses

Drug Generic name (Trade names)	Dosage	Nursing alert

A. Miscellaneous Antiarrhythmic Drug

| adenosine
(Adenocard) | **IV:** *Adults:* 6 mg, given as rapid IV bolus over 1–2 s. If no results, repeat 1–2 min later as 12-mg rapid bolus. The 12-mg dose may be repeated if required | • Monitor HR frequently (q15–30s) and ECG continuously throughout tx. Once conversion to normal sinus rhythm is achieved, transient arrhythmias may occur, but generally last a few seconds
• Monitor BP during tx
• Assess respiratory status (breath sounds, rate) following administration. Pts with hx of asthma may experience bronchospasm |

B. Class 1A Antiarrhythmic Drugs

| disopyramide
(Norpace, Rythmodan) | **Oral** (regular preparation): *Adults:* Initially, 100–200 mg q6h (range, 400–800 mg daily). For pts with renal or hepatic insufficiency, maint. dose of 100 mg with or without a loading dose of 150 mg at the following intervals: q8h (creatinine clearance, 30–40 mL/min); q12h (CrCl, 15–30 mL/min); or q24h (CrCl, < 15 mL/min). Pts of small stature or those with hepatic insufficiency, cardiomyopathy or cardiac decompensation also may require a smaller dose

(Prolonged-release): 300 mg q12h; 200 mg q12h in pts of small stature or those with moderate renal insufficiency. Do not use prolonged-release preparation in pts with severe renal insufficiency, cardiomyopathy or cardiac decompensation

Children (regular preparation): *< 1 year,* 10–30 mg/kg/day; *1–4 years,* 10–20 mg/kg/day; *4–12 years,* 10–15 mg/kg/day; *12–18 years,* 6–15 mg/kg/day | • A 1–10 mg/mL suspension can be prepared by adding the entire contents of disopyramide capsules to an appropriate volume of cherry syrup in an amber glass bottle. The suspension is stable for 1 month when refrigerated and should be thoroughly shaken before use. Administer on an empty stomach. Do not crush or chew prolonged-release tablets
• When changing from regular to prolonged release, give first dose 6 h after last regular dose
• May interfere with some lab tests (decreases blood glucose, increases BUN)
• Notify physician if P < 60 or > 120 bpm |
| procainamide
(Pronestyl, Procan) | *Note:* Reduce dosage in pts with impaired renal function

Oral (regular preparation): *Adults:* Initially, 250–500 mg q3–6h ATC. A 1-g loading dose produces effective serum concentrations rapidly. *Children:* 50 mg/kg daily in 4–6 divided doses | • When converting from IV to oral regimen, allow 3–4 h between last IV dose and first PO dose. Give on empty stomach with full glass of water. Do not crush or chew prolonged-release preparations

(cont'd on next page) |

Table 33.15 (continued)
The antiarrhythmics: Drug doses

Drug Generic name (Trade names)	Dosage	Nursing alert
B. Class IA Antiarrhythmic Drugs (cont'd)		
procainamide (Pronestyl, Procan) (cont'd)	Prolonged-release: *Adults:* For maintenance after initial tx with regular preparation, 500 mg to 1 g q6–8h or 50 mg/kg daily in divided doses at 6-h intervals **IV (slow):** *Adults:* 25–50 mg/min until arrhythmia is suppressed (max., 1 g). For maintenance, 2–4 mg/min. *Children:* 5–15 mg/kg given over 30 min	• Monitor CBC during first 3 months of tx. Prolonged-release preparations may leave a wax matrix deposit in the stool • Follow agency policy for direct IV administration. Continuous infusion: Use pump to control rate at 2–4 mg/min
quinidine sulfate	**Oral** (quinidine sulfate): *Adults:* 200–400 mg q4–6h. *Children:* 6 mg/kg q4–6h (quinidine gluconate): *Adults:* 324–972 mg q8–12h. As with quinidine sulfate, loading dose should be given if rapid antiarrhythmic response is required (quinidine polygalacturonate): *Adults:* 275 mg bid or tid	• A test dose of 200 mg may be administered to check for intolerance. Best on an empty stomach with a full glass of water; may be given with food if GI irritation occurs • Note that dosages of various forms are not interchangeable. Gluconate form is 62% quinidine; sulfate form is 83% quinidine • Periodically monitor hepatic/renal function, CBC, potassium serum levels during prolonged tx
C. Class IB Antiarrhythmic Drugs		
lidocaine HCl (Xylocaine, Xylocard)	**IV:** *Adults* (for ventricular arrhythmias): Loading dose, 50–100 mg given over 2–3 min. May be repeated in 5 min; or, 1–2 supplemental doses of 25–50 mg may be given at 5- or 10-min intervals (up to 300 mg in a 1-h period). Following loading dose, a solution is infused at a rate of 1–4 mg/min In pts ≥ 70 years and those with CHF, cardiogenic shock or hepatic disease, loading dose should be decreased by about one-half and the infusion rate should be reduced to 1–2 mg/min *Children:* 0.5–1 mg/kg q5min for a max. of 3 doses; or, a solution containing 5 mg/mL infused at a rate of 0.03 mg/kg/min **IM:** *Adults:* 300 mg (3 mL of a 10% solution) injected into the deltoid muscle	• IV administration requires constant cardiac monitoring. Lidocaine and its active metabolites accumulate in some pts during a constant maintenance infusion over 24–36 h. Monitoring for early evidence of toxicity should be carried out and the dose reduced if toxic effects appear. If symptomatic ventricular arrhythmias occur during the first 6 h of infusion, an additional smaller bolus may be given and the infusion rate increased. Only 1% and 2% solutions are used for IV. Follow agency policy for direct IV administration. Use infusion pump for continuous infusion at a rate of 1–4 mg/min • IM injections used only when continuous ECG monitoring not available. Use only deltoid muscle and aspirate to avoid IV injection

Table 33.15 (continued)
The antiarrhythmics: Drug doses

Drug Generic name (Trade names)	Dosage	Nursing alert
C. Class IB Antiarrhythmic Drugs (cont'd)		
mexiletine HCl (Mexitil)	**Oral:** *Adults:* Initially, 200 mg q8h. If rapid control is essential, an initial loading dose of 400 mg may be administered, followed by a 200-mg dose in 8 h. Dosage may then be increased or decreased by 50 mg or 100 mg with minimum of 2–3 days between adjustments. Usual maint. dose, 150–200 mg q8h. If adequate response is achieved with a dose of ≤ 200 mg q8h, the same total daily dose may be tried in divided doses q12h. If satisfactory response is not achieved and the drug is well tolerated, 400 mg may be given q8h or 450 mg q12h. Total dose should not exceed 1.2 g/day	• Mexiletine should be given with food or antacids • Carefully monitor response if pts switched from tid to bid. When switching from other antiarrhythmics, allow sufficient time for duration of action of previous drug
phenytoin (Dilantin)	**Oral:** *Adults:* 1 g on day 1; then 300–600 mg on days 2 and 3. Maint. dose, 300–400 mg/day in 1–4 divided doses. *Children:* Initially, 10–15 mg/kg in 2–3 doses over 24 h. Maint. dose, 5–10 mg/kg/day in 2–3 doses	• Give with food to reduce GI irritation. Chewable form must be chewed well before swallowing. Do not interchange tablets and capsules; doses are not equivalent • Periodically monitor CBC, hepatic/thyroid function during prolonged tx
tocainide HCl (Tonocard)	**Oral:** *Adults:* Initially, 400 mg q8h. Usual maint. dose, 1.2–1.8 g/day in 3 divided doses. Daily doses exceeding 2.4 g have been given infrequently. In pts who tolerate the drug when it is given tid, a bid schedule with careful monitoring may be tried. Smaller doses (< 1.2 g/day) may be required in pts with renal or hepatic insufficiency	• Give with food or milk to reduce GI irritation • Perform weekly blood counts during the first 3 months of tx and periodically thereafter
D. Class IC Antiarrhythmic Drugs		
flecainide acetate (Tambocor)	**Oral:** *Adults* (for supraventricular arrhythmias): Initially, 50 mg q12h. Dosage may be increased in 50-mg increments bid at 4-day intervals until efficacy is achieved (max. dose, 300 mg/day). For life-threatening ventricular tachycardia, initially, 100 mg q12h. Dose may be increased by 50 mg bid q4d until efficacy is achieved or to a max. of 400 mg/day. Maint. dose, 100 mg bid	• May be given with food • Plasma level monitoring (0.2–1 µg/mL) should guide dosage adjustments in pts with renal failure. Because of long half-life, full tx effects may take 3–5 days. Dosage adjustments should be made 3–4 days apart

(cont'd on next page)

Table 33.15 (continued)
The antiarrhythmics: Drug doses

Drug Generic name (Trade names)	Dosage	Nursing alert
D. Class IC Antiarrhythmic Drugs (cont'd)		
moricizine (Ethmozline)	**Oral:** *Adults* (for life-threatening ventricular arrhythmias): Usual dosage, 600–900 mg/day, given q8h in 3 equally divided doses. Within this range, dosage can be adjusted as tolerated in increments of 150 mg/day at 3-day intervals until desired effect is obtained. Pts with impaired hepatic or renal function: Initially, 600 mg/day or less	• Tx should be initiated in hospital with cardiac monitoring. Since antiarrhythmic effect of moricizine persists for more than 12 h, some responsive pts may be given the same total daily dose q12h to increase convenience and help ensure compliance. However, when higher doses are used, those receiving the drug q12h may experience more dizziness and nausea • Monitor pts with impaired hepatic or renal function closely before dosage adjustment. Due to long half-life, dosage adjustments should be 3 days apart • When substituting for another antiarrhythmic, allow sufficient time for duration of action of previous drug • Drug is found in breast milk
propafenone HCl (Rythmol)	**Oral:** *Adults:* Initially, 150 mg q8h. If arrhythmia is not controlled, dosage may be increased at 3- to 4-day intervals to 225 mg q8h and, if necessary, to 300 mg q8h	• Tx should be initiated in hospital with cardiac monitoring. Most serious effects occur within first 2 weeks of tx • Due to long half-life, dosage adjustments should be 3–4 days apart • Give with food
E. Class II Antiarrhythmic Drugs		
propranolol HCl (Inderal)	**Oral:** *Adults* (for arrhythmias): 10–30 mg tid or qid, ac and hs. For postmyocardial infarction: Initiate tx with a 20-mg dose. If no adverse reaction is noted, increase dose to 40 mg tid. After 1–2 weeks, increase dose to 60 mg tid. If necessary, dose may be increased to 80 mg tid	• Give with food. May be crushed, except for long-acting forms
esmolol HCl (Brevibloc)	*Consult detailed manufacturer's dosage instructions for this drug*	• Esmolol 2.5 g/10 mL ampoules are not for direct IV injection. These are concentrated solutions of a potent drug which must be diluted prior to injection. Esmolol should not be admixed with sodium bicarbonate or mixed with other drugs prior to dilution. Refer to manufacturer's instructions for dilution

Table 33.15 (continued)
The antiarrhythmics: Drug doses

Drug Generic name (Trade names)	Dosage	Nursing alert
F. Class III Antiarrhythmic Drugs		
amiodarone HCl (Cordarone)	**Oral:** *Adults* (for refractory ventricular arrhythmias): Initially, 800 mg to 1.6 g daily for 1–3 weeks, followed by 600–800 mg daily for 1 month. Thereafter, usual maint. dose is 400 mg/day. For supraventricular arrhythmias: 600 mg daily in 3 divided doses for 1 week, followed by 200–400 mg daily. Thereafter, lowest effective dose (often 200 mg/day) should be given to minimize side effects. A maint. dose of 200 mg on alternate days may be effective in some pts. For bradycardia-tachycardia syndrome (with a pacemaker in place): Initially, 200 mg bid, followed by 200–600 mg daily. *Children:* 3–20 mg/kg daily	• *Prior to tx:* Ophthalmic exam, thyroid function and potassium levels should be completed • Tx should be initiated with continuous cardiac monitoring • Divide oral dose and give with meals • High incidence of adverse effects. During initial tx, assist ambulation; peripheral neuropathy, tremors and abnormal gait are common • Instruct pt re: photosensitivity reactions; advise to use sunscreen, limit exposure • Amiodarone has a slow onset of action. Full tx response may not be evident for 1 week to 3 months, and effects may persist for 7–50 days or more after drug is discontinued
bretylium (Bretylol)	**IV:** For immediate control of life-threatening ventricular arrhythmias (esp. ventricular fibrillation): *Adults,* 5 mg/kg of undiluted drug, given rapidly. If fibrillation persists, dosage may be increased to 10 mg/kg and repeated prn. For immediate control of other ventricular arrhythmias: *Adults:* Contents of one ampoule should be diluted with at least 50 mL dextrose injection or sodium chloride injection and 5–10 mg/kg infused slowly over 8 min or more to avoid nausea; dose may be repeated in 1–2 h. For maintenance: *Adults:* A dilute solution may be infused continuously at a rate of 1–2 mg/min, or 5–10 mg/kg may be given by slow intermittent infusion q6h **IM:** *Adults:* 5–10 mg/kg. Subsequent doses may be given at 1- to 2-h intervals if the arrhythmia persists. Thereafter, this dosage is given q6–8h	• Bretylium should be used on a short-term basis, and BP and ECG should be monitored continuously during tx • Bretylium is eliminated by the kidneys as unchanged drug, thus dosage should be reduced in pts with impaired renal function • Dose should be reduced gradually over 3–5 days with continual cardiac monitoring • Notify physician if BP < 75 mm • Rotate IM sites and do not give more than 3 mL in one injection • Follow agency policy for direct IV administration. Use pump for continuous infusion
sotalol HCl (Betapace, Sotacor)	**Oral:** *Adults:* Usual initial dosage, 80 mg bid, which can be increased to 240 mg or 320 mg per day, divided bid or tid; 2–3 days with Q-T monitoring should be allowed between increments. Max. dosage, 480–640 mg/day. Lower dosage or increase interval between doses for pts with renal insufficiency	• Give on empty stomach; food reduces absorption • Confer with physician if P < 50 bpm *(cont'd on next page)*

Table 33.15 (continued)
The antiarrhythmics: Drug doses

Drug Generic name (Trade names)	Dosage	Nursing alert
G. Class IV Antiarrhythmic Drugs		
verapamil HCl (Calan, Isoptin)	**IV:** *Adults:* 5–10 mg (0.075–0.15 mg/kg) given over 2 min (or 3 min, in elderly pts). An additional 10 mg may be given if necessary in 30 min. For maintenance, infusions of 0.005 mg/kg/min have been employed. *Infants up to 1 year:* 0.1–0.2 mg/kg over 2 min, repeated if necessary in 30 min. *Children 1–15 years:* 0.1–0.3 mg/kg, repeated if necessary in 30 min. No more than 10 mg should be given as a single dose. **Oral:** *Adults:* 240–480 mg daily in 2 divided doses (prolonged-release form) or 3 or 4 divided doses (standard form)	• Give with food or milk. Do not crush or chew prolonged-release forms • Monitor BP, ECG continuously • Follow agency policy for direct IV administration. To minimize hypotensive effects, pts should remain lying for 1 h after IV dose

Response to Clinical Challenge

(To calculate infusion rate, refer to the chart below)

1. Given Mr. W.'s age, the loading dose should be approximately one-half the usual adult dose, or 25–50 mg given over 2–3 min.
2. The infusion dose of 1 mg/min is within recommended range for Mr. W.'s age.
3. To administer this dose using a concentration of 1 mg/mL (or 1 g in 1 L), the rate should be set at 60 mL/h (using an infusion pump to ensure accuracy).
4. The therapeutic window for lidocaine is 4.3 to 21.3 µmol/L. The major toxicities involve the central nervous and cardiovascular systems. Observe for drowsiness, paresthesias, twitching, respiratory depression and ECG changes.

Prepare a solution of 1 g in 1000 mL to produce a concentration of 1 mg/mL. Calculate the rate to deliver 1 mg/min.

Dose (mg/min)	1 mg/mL concentration	2 mg/mL concentration
1 mg/min	60 mL/h	30 mL/h
2 mg/min	120 mL/h	60 mL/h

Further Reading

Antiarrhythmic drugs. *AMA Drug Evaluations Subscriptions* 1993 (Winter):6.1–6.29.
Drugs for cardiac arrhythmias. *Medical Letter on Drugs and Therapeutics* 1992;33:55–60.

Antianginal Drugs

Topics Discussed
- Etiology of angina pectoris
- Definition of stable, unstable and variant (vasospastic) angina
- Drug treatment of angina pectoris
- For each drug discussed: Mechanism of action, pharmacologic effects, therapeutic uses, adverse effects
- Nursing management

Drugs Discussed
acebutolol (ass-eh-**byoo**-toe-lole)
amlodipine (am-**loe**-dip-een)
atenolol (at-**ten**-oh-lole)
diltiazem (dil-**tye**-ah-zem)
felodipine (fell-**oh**-dip-een)
isosorbide dinitrate (eye-soe-**sor**-byde dye-**nye**-trate)
isosorbide mononitrate (eye-soe-**sor**-byde mon-oh-**nye**-trate)
isradipine (iz-**rad**-ip-een)
metoprolol (met-**oh**-proe-lole)
nadolol (**nay**-doe-lole)
nicardipine (nye-**kar**-dip-een)
nifedipine (nye-**fed**-ip-een)
nitroglycerin (nye-tro-**gliss**-er-in)
pindolol (**pin**-doe-lole)
propranolol (proe-**pran**-oh-lole)
timolol (**tye**-moh-lole)
verapamil (ver-**ap**-ah-mil)

Clinical Challenge

Consider this clinical challenge as you read through this chapter. The response to the challenge appears on page 375.

Gladys is an 85-year-old woman, living alone in her home. She experiences an MI and recovers well following hospitalization, except for periods of vasospastic angina. She returns home with the following medications:

- Nitro-Dur® patch applied every morning, removed hs
- Nitrolingual® spray prn
- Diltiazem 60 mg PO tid

   One week after discharge, the physician changes the order to diltiazem prolonged-release capsules 60 mg bid.

   Gladys begins to experience more frequent angina and increases her use of nitro spray. Her usual daily routine is to retire between 20:00–21:00 and rise between 07:00–08:00. She is often awakened between 05:00–06:00 with angina.

1. Outline a teaching plan for Gladys at discharge.
2. What changes to her new dosage regime will you discuss with her physician?

Etiology of Angina Pectoris

Angina pectoris is a syndrome of paroxysmal left-sided chest pain. It is produced when the oxygen requirements of the heart exceed the oxygen supply.

Angina pectoris is a problem of regional ischemia. Not all areas of the heart are anoxic. The heart, more than other tissues, is particularly prone to the development of regional ischemia. Considering its resting metabolic rate, it is the most underperfused organ in the body. Unlike other tissues, which extract approximately 25% of the oxygen provided in arterial blood, the heart removes 75% of the oxygen perfusing coronary vessels. In contrast to other tissues — such as the skeletal muscles, in which a major increase in oxygen requirement can be satisfied by increasing both blood flow and the percentage of oxygen extracted from the blood — the heart must depend almost entirely on a significant increase in myocardial perfusion.

Angina pectoris may be divided into stable, unstable and variant angina.

In *stable angina* the cause of the problem is a reduction of blood flow to a particular area of the heart as a result of atherosclerosis. When the heart is required to work harder, regional ischemia develops. Patients who suffer from stable angina pectoris experience attacks when they are exposed to exercise, cold temperatures, cigarette smoke and excitement (including, alas, sexual excitement). Eating diverts blood flow to the gastrointestinal tract, away from the coronary blood vessels, and it too can precipitate an attack. These attacks often begin suddenly and stop abruptly.

Unstable angina is an intermediate syndrome between stable angina pectoris (in which the myocardial blood supply is temporarily inadequate, but there is no tissue death) and myocardial infarction (which is characterized by death of myocardial tissue). The term unstable angina cannot be used to label a specific clinical entity. Rather, it represents another pattern of presentation in the spectrum of coronary artery disease and may be added to the problems of a patient with stable exertional angina pectoris. Patients may range from having normal coronary anatomy to severe three-vessel involvement. Unstable angina may also represent the first manifestation of symptomatic ischemic heart disease. Its characteristics may include discrete episodes of severe ischemic chest pain that can occur at rest. Unstable angina will not be discussed further in this chapter, beyond stating that drug therapy involves the use of nitrates and beta blockers.

Variant (or *vasospastic*) *angina* is not caused by a fixed atherosclerotic narrowing of the vessel lumen but rather results from a coronary artery spasm. It often occurs when the patient is resting.

Drug Treatment of Angina Pectoris

The objectives in treating angina pectoris are twofold: (1) to stop an existing attack or prevent a new one from occurring and (2) to increase the exercise capacity of the patient. Drugs can do this by either increasing oxygen supply to the ischemic area(s) of the heart or by decreasing the oxygen requirements of the heart muscle.

In the case of stable angina, it is easier to decrease the oxygen requirements than to increase the oxygen supply to the heart. As previously explained, the cause of the problem in stable angina pectoris is a reduction in blood flow to a particular area of the heart as a result of atherosclerosis. It is exactly the nature of this problem that prevents drugs that dilate arterioles (precapillary resistance vessels) in other parts of the body from having the same effect in those vessels carrying blood to the ischemic area. Because these arterioles are atherosclerotic, they are hardened and cannot dilate. Thus, drugs such as the nitrates and the calcium channel blockers cannot dilate arterioles perfusing ischemic areas of the heart with stable angina because these vessels are incapable of dilating.

This is not to say, however, that nitrates and calcium channel blockers do not help patients with stable angina pectoris. Far from it; these drugs are quite effective. However, they owe their efficacy primarily to their ability to decrease the oxygen requirements of the heart. Exactly how they do this is explained in the sections that follow.

Beta blockers also prevent attacks of stable angina pectoris because they, too, reduce the oxygen requirements of the heart. In general, it may be stated that drugs that are effective in stable angina pectoris work primarily by decreasing the

Figure 34.1
Mechanism of action of antianginal drugs

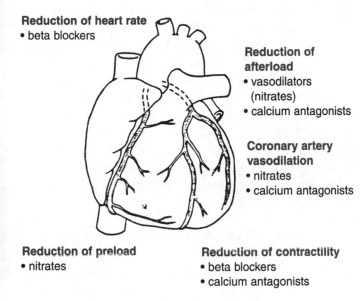

Reduction of heart rate
• beta blockers

Reduction of afterload
• vasodilators (nitrates)
• calcium antagonists

Coronary artery vasodilation
• nitrates
• calcium antagonists

Reduction of preload
• nitrates

Reduction of contractility
• beta blockers
• calcium antagonists

Source: Maclean D, Feely J. Calcium antagonists, nitrates and new antianginal drugs. *Br Med J* 1983;286:1127. Reproduced with permission.

oxygen requirement of the ischemic area of the heart.

The situation is very different with variant angina pectoris. In this case, atherosclerosis is not the cause of the pain. Rather, this form of angina is caused by coronary artery spasm (thus giving rise to its alternative name of vasospastic angina). Because the arterioles are not atherosclerotic, they will dilate when treated with drugs capable of relaxing blood vessels. Thus, both nitrates and calcium channel blockers (1) prevent the arteriole from going into spasm and (2) relax the arteriole that is in spasm. These classes of drugs are therefore effective in preventing and treating attacks of vasospastic angina pectoris.

Figure 34.1 depicts the mechanisms of action of antianginal drugs.

Nitrates

Mechanism of action and pharmacologic effects. Nitrates dilate veins (capacitance vessels), arteries (conductance vessels) and arterioles (precapillary resistance vessels) throughout the body. The effects of nitrates result from their actions on all three types of blood vessels.

By dilating veins, nitrates reduce venous

return, thereby decreasing left ventricular volume and intramyocardial tension. This has the effect of decreasing myocardial oxygen requirements because the major factor controlling the oxygen requirements of the heart is the degree to which it is stretched as it fills in diastole. By dilating the veins, and thereby lowering the filling pressure of the heart, nitrates reduce the amount of oxygen the heart needs.

An indirect result of venodilatation may be an increased oxygen delivery to the subendocardium. Blood flow to the subendocardium occurs primarily in diastole. Therefore, the reduction in left ventricular end-diastolic pressure induced by a nitrate reduces extravascular compression around the subendocardial vessels and favours a redistribution of coronary blood flow in this area. This effect of nitrates on the distribution of coronary flow is important because the subendocardium is particularly vulnerable to ischemia during acute attacks.

The ability of nitrates to relax the large epicardial arteries improves regional myocardial blood flow to ischemic areas. In patients with coronary artery disease, nitrates dilate both normal and diseased coronary arteries and collateral vessels and thus improve regional distribution of myocardial blood flow, even though the overall coronary blood flow may decrease because of the fall in central aortic pressure.

At higher doses, nitrates dilate peripheral arterioles to decrease peripheral resistance (afterload). Afterload is the pressure that the heart must contend with to pump blood throughout the body. If afterload increases, the heart must work harder and be supplied with more oxygen. A fall in afterload, on the other hand, makes the job of the heart easier, as it needs less oxygen to carry out its function. Thus, the reduction in afterload produced by nitrates decreases the oxygen requirements of the myocardium.

However, the ability of nitrates to dilate arterioles is a double-edged sword. Whereas it is true that decreasing the peripheral resistance reduces afterload and this is good, it is equally true that dilating peripheral arterioles reflexly increases heart rate. This increases the oxygen requirements of the heart and is not good. Fortunately, the increased oxygen demand created by tachycardia is not sufficient to override the beneficial effects of nitrates, and these drugs can be used either to terminate an existing attack or to prevent a new one.

Therapeutic uses. Various nitrate preparations are available to prevent or to terminate anginal attacks. Nitroglycerin, absorbed from the mouth, is the drug of choice to stop the pain of angina pectoris. Sublingual tablets will usually relieve pain within two minutes; their duration of action is approximately thirty minutes. Alternatively, nitroglycerin spray (Nitrolingual®) can be used under or on the tongue. This form of the drug is most popular and effective and may eventually replace sublingual tablets. If the patient can anticipate a situation that will stress the heart, nitroglycerin, placed under the tongue or sprayed on or under the tongue, can also prevent an attack of angina pectoris. However, the short duration of action of nitroglycerin sublingual tablets and spray makes them impractical for chronic prophylactic use.

Nitroglycerin is also used chronically to prevent attacks. When applied to the skin as an ointment (Nitro-Bid®, Nitrol®) or as patches (Transderm Nitro®, Nitrodisc®, Nitro-Dur®), nitroglycerin is absorbed through the stratum corneum. Because tolerance develops rapidly to the patches if they are applied on a twenty-four-hour basis, they should be applied for only twelve hours per day. Used this way, they provide effective long-term prophylaxis without the development of tolerance. Recipients of intermittent nitroglycerin therapy usually receive concomitant calcium channel blockers or beta blockers, or both, which reduce the risk of ischemic episodes during the nitrate-free period.

Buccal nitroglycerin (Nitrogard-SR®) contains nitroglycerin in an inert polymer matrix. The tablet is to be placed in the buccal cavity between the upper lip and gums. Dissolution of the tablet proceeds in a gradual, uniform manner. This formulation acts promptly, with an onset of action of one to two minutes. The tablet continues to release nitroglycerin into the circulation for a prolonged period, and exercise tolerance may be enhanced for up to five hours.

Isosorbide mononitrate (Monoket®, Ismo®) and isosorbide dinitrate (Isordil®, Sorbitrate®) protect the patient from angina attacks. Unfortunately, tolerance may also develop to these products. As for nitroglycerin patches, tolerance can be reduced by providing a nitrate-free interval — that is, the regular preparation may be taken two to three times daily during waking hours, or the prolonged-release preparation may be taken once or twice daily (e.g., at 08:00 and 14:00).

Adverse effects. Headache is the most commonly encountered adverse effect of the nitrates. This is due to vasodilatation of blood vessels in the scalp. The other adverse effects are dizziness and weakness, which may be attributed to postural hypotension produced when the drugs dilate capacitance vessels and allow blood to pool in the veins.

Tolerance may develop to nitrates. If this happens, the patient should discontinue taking the nitrate for a period of time, to allow the blood vessels to regain their responsiveness. To forestall the development of tolerance, patients should not receive nitrate therapy twenty-four hours a day.

Table 34.1 lists the clinically significant drug interactions with nitrates, while Box 34.1 outlines a patient teaching for these drugs.

Beta Blockers

Mechanism of action and pharmacologic effects. The pharmacology of beta blockers is presented in Chapter 30. These drugs block the beta

---

Table 34.1
Nitrates: Drug interactions

Drug	Interaction
Alcohol	• Nitroglycerin can produce additive hypotension; warn pts
Antidepressants, tricyclic	• TCAs can dry the mouth and decrease the dissolution of nitroglycerin tablets, resulting in reduced effect
Diazoxide	• Nitroglycerin and diazoxide can produce severe additive hypotension. Avoid concurrent use within 6 h
Diltiazem	• Nitroglycerin and diltiazem may produce additive hypotension. Avoid concurrent use

Box 34.1
Patient teaching: Nitrates

When should I take this medicine?

Take exactly as ordered by your physician. The sublingual tablets and spray are used to treat angina. Symptoms may include:

* pain, tightness, squeezing, heaviness or pressure in chest
* burning or feeling of indigestion
* pain between shoulder blades, down one or both arms or into the neck or jaw
* shortness of breath.

How should I take this medicine?

* When you begin to feel angina, sit down.
* *For sublingual tablet:* Place a tablet under your tongue and let it dissolve. You may experience a slight burning or tingling sensation as it dissolves. Do not swallow or chew the tablet. Do not drink anything until the taste of the medicine is gone.
* *For nitroglycerin spray:* Do not shake the canister. Hold it upright with your finger on the button and spray once into your mouth onto or under your tongue. Avoid inhaling or breathing the spray in through your nose.
* The pain should decrease within one minute. If it is not relieved in 5 min, use a second tablet or spray and remain resting. If you still have pain after another 5 min, take a third tablet or spray. Do not use more than 3 tablets or doses of spray in 15 min. If you still have angina, call your doctor and have someone take you to the nearest hospital Emergency Department.

How do I use the Nitro-Dur® patch?

* Apply the patch at the time prescribed by your doctor. Read the instructions on the label carefully. Be sure to choose an area of clean, dry skin with little or no hair. The area should be free from cuts, scars or irritation. Do not use lower arms or legs, as drug is not well absorbed from these areas. Use a different site every day. Wash hands after applying patch to remove any drug.
* Remove the patch at the time prescribed by your doctor. Grasp the edge of the patch and gently peel away from the skin. Wash area with soap and water and towel dry. Wash hands.
* You may shower with the patch in place.
* Keep the patch and all medicines out of the reach of children.

What benefits should I expect from using this drug?

* Besides relieving angina pain, nitrates can also be used to prevent angina. Learn what activities or situations may cause

angina for you. Prior to these activities (e.g., eating, exercise, stress, excitement, extreme changes in temperature), use a tablet or a dose of spray. This may prevent or minimize angina for up to one hour.

What unwanted effects are possible with this drug, and what can I do about them?

* All medicines can cause unwanted effects, but this does not mean that they will necessarily occur. Often, as your body gets used to the medicine, unwanted effects can lessen or disappear.
* Nitrates may cause a fast pulse, flushing of face and neck, nausea and vomiting. You should discuss these effects with your doctor.
* The medicine may make you feel dizzy or lightheaded when you get up. If so, you should change position slowly. Usually, this effect diminishes when you get used to the medicine.
* You may experience a headache after using a nitrate. If so, a mild pain reliever can be used.
* After you remove a patch, the skin may appear dry and red. This is normal. If the redness does not disappear within a few hours, discuss with your doctor.
* Call your doctor right away if you notice any of the following:
  − severe or prolonged headache
  − dry mouth
  − blurred vision
  − angina that is not relieved.

How should I store and carry my nitroglycerin tablets?

It is very important to store nitroglycerin correctly. The tablets lose their strength if they are exposed to heat, light or moisture. To make sure your tablets will work when you need them, you should:

* keep them in their original brown glass bottle
* store them in a cool, dry place (not the bathroom cupboard)
* remove cotton filler and reclose lid tightly
* write the date you opened the bottle on the label, and discard unused drug after 3 months
* separate 5–10 tablets into a second brown glass bottle and carry this with you at all times (do not count tablets in your hands; instead, pour some into the bottle cap, take what you need and return the others back into the bottle)
* keep a travelling supply of drug in your purse or outer pocket (away from body heat)
* be sure that family members know where you keep your supply.

adrenergic receptors in the heart. In response to the decrease in sympathetic nervous system stimulation of the heart, heart rate decreases, myocardial contractility falls and the oxygen requirements of the heart diminish.

Beta blockers differ in their abilities to block beta$_1$ receptors in the heart and beta$_2$ receptors on the peripheral blood vessels and bronchioles. Propranolol, nadolol and timolol are nonselective beta blockers, effectively preventing epinephrine and norepinephrine from stimulating all beta receptors in the body.

Atenolol and metoprolol are called cardioselective beta blockers because they block preferentially the beta$_1$ receptors in the heart, without having as pronounced an effect on beta$_2$ receptors.

Pindolol is a beta blocker with partial-agonist or intrinsic sympathetic activity (ISA). In contrast to the other beta blockers previously mentioned, this drug is not a true competitive inhibitor of beta receptors. Instead, it is a very weak beta stimulant that competes with the more potent chemicals epinephrine and norepinephrine at receptor sites, with a resulting reduction in beta-mediated responses. Thus, pindolol may not decrease resting heart rate as much as drugs with ISA.

Acebutolol combines the properties of the cardioselective beta blockers and beta blockers with ISA. It is a cardioselective partial agonist.

Therapeutic use. Beta blockers form the mainstay of prophylactic treatment of chronic stable angina pectoris. They are often used with a sustained-release nitroglycerin product or either isosorbide mononitrate or isosorbide dinitrate. The combination of a beta blocker with a nitrate is often more effective than either drug used alone. Furthermore, beta blockers prevent the reflex tachycardia that often accompanies nitrate therapy.

Beta blockers are contraindicated in the patient with congestive heart failure or bronchial asthma. They are also contraindicated in sinus bradycardia, heart block greater than first degree, cardiogenic shock and right ventricular failure secondary to pulmonary hypertension, unless the failure is due to a tachyarrhythmia treatable with the beta blocker. However, beta blockers are ideal drugs for patients suffering from both hypertension and angina pectoris.

Adverse effects. The major adverse effects of beta blockers result from inhibition of the sympathetic nervous system innervation of the heart. Heart rate and cardiac output fall as the cardiac sympathetic nerves are blocked. This may predispose the borderline patient to congestive heart failure. Thus, beta blockers are contraindicated in these patients. Other adverse effects of beta blockers and the drug interactions with these agents are presented in Table 30.4 (page 299).

Calcium Channel Blockers (Calcium Entry Blockers)

Mechanism of action and pharmacologic effects. Vasoconstriction depends upon the entry of small amounts of calcium into the vascular smooth muscle. The calcium enters the muscle cell through a special channel designed for it — the so-called calcium channel. Calcium channel blockers, also known as calcium entry blockers, block this entry of calcium into the vascular muscle and, as a result, prevent vasoconstriction.

All calcium channel blockers dilate coronary vessels, increasing oxygen supply to the patient with variant (vasospastic) angina pectoris. They differ, however, in other important respects. Amlodipine, felodipine, isradipine, nifedipine and nicardipine have the same basic chemical structure and are called dihydropyridines. These drugs are potent peripheral vasodilators. They decrease peripheral resistance and trigger a reflex increase in heart rate. This increase in heart rate is counterproductive to the reduction on myocardial oxygen requirements because an increase in heart rate, per se, increases the amount of oxygen the heart needs. However, this effect is more than offset by the other actions of these calcium channel blockers (see below), with the result that regional ischemia is reduced in the patient with angina pectoris.

Although all calcium channel blockers directly depress myocardial contractility, this effect is usually offset in the dihydropyridines by their marked ability to decrease peripheral resistance and decrease left ventricular afterload. Because dihydropyridine calcium channel blockers decrease peripheral resistance, and this results in a decrease in left ventricular afterload, these drugs reduce the oxygen requirements of the heart.

Verapamil is a potent myocardial depressant in isolated muscle preparations, but produces only a mildly decreased contractility in patients with normal cardiac function. The major antianginal effect of verapamil is due to peripheral vasodilatation, which decreases afterload and thus reduces myocardial oxygen demand. In addition, because verapamil is a myocardial depressant, and does not dilate peripheral vessels to the extent seen with the dihydropyridines, it does not increase heart rate. In fact, just the opposite happens. Verapamil produces mild bradycardia, increasing the amount of time spent in diastole, when most of the coronary perfusion occurs. Verapamil is also a potent inhibitor of coronary artery spasm. It thus increases myocardial oxygen delivery in patients with vasospastic angina.

Diltiazem is a less potent peripheral vasodilator than the dihydropyridines and a less potent negative inotrope and chronotrope than verapamil. Like verapamil and the dihydropyridines, diltiazem's antianginal effects result from both its ability to relax the peripheral arterioles, thereby reducing afterload and myocardial oxygen requirements, and its capacity to dilate both epicardial and subendocardial arteries and inhibit spontaneous coronary artery spasm, thus increasing oxygen delivery to heart muscle. Diltiazem may also reduce resting heart rate (although generally less than verapamil), which will also increase the time available for coronary perfusion.

Therapeutic uses. Calcium channel blockers alleviate the symptoms of variant angina by decreasing the oxygen requirements of the heart and increasing the oxygen supply. They are probably as effective as nitrates in treatment of variant angina.

In stable angina pectoris, calcium channel blockers reduce the frequency of attacks, decrease nitrate requirements and improve exercise performance. Their beneficial effect appears to be due primarily to reduced myocardial oxygen demand. A calcium channel blocker may be indicated in stable angina when nitrates are ineffective or poorly tolerated or when beta blockers are contraindicated or produce intolerable side effects. Calcium channel blockers also may be used as first-line therapy. Since these agents do not adversely affect airway resistance, they are preferred to beta blockers in

patients with bronchospastic disorders. They may also be better tolerated than beta blockers in patients with peripheral vascular disease, severe hypertriglyceridemia or unstable insulin-dependent diabetes mellitus. The calcium channel blockers may be used for angina after myocardial infarction, although in contrast to beta blockers, they do not appear to prevent recurrent infarction or death.

Adverse effects. The most common adverse effects of dihydropyridines result from their vasodilating action. These include headache, dizziness, lightheadedness and giddiness, flushing and heat sensation, peripheral edema and hypotension.

Diltiazem's most common adverse effects are nausea, swelling or edema, arrhythmia (A-V block, bradycardia, tachycardia and sinus arrest), headache, rash and fatigue. Diltiazem should be avoided in patients with sick sinus syndrome.

Adverse reactions to verapamil include bradycardia, transient asystole, hypotension, development or worsening of heart failure and development of rhythm disturbances, including A-V block and ventricular dysrhythmias, flushing, peripheral edema and pulmonary edema. CNS effects include dizziness, headache, fatigue, excitation, vertigo, syncope and tremor. Constipation, nausea, vomiting and gastrointestinal complaints are the most common adverse effects seen after oral administration. A smaller percentage of patients may experience bronchospasm and dyspnea, which are more prevalent following parenteral administration of verapamil.

The drug interactions for the calcium channel blockers are presented in Table 36.3 (page 394).

Nursing Management

Table 34.2 on the next page describes the nursing management of the patient receiving antianginal drugs. Dosage details of individual drugs are given in Table 34.3 (pages 376–379).

Table 34.2
Nursing management for antianginal drugs

Assessment of risk vs. benefit	Patient data	• Assess baseline data for P (rate and rhythm), BP and pattern of angina • *Age:* Many antianginals should be used cautiously in the elderly pt; reduce dose or increase interval between doses • Use cautiously in renal or hepatic disease • *Pregnancy:* Risk category C (animal studies show adverse effects to fetus but human data are unknown or insufficient); benefits may be acceptable despite risks
	Drug data	• *Nitrates:* Generally well tolerated except for flushing, headache and dizziness. Check for hx allergic reactions • *Calcium channel blockers:* Use cautiously with hypotension • *Beta blockers:* Avoid in pts with asthma • Check with pharmacist for potential drug interactions
Implementation	Rights of administration	• Using the "rights" helps prevent errors of administration
	Right route	• Give PO or sublingually. Some drugs are also available as a spray or transdermal patch. Check dosage forms carefully: may be available in regular and extended-release forms
	Right time	• See Table 34.3. Note variation in dosage schedules among drugs in this class • Nitroglycerin is often self administered; monitor the number of tablets used and replenish the supply
	Right technique	• Nitroglycerin tablets must be properly stored to prevent deterioration. Use a tightly sealed, dark-coloured container. Keep in a cool place; even body heat can cause deterioration. • Patches must be applied to clean, dry skin, preferably on a hairless area. Sites should be rotated and extremities should be avoided owing to poor absorption. Skin should be cleansed and inspected when patch is changed
	Nursing therapeutics	• *Protect safety of pt:* Drugs can cause hypotension and dizziness. Maintain clean environment and remind pt to rise slowly and request assistance if necessary • Administer analgesic prn for headache caused by nitrates • *Encourage pt to reduce risk factors:* Aavoid precipitating situations, reduce weight, follow regular exercise program, stop smoking, follow tx for any contributing diseases, such as hypertension
	Patient/family teaching	• Educate for proper use of drug (see Box 34.1) • Remind pts to check with physician or pharmacist before using other drugs. Alcohol should be limited or avoided as it increases vasodilatation (dizziness and hypotension) • Emphasize that pt should not suddenly discontinue any antianginal: severe, rebound angina may occur • Compliance and follow-up are essential factors in successful tx. Review principles of pt education in Chapter 3

Table 34.2 (continued)
Nursing management for antianginal drugs

Outcomes	Monitoring of progress
	Continually monitor:
	•Clinical response indicating tx success (reduction in incidence of angina, increased exercise tolerance)
	•Particularly at initiation of tx, be alert for signs/symptoms of adverse reactions; document and report immediately to physician
	•Sudden withdrawal of these drugs may precipitate severe angina. Do not miss any doses; confer with physician if withholding a dose for bradycardia or hypotension

Response to Clinical Challenge

1. Gladys should know how and when to apply and remove the patch, how to use the spray and when to seek emergency treatment. She should also know the importance of using all drugs as ordered and what to do if she misses a dose. Finally, you should review the common adverse effects, what she can do about them, how to minimize or prevent them and when to call the doctor.

2. Gladys does not currently enjoy good control of her angina, which is the vasospastic type. There may be two reasons for this. First, when she was converted to the long-acting form of diltiazem, she should have received a direct dosage conversion; that is, she was taking 60 mg tid and now should take 90 mg bid. The dosage should be adjusted. Second, Gladys is well covered during the day by the nitrate patch but experiences angina in the early morning. Perhaps the physician would consider reversing the use of the patch; that is, on for 12 h at night and off during the day. Alternatively, there are 3 dosages strengths of the patch; perhaps an increased dosage would be sufficient to improve control of Gladys's angina. The diltiazem should be increased first; if the problem persists, adjustments can be made with the patch.

Further Reading

Byers J. The use of aspirin in cardiovascular disease. *J Cardiovasc Nurs* 1993;8(1):1–18.

Drugs for angina pectoris. *Medical Letter on Drugs and Therapeutics* 1994;36:111.

Gleeson B. Teaching your patient about his antianginal drugs. *Nursing* 1991;21(2):65–72.

Gold ME. Pharmacology of the nitrovasodilators: antianginal, antihypertensive and antiplatelet actions. *Nurs Clin North Am* 1991;26:437–450.

Table 34.3
The antianginals: Drug doses

Drug Generic name (Trade names)	Dosage	Nursing alert
A. Nitrates		
nitroglycerin sublingual tablets (Nitrostat)	**Sublingual:** *Adults:* 0.15–0.6 mg; usual dose, 0.3–0.4 mg. If symptoms are not relieved by a single dose, additional or larger doses may be taken at 5-min intervals, but no more than 3 tablets should be used within a 15-min period	• Conventional sublingual nitroglycerin tablets gradually lose potency through volatilization; therefore, the drug must be packaged in glass containers with tightly fitting metal screw caps and with no more than 100 dose units in each container. The tablets should be dispensed in the original unopened container, which should be closed tightly after each use. They should not be exposed to heat, and the bulk of the supply should be refrigerated. In the hospital setting, a supply of tablets will be kept at the bedside. Check the supply to monitor the number of tablets used and to replenish the supply. The tablets should be held under the tongue until dissolved. Do not drink, eat or smoke until the tablet is dissolved completely.
nitroglycerin buccal spray (Nitrolingual Spray)	**Onto or under tongue:** With onset of acute attack, 1–2 metered doses (0.4 or 0.8 mg) of nitroglycerin. Optimal dose may be repeated 2x at 5- to 10-min intervals	• Pts should be instructed not to inhale. Dosage must be individualized and should be sufficient to provide relief without producing untoward reactions. During administration, pts should be at rest, ideally in the sitting position, and the canister kept vertical with the nozzle up. Opening of nozzle head should be kept as close to mouth as possible
buccal nitroglycerin (Nitrogard)	**Buccal:** *Adults:* Initially, 1 mg tid q5h during waking hours. If angina occurs while tablet is in place, dosage should be increased to next tablet strength	• Tablet should be placed between lip and gum above incisors or between cheek and gum. Onset of action may be increased by touching tablet with tongue
nitroglycerin sustained-release tablet (Nitrong SR, Nitrospan)	**Oral:** 1 tablet (2.6 mg) tid before breakfast, late afternoon ac, and hs. May be increased progressively up to 2 tablets tid	• Do not crush or chew tablet
nitroglycerin ointment 2% (Nitro-Bid, Nitrol)	**Topical:** Usual dose is 2.5–5 cm. Optimal dose is determined by starting with an application of 1.25 cm and increasing dose by 1.25 cm at a time until adverse effects (usually headache) occur or satisfactory response is obtained. Some pts may require as much as 10–12.5 cm and/or application q4h	• Apply ointment using dose-measured paper. Use paper to spread ointment onto skin (area should be clean, dry and preferably hairless). Do not rub in. Do not allow ointment to touch hands

Table 34.3 (continued)
The antianginals: Drug doses

Drug Generic name (Trade names)	Dosage	Nursing alert
A. Nitrates (cont'd) nitroglycerin patches (Transderm Nitro, Nitro-Dur)	**Topical** (starting dose): One 0.2-mg/h patch (10 cm^2) applied in a.m. If 0.2 mg/h (10 cm^2) is well tolerated, dose can be increased to 0.4 mg/h (20 cm^2) prn. A max. of 0.8 mg/h (40 cm^2) may be used	• Tolerance can be prevented or attenuated by use of an intermittent dosage schedule: daily patch on for 12–14 h, and a daily patch-off period of 10–12 h. Patch-free time should coincide with period in which angina pectoris is least likely to occur (usually at night). Watch pts carefully for increase of angina pectoris during patch-free period. Patches can be applied to all areas of skin except the distal extremities. Area should be clean, dry and preferably hairless. If hair is likely to interfere with patch adhesion or removal, clipping may be necessary prior to application. Take care to avoid areas with cuts or irritations
isosorbide-5-mononitrate (Monoket, ISMO)	**Oral:** *Adults* (for maintenance): 20 mg bid; first dose is taken on awakening and the second dose 7 h later	• Take on empty stomach with full glass of water for faster absorption
isosorbide dinitrate (Isordil, Sorbitrate)	**Oral:** *Adults:* Recomm. maint. dosage is 10–40 mg q6h (regular preparation) or 40–80 mg q8–12h (prolonged-release preparation). Risk of tolerance can be reduced by providing a nitrate-free interval, i.e., the regular preparation may be taken bid or tid during waking hours or the prolonged-release preparation may be taken od or bid at 08:00 and 14:00 **Sublingual:** *Adults:* 2.5–5 mg	• Check dosage form: available as sublingual, chewable and sustained-release. Chewable tab should be held in mouth for 2 min before swallowing. Do not crush or chew sustained-release tabs
B. Beta Blockers acebutolol HCl (Monitan, Sectral)	**Oral:** *Adults:* Initially, 400 mg daily in 2 divided doses. Increase gradually prn to control symptoms	• Take apical pulse prior to administration. Withhold dose if P<50 bpm and notify physician • May be given without regard to food
atenolol (Tenormin)	**Oral:** *Adults:* 50, 100 or 200 mg od. Increase dosage interval in pts with impaired renal function	• Give without regard to food • Take apical pulse. Withhold dose and notify physician if P<50 bpm
metoprolol tartrate (Betaloc, Lopresor, Lopressor)	**Oral:** *Adults:* Recomm. dosage is 100–400 mg/day in divided doses. Initially, 50 mg bid for first week. If needed, increase daily dose by 100 mg for second week. Usual maint. dose, 200 mg/day	• During initial tx, confer with physician if P<50 bpm

(cont'd on next page)

Table 34.3 (continued)
The antianginals: Drug doses

Drug Generic name (Trade names)	Dosage	Nursing alert
B. Beta Blockers (cont'd)		
nadolol (Corgard)	**Oral:** *Adults:* Initially, 40 mg od; may increase gradually by 40- to 80-mg increments at 3- to 7-day intervals until desired response is obtained. Usual maint. dose, 40–80 mg od. Increase dosage interval in pts with renal impairment	•Give without regard to food. May be crushed and mixed with food or fluid, if necessary
pindolol (Visken)	**Oral:** *Adults:* Initially, 5 mg tid with meals. If adequate response is not observed after 1–2 weeks, dosage may be increased. Usual maint. dose, 15 mg up to a max. of 40 mg/day	•Single daily dosing may be used when response is determined
propranolol HCl (Inderal)	**Oral** (regular preparation): *Adults:* Initially, 10–20 mg tid or qid. Increase gradually prn to control symptoms. For maintenance, most pts require at least 160–240 mg daily, usually given in 4 divided doses. Some pts require up to 400 mg daily. Administration bid may be effective in some pts with stable angina (Long-acting preparation): Initially, 80 mg od. May be increased gradually at 3- to 7-day intervals until optimal response is obtained. Average maint. dose, 160 mg od	•Check dosage form: available as regular tablets and sustained-release capsules. Best given with food. May crush tablets. Do not crush long-acting capsules
timolol maleate (Blocadren)	**Oral:** *Adults:* 10–30 mg bid	•May be given without regard to food
C. Calcium Channel Blockers (Calcium Entry Blockers)		
amlodipine besylate (Norvasc)	**Oral:** *Adults:* Initially, 5 mg od. After 1–2 weeks, dosage may be increased to a max. of 10 mg od. For geriatric pts and those with impaired renal function: Initially, 5 mg od; increase gradually prn. For hepatic dysfunction: Initially, 2.5 mg od	•May be given without regard to food
diltiazem HCl (Cardizem, Cardizem SR, Cardizem CD)	**Oral** (regular release preparation [Cardizem®]): *Adults:* Initially, 30 mg qid for stable angina, ac and hs. Increase gradually prn at 1–2 day intervals to 240 mg/day, given in 3 or 4 equally divided doses. *Cardizem SR®:* Intended for maint. tx in pts requiring 120–360 mg/day. Pts stabilized in this dosage range on regular Cardizem® may be changed to same daily dose of Cardizem-SR® divided into 2 equal doses and taken q12h. *Cardizem CD®:* Initially, 120–180 mg od.	•Check dosage form. Tablets may be given with food to reduce GI irritation. Tabs may be crushed; capsules must not be crushed or chewed

Table 34.3 (continued)
The antianginals: Drug doses

Drug Generic name (Trade names)	Dosage	Nursing alert
C. Calcium Channel Blockers (Calcium Entry Blockers) (cont'd)		
diltiazem HCl (Cardizem, Cardizem-SR, Cardizem-CD) (cont'd)	Max. dose, 360 mg od. Titration should be carried out over 7- to 14-day period. Pts controlled on diltiazem alone or in combination with other medications may be safely switched to Cardizem CD® capsules at the nearest equivalent total daily dose	
felodipine (Plendil, Renidil)	**Oral:** *Adults:* 10 mg od. Do not exceed 20 mg/day	• Extended-release formulation. Do not crush or chew
isradipine (Dynacirc)	**Oral:** *Adults:* Initially, 2.5 mg od for 2–4 weeks. Dosage may be increased in 5-mg increments every 2–4 weeks until optimal response is achieved. Max. dose, 20 mg od	• Food slows, but does not prevent, absorption
nicardipine (Cardene)	**Oral:** *Adults:* Initially, 20 mg tid. After 3 days, dose may be increased. Maint. dose, 20–40 mg tid. Sustained-release capsules: 30–60 mg bid	• Best on empty stomach. Check dosage form. Regular capsules can be crushed; do not crush or chew sustained-release capsules
nifedipine HCl (Adalat, Procardia, Adalat-XL, Procardia-XL)	**Oral** (regular preparation): *Adults:* Initially, 10 mg tid. Usual range, 10–20 mg tid. *(Extended-release [Adalat-XL®, Procardia-XL®]):* Initially, 30 or 60 mg od. Doses greater than 90 mg daily are not recommended. Pts controlled on regular preparation alone or in combination with beta blockers may be safely switched to extended-release preparation at nearest equivalent dose. Subsequent titration to higher or lower doses may be necessary and should be initiated as clinically warranted	• May be given with food if GI irritation occurs • Check dosage form. Do not crush or chew sustained-release tablets. Empty sustained-release tablet forms in stool are not significant
verapamil HCl (Calan, Isoptin)	**Oral:** *Adults:* 240–480 mg daily in 3 or 4 divided doses. Pts with severely impaired hepatic function should receive approximately 30% of this dose	• Give with food to reduce GI irritation

CHAPTER 35

Drugs Used in the Treatment of Peripheral and Cerebral Vascular Disorders

Topics Discussed
- Vasospastic disorders
- Chronic occlusive peripheral vascular disease
- For each drug discussed: Mechanism of action, pharmacologic effects, therapeutic uses, adverse effects
- Nursing management

Drugs Discussed
cyclandelate (sye-**klan**-deh-late)
nylidrin (**nye**-lih-drin)
pentoxifylline (pen-tok-**sif**-ih-lin)

Clinical Challenge

Consider this clinical challenge as you read through this chapter. The response to the challenge appears on page 382.

You are participating in a therapeutic drug review for a newly admitted patient to your continuing care facility. Mr. B. has been receiving a peripheral vasodilator for intermittent claudication.

One of the major goals for drug therapy is to use a drug regimen in which the benefits outweigh the risks. For the patient with chronic occlusive peripheral vascular disease, drug therapy has very little efficacy. State your arguments for and against continuing drug therapy for Mr. B.

Vasospastic Disorders

Vasospastic disorders result from a reduction in blood flow secondary to vasoconstriction. Regardless of whether vasoconstriction is precipitated by such factors as exposure to cold or emotional stress or occurs as a complication of collagen disease, arterial disease or other conditions, vasodilators may improve blood flow to ischemic areas, thereby providing relief. However, their usefulness is limited by two basic problems. First, they may decrease blood pressure, thereby reducing blood flow; second, they may dilate other vascular beds, thereby redirecting blood flow from the ischemic areas.

Drugs used to treat vasospastic disorders may (1) decrease central sympathetic tone (reserpine and methyldopa), (2) act on peripheral sympathetic nerve endings to reduce norepinephrine release (guanethidine), (3) block alpha$_1$ receptors on blood vessels (phenoxybenzamine), (4) stimulate beta$_2$ receptors on blood vessels (nylidrin) or (5) directly dilate blood vessels (calcium channel blockers and hydralazine). The pharmacology of reserpine, methyldopa and guanethidine was discussed in Chapter 30 and need not be repeated here. By the same token, the pharmacology of calcium channel blockers is presented in Chapters 34 and 36; hydralazine is also covered in Chapter 36. Phenoxybenzamine is no longer widely available and for this reason it, too, will not be discussed here. Only nylidrin will be presented specifically in this chapter.

Nylidrin (Arlidin®)

Nylidrin reputedly stimulates beta$_2$ receptors on blood vessels, thereby causing vasodilatation. It should be effective for the treatment of vasospastic disorders. However, there is little evidence to suggest that it is effective in Raynaud's phenomenon, cerebrovascular disorders or other conditions such as circulatory disorders of the inner ear. Patients taking the drug may experience dizziness, tachycardia, hypotension, nausea and vomiting.

Chronic Occlusive Peripheral Vascular Disease

Skeletal muscle blood flow is reduced by atherosclerosis. When this happens, intermittent claudication (lameness) may occur. Patients may experience no pain at rest but once they have walked a short distance, the pain of ischemia may force them to stop. The muscles in the leg(s) receive, under these conditions, inadequate blood flow to satisfy their metabolic requirements.

The effectiveness of drugs designed to relieve the symptoms of chronic occlusive peripheral vascular disease is limited. The products of anoxia and the increase in pCO$_2$ dilate blood vessels, if they are dilatable. This is the normal response of ischemic tissues in an attempt to increase blood flow. However, the blood vessels are often nondilatable because they are sclerotic and neither the products of anoxia nor vasodilator drugs will help.

A further complication of the use of vasodilators to treat chronic occlusive peripheral vascular disease is that these drugs will dilate those vessels that are still dilatable. These are, of course, healthy blood vessels perfusing tissues that are not ischemic. By decreasing peripheral vascular resistance in healthy parts of the body and not affecting it in damaged areas, vasodilators reduce the percentage of the cardiac output perfusing the tissues of concern and make the situation worse.

Little time will be spent discussing most of the drugs used to treat peripheral and cerebral vascular disorders. They work either by stimulating beta receptors in the vascular bed or by directly relaxing arterioles. Nylidrin is believed to be a beta$_2$ agonist. Isoxsuprine, cyclandelate and tolazoline are smooth muscle relaxants. It should be noted that these drugs can cause adverse effects: nausea, tremor, palpitations and tachycardia.

Pentoxifylline (Trental®)

Mechanism of action and pharmacologic effects. Pentoxifylline is discussed separately because, in contrast to the other drugs previously mentioned, evidence can be found to support its clinical effectiveness. The primary actions of pentoxifylline include increased erythrocyte flexibility, reduced blood viscosity and improved microcirculatory flow and tissue perfusion. As a result, orally administered pentoxifylline improves the supply of oxygen to ischemic muscles of the limbs.

Therapeutic uses. Pentoxifylline has been shown to be effective in the treatment of intermittent claudication. Most double-blind trials conducted in patients with moderate chronic obstructive arterial disease have demonstrated a significant improvement in walking performance in pentoxifylline-treated patients compared with those treated by placebo. Despite these most encouraging results, it is still not clear if pentoxifylline will improve the walking distance attained through an exercise regimen or if it will help the severely limited patient who cannot walk fifty metres.

Adverse effects. The most common adverse effects of pentoxifylline involve the gastrointestinal tract. Patients most often complain of nausea, vomiting, dyspepsia, abdominal discomfort and bloating. Other adverse effects include flushing, dizziness, lightheadedness and headache.

Table 35.1
Pentoxifylline: Drug interactions

Drug	Interaction
Anticoagulants, oral	• The activity of oral anticoagulants may be increased when combined with pentoxifylline
Antihypertensives	• Antihypertensive drugs may require lower doses in the presence of pentoxifylline
Hypoglycemics	• Hypoglycemic drugs may require a moderate adjustment in the dose when pentoxifylline is prescribed
Xanthines or sympathomimetics	• Xanthines or sympathomimetics, plus pentoxifylline, may cause excessive CNS stimulation

Table 35.1 lists the clinically significant drug interactions with pentoxifylline.

Nursing Management

Table 35.2 describes the nursing management of the patient receiving vasodilator drugs. Dosage details of individual drugs are given in Table 35.3 (page 384).

Response to Clinical Challenge

Arguments against using vasodilator therapy for chronic obstructive peripheral vascular disease:
• Drugs can cause significant adverse effects that interfere with ADL (nausea, headaches, hypotension, dizziness)
• Syncope or presyncope (near fainting or extreme dizziness) are common ADRs in elderly patients
• Drug efficacy is controversial: may dilate healthy vessels (which do not need drug treatment) and cannot dilate sclerotic vessels in the ischemic area; may also divert blood flow to other areas through venodilatation
• These drugs have significant drug interactions
• An exercise program and change in lifestyle may accomplish positive outcomes with fewer risks.

Arguments for using vasodilator therapy for chronic obstructive peripheral vascular disease:
• Pentoxifylline has research evidence for efficacy
• Patient may experience walking improvement which can improve quality of daily living.

Conclusion and recommendations:
Only pentoxifylline has research-based rationale for use in this patient. Daily activity and lifestyle programs should be used first. Drug should be avoided if drug interactions are significant or if patient is sensitive to xanthines (e.g., caffeine).

Table 35.2
Nursing management of the vasodilator drugs

Assessment of risk vs. benefit	Patient data	• Assess to establish baseline VS • *Pregnancy:* Risk category C (animal studies show adverse effects to fetus but human data are unknown or insufficient); benefits may be acceptable despite risks
	Drug data	• Physician should determine whether pre-existing condition warrants and will respond to vasodilator tx (sclerotic blood vessels will not dilate) • Pentoxifylline should not be used if pt is sensitive to xanthines (e.g., caffeine) • Several clinically significant drug interactions (see Table 35.1)
Implementation	Rights of administration	• Using the "rights" helps prevent errors of administration
	Right route	• Give PO
	Right time	• See Table 35.3. Drugs have short half-lives, thereby requiring regular, frequent administration for effectiveness
	Nursing therapeutics	• Provide pain control measures as required for leg pain • Monitor BP; hypotension increased if pt is also receiving antihypertensive tx • Drugs should be used with caution in older pts owing to risk of falls r/t dizziness/hypotension
	Patient/family teaching	• Instruct pt to enhance circulation through exercise program, smoking cessation, reduction in cholesterol • Advise pt to check with pharmacist/physician before taking any other medications • Instruct pt/family that short-term tx is of little benefit. Tx must be consistent and long-term • Caution pt regarding risks of dizziness and drowsiness
Outcomes	Monitoring of progress	*Continually monitor:* • Clinical response indicating tx success (reduction in signs/symptoms of cramping/pain in calf muscles, buttocks, thighs, feet). Note improvement in walking endurance. Benefits may not occur immediately • Be alert for signs/symptoms of adverse reactions: document and report immediately to physician

Table 35.3
Treatment of peripheral and cerebral vascular disorders: Drug doses

Drug Generic name (Trade names)	Dosage	Nursing alert
cyclandelate (Cyclospasmol)	**Oral:** *Adults:* Initially, 1.2–1.6 g/day in divided doses ac and hs. When clinical response occurs, reduce by decrements of 200 mg until a maint. dose of 400–800 mg/day in 2–4 divided doses is reached	• Monitor for effects and adverse reactions until stabilized • Give with meals or antacids
nylidrin HCl (Arlidin)	**Oral** (vasospastic tx adjunct): *Adults:* 3–12 mg tid or qid	• Nylidrin should not be initiated before a careful diagnosis of chronic brain syndrome or organic mental disorder is established since it is essential to identify the many treatable or reversible conditions or mental changes in those pts that will benefit from specific tx
pentoxifylline (Trental)	**Oral:** *Adults:* Initially, 400 mg bid. Usual maint. dose, 400 mg bid or tid. Max. dose, 400 mg tid	• Administer with meals to limit GI effects. Do not crush, break or chew tablets • Monitor BP carefully if antihypertensive drugs are used concurrently

CHAPTER 36

Antihypertensive Drugs

Topics Discussed

- Hypertension
- Diuretics
- Vasodilators
- Drugs that depress venous return
- Drugs that decrease cardiac output
- Central sympathetic inhibitors
- For all drugs discussed: Mechanism of action, pharmacological effects, therapeutic uses, adverse effects
- Pharmacologic approach to the treatment of hypertension
- Nursing management

Drugs Discussed

acebutolol (ass-eh-**byoo**-toe-lole)
amiloride (am-**mill**-oh-ryde)
amlodipine (am-**loe**-dip-een)
atenolol (at-**ten**-oh-lole)
benazepril (ben-**az**-eh-pril)
captopril (**kap**-toe-pril)
chlorthalidone (klor-**thal**-ih-doan)
cilazapril (sil-**az**-ah-pril)
clonidine (**klon**-ih-deen)
diazoxide (dye-az-**ox**-ide)
diltiazem (dil-**tye**-ah-zem)
doxazosin (dock-**saz**-oh-sin)
enalapril (en-**al**-ah-pril)
felodipine (fell-**oh**-dip-een)
fosinopril (foss-**in**-oh-pril)
furosemide (fyoor-**oh**-seh-myde)

guanadrel (**gwahn**-ah-drel)
guanethidine (gwahn-**eth**-ih-deen)
hydralazine (hy-**dral**-ah-zeen)
hydrochlorothiazide (hy-droe-khlor-oh-**thye**-ah-zyde)
indapamide (in-**dap**-ah-myde)
isradipine (is-**rad**-ih-peen)
labetalol (la-**bet**-ah-lole)
lisinopril (lyse-**in**-oh-pril)
losartan (loe-**sar**-tan)
methyldopa (meth-ill-**doe**-pah)
metolazone (me-**tole**-ah-zone)
metoprolol (met-**oh**-proe-lole)
nadolol (**nay**-doe-lole)
nicardipine (nye-**kar**-deh-peen)
nifedipine (nye-**fed**-ip-een)
nitroprusside (nye-troe-**pruss**-ide)
oxprenolol (ox-**pren**-oh-lole)
peridopril (per-ee-**doe**-pril)
pindolol (**pin**-doe-lole)
prazosin (**praz**-oh-sin)
propranolol (proe-**pran**-oh-lole)
quinapril (**kwin**-ah-pril)
ramipril (**ram**-ih-pril)
reserpine (res-**ser**-peen)
sotalol (**soe**-tah-lole)
spironolactone (speer-on-oh-**lak**-tone)
terazosin (ter-**az**-oh-sin)
timolol (**tye**-moe-lole)
triamterene (trye-**am**-ter-een)
verapamil (ver-**ap**-ah-mil)

Clinical Challenge

Consider this clinical challenge as you read through this chapter. The response to the challenge appears on page 400.

You are working as a public health nurse in a small community and are asked to present an educational session at the local library. The topic is "Know Your Blood Pressure."

Prepare an outline of the content and identify resources you will use. Be prepared to answer the following questions:

1. What will happen if I stop taking my blood pressure pills?
2. I am feeling fine: why do I have to take these pills?
3. If I take this drug and find out that I am pregnant, will my baby be harmed?
4. Why do I have to take two different pills to control my blood pressure?
5. How does alcohol affect blood pressure?

Hypertension

Hypertension is a major hazard to public health. Affecting the lives of millions, it is critically important in the pathogenesis of many cardiovascular diseases, including angina pectoris, acute myocardial infarction and congestive heart failure. Although the boundary between normotensive and hypertensive blood pressures is subject to debate, many authorities consider that blood pressures above 140/90 increase the risk of cardiovascular disease significantly. The reduction of elevated blood pressures by drugs lowers the risk of many of the complications of cardiovascular disease.

Approximately two-thirds of individuals over sixty-five years of age have hypertension. Many have *isolated systolic hypertension (ISH),* which is defined as a systolic blood pressure greater than or equal to 160 mm Hg and a diastolic of 90 mm Hg. This designation must be based on the average of two or more sitting readings on two or more occasions. Like hypertension, ISH is associated with increased risk for heart attack and stroke.

The past thirty years have seen the introduction of many drugs capable of reducing elevated blood pressures. With so many drugs available, it is important to select a drug, or combination of drugs, that best meets the needs of individual patients. In this regard, it is not only important to treat a patient with a drug or drugs that lower his

or her blood pressure, but equally vital to select the agent(s) that will improve the patient's quality of life.

Cardiac output (CO) and peripheral resistance (PR) are the two major determinants of blood pressure. Drugs that lower blood pressure reduce cardiac output or peripheral resistance, or both. These drugs work at the following anatomic sites:

- the kidneys, to increase salt and water loss and decrease blood volume (diuretics);
- the arterioles, to decrease PR (vasodilators);
- the veins, to decrease venous return and reduce CO (venodilators);
- the heart, to reduce CO (beta blockers);
- the sympathetic centres in the brain, to decrease sympathetic stimulation of the heart and blood vessels (central sympathetic inhibitors).

Figure 36.1 shows the sites of action of antihypertensive drugs.

Diuretics

Thiazides, Chlorthalidone and Metolazone

Mechanism of action and pharmacologic effects. Diuretics have become mainstays in the treatment of hypertension. Thiazides or chlorthalidone are used most frequently. Chlorthalidone

Figure 36.1
Sites of action of antihypertensive drugs

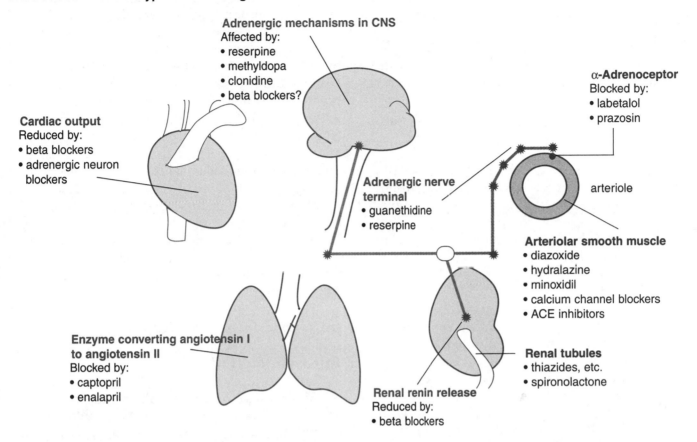

Source: Adapted from Simpson FO. Antihypertensive disease. In: Avery GS, ed. *Drug Treatment.* 2nd ed. Sydney/Auckland: ADIS Press; 1980:638.

(Hygroton®) and metolazone (Zaroxolyn®) are similar in action to the thiazides, with the exception that their effects are more prolonged.

The antihypertensive effects of these drugs cannot be attributed to a single action. Initially, they increase salt and water elimination, leading to a decrease in cardiac output. During chronic therapy, however, cardiac output increases to approach normal and peripheral resistance decreases. The antihypertensive effects of drugs during long-term therapy are due to a fall in peripheral resistance. Figure 36.2 illustrates the hemodynamic changes responsible for the antihypertensive effects of diuretic therapy.

Thiazides, chlorthalidone and metolazone decrease peripheral resistance by two separate mechanisms. First, they increase body water loss and decrease blood volume. As a result of less blood being forced through arterioles, peripheral resistance falls. Second, in an action unrelated to their effects on the kidneys, thiazides,

Figure 36.2
Hemodynamic changes responsible for the anti-hypertensive effects of diuretic therapy

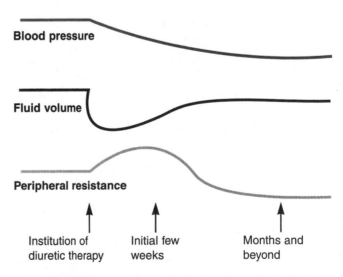

Source: Kaplan NM. The therapy of hypertension. In: Kaplan NM, ed. *Clinical Hypertension.* 4th ed. Baltimore: Williams and Wilkins; 1986:180. Reproduced with permission.

chlorthalidone and metolazone directly dilate pre-capillary resistance vessels (arterioles). This action accounts for much of their antihypertensive effects during chronic therapy.

It has been contended that the fall in body sodium produced by these diuretics accounts for their actions on resistance vessels. This cannot be the entire explanation, because loop diuretics produce a more profound loss of sodium but do not dilate arterioles.

Therapeutic uses. A thiazide or chlorthalidone is often used first in treating hypertension. Few differences can be found between the many available thiazides. Hydrochlorothiazide (HydroDIURIL®, Esidrix®) is the most frequently used. Chlorthalidone and metolazone have effects similar to those of thiazides but have longer durations of action.

Often, either a thiazide or chlorthalidone may suffice alone in patients with mild hypertension. If a second drug is necessary, a beta blocker or an ACE inhibitor can be added. To understand why either a diuretic plus a beta blocker, or a diuretic with an angiotensin-converting enzyme inhibitor (ACEI), is rational, the nurse must recognize that the fall in blood pressure produced by diuretics triggers an increase in sympathetic nervous system activity. The increased sympathetic drive stimulates vasoconstrictor alpha$_1$ receptors and releases renal renin. The newly released renin is converted first to angiotensin I and then to angiotensin II, a potent vasoconstrictor. Angiotensin II also releases aldosterone, which increases salt and water retention by the kidneys.

The release of renin is mediated by beta receptors in the kidney. The use of a beta blocker with a diuretic will reduce the renal secretion of renin and increase the antihypertensive response of the patient. An alternative approach is to give an ACEI with the diuretic. By blocking the angiotensin-converting enzyme, ACEIs inhibit the conversion of angiotensin I to angiotensin II, thereby reducing the vasoconstriction produced by angiotensin II and decreasing aldosterone secretion and salt and water retention.

Adverse effects. The adverse effects of the thiazides, chlorthalidone and metolazone, along with the nursing management, are presented in detail in Chapter 39. Hypokalemia, hyperglycemia, hyperuricemia and hyperlipidemia are the most frequently encountered adverse effects. Hypokalemia can be controlled by the concomitant administration of either a potassium salt, such as Slow-K® or Micro-K Extencaps®, or a potassium-sparing diuretic, such as triamterene (found in the product Dyazide®, which contains both triamterene and hydrochlorothiazide), amiloride (supplied in Moduret®, which provides both amiloride and hydrochlorothiazide), or spironolactone (provided in Aldactazide®, which contains both spironolactone and hydrochlorothiazide).

Diuretics also increase plasma cholesterol and triglyceride levels, and this is a matter of concern. However, the hyperlipidemic effects of these drugs can be diminished by administering lower doses (25 mg hydrochlorothiazide or 25 mg chlorthalidone per day).

The drug interactions of the thiazide diuretics are listed in Table 39.1 (page 436).

Furosemide (Lasix®)

Mechanism of action, pharmacologic effects and therapeutic use. Furosemide is a high-ceiling or loop diuretic, more potent than the thiazides, chlorthalidone or metolazone. In contrast to these drugs, furosemide does not dilate arterioles and therefore is not as effective as an antihypertensive. Because furosemide does not dilate arterioles, it should not be used routinely in treatment of hypertension. Rather, its use should be restricted to patients with renal damage who do not obtain adequate diuresis from hydrochlorothiazide or chlorthalidone.

Adverse effects. In general, furosemide's contraindications and adverse effects are similar to those of the thiazides and chlorthalidone (Chapter 39). However, because of its potent diuretic effects, furosemide has a greater potential for producing serious electrolyte disturbances. Hyponatremia, hypokalemia and hypovolemia are among the adverse effects of the drug. Other adverse effects include various forms of dermatitis, tinnitus and reversible deafness. Furosemide's drug interactions and nursing management are given in Tables 39.1 (page 436) and 39.4 (page 439), respectively.

Vasodilators

Angiotensin-Converting Enzyme Inhibitors (ACEIs)

Mechanism of action and pharmacologic effects. Renin, released from the kidney, is converted to angiotensin I, which in turn is changed to angiotensin II. Angiotensin II increases blood pressure in two ways. It constricts blood vessels and increases aldosterone secretion. As previously explained, the mineralocorticoid aldosterone retains fluid in the body and increases blood pressure. Figure 36.3 depicts the renin-angiotensin-aldosterone axis and its influence on blood pressure.

The ACEIs currently on the market include captopril (Capoten®), benazepril (Lotensin®), cilazapril (Inhibace®), enalapril (Vasotec®), fosinopril (Monopril®), lisinopril (Prinivil®, Zestril®), peridopril (Coversyl®), quinapril (Accupril®) and ramipril (Altace®). Captopril's action is depicted in Figure 36.4. Because ACEIs dilate arterioles but do not dilate veins, they reduce peripheral resistance without postural hypotension. ACEIs may also prevent the degradation of the vasodilator bradykinin and increase the production of vasodilator prostaglandins.

By decreasing aldosterone secretion, ACEIs promote the loss of salt and water. This action also plays a role in their antihypertensive effects.

Enalapril is de-esterified in the liver to the active chemical enalaprilat. Lisinopril is the lysine derivative of enalaprilat. It is absorbed more slowly than enalapril.

Quinapril is rapidly de-esterified after absorption to quinaprilat, its principal active metabolite. Following oral administration, peak plasma concentrations of quinapril occur within one hour. Peak plasma quinaprilat concentrations occur approximately two hours after an oral dose of quinapril.

Fosinopril is rapidly hydrolyzed following oral administration to its principal active metabolite, fosinoprilat. After the oral administration of fosinopril, approximately half of the absorbed dose is excreted in the urine and the remainder in the feces. Renal impairment reduces the percentage of

**Figure 36.3
Renin-angiotensin-aldosterone axis and blood pressure control**

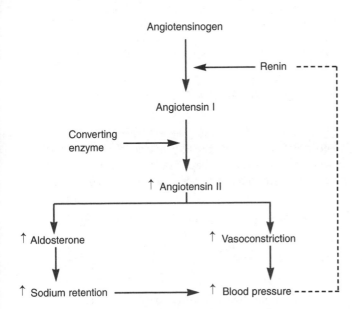

Source: Bristol-Myers Squibb. Reproduced with permission.

**Figure 36. 4
Effect of captopril on the renin-angiotensin-aldosterone axis**

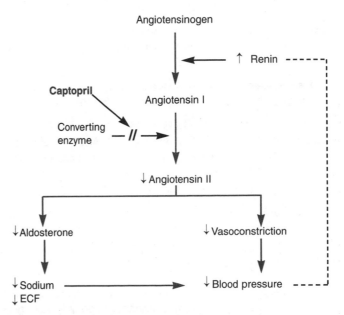

Source: Bristol-Myers Squibb. Reproduced with permission.

absorbed dose eliminated in the urine. However, a commensurate increase in fecal elimination takes place. By the same token, although hepatic insufficiency reduces the amount of drug eliminated in the feces, a commensurate increase in renal excretion occurs. For this reason, the elimination of fosinopril is said to be dual (urine and feces), balanced (approximately fifty percent by each route in patients with normal renal and hepatic function) and compensatory (one pathway picks up the slack in the face of impairment of the other). The age of the patient does not affect the pharmacokinetics of fosinopril.

Therapeutic uses. ACEIs represent a major advance in the development of antihypertensive therapy. As effective alone as beta blockers or diuretics, these drugs often produce fewer adverse effects than other antihypertensives. The alterations in blood chemistry, bradycardia, intermittent claudication, fatigue, cold extremities and decrease in libido produced by either diuretics and/or beta blockers are not experienced by patients receiving ACEIs. As a result, many patients taking ACEIs experience an increase in quality of life.

In addition to being effective alone, ACEIs can be used to complement the antihypertensive effects of a diuretic or a beta blocker. ACEIs also have an additive antihypertensive effect when combined with a calcium channel blocker.

Adverse effects. Overall, ACEIs may produce fewer adverse effects than many older antihypertensive drugs. Severe symptomatic hypotension can occur after the first dose of an ACEI. It is particularly prevalent in diuretic-treated patients who are salt depleted. This effect can be reduced, or prevented, if the diuretic is stopped, or its dose reduced, in the three to four days prior to treatment with an ACEI. In addition, patients should receive low doses of the ACEI. The dose can be increased gradually over the next few days.

A chronic, nonproductive cough is a common adverse effect of all ACEI. It occurs more frequently in women than in men, is especially bothersome when the patients is supine, and may necessitate drug withdrawal.

Generally, the adverse effects of ACEIs are usually mild and can be controlled by dosage reduction. However, some patients will discontinue an ACEI due to the dry, persistent, irritating

Table 36.1
ACE inhibitors: Drug interactions

Drug	Interaction
Allopurinol	• Allopurinol and captopril may increase the risk of Stevens-Johnson syndrome. Avoid concurrent use, especially in pts with renal failure
Anesthetics, halogenated	• Halogenated anesthetics (e.g., enflurane, halothane, isoflurane) can produce hypotension with ACEIs. Monitor BP
Diuretics	• Diuretics and an ACEI can produce a powerful hypotensive effect, possibly leading to postural hypotension. This can best be avoided by stopping the diuretic a few days before starting with low doses of the ACEI. Thereafter, it may be possible to reintroduce the diuretic and increase the dose of the ACEI slowly
Diuretics, potassium-sparing	• Potassium-sparing diuretics (e.g., amiloride, spironolactone, triamterene) increase the risk of hyperkalemia with ACEIs. Avoid concurrent use
Non-steroidal anti-inflammatory drugs	• NSAIDs can reduce the ability of ACEIs to dilate blood vessels
Potassium supplements	• Potassium supplements should not be used with ACEIs because ACEIs decrease aldosterone secretion, retaining potassium. Hyperkalemia can occur in pts receiving potassium supplements or potassium-sparing diuretics

cough. A small number experience serious adverse reactions, such as hyperkalemia, renal failure and angioedema, which can be fatal.

Table 36.1 lists the clinically significant drug interactions with ACEIs.

Nursing Management

Table 36.2 describes the nursing management of the patient receiving ACE inhibitors. Dosage details of individual drugs are given in Table 36.6 (pages 401–412).

Table 36.2
Nursing management of the ACE inhibitors (ACEIs)

Assessment of risk vs. benefit	Patient data	• Physician should determine whether hypertension exists with the average of two BP readings (sitting) taken on two occasions • Assess to establish baseline VS • *Pregnancy:* Risk category C in first trimester (animal studies show adverse effects to fetus but human data are unknown or insufficient; benefits may be acceptable despite risks). Risk category D in second and third trimesters (human fetal risk has been demonstrated)
	Drug data	• Drugs may be used alone or in combination with thiazide diuretics • *Some important drug interactions:* Confer with pharmacist • Serious adverse effects are rare, but include hyperkalemia, angioedema, renal failure and neutropenia
Implementation	Rights of administration	• Using the "rights" helps prevent errors of administration
	Right route	• Give PO
	Right time	• See Table 36.6. Note variation in dosage schedules among drugs in this class
	Nursing therapeutics	• Monitor BP closely during initiation of tx; be alert to first-dose hypotension

	Patient/family teaching	• Educate for management of hypertension through lifestyle and drug tx (Box 36.1)
		• Compliance and follow-up are essential factors in successful tx. Review principles of pt education in Chapter 3. Although hypertension can be controlled in most people, only about 20% actually receive adequate control. A major reason for this is lack of compliance. Clients fail to take antihypertensive drugs for many reasons:
		  – most have inadequate knowledge about the risks of their disease
		  – many are symptom-free and do not accept the seriousness of the risks
		  – many find the adverse effects difficult to cope with
		  – tx must be long-term; most hypertension occurs by age 30–40; drugs do not cure, only treat
		  – inadequate follow-up; need encouragement to remain on medication
		  – some drugs have a slow onset of action; results are not seen for 1–2 weeks; client may become discouraged

(cont'd on next page)

Table 36.2 (continued)
Nursing management of the ACE inhibitors (ACEIs)

Implementation (cont'd)	Patient/family teaching (cont'd)	• Pts/families should know warning signs/symptoms of possible toxicities of drugs. Report immediately: rash, mouth sores; fever, sore throat; swelling of hands or feet, face, eyes, lips or tongue; irregular heart beat, chest pain; dry cough, difficulty breathing; taste impairment • *Discuss possibility of pregnancy:* Advise pt to notify physician; discuss birth control methods. If pregnancy does occur, drug must be withdrawn ASAP
Outcomes	Monitoring of progress	*Continually monitor:* • Clinical response indicating tx success (reduction in BP without occurrence of undesirable effects) • Be alert for signs/symptoms of adverse reactions; document and report immediately to physician • Periodic lab tests may be considered (CBC, renal function)

Angiotensin II Receptor Antagonist: Losartan (Cozaar®)

Mechanism of action and pharmacologic effects. Losartan blocks the binding of angiotensin II to type 1 angiotensin II (AT-1) receptors in blood vessels and other tissues. As explained in our earlier discussion of ACE inhibitors, angiotensin II is a vasoconstrictor and stimulator of aldosterone secretion and is thought be important in the pathogenesis of hypertension. The ACEIs block the formation of angiotensin II from angiotensin I, but angiotensin I is also formed by other enzymes that are not blocked by ACEIs. In addition, ACEIs block the breakdown of bradykinin, resulting in alterations in prostaglandin metabolism. Angiotensin II receptor antagonists, therefore, inhibit the renin-angiotensin system more completely and more selectively than ACEIs.

Therapeutic uses. Losartan has been approved for oral treatment of hypertension. It is sold alone and in a fixed-dose combination with the diuretic hydrochlorothiazide (Hyzaar®). Like ACEIs, losartan has been less effective in black patients, tends to raise low serum potassium levels and, in some patients, decreases proteinuria. Unlike ACEIs, losartan lowers elevated serum uric acid levels.

Adverse effects. Except for a low incidence of dizziness, losartan has caused no adverse effects at a significantly higher rate than placebo in clinical trials. Few data are available, however, on the use of the drug in high-risk patients, such as those with decreased renal function or renal artery stenosis.

Cough, which has been a problem with ACEIs, does not appear to occur with losartan, probably because losartan's specificity in binding to receptors avoids effects on the kinin and prostaglandin systems. Angioedema, which can occur with ACEIs, also has not been reported with losartan. Except for occasional increases in serum aminotransferase activity, no clinically significant laboratory abnormalities have been detected.

Increases in serum potassium concentrations can occur, but hyperkalemia severe enough to require stopping the drug has not been reported.

Losartan should not be given to pregnant women because drugs that act on the renin-angiotensin system can cause fetal and neonatal injury and death.

Calcium Channel Blockers (Calcium Entry Blockers)

Mechanism of action and pharmacologic effects. Amlodipine (Norvasc®), diltiazem (Cardizem®), felodipine (Plendil®, Renedil®), isradipine (DynaCirc®), nicardipine (Cardene®), nifedipine (Adalat®, Procardia®) and verapamil (Isoptin®) are calcium channel blockers. These drugs are also referred to calcium entry blockers. Some of these drugs have previously been discussed as antianginal agents in Chapter 34.

The contractile process of vascular smooth muscle is dependent upon the movements of extracellular calcium into the cells through special ion channels. Amlodipine, diltiazem, felodipine, isradipine, nicardipine, nifedipine and verapamil selectively inhibit this transmembrane influx of calcium ions into vascular smooth muscle. As a result, the precapillary resistance vessels (arterioles) dilate and peripheral resistance falls.

Therapeutic uses. The introduction of calcium channel blockers for the treatment of hypertension represents a significant advance in the treatment of this disease. Similar to ACEIs, calcium channel blockers are effective vasodilators and not encumbered by many of the adverse effects commonly associated with the older drugs, such as diuretics, beta blockers and central sympathetic inhibitors.

If additional antihypertensive effects are required, a calcium channel blocker may be combined with a diuretic. In addition, amlodipine, felodipine, isradipine, nifedipine and nicardipine are often used with a beta blocker. However, verapamil and diltiazem have myocardial depressant effects and are not recommended in combination with beta blocker therapy.

Diltiazem, felodipine, nifedipine and verapamil are prepared in a extended-release formulations for the treatment of hypertension. Amlodipine is absorbed slowly and has a terminal elimination half-life of thirty-five to fifty hours. Thus, it does not require an extended-release formulation to work for twenty-four hours.

Adverse effects. Amlodipine, felodipine, isradipine, nifedipine and nicardipine are similar pharmacologically. Their adverse effects can include flushing, heat sensation or reddening of the skin, peripheral edema, fluid retention and swelling, palpitation or tachycardia, hypotension and syncope. Other adverse effects of these drugs include headache, tiredness and weakness, dizziness, light-headedness or giddiness, shakiness, nervousness and nausea or vomiting.

Diltiazem can produce bradycardia, dizziness, weakness, headache, flushing, dryness of the mouth and pedal edema. In addition, gastrointestinal disturbances and dermatological reactions have occurred with the drug. Diltiazem is contraindicated in patients with sick sinus syndrome, except in the presence of a functioning ventricular pacemaker; second- or third-degree A-V block; hypersensitivity to diltiazem; or severe hypotension (less than 90 mm Hg systolic pressure).

The most common adverse reactions with verapamil are constipation, dizziness and nausea. Because verapamil is a potent myocardial depressant with the ability to delay A-V conduction, it can produce bradycardia, A-V block, A-V dissociation, heart failure and pulmonary edema. Verapamil is contraindicated after acute myocardial infarction. It should not be given to patients with severe congestive heart failure and/or severe congestive dysfunction (unless secondary to a supraventricular tachycardia amenable to oral verapamil therapy); cardiogenic shock; severe hypotension; second- or third-degree A-V block; sick sinus syndrome; and marked bradycardia.

Table 36.3 on the next page lists the clinically significant drug interactions with calcium channel blockers.

Nursing Management

Table 36.4 (page 395) describes the nursing management of the patient receiving calcium channel blocker drugs. Dosage details of individual drugs are given in Table 36.6 (pages 401–412).

Directly Acting Arteriole Vasodilators

Hydralazine (Apresoline®)

Mechanism of action and pharmacologic effects. Hydralazine relaxes arteriolar smooth muscles by activating guanylate cyclase, resulting in the accumulation of cyclic guanosine monophosphate (cGMP). It has relatively little effect on veins. Thus, it decreases peripheral resistance and blood pressure without producing postural hypotension. Unfortunately, the fall in blood pressure triggers a reflex sympathetic response, resulting in an increase in heart rate and renin release and offsetting, in part, the primary hypotensive effects of the drug.

Hydralazine is metabolized in the liver.

Table 36.3
Calcium channel blockers: Drug interactions

Drug	Interaction
Amlodipine	
+ beta blockers	• Beta blockers may increase amlodipine's BP-lowering effects. Monitor pts carefully
Diltiazem	
+ beta blockers	• Beta blockers and diltiazem can lead to severe sinus bradycardia, hypotension and heart failure. Use with caution and monitor carefully
Felodipine	
+ cimetidine	• Cimetidine can increase the AUC and C_{max} of felodipine. It is recommended that low doses of felodipine be used when given concomitantly with cimetidine
+ phenytoin, carbamazepine, phenobarbital	• These drugs lower the maximum plasma concentration and AUC of felodipine. Consider alternative antihypertensive tx for these pts
Nicardipine	
+ beta blockers	• Beta blockers may have their antihypertensive effects increased by nicardipine
+ cimetidine	• Cimetidine increases nicardipine plasma levels. Pts receiving these two drugs concomitantly should be carefully monitored
+ digoxin	• Digoxin plasma levels may increase following concomitant tx with nicardipine. Pts should be monitored for increased digoxin levels
+ cyclosporin	• Cyclosporin plasma levels can increase when nicardipine is administered concomitantly. Plasma levels of cyclosporin should be monitored closely, and its dosage reduced accordingly in pts treated with nicardipine
Nifedipine	
+ antihypertensives	• Antihypertensive drugs may have their effects potentiated by nifedipine
+ beta blockers	• Beta blockers and nifedipine may occasionally provoke severe hypotension and overt heart failure in a susceptible pt with poor myocardial reserve
+ cimetidine	• Cimetidine may reduce the clearance of nifedipine
Verapamil	
+ antihypertensives	• Antihypertensive drugs may have their effects potentiated by verapamil
+ beta blockers	• Beta blockers, plus verapamil, can result in enhanced myocardial depression, hypotension, bradycardia, A-V blockade and asystole. These drugs should not be used concomitantly if left ventricular function is compromised
+ cimetidine	• Cimetidine may reduce the clearance of verapamil
+ digoxin	• Verapamil increases serum digoxin levels
+ rifampin	• Rifampin reduces the oral bioavailability of verapamil

Acetylation is the major route of inactivation. Patients may be divided into rapid acetylators and slow acetylators. During chronic therapy, hydralazine will accumulate in the slow acetylators unless lower doses are given.

Therapeutic uses. The use of hydralazine alone to treat hypertension is limited because of reflex tachycardia. It is often used together with a beta blocker and a diuretic, with the beta blocker preventing tachycardia and the diuretic increasing salt and water excretion. Hydralazine is contraindicated in patients with coronary artery disease, mitral valvular rheumatic heart disease and acute dissecting aneurysm of the aorta.

Adverse effects. Hydralazine's adverse effects include headache (due to vasodilatation), tachycardia, anginal symptoms, edema and heart failure. Patients may also experience anorexia, nausea,

Table 36.4
Nursing management of the calcium channel blockers

Assessment of risk vs. benefit	Patient data	•Physician should determine whether hypertension exists with the average of two BP readings (sitting) taken on two occasions •Assess to establish baseline VS •*Pregnancy:* Risk category C (animal studies show adverse effects to fetus but human data are unknown or insufficient: benefits may be acceptable despite risks)
	Drug data	•Drugs may be used alone or in combination with thiazide diuretics •*Some important drug interactions:* Confer with pharmacist •*Adverse effects/reactions:* See text
Implementation	Rights of administration	•Using the "rights" helps prevent errors of administration
	Right route	•Give PO. Check dosage forms; some have sustained-release preparations
	Right time	•See Table 36.6. Note variation in dosage schedules among drugs in this class
	Nursing therapeutics	•Monitor BP, P during tx. Check fluid I/O, body mass. Encourage pt to remain on drug tx; reduction in risk for heart disease or stroke is a valuable outcome even when weighed against adverse effects
	Patient/family teaching	•Educate for management of hypertension through lifestyle and drug tx (see Box 36.1) •Compliance and follow-up are essential factors in successful tx. Review principles of pt education in Chapter 3 •Pts/families should know warning signs/symptoms of possible toxicities of drugs. Report immediately: irregular heartbeat, difficulty breathing, pronounced dizziness, swelling of hands or feet •*Discuss possibility of pregnancy:* Advise pt to notify physician; discuss birth control methods
Outcomes	Monitoring of progress	*Continually monitor:* •Clinical response indicating tx success (reduction in BP without occurrence of adverse effects) •Be alert for signs/symptoms of adverse reactions; document and report immediately to physician •Periodic ECG monitoring may be required

dizziness and sweating. The most serious adverse effect of hydralazine is a lupus erythematosus-like syndrome, most often seen in slow acetylators. These patients must receive lower doses to prevent toxic levels of hydralazine from accumulating.

Table 36.5 on the next page lists the clinically significant drug interactions with hydralazine.

Alpha₁ Adrenergic Blockers

Mechanism of action and pharmacologic effects. Doxazosin (Cardura®), prazosin (Minipres®) and terazosin (Hytrin®) selectively block alpha₁ receptors and reduce peripheral resistance. In contrast to hydralazine, alpha₁

Table 36.5
Hydralazine: Drug interactions

Drug	Interaction
Diazoxide	• Diazoxide and hydralazine produce additive hypotensive effects
Monoamine oxidase inhibitors	• MAOIs should be used with caution in pts receiving hydralazine

adrenergic blocking drugs produce only a small increase in heart rate and little change in cardiac output and plasma renin levels. The drugs may also reduce total cholesterol and triglyceride concentrations. Doxazosin has also been shown to increase the ratio of high-density lipoprotein (HDL) to total cholesterol.

Therapeutic use. Doxazosin, prazosin and terazosin are indicated for mild to moderate hypertension. They are usually employed in a general treatment program in conjunction with a thiazide diuretic and/or other antihypertensive drugs.

Adverse effects. Alpha$_1$ adrenergic blockers dilate veins, reduce venous return and produce postural hypotension. Patients may complain of dizziness. Other adverse effects can include nausea, drowsiness, nasal congestion, palpitations, dry mouth, weakness and fatigue or malaise. For drug interactions and nursing management, consult Chapter 30.

Labetalol (Normodyne®, Trandate®)

Mechanism of action and pharmacologic effects. Labetalol blocks both alpha$_1$ and beta receptors. Although more potent as a beta blocker, labetalol's antihypertensive effects are due primarily to alpha$_1$ receptor antagonism, resulting in decreased peripheral resistance. The reflex tachycardia normally seen with arteriolar dilatation is prevented by the partial beta blockade. Bradycardia, usually seen with beta blocker therapy, does not occur with labetalol. Presumably the increase in sympathetic stimulation to the heart, secondary to vasodilatation, competes with the beta-blocking effects of the drug, the one offsetting the other.

Therapeutic uses. Labetalol is usually added to other therapeutic regimens, notably diuretic therapy. It may be tried alone as an initial agent in those patients in whom, in the judgment of the physician, treatment should be started with an alpha-beta blocker rather than a diuretic.

Adverse effects. The most serious adverse effects of labetalol reported are severe postural hypotension, jaundice and bronchospasm. Nausea and vomiting may also be experienced. Other adverse effects reported with labetalol include drug rash, paresthesias, muscular aches and pains, fatigue/malaise, headache and visual blurring.

Labetalol is contraindicated in uncontrolled congestive heart failure because sympathetic stimulation is a vital component supporting circulatory function in CHF, and inhibition with beta blockade carries the potential hazard of further depressing myocardial contractility and precipitating cardiac failure. Because of its ability to block both alpha$_1$ and beta receptors, the drug is also contraindicated in severe chronic obstructive lung disease, A-V block greater than first degree, cardiogenic shock and other conditions associated with severe and prolonged hypotension, and sinus bradycardia.

The drug interactions and nursing management for labetalol are presented in Tables 30.5 (page 300) and 30.10 (pages 304–305), respectively.

Diazoxide (Hyperstat®) and Sodium Nitroprusside (Nipride®)

Diazoxide and sodium nitroprusside are given parenterally to treat hypertensive crises. Diazoxide dilates arterioles primarily, and sodium nitroprusside relaxes both arterioles and veins. Although many physicians and nurses may encounter these drugs only rarely, one or both are usually stocked in all hospitals. Given to the patient suffering through a hypertensive crisis, either drug may be life-saving. Both drugs are contraindicated in compensatory hypertension, such as that associated with aortic coarctation or A-V shunt.

Drugs That Depress Venous Return

Guanethidine (Ismelin®)

Mechanism of action and pharmacologic effects. Guanethidine reduces the levels of norepinephrine in sympathetic nerve endings (see Chapter 30). It decreases venous return and reduces both heart rate and cardiac output. Guanethidine also dilates arterioles and reduces peripheral resistance. Because guanethidine blocks sympathetic innervation to the veins, it reduces venous return in the standing patient and produces orthostatic (postural) hypotension.

The decrease in cardiac output produced by guanethidine reduces renal blood flow and glomerular filtration rate. This can increase blood volume.

Therapeutic uses. Guanethidine is an effective antihypertensive drug. Concern over its adverse effects has relegated it to a position behind other antihypertensives. It is usually used with a diuretic, such as hydrochlorothiazide.

Adverse effects. The adverse effects of guanethidine are predictable on the basis of its mechanism of action. They include orthostatic (postural) hypotension, retrograde ejaculation, diarrhea, dyspnea, asthma and nasal stuffiness. Guanethidine does not cross the blood-brain barrier and sedation is thus not common.

The drug interactions and nursing management for guanethidine are presented in Tables 30.7 (page 302) and 30.10 (pages 304–305), respectively.

Reserpine (Serpasil®)

Reserpine is an adrenergic neuron blocker with mild antihypertensive activity (see Chapter 30). It is doubtful if many patients are started on this drug today. However, reserpine treatment is continued in many individuals who first received the drug years ago.

Reserpine crosses the blood-brain barrier and can cause severe depression. Once the depressant effects of reserpine have taken their toll, several drug-free weeks may be required before the patient returns to normal. Reserpine is contraindicated in mental depression, active peptic ulcer, ulcerative colitis, digitalis intoxication and aortic insufficiency. Drug interactions for reserpine and its nursing management are given in Tables 30.6 (page 301) and 30.10 (pages 304–305), respectively.

Drugs That Decrease Cardiac Output (Beta Blockers)

Mechanism of action and pharmacologic effects. Beta blockers are given to reduce beta$_1$-receptor mediated effects. By blocking beta$_1$ receptors, these drugs reduce cardiac output, thereby lowering blood pressure.

Propranolol (Inderal®), the prototype beta blocker, blocks both beta$_1$ and beta$_2$ receptors. By blocking beta$_2$ receptors on the bronchioles, it exposes the asthmatic or bronchitic patient to increased risk for bronchoconstriction. Blocking beta$_2$ receptors on blood vessels allows unopposed alpha$_1$ vasoconstriction, which may become clinically apparent especially in patients with Raynaud's phenomenon. Timolol (Blocadren®), nadolol (Corgard®) and sotalol (Sotacor®) are very similar to propranolol in their ability to block both beta$_1$ and beta$_2$ receptors. Both timolol and nadolol are used to treat hypertension. Sotalol also has Class III antiarrhythmic effects (see Chapter 33), and thus it can induce cardiac arrhythmias. Because of the proarrhythmic effects of sotalol, its use in patients with hypertension is limited to individuals who also require the drug for the treatment of ventricular arrhythmias.

The cardioselective beta blockers acebutolol (Monitan®, Sectral®), atenolol (Tenormin®) and metoprolol (Betaloc®, Lopresor®, Lopressor®) preferentially block beta$_1$ receptors, with less effect on beta$_2$ sites. As a result, these drugs have less effect on the bronchioles. However, this is largely of academic interest, because no beta blocker should be given to an asthmatic patient.

Cardioselective beta blockers are preferred in a diabetic patient. Normally, the hypoglycemic action of insulin is counterbalanced, in part, by the hyperglycemic effect of epinephrine — a beta$_2$-mediated effect. Nonselective beta blockers prevent this effect of epinephrine and accentuate the hypoglycemia produced by insulin. Acebutolol, atenolol and metoprolol may not prevent the beta$_2$ effects of epinephrine and thus are preferred. Both cardioselective and nonselective beta blockers reduce the tachycardia and tremor that may be early signs of hypoglycemia.

Patients who experience cold hands and feet following administration of propranolol, timolol or nadolol may prefer a cardioselective beta blocker. By blocking beta$_2$ receptors in peripheral arterioles, nonselective beta blockers predispose patients to alpha$_1$-receptor mediated vasoconstriction. If either acebutolol, atenolol or metoprolol is taken, vessel tone remains a balance between beta$_2$-receptor induced vasodilatation and alpha$_1$-receptor mediated constriction.

Pindolol (Visken®) and oxprenolol (Trasicor®) are beta blockers with partial-agonist or intrinsic sympathetic activity (ISA). They are not true competitive inhibitors of beta receptors. Instead, the drugs are very weak beta stimulants that compete with the more potent chemicals epinephrine and norepinephrine at receptor sites, with the result that they reduce beta-receptor mediated responses. Beta blockers with ISA may not reduce resting heart rate as much as other beta blockers.

Acebutolol (Monitan®, Sectral®) is a cardioselective partial agonist, exerting its ISA only on beta$_1$ receptors.

It is also possible to classify beta blockers on the basis of their lipid solubility. Propranolol, timolol, metoprolol, oxprenolol, pindolol and sotalol have significant lipid solubility and cross the blood-brain barrier readily. Nadolol, atenolol and acebutolol, on the other hand, have poor lipid solubility and are far less able to enter the brain. It has been argued that this gives the latter three a definite advantage because they may produce fewer CNS adverse effects.

Therapeutic uses. Beta blockers can be used as initial drugs in the treatment of hypertension. If a beta blocker alone proves inadequate, a diuretic such as hydrochlorothiazide or chlorthalidone may be added. Alternatively, a diuretic can be used first, with the beta blocker added when required. When the combination of a beta blocker and a diuretic fails to suffice, a vasodilator is usually added as a third drug.

Adverse effects. Bradycardia, fatigue, congestive heart failure and reduction in or loss of libido are the most obvious effects of a beta blocker. A block of beta$_2$ receptors in the bronchioles can produce bronchoconstriction in asthmatic patients. Beta blockers can precipitate cardiac failure in patients with CHF.

The other adverse effects of beta blockers include nausea, vomiting, constipation, diarrhea, depression, disturbed sleep and nightmares. Allergic reactions such as rashes, fever and purpura may also be seen. Finally, peculiar inflammatory reactions with fibrosis have been reported.

Beta blockers are contraindicated in bronchospasm, including bronchial asthma. Other contraindications to the use of beta blockers include allergic rhinitis during the pollen season, sinus bradycardia, A-V block greater than first degree, cardiogenic shock, right ventricular failure secondary to pulmonary hypertension, and CHF. The drug interactions and nursing management for beta blockers are given in Tables 30.4 (page 299) and 30.10 (pages 304–305), respectively.

Central Sympathetic Inhibitors

Clonidine (Catapres®)

Mechanism of action and pharmacologic effects. Clonidine stimulates alpha$_2$ receptors in the brain, thereby reducing norepinephrine release from the CNS sympathetic neurons (see Chapter 30). As a result of reduced sympathetic nervous system stimulation, renin release decreases and blood pressure falls.

Therapeutic uses. Clonidine is a very potent antihypertensive. It may be used concomitantly with other antihypertensive agents, such as diuretics or beta blockers.

Adverse effects. Some patients may experience an initial dry mouth and sedation. These effects are mild and usually diminish two to three weeks after the initiation of therapy. Should it become necessary to stop the drug, withdrawal should be achieved gradually over several days rather than abruptly, to prevent rebound hypertension. The drug interactions and nursing management for clonidine are given in Tables 30.8 (page 303) and 30.10 (pages 304–305), respectively.

Methyldopa (Aldomet®)

Mechanism of action and pharmacologic effects. Methyldopa reduces central sympathetic activity (see Chapter 30), decreases total peripheral resistance and reduces blood pressure. Cardiac output and blood flow are maintained. Because sympathetic reflexes are maintained fairly well when the patient stands, methyldopa does not produce the same degree of postural hypotension as guanethidine.

Therapeutic uses. Methyldopa is usually employed in a general treatment program in conjunction with a diuretic and/or other antihypertensive drugs, as needed. Methyldopa may also be used in the treatment of hypertensive crises.

Adverse effects. Methyldopa's adverse effects include sedation, edema, impotence and postural hypotension. Other adverse effects of the drug include nausea, vomiting, distention, constipation, flatus, diarrhea, colitis and mild dryness of the mouth. Drug fever, hepatic dysfunction, hemolytic anemia and lactation are seen rarely. Up to twenty-five percent of patients taking one gram of methyldopa daily for six months or more develop a positive Coombs' test. However, this has little clinical significance.

Methyldopa is contraindicated in patients with active hepatic disease. It should also not be used in persons in whom previous methyldopa therapy has been associated with liver disorders or hemolytic anemia.

The drug interactions and nursing management for methyldopa are given in Tables 30.9 (page 303) and 30.10 (pages 304–305), respectively.

Pharmacologic Approach to the Treatment of Hypertension

Drug therapy for mild to moderate hypertension should be attempted only after nonpharmacological measures (weight loss and reduction in dietary sodium intake) have failed. Weight loss by patients who are only slightly obese can reduce blood pressure significantly, independently of salt intake. With respect to salt, an intake in excess of approximately ten grams per day may aggravate hypertension, and dietary salt intake below normal intake levels may produce a small reduction in blood pressure. Furthermore, if drug therapy is required, reducing salt intake may increase the activity of antihypertensive drugs. Therefore, not only should excessive sodium intake be discouraged but further, mild sodium restriction (the "no added salt" diet, or less than five grams of sodium chloride daily) should be advised for hypertensive patients. As well, reducing dietary fat and increasing the ratio of polyunsaturated to saturated fat may also reduce blood pressure.

Mild hypertension may often be treated with one antihypertensive. More severe hypertension often may justify the use of two or more drugs. Two drugs, acting by different mechanisms, can often lower the blood pressure more than higher doses of each drug used alone. Drugs should be selected so that their mechanisms of action complement each other and reduce the consequences of the physiological response mechanisms evoked by each agent.

Hydrochlorothiazide or chlorthalidone may be adequate to treat patients with mild hypertension, with diastolic pressures between 90–100 mm Hg. However, because they increase both blood sugar and uric acid levels, diuretics should be avoided in patients with either diabetes or gout. Diuretics also increase renin release, and the resulting increase in angiotensin II and aldosterone levels may be sufficient to keep the patient hypertensive. If this happens, a beta blocker that will block beta$_1$ receptors in the kidney and the heart can be added to the therapeutic regimen. The beta blocker will reduce renin release and decrease cardiac output, resulting in a further decrease in blood pressure. Alternatively, an ACEI can be combined with the diuretic.

Some physicians elect to treat essential hypertension with a beta blocker first. A beta blocker should be avoided in patients with congestive heart failure, diabetes, asthma or peripheral vascular disease. Beta blockers decrease renal perfusion and may increase blood volume. In this situation a diuretic, such as hydrochlorothiazide, can be added to the beta blocker therapy. Alternative combination therapy involves the use of a calcium channel blocker, such as nifedipine, with the beta blocker.

More physicians are turning to an ACEI as the first drug of choice in the treatment of essential hypertension. These agents are effective peripheral vasodilators and appear to improve the overall quality of life more than diuretics, beta blockers or methyldopa. Furthermore, they are not contraindicated in diabetes or gout (as are diuretics), heart failure, diabetes, asthma, peripheral vascular disease (as are beta blockers) or depression or liver disease (as is methyldopa). Obviously, if a second drug is required, a diuretic represents the logical choice for combination therapy with an ACEI.

Calcium channel blockers are also popular drugs for the treatment of hypertension. Like ACEIs, calcium channel blockers may be used in conditions that contraindicate the administration of either a diuretic or a beta blocker.

Other vasodilators, such as hydralazine, doxazosin, prazosin or terazosin, are usually reserved for patients with moderate hypertension (diastolic pressures between 100–110 mm Hg). They are often added to a regimen consisting of a diuretic and a beta blocker. The beta blocker will reduce the reflex tachycardia produced by the vasodilator, and the diuretic will ensure that an increase in blood volume does not occur.

Methyldopa or clonidine may be used in place of the vasodilator in the patient with moderate hypertension. These drugs are effective antihypertensives and are usually combined with hydrochlorothiazide or chlorthalidone. Their selection over a vasodilator is determined largely on the basis of the clinical response of the particular patient to one drug or the other, or the adverse effects that are best tolerated. Contraindications to the use of methyldopa have already been mentioned. Clonidine should be avoided in patients who suffer from depression.

Adrenergic neuron-blocking drugs, such as guanethidine, are usually reserved for the severely hypertensive patient, with a diastolic pressure in excess of 110 mm Hg, whose hypertension is not controlled on other drugs. These agents are often added to pre-existing treatment regimens consisting of a diuretic and a vasodilator. The adverse effects of blocking all peripheral sympathetic nerve endings are often so galvanizing that many physicians are reluctant to resort to guanethidine unless all other agents have been tried.

Response to Clinical Challenge

Topic: Know Your Blood Pressure

Outline of content
You should explain the terms blood pressure and hypertension, how it is measured and what the numbers mean. You should include a brief explanation of the lifestyle factors that affect blood pressure.

Resources
Consider the library; local or provincial office of the Heart and Stroke Foundation. Look for patient education materials such as *Medication Teaching Aids* (Springhouse).

1. What will happen if I stop taking my blood pressure pills?
The blood pressure will rise again. Stopping suddenly can cause serious effects, as the blood pressure may rise very quickly.

2. I am feeling fine: why do I have to take these pills?
High blood pressure does not usually cause any symptoms by itself. However, it does increase the risk for heart disease and stroke, so it is important to treat it for your lifetime.

3. If I take this drug and find out that I am pregnant, will my baby be harmed?
If you are taking an ACEI then you must stop the drug, with physician's advice, immediately after confirming the pregnancy. These drugs must not be continued during the second/third trimesters of pregnancy. Other antihypertensive drugs can be used safely during pregnancy.

4. Why do I have to take two different pills to control my blood pressure?
For some people, two drugs are better than one. The combination of drugs may be more effective with fewer adverse effects than higher doses of either drug. Sometimes one drug may offset an adverse effect of the other.

5. How does alcohol affect blood pressure?
Alcohol dilates blood vessels and can lower the blood pressure. If you combine alcohol with pills, your blood pressure may fall too low and cause fainting, rapid pulse and other effects.

Box 36. 1
Patient teaching: Hypertension

What is hypertension?

Hypertension is the term for high blood pressure, which is the force of blood as it moves through the arteries. Normal blood pressure should be less than 140/90. The first number is called the systolic and measures the highest pressure in the artery with a heartbeat. The diastolic is the lower number and measures the pressure when the heart rests between beats. You can have your blood pressure measured by your health professional or learn to do this yourself with instruction.

How does lifestyle affect blood pressure?

Lack of activity, smoking, alcohol, stress and some dietary factors can all increase blood pressure. You can help to keep your blood pressure low with a healthy diet, by starting a regular exercise program, stopping smoking and limiting alcohol to 60 mL (2 oz) per day. A healthy diet should include plenty of fluids, limited sugar, caffeine, sodium (salt) and fat. Stress management is equally important.

What should I know about drug therapy?

• To control blood pressure, drug therapy must be long-term and consistent. Drugs do not cure the problem. Follow the directions and do not miss any doses. If you do forget to take a dose, take it as soon as you remember — but never take two doses together.
• You should know the adverse effects of your medication and how to reduce them, if possible. For example, to avoid the dizziness that can occur with lowered blood pressure, change positions slowly, avoid very hot baths and limit activity in hot weather. Do not stop taking the drug if you experience mild side effects: discuss first with your physician.
• Do not take any other medications without checking with your pharmacist or physician, and tell your dentist about the drugs you are taking.
• If you have any serious side effects, call your doctor immediately.
• If you intend to become pregnant, discuss first with your physician. If you do become pregnant, contact your physician immediately.

Table 36.6
The antihypertensives: Drug doses

Drug Generic name (Trade names)	Dosage	Nursing alert
A. Diuretics hydrochlorothiazide ((Esidrix, HydroDIURIL)	**Oral:** *Adults:* Initially, 12.5–25 mg/day. May be increased to 50 mg/day. *Children:* 1–2 mg/kg/day in 2 divided doses	• Administer in a.m. to prevent nocturia. May give with food or milk if GI irritation occurs. May crush and mix with food
chlorthalidone (Hygroton)	**Oral:** *Adults:* Initially, 12.5–25 mg/day. May be increased to 50 mg/day. *Children:* 0.5–2 mg kg/day	• As for hydrochlorothiazide
indapamide hemihydrate (Lozide, Lozol)	**Oral:** *Adults:* Initially, 1.25 mg/day. May be increased to 2.5–5 mg/day	• As for hydrochlorothiazide
metolazone (Zaroxolyn)	**Oral:** Initially, 2.5–5 mg/day; may be increased to 10 mg/day	• As for hydrochlorothiazide • Do not substitute prompt and extended-release tablets. Do not crush extended-release tablets
furosemide (Lasix)	**Oral:** *Adults:* Initially, 20–40 mg/day. If necessary, increase gradually. *Children:* 0.5–2 mg/kg/day in 2 doses	• As for hydrochlorothiazide

(cont'd on next page)

Table 36.6 (continued)
The antihypertensives: Drug doses

Drug Generic name (Trade names)	Dosage	Nursing alert
B. Potassium-Sparing Diuretics		
amiloride HCl (Midamor)	**Oral:** *Adults:* Initially, 5 mg/day. Usual max. dose, 10 mg/day	• As for hydrochlorothiazide
amiloride HCl 5 mg + hydrochlorothiazide 50 mg (Moduret)	**Oral:** *Adults:* Initially, 1/2 tablet daily. Adjust dosage in accordance with BP and serum potassium level	• As for hydrochlorothiazide
spironolactone (Aldactone)	**Oral:** *Adults:* Initially, 25 mg/day. May be increased to 100 mg/day in a single dose or 2 divided doses. *Children:* 1–2 mg/kg/day in 2 doses. Adjust in accordance with BP and serum potassium level	• As for hydrochlorothiazide
spironolactone 25 mg + hydrochlorothiazide 25 mg (Aldactazide 25/25) spironolactone 50 mg + hydrochlorothiazide 50 mg (Aldactazide 50/50)	**Oral:** Initially, 1 tablet containing 25 mg of each component daily. Increase to 50 mg of each component daily in a single dose or divided doses, if necessary. Adjust dosage in accordance with BP and serum potassium level	• As for hydrochlorothiazide
triamterene (Dyrenium)	**Oral:** *Adults:* Initially, 50 mg/day. May be increased to 150 mg/day in a single dose or 2 divided doses given pc. Max. daily dose, 300 mg. *Children:* 1–2 mg/kg/day in 2 doses. Adjust dosage in accordance with BP and serum potassium level	• Administer with food or milk to reduce GI irritation and increase bioavailability. Capsules may be opened and contents mixed with food or fluids
triamterene 50 mg + hydro-chlorothiazide 25 mg (Dyazide)	**Oral:** *Adults:* Initially, 1 capsule daily. May be increased to 2 capsules/day in single or divided doses. The dosage should be adjusted in accordance with BP and serum potassium level	• As for triamterene

Table 36.6 (continued)
The antihypertensives: Drug doses

Drug Generic name (Trade names)	Dosage	Nursing alert
C. Angiotensin-Converting Enzyme Inhibitors (ACEIs)		
captopril (Capoten)	**Oral:** *Adults:* Initially, 25 mg bid or tid, the dosage being increased if necessary after 1–2 weeks to 50 mg bid or tid	• Monitor BP after first dose (1–3 h) • Food reduces absorption by 30–40%. Tablets may be crushed but do not mix with food. May dissolve in water
benazepril HCl (Lotensin)	**Oral:** *Adults:* Initially, 10 mg (base) od. Maintenance: 20–40 mg (base)/day as a single dose or in 2 divided doses. In sodium- or water-depleted pts, or pts receiving diuretics, or pts with renal failure (CrCl < 30 mL/min per 1.73m^2): Initially, 5 mg	• Monitor BP after first dose: may cause precipitous drop. Discontinue diuretic tx 2–3 days prior to initiating drug. Absorption not affected by food. Keep pts who are sodium- or water depleted, pts with renal failure, or pts who are currently or have recently been on diuretic tx under supervision for at least 2 h after initial dose and watch for excessive hypotension
cilazapril (Inhibace)	**Oral:** Monotherapy: Initial dose is 2.5 mg od. Adjust dosage according to BP response, generally at intervals of at least 2 weeks. Usual dose range is 2.5–5 mg od	• To determine effectiveness of od dosing, monitor BP prior to daily dose. If possible, discontinue diuretics prior to initiating tx • Absorption is not affected by food
enalapril maleate (Vasotec)	**Oral:** *Adults:* Initial: 5 mg od; adjust dosage after 1–2 weeks according to clinical response. Maintenance: 10–40 mg/day, as a single dose or in 2 divided doses. For pts who are sodium- or water depleted as a result of prior diuretic tx, pts on current diuretic tx, or pts with renal failure (CrCl < 30 mL/min): Initially, 2.5 mg	• Absorption is not affected by food • Keep pts who are sodium- or water depleted, pts with renal failure, or pts who are currently or have recently been on diuretic tx under supervision for at least 2 h after initial dose and watch for excessive hypotension. To determine effectiveness, monitor BP prior to daily dose
fosinopril sodium (Monopril)	**Oral:** *Adults:* Initial: 10 mg od; adjust dosage according to clinical response. Maintenance: 20–40 mg od	• Monitor BP after first dose: precipitous drop may occur
lisinopril (Prinivil, Zestril)	**Oral:** *Adults:* Initial: 10 mg od; adjust dosage according to clinical response. Maintenance: 10–40 mg od. For pts who are sodium- or water depleted as a result of prior diuretic tx, pts on current diuretic tx, or pts with renal failure (CrCl < 30 mL/min): Initially, 2.5–5 mg. For pts with CrCl < 10 mL/min: Initially, 2.5 mg	• Absorption not affected by food • Keep pts who are sodium- or water depleted, have renal failure or who are currently/ have recently been receiving diuretic tx under medical supervision for at least 2 h after initial dose; watch for excessive hypotension. To determine effectiveness, monitor BP prior to daily dose

(cont'd on next page)

Table 36.6 (continued)
The antihypertensives: Drug doses

Drug Generic name (Trade names)	Dosage	Nursing alert
C. Angiotensin-Converting Enzyme Inhibitors (ACEIs) (cont'd)		
quinapril HCl (Accupril)	**Oral:** *Adults:* Initially, 10 mg (base) od. Adjust slowly, at 2-week intervals, according to clinical response. Maintenance: 10–20 mg od; max., 40 mg/day. For pts who are sodium- or water depleted as a result of prior diuretic tx, pts currently receiving diuretic tx or pts with renal failure (CrCl = 30–60 mL/ min): Initially, 5 mg. If CrCl = 10–30 mL/min, init. dose is 2.5 mg. Insufficient data for dosage recommendation in pts with CrCl < 10 mL/min	• Absorption not affected by food • Keep pts who are sodium- or water depleted, pts with renal failure or pts who are currently/have recently been receiving diuretic tx under supervision for at least 2 h after initial dose; watch for excessive hypotension. To determine effectiveness, monitor BP prior to daily dose
ramipril (Altace)	**Oral:** *Adults:* Initially, 2.5 mg od, the dosage being adjusted according to clinical response. Maintenance: 2.5–20 mg od or divided into 2 equal doses. For pts who are sodium- or water depleted as a result of prior diuretic tx, pts currently receiving diuretic tx or pts with renal failure (CrCl < 40 mL/min/1.73m²): Initially, 1.25 mg od. Titrate dosage slowly upward until adequate BP control is achieved or to a max. total daily dose of 5 mg. For pts with CrCl < 10 mL/min/1.73 m², max. dose is 2.5 mg/day	• Absorption not affected by food • Keep pts who are sodium- or water depleted, pts with renal failure or pts who are currently/have recently been receiving diuretic tx under supervision for at least 2 h after initial dose; watch for excessive hypotension. To determine effectiveness, monitor BP prior to daily dose
D. Angiotensin II Receptor Antagonist		
losartan potassium (Cozaar)	**Oral:** Initially, 50 mg od. For pts taking diuretics and those with hepatic impairment: Initially, 25 mg. Most pts require 50–100 mg/day, taken in 1–2 doses	• No dosage adjustment required for renal impairment or elderly pts. Lower doses for hepatic impairment
E. Calcium Channel Blockers (Calcium Entry Blockers)		
amlodipine besylate (Norvasc)	**Oral:** *Adults:* 5–10 mg od. For geriatric pts with impaired renal function: 5 mg od. Pts with impaired hepatic function: Initially, 2.5 mg	• Absorption not affected by food • Monitor pulse, BP, weight and fluid I/O
diltiazem HCl (Cardizem, Dilacor)	**Oral:** *Adults* (Cardizem CD® or Dilacor XR®): 180–240 mg od. Adjust after 14 days prn. Total daily dose ranges from 240–360 mg. (Cardizem SR®): Initially, 120–360 mg/day, administered in 2 equally divided doses	• As for amlodipine, plus do not crush or chew sustained-release forms. Do not substitute different dosage forms

Table 36.6 (continued)
The antihypertensives: Drug doses

Drug Generic name (Trade names)	Dosage	Nursing alert
E. Calcium Channel Blockers (Calcium Entry Blockers) (cont'd)		
felodipine extended-release (Plendil, Renedil)	**Oral:** *Adults:* Initially, 5 mg od. Adjust dosage prn, usually at intervals of not less than 2 weeks. Maintenance: 5–10 mg od. Usual adult prescribing limits: Up to 20 mg od. Geriatric pts may be more sensitive to effects of usual adult dose	• Monitor P, BP, weight, fluid I/O • Do not crush or chew tablet
isradipine (DynaCirc)	**Oral:** *Adults:* Initially, 2.5 mg bid, alone or in combination with a thiazide diuretic. Increase dosage prn, in increments of 5 mg/day at 2- to 4-week intervals. Usual adult prescribing limits: Up to 10 mg bid. Geriatric pts may be more sensitive to effects of usual adult dose	• Food reduces onset of action but not total bioavailability • Administer consistently at same time each day • Monitor P, BP, weight, fluid I/O
nicardipine HCl (Cardene)	**Oral:** Initially, 20 mg tid. Adjust dosage prn and as tolerated	• Food decreases absorption. Give 1 h ac or 3 h pc • Dosage adjustments should not be made more frequently than every 3 days
nifedipine (Adalat, Procardia)	**Oral:** *Adults:* Initially, 10 mg tid. Increase dosage gradually over a 7- to 14-day period as needed and tolerated. For hospitalized pts under close supervision, dosage may be increased by 10-mg increments over 4- to 6-h periods until symptoms are controlled. Daily dose, up to 180 mg (a total daily dose > 120 mg is rarely required). Geriatric pts may be more sensitive to effects of usual adult dose (Adalat-PA®): Initially, 10–20 mg bid. Usual adult dose, 20 mg bid. Increase prn to 40 mg bid. Do not exceed a max. of 80 mg/day (Adalat-XL® [extended-release] tablets): Initially, 30–60 mg od. Usual maint. dose, 60–90 mg od. Do not exceed max. dose of 120 mg od	• May be taken with food. Do not crush or chew sustained-release products • For hypertensive emergencies, instruct pt to bite the capsule and swallow contents. This has a faster onset of action than sublingual administration

(cont'd on next page)

Table 36.6 (continued)
The antihypertensives: Drug doses

Drug Generic name (Trade names)	Dosage	Nursing alert

E. Calcium Channel Blockers (Calcium Entry Blockers) (cont'd)

verapamil HCl (Isoptin)	**Oral:** *Adults:* Initially, 80–120 mg (HCl) tid. Increase dosage at daily or weekly intervals as needed and tolerated. An initial dose of 40 mg (HCl) tid is recommended in pts who may have increased response to verapamil (e.g., those with hepatic function impairment, elderly pts, pts with poor left ventricular function). Total daily adult dose usually ranges from 240–480 mg. Geriatric pts may be more sensitive to effects of usual adult dose (Isoptin-SR): Usual adult dose is 180–240 mg od each morning with food. If required, this dose may be increased up to 240 mg bid. Do not exceed total daily dose of 480 mg/day. Total daily dosages of 360 mg or 480 mg should be divided into morning and evening doses	• Administer with food to reduce GI irritation. Do not crush or chew sustained-release products

F. Directly Acting Arteriole Vasodilators

diazoxide (Hyperstat)	**IV:** *Adults:* Up to 150 mg, or 1–3 mg/kg. Repeat q5–15min if necessary to obtain desired response. Further doses may be administered q4–24h as needed to maintain desired BP until oral antihypertensive medication is effective, usually within 4–5 days. Usual adult prescribing limits: Up to 1.2 g/day *Pediatric:* 1–3 mg/kg, or 30–90 mg/m^2 of body surface, repeated in 5–15 min if necessary to obtain desired response. Further doses may be administered q4–24h as needed to maintain desired BP until oral antihypertensive medication is effective	• For direct IV, follow agency policy. Give over 30 s, undiluted, into peripheral vein • Parenteral administration should always be carried out cautiously, with continuous monitoring of BP and ECG. Pt should remain supine for 1 h after infusion. Monitor pt's ambulation closely and check standing BP to determine orthostatic hypotension • Protect solution from light. Solution should be clear and colourless. Do not use darkened solution
hydralazine HCl (Apresoline)	**Oral:** *Adults:* 10 mg qid for first 2–4 days, followed by 25 mg qid for the balance of first week. Maintenance: 50 mg qid for second and subsequent weeks; dosage should be adjusted to lowest effective level.	

Table 36.6 (continued)
The antihypertensives: Drug doses

Drug Generic name (Trade names)	Dosage	Nursing alert

F. Directly Acting Arteriole Vasodilators (cont'd)

Drug	Dosage	Nursing alert
hydralazine (Apresoline) (cont'd)	**(Oral/cont'd):** Geriatric pts may be more sensitive to effects of usual adult dose. Usual adult prescribing limits: Up to 300 mg/day (higher doses have been used in tx of CHF) **IV:** Initially, 5–10 mg by slow injection to avoid precipitous decrease in mean arterial pressure. In hypertensive crises, other than pre-eclampsia/eclampsia, initial doses of up to 40 mg have been used. If necessary, dose can be repeated after an interval of 20–30 min. Hydralazine may also be given by continuous IV infusion, beginning with a flow rate of 200–300 µg/min. Maint. flow rates must be determined individually, usually within the range of 50–150 µg/min	**•IV:** Parenteral administration of hydralazine should always be carried out cautiously and under strict medical supervision. BP and HR should be checked frequently (q5min). BP may begin to fall within a few minutes after injection, with an average max. decrease occurring in 10–80 min. Most pts can be transferred to oral hydralazine within 24–48 h
sodium nitroprusside (Nipride)	**IV infusion:** *Adults:* Initially, 0.3 µg (0.0003 mg) (sodium nitroprusside dihydrate) per kg per minute, adjusted every few minutes according to response; usual dose is 3 µg (0.003 mg) per kg per minute. Geriatric pts may be more sensitive to usual adult dose of nitroprusside. Max. dose for adults: Up to 10 µg (0.01 mg) per kg per minute for a max. of 10 min, or total dose of 3.5 mg/kg body weight (500 µg [0.5 mg] per kg of body weight during short-term infusions such as in controlled hypotension during surgery). To keep the steady-state thio-cyanate concentration below 1 mmol/L, the rate of a prolonged infusion should be no more than 3 µg/kg of body weight per minute (1 µg/kg of body weight per minute in anuric pts)	•Use infusion pump to ensure accuracy. Use dosage chart to calculate rate •Preparation of dosage form: Reconstitute by dissolving the contents of a 50-mg vial in 2–3 mL of 5% dextrose injection only and shaking gently to dissolve. Dilute further in 250–1000 mL of 5% dextrose injection and wrap container in a supplied opaque sleeve, aluminum foil or other opaque material to protect it from light (it is not necessary to wrap the infusion drip chamber or the tubing) •*Stability:* Solutions of nitroprusside should be freshly prepared and any unused portion discarded. A freshly prepared solution has a slight brownish tint and should be discarded if the colour is dark brown, orange or blue. Solution must be used within 24 h. No other medications should be added to infusion fluid containing nitroprusside. Sodium nitroprusside solution is rapidly degraded by trace contaminants, often with resulting colour changes. A change in colour to blue, green or bright red indicates reaction of nitroprusside ion with another substance, and the solution must be replaced and discarded

(cont'd on next page)

Table 36.6 (continued)
The antihypertensives: Drug doses

Drug Generic name (Trade names)	Dosage	Nursing alert
G. Alpha₁ Adrenergic Blockers		
doxazosin mesylate (Cardura)	**Oral:** *Adults:* Initially, 1 mg (base) od hs. Maintenance: Increase dosage gradually every 2 weeks to 2, 4, 8 and 16 mg to meet individual requirements and as tolerated. Increases in dose beyond 4 mg (base) increase likelihood of excessive postural effects including syncope, postural dizziness/vertigo and postural hypotension. Geriatric pts may be more sensitive to effects of usual adult dose	• Monitor BP and P 2–6 h after initial doses and with each dosage increase • Absorption is not affected by food
prazosin HCl (Minipress)	**Oral:** *Adults:* Starting dose, 0.5 mg with evening meal, then 09.5 mg bid–tid for at least 5 days. Maintenance: adjust gradually to meet individual requirements, most commonly 6–15 mg (base) per day in 2–3 divided doses. Geriatric pts may be more sensitive to effects of usual adult dose. Daily doses > 20 mg (base) usually do not have increased efficacy	• Monitor closely after first dose and during titration • May give at evening meal to minimize hypotension. Give with food
terazosin HCl (Hytrin)	**Oral:** *Adults:* Initially, 1 mg (base) od hs. Maintenance: Adjust dosage gradually to meet individual requirements, usually 1–5 mg (base) od. If the antihypertensive effect is not maintained for a full 24 h, bid dosing may be more effective. Geriatric pts may be more sensitive to effects of usual adult dose	• Monitor closely after first dose and during titration. Take BP prior to next dose to evaluate effectiveness
H. Alpha₁ Adrenergic and Beta Blocker		
labetalol HCl (Normodyne, Trandate)	**Oral:** *Adults:* Initially, 100 mg bid. Adjust in increments of 100 mg bid every 2–3 days until desired response is achieved. Maintenance: 200–400 mg bid. Labetalol may be administered in 3 divided daily doses if necessary because of adverse effects such as nausea or dizziness. In severe hypertension, doses of 1.2–2.4 g/day, in 2–3 divided doses, may be needed. Geriatric pts may have increased or decreased sensitivity to effects of usual adult dose	• **Oral:** Give with food to enhance absorption • Confer with physician if P<50/min. Monitor BP, weight, fluid I/O

Table 36.6 (continued)
The antihypertensives: Drug doses

Drug Generic name (Trade names)	Dosage	Nursing alert
H. Alpha₁ Adrenergic and Beta Blocker (cont'd)		
labetalol (Normodyne, Trandate) (cont'd)	**Repeated IV injections:** Initially, 20 mg by slow injection over 2 min. Additional injections of 40 or 80 mg can be given at 10-min intervals until desired supine BP is achieved or a total of 300 mg has been injected **Slow continuous IV infusions:** 2 mg/min. Consult manufacturer's instructions for preparation of infusion solution	• **IV:** Should be restricted to hospitalized pts. Keep pt supine during administration. Determine pt's ability to tolerate upright position, especially during 3 h postinjection. Monitor BP during and after completion of infusion or IV injections. Follow manufacturer's directions for preparation of IV infusion solution
I. Adrenergic Neuron Blockers		
guanethidine (Ismelin)	**Oral:** *Adults* (ambulatory): Initially, 10 mg or 12.5 mg od. Increase daily dosage by 10 mg or 12.5 mg at 5- to 7-day intervals prn. Maint. dose, 25–50 mg od. (Hospitalized): Initially, 25–50 mg od. Increase daily dosage by 25–50 mg at daily or every-other-day intervals prn. Geriatric pts may be more sensitive to effects of usual adult dose	• Monitor lying and standing BP during initial tx • Tablets may be crushed and mixed with fluid
reserpine (Serpasil)	**Oral:** *Adults:* 100–250 μg (0.1–0.25 mg) per day. Geriatric pts may be more sensitive to effects of usual adult dose	• Give with food or milk • Monitor mental status
J. Beta Blockers		
acebutolol HCl (Monitan, Sectral)	**Oral:** *Adults:* Initially, 100 mg bid. Adjust dosage weekly prn up to a max. of 400 mg bid	• Give without regard to food • Confer with physician if apical P<50 bpm or if dysrhythmia occurs
atenolol (Tenormin)	**Oral:** *Adults:* Initially, 25–50 mg od. Increase dosage to 50–100 mg/day after 2 weeks prn. Geriatric pts may have increased or decreased sensitivity to effects of usual adult dose. For pts with severe renal function impairment, consult manufacturer's dosage recommendations	• Give without regard to food. Tablets may be crushed • Confer with physician if apical P<50 bpm

Table 36.6 (continued)
The antihypertensives: Drug doses

Drug Generic name (Trade names)	Dosage	Nursing alert
J. Beta Blockers (cont'd)		
metoprolol tartrate (Betaloc, Lopresor, Lopressor)	**Oral:** *Adults:* Initially, 50 mg bid. Increase prn to 100 mg bid	• Give with meals. Do not crush or chew sustained-release preparations • Confer with physician if apical P<50 bpm. Monitor lying/sitting/standing BP during initial tx
nadolol (Corgard)	**Oral:** *Adults:* Initially, 80 mg od. Increase dosage in increments of 40–80 mg at 1-week intervals prn up to a total of 320 mg/day. Geriatric pts may have increased or decreased sensitivity to effects of usual adult dose. For pts with renal function impairment, consult manufacturer's information	• Give without regard to food. Tablets may be crushed • Confer with physician if apical P<50/min. Monitor lying/sitting/standing BP during initial tx
oxprenolol HCl (Trasicor)	**Oral:** *Adults:* Initially, 20 mg tid. Increase dosage in increments of 60 mg/day every 1–2 weeks prn. Dosage is usually in range of 120–320 mg/day. Usual max. dose, 480 mg/day. Once the optimal daily dose has been reached, bid dosing may be used. Geriatric pts may have increased or decreased sensitivity to effects of usual adult dose	• Give without regard to meals. Do not crush or chew sustained-release preparations • Confer with physician if apical P<50 bpm. Monitor lying/sitting/standing BP during initial tx
pindolol (Visken)	**Oral:** *Adults:* Initially, 5 mg bid. Increase in increments of 10 mg/day at 2- to 3-week intervals prn to a max. of 45 mg/day. Geriatric pts may have increased or decreased sensitivity to effects of usual adult dose	• Give without regard to food. May crush tablets • Confer with physician if apical P<50 bpm. Monitor lying/sitting/standing BP during initial tx
propranolol HCl (Inderal)	**Oral:** *Adults:* Initially, 2 equal doses of 40 mg. Increase prn in 1 week to 80 mg bid. If necessary, increase to 160 mg bid. For most pts, dosage is in range of 160–320 mg/day	• Give with food. Do not crush or chew long-acting tablets • Confer with physician if apical P<50 bpm. Monitor lying/sitting/standing BP during initial tx

Table 36.6 (continued)
The antihypertensives: Drug doses

Drug Generic name (Trade names)	Dosage	Nursing alert
J. Beta Blockers (cont'd)		
propranolol (Inderal) (cont'd)	Inderal-LA® (long acting): Intended for maint. tx in pts requiring doses in the range of 60–320 mg/day. Capsules are taken od, a.m. or p.m. Pts should be started and stabilized on regular tablets before considering long-acting capsules. When changing to Inderal-LA® from regular tablets, the need for a possible up-titration of dosage should be considered. Geriatric pts may have increased or decreased sensitivity to effects of usual adult dose	
timolol maleate (Blocadren)	**Oral:** *Adults:* Initially, 5–10 mg bid. Increase at 1-week intervals prn. Maintenance: Usually 20–40 mg/day; doses up to 60 mg/day divided into 2 doses may be necessary	• Give without regard to food. Tablets may be crushed • Confer with physician if apical P<50 bpm. Monitor lying/sitting/standing BP during initial tx
K. Central Sympathetic Inhibitors		
clonidine HCl (Catapres)	**Oral:** *Adults:* Initially, 100 µg (0.1 mg) bid. Increase by 100 or 200 µg (0.1 or 0.2 mg, respectively) per day every 2–4 weeks prn. Maintenance: 200–600 µg (0.2–0.6 mg) per day in divided doses. Severe hypertension in the urgent but not emergency situation (loading dose): 200 µg (0.2 mg), followed by 100 µg (0.1 mg) q1h until DBP is controlled or a total of 800 µg (0.8 mg) has been given; pt is then controlled on a normal maint. dose. Geriatric pts may be more sensitive to effects of usual adult dose	• **Oral:** Give last daily dose hs
	Transdermal: *Adults:* Initially, Catapres TTS-1® once weekly. After 1–2 weeks, dosage may be increased by adding another Catapres-TTS-1® or changing to a larger system. Max. dose is 2 Catapres-TTS-3® patches. Catapres-TTS-1®, -2®, -3®: Each patch delivers clonidine 0.1, 0.2 or 0.3 mg/day	• **Transdermal:** Apply to clean, dry, hairless, healthy site every 7 days. Rotate sites. Absorption is greatest from chest or upper arms

(cont'd on next page)

Table 36.6 (continued)
The antihypertensives: Drug doses

Drug Generic name (Trade names)	Dosage	Nursing alert
K. Central Sympathetic Inhibitors (cont'd)		
methyldopa (Aldomet)	**Oral:** *Adults:* Initially, 250 mg bid or tid for 2 days, then adjust, preferably at intervals of not less than 2 days, prn. Maintenance: 500 mg to 2 g/day, divided into 2–4 doses. Geriatric pts may be more sensitive to effects of usual adult dose and may require lower dose to prevent syncope. Usual adult prescribing limits: Up to 3 g/day	• Tolerance may develop within 2–3 months of initiating tx. Diuretic may be added. Monitor BP to determine continued effectiveness. Add dosage increases to hs dose due to sedation

Further Reading

Carruthers SG. Hypertension. In: Gray J, ed. *Therapeutic Choices*. Ottawa: Canadian Pharmaceutical Association; 1995.

Cusson J. Treating the elderly hypertensive. *Cardiol Consult* 1994;5(1):14–18.

Deglin J, Deglin S. Hypertension: current trends and choices in pharmacotherapeutics. *Clin Iss Crit Care Nurs* 1992;3(2):507–526.

Drugs for hypertension. *Medical Letter on Drugs and Therapeutics* 1995;37:45–50.

Glickstein J, ed. Hypertension in the elderly. *Focus on Geriatric Care & Rehabilitation* 1993;7(1):1–7.

Hogenson K. Acute postoperative hypertension in the hypertensive patient. *J Post Anesth Nurs* 1992;7(1):38–44.

Losartan for hypertension. *Medical Letter on Drugs and Therapeutics* 1995;37:57–58.

Drugs for the Treatment of Hypotension and Shock

Topics Discussed
- Drugs used to treat shock: Sympathomimetics and vasodilators
- For each drug discussed: Mechanism of action, pharmacological effects, therapeutic uses, adverse effects
- Nursing management

Drugs Discussed
adrenaline (ad-**ren**-ah-lin)
dobutamine (doe-**byoo**-tah-meen)
dopamine (**dope**-ah-meen)
epinephrine (ep-ih-**neff**-rin)
levarterenol (lev-ar-teh-**ray**-nol)
nitroglycerin (nye-troh-**gliss**-er-in)
nitroprusside (nye-troe-**pruss**-ide)
noradrenaline (nor-ad-**ren**-ah-lin)
norepinephrine (nor-ep-ih-**neff**-rin)

Clinical Challenge

Consider this clinical challenge as you read through this chapter. The response to the challenge appears on page 418 .

Your patient has recently arrived by ambulance following a serious accident. He has impaired renal function. He weighs approximately 70 kg. His vital signs indicate severe shock. A dopamine drip is commenced at 1 µg/min.

1. Why is dopamine the drug of choice?
2. How will you prepare the infusion?
3. At what rate will you set the infusion pump?
4. What parameters will you monitor?

Infusion Chart
Add 200 mg dopamine to 500 mL NS solution. Concentration: 400 µg/mL

µg/min	body weight (kg)					
	60	65	70	75	80	
1	9	10	11	11	12	mL/min
2	18	19	21	23	24	mL/min
3	27	29	31	34	36	mL/min

Shock is a condition of acute peripheral circulatory failure. It can result from the loss of circulatory control or circulating fluid. Therapy is aimed at correcting the hypoperfusion of vital organs. *Hypovolemic shock* is treated by volume replacement; *bacteremic shock* by intensive antibiotic therapy, corticosteroids and volume replacement. In addition, sympathomimetic drugs or vasodilators (which either increase cardiac output or alter peripheral resistance, or both) may be appropriate. This chapter discusses the use of sympathomimetics and vasodilators in shock.

In discussing tissue perfusion during hypotension and shock, the heart, brain and kidneys deserve special comment. The major factor regulating blood flow through the coronary and cerebral vessels is the mean diastolic pressure. In the presence of hypotension, myocardial and cerebral perfusion are compromised. In this situation, sympathomimetics that increase blood pressure will improve the perfusion of both organs. Sympathomimetics can be used without concern that they might constrict the blood vessels in the heart and brain. The calibre of these vessels is determined by the metabolic needs of the tissue, not by stimulation of adrenergic receptors.

The heart differs from the brain in one important aspect. Although the heart normally uses an aerobic metabolic pathway, it can operate for a short time anaerobically. The brain needs oxygen for its metabolism and is particularly susceptible to the consequence of acute hypotension and shock.

In contrast to the heart and brain, the kidney extracts only a relatively small amount of the oxygen provided to it under resting conditions, which means it can withstand, within limits, a reduction in blood flow by extracting a higher percentage of the oxygen supplied. However, sympathetic stimulation causes renal vasoconstriction. Adrenergic vasoconstrictors also reduce blood flow, possibly leading to renal ischemia.

Sympathomimetics

Sympathomimetics are used to improve tissue perfusion. They stimulate (1) alpha$_1$ receptors, to increase venous return and peripheral resistance, (2) beta$_1$ receptors, to increase heart rate and cardiac output (if venous return is adequate) or (3) dopamine receptors, to dilate the renal and splanchnic beds. The pharmacologic actions of these drugs are described in detail in Chapter 29. Readers are encouraged to refer to this chapter if additional information is required on any of the drugs presented below.

Epinephrine, Adrenaline (Adrenalin®)

Mechanism of action and pharmacologic effects. Epinephrine stimulates beta$_1$ receptors in the heart and increases both heart rate and cardiac output. In small doses it dilates precapillary resistance vessels (arterioles) in skeletal muscles (beta$_2$ receptors) and constricts capacitance vessels (veins), an alpha$_1$-receptor mediated effect. The result is a decrease in peripheral resistance and an increase in venous return. Larger doses stimulate alpha$_1$ receptors on precapillary resistance vessels, producing a generalized vasoconstriction and an increase in peripheral resistance. Epinephrine also dilates the bronchioles.

Therapeutic uses. Histamine, released from mast cells during anaphylactic shock, constricts bronchioles and dilates blood vessels. Epinephrine is the drug of choice for the treatment of anaphylactic shock because it prevents or reverses histamine-induced bronchoconstriction and vasodilatation. These actions are consistent with the pharmacologic properties of epinephrine. By stimulating beta$_2$ receptors epinephrine prevents, or reverses, a histamine-induced bronchoconstriction. The ability of therapeutic doses of epinephrine to stimulate alpha$_1$ receptors enables it to reverse the histamine-induced vasodilatation.

Epinephrine should be given with caution to elderly patients and to those with cardiovascular disease, hypertension, diabetes or hyperthyroidism. It must be used with extreme caution in patients with long-standing bronchial asthma and emphysema who have developed degenerative heart disease. Epinephrine is contraindicated in patients with organic brain damage, cardiac dilatation or coronary insufficiency.

Adverse effects. Epinephrine's adverse effects include anxiety, headaches, fear, palpitations, weakness and precordial pain. These are more prevalent in hyperthyroid patients. The drug interactions and nursing management for epinephrine are given in Tables 29.3 (page 287) and 29.5 (pages 289–290), respectively.

Levarterenol, Norepinephrine, Noradrenaline (Levophed®)

Mechanism of action and pharmacologic effects. Levarterenol stimulates alpha$_1$ receptors, constricting both capacitance and precapillary resistance vessels. The resulting increase in blood pressure activates the carotid sinus and aortic arch pressor receptors to stimulate reflexly the vagus nerve. The result is a fall in heart rate and cardiac output. Although levarterenol stimulates beta$_1$ receptors in the heart and might be thought to increase heart rate, this effect is not sufficient to override reflex stimulation of the vagus.

Therapeutic uses. Levarterenol is indicated for the maintenance of blood pressure in acute hypotensive states, surgical and nonsurgical trauma, central vasomotor depression and hemorrhage. Its use in patients who are hypotensive from blood volume deficit is contraindicated, except as an emergency measure to maintain coronary and cerebral artery perfusion until blood volume replacement can be completed.

Adverse effects. Because of its ability to produce marked vasoconstriction, levarterenol can cause tissue necrosis at the site of injection. This danger is minimized by administering the drug through a catheter into a deeply seated vein and changing the infusion site when prolonged treatment is required. Phentolamine (Regitine®, Rogitine®) can be injected to overcome the effects of extravasation.

The drug interactions and nursing management for levarterenol are given in Tables 29.3 (page 287) and 29.5 (pages 289–290), respectively.

Dobutamine (Dobutrex®)

Mechanism of action and pharmacologic effects. Dobutamine stimulates beta$_1$ receptors, with relatively less effect on beta$_2$ receptors and alpha receptors. Dobutamine does not stimulate dopaminergic receptors. Moderate doses of dobutamine increase myocardial contractility and cardiac output. The drug may also reduce peripheral resistance and ventricular filling pressure when administered in moderate doses. Large doses of dobutamine increase heart rate and blood pressure.

Therapeutic uses. Dobutamine is indicated for the treatment of adults with cardiac decompensation due to depressed contractility resulting from organic heart disease or following cardiac surgical procedures in which parenteral therapy is necessary for inotropic support. It is contraindicated in dobutamine hypersensitivity, pheochromocytoma, idiopathic hypertrophic subaortic stenosis, uncorrected tachycardia or ventricular fibrillation.

Adverse effects. A 10- to 20-mm Hg increase in systolic blood pressure and an increase in heart rate of 5–15 beats/min have been noted in most patients. About 5% of patients have increased premature ventricular beats during infusion. Precipitous decreases in blood pressure associated with dobutamine therapy have been reported. Less common cardiovascular effects include cardiac awareness, transient bigeminy, bradycardia, angina and palpitations. The other adverse effects of dobutamine include headache, anxiety, fatigue, paresthesia, nausea, vomiting and shortness of breath.

The drug interactions and nursing management for dobutamine are given in Tables 29.3 (page 287) and 29.5 (pages 289–290), respectively.

Dopamine (Dopastat®, Intropin®)

Mechanism of action and pharmacologic effects. The effect of dopamine is dose dependent. In doses less than 5 µg/kg/min it stimulates dopaminergic receptors in the renal and mesenteric beds to produce vasodilatation and increase renal and mesenteric blood flow. Doses of 5–10 µg/kg/min also increase renal and mesenteric blood flow, while at the same time stimulating beta$_1$ receptors to increase myocardial contractility, heart rate and cardiac output. At doses above 10 µg/kg/min, dopamine produces a generalized alpha$_1$-receptor mediated vasoconstriction and a reduction in renal blood flow.

Therapeutic uses. Dopamine is used to increase cardiac output and improve renal blood flow in shock due to myocardial infarction, sepsis and trauma, as well as in acute renal failure, open heart surgery and chronic congestive heart failure. Because it can dilate renal vessels, dopamine is preferred over other sympathomimetics in patients with impaired renal function.

Adverse effects. Dopamine can produce tachyarrhythmias, anginal pain, CNS stimulation, nausea, vomiting and headache. It may also increase myocardial oxygen consumption in patients with cardiogenic shock. However, it is less likely than norepinephrine to cause necrosis following extravasation. Phentolamine (Regitine®, Rogitine®; 5–10 mg in 10 mL) can be used to infiltrate the site if extravasation occurs. Patients with pre-existing vascular disease may be particularly sensitive to dopamine's vasoconstrictive effects.

The drug interactions and nursing management for dopamine are given in Tables 29.3 (page 287) and 29.5 (pages 289–290), respectively.

Vasodilators

Vasodilators are used in patients with severe pump failure following acute myocardial infarction and individuals with refractory chronic congestive heart failure. Vasodilators increase cardiac output by reducing peripheral resistance (afterload reduction). They also relieve pulmonary congestion by increasing venous capacitance (preload reduction), and limit the extent of ischemic damage by reducing myocardial oxygen demand and increasing myocardial oxygen supply.

Sodium Nitroprusside (Nipride®, Nitropress®)

Mechanism of action and pharmacologic effects. Nitroprusside dilates venous and arterial beds. Because it has a greater effect on afterload than nitroglycerin, nitroprusside is more likely to increase cardiac output. However, because its primary action on the coronary circulation is on the resistance rather than the conductance vessels, intravenous nitroprusside can cause coronary steal.

The effects of nitroprusside are almost immediate and end quickly once the infusion is stopped. The brief duration of action of nitroprusside's action is due to its rapid metabolism to thiocyanate.

Therapeutic uses. Nitroprusside can be used to treat severe persistent pump failure in patients with markedly reduced cardiac output and increased peripheral vascular resistance. The drug is particularly valuable in patients with severe acute decompensated chronic congestive heart failure, refractory to digoxin and diuretics. It should not be used in the treatment of compensatory hypertension, e.g., A-V shunt or coarctation of the aorta.

Adverse effects. Nitroprusside may produce hypotension and tachycardia. Prolonged infusion of nitroprusside can lead to the accumulation of thiocyanate. Blood thiocyanate levels should be determined daily if nitroprusside is infused for more than seventy-two hours. In addition, the prolonged infusion of nitroprusside may lead to high levels of blood cyanide and cyanide toxicity.

Nitroglycerin (Nitro-Bid IV®, Nitrostat IV®, Tridil®)

Nitroglycerin dilates both arterial and venous vessels, with its effect being greater on the venous side. Intravenous nitroglycerin relieves pulmonary congestion, decreases myocardial oxygen consumption and reduces ST-segment elevation. It can thus be used to decrease myocardial ischemia and improve hemodynamics in severe left ventricular dysfunction complicating acute myocardial infarction. Its primary use is in patients with recurrent ischemic pain or marked elevation of left ventricular filling pressure and pulmonary edema.

The major adverse effects of intravenous nitroglycerin include symptomatic hypotension, reflex tachycardia, paradoxical increase of angina pain and palpitations. CNS adverse effects include transient headache, weakness, dizziness, apprehension and restlessness. Patients may also experience nausea, vomiting and abdominal pain. Methemoglobinemia may also be produced.

Table 37.1 lists the clinically significant drug interactions with intravenous nitroglycerin.

Nursing Management

Table 37.2 describes the nursing management of the patient receiving emergency drug treatment for shock. Dosages for individual drugs are given in Table 37.3 (pages 419–420).

Table 37.1
IV nitroglycerin: Drug interactions

Drug	Interaction
Ethanol	• Ethanol plus nitrates may lead to more profound hypotension
Long-acting nitrates	• The chronic administration of long-acting nitrates can produce tolerance to nitroglycerin

Table 37.2
Nursing management for drug treatment of shock and hypotension

Assessment of risk vs. benefit	Patient data	• Physician should determine any contraindications such as those described with adverse effects (see text). Particularly, assess for CV disease, diabetes, hyperthyroidism, glaucoma • Assess to establish baseline VS, including BP, apical and peripheral P, R, ECG, urinary output • *Pregnancy and lactation:* Safety not established. Should be used only if benefits outweigh risks
	Drug data	• Response depends on specificity of action on adrenergic receptors, e.g.: epinephrine — α_1, β_1, β_2; norepinephrine — α_1; dopamine — dopaminergic receptors in kidney, β_1, α_1; dobutamine — β_1 mainly, weaker β_2 • Actions and adverse effects are dose related; increasing dose may cause increased response at other receptors
Implementation	Rights of administration	• Using the "rights" helps prevent errors of administration
	Right route	• Give mainly by IV route; epinephrine may also be given SC/IM. Check available form carefully; e.g., suspension may be given SC but not IM or IV
	Right dose	• All drugs in this class are potent. Check doses very carefully, e.g., may be ordered as µg/kg and available supply may state mg/mL. Epinephrine is supplied as 1% (1:100), 0.1% (1:1000) and 0.01% (1:10 000) solutions
	Right time	• Many of these drugs are used in emergency situations and titrated to pt's response. For IV route, use infusion pump to control rate. *Note:* Drug interactions can be serious (causing hypertension, hypotension, cardiac arrhythmias, hyperglycemia). Check complete drug regimen with physician or pharmacist
	Right technique	• For infusion, follow manufacturer's instructions for reconstitution and compatibility. Most are compatible with variety of solutions but norepinephrine should be given with dextrose. Normal saline alone is not recommended • IV should be given in central line or large vein; powerful vasoconstricting action may cause venous damage. If drug extravasates into surrounding tissue, can cause ischemia and necrosis. Observe site frequently; if extravasation occurs, affected area should be infiltrated with 10–15 mL of saline solution containing 5–10 mg of phentolamine (see Chapter 29) • Always check solution; do not use if discoloured or contains a precipitate. Check stability: may be stable at room temperature for 24–48 h

(cont'd on next page)

Table 37.2 (continued)
Nursing management for drug treatment of shock and hypotension

Implementation (cont'd)	Patient/family teaching	• In general, pt's condition is not conducive to elaborate teaching. However, reassurance and explanation are appropriate
Outcomes	Monitoring of progress	*Note: Because of the serious nature of the indications for use of these drugs, constant monitoring and titration of dose is required* • Monitoring includes: BP, HR, ECG, R, CNS status, peripheral perfusion, renal output and hemodynamic parameters (measurements of cardiac output, preload, afterload). Blood gases and electrolytes may also be monitored frequently

Response to Clinical Challenge

1. Dopamine can dilate renal vessels and is preferred over other sympathomimetics in patients with impaired renal function.
2. To prepare the infusion, add 200 mg dopamine to 500 mL NS solution to produce a solution with a concentration of 400 µg/mL.
3. Use the infusion chart to calculate the rate (in mL/min) for a 70-kg man for 1 µg/min. The initial rate is 11 mL/min.
4. Continuous monitoring of BP, apical P (including rate, rhythm and quality) and R, q5–15min. Monitor urine output and peripheral pulses frequently. Continuous ECG monitoring must be used.

Infusion Chart
Add 200 mg dopamine to 500 mL NS solution.
Concentration: 400 µg/mL

µg/min	body weight (kg)					
	60	65	70	75	80	
1	9	10	11	11	12	mL/min
2	18	19	21	23	24	mL/min
3	27	29	31	34	36	mL/min

Further Reading

Fallaen EL. Acute and postmyocardial infarction. In: Gray J, ed. *Therapeutic Choices*. Ottawa: Canadian Pharmaceutical Association; 1995: 134–145.

Table 37.3
Treatment of hypotension and shock: Drug doses

Drug Generic name (Trade names)	Dosage	Nursing alert
A. Sympathomimetics		
epinephrine, adrenaline (Adrenalin)	Anaphylactic shock: **SC (preferred); IM:** Initial dose (repeated q20–30 min prn, up to 3 doses): *Adults:* 0.3–0.5 mL 1/1000 epinephrine solution. *Children:* 0.01 mL/kg 1/1000 epinephrine solution (max., 0.3 mL) Cardiogenic shock: **IV:** *Adults:* 0.5–1.0 mg (5–10 mL 1:10 000 solution) q3min during CPR. Larger doses have been used in pts who did not respond to standard tx	• Read label carefully; drug is supplied in different dosage strengths. Use tuberculin syringe for accuracy • Massage IM/SC site well to enhance absorption. Rotate sites. Do not use solutions if brownish/pinkish. Store protected from light. Use pediatric solution of 1:100 000 for children
levarterenol, norepinephrine bitartrate, noradrenaline (Levophed)	**IV infusion:** *Adults:* Initially, 0.5–1 µg (base) per minute; adjust dosage gradually to achieve desired BP. Maintenance: 2–12 µg (base) per minute. *Note:* Pts with refractory shock may require dose up to 30 µg (base) per minute Usual pediatric dose: Vasopressor — **IV infusion:** 0.1 µg (base) per kg body weight per minute; adjust dosage gradually to achieve desired BP, up to 1 µg/kg body weight per minute	• If whole blood or plasma is indicated to increase blood volume, it should be administered separately (e.g., use of a Y-tube and individual flasks, if given simultaneously) • Norepinephrine is administered only by IV infusion. SC or IM administration is not recommended because of the potent vasoconstrictor effect. Dilute 1 mg in 250 mL D5W or 5% in normal saline (concentration of 4 µg/mL). Do not mix in normal saline alone. Do not use solution if discoloured or has precipitate. Use infusion pump and chart to ensure accurate rate
dobutamine HCl (Dobutrex)	**IV infusion:** *Adults* (for pts with acute MI): 8–24 µg/kg/min	• Follow manufacturer's instructions for reconstitution. Use infusion pump and chart to ensure accuracy • Solution stable for 24 h at room temperature. Slight pink colour to solution does not affect potency. Monitor site frequently
dopamine HCl (Dopastat, Intropin)	**IV infusion:** *Adults:* 2–5 µg/kg/min. In more seriously ill pts, an initial infusion rate of 5 µg/kg/min may be increased gradually to 5–10 µg/kg/min, and rarely, to 20–30 µg/kg/min	• Follow manufacturer's instructions for reconstitution. Use infusion pump and chart to ensure accuracy • Solution stable 24 h at room temperature. Discard solution if cloudy or discoloured. Monitor site frequently

(cont'd on next page)

Table 37.3 (continued)
Treatment of hypotension and shock: Drug doses

Drug Generic name (Trade names)	Dosage	Nursing alert
B. Vasodilators		
sodium nitroprusside (Nipride, Nitropress)	**IV infusion:** For severe, persistent pump failure in pts with markedly reduced cardiac output and increased peripheral vascular resistance: *Adults/adolescents:* Initially, a dilute solution is infused at rate of 16 µg/min. Subsequent infusion rate should be determined by hemodynamic monitoring	•Use infusion pump to ensure accuracy. Use dosage chart to calculate rate •*Preparation of dosage form:* Reconstitute by dissolving contents of a 50-mg vial in 2–3 mL of 5% dextrose injection only and shaking gently to dissolve. Dilute further in 250–1000 mL of 5% dextrose injection and wrap container in supplied opaque sleeve, aluminum foil or other opaque material to protect it from light (it is not necessary to wrap the infusion drip chamber or the tubing). Monitor site frequently •*Stability:* Follow manufacturer's instructions for reconstitution. Solutions of nitroprusside should be freshly prepared and any unused portion discarded. A freshly prepared solution has a slight brownish tint and should be discarded if the colour is dark brown, orange or blue. Solution must be used within 24 h. No other medications should be added to infusion fluid containing nitroprusside. Sodium nitroprusside solution is rapidly degraded by trace contaminants, often with resulting colour changes. A change in colour to blue, green, or bright red indicates reaction of nitroprusside ion with another substance, and the solution must be replaced and discarded
nitroglycerin (Nitro-Bid IV, Nitrostat IV, Tridil)	**IV infusion:** For severe resistant, chronic heart failure: *Adults:* Initially, 5 µg/min of dilute solution. Dosage may be increased by 5 µg/min q3–5min as required. If no response is observed with dose of 20 µg/min, increments of 10 µg/min (and later, 20 µg/min) may be used	•Use infusion pump and chart to ensure accuracy. Solution stable 48 h at room temperature. Standard infusion sets (PVC) absorb up to 80% of the drug. Use glass bottles and special tubing provided by the manufacturer

Drugs and Water Balance

Unit 7 begins with a discussion of water, electrolytes and acid-base balance (Chapter 38). Although it may seem unusual to consider water, sodium, potassium, calcium, magnesium and hydrogen as drugs, alterations in the amounts of any of these substances in the body can have profound effects on our ability to carry out normal biologic functions. In the face of either an excess or deficit in their levels, appropriate steps must be taken to restore normal concentrations.

Chapters 39 and 40 carry us into the area of renal pharmacology. In addition to eliminating sodium, chloride, water and body wastes, the kidney works in concert with the cardiovascular system to regulate blood pressure and cardiac function. Kidney failure leads to the accumulation of salt and water in the extracellular spaces of the body and can precipitate hypertension and congestive heart failure. The kidney is also responsible for the secretion of renin, which is subsequently converted into the vasopressor chemical angiotensin II. Diuretics (Chapter 39) increase the renal excretion of sodium, chloride and water. They form an important component of the treatment of heart failure, hypertension and renal disease. Vasopressin (the antidiuretic hormone; Chapter 40) decreases the excretion of water and is essential in the treatment of diabetes insipidus.

Finally, Chapter 41 reviews the use of drugs in urologic disorders. These conditions are unrelated to kidney dysfunction, arising instead from problems in the bladder or prostate. Nurses should be familiar with drugs used to treat adult incontinence, childhood enuresis and benign prostatic hypertrophy.

Water, Electrolytes and Acid-Base Balance

Topics Discussed
- Dehydration and water intoxication
- Hyponatremia and hypernatremia
- Hypokalemia and hyperkalemia
- Hypocalcemia and hypercalcemia
- Hypomagnesemia and hypermagnesemia
- Hydrogen ion concentration, acidosis and alkalosis
- Nursing management

Body water may be classified according to whether it occupies intracellular or extracellular compartments. Extracellular water is composed of interstitial water and plasma. Electrolytes are dissolved in these water compartments; they contribute to the osmolality, pH and volume of liquid found at each site. Under normal conditions the kidneys and lungs combine to control electrolyte concentrations and water volume in the body. However, conditions may arise that alter either water volume or concentrations of electrolytes, or both. When this occurs, prompt attention may be required to prevent irreparable damage.

This chapter discusses the conditions that alter water and/or electrolyte balance in the body and the measures that can be taken to restore them to normal.

Total body water varies from 50% of body mass/weight in obese adults to 70% in lean adults. Major differences exist in both the volume and content of the intracellular and extracellular water compartments. Approximately 55% of the total body water is found intracellularly and 35% extracellularly. The remaining 10% can be divided between inaccessible bone water (7.5%) and transcellular water (2.5%) compartments. These latter compartments will not be discussed further, as they play little role in the maintenance of osmolality and pH.

The composition of electrolytes and protein in plasma water is given in Table 38.1. Sodium is the major cation found in plasma. Chloride and bicarbonate are the anions existing in highest concentrations. Potassium levels are low in plasma. The plasma concentrations of these electrolytes differ only slightly from their levels interstitially.

Potassium and magnesium are the major cations in the intracellular water. The prominent anions are phosphate and protein. Little sodium chloride and bicarbonate are found intracellularly. Table 38.2 presents the concentrations of electrolytes in intracellular water of muscle tissue. They represent the approximate levels of electrolytes within other tissues.

The difference in the concentrations of sodium and potassium in the extracellular and intracellular water compartments is the result of the active transport of sodium out of, and potassium into, the cells. Osmotic pressure is the major factor responsible for the transport of water from one

Table 38.1

Composition of electrolytes and protein in plasma (mmol/L or mEq/L)

Cations		Anions	
Sodium	135–145	Chloride	98–106
Potassium	3.5–5.0	Bicarbonate	24–28
Calcium	4.5–5.5	Phosphate; sulfate	2–5
Magnesium	1.5–2.0	Organic anions	3–6
		Protein	15–20

Table 38.2
Composition of electrolytes and protein in muscle intracellular water (mmol/L or mEq/L)

Cations		Anions	
Sodium	10	Bicarbonate	10
Potassium	150	Phosphate; sulfate	150
Magnesium	40	Protein	40

compartment to the other. An increase in sodium concentration in the body, together with its inability to enter body cells in high amounts, will draw water from the intracellular compartment into the extracellular space. By the same token, the accumulation of higher concentrations of potassium within cells causes water to diffuse from the extracellular compartment into the intracellular water space.

Dehydration and Water Intoxication

Dehydration

Dehydration is a water deficit that occurs either as a result of inadequate intake or increased loss of water. The former is most often encountered in unconscious patients or patients with esophageal or pyloric obstruction who are unable to ingest water. Water depletion results from such situations as fever, a hot environment, low levels of antidiuretic hormone (ADH) secretion or insensitivity of the kidney to the actions of ADH (see Chapter 40). Other causes of increased water loss include renal disease, impaired capacity to reabsorb water (secondary to potassium depletion) and intensive diuretic treatment.

Water deficit is treated by administering water. It can be given alone or with electrolytes. If it is required alone, water can be given with 2.5% to 5% dextrose. The latter substance, a sugar, is oxidized in the body to produce water. Two to three litres of water can be given per day if renal function is normal. In the face of dehydration with increased serum sodium concentration, water can be given to restore the normal osmolality of the serum.

Water Intoxication

Water intoxication is water excess that occurs if intake exceeds elimination. The most common causes are the parenteral administration of large volumes of water or reduced elimination of water due to renal insufficiency, congestive heart failure or liver disease accompanied by ascites.

Water excess is treated by restricting its intake. If severe water intoxication is present, the patient may be given a hypertonic solution of sodium chloride to increase water movement from the intracellular to the extracellular space and decrease intracellular water volume.

Hyponatremia and Hypernatremia

Hyponatremia

Hyponatremia occurs when the plasma sodium concentration falls below 130–135 mmol/L (mEq/L). This can occur as a result of loss of sodium or retention of water. In either case, the concentration of sodium in the plasma falls. In the first situation a marked loss of sodium can result from the overenthusiastic application of diuretic therapy. Other causes of sodium loss include excessive sweating, increased level of gastrointestinal secretions and renal or adrenocortical insufficiency.

When hyponatremia is the result of water retention instead of sodium loss, it is called *dilutional hyponatremia*. Water may be retained in large quantities following the use of ADH. Chronic severe heart failure, cirrhosis of the liver with ascites and the nephrotic syndrome may also result in water retention.

The treatment of hyponatremia depends on its etiology. If hyponatremia is a result of a sodium deficit, it may be treated by the administration of sodium chloride, with or without sodium bicarbonate. Moderate deficits in adults are usually handled by administering 0.9% sodium chloride, which contains 155 mmol or mEq of sodium and chloride per litre. Ringer's solution may also be used, with or without lactate. More severe sodium deficits usually require 3% or 5% solutions of sodium chloride, which contain 513 and 855 mmol (mEq) per litre, respectively. If water retention is the cause of the hyponatremia, water intake should be reduced. Sodium should not be administered in dilutional hyponatremia, as the total body sodium is normal or even elevated.

Hypernatremia

Hypernatremia is defined as serum or plasma sodium levels above the normal range. This usually means concentrations of sodium in excess of 150 mmol/L (mEq/L). The increased sodium levels may be a result of either an increased sodium intake without a commensurate increase in water, or a loss of water, without a corresponding increase in sodium elimination. On nursing assessment, evidence of hypernatremia will be displayed as CNS disturbances (confusion, stupor, coma), poor skin turgor and (possibly) postural hypotension (if the hypernatremia is due to water loss).

Hypernatremia resulting from an increase in sodium intake may be treated by reducing the amount of sodium provided to the patient. Diuretics may also be used to hasten sodium elimination. However, in this case, the water lost as a result of the diuretic must be replaced. If hypernatremia is due to a deficit of water, it is treated by administering water.

Hypokalemia and Hyperkalemia

Hypokalemia

Hypokalemia occurs when serum potassium levels fall below 3.5 mmol/L (mEq/L). A fall in serum potassium usually indicates a decrease in total body potassium. However, this is not always the case. Acute alkalosis, treatment with insulin or stimulation of beta receptors may lower serum potassium values without decreasing the total body potassium content. By the same token, total body potassium may fall without producing a decrease in serum potassium concentrations. This can be explained by the fact that most body potassium is found intracellularly, not extracellularly.

It is not possible in this text to list and explain all the possible causes of a total body potassium deficit. In short, they include reduced potassium

intake or increased potassium elimination. In the first instance, conditions such as starvation, upper gastrointestinal obstruction, steatorrhea and regional enteritis will decrease potassium intake. Increased potassium loss may occur through the gastrointestinal tract if emesis or diarrhea occurs, or via the kidneys, in conditions involving congenital tubule malfunction or diuresis from diabetes or diuretics. Metabolic alkalosis, burns and increased secretion of adrenocortical hormones may also increase potassium loss. The administration of large amounts of sodium chloride without potassium will increase potassium loss as it is exchanged for some of the increased sodium presented to the renal distal convoluted tubules.

Hypokalemia can be treated by administering potassium, either orally or parenterally. Potassium is toxic and care must be taken to prevent hyperkalemia. The kidneys are the main route for the elimination of potassium and their status must be assessed prior to beginning potassium therapy.

Hypokalemia is common when thiazide or loop diuretics are used (see Chapter 39). Potassium-sparing diuretics are often combined with these drugs to minimize their hypokalemic effects. An alternative approach to prevent hypokalemia is the administration of sustained-release potassium chloride preparations. Slow-K® and Micro-K Extencaps® contain 600 mg (8 mmol [mEq] of K+) per tablet or capsule, respectively. Klotrix® and K-Tabs® contain 750 mg of potassium chloride (equivalent to 10 mmol [mEq] of K+). K-Lyte® effervescent tablets contain 25 mmol (mEq) or 50 mmol (mEq) potassium as the bicarbonate and citrate salts.

The dosage of potassium must be individualized according to the patient's needs. Approximately 20–40 mmol (mEq) of potassium is given to prevent hypokalemia. Potassium depletion is treated with approximately 40 mmol (mEq) to a maximum of 100 mmol (mEq) per day. In general, a daily dose exceeding 60 mmol (mEq) of potassium should not be required. Potassium salts should be administered with milk or after meals in two or three divided doses per day to minimize gastric irritation and too-rapid absorption. Nausea, vomiting, diarrhea and abdominal cramps are the most frequent adverse effects.

Hyperkalemia

Hyperkalemia denotes a serum potassium concentration above 5 mmol/L (mEq/L). It is caused by either increased potassium intake or decreased potassium elimination. Excessive potassium administration, either parenterally or orally, can cause hyperkalemia. Kidney failure reduces potassium elimination and can produce hyperkalemia. Other causes include the release of intracellular potassium in burns, severe infections and crush injuries. In these situations potassium moves from the intracellular to extracellular water compartments and serum potassium levels increase. Metabolic acidosis also causes potassium to move from the intracellular water to the extracellular compartment.

The major consequence of hyperkalemia is its deleterious effect on heart function. Depending on the degree of hyperkalemia, minor alterations in conduction may proceed through a lengthening of A-V conduction to a depression of impulse generation and conduction in all heart tissue. Asystole is the eventual outcome. This may be preceded by ventricular tachycardia and/or fibrillation. Plasma potassium levels of 5–7 mmol/L (mEq/L) produce major depression in heart function.

Potassium is withheld from patients with hyperkalemia. A potassium exchange resin, sodium polysterene sulfonate (Kayexalate®), may be given either orally or by enema. It is less effective when given rectally. This material retains potassium in the gastrointestinal tract and is eliminated in the feces.

If hyperkalemia is very severe and an emergency arises, insulin or calcium may be given intravenously. Insulin causes a deposition of potassium in the liver, thereby lowering plasma potassium levels. Calcium has the opposite actions to those of potassium on the heart and serves as an antagonist. Sodium bicarbonate, given intravenously, raises the pH of the extracellular fluid and, as a result, causes potassium to move from extracellular water into intracellular water. The resulting fall in serum potassium reduces its effect on the heart. Hemodialysis may be used in patients with renal insufficiency.

Hypocalcemia and Hypercalcemia

Approximately 2% of the body's mass is calcium. Only 1% of this amount of calcium is in solution in body fluids. The normal total plasma or serum concentration of calcium ranges between 4.5–5.5 mmol/L (mEq/L). Levels above 5.8 mmol/L (mEq/L) are classified as hypercalcemia, and concentrations below 4.5 mmol/L (mEq/L) constitute hypocalcemia.

Hypocalcemia

The causes of hypocalcemia include hypoparathyroidism, chronic renal insufficiency and malabsorption syndromes. Hypocalcemia may produce rickets and osteomalacia. Calcium is an essential ion for many enzymes. It is important in membrane function and plays a vital role in neuromuscular function.

The treatment of hypocalcemia involves correcting the primary disease causing the low plasma levels. Thus, hypoparathyroidism is treated with vitamin D and calcium. This is discussed in more detail in Chapter 64. If tetany is present, calcium gluconate in a 10% solution can be given intravenously. A variety of different calcium salts are available for oral administration to treat less severe symptoms. These include calcium chloride, calcium lactate, calcium gluconate and calcium carbonate.

Hypercalcemia

Hypercalcemia also alters neuromuscular function. However, in contradistinction to hypocalcemia, which causes skeletal muscle hyperirritability, hypercalcemia produces muscle weakness as excitability is diminished.

If possible, the cause of hypercalcemia should be treated. Hypercalcemia is caused by hyperparathyroidism, bone neoplasms, sarcoidosis, multiple myeloma and vitamin D intoxication. Symptomatic hypercalcemia carries a high mortality rate and must be treated quickly. Calcium excretion can be increased by the use of diuretics. Obviously water, sodium, potassium and possibly also magnesium may need to be replaced when large diuretic doses are administered. Once the primary disease is treated, diuretic therapy may be discontinued. If hypercalcemia is a result of sarcoidosis or neoplasm activity, corticosteroid therapy, such as prednisone, may be used.

Hypomagnesemia and Hypermagnesemia

Magnesium is an ion that receives relatively little attention when compared with sodium, potassium and calcium. However, aberrations in magnesium plasma concentrations can cause alterations in body function. Magnesium is essential to the action of many enzymes. Peripherally, it blocks the release of acetylcholine and decreases neuromuscular excitability. Normal plasma magnesium levels vary from 1.5–2.5 mmol/L (mEq/L).

Hypomagnesemia

Hypomagnesemia may be seen following starvation, diarrhea, malabsorption and primary aldosteronism. It may also be present in the alcoholic patient or following enthusiastic diuretic therapy. Hypoparathyroidism can produce hypomagnesemia. The ingestion of large doses of calcium and vitamin D will also lower plasma magnesium levels.

The treatment of hypomagnesemia involves administering magnesium chloride or magnesium sulfate parenterally in a dose of 10–40 mmol (mEq) per day initially to overcome the severe deficiency. Thereafter, a maintenance dose of 10 mmol (mEq) per day can be given.

Hypermagnesemia

Magnesium is eliminated from the body by the kidneys. Hypermagnesemia occurs when renal function is impaired and the body cannot eliminate the magnesium absorbed from food. Elevated plasma magnesium levels produce central and peripheral nervous system depression. Deep tendon reflexes are decreased if plasma magnesium levels exceed 4 mmol/L (mEq/L). In addition, changes in heart function may appear if the concentration of the ion reaches 10–15 mmol (mEq/L). These include an increase in the P-R interval, broadened QRS complexes and elevated T waves. However, death is usually not due to depressed cardiac

function. Rather, it results from respiratory muscle paralysis because of the decreased release of acetylcholine at the motor end-plates. Respiratory paralysis is a potential hazard as plasma magnesium levels reach 12–15 mmol/L (mEq/L).

Treatment involves administration of calcium to antagonize the effects of magnesium on skeletal muscle, and extracorporeal or peritoneal dialysis to clear magnesium from the body. Nursing evaluation focusses on monitoring the effectiveness of the treatment in removing excess magnesium and on identification of early indications of hypomagnesemia.

Hydrogen Ion Concentration, Acidosis and Alkalosis

Food metabolism results in the production of the strongly acidic anions phosphate and sulfate. In addition, lactic acid and acetoacetic acid are formed as a result of the metabolism of fat and carbohydrates. Under normal circumstances these acids are buffered in the body and the hydrogen ion concentration, or pH, of the body fluids does not change. Both the kidneys and the lungs play a vital role in regulating body pH. The kidney eliminates both bicarbonate and hydrogen ions. The lungs expire carbon dioxide, thereby lowering the concentration of carbonic acid in the body.

Nursing assessment parameters related to acidosis and alkalosis are briefly summarized in Table 38.3. Detailed information related to the relevant nursing actions and responsibilities is beyond the scope of this book. Readers seeking such information are advised to consult a medical-surgical nursing text.

Respiratory Acidosis

Respiratory acidosis results from the failure of the lungs to eliminate CO_2. As a result, carbon dioxide partial pressure (pCO_2) rises in the alveoli and arterial blood. The usual causes include asthma, emphysema, suppression of the respiratory centre by drugs or CNS disease, weakness of the respiratory muscles or inadequate ventilation during anesthesia.

Treatment involves improving ventilation. This can be done with bronchodilators (see Chapter 69)

Box 38.1
Signs and symptoms of water and electrolyte imbalance

Imbalance	Signs/symptoms
Water deficit	Thirst, dehydrated appearance, dry skin, dry mucous membranes, flushed skin, increased HR, oliguria, concentrated urine (specific gravity > 1.03) and hyperpnea. Additional observations will include weight loss, fever, lowered BP and postural hypotension. Pushed to the extreme, hallucinations, delirium and coma occur
Water intoxication	Polyuria, progressive deterioration in LOC (lethargy, confusion, stupor, coma), neuromuscular hyper-excitability (increased reflexes, muscular twitching, convulsions), headache, GI disturbances (nausea, vomiting, cramps), high skin turgor, edema
Hyponatremia	Muscle weakness, leg cramps, dry mouth, dizziness and GI disturbances (nausea, vomiting, cramps)
Hypernatremia	CNS disturbances (confusion, stupor, coma), poor skin turgor and, possibly, postural hypotension (if hypernatremia is due to water loss)
Hypokalemia	Impaired neuromuscular function, including postural hypotension, weakness, flaccid paralysis and difficulty breathing; progressive disturbances of mental functioning (lethargy, irritability, confusion); abnormal myocardial function (arrhythmias, CHF, heart block, cardiac arrest); and progressive GI disorders (anorexia, intestinal distention, paralytic ileus)
Hyperkalemia	Irritability (progressive from CNS irritability through muscular irritability to cardiac arrhythmias if untreated), GI disturbances (nausea, intestinal colic, diarrhea), neuromuscular disruptions (weakness, flaccid paralysis, dysphasia), oliguria or anuria
Hypocalcemia	Muscle hyperirritability (which can proceed to tetany and convulsions), alterations in ECG, with lengthening of Q-T interval and prolongation of S-T segment (owing to decreased myocardial contractility), stridor and dyspnea, abdominal cramps, urinary frequency and diplopia
Hypercalcemia	Increase in myocardial contractility and ventricular extra beats, possibly proceeding to idioventricular rhythm; polyuria, with accompanying thirst; anorexia and vomiting; occasionally, constipation; stupor and coma
Hypomagnesemia	Neuromuscular irritability and contractability (hyperactive reflexes, facial twitching, tetany, convulsions) and progressive psychological disorders (hallucinations, delusions, confusion)
Hypermagnesemia	Central and peripheral nervous system depression, decreased deep tendon reflexes, increased P-R interval, broadened QRS complexes, elevated T waves, respiratory paralysis (levels reach 12–15 mmol/L [mEq/L])

or mechanical aids. If drugs are responsible for the respiratory depression, steps should be taken to reverse their effects. In the case of anesthetics or most other CNS depressants, this may mean simply reducing the dose or stopping treatment. Narcotics may be reversed by the use of specific antagonists, such as naloxone (Narcan®). If respiratory acidosis is severe, it may be necessary to infuse sodium bicarbonate to correct the pH quickly.

Respiratory Alkalosis

Respiratory alkalosis occurs when the pCO_2 falls due to hyperventilation. As a result, the pH of the extracellular fluid increases. The most common cause of hyperventilation is anxiety or fear. Although the body responds to the decrease in pCO_2 by excreting more bicarbonate base via the kidneys, this process occurs too slowly to attenuate the effects of hyperventilation. The increase in pH can produce increased neuromuscular irritability, asterixis and tetany. Treatment of spontaneous hyperventilation due to anxiety can involve administration of antianxiety drugs. The immediate problems of tetany can be handled by having the patient breathe into a bag. By inhaling the expired CO_2 the patient will increase the pCO_2 and terminate the respiratory alkalosis.

Metabolic Acidosis

Metabolic acidosis is caused by the overproduction of acid. This occurs in severe diabetes mellitus accompanied by ketosis. The excessive loss of base, such as is seen when bicarbonate is eliminated in large amounts in diarrhea, can also produce acidosis. Renal insufficiency reduces the capacity of the kidney to excrete hydrogen ions and this, too, may cause metabolic acidosis. In addition, kidney failure limits the ability of the body to excrete phosphate and sulfate. This, combined with the increased loss of sodium due to the failure of the kidney to exchange it for hydrogen ions, increases metabolic acidosis.

Treatment of metabolic acidosis involves correcting the specific condition causing the acidosis. Thus, diabetes is treated with insulin and electrolytes, such as sodium, potassium and bicarbonate, together with water replacement. In renal insufficiency, water and electrolyte deficits are corrected. If serum phosphate levels are high, aluminum-containing preparations can be given orally to reduce phosphate absorption from the gastrointestinal tract. Hyperkalemia, if present, can be treated as described earlier.

Metabolic Alkalosis

Metabolic alkalosis can result from the loss of gastric acid or the ingestion of large amounts of sodium bicarbonate. It can also occur as a result of potassium deficiency. As indicated in Chapter 39, potassium and hydrogen are secreted in the distal convoluted tubules and collecting ducts of the nephron in exchange for the reabsorption of sodium. In the face of low potassium levels, increased quantities of hydrogen are exchanged for sodium and metabolic alkalosis can ensue.

Metabolic alkalosis is treated by replacing either chloride, if its loss from the stomach is the cause of alkalosis, or potassium, if its deficiency precipitated the increased renal elimination of hydrogen ions. Obviously, water and other electrolytes should also be replaced if their levels are low.

Nursing Management

Box 38.1 on the previous page summarizes the signs and symptoms of water and electrolyte imbalance, while the nursing management for these conditions is described in Table 38.3.

Further Reading

Graves L III. Disorders of calcium, phosphorus and magnesium. *Crit Care Nurs Q* 1990;13(3):3.

Janusek LW. Metabolic acidosis: pathophysiology, signs and symptoms. *Nursing* 1990;20(7):52.

Janusek LW. Metabolic alkalosis: pathophysiology and the resulting signs and symptoms. *Nursing* 1990;20(6):52.

Metheny NM. Why worry about IV fluids? *Am J Nurs* 1990(6):50.

Nacker JG, Brubakken KM. Accuracy of infusing IV fluids: a QA approach. *J Intrav Nurs* 1990;13(1):23.

Thomason SS. Using a Groshong central venous catheter. *Nursing* 1991;21(10):58.

Yarnell RP, Craig MP. Detecting hypomagnesemia: the most overlooked electrolyte imbalance. *Nursing* 1991;21(7):55.

Table 38.3
Nursing management for water, electrolytes and acid-base balance

Assessment of risk vs. benefit	Patient data	•Baseline data are essential to determine the state of balance with respect to water and electrolytes. Observations include fluid I/O, lab results and signs/symptoms of deficit or excess of electrolytes
	Drug data	•Tx of choice involves replacement with fluids and/or electrolytes. Nurses should become familiar with all PO and IV preparations of fluids and electrolytes
Implementation	Rights of administration	•Using the "rights" helps prevent errors of administration
	Right route	•Fluids and electrolytes can be administered PO and IV. Dietary intake should also be considered
	Right time	•PO doses of calcium should be given 1 h pc to improve absorption
	Right technique	•*(Potassium replacement will be discussed as an example)* Oral solutions should be diluted in strongly flavoured drinks to disguise taste and decrease gastric irritation. Should be taken with meals or pc to reduce gastric upset •Potassium chloride, given parenterally in saline or glucose solutions, must be highly diluted and well mixed to prevent "crowning" of KCl in the IV bag. The max. rate should not exceed 20 mmol (mEq) per hour. An infusion pump and frequent monitoring should be used to ensure accuracy. Similarly, IV calcium should be administered at a slow, controlled rate
	Nursing therapeutics	•Local irritation at the site can be alleviated by reducing the rate or diluting the drug further •Dietary supplements to replace electrolytes should be used whenever possible
	Patient/family teaching	•Instruct pts/families regarding IV tx in general (restricted movement, how IV and pump work, need for frequent observation). Remind them to report unusual reactions and changes in symptoms •If pt continues to receive potassium supplements, review proper administration; powders and solutions should be dissolved in cold water or juice. Drink slowly. Do not crush or chew controlled-release tablets or capsules
Outcomes	Monitoring of progress	*Continually monitor:* •Indications of positive response to tx (i.e., imbalance is corrected) as well as adverse reactions such as side effects of the fluid or electrolyte or overcorrection resulting in excess (see Box 38.1, page 427)

Diuretics

Topics Discussed
● Reabsorption of sodium, chloride and water from the nephron
● Sites of action of diuretics within the nephron
● Groups of diuretics
● For each drug group discussed: Mechanism of action and pharmacologic effects, therapeutic uses, adverse effects
● Nursing management

Drugs Discussed

Thiazide and Thiazide-Like Diuretics:
bendroflumethiazide (ben-droe-flew-meh-**thye**-ah-zide)
chlorothiazide (klor-oh-**thye**-ah-zide)
chlorthalidone (klor-**thal**-ih-doan)
hydrochlorothiazide (hye-droe-klor-oh-**thye**-ah-zide)
indapamide (in-**dap**-ah-mide)
methyclothiazide (meh-thee-klo-**thye**-ah-zide)
metolazone (meh-**tole**-ah-zone)

Loop Diuretics:
bumetanide (byoo-**met**-ah-nide)
ethacrynic acid (eth-ah-**krin**-ik)
furosemide (fur-**oh**-seh-mide)

Potassium-Sparing Diuretics:
amiloride (am-**ill**-oh-ride)
spironolactone (speer-oh-no-**lack**-tone)
triamterene (trye-**am**-ter-een)

Osmotic Diuretics:
mannitol (**man**-ih-tol)

Clinical Challenge

Consider this clinical challenge as you read through this chapter. The response to the challenge appears on page 440.

An elderly man with a history of significant alcohol use is given diuretics for the treatment of pulmonary edema. He also has diabetes which has been controlled by oral medications and diet. His condition improves and he is discharged.

The following week he goes fishing and experiences weakness, fatigue and a generalized rash on his face and arms. The metatarsal joint on his left foot is red, swollen and painful. His blood work indicates:

Na: 137 mmol/L
Cl: 105 mmol/L
K: 4.5 mmol/L
WBC, RBC and HCT: Normal
Blood glucose: 9 mmol/L
Uric acid: 0.83 mmol/L
BP lying: 120/80; standing: 110/80
Radial pulse: 86, irregular rhythm

1. Which patient data indicate increased risk for adverse reactions to diuretics?
2. What questions would you ask prior to contacting the physician? What other investigation should be conducted?
3. What are the possible explanations for this patient's signs and symptoms?

Reabsorption of Sodium, Chloride and Water from the Nephron

Diuretics increase the rate of urine formation by reducing the ability of nephrons to reabsorb water. They are used primarily to decrease extracellular fluid volume. Before discussing the mechanisms of action of diuretics, it is essential to review the role of the nephron in the reabsorption of sodium, chloride and water. Particular attention is paid to sodium and chloride because they are the major electrolytes found in extracellular fluid. When these electrolytes are reabsorbed from the nephron, water is also returned to the body. When they are lost in urine, they carry with them water molecules. All major diuretics decrease, in one way or another, the renal reabsorption of sodium and chloride, thereby promoting the excretion of water.

The following discussion of the physiology of the kidney is tortuous, and for this the authors apologize. However, there is no simple way to lead the reader through the nephron. Figure 39.1 and Table 39.1 on the next page should help to illustrate points raised in the text.

The functional unit of the kidney is the nephron. It is composed of the glomerulus, the proximal convoluted tubule, the loop of Henle, the distal convoluted tubule and the collecting duct. The initial process in urine formation is the filtration of plasma by renal glomeruli. The glomerular filtration rate (GFR) in normal humans is approximately 120 mL/min. Sodium and chloride are filtered through the glomeruli and their concentrations in the glomerular filtrate reflect their plasma levels.

Following the filtration of plasma by renal glomeruli, most of the sodium, chloride and water is reabsorbed from subsequent sections of the nephron. Under normal conditions, approximately 99% to 99.5% of the sodium, chloride and water filtered through renal glomeruli is reabsorbed into the systemic circulation from subsequent sections of the nephron. Any decrease in the percentage of material reabsorbed, regardless of how small it may appear in relation to the quantities filtered, may significantly increase the amount of urine voided. For example, a decrease in the amount of sodium and chloride reabsorbed from 99.5% to 98.0% will cause a fourfold increase in urine production.

The mechanics of salt and water reabsorption differ depending on the section of the nephron involved. Approximately eighty percent of the glomerular filtrate is reabsorbed in the proximal convoluted tubule. This section of the nephron is permeable to water. As a result, when glucose, amino acids, phosphate and sodium are actively reabsorbed from the proximal convoluted tubule, water is drawn along with them to maintain the isotonicity of the fluid remaining in the lumen. Chloride is also reabsorbed passively in the proximal tubule. Chloride carries a negative charge and it accompanies positively charged sodium to maintain electrical neutrality.

The medulla of the kidney is hypertonic. Water descending down the loop of Henle is drawn into the hypertonic medulla in response to the higher osmotic pressure in this portion of the kidney. The descending loop of Henle is not permeable to sodium and chloride. These ions do not leave and, as a result, the liquid remaining in the tubule at the bend of the loop of Henle is hypertonic.

The ascending loop of Henle has characteristics opposite to those of the descending limb. It is permeable to sodium and chloride but impermeable to water. As fluid travels up the ascending loop, chloride is actively reabsorbed into the medulla of the kidney, with sodium accompanying it to maintain electrical neutrality. Water is not reabsorbed because, as just stated, the ascending limb of Henle's loop is impermeable to it.

Before proceeding further on our safari through the nephron, let us pause for a moment to investigate the reasons for, and the consequences of, the aforementioned hypertonicity of the renal medulla. One reason is the previously described selective reabsorption of sodium and chloride from the ascending limb of the loop of Henle. The second reason is the reabsorption of urea from the collecting ducts into the medullary tissue. It may seem a little premature to digress and consider the collecting ducts at the end of our golden stream while we are still working our way up Henle's loop. However, if readers will cast their eyes to a point just before our river empties into the Bay of Bladder, they will see that urea is absorbed into the renal medulla at this point.

Now that we have established the reasons for

the hypertonic medulla, what are its consequences? Stated simply, the hypertonic medulla provides the kidney with its final opportunity to concentrate urine. Under the influence of the antidiuretic hormone (ADH, vasopressin), water is drawn out of the collecting ducts into the hypertonic renal medulla and then reabsorbed into the blood. If anything, such as a loop diuretic, reduces the hypertonicity of the medulla, the ability of the nephron to concentrate urine is diminished and the kidney excretes increased quantities of this fluid.

Returning now to our story, we pick up our fluid as it emerges from the renal medulla and travels up the ascending limb of the loop of Henle through the renal cortex. Here too, sodium and chloride are reabsorbed, and water is retained within the lumen. However, in contrast to the medulla, the renal cortex is not hypertonic. Blood flow through the renal cortex is greater than that through the medulla. As a consequence, the reabsorbed salt is not trapped but instead is rapidly removed from the kidney. The significance of this fact will become apparent soon.

The reabsorption of sodium and chloride, together with the retention of water in the tubular

Table 39.1
Percentage of water and sodium remaining at different points in the nephron

	% H₂O remaining	% Sodium remaining
End of proximal tubule	20	20
End of loop of Henle	14	7
End of distal tubule	2–5	1–5
Excreted urine	0.1–1	0–1

Figure 39.1
Reabsorption of electrolytes and water from the nephron

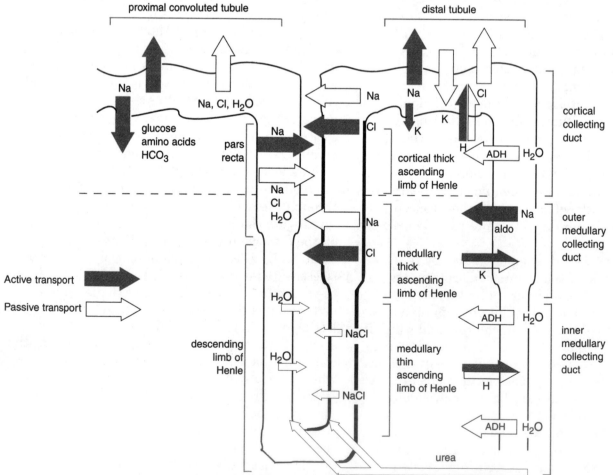

Source: Jacobson HR, Kokko JF. Diuretics: sites and mechanisms of action. *Ann Rev Pharmacol Toxicol* 1976;16:201–214. Reproduced with permission.

lumen, results in the dilution of water, with the result that a hypotonic fluid is presented to the distal convoluted tubule. Within the distal convoluted tubule, sodium, chloride and water reabsorption continues, with electrolyte transport occurring actively and water following in a passive manner.

In addition, an exchange of ions occurs in the last section of the distal tubule and collecting ducts. Under the influence of the mineralocorticoid aldosterone, sodium is reabsorbed in exchange for potassium and hydrogen, which are secreted into the lumen. This aspect of renal function has great clinical significance. All thiazide and loop diuretics reduce the reabsorption of sodium before it reaches the distal convoluted tubule. The higher levels of sodium in the fluid presented to the distal tubule cause an increase in sodium-potassium exchange. The increase in potassium secretion and excretion can produce hypokalemia. This will be discussed in more detail shortly.

The final process in the formation of urine has been referred to above. It occurs as fluid passes down the renal collecting ducts through the hypertonic medulla. The permeability of the collecting ducts to water is controlled by the secretion of the antidiuretic hormone (ADH, vasopressin) by the pituitary. When ADH is secreted, the collecting ducts are permeable to water, which is drawn from the lumen by the hypertonic medulla into medullary tissue and subsequently reabsorbed into the general circulation. In the absence of ADH, water cannot pass through the collecting ducts into the medulla. As a result, the concentration of urine does not occur. In this case an increased amount of urine is presented to the bladder.

Most readers have experienced the full bladder that accompanies ingestion of ethanol. The explanation behind this phenomenon can be found in the fact that alcohol depresses the release of ADH by the pituitary, bringing with it diuresis. Another consequence is secondary dehydration. Think back and remember how much water you drank the "day after."

Sites of Action of Diuretics within the Nephron

It is pertinent now to consider the possible sites where diuretics may act (Figure 39.2). Because the majority of the glomerular filtrate is reabsorbed from the proximal convoluted tubule (site I), students cannot be faulted if they conclude that drugs which reduce the percentage of salt and water reabsorbed from the proximal convoluted tubule produce a marked diuresis. However, this is not the case, because salt and water retained in the proximal convoluted tubule are reabsorbed in the subsequent portions of the nephron.

On the other hand, drugs that inhibit the reabsorption of sodium and chloride from the medullary component of the ascending limb of the loop of Henle (site II) are most effective. Because they reduce the hypertonicity of the renal medulla, these drugs, called *loop diuretics* or *high-ceiling diuretics,* impair the ability of the nephron to concentrate urine in the collecting ducts.

Drugs that block the reabsorption of sodium and chloride in the cortical diluting segment (site III) will also produce marked diuresis. However, they are not as effective as the loop diuretics

Figure 39.2
Sites of sodium reabsorption and diuretic action in the nephron

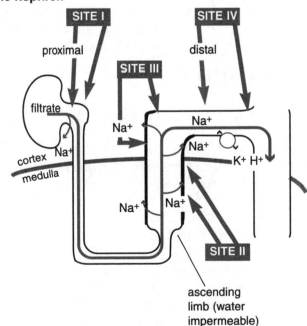

I = proximal tubule; II = ascending limb of Henle's loop; III = cortical diluting site; IV = distal Na+/K+H+ exchange site.

Source: Lant AF, Wilson GM. Modern diuretic therapy. *Excerpta Medica;* 1974. Reproduced with permission.

because they modify neither the hypertonicity of the renal medulla nor the concentrating ability of the collecting ducts.

By the time urine reaches the distal convoluted tubule (site IV), very little sodium and chloride remain to be reabsorbed. Therefore, drugs that block sodium and chloride reabsorption only in the distal convoluted tubule have limited effectiveness as diuretics. They are important, however, in reducing the renal secretion, and subsequent excretion, of potassium. Remember that potassium is normally exchanged for some of the sodium arriving in the distal convoluted tubules and collecting ducts. Potassium-sparing diuretics act in the distal convoluted tubules and collecting ducts to reduce this exchange. They are often used together with a loop diuretic or a drug that acts at site III to reduce the increased potassium-sodium exchange that would normally occur as a result of increased concentrations of sodium arriving in the distal segments of the nephron.

The reabsorption of water from the collecting ducts depends on the secretion of ADH. Patients with diabetes insipidus (Chapter 40) are deficient in this hormone and excrete large amounts of water. Few drugs depress ADH secretion. The effects of ethanol have already been mentioned. However, its other actions make it impractical to use on a long-term basis as a diuretic.

Groups of Diuretics

Thiazides and Their Analogues

Chlorothiazide (Diuril®) et al., Chlorthalidone (Hygroton®), Metolazone (Zaroxolyn®) and Indapamide (Lozide®, Lozol®)

Mechanism of action and pharmacologic effects. Thiazides were introduced in the mid-1950s. Chlorothiazide (Diuril®) was the first drug on the market and it was rapidly followed by many others, such as hydrochlorothiazide (Hydro-DIURIL®, Esidrix®), hydroflumethiazide (Naturetin®) and cyclothiazide (Anhydron®). Qualitatively, all thiazides are identical. They differ only in the doses required to produce diuresis. Hydrochlorothiazide is currently the most popular member of the group.

Two additional drugs, chlorthalidone (Hygroton®) and metolazone (Zaroxolyn®), have actions very similar to those of the thiazides. They differ from thiazides only in the fact that they have longer durations of action and are therefore given less often.

Thiazides, chlorthalidone and metolazone block sodium and chloride reabsorption in the cortical diluting segment of the loop of Henle and in the proximal section of the distal convoluted tubule. As a result, water is also retained in the lumen of the nephron because of the osmotic drawing power of sodium and chloride. By blocking sodium reabsorption, thiazides, chlorthalidone and metolazone also increase potassium secretion. With more sodium arriving at the latter sections of the distal convoluted tubules and collecting ducts, increased quantities of potassium are secreted into the tubular lumen, in exchange for sodium, which is reabsorbed from the lumen into the systemic circulation. As a result of the increased excretion of potassium, serum potassium levels can fall and the patient may become hypokalemic.

The thiazides, chlorthalidone and metolazone decrease the renal excretion of uric acid, thereby increasing its concentration in plasma and predisposing patients to gout.

These diuretics may also induce hyperglycemia and aggravate pre-existing diabetes mellitus. The exact mechanism by which they produce this effect is still in doubt. It has been postulated that they inhibit the pancreatic release of insulin and block the peripheral utilization of glucose.

Indapamide, like the thiazides, chlorthalidone and metolazone, is an orally effective diuretic. It has been claimed that indapamide does not increase serum cholesterol and has a minimal impact on potassium. However, indapamide can cause potassium loss (although possibly less than high doses of thiazides) and significant hypokalemia.

Therapeutic uses. Thiazide and thiazide-like diuretics are used, together with salt restriction, to treat edema. Their efficacy depends on the condition being treated. These drugs are used in the treatment of ascites, particularly when it is secondary to cirrhosis. They may eliminate the need for paracentesis or reduce the number of occasions this procedure is performed. Thiazides, chlorthalidone or metolazone may correct edema in chronic renal disease, if enough nephrons remain functional. However, if a significant number of nephrons have been destroyed, a loop diuretic may be required (see below). Diuretic therapy has often been disappointing in the treatment of the nephrotic syndrome. Thiazides, chlorthalidone and metolazone are contraindicated in anuria. They should be discontinued if increasing azotemia and oliguria occur during treatment of severe progressive renal disease.

The treatment of hypertension with diuretics is discussed in Chapter 36. Thiazides or chlorthalidone are usually the drugs of choice because they decrease blood volume and dilate arterioles. Metolazone may have similar actions. Although loop diuretics are more effective, they do not dilate arterioles and usually are less effective in hypertension.

The use of diuretic therapy in the treatment of congestive heart failure is discussed in Chapter 32; diuretics are appropriate first-line agents for all grades of cardiac failure when sinus rhythm is present. They are usually sufficient alone in mild heart failure. When the patient is afflicted with more severe heart failure, diuretics are usually given with other drugs, such as a vasodilator or digoxin, or both.

Adverse effects. Thiazides, chlorthalidone or metolazone can produce hypovolemia, hyponatremia and hypokalemia. In addition, they can precipitate attacks of gout because they reduce the elimination of uric acid by the kidney. These drugs also produce hyperglycemia and aggravation of pre-existing diabetes mellitus.

Other adverse reactions are anorexia, gastric irritation, nausea, vomiting, cramping, diarrhea, constipation, jaundice and pancreatitis. Patients may experience CNS effects (dizziness, vertigo, paresthesias, headache, xanthopsia). Hypersensitivity reactions include purpura, photosensitivity, rash, urticaria, necrotizing angiitis, fever, respiratory distress (including pneumonitis) and anaphylactic reactions. Leukopenia, thrombocytopenia, agranulocytosis, aplastic anemia and hemolytic anemia have also been reported. In spite of this list, these drugs are generally considered to be quite safe when used in normal therapeutic doses.

Loop Diuretics

Furosemide (Lasix®), Ethacrynic Acid (Edecrin®) and Bumetanide (Burinex®)

Mechanism of action and pharmacologic effects. Loop (or high-ceiling) diuretics inhibit the reabsorption of sodium and chloride in the ascending limb of the loop of Henle as it passes through the renal medulla. The resulting reduction in the hypertonicity of the renal medulla impairs the concentrating ability of the collecting ducts. As a consequence, loop diuretics are the most potent of the diuretics, surpassing the effects produced by thiazides, chlorthalidone and metolazone.

Because loop diuretics increase the concentration of sodium presented to the distal convoluted tubules and collecting ducts, they also promote greater sodium-potassium exchange. Thus, potassium excretion is increased, and patients may experience hypokalemia.

Therapeutic uses. The major therapeutic use of loop diuretics is to treat edema in patients with severe edema or renal impairment where the thiazides, chlorthalidone or metolazone may be ineffective. Furosemide is the most popular drug. Loop diuretics are sometimes used for the treatment of hypertension in place of a thiazide, chlorthalidone or metolazone. Often this is not appropriate because loop diuretics do not dilate arterioles and are not as effective as the thiazides, chlorthalidone or metolazone in lowering blood pressure.

Loop diuretics are contraindicated in the presence of complete renal shutdown. If increasing azotemia and oliguria occur during treatment of severe progressive renal disease, the loop diuretic should be discontinued. In hepatic coma and conditions producing electrolyte depletion, loop diuretic therapy should not be instituted until the underlying condition has been corrected or ameliorated. These drugs are also contraindicated in severe hypokalemia, hypovolemia or hypotension. Because furosemide has the potential to displace bilirubin from plasma albumin, it is contraindicated in newborns with jaundice or infants with conditions that might induce hyperbilirubinemia or kernicterus.

Adverse effects. Electrolyte depletion is a major concern with the use of these drugs. This

Table 39.2
Thiazide, thiazide-like and loop diuretics: Drug interactions

Drug	Interaction
Alcohol	• Acute ingestion of alcohol may lead to an additive antihypertensive effect with thiazide, thiazide-like or loop diuretics
Amphotericin B	• Amphotericin B and thiazide, thiazide-like or loop diuretics have additive hypokalemic effects
Anesthetics, general	• Diuretics may potentiate the actions of general anesthetics
ACE inhibitors	• ACEIs and a diuretic can produce a powerful hypotensive effect in CHF patients. This can best be avoided by stopping the diuretic a few days before starting with low doses of the ACEI. Thereafter, it may be possible to reintroduce the diuretic and increase the dose of the ACEI slowly
Antihypertensive drugs	• Antihypertensive drugs and thiazide, thiazide-like or loop diuretics have additive antihypertensive effects
Cholestyramine and colestipol	• Cholestyramine and colestipol decrease the absorption of diuretics
Corticosteroids	• Corticosteroids can have their potassium-lowering effects potentiated by a diuretic
Digoxin (and other cardiac glycosides)	• Diuretic-induced hypokalemia increases the risk of cardiac glycoside toxicity
Insulin and oral hypoglycemics	• Insulin and oral hypoglycemics may require higher doses because diuretics can increase blood sugar
Lithium	• Lithium levels and lithium-induced toxicities can be increased by diuretics
Neuromuscular blocking drugs	• Diuretics may potentiate the actions of neuromuscular blocking drugs
Nitrates	• Nitrates and a thiazide, thiazide-like or loop diuretic may produce additive antihypertensive effect
Nonsteroidal anti-inflammatory drugs	• NSAIDs may inhibit the actions of diuretics
Penicillins — antipseudomonal	• Mezlocillin, piperacillin or ticarcillin plus a thiazide, thiazide-like or loop diuretics have an additive hypokalemic effects

manifests as weakness, dizziness, lethargy, leg cramps, sweating, bladder spasms, anorexia, vomiting and/or mental confusion. Loop diuretics reduce uric acid secretion in the proximal convoluted tubules, predisposing patients to increased plasma uric acid levels and attacks of gout. Various forms of dermatitis and skin rashes have occurred with these drugs. Cases of vertigo, tinnitus and reversible deafness have also been reported.

Ethacrynic acid has also been reported to affect adversely the gastrointestinal tract, with symptoms of anorexia, malaise, abdominal discomfort or pain, dysphagia, nausea, vomiting and diarrhea.

Bumetanide produces similar electrolyte changes to those caused by furosemide or ethacrynic acid. It may also cause azotemia, hyperuricemia and rarely, impaired glucose tolerance.

Large doses may cause myalgia in patients with renal failure. Nausea, vomiting, abdominal pain and rashes have also been reported with bumetanide.

Table 39.2 lists the clinically significant drug interactions with thiazide, thiazide-like and loop diuretics.

Potassium-Sparing Diuretics

Spironolactone (Aldactone®)

Mechanism of action and pharmacologic effects. Spironolactone is similar in structure to aldosterone and acts as a competitive inhibitor of the mineralocorticoid in the distal convoluted tubules and collecting ducts. As a result, it prevents the aldosterone-induced loss of potassium.

Therapeutic uses. Spironolactone may be given to treat conditions of excessive aldosterone levels, such as primary aldosteronism or cirrhosis accompanied by edema or ascites, or both. Spironolactone is used in the treatment of congestive heart failure in which edema and sodium retention are only partially responsive to, or intolerant of, other therapeutic measures. It does not affect the basic pathologic process of the nephrotic syndrome but may be used for inducing a diuresis in patients not responding to glucocorticoids or other diuretics.

The drug is most often combined with a thiazide, chlorthalidone, metolazone, furosemide or ethacrynic acid to prevent hypokalemia produced by these compounds. A popular product, marketed under the trade name Aldactazide®, contains a fixed ratio of either 25 mg of hydrochlorothiazide and 25 mg of spironolactone or 50 mg of hydrochlorothiazide plus 50 mg of spironolactone. The use of spironolactone in the treatment of hypertension is discussed in Chapter 36.

Spironolactone is contraindicated in anuria, acute renal insufficiency, significant impairment of renal function and hyperkalemia. It should not be used with potassium supplements.

Adverse effects. In addition to hyperkalemia, the most common adverse effects for which nurses must evaluate patients using spironolactone include gynecomastia and gastrointestinal symptoms, such as nausea, cramping and diarrhea. Concern has surfaced over the use of spironolactone with the report of carcinoma of the breast in both men and women receiving the drug. At the present time no cause-and-effect relationship between the use of the drug and the appearance of the carcinoma has been established. Other adverse effects of spironolactone include drowsiness, dizziness, lethargy, headache, maculopapular or erythematous cutaneous eruptions, urticaria, mental confusion, drug fever, ataxia, mild androgenic effects including hirsutism, irregular menses, deepening of the voice, amenorrhea, postmenopausal bleeding, alterations in libido and sweating. These are usually reversible if the drug is discontinued.

Triamterene (Dyrenium®) and Amiloride (Midamor®)

Mechanism of action and pharmacologic effects. Triamterene and amiloride act directly on tubular transport in the distal convoluted tubules and collecting ducts to inhibit the reabsorption of sodium and the secretion of potassium. They work independently of aldosterone and are not competitive inhibitors of the mineralocorticoid.

Therapeutic uses. Either drug may be used alone. Triamterene is indicated for the treatment of edema associated with congestive heart failure, hepatic cirrhosis, nephrotic syndrome, idiopathic edema, steroid-induced edema and edema due to secondary hyperaldosteronism. The indications for the use of amiloride are much the same. However, their major clinical use is in combination with a thiazide, chlorthalidone, metolazone or a loop diuretic to reduce or prevent the hypokalemia produced by these agents. A most popular product, marketed under the trade name Dyazide®, contains a fixed ratio of 50 mg triamterene and 25 mg hydrochlorothiazide. The product Moduret® contains 5 mg amiloride and 50 mg hydrochlorothiazide.

Triamterene and amiloride are contraindicated in the presence of elevated serum potassium levels, anuria, acute renal failure and severe or progressive renal disease. Triamterene should not be used in severe or progressive hepatic dysfunction, or given to nursing mothers. Amiloride should not be given to patients with diabetic nephropathy. Neither drug should be used with potassium supplements.

Adverse effects. Hyperkalemia is the major adverse effect of triamterene and amiloride; relatively few other adverse effects are seen. The most common are nausea, vomiting, leg cramps and dizziness. Amiloride produces adverse CNS effects in about ten percent of patients. These include headache, dizziness, confusion, insomnia, depression, somnolence and decreased libido.

Table 39.3 on the next page lists the clinically significant drug interactions with potassium-sparing diuretics.

Table 39.3
Potassium-sparing diuretics: Drug interactions

Drug	Interaction
Alcohol	• Acute ingestion of alcohol may lead to an additive antihypertensive effect with a potassium-sparing diuretic
Amantadine	• Triamterene increases the circulating levels of amantadine
ACE inhibitors	• An ACEI and a potassium-sparing diuretic can lead to hyperkalemia
Anticoagulants	• Spironolactone may decrease the effects of anticoagulants
Antihypertensive agents	• Antihypertensive drugs plus a potassium-sparing diuretic can led to an additive antihypertensive effect
Cimetidine	• Cimetidine increases the effects of triamterene
Cyclosporin	• Cyclosporin plus a potassium-sparing diuretic can lead to hyperkalemia
Indomethacin	• Increased risk of nephrotoxicity if indomethacin and triamterene are used together
Lithium	• Lithium plasma levels and toxicities may increase if lithium is used concomitantly with a potassium-sparing diuretic
Nitrates	• Nitrates plus a potassium-sparing diuretic can lead to an additive antihypertensive effect
Nonsteroidal anti-inflammatory drugs	• NSAIDs may decrease the antihypertensive effect of potassium-sparing diuretics and increase the risk of renal reactions with spironolactone
Potassium supplements	• Potassium supplements and a potassium-sparing diuretic can lead to hyperkalemia

Osmotic Diuretics

Mannitol (Osmitrol®)

Mechanism of action and pharmacologic effects. Osmotic diuretics, such as mannitol, are pharmacologically inert nonelectrolytes that are freely filtered by the renal glomerulus and not reabsorbed from the nephron. When the diuretic is excreted in urine, it carries with it an amount of water equivalent to its osmotic drawing power.

Therapeutic uses. Mannitol is the osmotic diuretic used most extensively. It must be injected and is available alone and in combination with sodium chloride. The drug is used to increase urine production when the renal filtration rate is acutely reduced. In this situation a higher percentage of sodium, chloride and water are reabsorbed. Loop diuretics and the thiazides may prove ineffective because they cannot reduce the reabsorbing capacity of the nephron for sodium and chloride sufficiently to increase urine flow. Osmotic diuretics may prove effective in this situation.

Mannitol is also employed for the reduction of cerebrospinal fluid pressure and volume. In this situation, the drug increases plasma osmolality, with the result that water diffuses from the cerebrospinal fluid into the plasma to be excreted by the kidneys.

Adverse effects. A major adverse effect of mannitol is an increase in the extracellular fluid volume. By administering a large volume of hypertonic mannitol, which distributes throughout the extracellular space, fluid is drawn from the cells into the extracellular compartment. Hypersensitivity reactions, diverse in nature, have been reported with mannitol.

Nursing Management

Table 39.3 describes the nursing management of patients receiving diuretic therapy. Doses of individual drugs are given in Table 39.5 (pages 441–444).

Table 39.3
Nursing management of the diuretics

Assessment of risk vs. benefit	Patient data	• Assess to establish baseline VS, general state of health. Include fluid I/O, BP (lying and standing), P, R, electrolyte levels, body mass/weight, as well as site and extent of edema. Liver or kidney disease, low serum potassium or sodium levels or diabetes should be known before tx is commenced • *Pregnancy:* Risk category varies among drugs in the class. Many are category B or C. Benefits may be acceptable despite risks. Thiazide diuretics should be avoided during pregnancy and breast feeding
	Drug data	• Generally tolerated
Implementation	Rights of administration	• Using the "rights" helps prevent errors of administration
	Right route	• Give IV and PO
	Right time	• See Table 39.5. Note variation in dosage schedules among drugs in this class. Generally, diuretics are given in a.m. to prevent nocturia; however, those pts whose lifestyles involve limited access to toilet facilities (e.g., crane operators, bus drivers) should take their medication at a time most convenient to their activities
	Right technique	• IV administration requires knowledge of correct diluent and IV solution, correct dilution and rate of administration. Always refer to manufacturer's or agency's instructions for this route
	Nursing therapeutics	• Provide bathroom access. Limit fluid intake as appropriate • Promote balanced dietary intake of sodium and potassium • Interventions will vary with indication for drug use, e.g., tx of edema r/t CHF vs. tx of hypertension
	Patient/family teaching	• Compliance and follow-up are essential factors in successful tx; review principles of patient education in Chapter 3 • Instruct pts/families regarding dietary sources of potassium and sodium. Potassium-rich foods include dried fruits (dates, raisins), bananas, apricots and other fruits and juices. Pts/families should know warning signs/symptoms of possible toxicities of these drugs. Report immediately: rash, muscle weakness or cramps, tinnitus, numbness or tingling of extremities, nausea or dizziness • Warn pts to limit alcohol; increased risk of orthostatic hypotension • *Discuss possibility of pregnancy:* Advise pt to notify physician; discuss birth control methods
Outcomes	Monitoring of progress	*Continually monitor:* • Clinical response indicating success (reduction in signs/symptoms) • Signs/symptoms of adverse reactions; document and report immediately to physician. Especially watch for hypokalemia, glucosuria and hyperglycemia, hyperuricemia and gout, and hyponatremia (see Chapter 38). Blood tests to monitor electrolytes may be ordered periodically

Response to Clinical Challenge

1. The patient's age, alcohol use and diabetes increase his risk for adverse reactions to diuretics.

2. His blood work indicates normal electrolytes, blood cells and hydration.

His blood glucose is elevated (normal, 3.6–6.1 mmol/L), which may indicate poor control of his diabetes or hyperglycemia caused by the diuretic. It may also be related to his age (glucose increases slightly). Determine whether this was a spot or fasting blood sugar and what his diet was prior to the test. Review his history regarding usual blood sugar levels. Ask regarding use of his hypoglycemic medications; recent alcohol use.

His uric acid level is elevated (normal for adult male, 0.15–0.48 mmol/L). The inflamed, painful foot could indicate gout induced by the diuretic. Explore whether this has occurred before.

His BP is within normal limits, with a slight drop upon standing.

His radial pulse is abnormal. Take an apical rate for one minute.

Complete a respiratory assessment and determine whether pulmonary edema has returned.

Examine his skin rash for appearance, pruritus and location.

Thoroughly review all medications he is currently taking, including OTCs, herbal remedies and new as well as old prescriptions.

3. Possible explanations for this patient's signs and symptoms include:
- exacerbation of pulmonary edema due to medication failure or missed doses, causing weakness and fatigue
- photosensitivity reaction (if rash occurs only on exposed skin)
- drug-induced gout reaction
- drug-induced hyperglycemia (due to diuretic or to missed doses of hypoglycemic agent); dietary or activity changes
- drug interactions (diuretics and digoxin can cause dysrhythmias).

Further Reading

Berndt WO, Stitzel RE. Water, electrolyte metabolism and diuretic drugs. In: Craig CR, Stitzel RE, eds. *Modern Pharmacology*. 4th ed. Boston: Little, Brown; 1994:211–228.

Byers J, Goshorn J. How to manage diuretic therapy. *Am J Nurs* 1995;95(1):38.

Jackson EK. Diuretics. In: Hardman JG, Limbird LE, eds. *Goodman and Gilman's The Pharmacological Basis of Therapeutics*. 9th ed. New York: Pergamon; 1996:685–714.

Table 39.5
The diuretics: Drug doses

Drug Generic name (Trade names)	Dosage	Nursing alert
A. Thiazide and Thiazide-Like Diuretics		
bendroflumethiazide (Naturetin)	**Oral:** For edema: *Adults:* Initially, average dose, 5 mg od in a.m.; up to 20 mg may be given od or divided into 2 doses. Maintenance, 2.5–15 mg. For hypertension: Initially, 5–20 mg daily; maintenance, 2.5–15 mg/day	• Administer in a.m. to prevent nocturia • Advise use of sunblock to prevent photosensitivity reaction
chlorothiazide (Diuril)	**Oral:** *Adults* (diuretic): 250 mg q6–12h; (antihypertensive): 250 mg to 1 g/day, as a single dose or in divided daily doses. Geriatric pts may be more sensitive to effects of usual adult dose. *Children up to 6 months of age:* 10–30 mg/kg/day, as a single dose or in 2 divided daily doses. *Children 6 months of age and over:* 10–20 mg/kg/day, as a single dose or in 2 divided daily doses	• Administer with food to enhance absorption and in a.m. to prevent nocturia. Do not give more than 250 mg in single dose • Advise use of sunblock to prevent photosensitivity reaction
chlorthalidone (Hygroton, Thalitone)	**Oral:** *Adults:* 25–100 mg/day or 100 mg qod or 3x weekly. *Children:* 2 mg/kg 3x weekly	• As for bendroflumethiazide
hydrochlorothiazide (HydroDIURIL, Esidrix, Oretic)	**Oral:** *Adults:* 25–100 mg/day in 1–2 doses (up to 200 mg/day). As a diuretic, may be given qod or 3–5 days/week. *Children > 6 months:* 1–2 mg/kg (30–60 mg/m²/day) in 1–2 divided doses. *Children < 6 months:* Up to 3.3 mg/kg/day in 2 divided doses	• Administer with food to reduce GI irritation and in a.m. to prevent nocturia • Advise use of sunblock to prevent photosensitivity reaction • Monitor insulin requirements in pts with diabetes
indapamide hemihydrate (Lozide, Lozol)	**Oral:** 2.5 mg/day taken in the a.m. as a single dose	• Give in a.m. to prevent nocturia • Advise use of sunblock to prevent photosensitivity reaction
methyclothiazide (Aquatensen, Enduron)	**Oral:** *Adults* (diuretic): 2.5–10 mg od or qod for 3–5 days/week; (antihypertensive): 2.5–5 mg od. Geriatric pts may be more sensitive to effects of usual adult dose. *Children:* 50–200 µg (0.05–0.2 mg) per kg	• As for indapamide
metolazone (Zaroxolyn)	**Oral:** *Adults* (for hypertension): 2.5–5 mg/day; (for edema): 5–20 mg/day	• Do not substitute prompt tablets for extended-release forms • Give in a.m. to prevent nocturia • Advise use of sunblock to prevent photosensitivity reaction

(cont'd on next page)

Table 39.5 (continued)
The diuretics: Drug doses

Drug Generic name (Trade names)	Dosage	Nursing alert
B. Loop Diuretics		
bumetanide (Burinex)	**Oral:** *Adults:* 0.5–2 mg/day (up to 10 mg/day; larger doses may be required in renal insufficiency) **IV:** *Adults:* 0.5–1.0 mg; may give 1–2 more doses q2–3h (not to exceed 10 mg/24 h). In severe renal impairment, an infusion of 12 mg over 12 h has been used	• **PO:** Give dose with food to reduce GI irritation • **IV:** For direct IV, follow agency policy. For intermittent infusion, use compatible solution, infuse at ordered rate using a pump to ensure accuracy. Use reconstituted solution within 24 h. Continuous infusion generally not recommended
ethacrynic acid (Edecrin)	**Oral:** *Adults:* Day 1: 50 mg (single dose) pc. Day 2: 50 mg bid pc. Day 3: 100 mg in a.m. and 50–100 mg after lunch or evening meal, depending upon response to the a.m. dose. *Children:* Initially, 25 mg. Careful stepwise increments in dosage of 25 mg should be made to achieve effective maintenance	• Give following food to reduce GI irritation • Dosage must be regulated carefully to prevent a more rapid or substantial loss of fluid or electrolyte than is indicated or necessary. Discontinue drug if severe diarrhea occurs
furosemide (Lasix)	**Oral/IM/IV:** *Adults:* 20–80 mg/day initially (up to 600 mg may be necessary; doses up to 1 g/day have been used in CHF and renal failure). When maintenance dose is determined, dose may be given qod or 2–3x weekly. *Children:* 1–2 mg/kg/day initially (up to 6 mg/kg/day); may be increased at 6- to 8-h intervals	• Give with food to reduce GI irritation and in a.m. and early afternoon to prevent nocturia. Store tablets in dark container • **IV:** For direct IV, follow agency policy. For intermittent infusion, reconstitute according to manufacturer's instructions. Infuse at a rate not to exceed 4 mg/min. Use infusion pump for accuracy. Discard discoloured tablets and IV solution. Use reconstituted IV solution within 24 h
C. Potassium-Sparing Diuretics		
amiloride HCl (Midamor)	Amiloride: **Oral:** *Adults* (diuretic or antihypertensive): 5–10 mg/day as a single dose. Geriatric pts may be more sensitive to effects of usual adult dose	• Give with food to reduce nausea. Give in a.m. to prevent nocturia
amiloride HCl [5 mg] + hydrochlorothiazide [50 mg] (Moduret)	Amiloride + hydrochlorothiazide: **Oral:** *Adults* (diuretic or antihypertensive): 1–2 tablets/day. Geriatric pts may be more sensitive to effects of usual adult dose	

Table 39.5 (continued)
The diuretics: Drug doses

Drug Generic name (Trade names)	Dosage	Nursing alert
C. Potassium-Sparing Diuretics (cont'd)		
spironolactone (Aldactone)	Spironolactone: **Oral:** *Adults* (diuretic; edema due to CHF, hepatic cirrhosis or nephrotic syndrome): Initially, 25–200 mg/day in 2–4 divided doses for at least 5 days; (antihypertensive): Initially, 50–100 mg/day as a single daily dose or in 2–4 divided doses for at least 2 weeks, followed by gradual dosage adjustment q2weeks prn up to 200 mg /day. Primary hyperaldosteronism: 100–400 mg/day in 2–4 divided daily doses prior to surgery; smaller doses may be used for long-term maintenance in pts unsuitable for surgery. Geriatric pts may be more sensitive to effects of usual adult dose	•Protect drug from light •Give with food to enhance absorption
spironolactone [25 mg] + hydrochlorothiazide [25 mg] or spironolactone [50 mg] + hydrochlorothiazide [50 mg] (Aldactazide, Spirozide)	Spironolactone + hydrochlorothiazide: **Oral:** *Adults* (diuretic; edema due to CHF, hepatic cirrhosis, nephrotic syndrome): Daily dosage of 2–4 tablets aldactazide 25 mg or 1–2 tablets aldactazide 50 mg in single or divided doses should be adequate for most pts, but may range from 2–8 tablets aldactazide 25 mg daily or 1–4 tablets aldactazide 50 mg. *Children* (edema): Usual daily maint. dose of aldactazide should be that which provides 1.65–3.3 mg spironolactone/kg. Essential hypertension: Daily dosage of 2–4 aldactazide 25 mg or 1–2 aldactazide 50 mg in single or divided doses will be adequate for most pts, but may range from 2–8 tablets aldactazide 25 mg or 1–4 tablets of aldactazide 50 mg	
triamterene (Dyrenium)	Triamterene: **Oral:** *Adults* (for edema): 100 mg bid pc. Max. dose, 300 mg/day. *Children:* 2–4 mg/kg/day in divided doses	•Give following food to prevent nausea •Advise use of sunblock to prevent photosensitivity reaction
triamterene [50 mg] + hydrochlorothiazide [25 mg] (Dyazide)	Triamterene + hydrochlorothiazide: **Oral:** *Adults* (for edema): Initially, 1 tablet bid pc. Maintenance: 1 tablet daily. For hypertension: Initially, 1 tablet bid pc. Increase or decrease dosage prn. If 2 or more tablets/ day are needed, give in divided doses. Max. daily dose should not exceed 4 tablets	

(cont'd on next page)

Table 39.5 (continued)
The diuretics: Drug doses

Drug Generic Name (Trade Names)	Dosage	Nursing Alert
D. Osmotic Diuretic		
mannitol (Osmitrol)	**IV:** For edema, oliguric renal failure: *Adults:* 50–100 g as a 5–25% solution. May precede with a test dose of 0.2 g/kg over 3–5 min. *Children:* 0.25–2 g/kg as a 15–20% solution over 2–6 h. May precede with a test dose of 0.2 g/kg over 3–5 min For reduction of intracranial or intraocular pressure: *Adults:* 0.25–2g/kg as 15–25% solution over 30–60 min. *Children:* 1–2 g/kg (30–60 g/m^2) as a 15–20% solution over 30–60 min. (500 mg/kg may be sufficient in small or debilitated pts) For diuresis in drug intoxication: *Adults:* 50–200 g as a 5–25% solution titrated to maintain urine flow of 100–500 mL/h. *Children:* Up to 2 g/kg (60 g/m^2) as a 5–10% solution	• Carefully monitor VS, fluid I/O, CVP and serum electrolytes during infusion • To redissolve crystallized solution, warm bottle using a hot water bath, shake vigorously and allow to cool before administration. Use infusion pump for intermittent or continuous infusion. Direct injection not recommended. Observe site frequently for extravasation. Use an in-line filter for solutions >15% concentration

Drugs That Increase the Renal Conservation of Water

Topics Discussed
- Diabetes insipidus
- Drugs used to treat diabetes insipidus: Mechanism of action, pharmacologic effects, therapeutic uses, adverse effects
- Nursing management

Drugs Discussed
antidiuretic hormone (an-tee-die-yur-**et**-tick)
chlorothiazide (klor-oh-**thye**-ah-zyde)
desmopressin (des-moe-**press**-in)
hydrochlorothiazide (hye-droe-klor-oh-**thye**-ah-zyde)
vasopressin (vass-oh-**press**-in)

Diabetes Insipidus

Diabetes insipidus is a disease of impaired renal conservation of water due either to an inadequate secretion of vasopressin from the neurohypophysis (in the case of central or cranial diabetes insipidus) or to an insufficient renal response to vasopressin (in the case of nephrogenic diabetes insipidus).

Patients with diabetes insipidus excrete large volumes — more than 30 mL/kg per day — of dilute (< 200 mOsm/kg) urine and, if their thirst mechanism is functioning normally, are polydipsic. In contrast to the sweet urine excreted by patients with diabetes mellitus, urine from patients with diabetes insipidus is tasteless (hence the name, insipidus).

Central diabetes insipidus can be distinguished from nephrogenic diabetes insipidus by the administration of desmopressin, a vasopressin analogue. This drug increases urine osmolality in patients with central diabetes insipidus, but has little or no effect in patients with nephrogenic diabetes insipidus.

Drugs Used to Treat Diabetes Insipidus

Vasopressin (Antidiuretic Hormone, ADH)

Mechanism of action and pharmacologic effects. Vasopressin, also called the antidiuretic hormone (ADH), is secreted by the posterior pituitary gland in response to an increase in plasma osmolality or a decrease in extracellular volume. Its actions on the kidney have been described in Chapter 39. Briefly, vasopressin increases the permeability of the collecting ducts to water and thereby enables the kidney to conserve water in the face of dehydration.

When the tubular fluid reaches the collecting ducts it is hypotonic because of the reabsorption of sodium and chloride in the ascending limb of the loop of Henle. If a patient is well hydrated, vasopressin secretion is low, the collecting duct is impermeable to water and a large volume of hypotonic urine is voided. However, if the extracellular

Table 40.1
Vasopressin: Drug interactions

Drug	Interaction
Alcohol	•All these drugs may decrease the antidiuretic effects of vasopressin and its analogues
Carbamazepine	
Chlorpropamide	
Clofibrate	
Demeclocycline	
Fludrocortisone	
Heparin	
Lithium	
Norepinephrine	
Drugs that affect BP	•Vasopressin is a vasoconstrictor and will modify the actions of other drugs that affect BP

fluid volume is low, or the osmolality of the plasma is high, vasopressin is secreted and water reabsorption occurs from the collecting ducts.

In addition to its actions on water retention, vasopressin has a pronounced vasoconstrictor effect, affecting all parts of the vascular system. This effect is seen with doses of vasopressin greater than those necessary for maximal water conservation. The increase in blood pressure is not mediated through the autonomic nervous system; thus, it cannot be blocked by adrenergic receptor blockers or sympathetic denervation.

Therapeutic uses. A major therapeutic use of vasopressin is the treatment of diabetes insipidus. In this condition, vasopressin therapy provides effective and immediate treatment and urine volume returns to normal.

Vasopressin is a polypeptide containing eight amino acids. If given orally, it is rapidly inactivated within the gastrointestinal tract. To be effective, vasopressin must be given parenterally or by insufflation. Vasopressin is available for intramuscular or subcutaneous administration in both aqueous solution or peanut oil suspension. The effects of the water-soluble form of vasopressin (Pitressin®) last only a few hours. Desmopressin acetate (DDAVP®) is a vasopressin analogue formulated in an isotonic aqueous solution for parenteral or intranasal administration (see Box 40.1 for a sample patient teaching; Box 41.1, page 455, describes an alternative technique).

Box 40.1
Patient teaching: Intranasal use of desmopressin acetate spray

1. Gently blow your nose.
2. Remove the protective cap from the bottle.
3. The very first time the spray is used, prime the pump by pressing down downwards on the white collar, using your index and middle fingers while supporting the base of the bottle with your thumb. Press down four times or until an even spray appears. The spray is now ready for use.
4. While sitting or standing, tilt your head backward slightly and carefully insert the nasal applicator into one nostril.
5. For each spray your physician has instructed you to take, press firmly downwards once on the white collar using your index and middle fingers while supporting the base of the bottle with your thumb. Hold your breath as you administer the dose.
6. If more than 1 spray is prescribed by your physician, repeat steps 4 and 5 above for the other nostril. Alternate nostrils for each additional spray.
7. Replace the protective cap on the bottle.
8. Store in the refrigerator at 2–8°C (36–46°F) but do not freeze. May be kept at room temperature, 15–25°C (59–77°F) for up to 3 months.

Adverse effects. The vasoconstrictor effects of vasopressin may reduce myocardial perfusion. Patients suffering from coronary artery disease should therefore receive only small doses of this drug. Parenteral therapy is contraindicated in patients with cardiovascular and renal disease with hypertension, advanced arteriosclerosis, coronary thrombosis, angina pectoris, epilepsy or toxemia of pregnancy. The other adverse effects of vasopressin include facial pallor, headaches and increased uterine activity.

Several drugs have been shown to interact with vasopressin. Indomethacin, chlorpropamide and acetaminophen enhance the effects of the hormone. Lithium carbonate and methoxyflurane antagonize the effects of vasopressin on the kidney and can produce a vasopressin-resistant polyuria. The ability of demeclocycline to block the actions of vasopressin has led to its use in the treatment of patients with water intoxication due to high levels of vasopressin.

Table 40.1 lists the clinically significant drug interactions with vasopressin and its analogues.

Thiazides

The pharmacology of the thiazides and their nursing process were presented in Chapter 39. In view of their diuretic properties, it might seem unusual (to say the least) to include thiazides in a chapter dealing with drugs that increase the conservation of water. However, by producing mild volume depletion, thiazides enhance proximal tubular reabsorption of glomerular filtrate. This action reduces delivery of water to the distal parts of the nephron that are dependent on the secretion of vasopressin for water reabsorption. As a result, the consequences of a reduction in secretion of vasopressin are not so readily apparent.

Chlorothiazide (Diuril®) and hydrochlorothiazide (Esidrix®, HydroDiuril®) are the two drugs used most often. They are employed primarily in the treatment of nephrogenic diabetes insipidus. The usual doses of chlorothiazide or hydrochlorothiazide are 1–1.5 g or 50–150 mg, respectively, in daily divided doses. Thiazides are not effective unless dietary sodium is restricted.

The clinically significant drug interactions for thiazides are presented in Table 39.2 (page 436).

Nursing Management

Table 40.2 page describes the nursing management of patients receiving antidiuretic therapy. Doses of individual drugs are given in Table 40.3 (page 449).

Table 40.2
Nursing management of the antidiuretics

Assessment of risk vs. benefit	Patient data	• Assess for baseline BP, weight, fluid I/O, specific gravity of urine, skin turgor and frequency of urination prior to first dose • *Pregnancy:* Risk category unknown
	Drug data	• Vasopressin is used for diabetes insipidus only • Desmopressin is used for diabetes insipidus and is also given IV for tx of hemorrhage due to certain types of hemophilia and von Willebrand's disease. Has also been used for nocturnal enuresis. Dosage and route will vary according to indication for use

(cont'd on next page)

Table 40.2 (continued)
Nursing management of the antidiuretics

Implementation	Rights of administration	• Using the "rights" helps prevent errors of administration
	Right route	• Vasopressin is given IV, SC and IM. Desmopressin is given by the intranasal, SC and IV routes. Do not confuse the drugs or their dosages
	Right dose	• Note that IV route is 10x more effective than intranasal route. Therefore. intranasal dose is 10x greater than the IV dose
	Right technique	• IV administration requires knowledge of correct diluent and IV solution, correct dilution and rate of administration. Always refer to manufacturer's instructions for this route. Check agency policy regarding direct IV administration
	Nursing therapeutics	• Chronic intranasal use for more than 6 months may cause tolerance. Careful increase in dosage may be required • Dosage is parenteral according to urine osmolality. Frequent monitoring of urine specific gravity may be required
	Patient/family teaching	• Instruct for intranasal use (see Box 40.1, page 446) • Pts/families should report adverse effects or an increase in symptoms to physician
Outcomes	Monitoring of progress	*Continually monitor:* • Clinical response indicating tx success (reduction in signs/symptoms) • Fluid I/O, urine osmolality • Signs/symptoms of adverse reactions. Document and report immediately to physician

Table 40.3
The antidiuretics: Drug doses

Drug Generic name (Trade names)	Dosage	Nursing alert
A. Antidiuretic Hormone: Vasopressin		
desmopressin acetate (DDAVP)	**IV/SC:** *Adults:* 0.5–1 mL (4 µg/mL) daily in 2 divided doses; a.m. and p.m. doses should be adjusted separately on the basis of changes in urine volume osmolality and control of nocturia **Intranasal:** *Adults:* 0.1 mL bid (range, 0.1–0.4 mL daily as a single dose or divided into 2 or 3 doses). *Children 3 months to 12 years:* 0.05–0.3 mL daily as a single dose or in 2 divided doses. Solution for intranasal administration contains 0.1 mg/mL	• For direct IV, follow agency policy. For intermittent IV, dilute dose in 50 mL 0.9% NaCl and infuse over 15–30 min • Instruct pt re: intranasal administration. Only 10–20% drug absorbed by nasal route
vasopressin (Pitressin Synthetic)	**IM/IV/SC:** *Adults:* 5–10 U (0.25–0.5 mL) tid or qid. *Children:* 2.5–10 U (0.125–0.5 mL) tid or qid	• Shake suspension thoroughly to ensure even dispersement. Rotate injection sites. Give 1–2 glasses of water at time of administration to reduce adverse effects of nausea, abdominal cramps
B. Thiazide Diuretics		
chlorothiazide (Diuril)	**Oral:** *Adults:* 500 mg to 1 g od or bid	• Administer with food to enhance absorption and in a.m. to prevent nocturia. Do not give more than 250 mg in single dose • Advise use of sunblock to prevent photosensitivity reaction
hydrochlorothiazide (Esidrix, HydroDIURIL)	**Oral:** *Adults* (hypertension): 25–50 mg od or bid. (Edema): 25–100 mg od or bid	• Administer with food to reduce GI irritation and in a.m. to prevent nocturia • Advise use of sunblock to prevent photosensitivity reaction • Monitor insulin requirements in pts with diabetes

Drugs Used in Urologic Disorders

Topics Discussed
● Incontinence in adults
● Childhood enuresis
● Benign prostatic hyperplasia (BPH)
● Nursing management

Drugs Discussed
bethanechol (beth-**ayn**-eh-kole)
desmopressin (des-moe-**press**-in)
dicyclomine (dye-**sye**-clo-meen)
doxazosin (dock-**saz**-oh-sin)
estrogens (conjugated) (**ess**-troe-jenz)
finasteride (fin-**ass**-teh-ride)
flavoxate (flav-**ocks**-ate)
imipramine (im-**ip**-rah-meen)
oxybutynin (ox-ee-**byoo**-tin-in)
phenylpropanolamine (fen-il-proe-pan-**ole**-ah-meen)
prazosin (**praz**-oh-sin)
propantheline (proe-**pan**-the-leen)
pseudoephedrine (syoo-doe-eh-**fed**-rin)
terazosin (ter-**az**-oh-sin)

Incontinence in Adults

Incontinence is the involuntary loss of urine. The condition represents a failure in the storage phase of bladder function. Incontinence may be classified as overflow incontinence, stress incontinence, urge incontinence, functional incontinence and developmental or maturational incontinence.

Overflow Incontinence

Overflow incontinence is the leakage of urine due to an overdistended bladder, commonly caused by outlet obstructions (e.g., prostatic hyperplasia) or neurogenic causes (e.g., multiple sclerosis).

Patients with significant urinary retention leading to overflow incontinence require either surgical removal of an obstructing lesion, or continuous or intermittent catheter drainage of the bladder. Intermittent catheterization is generally preferred if the patient is willing and able to learn and perform the required procedures regularly.

Pharmacologic approaches include bethanechol to stimulate bladder contraction and alpha adrenergic blockade (e.g., prazosin, terazosin, doxazosin) to relax the smooth muscle of the urethra (and prostatic capsule, in men). These drugs have previously been discussed in Chapters 27 (bethanechol) and 30 (alpha adrenergic blockers).

Bethanechol is not felt to be effective on a chronic basis. However, it may be helpful when given subcutaneously during bladder retraining after an overdistention injury to the bladder that causes a transient period of bladder muscle dysfunction. Alpha adrenergic blockers have been shown to provide some, albeit temporary, relief of symptoms associated with benign prostatic obstruction. These agents are not effective, however, in improving bladder emptying when obstruction has progressed to cause significant urinary retention (postvoid residual > 200 mL).

Stress Incontinence

Stress incontinence is loss of urine due to an increase in intra-abdominal pressure (e.g., cough, exercise). It is more common in women. Weakness in pelvic musculature (e.g., due to childbirth) is the primary cause.

Behavioural therapies are generally the initial approach to the patient with stress incontinence. These include pelvic muscle (Kegel) exercises and timed voiding to avoid a full bladder. When relevant, weight loss, smoking cessation and cough suppression may also be indicated. Several techniques have been used to enhance behavioural therapies for stress incontinence, including biofeedback, electrical stimulation and vaginal cones (weights for pelvic muscle strengthening).

Pharmacologic treatment may be used alone or in combination with behavioural therapy and consists of an alpha adrenergic agent — e.g., phenylpropanolamine or pseudoephedrine — with or without conjugated estrogens.

Urge Incontinence

Urge incontinence is the leakage of moderate to large amounts of urine due to inability to delay voiding when an urge is perceived. Causes include bladder wall hyperactivity or instability and CNS disorders (e.g., parkinsonism, stroke).

Urge incontinence is generally managed by a combination of behavioural therapy and pharmacologic treatment. Behavioural therapies include bladder training and pelvic muscle exercises. Pharmacologic treatment involves the use of bladder relaxant medications, almost all of which have significant anticholinergic activity (see Chapter 28). Drugs commonly prescribed include dicyclomine, flavoxate, oxybutynin and propantheline. Tricyclic antidepressants, such as imipramine, also have significant anticholinergic effects, and these drugs have also been used to treat urge incontinence.

Dry mouth is the most common adverse effect, but other anticholinergic effects, such as constipation and blurred vision, can also occur.

Functional Incontinence

Functional incontinence is loss of urine because of the inability to get to a toilet. Causes may include physical or cognitive disabilities and environmental barriers. The condition may also occur in those with normal neuromuscular anatomy whose mechanism of voiding is functionally disturbed.

Incontinent patients with prominent impairments of cognitive and/or physical functioning require caregiver assistance for the management of their incontinence. Various types of simple toileting procedures, such as prompted voiding, habit training and scheduled toileting, are very effective in some of these patients but require consistent implementation by caregivers.

Childhood Enuresis

The clinical definition of childhood enuresis is childhood bladder incontinence that is bothersome to the child and to the parents. It is not until age five or six years that ninety percent of children maintain nighttime dryness. Daytime incontinence is less common than is nocturnal enuresis.

The options available for the treatment of childhood enuresis are:

• Reassurance of patient and parents that there is no medical, psychologic or parenting problem, and advice to let time take its course. (The spontaneous enuresis rate is fifteen percent per year.)
• Tricyclic antidepressant drugs, such as imipramine, to relax the bladder. These drugs are twice as effective as placebo, but have a fairly high relapse rate unless tapered slowly.
• Conditioning systems, such as an alarm attached to the child's pajamas. These systems are effective, yet also have a high relapse rate. They can be reinstituted as necessary.
• Intranasal desmopressin (DDAVP®) (see Chapter 40 and Box 41.1, page 452). While this drug is effective against nocturnal enuresis in short-term trials, it is expensive and has a high relapse rate. Its use should be reserved for temporary settings such as summer camps.

Nursing Management

For the nursing management of cholinergic drugs, refer to Tables 27.1 (page 267) and 27.3 (pages 269–270). The nursing management of anticholinergic drugs appears in Table 28.2 (page 278), while that for tricyclic antidepressants is given in Table 46.9 (page 535).

Doses for individual drugs discussed in this chapter are given in Table 41.1 (pages 453–455).

Benign Prostatic Hyperplasia

Benign prostatic hyperplasia (BPH) is a disease of elderly males. Among the 40-year-old men who survive to 80 years of age, 78% will present with symptoms of BPH and 30% to 40% will undergo prostatectomy.

The cause of BPH remains unclear, but it appears that the abnormal prostate size is due to a decreased rate of cell death rather than an increased rate of cell replication. This phenomenon is thought to be under the control of estrogens and dihydrotestosterone. Estradiol is also thought to stimulate stromal and collagen synthesis with resultant stromal hyperplasia.

The symptoms of BPH are multiple and may include urgency, frequency, nocturia, decreased force of the urinary stream, hesitancy, a feeling of incomplete emptying, urge incontinence and urinary retention.

Strong indicators for therapeutic intervention include azotemia with chronic urinary retention, hydronephrosis, overflow incontinence, large postvoid residuals, urinary tract infection and severe hematuria resulting in urinary clot retention or the need for transfusion. Moderate indicators include acute urinary retention, severe obstructive symptoms, and poor urine flow rate (< 10 mL/s).

Surgery in the form of transurethral resection (TURP) and open prostatectomy remains a mainstay of treatment. Both methods debulk the prostate by surgically removing the adenoma. The medical treatment of benign prostatic hyperplasia uses pharmacologic agents that reduce the muscle tone of the prostate or the tissue bulk of the gland. Alpha$_1$ adrenergic blockade and androgen ablation form the basis for drug therapy.

Alpha$_1$ Adrenergic Blockers

The pharmacology of alpha$_1$ adrenergic blockers is presented in detail in Chapter 30. Terazosin (Hytrin®) and doxazosin (Cardura®) are the most commonly used agents to block alpha$_1$ muscular activity in the bladder neck, prostate and prostatic capsules, reducing the dynamic component to bladder outlet obstruction. Over a period of weeks, this may improve urinary flow rates and symptom scores.

Since both drugs cause systemic vasodilatation, they must be started at a very low dosage and gradually increased until symptomatic improvement or intolerance occurs. Postural hypotension occurs in about four percent of patients. The drug interactions of these drugs are given in Table 30.1 (page 295).

5-Alpha-Reductase Inhibitors

Finasteride (Proscar®) inhibits the enzyme 5-alpha-reductase, which blocks the metabolism of testosterone to dihydrotestosterone. The effect of this action is to decrease intraprostatic dihydrotestosterone and progressively reduce prostatic volume. This decreases the static component of bladder outlet obstruction over a period of weeks to months and may be accompanied by an improvement in urinary flow rates and symptom scores.

Because of the site specificity of finasteride, the drug produces a low incidence of adverse effects (e.g., 3% to 4% sexual dysfunction) and little risk of drug interactions. Finasteride decreases prostatic-specific antigen (PSA) by approximately 50% in men with BPH and may partially suppress serum PSA in men with prostate cancer.

Box 41.1
Patient teaching: Intranasal administration of DDAVP

Medication may be supplied as a nasal spray or as a solution with a flexible, calibrated catheter (rhinyle). For instructions with spray, see Box 40.1, page 446. Instructions for using solution and rhinyle follow:

1. Pull plastic tag on nexk of bottle and tear off security seal.
2. Remove plastic cap and save to reclose bottle.
3. Insert rhinyle (catheter tube) into solution; squeeze plastic teat and draw solution into the tube until it reaches desired mark.
4. Insert one end of the tube into the nostril, place the other end of the tube into the mouth, tilt head back and blow to deposit solution deep into nasal cavity.
5. Rinse tube with water after each use.
6. Reclose bottle with cap.

Refer to package insert for detailed instructions and illustrations.

Table 41.1
Treatment of urologic disorders: Drug doses

Drug Generic name (Trade names)	Dosage	Nursing alert
A. Drugs for Overflow Incontinence		
1. Direct-Acting Cholinergics		
bethanechol chloride (Urecholine)	**SC:** Usually 5 mg, but some pts may respond to as little as 2.5 mg **Oral:** For pts with lesions above the sacral reflex arc and coordinated bladder and sphincter function, initially 25 mg q6h. Increase or decrease prn (usual adult dose is 50–100 mg qid). Drug should be discontinued if reflex voiding is established	• Oral and SC doses are not interchangeable. Give PO on empty stomach. Do not give IM or IV • Do not use solution if discoloured or has a precipitate
2. Alpha₁ Adrenergic Blockers		
prazosin HCl (Minipres)	**Oral:** *Adults:* Initially, 1 mg hs, then 1 mg tid. Dose may be increased at weekly intervals by 1 mg/dose prn	• Monitor; first dose can cause orthostatic hypotension within 30 min to 2 h. Give first dose hs to minimize risk
terazosin HCl (Hytrin)	**Oral:** *Adults:* Initially, 1 mg hs; increase gradually to 10 mg/day as single dose hs for 3–7 days	• Give hs to reduce risks associated with hypotension
B. Drugs for Stress Incontinence		
1. Alpha₁ Adrenergic Agonists		
phenylpropanolamine HCl (Propagest)	**Oral:** *Adults:* 50–75 mg tid. A single 75-mg prolonged-release preparation each a.m. may be adequate	• Time last dose in early evening to minimize insomnia. Do not substitute prompt with time-release form. Do not crush or chew time-release form
pseudoephedrine HCl (Sudafed, Novafed)	**Oral:** *Adults:* 30–60 mg qid. Prolonged-release formulation: 20 mg bid	• As for phenylpropanolamine
2. Estrogen Therapy		
conjugated estrogens	**Vaginal:** 1 g 2–3x/week. **Oral:** 0.3–0.625 mg/day	• Give oral dose with food to reduce nausea • Instruct re: vaginal administration and hygiene

Table 41.1 (continued)
Treatment of urologic disorders: Drug doses

Drug Generic name (Trade names)	Dosage	Nursing alert
C. Drugs for Urge Incontinence		
1. Anticholinergic Drugs		
dicyclomine HCl (Bentyl, Formulex)	**Oral:** *Adults:* 10–20 mg tid or qid	• Dose is titrated according to pt's response • Give on empty stomach
flavoxate HCl (Urispas)	**Oral:** *Adults/children > 12 years:* 100–200 mg tid or qid	• Older pts may require lower doses
oxybutynin chloride (Ditropan)	**Oral:** *Adults:* 5 mg bid or tid. Max. dose, 5 mg qid	• May be given with food if nausea occurs • Store drug in tightly closed container • Tolerance may develop. Drug may be discontinued briefly and restarted if necessary
propantheline bromide (Pro-Banthine)	**Oral:** *Adults:* Initially, 15 mg q4–6h. Increase prn by 15 mg/dose at weekly intervals	• Give on empty stomach • Older pts usually require smaller doses
2. Tricyclic Antidepressants		
imipramine HCl (Tofranil)	**Oral:** *Adults:* 10–25 mg tid or qid. *Elderly:* 10 mg tid or qid	• Give with food to reduce GI irritation
D. Drugs for Childhood Enuresis		
1. Tricyclic Antidepressants		
imipramine HCl (Tofranil)	**Oral:** For nocturnal enuresis: *Children 6–12 years,* 25 mg/day. Increase to 50 mg prn. *Children > 12 years,* up to 75 mg/day	• Drug may be administered after the evening meal or up to 1 h before bedtime
2. Antidiuretic Hormone Therapy		
desmopressin acetate (DDAVP)	**Intranasal:** Initially, 20 µg (10 µg in each nostril) 1 h before sleep. Increase up to 40 µg/day, if there is no improvement after 2 weeks	• Instruct pt re intranasal administration (see Box 40.1, page 446, and Box 41.1, page 452). Draw solution into flexible calibrated catheter, insert one end into nostril, blow on the other end to deposit into nostril cavity. Rinse tube after each use. Cold or rhinitis will reduce absorption

Table 41.1 (continued)
Treatment of urologic disorders: Drug doses

Drug Generic name (Trade names)	Dosage	Nursing alert
E. Drugs for Benign Prostatic Hyperplasia (BPH)		
1. Alpha₁ Adrenergic Blockers		
doxazosin mesylate (Cardura)	**Oral:** 4–12 mg qhs	• Give hs to minimize risks with drowsiness or low BP
prazosin HCl (Minipres)	**Oral:** 1 mg hs, then 1 mg tid. Dose may be increased at weekly intervals by 1 mg/dose prn. Max. dose, 3–4 mg tid	• As previously described for prazosin under Drugs for Overflow Incontinence, (A) above
terazosin HCl (Hytrin)	**Oral:** 1 mg/day hs; increase gradually to 10 mg/day given as a single dose hs for 3–7 days	• As previously described for terazosin under Drugs for Overflow Incontinence, (A) above
2. 5-Alpha-Reductase Inhibitors		
finasteride (Proscar)	**Oral:** *Adults:* 5 mg/day. At least 6–12 months of tx may be necessary	• Give without regard to food • Women who are pregnant should not handle the crushed drug, which may be absorbed and cause damage to male fetus

Further Reading

Feldman W. Childhood enuresis. In: Rakel RE, ed. *Conn's Current Therapy*. Philadelphia: W.B. Saunders; 1993:660–661.

Ouslander JG. Urinary incontinence. In: Rakel RE, ed. *Conn's Current Therapy*. Philadelphia: W.B. Saunders; 1993:661–664.

Timmons SL, Webster GD. Benign prostatic hyperplasia. In: Rakel RE, ed. *Conn's Current Therapy*. Philadelphia: W.B. Saunders; 1993: 677–680.

Drugs and the Blood

The importance of the blood for the transport of drugs to body tissues has been mentioned. However, blood is more than just a vehicle in which drugs are dissolved, or a highway on which they are carried throughout the body. Blood is also a tissue and like all other tissues it, too, is subject to human frailty.

Unit 8 discusses the use of drugs to treat disorders of the blood. Blood physiol-ogy includes the role of blood in transport of lipoproteins and oxygen and the means by which blood coagulates. Accordingly, the authors have chosen to discuss the use of antihyperlipidemic drugs in Chapter 42.

Chapter 43 deals with the use of iron, folic acid and vitamin B_{12} in the treatment of anemias. Finally, Chapter 44 discusses the use of anticoagulant and antiplatelet drugs, as well as fibrinolytic agents and vitamin K.

Antihyperlipidemic Drugs

Topics Discussed
- Atherosclerosis
- Classification of plasma lipoproteins
- Origins of various lipoproteins
- Causes of hyperlipidemias
- Drug treatment of hyperlipidemias
- Nursing management

Drugs Discussed

Drugs Affecting Primarily VLDL:
bezafibrate (bez-ah-**fye**-brayt)
clofibrate (kloe-**fye**-brayt)
fenofibrate (fen-oh-**fye**-brayt)
gemfibrozil (gem-**fye**-broe-zil)

Drugs Affecting Primarily LDL:
cholestyramine (kole-es-**tir**-ah-meen)
colestipol (koe-**less**-tih-pol)
fluvastatin (flew-vah-**stat**-in)
lovastatin (loe-vah-**stat**-in)
niacin (**nye**-ah-sin)
pravastatin (prav-ah-**stat**-in)
probucol (**proe**-byoo-kole)
simvastatin (sim-vah-**stat**-in)

Atherosclerosis

Myocardial infarction (MI), caused by atherosclerosis, is the most common cause of death in the Western world. At least three factors have been implicated in the development of atherosclerosis: hypertension, smoking and high plasma lipid levels. Individuals with high plasma lipid levels are more likely to suffer a myocardial infarct, and reduction in elevated plasma lipids decreases the

Clinical Challenge

Consider this clinical challenge as you read through this chapter. The response to the challenge appears on page 467.

As an occupational health nurse, you are often asked about risk factors for heart disease. A 47-year-old man, who smokes and has a sedentary job, is concerned about his risk because both his father and brother have had heart attacks. He thinks that they had elevated cholesterol and wonders if this is a "family thing." He is interested in the wellness clinic at work and thinks he could start a new lifestyle for better health. He asks you the following questions:

1. What pills could he take to reduce his risks?
2. What diet should he follow?
3. What blood tests should he have, and how often?
4. What advice do you have regarding his general lifestyle?

risk. Drugs are used to lower plasma lipids with the intent of preventing myocardial infarcts.

Classification of Plasma Lipoproteins

The plasma lipids implicated in the development of atherosclerosis are cholesterol and the triglycerides. Insoluble in the plasma, they form complexes with proteins and phospholipids and are carried in the plasma as lipoproteins. Two techniques have been used to classify plasma lipoproteins. Nurses should understand the value of these tests in diagnosing plasma lipoprotein abnormalities.

Ultracentrifugation

One method of classifying lipoproteins involves drawing a plasma sample and subjecting it to ultracentrifugation. The denser lipoproteins are found at the bottom of the centrifuge tube and the lighter ones near the top. The *lipoprotein fractions* are constituted as follows:

• *Chylomicrons,* which consist of 80% to 90% triglycerides and remain at the top of the centrifuge tube. Chylomicrons are formed in the intestine from food containing fatty acids that have more than twelve carbons.
• The next band of lipoproteins in the centrifuge tube are the *very low-density lipoproteins* (VLDL, pre-beta lipoproteins), which consist of 50% to 70% triglycerides and 20% cholesterol. VLDL are formed in the liver from free fatty acids, cholesterol and carbohydrate.
• *Intermediate-density lipoproteins* (IDL, broad-beta lipoproteins) are formed by the catabolism of VLDL and are intermediate products in the formation of low-density lipoproteins (LDL). As intermediates between VLDL and LDL they contain, percentage-wise, lesser amounts of triglycerides and more cholesterol than VLDL, but greater amounts of triglycerides and less cholesterol than LDL. IDL are not found in high concentrations in plasma, unless their subsequent catabolism is delayed.
• More dense than the VLDL and the IDL, and thus found farther down the centrifuge tube, is the band of *low-density lipoproteins* (LDL, beta lipoproteins), which contains mainly cholesterol. LDL are formed by the removal of triglycerides from VLDL.
• *High-density lipids* (HDL, alpha lipoproteins) are found near the bottom of the centrifuge tube. They contain 20% cholesterol and 8% triglycerides; phospholipids and proteins constitute the remaining 72%. An inverse relationship exists between plasma HDL levels and the incidence of coronary heart disease in subjects over age fifty.

Electrophoresis

A second method of differentiating between the various plasma lipoprotein complexes utilizes electrophoresis. If a plasma sample is placed on an electrophoresis plate and subjected to an electrical charge, the different lipoproteins can be separated on the basis of their ability to move in an electrical field into the following fractions:

• The fastest-moving fraction can be found the farthest distance down the plate. This is called the *alpha lipoprotein fraction* and is composed of HDL.
• The next fraction, called the *beta lipoprotein fraction,* moves more slowly than the alpha fraction. The beta lipoprotein band on the electrophoresis plate contains LDL.
• Moving more slowly than the beta fraction are the *pre-beta lipoproteins.* They are found between the beta band and the origin where the plasma sample was applied to the plate. The pre-beta band is composed of VLDL.
• Finally, one lipoprotein band does not migrate in an electrical field. This band is found at the origin. It is composed of *chylomicrons.*

Table 42.1 summarizes the comparative classification of lipoproteins.

Table 42.1
Classification of lipoproteins

Ultracentrifugation		Electrophoresis
1. Chylomicrons, found near the top of the tube. Contain 80%–90% triglycerides (TG)	=	Band that remains at the origin of the electrophoresis plate
2. VLDL, containing 50%–70% TG and cholesterol	=	Pre-beta band; moves slowly down the electrophoresis plate
3. LDL, responsible for 75% of cholesterol found in plasma	=	Beta band; moves farther down the electrophoresis plate than the pre-beta band
4. HDL, containing about 20% cholesterol and 8% TG. An inverse relationship exists between HDL levels and incidence of coronary heart disease in subjects over 50	=	Alpha lipoproteins; move farthest down the electrophoresis plate

Origins of the Various Lipoproteins

The formation of the various lipoprotein complexes is shown in Figure 42.1. Chylomicrons are formed in the intestine from food and contain mainly triglycerides. They are synthesized from fatty acids having more than twelve carbons, and smaller amounts of cholesterol. Once chylomicrons reach the plasma, their triglycerides are released by the enzyme lipoprotein lipase and stored as fat or converted to fatty acids.

VLDL are formed in the liver from free fatty acids, cholesterol and carbohydrate. The VLDL are subsequently stripped of some of their triglycerides and converted to intermediate-density lipoproteins or remnants. As the intermediate-density proteins lose more triglycerides they are converted to LDL, which contain mainly cholesterol.

Causes of Hyperlipidemias

Hyperlipidemias may be of exogenous or endogenous origin. Exogenous hyperlipidemia results from the ingestion of a meal high in content of fatty acids having twelve or more carbons. The chylomicrons formed are released into the circulation by the intestinal lymphatics. Exogenous hyperlipidemia can be reduced by eating food containing fatty acids having fewer than twelve carbons, because these are absorbed directly into the portal circulation and carried to the liver.

Figure 42.1
Physiology of lipid transport in humans

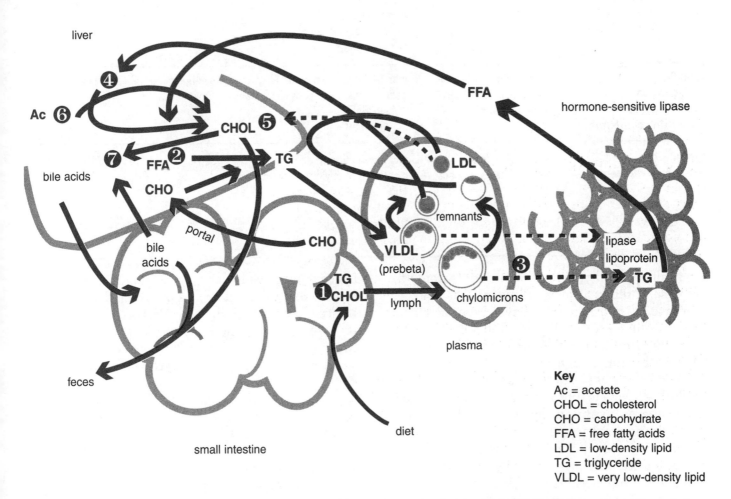

Source: Hazzard WR. (1976), A pathophysiologic approach to managing hyperlipemia. *Am Fam Phys* 1976;14(2):78–87. Reproduced with permission.

Table 42.2
Types of hyperlipoproteinemia

	Lipoprotein charac-teristics of plasma	Metabolic defect	Appearance of fasting plasma after standing overnight at 4°C	Cholesterol/triglyceride ratio
Type I **Exogenous** **hyperlipidemia** **(hyperchylomicronemia)**	Major incr. in chylo-microns. Us. decr. LDL, VLDL, HDL	Decr. chylomicron clearance due to deficiency of lipoprotein lipase or abnormality of apo-CII	Creamy supernatant w. clear infranate	< 0.2/1
Type IIa **Hyperbetalipoproteinemia** **(hypercholesterolemia)**	Incr. LDL; normal VLDL; absence of chylomicrons	Incr. LDL synthesis, decr. clearance due to deficiency of or defect in LDL receptors	Clear	> 1.5/1
Type IIb **Combined hyperlipidemia** **(mixed hyperlipidemia)**	Incr. LDL; incr. VLDL; absence of chylomicrons	Same defect as type IIa but also incr. VLDL	No creamy layer on top but infranate may range from clear to turbid	Variable
Type III **Broad-beta** **(dysbetalipoproteinemia)**	Incr. IDL; poss. presence of chylomicrons	Incr. IDL production or decr. clearance. Incr. total plasma apo-E plus deficiency of apo-E-III. Possible deficiency of hepatic lipase	Faint creamy supernatant w. turbid infranate	Range 0.3/1–2.0/1, with 1/1 often found
Type IV **Endogenous** **hyperlipidemia** **(hypertriglyceridemia)**	Incr. VLDL; normal or decr. LDL; absence of chylomicrons	Incr. VLDL production or decr. clearance or both. Possible abnormal apo-I/C-III complex	No creamy supernate, clear to turbid infranate	Variable
Type V **Mixed hyperlipidemia**	Incr. VLDL; incr. chylomicrons; normal or decr. LDL	Incr. production or decr. clearance of chylomicrons and VLDL. Possible imbalance between apo-CII and CIII, as well as possible abnormal apo-E	Clear supernate and turbid infranate	0.15/1–0.6/1

Endogenous hyperlipidemia results from an increase in the synthesis of lipoproteins or a decrease in their rate of removal from the plasma. Excessive hepatic triglyceride and VLDL synthesis in the liver is the most common cause of hyper-triglyceridemia. Triglyceride synthesis is stimulated by caloric excess, dietary carbohydrates, ethanol, estrogens and hyperinsulinism secondary to peripheral insulin antagonism, such as is seen in obesity and corticosteroid excess. Endogenous hypertriglyceridemia may also be genetic in origin.

Lipoprotein lipase is responsible for the removal of triglycerides from VLDL and chylomicrons. A defect in this enzyme is the most common cause of massive hypertriglyceridemia. Both insulin and thyroxin are required for the maintenance of lipoprotein lipase activity. Uncontrolled diabetes mellitus and hypothyroidism are the leading causes of severe hypertriglyceridemia. Treatment with insulin or thyroid hormone reverses the condition.

Endogenous hypercholesterolemia can result from overproduction of cholesterol in the liver. This condition is associated with obesity and genetic abnormalities and can result in premature coronary heart disease.

The hyperlipoproteinemias can be classified into five types, as shown in Table 42.2.

Table 42.3
Bezafibrate: Drug interactions

Drug	Interaction
Anticoagulants, oral	• Caution should be exercised when oral anticoagulants are given with bezafibrate. The dosage of anticoagulants should be reduced up to 50% to maintain the prothrombin time (PT) at the desired level to prevent bleeding complications. Careful frequent (e.g., weekly) monitoring of PT is recommended until it has been definitely determined that the prothrombin level has been stabilized
Cholestyramine and colestipol	• Cholestyramine and colestipol can reduce the absorption of bezafibrate
Estrogens	• Since estrogens may lead to a rise in lipid levels, the prescribing of bezafibrate in pts taking estrogens or estrogen-containing contraceptives must be critically considered on an individual basis
MAOIs (with hepatotoxic potential)	• These drugs should not be used with bezafibrate
Statins and cyclosporine	• Severe myositis and rhabdomyolysis have occurred when a statin or cyclosporine was administered with a fibrate

Drug Treatment of Hyperlipidemias

Initial treatment for hyperlipidemia should include a specific diet, weight reduction and an exercise program. For patients with diabetes mellitus good diabetic control must be maintained. Drug therapy is often not recommended until diet and exercise have been tried for two to three months. The institution of drug therapy should not mean that non-drug therapy can be discontinued. Nonpharmacologic means of controlling hyperlipidemias must remain an integral part of the treatment regimen.

Drugs Affecting Primarily VLDL: The Fibrates

Bezafibrate (Bezalip®)

Mechanism of action and pharmacologic effects. The fibrates, including bezafibrate, lower elevated serum lipids by decreasing the LDL fraction rich in cholesterol and the VLDL fraction rich in triglycerides. In addition, the fibrates increase the HDL cholesterol fraction.

Bezafibrate is rapidly and almost completely absorbed from the standard 200-mg immediate-release tablet. Bezafibrate is also available in a 400-mg sustained-release tablet that has approximately seventy percent of the bioavailability of the standard tablet.

Therapeutic uses. Bezafibrate is indicated as an adjunct to diet and other therapeutic measures for treatment of patients with hypercholesterolemia types IIa and IIb to regulate lipid and apoprotein levels.

Adverse effects. The most common adverse reactions of bezofibrate involve the gastrointestinal tract and the skin. These include epigastric distress, flatulence, nausea, diarrhea, constipation, pruritus, urticaria and erythema.

Table 42.3 lists the clinically significant drug interactions with bezafibrate.

Clofibrate (Atromid-S®)

Mechanism of action and pharmacologic effects. The main effect of clofibrate is to reduce VLDL. Clofibrate stimulates lipoprotein lipase to increase VLDL triglyceride removal from the circulation. The elevated plasma level of LDL is also reduced in responsive patients.

Therapeutic uses. Clofibrate is used in the treatment of hyperlipidemias characterized by an increase in VLDL. It is claimed to be particularly

Table 42.4
Clofibrate: Drug interactions

Drug	Interaction
Anticoagulants, oral	• Oral anticoagulants may demonstrate increased effect in the presence of clofibrate. The dosage of the oral anticoagulant should be reduced to 50% to maintain PT at desired levels
Antidiabetic drugs, oral	• Oral antidiabetic drugs may demonstrate increased effect in the presence of clofibrate
Furosemide	• Furosemide and clofibrate may compete for plasma albumin binding sites, resulting in painful or stiff muscles and marked diuresis

effective in type III hyperlipoproteinemias because it stimulates the degradation of beta VLDL particles. Its clinical efficacy is still disputed.

Clofibrate is contraindicated in pregnancy. It should not be given to nursing mothers because it can be excreted in milk. Clofibrate should also not be given to patients with renal disease.

Adverse effects. Although clofibrate is fairly well tolerated, adverse effects have been reported, including weight gain, alopecia, leukopenia, nausea, dysphagia and allergic reactions.

Table 42.4 lists the clinically significant drug interactions with clofibrate.

Fenofibrate (Lipidil®, Lipidil Micro®)

Mechanism of action and pharmacologic effects. Fenofibrate lowers elevated serum lipids by decreasing the LDL and VLDL fractions. In addition, the drug increases the HDL cholesterol fraction. Fenofibrate appears to have a greater depressant effect on VLDL than on LDL. Therapeutic doses produce variable elevations of HDL cholesterol, a reduction in the content of total LDL cholesterol and a substantial reduction in the triglyceride content of VLDL.

Therapeutic uses. Fenofibrate is used as an adjunct to diet and other therapeutic measures to treat patients with mixed hyperlipidemias or high serum triglyceride levels. The drug is contraindicated in the presence of hepatic or renal dysfunction, including primary biliary cirrhosis, and in pre-existing gallbladder disease. It should not be used in pregnant or lactating patients.

Fenofibrate is available in two formulations. Lipidil® is a standard-release capsule designed to be taken three times daily. Lipidil Micro® capsules contain micronized fenofibrate, which increases the drug's absorption and reduces both frequency of administration (from three times daily to once daily) and total daily dose (from 300 mg to 200 mg).

Adverse effects. Fenofibrate can cause epigastric distress, flatulence, abdominal pain, nausea, diarrhea and constipation. It can also cause erythema, pruritus and urticaria. Musculoskeletal adverse effects include muscle pain, weakness and arthralgia. CNS effects can include headache, dizziness and insomnia. Decreased libido, hair loss and weight loss have also been reported.

Table 42.5 lists the clinically significant drug interactions with fenofibrate.

Table 42.5
Fenofibrate: Drug interactions

Drug	Interaction
Anticoagulants, oral	• Oral anticoagulants may demonstrate increased effect in the presence of fenofibrate. The dosage of t he oral anticoagulant should be reduced to maintain PT at desired levels
Lovastatin	• Lovastatin plus gemfibrozil has produced severe myositis. Gemfibrozil is chemically related to fenofibrate. It is not known whether the same interaction occurs with fibrates other than gemfibrozil

Table 42.6
Gemfibrozil: Drug interactions

Drug	Interaction
Anticoagulants, oral	• Oral anticoagulants must be administered with caution to pts taking gemfibrozil. The dosage of the anticoagulant should be reduced to maintain the PT at the desired level to prevent bleeding complications. Frequent prothrombin determinations are advisable until it has been determined that the prothrombin level has stabilized
Lovastatin	• Lovastatin and gemfibrozil used together have been reported to produce severe myositis with markedly elevated serum creatinine kinase (CK) and myoglobinuria (rhabdomyolysis). When myoglobinuria is severe, acute renal failure may ensue. Therefore, lovastatin should not be used concomitantly with gemfibrozil

Gemfibrozil (Lopid®)

Mechanism of action and pharmacologic effects. Gemfibrozil inhibits peripheral lipolysis and decreases the hepatic extraction of free fatty acids. These effects reduce hepatic triglyceride production. As a result, gemfibrozil produces a greater fall in VLDL than LDL. Gemfibrozil may also increase HDL cholesterol.

Therapeutic uses. Gemfibrozil is indicated as an adjunct to diet and other therapeutic measures in the management of patients with type IV hyperlipidemia who are at high risk for sequelae and complications from their hyperlipidemia. If a significant serum lipid response is not obtained in three months, gemfibrozil should be discontinued. Gemfibrozil is contraindicated in the presence of hepatic or renal dysfunction, including primary biliary cirrhosis. It is also contraindicated in patients with pre-existing gallbladder disease. *Strict birth control procedures must be exercised by women of childbearing potential.* If pregnancy occurs, gemfibrozil must be discontinued. Women who are planning pregnancy should discontinue gemfibrozil several months prior to conception.

Adverse effects. The incidence of adverse effects with gemfibrozil is low. Nausea, vomiting, abdominal and epigastric pain appear to be the most common effects, with approximately five percent of patients encountering these problems.

Table 42.6 lists the clinically significant drug interactions with gemfibrozil.

Drugs Affecting Primarily LDL

The Resins: Cholestyramine (Questran®) and Colestipol HCl (Colestid®)

Mechanism of action and pharmacologic effects. Cholestyramine and colestipol hydrochloride are nonabsorbed resins that sequester bile acids in the intestine, preventing their absorption. The liver responds to the lowered levels of bile acids by increasing the conversion of cholesterol to bile acids. This has the effect of lowering cholesterol levels, while increasing LDL receptor activity and apoprotein B catabolism. Unfortunately, the decrease in LDL is offset, at least in part, by a compensatory increase in cholesterol synthesis in the liver and intestine.

Therapeutic uses. Cholestyramine and colestipol are used to treat hyperlipidemias characterized by an increase in beta lipoproteins or LDL. They are used in conditions where the increase is seen only in LDL or in situations where the increase in LDL is also accompanied by a rise in pre-beta lipoproteins or VLDL. Cholestyramine is a drug of choice for type IIa hyperlipidemia (hyperbetalipoproteinemia). When used with dietary control, cholestyramine reduces LDL an additional 20% to 40%.

Adverse effects. The adverse effects of cholestyramine and colestipol hydrochloride include abdominal discomfort, bloating, nausea, dyspepsia, steatorrhea and possibly either constipation or diarrhea.

Table 42.7 on the next page lists the clinically significant drug interactions with cholestyramine and colestipol.

Table 42.7
Cholestyramine and colestipol: Drug interactions

Drug	Interaction
Acidic drugs (including warfarin, phenylbutazone, digoxin, thiazides, phenobarbital and thyroid hormones)	• Acidic drugs bind to cholestyramine and colestipol in the GI tract. As a result, cholestyramine and colestipol can block their absorption
Fat-soluble vitamins	• Absorption of fat-soluble vitamins is blocked by cholestyramine and colestipol
Tetracyclines	• Absorption of tetracyclines is blocked by cholestyramine and colestipol

HMG-CoA Reductase Inhibitors: The Statins — Fluvastatin (Lescol®), Lovastatin (Mevacor®), Pravastatin (Pravachol®) and Simvastatin (Zocor®)

Mechanism of action and pharmacologic effects. Fluvastatin, lovastatin, pravastatin and simvastatin inhibit 3-hydroxy-3-methylglutaryl-coenzyme A (HMG-CoA) reductase. This enzyme catalyzes the conversion of HMG-CoA to mevalonate, which is an early and rate-limiting step in the biosynthesis of cholesterol. The four drugs reduce LDL synthesis and increase LDL catabolism as a result of the induction of LDL receptors. They may also increase HDL levels.

Therapeutic uses. Fluvastatin, lovastatin, pravastatin and simvastatin are indicated as adjuncts to diet for the reduction of elevated total and low-density lipoprotein cholesterol levels in patients with primary hypercholesterolemia (types IIa and IIb; see Table 42.2), when the response to diet and other measures alone has been inadequate. Types IIa and IIb hyperlipoproteinemia are characterized by elevated serum cholesterol levels, in association with normal triglyceride levels (type IIa) or elevated serum cholesterol levels plus increased triglyceride levels (type IIb).

Lovastatin is contraindicated in patients with active liver disease with unexplained persistent elevations of serum transaminase levels. It is recommended that liver function tests be performed at baseline and every four to six weeks during the first fifteen months of therapy with lovastatin, and periodically thereafter. If the transaminase levels show evidence of progression, particularly if they rise to three times the upper limit of normal and are persistent, the drug should be discontinued.

The contraindications to the use of fluvastatin, pravastatin and simvastatin include acute liver disease or unexplained persistent elevations of serum transaminases.

Adverse effects. Fluvastatin's adverse effects are usually mild and transient and similar in incidence to placebo. In the controlled clinical trials and their open extensions, one percent of patients were discontinued because of adverse experiences attributable to fluvastatin. The incidence was slightly less for patients receiving fluvastatin compared with those receiving placebo. Common adverse experiences possibly attributable to fluvastatin at the recommended dose range of 20–40 mg/day include dyspepsia (6.6%), diarrhea (3.2%), abdominal pain (3.9%) and nausea (1.6%).

Lovastatin is generally well tolerated, and adverse reactions are usually mild and transient. The most frequently encountered involve the GI tract (constipation, diarrhea, dyspepsia, flatus, abdominal pain or cramps, heartburn and nausea). Muscle cramps and myalgia are sometimes observed. Headache has been reported in 9% to 10% of patients taking the drug. Transient elevations of creatinine phosphokinase (CK) are commonly seen in lovastatin-treated patients but have usually been of no clinical significance. Rhabdomyolysis has occurred rarely. Lovastatin therapy should be discontinued if marked elevation of CK levels occurs, and appropriate therapy should be instituted.

Simvastatin's adverse effects include constipation, flatulence, nausea, headache and abdominal pain. Elevations of creatinine phosphokinase levels three or more times the normal values on one or more occasions have been reported in approximately five percent of patients taking simvastatin. This

Table 42.8
Fluvastatin: Drug interactions

Drug	Interaction
Cholestyramine	• Cholestyramine decreases fluvastatin absorption
Cimetidine, ranitidine, omeprazole	• Concomitant administration of fluvastatin with cimetidine, ranitidine and omeprazole results in a significant increase in the plasma level of fluvastatin
Gemfibrozil, fenofibrate, niacin	• Myopathy, including rhabdomyolysis, has occurred in patients who were receiving coadministration of other HMG-CoA reductase inhibitors with fibric acid derivatives and niacin, particularly in subjects with pre-existing renal insufficiency
Rifampin	• Administration of fluvastatin to subjects pretreated with rifampin results in a reduction in plasma levels of fluvastatin and an increase in its plasma clearance

is attributable to the noncardiac fraction of CK. Myopathy has been reported rarely. In clinical trials, marked persistent increases (to more than three times the upper limit of normal) in serum transaminases have occurred in one percent of adult patients who received simvastatin. It is recommended that liver function tests be performed at baseline, and periodically thereafter, in all patients. If the transaminase levels show evidence of progression, particularly if they rise to three times the upper limit of normal and are persistent, simvastatin should be discontinued. Simvastatin should be used with caution in patients who consume substantial quantities of alcohol and/or have a history of liver disease.

Liver function tests should be performed at baseline and periodically thereafter in all patients taking pravastatin. Special attention should be given to patients who develop increased transaminase levels. Liver function tests should be repeated to confirm an elevation and subsequently monitored at more frequent intervals. If increases in alanine aminotransferase (ALAT) and aspartate aminotransferase (ASAT) equal or exceed three times the upper limit of normal and persist, therapy should be discontinued. In view of these concerns, it is not surprising that caution should be exercised when pravastatin is administered to patients with a history of liver disease or heavy alcohol ingestion.

As previously explained, HMG-CoA reductase inhibitors, including pravastatin, have been associated with elevations of creatinine kinase. Myalgia has been associated with pravastatin therapy. Interruption of therapy with pravastatin should be considered in any patient with an acute, serious

Table 42.9
Lovastatin: Drug interactions

Drug	Interaction
Anticoagulants, oral	• Oral anticoagulants may interact with lovastatin. Careful monitoring of PT is recommended
Cholestyramine and colestipol	• Cholestyramine and colestipol may produce additive effects with lovastatin
Gemfibrozil and niacin	• Gemfibrozil and niacin may increase the incidence of myopathy with lovastatin. In clinical trials the incidence of myopathy within one year of starting tx with gemfibrozil plus lovastatin, or niacin plus lovastatin, was 5% and 2%, respectively. It is not known whether the same phenomenon occurs with concomitant use of lovastatin with fibrates other than gemfibrozil
Immunosuppressants	• Immunosuppressants increase the incidence of myopathy with lovastatin. In clinical trials, about 30% of pts receiving immunosuppressive tx, including cyclosporine, developed myopathy within a year after starting tx with lovastatin

Table 42.10
Pravastatin: Drug interactions

Drug	Interaction
Antacids	• Antacids reduce the bioavailability of pravastatin. The clinical significance is probably minimal
Cholestyramine and colestipol	• Cholestyramine and colestipol may reduce the absorption of pravastatin. Give pravastatin at least 1 h before or 4 h after either drug
Cimetidine	• Cimetidine increases the bioavailability of pravastatin. The clinical significance is probably minimal
Immunosuppressive drugs, fibrates, erythromycin, niacin	• When administered concomitantly with lovastatin, these drugs increase the risk for myopathy or rhabdomyolysis associated with lovastatin. Because of the similarities between pravastatin and lovastatin, concomitant use of these drugs with pravastatin should be considered carefully

condition, suggestive of a myopathy or having a risk factor predisposing to the development of renal failure or rhabdinomyolysis, such as severe acute infection, hypotension, major surgery, trauma, severe metabolic, endocrine or electrolyte disorders and uncontrolled seizures.

Tables 42.8, 42.9, 42.10 and 42.11 list the clinically significant drug interactions with fluvastatin, lovastatin, pravastatin and simvastatin, respectively.

Miscellaneous Drugs

Niacin (vitamin B$_3$). Niacin decreases both VLDL and LDL cholesterol and increases HDL cholesterol. It may be effective in all types of hyperlipoproteinemia except type I. Niacin may produce a greater fall in triglycerides in patients with type V hyperlipoproteinemia than other drugs.

Flushing occurs in almost all patients when treatment with niacin is started. Although this effect often subsides, 10% to 15% patients experience it throughout the duration of therapy. Other adverse effects include pruritus, dry skin with scaling, and acanthosis nigrans. Gastrointestinal effects attributed to niacin include nausea, vomiting, flatulence and diarrhea. Reactivation of peptic ulcer is a more serious GI effect. Other serious reactions to niacin include impaired glucose tolerance, hyperuricemia and liver dysfunction, including cholestatic jaundice. Liver tests should be performed periodically.

Probucol (Lorelco®). Probucol reduces elevated cholesterol levels. It is used in the treatment of patients with elevated LDL and combined hyperlipidemias. Probucol's adverse effects are diarrhea, flatulence, abdominal pain and nausea.

Table 42.12 lists the clinically significant drug interactions with probucol.

Nursing Management

The nursing management of patients receiving antihyperlipidemic drugs is described in Table 42.13 (page 468). Dosages of individual drugs are given in Table 42.14 (pages 469–470).

Table 42.11
Simvastatin: Drug interactions

Drug	Interaction
Cholestyramine	• Cholestyramine appears to have additive cholesterol-lowering effects with simvastatin
Immunosuppressive drugs, fibrates, erythromycin, niacin	• When administered concomitantly with lovastatin, these drugs increase the risk for myopathy or rhabdomyolysis associated with lovastatin. Because of the similarities between simvastatin and lovastatin, concomitant use of these drugs with simvastatin should be considered carefully

Table 42.12
Probucol: Drug interactions

Drug	Interaction
Clofibrate	•Clofibrate and probucol are not recommended concomitantly because an increase in serum triglycerides can occur

Response to Clinical Challenge

Hyperlipidemias are known to be associated with increased risk for CAD, as are several other factors including smoking, sedentary lifestyle, obesity, hypertension, diabetes and family history. This man presents several risks that can be reduced by commitment to lifestyle changes.

Proper encouragement and information can give him the tools he needs to make such changes. Your responses should include the following points:

1. His physician should assess whether he might benefit from one of the drugs in this class. The drug would be selected based on his blood profile and his history.
2. There are several important principles to share regarding diet. He might want to consult a dietitian or read further from sources in a local library or health clinic. Inform him of the following guidelines:
• total dietary fat should not exceed 30% of daily caloric intake
• saturated fats should be limited to 10% or less of caloric intake
• total daily intake of cholesterol should be < 300 mg
• alcohol should be limited or avoided (owing to caloric intake and possible interactions with some drugs in this class).
3. His physician will order tests to determine his lipid profile and may also order tests of liver and renal function, depending on client history and symptoms. If drug therapy is initiated, he will require initial and periodic monitoring of lipid levels.
4. Explore his beliefs about such lifestyle issues as smoking and exercise/activity level. Ask whether he has stopped smoking previously and what assistance he would prefer to stop now. Provide information on smoking cessation programs, if desired.

Discuss opportunities for daily activity/exercise. Ask if he would like to include his father (brother, workmate) in his new lifestyle program. Arrange a discussion with his family physician or clinic doctor to plan the program.

Further Reading

Choice of cholesterol-lowering drugs. *Medical Letter on Drugs and Therapeutics* 1991;33:1–4.

Witztum JL. Drugs used in the treatment of hyperlipoproteinemias. In: Hardman JG, Limbird LE, eds. *Goodman and Gilman's The Pharmacological Basis of Therapeutics*. 9th ed. New York: Pergamon; 1996:875–897.

Table 42.13
Nursing management of the antihyperlipidemics

Assessment of risk vs. benefit	Patient data	• Physician should determine risk factors including liver and renal function, history of peptic ulcer, gout or diabetes. Baseline lab tests of total cholesterol, LDL-C, HDL-C and triglycerides (VLDL) • *Pregnancy:* Risk category varies. Some drugs in this class are category B (animal studies may or may not have shown risk; no risk has been shown in human studies, or insufficient data in pregnant women), while others are category X (human fetal risk has been clearly documented; use must be avoided during pregnancy)
	Drug data	• Select drugs based on pt's lipid profile • *Some serious drug interactions:* Confer with pharmacist • Although generally well tolerated, some serious adverse effects can occur including hepatic disease, myopathy and allergic reactions
Implementation	Rights of administration	• Using the "rights" helps prevent errors of administration
	Right route	• Give PO
	Right time	• See Table 42.14. Note variation in dosage schedules among drugs in this class
	Right technique	• Follow instructions for mixing powders. Do not crush time-release forms
	Nursing therapeutics	• Emphasize importance of lifestyle factors in contributing to the risks for coronary artery disease (CAD). Verify dosage time prior to administration: i.e., some should be with food while others in this class must be taken on an empty stomach
	Patient/family teaching	• Compliance and follow-up are essential factors in successful tx. Review principles of patient education in Chapter 3 • Explain that successful response may require lifelong tx • Instruct regarding management of common side effects such as constipation. (For lifestyle changes, see Response to Clinical Challenge, page 467) • Pts/families should know warning signs/symptoms of possible toxicities of drugs. Report immediately: unusual bleeding or bruising, unexplained muscle pain or weakness, dark urine or jaundice, blurred vision • Warn pts to avoid alcohol (increased risk of hepatotoxicity) • *Discuss possibility of pregnancy:* Advise pt to notify physician; discuss birth control methods
Outcomes	Monitoring of progress	*Continually monitor:* • Clinical response indicating tx success (reduction in cholesterol levels) • Signs/symptoms of adverse reactions; document and report immediately to physician

Table 42.14
The antihyperlipidemics: Drug doses

Drug Generic name (Trade names)	Dosage	Nursing alert
A. Drugs Affecting Primarily VLDL: The Fibrates		
bezafibrate (Bezalip)	**Oral:** *Adults:* Immediate-release tablets: 200 mg tid. In hypertriglyceridemia, dosage may be reduced to 200 mg bid. Sustained-release tablets: 400 mg od	• For all fibrates (bezafibrate, clofibrate, fenofibrate, gemfibrozil): Monitor. If no benefit after 3 months, drug should be discontinued. For clofibrate, monitor renal and liver function
clofibrate (Atromid-S)	**Oral:** *Adults:* 1 g bid	• Give with meals
fenofibrate (Lipidil, Lipidil Micro)	**Oral:** *Adults:* Regular fenofibrate capsules (Lipidil®) 100 mg tid with meals. Max., 400 mg/day. Micronized fenofibrate capsules (Lipidil Micro®): 200 mg od t	• Give with main meal
gemfibrozil (Lopid)	**Oral:** *Adults:* 600 mg bid	• Give 30 min before breakfast and dinner
B. Drugs Affecting Primarily LDL		
1. Resins		
cholestyramine resin (Questran)	**Oral:** *Adults:* 4 g 1–6x daily	• Sprinkle powder into large glass of water, milk or juice. Let stand for a few minutes, then stir. After drinking, pt should add additional liquid to mix any remaining residue to ensure that entire dose has been taken • All other drugs must be taken 1 h before or 4 h after to prevent reduction in their absorption
colestipol HCl (Colestid)	**Oral:** *Adults* (granules): 5–30 g/day, given once or in divided doses. Increments of 5 g/day may be instituted no more frequently than at 1-month intervals. (Tablets:) 2–16 g/day, given once or in divided doses. Increments of 2 g once or twice daily may be instituted no more frequently than at 1-month intervals	• As for cholestyramine

(cont'd on next page)

Table 42.14 (continued)
The antihyperlipidemics: Drug doses

Drug Generic name (Trade names)	Dosage	Nursing alert
B. Drugs Affecting Primarily LDL (cont'd)		
2. HMG-CoA Reductase Inhibitors (Statins)		
fluvastatin sodium (Lescol)	**Oral:** *Adults:* Initially, 20 mg od hs. Range, 20–80 mg/day	• May be taken without regard to food. More effective when taken hs
lovastatin (Mevacor)	**Oral:** *Adults:* Initially, 20 mg/day given as single dose with evening meal. Adjustments should be made at intervals of not less than 4 weeks, to a max. of 80 mg/day given as single or divided doses (a.m. or p.m.)	• Most effective if taken with evening meal • Store in light-resistant container
pravastatin sodium (Pravachol)	**Oral:** *Adults:* Initially, 10–20 mg od hs. If serum cholesterol is markedly elevated (e.g., total cholesterol > 7.75 mmol/L [300 mg/dL]), dosage may be initiated at 40 mg/day. Range, 10–40 mg od hs	• Most effective when taken hs • May be taken without regard to food
simvastatin (Zocor)	**Oral:** *Adults:* Initially, 10 mg/day given as single dose hs. Adjustments should be made at intervals of not less than 4 weeks, to a max. of 40 mg/day given hs	• Best absorbed and most effective when taken hs
3. Miscellaneous Drugs		
Niacin, vitamin B$_3$	**Oral:** *Adults:* Initially, 100 mg tid; increase gradually over 6–8 weeks to 1.5–3 g/day, given in 3–4 divided doses	• Give with milk or meals to reduce GI irritation. Do not crush or chew time-release form
probucol (Lorelco)	**Oral:** *Adults:* 500 mg bid, with morning and evening meals	• Give with food to enhance absorption

Antianemic Drugs

Topics Discussed
- Body iron requirements
- Oral iron preparations
- Parenteral iron preparations
- Acute iron toxicity
- Folic acid and vitamin B_{12} deficiency
- Nursing management

Drugs Discussed

Oral Iron-Containing Preparations:
ferrous sulfate (fer-us **sul**-fate)
ferrous gluconate (**glue**-koe-nate)
ferrous succinate (**suck**-sin-ate)
ferrous fumarate (**fume**-ar-ate)

Parenteral Iron-Containing Preparations:
iron dextran (**dex**-tran)
iron sorbitex (**sore**-bih-tex)
iron sorbitol (**sore**-bih-tawl)

deferoxamine (def-air-**ox**-ah-meen)

folic acid (**foal**-ic)
vitamin B_{12}
cyanocobalamin (sye-an-oh-koe-**bal**-ah-min)

Clinical Challenge

Consider this clinical challenge as you read through this chapter. The response to the challenge appears on page 477.

Mary, a 25-year-old pregnant woman, visits the clinic with her 2-year-old son to attend community prenatal classes.

What information will she learn about iron and folic acid supplements during pregnancy? Specifically:

1. What is the daily iron requirement during pregnancy? How much iron must be ingested from food sources to supply this amount of iron?
2. What are good food sources of iron?
3. What are the pros and cons of using iron supplements?
4. What is the daily recommended supplement for folic acid during pregnancy?
5. What safety issues should be discussed with Mary?

Body Iron Requirements

Iron Metabolism

Although iron absorption may occur throughout the gastrointestinal tract, most takes place from the duodenum. Usually the amount of iron absorbed equals the quantity eliminated by the kidneys. Iron absorption increases in response to iron-deficiency anemia or pyridoxine deficiency. It is also increased during the latter months of pregnancy. Normally, between 5% to 10% of the iron ingested in food is absorbed. This increases to approximately 20% in iron-deficient subjects given normal amounts of iron in the diet.

Once absorbed, iron is usually carried in the blood bound to the transport alpha$_1$-globulin protein, transferrin. This protein is usually about one-third saturated with iron and, as a result, if more iron is absorbed it, too, can be carried on the transferrin. A decrease in plasma iron level, together with an increase in the iron binding capacity, is encountered in iron deficiency. Hemosiderosis and hemochromatosis, on the other hand, present pictures of high levels of plasma iron, with transferrin being almost completely saturated.

The quantity of iron in the body varies according to the age of the individual. At birth it ranges from 200–300 mg, depending on the weight of the child. Thereafter, it builds slowly to 2–6 g in adults.

Iron is present in many forms in the body. Hemoglobin accounts for approximately 70% of the total body iron. Myoglobin, the heme protein of skeletal and cardiac muscle, amounts to about 3% of total body iron. Approximately 25% of body iron is found in the storage forms of ferritin and hemosiderin. Although transferrin is important in the transport of iron in plasma, it accounts for only 0.1% of the body iron content. In addition to its role in the transport of oxygen in the blood, iron is important in many enzyme functions, such as those mediated by cytochrome-c catalase. The amounts of iron needed for these functions are very small, and parenchymal iron accounts for only 0.2% of the total body content.

Iron is transferred from transferrin to specific receptor sites on the membrane of erythrocyte precursors, after which it is incorporated into the protoporphyrin molecule to form heme. Heme is subsequently coupled with globin to form the oxygen-carrying material hemoglobin. The normal erythrocyte has a lifespan of approximately 120 days. About 21.5 mg of iron, or 6.25 g of hemoglobin, turn over each day.

The capacity of the body to eliminate iron is limited. Only 0.5–1 mg of iron is lost each day by adult males and nonmenstruating females from the 21.5 mg liberated from erythrocytes. The remainder is reutilized. Menstruating females may lose an additional 0.5–0.6 mg of iron daily.

Dietary iron requirements vary throughout life. In the adult, they approximate the daily loss. During periods of growth, menstruation or pregnancy, the requirements for iron are greater. Table 43.1 presents the estimated dietary iron requirements for men and women at different ages.

Table 43.1
Daily iron requirements*

	Iron need for erythropoiesis (mg/day)	Food iron requirement (mg/day)
Infants	0.5–1.5	1.5 mg/kg**
Children	0.4–1	4–10
Adolescents	1–2	10–20
Menstruating women	1–2	7–20
Pregnant women	2–5	20–50†
Normal men and nonmenstruating women	0.5–1	5–10

* Modified slightly from report of the ad hoc Committee of the Council on Foods and Nutrition of the American Medical Association.

** To a maximum of 1.5 mg daily.

† This amount of iron cannot be provided in the diet and requires supplementation with medicinal iron.

Source: Fairbanks VF, Fahey JL, Beutler E. *Clinical Disorders of Iron Metabolism.* New York: Grune & Stratton; 1971. Reproduced with permission.

Although dietary iron should provide most men and postmenopausal women in North America with sufficient iron, adolescent girls and, to a lesser degree, mature premenopausal women may require iron supplementation. Infants between six and twenty-four months of age and pregnant women also require additional iron.

Iron-Deficiency Anemia

The expression iron-deficiency anemia is almost as much a part of North Americana as hot dogs, beer and baseball. The intellect of the public is constantly insulted with ads for one or another "iron tonic." It is apparent from the preceding discussion that most people obtain sufficient iron from their diet. Furthermore, iron deficiency does not always produce anemia. Small decreases in total body iron may have no effect on hemoglobin.

Progressing in severity, iron deficiency may (1) decrease only the iron stores without lowering serum iron concentration, (2) deplete the iron stores and produce a fall in serum iron levels insufficient to cause anemia or (3) deplete the iron stores and produce a fall in serum iron concentration of sufficient magnitude to produce anemia. The red cells in iron deficiency are usually hypochromic and microcytic.

Iron deficiency is a symptom rather than a disease. It is caused by either the inadequate absorption or the increased elimination of iron. The presence of iron-deficiency anemia in adult males or postmenopausal women indicates significant blood loss, and these patients should be investigated to determine its cause. Excessive menstrual flow or multiple pregnancies are the most common causes of iron-deficiency anemia in women of childbearing age. Iron provided by the diet may be inadequate to meet the growth needs of infants and children. Other causes of inadequate iron absorption include diseases or surgical alterations of the gastrointestinal tract.

Oral Iron Preparations

Therapeutic Uses and Adverse Effects

Many iron-containing products are available, and there is little to choose among them. The correct product for a particular patient is the one that he or she can tolerate best. Iron may cause nausea, abdominal cramps and either diarrhea or constipation. Patients may be obliged to try several different salts of iron before they find the one they tolerate best. Generally speaking, gastric intolerance is closely related to the iron content of each salt. Products that produce a reduced incidence of gastrointestinal distress usually contain less iron.

Several sustained-release formulations of iron are available that are designed to release iron slowly as the tablet progresses down the GI tract. This type of formulation should produce less GI irritation. Unfortunately, many sustained-release tablets may not allow for optimal absorption because iron is best absorbed from the duodenum. These products are best reserved for patients who have demonstrated intolerance to standard iron-containing tablets.

After selecting the iron salt most compatible with the continued gastrointestinal peace of the patient, the next question is how much and for how long. At maximum rates of red cell formation during the treatment of iron-deficiency anemia, about 40–60 mg of iron are necessary for optimum hemoglobin production in adults. Allowing for 20% absorption in iron-deficient patients, approximately 200–300 mg of iron should be required on a daily basis for maximum hemoglobin production. However, hemoglobin production seldom continues at maximum rates for long periods of time. As a result, 180–240 mg of iron daily should suffice to produce an optimal response of a 1% increase in hemoglobin concentration per day.

Ferrous sulfate is the standard iron salt against which all other preparations should be compared. It is usually prepared in 300-mg tablets. Many physicians and nurses feel that ferrous sulfate is the most irritating of all iron salts. This may be due to the fact that it contains more iron per milligram of salt than most of its competitors.

Ferrous gluconate is a popular iron salt because it produces less gastric irritation than ferrous sulfate. However, 300 mg of ferrous gluconate contains only 35 mg of iron compared with the 60 mg in ferrous sulfate. This can explain its reduced incidence of gastric intolerance.

Ferrous fumarate contains 33% iron, with a 200-mg tablet providing 65 mg of the element. Although it is popular with some people, there seems to be little reason for selecting it over the cheaper ferrous sulfate.

Ferrous succinate contains 35% iron and is usually provided in 100-mg tablets. It is usually more expensive than ferrous sulfate and there is little evidence to suggest that it is superior, either in efficacy or in reduced gastrointestinal adverse effects.

Table 43.2 lists the clinically significant interactions with oral iron preparations.

Table 43.2
Oral iron preparations: Drug interactions

Drug	Interaction
Antacids	• Antacids, given concomitantly with oral iron preparations, decrease iron absorption
Tetracyclines	• The absorption of tetracyclines is reduced by iron

Parenteral Iron Preparations

Therapeutic Uses and Adverse Effects

Parenteral iron is required for patients who are unable to tolerate oral iron or absorb it from the GI tract. Patients with chronic inflammatory bowel disease or colostomies may be unable or unwilling to ingest iron. Idiopathic or postresection malabsorption syndromes may be another indication for parenteral iron because patients with these problems may be unable to absorb iron from oral sources. Very occasionally, some patients with severe iron deficiency discovered late in pregnancy may qualify for parenteral iron treatment. Patients suffering from severe uncontrollable GI bleeding may also receive parenteral iron.

Parenteral iron has advantages and drawbacks. Although one can correct iron deficiency quickly with parenteral iron therapy, the ability of the body to eliminate iron is limited. Care must be taken to calculate the dose accurately to avoid iron overload, with consequent hepatic damage.

Iron dextran (Imferon®) is a parenterally formulated complex of ferric hydroxide and low molecular weight dextran that can be given either intramuscularly or intravenously. Iron sorbitol–citric acid complex (iron sorbitex) injection (Jectofer®) must be administered intramuscularly only. When iron is administered IM, the needle should be inserted into the muscle using the Z-track method, as shown in Figure 43.1.

Acute Iron Toxicity

Nurses may encounter children who have accidentally swallowed large numbers of iron tablets. This is a relatively common occurrence because iron is often prescribed for young mothers and also may be obtained without prescription in a variety of over-the-counter products. Depending on the size of the child, as few as ten to thirty tablets have been reported to produce death.

The irritant effects of iron on the GI tract have already been mentioned. When large amounts are consumed, iron can produce a necrotizing gastroenteritis. Bleeding and transudation into the lumen can occur. Shock may ensue as a result of fluid loss or vasodilatation. The latter effect has been attributed either to the actions of large amounts of

**Figure 43.1
Z-track injection method**

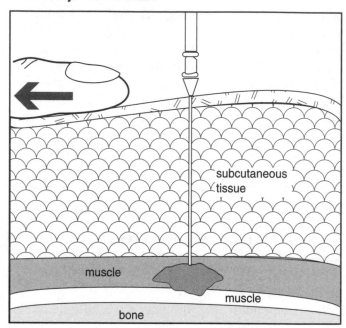

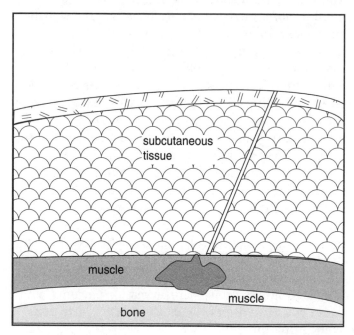

ferritin on the blood vessels or the consequences of bacterial toxins crossing the damaged intestine.

Initially, the patient may experience acute enteritis and shock. This is evidenced by vomiting and diarrhea together with dyspnea and lethargy. After this initial period, which may last from one to six hours, the patient may recover. However, some subjects proceed to metabolic acidosis and coma. First-aid treatment should include attempts to have the subject vomit. Gastric lavage may be attempted in a hospital setting (gavage with 5% sodium bicarbonate to form an insoluble nonabsorbable complex).

Deferoxamine (Desferal®)

Deferoxamine (Desferal®) is a material that chelates with iron to make a nontoxic complex. It can be given intramuscularly or intravenously to reverse the effects of systemic iron toxicity. However, deferoxamine can be toxic in its own right and should be used only if symptoms of systemic iron poisoning appear.

The adverse effects of deferoxamine include allergic skin reactions (urticaria, generalized erythema), hypotension, tachycardia, shock, dizziness, convulsions, abdominal discomfort, diarrhea, thrombocytopenia, blurred vision, impaired hepatic and renal function, dysuria and pyrexia. In the presence of a nursing assessment that reveals a current pregnancy, anuria or history of pyelonephritis or other kidney disease, the danger of using this medication must be weighed against the risk of fatality due to iron toxicity. Only fully dissolved medication should be administered and at the specific infusion rate specified by the physician.

Nursing evaluation should monitor vital signs and fluid intake and output for evidence of adverse reactions (fever, hypotension, shock). Reddish-coloured urine following administration of deferoxamine indicates high serum iron levels and the necessity for continuing therapy. Long-term therapy necessitates careful monitoring of ophthalmic function, since deferoxamine has been shown to cause blurred vision and cataracts.

Table 43.3 lists the clinically significant drug interactions with deferoxamine.

Folic Acid and Vitamin B$_{12}$ Deficiency

Discussion of the actions of folic acid and vitamin B$_{12}$ follows logically that of iron. A deficiency in any of the three can cause anemia. However, in the case of iron deficiency, the anemia is usually hypochromic and microcytic, whereas folic acid or vitamin B$_{12}$ deficiency produces hyperchromic megaloblastic anemia. Both folic acid and vitamin B$_{12}$ are essential for the synthesis of deoxyribonucleic acid (DNA) in the nucleus of cells. In their absence cell mitosis stops. The consequences of vitamin B$_{12}$ deficiency exceed those of a lack of folic acid. Although both conditions produce similar changes in bone marrow, a lack of vitamin B$_{12}$ produces pernicious anemia, a condition marked by megaloblastic anemia, GI symptoms (including glossitis and dyspepsia) and neurological abnormalities.

Folic Acid

Metabolism. Folic acid is widely distributed in animal and vegetable foods. Although the conjugated form of the vitamin found in food is less readily absorbed than folic acid in tablets, humans can usually absorb sufficient amounts in their diet to meet the needs of the body. The chemical is absorbed in the first third of the small intestine. Its absorption may be inadequate in patients with diseases of the small intestine. Once absorbed, folic acid is distributed throughout the body and eliminated by the kidneys. When normal amounts are ingested, only small amounts of folic acid are lost in the urine. As the dose is increased, more of it may find its way through the nephrons.

The healthy adult requires about 50 µg of folic acid daily, which is usually supplied by the diet. During pregnancy the requirements for folic acid increase to 100–200 µg per day and may exceed the dietary supply. Supplemental folic acid is usually given at this time.

Table 43.3
Deferoxamine: Drug interactions

Drug	Interaction
Ascorbic acid	• Ascorbic acid (administered in a dose of 1 mg per 1 mg deferoxamine) for 3 or more days before deferoxamine, doubles iron excretion

As mentioned earlier, folic acid is essential for the synthesis of DNA by the nucleus of cells. In its absence the DNA content of cell nuclei falls and the ability of cells to divide by mitosis is reduced. This is seen first in rapidly dividing cells, such as those responsible for the formation of new erythrocytes.

Therapeutic uses. Supplemental folic acid is administered when inadequate amounts of the vitamin are absorbed, as a result of either a dietary deficiency or a malabsorption syndrome. The former situation is not common because of widespread distribution of the vitamin in food. It is seen more often in chronic alcoholics and the elderly who may fail to eat a balanced diet. The latter condition occurs following partial gastrectomy or diseases of the small intestine, such as tropical sprue, steatorrhea or celiac disease. Regional ileitis, irradiation damage and intestinal tuberculosis are other causes of folic acid malabsorption.

The replacement of folic acid in the diet of patients who fail to eat adequate amounts of food requires only 100–200 µg daily. Larger quantities, in the range of 0.5–1 mg (500–1000 µg) daily, are warranted for patients with malabsorption problems.

Increased requirement for folic acid during pregnancy has already been mentioned. Failure to provide patients with adequate amounts of folic acid during pregnancy may result in megaloblastic anemia. Not surprisingly, this condition is more prevalent in less developed countries and poorer areas of North America. Occurring during the third trimester, and more often during twin pregnancies, folic acid deficiency results from the increased fetal requirements placed on the mother. The dose of folic acid required during pregnancy is similar to that recommended for malabsorption syndromes — 0.5–1 mg daily.

Table 43.4 lists the clinically significant drug interactions with folic acid.

Vitamin B_{12}

Metabolism. Vitamin B_{12}, or cyanocobalamin, is found only in food of animal origin. Its absorption in the lower part of the ileum depends upon the secretion of a glycoprotein, called the intrinsic factor, by the parietal cells of the fundus and body of the stomach. In the absence of the intrinsic factor, very little vitamin B_{12} is absorbed and pernicious anemia occurs. Once absorbed, vitamin B_{12} is stored in the liver and eliminated in the bile.

Daily requirements for vitamin B_{12} are minute. The normal diet provides from 1–85 µg daily, with the amount lost in the bile being only 1 µg every twenty-four hours. The amount stored in the body is about 5 mg. It follows from these figures that several years free of vitamin B_{12} are required before a patient develops a deficiency of clinical significance.

In some ways the actions of vitamin B_{12} and folic acid overlap. Both chemicals are required for the synthesis of DNA. As a result, patients with pernicious anemia demonstrate a megaloblastic anemia similar to that described previously for folic acid deficiency. However, the consequences of pernicious anemia involve also the neurological and gastrointestinal systems.

The neurological signs of vitamin B_{12} deficiency include degenerative changes of the dorsal and lateral columns of the spinal cord and peripheral nerves. As a result, patients experience disturbances of vibratory sense, proprioception and pyramidal tract function. In addition, mental disturbances, ranging from mood swings to psychosis, may appear. Optic atrophy can also occur.

The consequences of vitamin B_{12} deficiency on the gastrointestinal system include glossitis and

---

Table 43.4
Folic acid: Drug interactions

Drug	Interaction
Antiepileptics	• Carbamazepine, mephobarbital, phenytoin and primidone can inhibit folic acid absorption. Phenytoin's actions may also be reduced by folic acid
Oral contraceptives	• Oral contraceptives may rarely reduce folic acid absorption. If supplemental folic acid is not provided, megaloblastic anemia may occur

dyspepsia. They reflect gastric mucosal atrophy and result from the inability of normally rapidly developing cells to form sufficient DNA for mitosis.

Vitamin B_{12} injection reverses these effects. Folic acid will treat the megaloblastic anemia but has no effect on the other consequences of vitamin B_{12} deficiency. For this reason, it should not be used to treat megaloblastic anemia until it is clear that a vitamin B_{12} deficiency is not the cause of the anemia. If folic acid is used inappropriately to treat a megaloblastic anemia due to vitamin B_{12} deficiency, the physician and nurse may be lulled into a false sense of security by the improvement in the blood picture while the GI and neurological systems continue to deteriorate.

Therapeutic uses. Vitamin B_{12} is used to treat pernicious anemia and other vitamin B_{12} deficiency states. The effects of vitamin B_{12} are often rapid. Mental symptoms often improve within hours and the megaloblastic anemia disappears in a few weeks. The neurologic effects respond more slowly. Peripheral neuropathy usually disappears and subacute degeneration of the spinal cord stops, but improvement is slow.

Vitamin B_{12} can be given orally to the very unusual patients (generally, strict vegetarians, or vegans) in whom symptoms are due to dietary deficiency, not an absence of the intrinsic factor. The dosage range for oral therapy is 1–25 µg/day, accompanying meals. If patients are unwilling to take oral vitamin B_{12} daily to replace the quantity normally consumed in the diet, monthly injections can be given.

Nursing Management

Table 43.5 on the next page describes the nursing management of patients receiving antianemic drugs. Dosages of individual drugs are given in Table 43.6 (pages 479–480).

Response to Clinical Challenge

1. The daily iron requirement during pregnancy is 2–5 mg/day. To supply this amount of iron, 20–50 mg of iron must be ingested from food sources. Since the diet cannot supply this much, supplements are required.
2. Good food sources of iron include cereals, dried beans and peas, leafy green vegetables, dried fruits, lean red meats and organ meats.
3. The pros and cons of using iron supplements are similar to those for using any drugs: the benefits must outweigh the risks. Supplements should be used only if the diet cannot supply the required amounts of iron. Generally, iron is well tolerated except for GI effects such as constipation or nausea. However, excess use can cause serious toxicity and overdose in children can be fatal without urgent treatment.
4. The daily recommended supplement for folic acid during pregnancy 100–200 µg per day.5. For safety of her 2-year-old, Mary must keep the supply of iron out of reach and teach her son that this is a medication that should not be taken without permission. Unfortunately, iron pills may look like candy. Children should be taught that they are drugs.

Table 43.5
Nursing management of antianemic drugs

Assessment of risk vs. benefit	Patient data	• Physician should determine the necessity for iron supplementation through baseline lab tests of hemoglobin, HCT and reticulocyte values. Ferritin levels may also be determined. Hx of peptic ulcer or ulcerative colitis should be determined • Pts may self-medicate with iron to treat lethargy or low energy. They should be encouraged to discuss the use of supplements with a health professional
	Drug data	• Drug products are similar in action and side effects. However, the choice of salt may alter the degree of absorption, as well as the incidence of gastric reactions. Pts may need to try more than one product to find the most suitable
Implementation	Rights of administration	• Using the "rights" helps prevent errors of administration
	Right route	• Give IV, IM and PO
	Right time	• Give oral products with food to prevent GI irritation. May be taken with citrus juice to facilitate absorption but should not be taken with milk or antacids • Liquid iron preparations stain teeth and should be well diluted and taken through a straw. Pt should rinse mouth well after. Brushing with 3% hydrogen peroxide may remove stains
	Right technique	• **IM:** Following test dose, inject deeply into buttocks using Z-track method (Fig. 43.1, page 474). Use a 5-cm, 22-gauge needle and change needle after drawing up solution to prevent tissue staining, which may be permanent. Do not massage site • **Direct IV:** Follow agency policy. Give test dose of 25 mg over 5 min. If no reaction, give undiluted at a rate of 50 mg over 1 min. For continuous infusion, conduct test dose and if no reaction, administer slowly over 4–12 h
	Nursing therapeutics	• Give test doses for IV and IM routes and observe carefully to detect adverse or allergic reactions. During initial IV administration, monitor VS closely
	Patient/family teaching	• Educate re: time of administration, dietary sources of iron and importance of storing drug out of reach of children. The lethal dose for children has been reported as low as 60 mg. Pts/families should know warning signs/symptoms of iron toxicity. Seek urgent tx
Outcomes	Monitoring of progress	*Continually monitor:* • Clinical response indicating tx success (reduction in signs/symptoms such as fatigue, lethargy) • Signs/symptoms of adverse reactions; document and report immediately to physician • Periodic blood tests to monitor tx effectiveness

Table 43.6
The antianemics: Drug doses

Drug Generic name (Trade names)	Dosage	Nursing alert
A. Oral Iron-Containing Preparations		
ferrous sulfate (Feosol, Fer-In-Sol, Fer-Grad, Ferro-Gradument, Fesofo, Mol-Iron, among others)	**Oral:** *Adults:* Initially, 30–60 mg elemental iron; increase prn in 30-mg increments to max. 180 mg/day in 3–4 doses. *Children 6–12 years:* 24–120 mg (3 mg/kg) elemental iron per day in 3–4 divided doses; *2–5 years:* 15–45 mg (3 mg/kg) of elemental iron per day in 3–4 divided doses; *6 months to 2 years:* up to 6 mg/kg/day of elemental iron in 3–4 divided doses. *Infants:* 10–25 mg of elemental iron per day given in 3–4 divided doses. Consult product monograph for individual product	• Best absorption occurs if taken on empty stomach but may be taken with food if GI irritation occurs. However, avoid dairy products, whole-grain breads, coffee and tea at same time as iron salts • Take with full glass of liquid. Do not crush or chew coated tablets. Dilute liquid preparations and use straw to avoid staining teeth. Best to use water or juice. Do not use milk
ferrous gluconate (Fergon)	(Prophylactic) **Oral:** *Adults:* 325 mg/day. *Children > 2 years:* 8 mg/kg/day. (Therapeutic) *Adults:* 325–650 mg qid. Sustained-release capsules may be given bid	• As for ferrous sulfate
ferrous fumarate (Feostat, Feroton, Ferrofume, Fersamet, Hematon, Toleron)	(Prophylactic) **Oral:** *Adults:* 200 mg/day. *Children:* 3 mg/kg/day. (Therapeutic) *Adults:* 200 mg tid or qid. Controlled-release may be given bid. *Children:* 3–6 mg/kg tid	• As for ferrous sulfate
ferrous succinate (Cerevon)	**Oral:** *Adults/children > 12:* 100–300 mg [35–105 mg elemental Fe] daily	• As for ferrous sulfate
B. Parenteral Iron-Containing Preparations		
iron dextran (Imferon)	**IM/IV:** Dosage is highly individualized. Consult manufacturer's information for details	• **IM:** Give test dose of 0.5 mL (25 mg). If no reaction occurs within 1 h, proceed with daily dose. Inject into buttocks using Z-track method (Fig. 43.1, page 474) • **IV:** Dilute in 250 mL to 1 L normal saline. Infuse test dose of 25 mg over 5 min. If no reaction within 5 min, infuse slowly over 4–12 h. Observe site frequently

(cont'd on next page)

Table 43.6 (continued)
The antianemics: Drug doses

Drug Generic name (Trade names)	Dosage	Nursing alert
B. Parenteral Iron-Containing Preparations (cont'd)		
iron sorbitol–citric acid complex, iron sorbitex (Jectofer)	**IM:** *Adults/adolescents:* Deficiency (tx): 1.5 mg elemental iron/kg/day. Give drug qd or qod until Hgb values are normal. To increase Hgb by 1 g/100 mL: 200 mg elemental iron for women and 250 mg for men. To replenish iron stores, an additional 250–1000 mg elemental iron is needed. Usual adult prescribing limits: 100 mg/day *Pediatric dose:* Deficiency (tx): To restore Hgb and replenish iron stores: 1.5 mg of elemental iron/kg/day. Give drug qd or qod until Hgb values are normal	• IM: Inject deep into large muscle using Z-track method (Fig. 43.1, page 474). Do not give IV
C. Iron Antidote		
deferoxamine (Desferal)	(For acute iron intoxication) **IM:** Initially, 90 mg/kg. May be followed by 45 mg/kg q4–12h prn. Max. single dose in children should not exceed 1 g (2 g in adults). In general, not more than 6 g should be given in 24 h (For shock and signs of CV collapse) **IV:** Infusion rates should be adjusted to severity of poisoning. Rate of infusion should not exceed 15 mg/kg/h	• **IM** (preferred route): Reconstitute with sterile water for injection. Stable for 1 week if protected from light. Inject deep and massage well. Warn pt that injection may cause transient but severe pain • **IV:** Reconstitute, then dilute further in NS, D5W, or lactated Ringer's and infuse at a rate not exceeding 15 mg/kg/h. IV route is only for pts in shock
D. Vitamin Preparations for the Treatment of Anemia		
folic acid (Folvite)	**PO/IM/IV/SC:** (For anemia) *Adults/children:* 0.25–1.0 mg/day. (Pregnancy/lactation) *Adults:* 0.8–1.0 mg/day. (Dietary supplement) *Adults/children:* 0.1–1.0 mg/day	• Oral route is preferred. If IM route is used, give deep injection. For direct IV route, follow agency policy
vitamin B$_{12}$, cyanocobalamin (Betalin 12 Crystalline, Redisol, Rubramin, Ruvite, Sytobex)	**Oral:** *Adults:* 1–25 µg/day. *Children < 1 year:* 0.3 µg/day. *Children > 1 year:* 1 µg/day **IM/SC:** *Adults:* 100µg/day for 6–7 days, then 100 µg qod for 7 more doses, then 100 µg every 3–4 days for 2–3 more weeks initially, then 100–200 µg every month. Flushing dose for Shilling test: 1000 µg **IM/IV:** *Children:* 30–50 µg/day for 2 weeks or more (total dose, 1–5 mg) initially, then 100 µg monthly	• If administered PO, give with meals to increase absorption • Store parenteral solution at room temperature. Protect from light and heat

Anticoagulant and Antiplatelet Drugs, Fibrinolytic Agents and Vitamin K

Topics Discussed
- Thromboses and emboli
- Anticoagulant drugs
- Antiplatelet drugs
- Fibrinolytic drugs
- Fibrinolytic inhibitors
- Vitamin K_1, vitamin K_2 and menadione
- Nursing management

Clinical Challenge

Consider this clinical challenge as you read though this chapter. The response to the challenge appears on page 496.

Jayne, a 43-year-old teacher, is brought to the Emergency Department by her distraught husband. He states that she began feeling ill after supper, complaining of indigestion and back pain. Shortly after, she became very pale, diaphoretic, dyspneic and nauseated, and had difficulty answering his questions.

He drove her to the nearest hospital, where the Emergency physician ordered an ECG and blood work. The doctor also consulted with a cardiologist who recommended immediate treatment with a fibrinolytic agent. *(cont'd on next page)*

Drugs Discussed

Injectable Anticoagulants:
enoxaparin (ee-nox-ah-**par**-in)
dalteparin (dal-teh-**par**-in)
heparin (**hep**-ah-rin)

Oral Anticoagulants:
dicumarol (dye-**koom**-ah-rol)
warfarin (**war**-fa-rin)

Antiplatelet Drugs:
acetylsalicylic acid; ASA (ass-ee-til-sal-ih-**sill**-ik)
dipyridamole (dye-peer-**id**-ah-mole)
sulfinpyrazone (sul-fin-**peer**-ah-zone)
ticlopidine (tye-**cloe**-pid-een)

Fibrinolytic Drugs:
alteplase (**al**-teh-playse)
streptokinase (strep-toe-**kye**-nase)
urokinase (yoor-oh-**kye**-nase)

Fibrinolytic Inhibitors:
aminocaproic acid (am-ee-noe-kah-**proe**-ik)
aprotinin (ap-**roe**-tin-in)

Vitamin K Products:
vitamin K_1 (phytonadione) (fye-toe-**nad**-ee-own)
vitamin K_2 (menaquinone) (men-ah-**kwin**-own)
vitamin K_3 (menadione) (men-a-**die**-own)
menadiol (men-a-**die**-awl)

Thromboses and Emboli

Three groups of drugs can be used in the management of thromboses and emboli. These are (1) anticoagulants, which inhibit the formation of fibrin, (2) antiplatelet drugs, which reduce platelet adhesion and/or aggregation and (3) fibrinolytic and thrombolytic agents, which digest fibrin (Table 44.1). This chapter discusses all three groups. In addition, the use of vitamin K is discussed because of its importance in the process of coagulation.

Formation of Venous and Arterial Thromboses

Venous and arterial thromboses have different causes. Venous thrombi usually form in regions of slow or disturbed blood flow. They begin as small deposits in either the venous sinuses of the deep veins of the legs or of the valve cusp pockets. Coagulation of the blood plays a major role in the formation and extension of venous thrombi.

Arterial thromboses are formed after damage to the endothelium of the artery allows platelets to adhere to the vessel wall, serving as the focus for thrombus formation. The adhesion of a few platelets to the vessel wall is followed by the aggregation of increased numbers of thrombocytes. Fibrin, formed by coagulation, subsequently encases the platelets, giving rise to a platelet-fibrin plug. Because blood flow in the arteries is rapid, arterial thrombi stay close to vessel walls and have been termed *mural thrombi*.

A mural thrombus may either remain at its original site or be sheared away by the rapid blood flow to locate in other parts of the body. If it remains at its site of origin, the mural thrombus can serve as a focus for further platelet aggregation. In that case, a platelet-fibrin plug may be formed, which becomes incorporated into the vessel wall to produce atherosclerosis-like lesions.

These vascular problems are treatable by different types of drugs. Anticoagulants are employed

---

Table 44.1
Antithrombotic drugs

Anticoagulants
1. **Warfarin and other oral anticoagulants** — reduce the activity of vitamin K-dependent clotting factors II, VII, IX and X
2. **Heparin** — increases the activity of antithrombin III and so potentiates the naturally occurring plasma inhibitor of activated factors IX, X, XI and of thrombin
3. **Low-molecular-weight heparins** (dalteparin and enoxaparin) — more potent antithrombotics than heparin, with decreased potential to cause hemorrhage compared with heparin
4. **Ancrod** — converts fibrinogen to an unstable form of fibrin, the plasma fibrinogen level being markedly reduced

Antiplatelet agents
5. **Drugs that inhibit some platelet functions** (e.g., ASA, sulfinpyrazone, dipyridamole, ticlopidine, possibly dextran)

Fibrinolytic agents
6. **Streptokinase** — activates plasminogen to form plasmin indirectly (via the formation of an activator complex with plasminogen or plasmin)
7. **Urokinase** — activates plasminogen to form plasmin directly
8. **Altepase** — recombinant tissue plasminogen activator (TPA) that lyses (dissolves) clots without having a significant effect on circulating plasminogen

Fibrinolytic inhibitors
9. **Aminocaproic acid, aprotinin** — competitively inhibit plasminogen activation and noncompetitively inhibit plasmin; aprotinin also has vasoactive properties

Figure 44.1
Human blood coagulation and fibrinolytic enzyme system

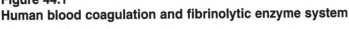

Blood coagulation meachanism   **Fibrinolytic enzyme system**

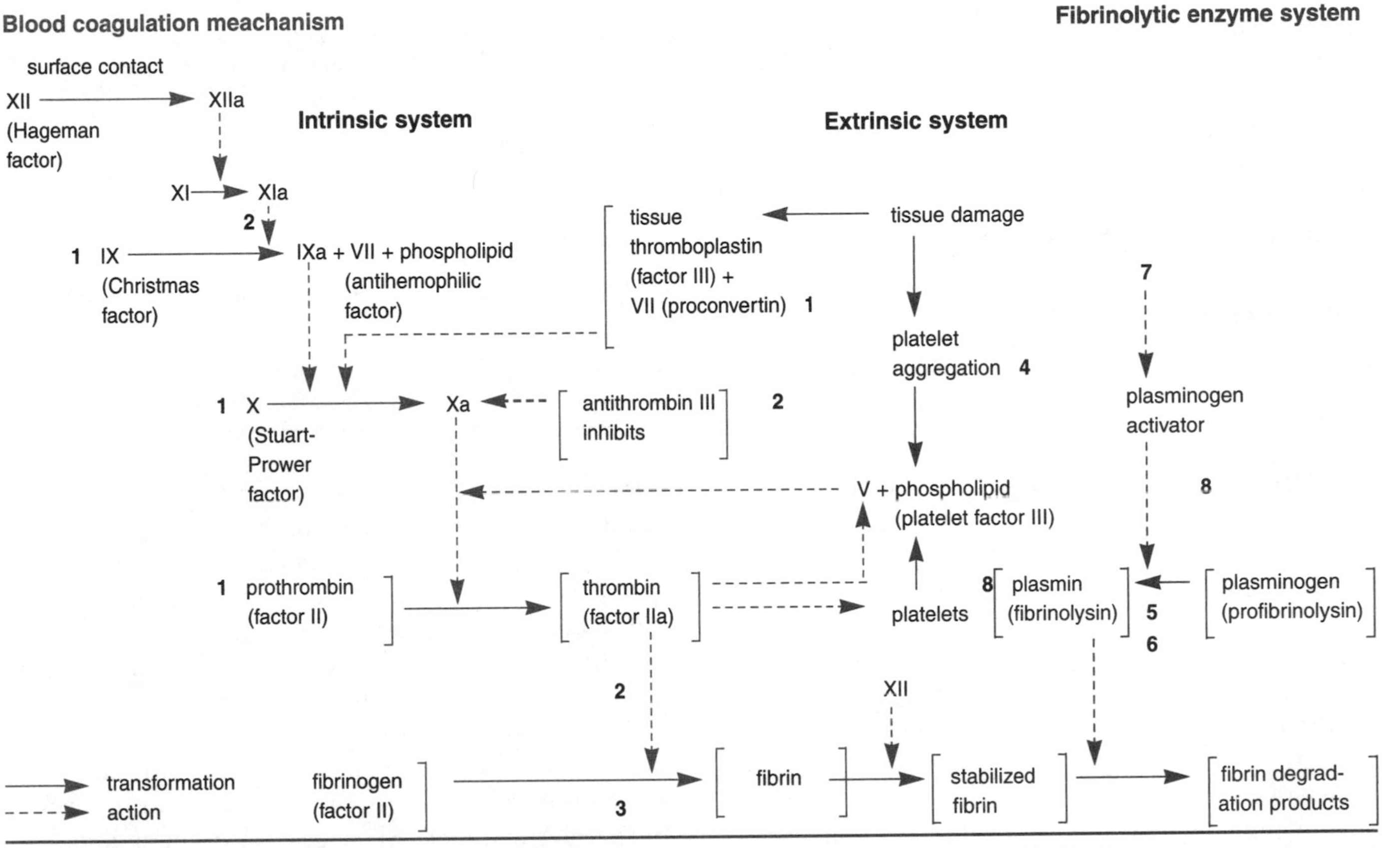

Note: For simplicity and clarity, the role of calcium in the activation reactions of coagulation factors is not included in this diagram. Calcium is not required for the activation of factor XII or for action of factor XI.

Source: Gallus AS, Hirsh J. Antithrombotic drugs: part 1. *Drugs* 1976;12:41–68. Reproduced with permission.

to prevent thrombus formation in the veins, where blood coagulation plays an important role. Antiplatelet drugs are used to stop microemboli forming in the arteries and arterioles, where platelet adhesion is involved.

The various types of antithrombotic drugs are listed in Table 44.1.

Anticoagulant Drugs

Blood coagulation is a complex process (see Figure 44.1). Clotting can be precipitated either by contact activation through the intrinsic system or by the traumatic release of tissue thromboplastin via the extrinsic system. The importance of vitamin K is evident from the fact that clotting factors II, VII, IX and X depend upon it for their synthesis.

Heparin

Mechanism of action and pharmacologic effects. Heparin is a very potent anticoagulant. It works by means of a plasma cofactor, the heparin cofactor or antithrombin III, which neutralizes several activated clotting factors: XIIa, kallikrein, XIa, IXa, Xa, IIa and XIIIa. Heparin must be injected to be effective. Once it is injected its effects are immediate but fleeting, with fifty percent of the drug being dissipated within the first hour.

Heparin also decreases plasma turbidity normally seen after the ingestion of a fat-containing meal. This effect is attributed to a release of a lipase from capillary walls that breaks down chylomicrons and free fatty acids in plasma. At the present time it is not clear whether this action of heparin has any therapeutic significance.

Table 44.2
Heparin: Drug interactions

Drug	Interaction
Anticoagulants, oral	• Heparin administration may prolong the prothrombin time (PT) in pts receiving oral anticoagulants. Blood for testing PT should not be drawn within 4–5 h of IV heparin administration and 12–24 h after the SC dose of heparin
Antihistamines	• Antihistamines may partially counteract the effects of heparin
Dextran	• Dextran and heparin may act synergistically
Ethacrynic acid	• Ethacrynic acid increases the incidence of heparin-induced GI bleeding
Salicylates and other NSAIDs	• Salicylates and other NSAIDs may induce bleeding and should be used with caution in pts receiving heparin
Tetracycline antibiotics	• Tetracycline antibiotics may partially counteract the anticoagulant effects of heparin

Therapeutic uses. The clinical uses of heparin are based on its ability to prevent new clot formation and limit the propagation of existing thrombi. The drug also has the advantage of rapid onset of anticoagulant action. Lower doses are used to prevent a thrombosis and higher doses to treat an established thrombosis. Heparin is the preferred anticoagulant during pregnancy.

The routes of administration and doses for heparin are summarized in Table 44.10 at the end of this chapter. These dosages, however, are only estimates and should be altered in accordance with the results of coagulation tests, such as whole blood clotting time, thrombin time or activated partial thromboplastin time (aPTT). If an oral anticoagulant is also used, a prothrombin test should be performed as well. When heparin is given continuously intravenously, the coagulation test should be performed about every four hours in the early stages of treatment. If heparin is given intermittently, a coagulation test is performed before each injection. Once the dosage range has been stabilized, daily coagulation tests are generally satisfactory.

Heparin is contraindicated in the presence of hemophilia, severe clotting disorders and uncontrollable bleeding. It is also contraindicated in patients with severe liver damage, those in shock and those who are hypersensitive to the drug. The administration of large doses of heparin should be delayed four hours postoperatively.

Adverse effects. Bleeding is the major complication of heparin therapy. In addition, patients receiving more than 15 000 USP units per day on a long-term basis may develop osteoporosis. A small number of patients receiving heparin develop a thrombocytopenia of unknown origin; thus, platelet counts should be performed during heparin therapy. In many cases the adverse effects can be terminated simply by stopping the drug.

If it is necessary to inhibit heparin's effects immediately, protamine sulfate can be administered. Protamine sulfate binds to heparin to form an inactive complex. Because protamine is itself an anticoagulant, it must not be administered in excess of the amount required to neutralize heparin. Each milligram of protamine neutralizes approximately 90 USP units of heparin activity derived from lung tissue or about 115 USP units of heparin activity derived from intestinal mucosa. Protamine should be given by very slow intravenous infusion in doses not to exceed 50 mg of protamine in any ten-minute period. Too-rapid administration of protamine can cause severe hypotensive anaphylactoid-like reactions. Facilities to treat shock should be available. Because of the anticoagulant effect of protamine, it is unwise to give more than 100 mg over a short period unless a larger requirement is certain.

Table 44.2 lists the clinically significant drug interactions with heparin.

Protocol of intravenous heparin therapy. Some hospitals use a standard protocol for heparin administration. Recognizing the wide variability of response to this drug, a protocol describes the steps to initiate therapy and to monitor the

Table 44.3
Heparin protocol

aPTT (s)	Stop infusion for (min)	Rate change	Repeat aPTT
<45	0	+6 mL/h	4–6 h
46–54	0	+3 mL/h	4–6 h
55–85	0	0	in a.m.
86–110	30	–3 mL/h	4–6 h after restarting heparin
>110	60	–6 mL/h	4–6 h after restarting heparin

individual patient's response to each dose. Table 44.3 outlines one example of such a protocol.

• **Step 1:** Initiate therapy with a bolus/loading dose of 5000 U heparin IV.
• **Step 2:** Infuse, using standard heparin infusion of 25 000 U in 500 mL D5W. Run at the prescribed rate, using an infusion pump (see Table 44.3).
• **Step 3:** Monitor aPTT and adjust infusion rate accordingly. The desired aPTT level is 55–85 s. For example, if the infusion has been running at 30 mL/h and the aPTT value is 90 s, stop the infusion for 30 min and recommence at a reduced flow rate of 27 mL/h. Repeat aPTT in 4–6 h.

Low-Molecular-Weight Heparins: Dalteparin (Fragmin®) and Enoxaparin (Lovenox®)

Mechanism of action and pharmacologic effects. Low-molecular-weight heparins are derived from unfractionated heparin by various depolymerization methods. These drugs differ from unfractionated heparins in their high ratio of antifactor Xa to antifactor IIa (antithrombin) activity, which could produce a more favourable ratio of antithrombotic effect to bleeding complications. Other possible advantages of low-molecular-weight heparins compared with unfractionated heparin are greater bioavailability after subcutaneous injection and longer half-life. The longer half-life permits fewer doses per day, and the improved bioavailability leads to more predictable plasma heparin concentrations, permitting subcutaneous administration of fixed dosages without monitoring plasma antifactor Xa activity or aPTT.

Dalteparin (Fragmin®) and enoxaparin (Lovenox®) are low-molecular-weight heparins. They differ significantly from heparin. Heparin has antithrombotic actions, but it is also a potent anticoagulant; dalteparin and enoxaparin preferentially reduce thrombus formation. Compared with heparin, they have reduced anticoagulant effect. As a result, dalteparin and enoxaparin are less likely to cause hemorrhage than heparin.

Therapeutic uses. Dalteparin and enoxaparin are used for the prophylaxis of thromboembolic disorders (deep vein thrombosis) and in conjunction with surgery. Because they are more potent antithrombotic drugs than anticoagulants, dalteparin and enoxaparin decrease the possibility of thrombus formation postsurgery and have reduced likelihood of causing hemorrhage, compared with heparin.

Table 44.4
Dalteparin and enoxaparin: Drug interactions

Drug	Interaction
Anticoagulants, oral Inhibitors of platelet aggregation NSAIDs Preparations containing ASA or dextran	•Because of the possibility of interaction with blood clotting mechanisms, caution should be exercised if dalteparin or enoxaparin is combined with any of these drugs

Dalteparin and enoxaparin are contraindicated in acute or subacute septic endocarditis, allergy to heparin, active bleeding or history of thrombocytopenia. These drugs should be used cautiously during menses, hepatic and renal disease. Protamine can be used as an antidote.

Adverse effects. As with any antithrombotic treatment, hemorrhage can occur. The incidence of hemorrhage with enoxaparin treatment has been low.

Table 44.4 on the previous page lists the clinically significant drug interactions with dalteparin and enoxaparin.

Nursing management. Table 44.5 describes the nursing management of the patient receiving parenteral anticoagulant drugs. Dosage details for individual drugs are given in Table 44.10 (pages 497–501).

Oral Anticoagulants

Mechanism of action and pharmacologic effects. Warfarin is the oral anticoagulant preferred by the great majority of physicians and thus is the only oral anticoagulant whose dose is provided in Table 44.10. Dicumarol is occasionally used. Oral anticoagulants are similar in structure to vitamin K. They competitively inhibit the action of vitamin K and reduce the synthesis of factors II, VII, IX and X in the liver. In contrast to the immediate onset of action of heparin, the effects of oral anticoagulants are delayed until the coagulation factors formed prior to treatment disappear. This usually requires thirty-six to forty-eight hours.

The goal of anticoagulant therapy is to reduce coagulability to the degree that thrombosis does not occur, but not so low as to cause hemorrhage. Traditionally, the prothrombin time (PT) ratio (i.e., the comparison of the patient's PT to a control PT) was used to monitor anticoagulant therapy. However, there is considerable variation in PT values between laboratory procedures, resulting in confusion for interpretation. Today, results are reported in terms of an international normalized ratio (INR). The observed PT is corrected depending on the reagent used in the testing. For most situations, the target INR is 2–3; however, in some situations, the target may be as high as 4.5, for example, with a recurrent embolism.

Heparin can influence PT values; therefore, blood tests should be drawn at least 5 h after intravenous heparin and 24 h following subcutaneous injection of heparin.

Therapeutic uses. Oral anticoagulants are used to prevent the formation of new fibrin thrombi and reduce the extension of already formed clots. In the treatment of an acute deep venous thrombosis, heparin is used first, followed by three to six months of therapy with an oral anticoagulant. Low-dose heparin has been shown to be effective in preventing thrombosis before and after surgery in certain high-risk patients. Patients with rheumatic valve disease experience a lower incidence of pulmonary or systemic emboli if treated with an oral anticoagulant. Oral anticoagulants have likewise been used in patients recovering from myocardial infarcts, but evidence for their efficacy is not conclusive. They are also given to patients suffering from cerebrovascular disease to reduce the incidence of transient cerebral ischemic attacks (TIAs).

At the earliest signs of bleeding, the oral anticoagulant should be withdrawn. Conditions associated with increased risk include severe to moderate hepatic or renal insufficiency, infectious diseases or disturbances of intestinal flora, moderate to severe hypertension, and surgery or trauma resulting in large exposed raw surfaces. Congestive heart failure may increase sensitivity to oral anticoagulants.

Adverse effects. Hemorrhage is the major adverse effect of oral anticoagulants. Although bleeding may occur anywhere in the body, the gastrointestinal tract is the most common site. Patients with undiagnosed peptic ulcers or GI neoplasms are at greater risk. Intracerebral hemorrhage is another major cause of death. Sudden neurologic or psychiatric problems are of concern and should be reported to the physician because of the risk for subdural hematoma. Hemorrhages are treated by stopping the drug and administering vitamin K_1. In emergencies, plasma derivatives containing vitamin K-dependent clotting factors can be given.

Other adverse effects of oral anticoagulant drugs include rashes, diarrhea, pyrexia, neutropenia, thrombocytopenia, agranulocytosis, hepatitis and nephritis.

Table 44.5
Nursing management of the parenteral anticoagulants

Assessment of risk vs. benefit	Patient data	• Physician should determine which anticoagulant will be most effective. Baseline lab tests of aPTT and CBC, platelet counts may be required • *Pregnancy:* Risk category C (animal studies show adverse effects to fetus but human data are unknown or insufficient); benefits may be acceptable despite risks. Should be used with extreme caution in the last trimester and postpartum
	Drug data	• *Some serious drug interactions:* Confer with pharmacist • Most serious adverse effects are bleeding and thrombocytopenia. Occasionally, allergic reactions may occur (chills, fever, pruritus, urticaria, asthma or anaphylaxis)
Implementation	Rights of administration	• Using the "rights" helps prevent errors of administration
	Right route	• Give IV and SC
	Right dose	• Check vial carefully. Heparin is prepared in various strengths, e.g., as dilute as 10 U/mL and as concentrated as 40 000 U/mL. Dalteparin is available in two strengths
	Right time	• See Table 44.10. Note variation in dosage schedules among drugs in this class, depending on indication for use
	Right technique	• IV administration requires knowledge of correct diluent and IV solution, correct dilution and rate of administration. Always refer to manufacturer's instructions for this route. Rate must be carefully controlled; an infusion pump is recommended. For SC route, inject deep, with a 25- to 26-gauge, 1/2" or 5/8" needle into abdominal fat layer. Do not inject within 5 cm of umbilicus or scarred area. Rotate injection sites. Do not massage site. Never give IM
	Nursing therapeutics	• Provide physical care cautiously to minimize risk of bruising. Avoid all IM injections owing to risk of hematoma; request alternative routes for other medications. Inquire regarding menses
	Patient/family teaching	• Pt's need for information may be influenced by length of time required for tx. Compliance and follow-up are essential factors in success; review principles of pt education in Chapter 3 • Pts/families should know warning signs/symptoms of possible toxicities of drugs. Report immediately: unusual bleeding or bruising, signs of allergic reaction • *Discuss possibility of pregnancy:* Advise pt to notify physician; discuss birth control methods
Outcomes	Monitoring of progress	*Continually monitor:* • Clinical response indicating tx success (evidenced by aPTT or platelet count) • Signs/symptoms of adverse reactions; document and report immediately to physician • Blood tests to monitor aPTT and platelet count (daily or weekly) for heparin only; not required for low-molecular-weight heparins such as dalteparin and enoxaparin

Many drugs interact with oral anticoagulants. Some influence the ability of anticoagulants to antagonize vitamin K in the body; others alter their absorption, distribution or elimination. It is beyond the scope of this text to discuss all drugs that have been shown to interact with oral anticoagulants.

Table 44.6 lists the clinically significant drug interactions with oral anticoagulants. Collaboration and consultation with a pharmacist will ensure nurses access to the most current information on drug interactions.

Nursing management. Table 44.7 (page 490) describes the nursing management of the patient receiving oral anticoagulant drugs. Dosage details of individual drugs are given in Table 44.10 (pages 497–501).

Box 44.1
Patient teaching: Oral anticoagulants

✔ Avoid high-risk activities that may cause injury.
✔ Use a soft toothbrush.
✔ Shave with an electric razor.
✔ Limit intake of foods high in vitamin K (which counters anticoagulant activity). These include dark, green vegetables; cheeses and milk; fish and pork.

Antiplatelet Drugs

The pathogenesis of arterial thrombi was presented in the initial paragraphs of this chapter. To review briefly: A few platelets adhere to the damaged section of a blood vessel and secrete chemicals that allow other platelets to aggregate around the original thrombocytes. This triggers blood coagulation, and soon the platelets are encased in fibrin. The fast flow of blood in the arteries may shear some of the platelet-fibrin mass free of the vessel wall to be carried away in the circulation. At this time the platelet-fibrin mass may completely disintegrate, with the individual platelets returning to their original form. It is also possible,

however, that the small platelet-fibrin mass may not disintegrate. Instead, it may be carried to a very small blood vessel, where it can lodge and block the microcirculation to a small area of the body (see Figure 44.2).

Microemboli blocking the blood flow to small areas of the heart have been blamed for starting cardiac arrhythmias. In the brain they have been accused of producing transient ischemic attacks (TIAs), uniocular visual loss and cerebrovascular accidents. For these reasons, it is in the patient's best interest to deter platelets from adhering to damaged walls or arteries. It should also be noted that if a platelet-fibrin plug is not sheared from

Figure 44.2
Microcirculation obstruction

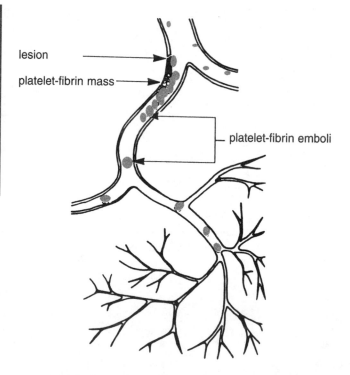

The microcirculation of an organ can be obstructed by emboli arising from mural thrombi composed of platelets and fibrin. Intravascular platelet aggregates may have a similar effect. Obstruction of the microcirculation is known to occur in transient attacks of monocular blindness and cerebral ischemia, and may also be responsible for kidney damage associated with atherosclerotic lesion of the aorta above the renal arteries, and some cases of myocardial infarction.

Source: Mustard JF, Packham MA. Platelets, thrombosis and drugs.

Table 44.6
Oral anticoagulants: Drug interactions

Drug	Interaction
Allopurinol	• Allopurinol may inhibit the metabolism and prolong the action of oral anticoagulants
Aminoglycoside antibiotics	• Aminoglycoside antibiotics may reduce vitamin K production by gut bacteria, thus enhancing the effect of oral anticoagulants
Anabolic steroids	• Anabolic steroids increase pts' sensitivity to oral anticoagulants
Antidiabetics, oral	• Oral antidiabetics may interact in different ways with oral anticoagulants. Dicumarol may inhibit the metabolism of tolbutamide and increase serum chlorpropamide levels. Tolbutamide may displace dicumarol from plasma protein binding, increasing its effects
Barbiturates	• Barbiturates may increase the metabolism of coumarin anticoagulants as well as decreasing GI absorption of dicumarol. Starting or stopping barbiturates may require readjustment of anticoagulant dosage
Carbamazepine	• Carbamazepine may increase warfarin metabolism
Chloral hydrate	• Chloral hydrate gives rise to trichloroacetic acid as a major metabolite which may displace warfarin from plasma protein binding sites
Cholestyramine	• Cholestyramine may impair both anticoagulant and vitamin K absorption. Giving warfarin at least 6 h after cholestyramine avoids the impaired absorption. If concurrent use is necessary, pts should be monitored more frequently
Clofibrate	• Clofibrate may enhance the effect of warfarin on vitamin K-dependent clotting factor synthesis and/or turnover of vitamin K
Contraceptives, oral	• Oral contraceptives may increase the activity of certain clotting factors in the blood and increase dosage requirements for oral anticoagulants
Corticosteroids	• Corticosteroids produce hypercoagulability of the blood and may antagonize the actions of oral anticoagulants
Dextrothyroxine	• Dextrothyroxine enhances the rate of factor II degradation. Avoid concomitant use, if possible
Ethacrynic acid	• Ethacrynic acid displaces warfarin from plasma albumin binding sites
Ethanol	• Ethanol may increase the activity of oral anticoagulants, but heavy drinkers metabolize warfarin faster than normal individuals. Pts taking oral anticoagulants should avoid consuming large amounts of ethanol
Glucagon	• Glucagon may increase the hypoprothrombinemic response to warfarin
Glutethimide	• Glutethimide increases the metabolism of oral anticoagulants
Griseofulvin	• Griseofulvin may inhibit the effect of warfarin
Heparin	• Heparin may prolong further the PT in pts receiving oral anticoagulants
Indomethacin	• Indomethacin can produce ulcers as well as inhibit platelet function. Perform more frequent PTs
Metronidazole	• Metronidazole may inhibit the metabolism of warfarin and increase its pharmacologic activity. Avoid concomitant use, if possible
NSAIDs	• NSAIDs may displace warfarin from plasma albumin binding sites, thereby increasing its activity
Phenylbutazone and oxyphenbutazone	• Phenylbutazone and oxyphenbutazone may inhibit the metabolism of warfarin, as well as produce GI ulceration and impair platelet function. Avoid concomitant use
Phenytoin	• Phenytoin can have its metabolism inhibited and its duration of action increased by dicumarol, and possibly also phenprocoumon. Phenytoin may stimulate the metabolism of dicumarol as well as displace dicumarol from its plasma protein binding sites. In addition, phenytoin may prolong PT in some pts. Avoid concomitant use of these drugs. Warfarin is the oral anticoagulant of choice in pts receiving phenytoin
Quinidine	• Quinidine may produce additive effects with oral anticoagulants
Rifampin	• Rifampin increases warfarin metabolism
Salicylates	• Large doses of salicylates may reduce plasma prothombin levels and displace oral anticoagulants from plasma protein binding sites. Salicylates are usually not recommended for pts receiving oral anticoagulants
Thyroid preparations	• Thyroid preparations increase catabolism of vitamin K-dependent clotting factors
Vitamin K	• Vitamin K antagonizes the effects of oral anticoagulants. A sudden increase in the intake of leafy vegetables or other foods high in vitamin K content will modify the hypoprothrombinemic response to oral anticoagulants

Table 44.7
Nursing management of the oral anticoagulants

Assessment of risk vs. benefit	Patient data	• Physician should determine which anticoagulant will be most effective. Baseline lab tests of PT and CBC, platelet counts may be required • *Pregnancy:* Risk category unknown; benefits may be acceptable despite risks. Should be used with extreme caution in the last trimester and postpartum
	Drug data	• *Some serious drug interactions:* Confer with pharmacist • Most serious adverse effects are bleeding and thrombocytopenia
Implementation	Rights of administration	• Using the "rights" helps prevent errors of administration
	Right route	• Give PO
	Right time	• See Table 44.10. Note variation in dosage schedules among drugs in this class
	Nursing therapeutics	• Provide physical care cautiously to minimize risk of bruising. Avoid all IM injections owing to risk of hematoma. Request alternative routes for other medications. Inquire regarding menses
	Patient/family teaching	• Pt's need for information may be influenced by length of time required for tx • Compliance and follow-up are essential factors in success; review principles of pt education in Chapter 3. Box 44.1 (page 488) summarizes points that pts need to know • Pts/families should know warning signs/symptoms of possible toxicities of drugs. Report immediately: unusual bleeding or bruising; nosebleed; black, tarry stools; hematuria; excessive menstrual flow • Stress importance of informing dentist of use of anticoagulants, wearing a medical alert warning, and regular follow-up visits with lab work • Pts should discuss the use of all OTCs or alcohol with physician or pharmacist • *Discuss possibility of pregnancy:* Advise pt to notify physician; discuss birth control methods
Outcomes	Monitoring of progress	*Continually monitor:* • Clinical response indicating tx success (evidenced by PT and INR) • Signs/symptoms of adverse reactions; document and report immediately to physician • PT and INR (blood tests daily or weekly)

the wall by the force of the circulation it will enlarge until it occludes blood flow at its original site or provides a focus for subsequent atherosclerosis formation.

At the present time, four drugs are being studied actively for their effects on platelet adhesion and/or aggregation. They are acetylsalicylic acid (ASA), sulfinpyrazone, dipyridamole and ticlopidine. The first three have been on the market for other clinical indications for several years. ASA is a tried-and-true analgesic/anti-inflammatory agent, used to relieve mild to moderate pain, inflammation or both. Sulfinpyrazone (Anturan®, Anturane®) was introduced as a uricosuric drug to treat gout. Dipyridamole (Persantine®) was originally used to prevent angina pectoris attacks.

Acetylsalicylic Acid, ASA (Aspirin®)

Mechanism of action and pharmacologic effects. ASA inhibits platelet aggregation by inactivating cyclo-oxygenase, the enzyme responsible for synthesizing the prostaglandin-like substance thromboxane-A_2 in platelets (Figure 44.3). Thromboxane-A_2 promotes platelet aggregation. ASA's effects are irreversible, lasting for the lifetime of the platelet (seven to ten days).

Therapeutic uses. ASA is used to reduce the risk of recurrent TIAs or stroke in patients who have had transient ischemia of the brain due to fibrin platelet emboli. At present, there is no evidence that ASA is a benefit in the treatment of completed strokes. ASA can also be used to reduce the adhesive properties of platelets in patients with diseased arteries, artificial blood vessel shunts and heart valves, and in patients with spontaneous platelet aggregation syndromes. The drug can also be used in the prophylaxis of venous thromboembolism after total hip replacement. Finally, ASA has been shown to be effective in reducing the risk of morbidity and death in patients who have recently suffered a myocardial infarction.

Figure 44.3
Conversion of arachidonic acid to prostaglandins

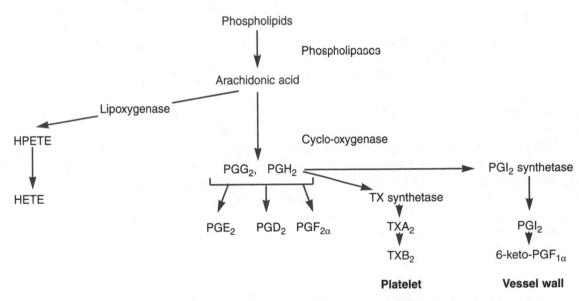

Arachidonic acid can be converted to prostaglandin G_2 (PGG$_2$) by cyclo-oxygenase. PGG$_2$ gives rise to PGH$_2$. In platelets, PGH$_2$ is converted to thromboxane-A_2 (TXA$_2$), PGD$_2$, PGE$_2$ and PGF$_{2\alpha}$. TXA$_2$ is rapidly converted to TXB$_2$. In the vessel wall, PGH$_2$ is converted to prostacyclin (PGI$_2$), an unstable compound that gives rise to 6-keto-PGF$_{1\alpha}$. In platelets, arachidonic acid can also be acted upon by lipoxygenase, giving rise to HPETE, which is converted to HETE.

Source: Mustard JF. Prostaglandins in disease: modification by acetylsalicylic acid. In: Barnett HJM, Hirsh J, Mustard JF, eds. *Acetylsalicylic Acid: New Uses for an Old Drug.* New York: Raven Press; 1982:1. Reproduced with permission.

Adverse effects. The pharmacology of ASA is detailed in Chapter 53. Readers are encouraged to refer to this chapter for the adverse effects of ASA before participating in the management of patients receiving the drug for its antiplatelet effects.

Sulfinpyrazone (Anturan®, Anturane®)

Mechanism of action and pharmacologic effects. Sulfinpyrazone prevents platelet adhesion by inhibiting the release reaction. The release reaction is a response of platelets to a stimulus that leads to a loss of biologically active material from platelets into the vascular bed. As release of these materials is essential for platelet aggregation and thrombus formation, inhibition of the release reaction will reduce or prevent these processes.

Therapeutic uses. Sulfinpyrazone is indicated in clinical states in which abnormal platelet behaviour is a causative or associated factor, as demonstrated by: amaurosis fugax (TIAs), thromboembolism associated with vascular and cardiac prostheses, recurrent venous thrombosis, and arteriovenous shunt thrombosis. The drug is also approved for prophylactic use after myocardial infarction.

Adverse effects. Sulfinpyrazone's adverse effects and drug interactions are discussed in Chapter 55 and Table 55.4 (page 659), respectively.

Dipyridamole (Persantine®)

Dipyridamole appears to block platelet aggregation, but its mechanism of action is still not clear. When tested in patients with cerebral vascular disease, dipyridamole had no effect. Similar results were obtained when the drug was given to patients with coronary artery disease. In one study,

patients given dipyridamole plus ASA had significantly fewer fatal and nonfatal myocardial infarcts than placebo-treated patients. Dipyridamole, together with warfarin, has been shown to reduce platelet adhesion or aggregation in patients with mitral valve replacement.

Oral dipyridamole may cause headache or gastric irritation at high dosage levels. An intravenous bolus of dipyridamole may be associated with chest pain/angina, headache and/or dizziness.

Ticlopidine (Ticlid®)

Mechanism of action and pharmacologic effects. Ticlopidine inhibits platelet aggregation. It causes a time- and dose-dependent inhibition of platelet aggregation and release of platelet factors, as well as a prolongation of bleeding time.

Therapeutic uses. Ticlopidine is indicated for reduction of the risk of first or recurrent stroke for patients who have experienced at least one of the following events: complete thromboembolic stroke, minor stroke, reversible ischemic neurological deficit, or transient ischemic attack including transient monocular blindness.

Adverse effects. Most adverse effects are mild, transient and occur early in the course of treatment. The most frequent include diarrhea, nausea, dyspepsia and gastrointestinal pain. However, slightly more than two percent of ticlopidine-treated patients in clinical trials developed neutropenia. All patients should have a white blood cell count with a differential count and a platelet count performed every two weeks for the first three months of therapy. Prolongation of bleeding time occurs in subjects treated with ticlopidine.

Table 44.8 lists the clinically significant drug interactions with ticlopidine.

Table 44.8
Ticlopidine: Drug interactions

Drug	Interaction
Anticoagulants	• Anticoagulants should be avoided with ticlopidine as tolerance and safety of simultaneous administration has not been established

Fibrinolytic Drugs

Three fibrinolytic, or thrombolytic, drugs have been studied during the past few years. They are urokinase, found in human urine; streptokinase (Kabikinase®, Streptase®), produced by beta-hemolytic streptococci; and alteplase, also known as tissue plasminogen activator (TPA) (Activase®).

Streptokinase (Streptase®)

Mechanism of action and pharmacologic effects. Blood contains plasminogen. When plasminogen is activated it releases plasmin, which lyses (dissolves) fibrin clots. Streptokinase activates the plasminogen-plasmin system, giving rise to increased amounts of plasmin. Streptokinase is administered to remove formed thrombi or emboli.

Therapeutic uses. Indications for the use of streptokinase include pulmonary embolism, deep vein thrombosis, arterial thrombosis and embolism, arteriovenous cannula occlusion and coronary artery thrombosis. Streptokinase treatment of coronary thrombosis should be instituted as soon as possible after the onset of symptoms of acute myocardial infarction, preferably within six hours.

Streptokinase is contraindicated in patients with a predisposition to bleeding. Because thrombolytic therapy increases the risk of bleeding, streptokinase is contraindicated in active internal bleeding, recent cerebrovascular accident (within two months), intracranial or intraspinal surgery and intracranial neoplasm.

Adverse effects. Hemorrhage is a danger when streptokinase is used. Aminocaproic acid (Amicar®) is an antidote for overdose of a fibrinolytic agent. It should be given in a loading dose of 5 g, either orally or intravenously by slow infusion, followed by 1–1.25 g/h until bleeding is controlled. Streptokinase also depletes the blood of its normal pool of plasminogen. As a result, spontaneous thrombosis can occur after the effects of streptokinase disappear. To prevent secondary clot formation, heparin should be given immediately after the effects of the fibrinolytic agent cease, followed by oral anticoagulants for seven days, during which time the blood plasminogen levels return to normal.

Because streptokinase is a bacterial protein elaborated by group C beta-hemolytic streptococci, it can produce allergic reactions. Reactions attributed to possible anaphylaxis have been observed rarely in patients treated with streptokinase. These range in severity from minor breathing difficulty to bronchospasm, periorbital swelling, or angioneurotic edema. Other, milder allergic effects such as urticaria, itching, flushing, nausea, headache and musculoskeletal pain have been observed. Approximately thirty-three percent of patients treated with streptokinase have shown increases in body temperature of greater than 0.83°C. Symptomatic treatment is usually sufficient to alleviate discomfort. The use of acetaminophen rather than ASA is recommended.

Urokinase

Mechanism of action and pharmacologic effects. Urokinase rapidly converts plasminogen to plasmin. Fibrinolytic activity disappears from the blood within one to two hours after the termination of an infusion of urokinase.

Therapeutic uses. Urokinase is indicated for the treatment of pulmonary embolism and coronary artery thrombosis.

Adverse effects. An overdose of urokinase may result in severe hemorrhage. Therapy should be discontinued if there is bleeding, and fresh whole blood or fresh-frozen plasma should be administered. If these measures fail to control bleeding, the use of aminocaproic acid is suggested.

Alteplase, Tissue Plasminogen Activator, TPA (Activase®)

Mechanism of action and pharmacologic effects. Recombinant tissue plasminogen activator (TPA) is a synthetic fibrinolytic protein that activates plasminogen or converts plasminogen to plasmin specifically in the presence of fibrin. The clot selectivity of TPA enables it to lyse clots without having a significant effect on circulating plasminogen. TPA has a half-life of about five minutes, compared to about twenty-three minutes for streptokinase.

Therapeutic uses. TPA's current indications are for the lysis of suspected occlusive coronary artery thrombi associated with evolving transmural myocardial infarction, and the improvement of ventricular function and reduction in the incidence of congestive heart failure associated with acute myocardial infarction.

The immediate benefits of TPA treatment include a prompt reperfusion and restoration of coronary artery patency in patients with total coronary artery occlusion. Electrocardiographic changes in cardiac enzymes and alterations in the pattern of chest pain indicate that rapid perfusion afforded by TPA may limit the size of the infarct.

Adverse effects. Bleeding is the most significant adverse effect with TPA. In most cases, bleeding has been minor. Contraindications include active internal bleeding, history of cerebrovascular accident, recent intracranial or intraspinal surgery or trauma (within two months), intracranial neoplasm, arteriovenous malformation or aneurysm, known bleeding diathesis, or severe uncontrolled hypertension.

Nursing Management

Table 44.9 describes the nursing management of the patient receiving fibrinolytic drugs. Dosage details of individual drugs are given in Table 44.10 (pages 497–501).

Fibrinolytic Inhibitors: Hemostatic Agents

Aminocaproic Acid

Mechanism of action and pharmacologic effects. Aminocaproic acid acts as a competitive inhibitor for the binding of plasminogen and plasmin to fibrin. As a result, fibrinolysis is inhibited.

Therapeutic uses. Aminocaproic acid is indicated for the treatment of excessive bleeding that results from systemic hyperfibrinolysis and urinary fibrinolysis. It is also indicated as an adjunct in replacement therapy in hemophiliac patients undergoing tooth extractions.

Adverse effects. The most common untoward effects of aminocaproic acid are nausea, diarrhea and vomiting.

Aprotinin

Mechanism of action and pharmacologic effects. Aprotinin is a potent and effective proteinase inhibitor extracted from bovine lung tissue. The drug is comparable to aminocaproic acid in its inhibitory action on plasmin activator. Aprotinin also directly inhibits plasmin.

Therapeutic uses. Aprotinin is indicated for the treatment of patients suffering from conditions caused by excessive fibrinolysis. These conditions occur in surgery (including open heart surgery and prosthetic surgery) and pathologic obstetrical bleeding conditions, such as abruptio placentae.

Adverse effects. Aprotinin is well tolerated at recommended dosages. However, allergic reactions such as flushing, tachycardia, itching, rash and urticaria have been reported, as well as dyspnea, sweating, palpitations and nausea. Anaphylactic reactions are rare.

Vitamin K$_1$, Vitamin K$_2$, and Menadione

Mechanism of action and pharmacologic effects. Although vitamin K is not a single chemical, it is often convenient to refer to it as such, as in "vitamin K deficiency." Such loose terminology is acceptable so long as we recognize the fact that there are two naturally occurring substances, vitamin K$_1$ (phytonadione) and vitamin K$_2$ (menaquinone), which stimulate the hepatic synthesis of vitamin K-dependent clotting factors. Both vitamin K$_1$ and vitamin K$_2$ are found in plant leaves and vegetable oils and synthesized in large quantities by bacteria in the intestinal tract. In addition to these naturally occurring substances, the synthetic chemical menadione (sometimes called vitamin K$_3$) is included in the general term "vitamin K."

Vitamins K$_1$ and K$_2$ are well absorbed from the gastrointestinal tract if bile salts are present.

Table 44.9
Nursing management of fibrinolytic drugs

Assessment of risk vs. benefit	Patient data	• Physician should determine which fibrinolytic will be most effective. Drugs must be used within a brief period (4–24 h) to be effective • Recent use of anticoagulants and antiplatelet drugs, including ASA, may increase risks of drug tx. Active bleeding, recent surgery or severe hypertension may contraindicate use of these drugs • *Pregnancy:* Risk category C (animal studies show adverse effects to fetus but human data are unknown or insufficient); benefits may be acceptable despite risks. Should be avoided postpartum
	Drug data	• *Some serious drug interactions:* Confer with pharmacist • Bleeding is the most serious adverse effect. Occasionally, allergic reactions may occur (chills, fever, pruritus, urticaria, asthma or ana-phylaxis). Have emergency equipment available
Implementation	Rights of administration	• Using the "rights" helps prevent errors of administration
	Right route	• Give IV
	Right dose	• Check instructions for reconstitution and flow rate carefully
	Right technique	• IV administration requires knowledge of correct diluent and IV solution, correct dilution and rate of administration. Always refer to manufacturer's instructions for this route. Rate must be carefully controlled; an infusion pump is recommended. For reconstitution, do not use diluents with preservatives and do not shake; these actions will reduce the activity of the drug
	Nursing therapeutics	• Provide physical care cautiously to minimize risk of bruising. Avoid IM injections and other invasive procedures. Bedrest is essential during tx • Monitor VS, temp carefully during administration. Observe for bleeding q15min during first hour of tx, then q30min during next 8 h
	Patient/family teaching	• Pts/families should know risk of bleeding associated with use of fibrinolytic drugs. Informed consent is essential
Outcomes	Monitoring of progress	*Continually monitor:* • Clinical response • Signs/symptoms of adverse reactions; document and report immediately to physician

Vitamin K_1 is also formulated for subcutaneous, intramuscular or intravenous administration. Menadione does not require bile for absorption. It is also available as a water-soluble salt, mena-dione sodium bisulfite, for parenteral administra-tion. Menadiol tetrasodium diphosphate (Kappadione®, Synka-Vite®) is another water-soluble salt of menadione, intended for oral or parenteral administration.

Therapeutic uses. Vitamin K is given to treat a deficiency resulting from its inadequate intake, absorption or utilization. It is also given to antagonize the actions of oral anticoagulants.

Vitamin K may be given during the first days of life to newborn infants, who have only 20% to 40% of adult levels of prothrombin. For prophylaxis and treatment of hemorrhagic diseases of the newborn, the water-soluble vitamin K analogues are not as safe as phytonadione. Doses of menadiol sodium diphosphate in excess of 10 mg have been associated with hyperbilirubinemia in infants.

Patients with intrahepatic or extrahepatic biliary obstruction may not absorb naturally occurring forms of vitamin K. Treatment with oral vitamin K_1 plus bile salts will usually correct the problem. Vitamin K_3 does not require bile for absorption. Broad-spectrum antibacterials can kill vitamin K-producing bacteria in the colon, leading to hypoprothrombinemia and hemorrhage. Treatment with vitamin K can reverse the hypoprothrombinemia. Hepatocellular disease may produce hypoprothrombinemia. Vitamin K is of no value in this condition because the problem lies in the inability of the liver to synthesize clotting factors, even in the presence of adequate amounts of the vitamin.

Menadiol sodium diphosphate should not be administered to a pregnant woman during the last few weeks of pregnancy. The drug should also not be administered to infants.

Adverse effects. As might be expected, the administration of a vitamin K product may cause temporary refractoriness to anticoagulant therapy. An overdose of vitamin K in an infant can produce hemolytic anemia or kernicterus.

Response to Clinical Challenge

1. This class of drug will be given by the IV route.
2. Observations for any signs/symptoms of bleeding must be made prior to and during infusion. It is also important to be alert for any signs of allergic reactions.
3. These drugs must be reconstituted in accordance with the manufacturer's instructions. In general, it is important to use diluent that does not contain preservatives and to avoid agitation of the solution. Failure to follow these directions can result in inactivation of the drug. For the infusion of these agents, use of a pump and in-line filters is recommended.
4. Fibrinolytic agents are most effective when given within 4–24 h after the initial clot formation.
5. The major risk of drug treatment is bleeding. This can be very serious, depending on the site and severity. Aminocaproic acid is an antidote. The other risk is for allergic responses.
6. To treat Jayne's nausea, it is important to use the oral route if possible. The IM route is contraindicated owing to the risk for hematoma.

Further Reading

Coller BSC. Platelets and thrombolytic therapy. *N Engl J Med* 1990;322:33–42.

Dalteparin — another low-molecular-weight heparin. *Medical Letter on Drugs and Therapeutics* 1995;37:115–116.

Enoxaparin — a low-molecular-weight heparin. *Medical Letter on Drugs and Therapeutics* 1993;35:75–76, 98.

Table 44.10

Anticoagulant and antiplatelet drugs, fibrinolytic agents and vitamin K: Drug doses

Drug Generic name (Trade names)	Dosage	Nursing alert
A. Injectable Anticoagulant Drugs		
heparin	*Therapeutic anticoagulation: Dose depends on results of PT* **Intermittent IV bolus:** *Adults:* 10 000 U, followed by 5000–10 000 U q4–6h. *Children:* 50 U/kg, followed by 50–100 U/kg q4h **IV infusion:** *Adults:* 5000 U (35–70 U/kg), followed by 20 000–40 000 U infused over 24 h (approx. 1000 U/h). *Children:* 50 U/kg, followed by 20 000 U/m²/24h **SC:** *Adults:* 5000 U IV, followed by initial SC dose of 10 000–20 000 U, then 8000–10 000 U q8h, or 15 000–20 000 U q12h Prophylaxis of thromboembolic events: **SC:** *Adults:* 5000 U q8–12h. (May be started 2 h prior to surgery.) **IV:** *Adults/children:* 10–100 U *Heparin lock procedure:* Inject 0.5–1 mL (10–100 U) q8–12h or after each medication infusion. To prevent incompatibility of heparin with medication, flush hep lock set with sterile water or normal saline for injection before and after administration of medication	• *Do not give IM:* Danger of hematoma. Avoid other injections while receiving heparin tx (except low-dose prophylaxis) • **SC:** Inject deeply and slowly, preferably in lower abdomen. Do not aspirate or massage site. Rotate sites. Observe site for bleeding • **IV:** For direct IV, follow agency policy. For continuous infusion, use protocol. Heparin lock: Follow agency policy or heparin lock procedure
dalteparin sodium (Fragmin)	*General surgery with associated risk of thromboembolic complications:* **SC:** 2500 IU 1–2 h before operation and thereafter 2500 IU each a.m. until pt is mobilized (in general, 5–7 days or longer) *General surgery associated with other risk factors and elective hip surgery:* **SC:** 5000 IU the evening before operation and 5000 IU on following evenings. Continue until pt is mobilized (in general, 5–7 days or longer) *Treatment of acute deep venous thrombosis:* **SC:** 100 IU/kg bid or 100 IU/kg over 12 h as continuous IV infusion For other conditions of use, consult manufacturer's recommended dosages	• Using a 25- or 26-gauge 1/2"–5/8" needle, inject deeply and slowly, preferably in lower abdomen. Do not aspirate or massage site. Rotate sites. Observe sites for hematoma. Antidote: Protamine sulfate (1 mg protamine = 100 IU dalteparin)

Table 44.10 (continued)
Anticoagulant and antiplatelet drugs, fibrinolytic agents and vitamin K: Drug doses

Drug Generic name (Trade names)	Dosage	Nursing alert
A. Injectable Anticoagulant Drugs (cont'd)		
enoxaparin (Lovenox)	**SC** (in the abdomen): *Adults:* Begin within first 24 h following orthopedic surgery, as soon as primary hemostasis has been established. Give 1 syringe q12h, equivalent to 30 mg enoxaparin bid. Usual duration of treatment, 7–14 days	• **SC:** Give deep, inject slowly. Do not massage site. Rotate sites
B. Oral Anticoagulant Drugs		
warfarin sodium (Athrombin-K, Coumadin, Warfilone, Warnerin)	**Oral:** *Adults:* 10 mg/day for 2–4 days, then adjust daily dose per results of PT (range, 2–10 mg/day). Initiate tx with lower doses in elderly or debilitated pts	• Give at same time each day. Dose adjusted according to PT
C. Antiplatelet Drugs		
acetylsalicylic acid, ASA (Aspirin)	**Oral:** Platelet antiaggregant: Optimal dose has not been determined. The following doses have been shown to be effective. Secondary prevention of myocardial infarction: 162.5–1500 mg/day; prevention of occlusion of coronary artery grafts: 100–975 mg/day; secondary prevention of TIAs: 1300 mg/day in 2–4 divided doses. For prevention of preeclampsia: 60–100 mg/day	• Give with food to reduce GI irritation. Do not crush or chew enteric-coated tablets. Do not take with antacids. Chewable tablets may be chewed, swallowed whole or crushed and mixed with food or liquid. ASA prolongs bleeding time for 4–7 days
dipyridamole (Persantine)	**Oral:** *Adults* (thromboembolic disease): 100 mg qid, 1 h ac	• Although absorbed faster on an empty stomach, dipyridamole may be taken with food if GI irritation occurs. May be crushed and mixed with food, if necessary
sulfinpyrazone (Anturan, Anturane)	**Oral** (for TIAs, thromboembolism associated with vascular and cardiac prostheses, recurrent venous thrombosis, arteriovenous shunt thrombosis): 600–800 mg/day in 3–4 divided doses	• Give with food or antacid to reduce GI irritation
ticlopidine HCl (Ticlid)	**Oral:** *Adults:* 250 mg bid with food	• Give with food to enhance absorption and reduce gastric irritation

Table 44.10 (continued)
Anticoagulant and antiplatelet drugs, fibrinolytic agents and vitamin K: Drug doses

Drug Generic name (Trade names)	Dosage	Nursing alert
D. Fibrinolytic Drugs		
alteplase, tissue plasminogen activator, TPA (Activase, rt-PA)	**IV:** *Adults:* Usually, 100 mg administered as 60 mg (34.8×10^6 IU) in the first hour (of which 6–7 mg is administered as bolus over the first 1–2 min and the remainder is administered by continuous infusion), 20 mg (11.6×10^6 IU) by continuous infusion during the second hour and 20 mg (11.6×10^6 IU) by continuous infusion over the following 1–4 h. For smaller pts (< 65 kg), a dose of 1.25 mg/kg may be warranted. Max. dose, 120 mg (69.6×10^6 IU)	• At initiation of tx, start two IV lines: one for TPA, another for other infusions • Follow instructions for reconstitution; do not shake. Mix only with sterile water with preservatives. Solution stable for 8 h (at room temp). Use infusion pump to ensure accurate administration rate • Avoid IM injections during tx, if possible
streptokinase (Streptase)	*Adults* (for all indications): Myocardial infarction: **IV:** 1 500 000 IU. Intracoronary: 20 000 IU bolus, followed by 2000 IU/min infusion for 60 min (140 000 IU total dose). Deep vein thrombosis, pulmonary emboli, arterial embolism or thromboses: **IV:** 250 000 IU loading dose, followed by 100 000 IU/h for 24 h for pulmonary emboli, 72 h for recurrent pulmonary emboli or deep vein thrombosis. Arteriovenous cannula occlusion: 100 000–250 000 IU into each occluded limb of cannula; clamp for 2 h, then aspirate	• Do PT and aPTT prior to infusion • Reconstitute with normal saline or dextrose and gently swirl to mix. Do not shake. Further infuse and administer using infusion pump for accuracy. Stable for 24 h. Use an in-line filter
urokinase (Abbokinase)	Lysis of coronary thrombi, MI: **Intracoronary:** *Adults:* 6000 IU/min for up to 2 h (preceded by 2500–10 000 U of heparin IV). Pulmonary emboli, deep vein thrombosis: **IV:** 4400 IU/kg loading dose over 10 min followed by 4400 IU/kg/h for 12 h. Occluded IV catheters, into catheter: 1–1.8 mL of 5000 IU/mL solution injected into catheter, then aspirated; may repeat q5min for 30 min. If no result, may cap and leave in catheter for 30–60 min, then aspirate	• Reconstitute with sterile water for injection, without preservatives. Dilute further, for infusion, using an in-line filter and pump • To free an occluded cannula or IV catheter, inject 1 mL slowly, clamp for 5 min, then aspirate. If no result, reclamp for 5 min and carefully aspirate. If continually unsuccessful after 30 min, clamp for 30–60 min and try again. A second dose may be needed

(cont'd on next page)

Table 44.10 (continued)
Anticoagulant and antiplatelet drugs, fibrinolytic agents and vitamin K: Drug doses

Drug Generic name (Trade names)	Dosage	Nursing alert

E. Fibrinolytic Inhibitors, Hemostatic Agents

Drug	Dosage	Nursing alert
aminocaproic acid (Amicar)	Acute bleeding syndromes due to elevated fibrinolytic activity: **Oral:** *Adults:* 5 g first hour, followed by 1–1.25 g q1h for 8 h or until hemorrhage is controlled, or 6 g/24 h after prostate surgery **IV:** *Adults:* 4–5 g over first hour, followed by 1 g/h for 8 h or until hemorrhage is controlled, or 6 g/24 h after prostate surgery (not > 30 g/day). **Oral/IV:** *Children:* 100 mg/kg or 3 g/m^2 over first hour, followed by continuous infusion of 33.3 mg/kg/h or 1g/m^2/h (total dose not > 18 g/m^2/24 h) Subarachnoid hemorrhage: **Oral:** *Adults:* 3 g q24h (36 g/day). If no surgery is performed, continue for 21 days after bleeding stops, then decrease to 2 g q2h (24 g/day) for 3 days, then 1 g q2h (12 g/day) for 3 days	• Use infusion pump to ensure accuracy. Follow manufacturer's instructions for reconstitution. Calculate dosages and flow rate carefully
aprotinin (Trasylol)	**IV** (hemorrhage due to hyperfibrinolysis): *Adults:* Owing to slight risk of allergic reactions, a 1-mL (10 000-KIU) initial dose should always be administered at least 10 min prior to remainder of dose. After the uneventful administration of the initial 1-mL dose, tx dose may be given. Initial dosage, 200 000–500 000 KIU, of which 200 000 should be given by IV injection (at a rate not to exceed 5 mL/min); the rest, if necessary, by slow infusion. Administration should be continued up to 1 000 000 KIU/day until hemorrhage has been arrested. Before infusion, aprotinin may be diluted with 5% dextrose or physiologic saline solution. The duration of tx should not exceed 5 days	• Administer test dose and monitor closely • Administer through a central line. Pt should remain supine during infusion • Use immediately after opening vial. Discard if solution is cloudy or contains precipitate

Table 44.10 (continued)
Anticoagulant and antiplatelet drugs, fibrinolytic agents and vitamin K: Drug doses

Drug Generic name (Trade names)	Dosage	Nursing alert
E. Vitamin K Products		
vitamin K_1, phytonadione (Aqua Mephyton, Konakion, Mephyton)	**Oral** (for anticoagulant overdose and other hypoprothrombinemic states): *Adults/children,* 2.5–25 mg; rarely, doses as large as 50 mg may be needed **IM** (for prophylaxis of hemorrhagic disease in newborn): 0.5–1 mg immediately after birth. **IM/SC** (for tx of hemorrhagic disease in newborn): 1 mg **IV:** Use only when other routes are not feasible and risk is justified. Rate of injection should not exceed 1 mg/min. For mild overdosage of oral anticoagulants: Initially, 0.5–5 mg. For moderate to severe hemorrhage: Up to 10 mg in divided doses. For other hypoprothrombinemic states: 2.5–25 mg	• Because of potential for severe allergic reactions, IV route should be used only when other routes are not feasible and risk is justified • Rate of injection should not exceed 1 mg/min • Frequency of administration and number of additional doses should be determined by the prothrombin time (PT) or the pt's condition. Monitor closely. Have emergency equipment nearby • Dilute with NS or D5W and protect container from light (i.e., with aluminum foil or brown paper bag) • IM injections for infants and small children should be given into anterior lateral thigh. The gluteus maximus site may be used for preteens and older individuals
menadione (Vitamin K_3)	**Oral:** 2–10 mg daily	• Monitor PT to determine effectiveness
menadiol sodium diphosphate (Synkavite)	**Oral:** *Adults* (for secondary hypoprothrombinemia): 5–10 mg daily **SC/IM/IV:** *Adults* (for management of hypoprothrombinemic hemorrhagic states): 5–15 mg od or bid. *Children:* 5–10 mg od or bid. Doses may be repeated if prothombin levels do not return to normal	• IV infusion should not exceed 1 mg/min • Monitor PT to determine effectiveness

Psychopharmacology

The importance of drugs affecting the brain cannot be minimized. The brain controls mood, motor function and the appreciation of pain, to mention but three functions.

The importance of antipsychotic drugs in our society today is reflected in our decision to discuss them first (Chapter 45). Chapter 46 continues with a discussion of the mood-altering drugs used to combat depression and manic depressive illness, while Chapter 47 deals with anxiolytics, sedatives and hypnotics. Finally, Chapter 48 considers the alcohols and drug therapy for alcoholism.

The use of psychoactive drugs must be considered in the context of their overall effects, both beneficial and adverse. Too often, we hear advocates of either persuasion espouse the view that these drugs are the salvation of the human race or a tool of the devil. Both positions are, of course, extreme.

Psychoactive drugs have their place in modern medicine. Many patients are permitted to live more normal lives than would have heretofore been possible. However, these drugs are not without their bad side. They can and do produce adverse effects that can reduce a patient's quality of life and decrease compliance. Nurses should be aware of both the good and the bad with regard to the psychoactive drugs so that they may be capable of detecting any drug-induced effects in their patients.

CHAPTER 45

Antipsychotic Drugs

Topics Discussed
- Typical antipsychotic drugs
- Atypical antipsychotic drugs
- For all drugs discussed: Mechanism of action and pharmacologic effects, therapeutic uses, adverse effects
- Antipsychotic drugs in the treatment of agitation and aggression
- Nursing management

Drugs Discussed

Typical Antipsychotic Drugs:
chlorpromazine (klor-**proe**-mah-zeen)
fluphenazine (floo-**fen**-ah-zeen)
flupenthixol (floo-pen-**thix**-awl)
fluspirilene (flo-**spy**-rih-leen)
haloperidol (ha-loe-**pair**-ih-dole)
loxapine (**lox**-ah-peen)
mesoridazine (mes-oh-**rid**-ah-zeen)
perphenazine (per-**fen**-ah-zeen)
pimozide (**pye**-moe-zyde)
pipotiazine (pip-oh-**tye**-ah-zeen)
prochlorperazine (proe-klor-**pair**-a-zeen)
promazine (**proe**-mazz-een)
thioridazine (thye-oh-**rid**-ah-zeen)
thiothixene (thye-oh-**thix**-een)
trifluoperazine (trye-floo-oh-**pair**-ah-zeen)

Atypical Antipsychotic Drugs
clozapine (**cloz**-ah-peen)
olanzapine (oh-**lanz**-ah-peen)
risperidone (ris-**speer**-ih-doan)

Clinical Challenge

Consider this clinical challenge as you read through this chapter. The response to the challenge appears on page 514.

Ken, a 20-year-old single, Caucasian male, is brought to the Emergency Department by friends. Symptoms include auditory hallucinations, delusions, aggressiveness and persecutory illusions. He had one previous hospitalization 18 months ago and was treated with haloperidol. Owing to adverse reactions, the drug was discontinued. He is not presently taking any medications.

Biophysical assessment: height, 170 cm; weight, 71 kg; BP, 120/80; P, 70-80, regular. No history of renal, liver or cardiovascular disorders.

Psychological assessment: lives alone; parents live in city, believe that Ken might do better living alone ("It might make him grow up and take care of himself"). Friends confirm Ken's frequent and excessive use of alcohol over the past 2 years.

Medical diagnosis: schizoaffective illness; alcohol abuse.

Medical order: chlorpromazine 50 mg PO stat, then CPZ 100 mg PO tid. One week later: CPZ 125 mg PO tid; 3 weeks later: CPZ 125 mg PO in a.m. and 300 mg PO hs. *(cont'd on next page)*

Clinical Challenge *(cont'd)*

Charting highlights:

• On admission, Ken was very restless, agitated and verbally abusive to everyone. Describes voices telling him that someone is going to hurt him. Participates in ward activities for only short time before losing temper or becoming too restless. Laughs inappropriately. Requires time-out for verbal aggressiveness. Sleeps very short periods during the night.

• One week later: has joined communication group and is participating in other ward activities. Denies hallucinations/delusions. Becomes easily bored and demonstrates few skills in coping with frustration. Still requires time-out and prn medication for agitation. BP and P stable.

• Three weeks later: participating in activities for sustained periods. No time-out required. Drowsy and lethargic much of the day. Discharge planning and a week-end pass with parents. Does not want to return home with them. No drinking during pass but states that having a drink is harmless fun.

Appropriate behaviour and participation. Has gained 2 kg; drinking apple juice frequently. Discharged to outpatient medication clinic. Will attend weekly education sessions and family program. Ordered flupenthixol decanoate (Fluanxol®).

1. Which drugs are most likely to be successful for Ken?
2. Describe flupenthixol's usual therapeutic effects. Why is Ken receiving this drug?
3. List nursing diagnoses (actual and potential): those related to drug outcome; those related to reducing side effects; those related to education.
4. Describe the injection technique for flupenthixol.

The appearance of chlorpromazine in France in the early 1950s heralded the introduction of antipsychotic drugs. Originally called major tranquilizers, these chemicals are now classified as antipsychotic (or neuroleptic) drugs, a term that more adequately describes their therapeutic effects. They are used to treat schizophrenia and other psychoses, including mania and paranoia. Box 45.1 summarizes the characteristics of schizophrenia.

Chlorpromazine was soon followed on the market by other antipsychotics, and the number of patients in mental hospitals dropped sharply. A cure for psychoses seemed at hand. However, this euphoria dissipated when the rates of readmission to hospitals increased and the toxicities of the drugs became better known. It is now recognized that typical antipsychotic drugs aid a great number of mentally ill patients. They do not, however, provide a cure. Indeed, not all patients respond to the drugs, and the possible benefits from their use must be weighed against their adverse effects.

Antipsychotic drugs can be divided into two major groups. The older drugs, now known as "typical or traditional antipsychotic drugs," treat the positive symptoms of schizophrenia. Typical antipsychotic drugs have not been demonstrated to be effective against the negative symptoms of schizophrenia (see Box 45.1 for positive and negative symptoms).

Typical antipsychotic drugs can induce *extrapyramidal symptoms* (EPS; i.e., deficits in postural, static, supporting and locomotor mechanisms) in 75% to 90% of patients, and this is the principal cause of noncompliance and relapse.

Box 45.1
Characteristics of schizophrenia

Definition
A chronic psychotic illness that emerges during adolescence or early adulthood. Symptoms include thought disorders and a reduction in pt's ability to comprehend reality

Positive vs. negative symptoms
Symptoms can be categorized as positive or negative. Positive symptoms are exaggerated or distorted function (e.g., agitation, tension, delusions, hallucinations, incoherent speech). Negative symptoms include losses or diminished function (e.g., emotional and social withdrawal, blunted affect, poverty of speech content, lack of initiative, motor retardation)

Acute episodes
Delusions and hallucinations become prominent. Delusions can be religious, grandiose or persecutory.

Auditory hallucinations, which may consist of voices that argue or comment on or about behaviour, are more common than visual hallucinations. The pt may feel that he or she is being controlled by external influences. The pt's misperception of reality and disordered thinking may make rational conversation impossible and result in hostile or uncooperative behaviour. Pts may neglect self-care because of impaired skills. Their sleeping and eating patterns may also be altered

Long-term course
The course of the illness includes both acute episodes and remissions. For some pts the long-term course results in a decline of mental status and functioning, whereas others may stabilize. The maintenance of appropriate drug tx can reduce acute relapse; however, such tx may not reduce the risk of long-term deterioration

---

Because of the seriousness of antipsychotic-induced EPS, this chapter contains a lengthy discussion of these reactions. Treatment often involves the use of antiparkinsonian drugs, which are discussed in Chapter 50.

Clozapine, risperidone and olanzapine are newer drugs, often called "atypical antipsychotics." For many patients, they provide a significant improvement in drug therapy. These drugs treat the positive and negative symptoms of schizophrenia, while sparing patients the extrapyramidal adverse effects caused by the older, typical antipsychotics. Because of the differences in the pharmacologic profiles of the typical and atypical antipsychotic drugs, each group will be discussed separately.

Typical or Traditional Antipsychotic Drugs

Mechanism of Action and Pharmacologic Effects

Typical antipsychotic drugs block dopamine D_2, histamine H_1, muscarinic and alpha$_1$ adrenergic receptors (Figures 45.1 and 45.2 on pages 506 and

507, respectively). As a result they produce a variety of effects, both desirable and undesirable. Nurses will remember the reasons for each drug-induced effect if they can associate the effect to the blockade of a specific group of receptors.

1. Block of Dopamine D_2 Receptors in the Brain

Antipsychotic actions. The ability of typical antipsychotics to block dopamine receptors in the brain lies at the root of their beneficial actions, and many of their major adverse effects. Typical antipsychotic drugs block D_2 receptors in the mesolimbic-mesocortical area of the brain. It is believed that this action plays a major role controlling the positive symptoms of schizophrenia.

Extrapyramidal effects. The extrapyramidal actions of typical antipsychotics, such as parkinsonian effects, dystonic reactions, akathisia and tardive dyskinesia, result from a blockade of D_2 receptors in the nigrostriatal pathway. Dopamine is essential for normal motor function. By blocking its actions in the basal ganglia in the brain, antipsychotics modify motor activity to produce EPS.

**Figure 45.1
Dopamine-blocking actions of antipsychotic
(neuroleptic) drugs**

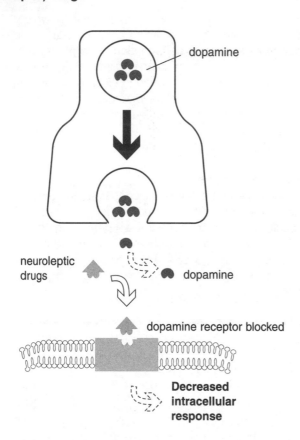

Source: Harvey RA, Champe PC. *Lippincott's Illustrated Review: Pharmacology.* New York: J.P. Lippincott; 1992. Reproduced with permission.

Hypersecretion of prolactin. The hypersecretion of prolactin produced by typical antipsychotics is due to a block of D_2 receptors in the pituitary. This gland has D_2 receptors that mediate the effects of the prolactin inhibitory factor (PIF). Blocking D_2 receptors increases prolactin release, which can result in amenorrhea, infertility and impotence.

Antiemetic action. Stimulation of D_2 receptors in the chemoreceptor area of the medulla oblongata area of the brain plays a pivotal role in the nausea and vomiting produced by many drugs and chemicals. The antiemetic action of many typical antipsychotics results from a block of these receptors.

2. Block of Histamine$_1$ (H$_1$) Receptors

Higher dose phenothiazines, such as chlorpromazine, are more likely to produce pronounced sedation. This may be due, at least in part, to a block of histamine$_1$ (H$_1$) receptors. Nurses who have taken any of the older antihistamines, such a diphenhydramine (Benadryl®), will recognize the sedation produced by these drugs and can associate this effect with the action of some typical antipsychotics.

3. Block of Muscarinic Receptors

The ability of typical antipsychotics to block muscarinic receptors in the body (see Chapter 28) explains the generalized inhibition of parasympathetic function experienced by patients. The effects encountered most frequently are dry mouth, constipation, urinary retention and cycloplegia.

4. Block of Alpha$_1$ Adrenergic Receptors

By blocking alpha$_1$ adrenergic receptors, some typical antipsychotic drugs dilate both arterioles and veins (see Chapter 30). This results in both a decrease in peripheral resistance and reduction in venous return. As a result, drugs such as chlorpromazine decrease blood pressure and produce orthostatic hypotension.

Chemically, typical or traditional antipsychotics may be classified as phenothiazines, thioxanthenes, butyrophenones, dibenzoxazepines and dibenzodiazepines. These drugs all block the same receptors (see Figures 45.1 and 45.2). They differ, however, in their relative potencies on individual groups of receptors. For example, chlorpromazine is more likely to block H$_1$ receptors and sedate patients. However, compared with haloperidol, chlorpromazine is not as potent an antagonist of D_2 receptors in the nigrostriatal pathway and, as a result, is less likely to produce EPS. Table 45.1 lists the common antipsychotics by potency.

When used in doses capable of blocking D_2 receptors in the mesolimbic-mesocortical area of the brain, all typical antipsychotics should be equally effective, and generally speaking, they are so. Therefore, drug selection is based more on the side-effect profile of each agent. The best drug for a particular patient is the one that has the adverse effects the patient is most willing to accept.

Figure 45.2
Blocking actions of antipsychotic (neuroleptic) drugs

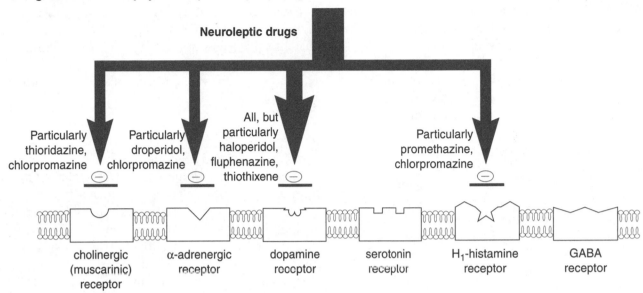

Besides dopaminergic receptors, antipsychotic drugs also block at adrenergic, cholinergic and histamine-binding receptors.

GABA = γ-aminobutyric acid

Source: Harvey RA, Champe PC. *Lippincott's Illustrated Review: Pharmacology.* New York: J.P. Lippincott; 1992. Reproduced with permission.

Table 45.1
Relative potency of the antipsychotics

Generic name (Trade name)*

High-potency
acetophenazine (Tindal)
flupenthixol (Fluanxol)
fluspiralene (IMAP)
fluphenazine (Modecate)
fluphenazine (Moditen)
fluphenazine (Prolixin)
haloperidol (Haldol)
perphenazine (Trilafon)
pimozide (Orap)
pipotiazine (Piportil)
respiridone (Risperdal)
thiothixene (Navane)

Low-potency
chlorpromazine (Largactil)
mesoridazine (Serentil)
promazine (Sparine)
thioridazine (Mellaril)

Mid-potency
clozapine (Clozaril)
loxapine (Loxapac)

*Further trade names, together with dosages, are listed in Table 45.9 (pages 519–522).

Therapeutic Uses

Psychoses are the major indications for use of these drugs. Antipsychotic drug therapy is the most effective treatment for the acute-onset phase in schizophrenia or schizophreniform disorder. These drugs may also be very helpful in the prevention or recurrence of acute schizophrenic disturbances. Typical or traditional antipsychotic agents are less effective in the chronic phase of schizophrenia, particularly with such negative symptoms as anergia, low motivation and flat affect. However, these drugs are used to treat other psychoses, including mania and paranoia.

In the hospital setting, usually three weeks or more of treatment are required before significant effects are seen. The question of duration of therapy is still controversial. Although discontinuing the drug to minimize or abolish adverse effects is appealing, many patients relapse when this is done and may require lifelong therapy. For others, intermittent therapy may be a means of managing the condition while reducing drug-related toxicities. Each patient must be managed on a protocol that best meets his or her clinical problem.

The question of drug selection is very important. Despite differences in potency, all typical antipsychotic drugs are equally effective in equivalent doses. The drug of choice is usually the one the patient can best tolerate. High-potency drugs are more likely to produce EPS, while low-potency agents are more likely to produce sedation and hypotension. Patients should receive the lowest possible dose to maintain therapeutic response.

For patients with bipolar affective disorders, typical antipsychotic drugs are often combined with lithium, both to treat the acute manic episode and to prevent recurrences. Chlorpromazine or haloperidol are used most often.

Organic mental syndromes, manifested as either delirium or dementia, can be treated with typical antipsychotic drugs. In delirium, short-term antipsychotic therapy may be required for patients with specific, identifiable behavioural problems until the medical cause for the delirium can be diagnosed and treated. Chronic intermittent therapy is warranted in patients with dementia whose structural brain changes cannot be rectified but whose behavioural symptoms can be modified.

Anxiety is normally not an indication for the use of antipsychotics. Their adverse effects dictate that they be used only when safer drugs, notably the benzodiazepines, have failed.

Nausea and vomiting resulting from the use of anticancer drugs, radiation, estrogens, tetracyclines and narcotics, and from uremia, can be treated with typical antipsychotic drugs. Only thioridazine seems devoid of antiemetic effects. Antipsychotics do not appear effective in controlling motion sickness.

At least two antipsychotic drugs, haloperidol and pimozide, may help minimize the symptoms of Tourette's syndrome — a rare, inherited disorder characterized by severe motor tics, spontaneous grunts and barking cries or involuntary outbursts of obscene language.

Chlorpromazine may be used to treat hiccoughs, though its mechanism of action in this condition is not known.

Adverse Effects

Typical antipsychotic drugs are characterized by a high therapeutic index with respect to mortality, but adverse effects occur routinely at therapeutic doses. Overdose is seldom fatal in adults, and most adverse reactions are not life-threatening. However, the characteristic neurologic adverse effects of these drugs are particularly troublesome; they often limit the tolerated dose and may interfere with therapeutic effects and compliance. Close and critical observation is essential to monitor the patient's progress and detect adverse reactions promptly.

The adverse effects of typical antipsychotic drugs include the following:

1. CNS Depression

This action may be due to a block of H_1 receptors. Sedation is common after the use of all typical antipsychotic drugs and is especially pronounced after large doses of the low-potency phenothiazines (see Table 45.1). It can be minimized by reducing the dose or substituting a less sedating drug. However, sedation decreases during long-term treatment, and many patients become tolerant to this effect. Daytime somnolence can be minimized by giving a single dose at bedtime.

2. Anticholinergic Effects

The ability of typical antipsychotics to block muscarinic receptors can lead to loss of accommodation, dry mouth, retention or difficulty in urinating and constipation. Muscarinic block may also cause a toxic-confusional state. Toxic delirium generally occurs with agents that have a pronounced anticholinergic effect and may be difficult to differentiate from deterioration in schizophrenia.

3. Alpha$_1$ Adrenergic Receptor Blockade

The consequences of this action may include orthostatic hypotension, impotence, and failure to ejaculate. Orthostatic hypotension is more prevalent with high-dose (low-potency) antipsychotics, such as chlorpromazine, thioridazine, and chlorprothixene.

4. Inhibition of Dopamine$_2$ (D$_2$) Pituitary Receptors

As previously explained, the pituitary has D_2 receptors that mediate the effects of the prolactin inhibitory factor (PIF). Blocking D_2 receptors increases prolactin release. Because typical antipsychotic drugs block pituitary D_2 receptors, they can cause amenorrhea, infertility and impotence.

5. Hypersensitivity Reactions

These include obstructive jaundice in 2% to 4% of patients treated with typical antipsychotic drugs. Blood dyscrasias, manifested as leukopenia, leukocytosis and eosinophilia, are also classified as hypersensitivity reactions.

6. Skin Pigmentation

This is seen most often with chlorpromazine and other low-potency drugs and is apparently the result of the accumulation of the antipsychotic and its metabolites in the skin. In extreme cases, involving the deposition of pigment in the lens and cornea, vision can be impaired. Pigment deposits tend to disappear slowly once drug treatment is stopped. Photosensitivity, most common with long-term chlorpromazine treatment, usually appears in the form of hypersensitivity to the sun and severe sunburn. (See Box 45.2 on the next page for a sample patient teaching on protecting the skin from photosensitivity.) Dermatitis can occur in health personnel who must handle the drug. Caution should be used.

7. Neuroleptic Malignant Syndrome (NMS)

This is a rare, but serious syndrome that carries the risk of mortality, and is more prevalent in men. Its cause is not known. A decade ago, one in five patients who suffered through NMS died. Today, however, that risk has been reduced to four percent, as a result of early recognition. Symptoms include tachycardia, sweating, rigidity, fever, fluctuations in blood pressure, seizure or coma. If NMS is not treated, respiratory failure or cardiovascular collapse may be the fatal outcome. Treatment includes stopping the antipsychotic drug and starting supportive measures for hyperthermia. Drug therapy with dantrolene or bromocriptine may also be used. Resuming antipsychotic drug therapy carries the risk of recurrence.

8. Extrapyramidal Symptoms (EPS)

Because of the importance of EPS, they have been left until last to facilitate a thorough discussion. Dopamine and acetylcholine are physiological antagonists in the striatum of the brain, with dopamine acting as an inhibitor and acetylcholine as an excitatory neurotransmitter. Because typical antipsychotics block dopamine D_2 receptors, they disturb the normal balance between acetylcholine and dopamine in the brain. As a result, the excitatory effects of acetylcholine are seen unfettered by the inhibitory actions of dopamine. The EPS of typical antipsychotics can be divided into the direct and indirect consequences of the block of D_2 receptors.

A. Direct effect of the block of dopamine receptors.

Parkinsonian effects — involve a decrease or slowing of voluntary movements associated with masked facies, tremor at rest, and a decrease in reciprocal arm movements when walking. Seen in about thirteen percent of patients treated with antipsychotic drugs, parkinsonian effects may occur as early as five days or as late as one month after treatment begins. Reducing the dose of the antipsychotic or adding an anticholinergic-antiparkinsonian drug, such as benztropine or trihexyphenidyl, decreases the severity of the parkinsonian syndrome. (See Chapter 50 for further information on the treatment of parkinsonism.)

Dystonic reactions — include facial grimacing, torticollis, oculogyric crisis, difficulty in speech and swallowing and uncoordinated, spastic movements of the body and limbs. The incidence of dystonic reactions is twelve percent in patients treated with typical antipsychotic drugs. These effects usually occur within one to five days of starting therapy. Treatment involves the use of an anticholinergic-antiparkinsonian drug.

Akathisia — is the inability to sit quietly. It is characterized as restlessness, pacing and insomnia. Seen in 37% of patients treated with typical antipsychotics, akathisia varies in onset from the first week of therapy to as late as two months. An anticholinergic-antiparkinsonian drug should reduce the symptoms.

B. Indirect effects of the block of dopamine receptors.

Tardive dyskinesia — occurs in 10% to 40% of patients receiving long-term typical antipsychotic drug therapy and results indirectly from a block of dopamine receptors. The block of dopamine D_2

Box 45.2
Patient teaching: Protecting your skin from photosensitive reactions

Exposure to the sun, or even to fluorescent lights, may make your condition worse. Excessive exposure, in fact, may cause rashes, fever, arthritis and even damage to the organs inside your body.

You needn't spend your waking hours in the dark to be safe, though. Just follow the precautions below.

✔ Prepare for going outdoors
Wear a wide-brimmed hat or visor to shield yourself from the sun's rays. Protect your eyes by wearing sunglasses. Put on a dark, densely woven, long-sleeved shirt and trousers to filter out harmful rays.

Buy a sunscreen containing PABA (para-aminobenzoic acid) with a skin protection factor (SPF) of 8 to 15. If you're allergic to PABA, choose a PABA-free product offering equivalent sun protection.

Before you go outside (at least half an hour beforehand), rub the sunscreen onto unprotected parts of your body, such as your face and hands. Read the label to determine how often to reapply it. Usually, you'll reapply the sunscreen after swimming or perspiring.

✔ Avoid strong sunlight
Try to stay indoors during the most intense hours of sunlight, from 10 a.m. to 2 p.m. The ideal time to garden, take a walk, play golf or do any other outdoor activity is just after sunrise or just before sunset.

✔ Remove fluorescent light
At home, replace any fluorescent fixtures or bulbs with incandescent ones. At work, though, avoiding fluorescent light may be difficult. Consider asking your supervisor about moving to a work area closer to a window, so you can use natural light. If you have a fluorescent light above your desk, turn it off and request a lamp that uses incandescent bulbs.

✔ Be careful with soaps and drugs
Certain toiletries, including deodorant soaps, may increase your skin's sensitivity to light.

Try switching to nondeodorant or hypoallergenic soaps. Certain drugs, including tetracyclines and phenothiazines, also make you more sensitive to light.

Always check with your doctor or pharmacist before taking any new medication.

✔ Recognize and report rashes
Be alert for the key sign of a photosensitivity reaction: a red rash on your face or other exposed area. If you discover a suspicious rash or other reaction to light, call your doctor. Remember, prompt treatment can prevent damage to the tissues beneath your skin.

Source: Medication Teaching Aids. Philadelphia: Springhouse; 1994. Reproduced with permission.

---

receptors by typical antipsychotics increases both the turnover and stores of dopamine within nerve endings. In time, the block of D_2 receptors also results in formation of new and supersensitive D_2 receptors. Tardive dyskinesia results from the overstimulation of these new D_2 receptors. It is characterized by involuntary movement, lateral jaw movements, and fly-catching movements of the tongue. Choreiform-like movements, characterized by quick, jerky, purposeless movements of the extremities, may also occur. Because tardive dyskinesia is caused by overstimulation of new supersensitive D_2 receptors and not cholinergic predominance, it does not respond to anticholinergic-antiparkinsonian drugs.

Tardive dyskinesia may occur within the first year of treatment or take considerably longer to appear. The risk increases with duration of treatment and the use of high-potency drugs.

Table 45.2 lists the clinically significant drug interactions with typical or traditional antipsychotic drugs.

Atypical Antipsychotic Drugs

Clozapine, risperidone and olanzapine are often referred to as "atypical antipsychotics" because their pharmacologic and therapeutic effects differ significantly from those previously described for the typical or traditional antipsychotics. For many patients, these drugs provide relief previously not available with the older drugs. Further, atypical antipsychotics do not appear to cause EPS, including tardive dyskinesia, and this is a substantial improvement over the older drugs.

Table 45.2
The traditional antipsychotics: Drug interactions

Drug	Interaction
Antacids	• Antacids may inhibit the absorption of orally administered phenothiazines
Anticholinergics	• Anticholinergics decrease phenothiazine absorption
CNS depressants	• CNS depressants may have their effects increased by antipsychotics
Hypotensives	• Hypotensives may have additive effects with phenothiazines
Levodopa and other dopamine receptor agonists	• Levodopa and dopamine receptor agonists, such as bromocriptine, have their effects reduced by typical antipsychotics because of the ability of the latter drugs to block D_2 receptors in the CNS

Clozapine (Clozaril®)

Mechanism of action and pharmacologic effects. Clozapine differs significantly from the typical or traditional antipsychotics in the fact that it is a relatively poor dopamine D_2 receptor blocker. Clozapine has the least affinity of any antipsychotic drug for D_2 receptors found in the caudate nucleus, and this fact probably accounts for the fact that it does not produce EPS. The drug differs further from the older antipsychotics in its blockade of dopamine D_4 receptors, and this action presumably explains its antipsychotic actions.

Therapeutic uses. Clozapine is effective in controlling both positive symptoms (e.g., irritability, hallucinations, delusions) and negative symptoms (e.g., social disinterest or incompetence, poor personal hygiene) of schizophrenia and other psychoses. A beneficial effect is often observed within two weeks, with further gradual improvement over many weeks. Compared with other antipsychotic drugs, clozapine appears to be particularly useful in the treatment of severely disturbed, treatment-refractory patients, in whom it has a 40% to 60% success rate. Clozapine also may be effective in otherwise unresponsive psychotic mood or schizoaffective disorders. In addition, because of the very low risk for most EPS with this drug, a trial of clozapine is clearly indicated for patients in whom EPS (including tardive dyskinesia) are severe and intolerable with other agents.

Unfortunately, clozapine presents a risk for agranulocytosis (see Adverse Effects), and this limits its use to treatment-resistant patients who are unresponsive to, or cannot tolerate, the other drugs. Currently, clozapine is administered only through treatment systems that are managed by Novartis (formerly Sandoz) Pharmaceuticals. These distribution systems are designed to ensure weekly monitoring of white blood cell counts.

Adverse effects. The most significant reaction associated with clozapine therapy is agranulocytosis, which occurs in 1% to 2% of patients, usually in the first six months of treatment. Although this reaction also occurs with other antipsychotic drugs, it is more prominent with clozapine and did result in several deaths before careful monitoring procedures were defined and implemented in Canada, the United States and the United Kingdom. The manufacturer has worked closely with health authorities in each country to ensure that clozapine is used in a safe and efficacious manner. Clients must have a normal white blood cell count and differential count prior to starting clozapine therapy. Subsequently, a WBC count and differential count must be carried out at least weekly throughout treatment and for at least four weeks after the discontinuation of clozapine.

Besides agranulocytosis, clozapine has been associated with drowsiness or sedation (40%), hypersalivation (30%), tachycardia (25%; persistent in 10%), dizziness (20%) and orthostatic hypotension (9%). Weight gain and transient fever can occur. Seizures have been estimated to occur in association with clozapine use at a cumulative incidence at one year of approximately five percent. Because of the risk for seizure associated with clozapine use, clients should be advised not to engage in any activity where sudden loss of consciousness could cause serious injury to themselves

Table 45.3
Clozapine: Drug interactions

Drug	Interaction
Benzodiazepines and other psychotropic drugs	• Caution is advised when one of these drugs is given with clozapine because these pts may be at increased risk for circulatory collapse accompanied by respiratory and/or cardiac arrest
Bone marrow suppressants	• Clozapine should not be used with other agents having a known potential to suppress bone marrow function. In particular, concomitant use of long-acting depot antipsychotic drugs should be avoided because these medications, which may potentially be myelosuppressive, cannot be rapidly removed from the body
Cimetidine	• Cimetidine inhibits the metabolism of many drugs and may increase plasma levels of clozapine, potentially resulting in adverse effects
CNS active drugs	• Alcohol, MAOIs, CNS depressants (including narcotics, antihistamines and benzodiazepines), anticholinergics and some antihypertensive agents may have their effects enhanced by clozapine
Epinephrine	• Administration of epinephrine to clozapine-treated pts should be avoided in the tx of drug-induced hypotension because clozapine can reverse the effect of epinephrine, with a further fall in BP
Fluoxetine	• Fluoxetine can increase both plasma levels and toxicity of clozapine
Phenytoin	• Phenytoin can increase the metabolism of many drugs. It can decrease clozapine plasma levels, resulting in decreased effectiveness of a previously effective clozapine dose
Drugs highly bound to plasma proteins	• Clozapine is highly bound to serum protein and should not be administered to a pt taking similar drug(s) (e.g., warfarin, digitoxin). Adverse effects may result from the displacement of protein-bound clozapine and/or the displacement of the other drugs

or others (e.g., driving, operating heavy machinery, swimming, climbing).

Table 45.3 lists the clinically significant drug interactions with clozapine.

Risperidone (Risperdal®)

Mechanism of action and pharmacologic effects. Clinical studies demonstrated that combining a typical antipsychotic that blocks dopamine D_2 receptors with a drug that blocks serotonin 5-HT_2 receptors increases the therapeutic effect of the antipsychotic while reducing its EPS. This work led to the development of risperidone, the first antipsychotic that effectively inhibits both D_2 and 5-HT_2 receptors. The balanced antagonism of both types of receptors is believed be the basis for risperidone's superior therapeutic efficacy and its reduced potential for inducing EPS.

Risperidone also inhibits alpha$_1$ adrenergic receptors and H_1 histaminergic receptors. As a result of its inhibition of alpha$_1$ receptors, risperidone can produce a dose-related fall in blood pressure and reflex tachycardia.

Risperidone changes sleep architecture by promoting deep slow-wave sleep, thereby improving sleeping patterns. This effect is most likely due to risperidone's blockade of serotonin receptors.

Substantial and sustained elevations in serum prolactin levels are induced by risperidone, and it appears that tolerance to hyperprolactinemia does not occur. However, the condition is reversible upon withdrawal of risperidone.

Therapeutic uses. Risperidone is used for the management of manifestations of schizophrenia. In controlled clinical trials, risperidone was found to improve both positive and negative symptoms. This latter point is most significant and, along with its increased safety, serves to set risperidone apart from the typical antipsychotics.

Adverse effects. Asthenia (weakness), sedation and difficulty in concentrating have been the most common adverse effects associated with risperidone. Orthostatic hypotension and reflex tachycardia can occur initially, especially in the elderly. Elevation of serum prolactin levels, weight gain and sexual dysfunction have been reported.

Table 45.4
Risperidone: Drug interactions

Drug	Interaction
Alcohol, CNS depressants and some antihypertensive drugs	• Risperidone may enhance the effects of these drugs
Carbamazepine and other drugs that increase drug metabolism	• Carbamazepine has been shown to decrease substantially the plasma levels of risperidone and its active metabolite 9-hydroxy-risperidone. Similar effects may be observed with other hepatic enzyme inducers. Consequently, in the presence of carbamazepine or other hepatic inducers, the dose of risperidone may have be adjusted. On discontinuation of these drugs, the dosage of risperidone should be re-evaluated and, if necessary, decreased
Hypotensive drugs	• Because of its potential for inducing hypotension, risperidone may enhance the hypotensive effects of other drugs with this potential
Levodopa and dopamine agonists	• Risperidone may antagonize the effects of these drugs

The incidence of EPS is dose dependent, but in patients taking recommended doses of risperidone the incidence has been only slightly higher than with placebo. Neither tardive dyskinesia nor agranulocytosis have been reported.

Table 45.4 lists the clinically significant drug interactions with risperidone.

Olanzapine (Zyprexa®)

Mechanism of action and pharmacologic effects. Olanzapine selectively modulates dopaminergic pathways implicated in schizophrenic psychopathology. This drug produces a selective inhibition of mesolimbic dopaminergic pathways — an effect generally associated with antipsychotic activity. Because olanzapine does not inhibit nigrostriatal dopaminergic activity, its EPS are kept to a minimum. This low incidence of side effects is also due to olanzapine's greater affinity for serotonin$_{2A}$ (5-HT$_{2A}$) over dopamine$_2$ (D$_2$) receptors.

Therapeutic uses. Olanzapine appears to control the positive, negative and affective (mood) symptoms of schizophrenia. Similar to the other atypical antipsychotics, olanzapine demonstrates fewer EPS. Moreover, the drug does not elevate prolactin levels as much as haloperidol does. Further, olanzapine has not been associated with the agranulocytosis sometimes seen with clozapine.

Adverse effects. In general, olanzapine has been well tolerated in clinical trials. Somnolence appears to be its most frequent adverse effect (in 25% of patients). Other possible effects include dizziness, headache, agitation and rhinitis. Olanzapine has not been reported to affect sexual function. The drug also appears to have an excellent cardiovascular safety profile (minimal changes in resting vital signs, orthostatic blood pressure and ECG).

Table 45.5 lists the clinically significant drug interactions with olazapine.

Table 45.5
Olanzapine: Drug interactions

Drug	Interaction
Carbamazepine and smoking	• The metabolism of olanzapine may be induced by concomitant smoking or by carbamazepine tx
CNS depressants (including alcohol)	• Given the somnolence that olanzapine can produce, cautions should be used when it is given in combination with CNS depressants

Antipsychotic Drugs in the Treatment of Agitation and Aggression

While psychotropic drugs may be warranted in the treatment of anxiety, agitation or aggression associated with psychiatric disorders or organic brain syndromes, these drugs should always be used with great caution. Older patients presenting with any type of dementia may exhibit behaviours that indicate underlying anxiety, depression, confusion or cognitive disturbances. For some, delusions and hallucinations accompany the disorder; agitation and aggression may also occur. These behaviours are of concern to family and patient and to caregivers in all clinical settings.

The general principles that direct the decision to use drugs for such situations are the same as for all drug therapy: (1) an accurate diagnosis must be made, and (2) the choice of drug and the consequences for the patient's behaviour are reasonably certain to outweigh the risks of the drug and the probability of improvement by other measures.

Assessment of risk versus benefit can be achieved by answering several questions:

- What is the primary diagnosis?
- What are the concurrent problems?
- What drug is recommended, and what is the rationale for the choice?
- What will the outcome be if the drug is not used? What alternatives to drug therapy should be explored?
- How will the recommended drug interact with others the patient currently receives?
- What is the predicted interaction between the drug and the present disease state(s)?
- What are the potential adverse effects and reactions?
- Do the potential benefits outweigh the risks?

The first question relates to the accuracy of the diagnosis. The term dementia alone is inadequate; one must explore the underlying possibilities of anxiety, fear, depression, pain, agitation or aggression. If drug treatment is chosen, the agent must be efficacious in alleviating the underlying problem. The remaining questions are best illustrated in Tables 45.6 and 45.7, which present two case studies, each with a different outcome.

Box 45.3
Assessment of delirium

D	**D**rugs? depression?
E	**E**motional trauma, environment, electrolytes?
L	**AL**cohol? listen (to pt and family)
I	**I**nfection? injury?
R	**R**enal/respiratory disease?
I	**I**mpaired vision/hearing?
U	**U**nderlying nutritional deficiencies?
M	**M**etabolic factors?

Nursing Management

Table 45.8 (pages 516–517) describes the nursing management of the patient receiving antipsychotic drugs. Dosage details for individual drugs are given in Table 45.9 (pages 518–522).

Response to Clinical Challenge

1. The typical or traditional antipsychotic drugs are most likely to be successful because they treat the positive symptoms of schizophrenia, exhibited by Ken on admission.
2. Ken is receiving this drug to reduce his hallucinations and aggressiveness and to improve his sleep patterns. The goals of drug therapy are to reduce the acute episode, prevent recurrences and maintain the patient's highest level of functioning.
3. *Nursing diagnoses related to drug outcome:* individual ineffective coping; altered thought processes

Diagnoses related to reducing side effects: potential activity intolerance; potential altered body temperature; potential altered cardiac output; potential for injury; impaired physical mobility; sensory/perceptual alterations (visual); potential for altered urinary patterns: retention; potential for altered bowel patterns: constipation

Diagnoses related to education: knowledge deficit regarding drug regime and observations to note and report.
4. For injection technique for flupenthixol, see Box 45.4 (page 517).

Table 45.6
Case study: Choosing drug therapy

Assessment
- What is the primary dx?
- What are the concurrent problems?

Example

Helen, a 79-year-old woman living with her 83-year-old husband, has shown s/s of dementia during the past year. Her dx includes hypertension (managed with current drug tx), osteoarthritis of both knees, occasional episodes of heartburn. She has indicated paranoid thinking over the past week, becoming hostile towards strangers, accusing her daughter of stealing her money, and refusing to let her family physician examine her. The family is upset but supportive and want her to remain at home.

- What drug is recommended; rationale?
- What will be the outcome if not drug is used? What alternatives to drug tx should be (have been) explored?

Antipsychotics may be useful in alleviating the paranoia. The high-potency, dopamine-specific drugs have fewer sedative and anticholinergic effects but greater risk of EPS. Helen also requires assessment and tx of her knee pain. If drug tx is not used, there is a risk of increasing hostility, agitation and aggression. Paranoid thinking is frightening to Helen and her family. Assessment of possible underlying causes must also be completed.

- How will the potential drug interact with others the pt currently receives?

Antipsychotics may interact with antihypertensive drugs by causing excessive hypotension. If analgesic is ordered, risk for potential interaction should also be considered.

- What is the predicted interaction between the drug and the present disease states?

Antipsychotics may further reduce Helen's BP; pt will require monitoring.

- What are the potential adverse effects/reactions?

EPS; Helen must be closely monitored.

- Do the potential benefits outweigh the risks?

Helen will require closer monitoring of her BP and symptoms but may avoid hospitalization and/or injury to self or others. The decision rests with Helen, her family and physician. The potential benefits meet the criteria that drug tx is more likely to be effective than other measures at this time.

Table 45.7
Case study: Choosing alternative therapy

Assessment
- What is the primary dx?
- What are the concurrent problems?

Example

Fred, an 84-year-old in-patient, has shown increasingly agitated, disruptive and aggressive behaviour. His dx is dementia with past hx of depression, UTI and MI. Presently, he is anxious at mealtimes, refuses to bathe and rises several times at night. He has become incontinent. Recently, an hs sedative and day-time anxiolytic have been prescribed. The team is considering adding an antipsychotic drug.

- What drug is recommended; rationale?
- What will be the outcome if not drug is used? What alternatives to drug tx should be (have been) explored?

First, Fred requires a thorough assessment for underlying causes for his agitation. Drug tx is not recommended at this time until a dx is confirmed. Behavioural approaches are indicated to assist him with his anxiety and agitation regarding care and sleep disturbance.

- How will the potential drug interact with others the pt currently receives?

Reassess the use of the sedative; anxiolytic medications may be contributing to delirium.

- What is the predicted interaction between the drug and the present disease states?

A delirium, superimposed over the dementia, is challenging to diagnose. Drugs can contribute to the confusion and should be avoided. (See Box 45.3.)

- What are the potential adverse effects/reactions?

The most serious effect of drug tx at this time is misdiagnosis, leading to further inappropriate tx.

- Do the potential benefits outweigh the risks?

The recommended action should include: discontinuing the sedative and anxiolytic; assessment and tx of all underlying causes (e.g., possible recurrence of UTI) and behavioural strategies.

Table 45.8
Nursing management of the antipsychotics

Assessment of risk vs. benefit	Patient data	• Choice of drug depends on pt status and ability to tolerate usual adverse effects. Obtain baseline measures of BP (lying and standing) for all antipsychotic drugs. Blood tests (CBC) required for clozapine. Cautious use for elderly pts, glaucoma or hx of CV disease
		• *Pregnancy:* Risk category C (animal studies show adverse effects to fetus but human data are unknown or insufficient); benefits may be acceptable despite risks
	Drug data	• Choose drug depending on symptoms. Blood test (CBC) may be required • *Some serious drug interactions:* Confer with pharmacist • Most serious adverse effects are EPS, anticholinergic effects, agranulocytosis
Implementation	Rights of administration	• Using the "rights" helps prevent errors of administration
	Right route	• Give PO (most usual route) or IM; occasionally by IV
	Right time	• See Table 45.9. Note variation in dosage schedules among drugs in this class
	Right technique	• Most drugs in this class can cause contact dermatitis. Handle with care; avoid exposure to skin. If necessary, wear disposable gloves • IM administration should be deep into well-developed muscle mass, usually the gluteus. Do not mix with any other drugs. For depot injection, see Box 45.4 • IV administration requires knowledge of correct diluent and IV solution, correct dilution and rate of administration. Always refer to manufacturer's instructions for this route. Care must be taken to avoid extravasation because of tissue irritation
	Nursing therapeutics	• Injection usually stings; pain may be reduced by diluting solution with NS providing that total volume for injection does not exceed 3 mL. Gentle massage may help • Do not interchange dosage forms, e.g., hydrochloride, decanoate or enanthate • Compliance can be a major issue
	Patient/family teaching	• Pt's need for information may be influenced by serious illness, symptoms and ability to attend to information. Timing of teaching is important • Compliance and follow-up are essential factors in successful tx. Review principles of pt education in Chapter 3 • Pts/families should know warning signs/symptoms of possible toxicities of drugs. Report immediately: fever, sore throat, infection, signs of movement disorders (EPS) or NMS • Warn pts to avoid alcohol • *Discuss possibility of pregnancy:* Advise pt to notify physician; discuss birth control methods • A sample teaching outline is included in Box 45.5 (page 518)

Table 45.8 (continued)
Nursing management of the antipsychotics

Outcomes	Monitoring of progress	*Continually monitor:*

Continually monitor:
- Clinical response indicating tx success. For pts with psychosis, there should be an observed reduction in signs/symptoms such as decreased emotional and psychomotor activity, paranoia, hallucinations or delusions, reduced hostility, more purposeful behaviour and rational thought processes. When drug is used for troublesome s/s accompanying dementia, pt should display less aggression and hostility as well as reduced delusions or hallucinations
- Signs/symptoms of adverse reactions; document and report immediately to physician. Be particularly alert for EPS
- Blood tests to monitor WBC will be ordered weekly for clozapine and periodically for other drugs

---

Box 45.4
Depot injections of antipsychotics

Benefits

✔ Long-acting antipsychotics are well suited for long-term tx

✔ With depot injection there is lower rate of relapse

✔ Maintains steady drug levels from dose to dose

✔ Risk of adverse effects is reduced owing to total dose-per-unit-time level, which is lower with depot than with PO tx

Factors that contribute to injection-site complications
1. **Drug.** Fluspirilene (2 mg/mL ≠ 10 mg/mL aqueous base) is more likely to cause tissue damage than fluphenazine enanthate or decanoate or haloperidol decanoate (oily bases).

2. **Volume.** Volumes > 3 mL are associated with more tissue damage.

3. **Site.** Correct client positioning, proper site selection and rotation can reduce complications. The dorsogluteal (gluteus medius) is recommended because of large muscle mass and sustained rate of absorption Ventrogluteal (gluteus minimus) should be used for obese patients, as there is less subcutaneous fatty tissue overlying this muscle. Client should be positioned prone with feet turned in to relax gluteal muscle. If standing, client should bear most weight on opposite leg with toes turned inward (this also relaxes the gluteal muscle). Visually observe and palpate site. Look for indurations of twitching.

4. **Equipment.** Correct needle gauge and length are essential. Use appropriate equipment for the medication to ensure that drug enters muscle and not subcutaneous tissue (22-gauge for aqueous base; 21-gauge for oily base; 1.5", 2" or 2.5" needle, depending on pt size).

Procedure
1. **Calculate dosage.** Draw up medication just before administration, as it may interact with syringe if left standing for a long period of time.

2. **Draw 0.1–0.2 mL of air into syringe.** The air bubble will clear the needle bore of medication at the end of the injection procedure (0.25 mL of air is harmless to tissue).

3. **Aspirate.** If no blood appears, inject drug and air bubble slowly. (With all oily solutions, it is important to aspirate before injection to prevent inadvertent intravascular injection).

4. **Change needle.** Medication on outside of needle will cause tissue irritation.

Note: A test dose of 0.25 mL should be given. If well tolerated, then routine injection may be used.

The preparation of the dose will influence its duration of action (e.g., fluphenazine hydrochloride is given q6–8h; fluphenazine enanthate, q 1–3 weeks; fluphenazine decanoate, q 4–6 weeks).

Box 45.5
Patient teaching: Antipsychotics

✔ Discuss the purpose of drug tx with pts and their families. Distinguish between positive and negative signs/symptoms accompanying schizophrenia. When drugs are used for dementia, families need to understand that drug tx alone cannot improve thinking ability but can alleviate thought disorders such as delusions and hallucinations and may reduce aggressive behaviour

✔ Describe drug onset and duration of action. Advise pts that symptoms may not be immediately relieved but that improvement should be noted within a few days. (Titrate dosage according to response and side effects. Maximum benefits may not be reached for several weeks)

✔ Review drug schedule, including what to do if a dose is missed and the importance of taking these drugs with food or fluids to reduce GI irritation. Use of calendars, dosettes or other aids may help pt to remember drug schedule

✔ Pts will appreciate knowing which side effects to expect and actions to alleviate these symptoms (e.g., bowel routine to reduce constipation; sugarless gum, sour hard candy or mouthwash for dry mouth). Measures to prevent photosensitivity are important (see Box 45.2, page 510)

✔ Teach actions r/t hypotensive effects: e.g., rising slowly, avoiding hot showers or prolonged standing may reduce dizziness. Until response to drug is known, pts should avoid dangerous activities (e.g., driving, operating machinery)

✔ Emphasize importance of regular follow-up visits

Table 45.9
The antipsychotics: Drug doses

Drug Generic name (Trade names)	Dosage	Nursing alert
A. Typical Antipsychotics		
1. Low-Potency Phenothiazines chlorpromazine (Largactil, Thorazine)	**Oral:** *Adults:* 10–25 mg 2–4x daily; increase by 20–50 mg/day q3–4days (usual dose, 200 mg/day; up to 1–2 g/day). Extended-release capsules may be given 1–3x daily. *Children:* 0.55 mg/kg q4–6h. Reduce dosages for elderly **IM:** *Adults:* 25–50 mg initially; may be repeated in 1 h. Increase to max. of 400 mg q3–12h if needed (up to 1–2 g/day). *Children > 6 months:* 0.55 mg/kg (15 mg/m^2) q6–8h (not to exceed 40 mg/day in children 6 months to 5 years, or 75 mg/day in children 5–12 years)	• Handle drug with care to prevent contact dermatitis • **Oral:** Give with food or liquid to reduce irritation. Dilute concentrate in 120 mL of any liquid just prior to administration • **Parenteral:** Pt should remain lying for 30 min due to risk of hypotension. Give deep IM to reduce pain. May be diluted with NaCl or procaine, if ordered. Do not use if solution contains precipitate
mesoridazine (Serentil)	**Oral:** Schizophrenia: 75–400 mg daily. Usual dose: 150 mg/day in divided doses. Mental retardation and chronic brain syndrome: 75–300 mg daily. Usual dose: 100 mg/day in divided doses	• Give with food or milk to reduce gastric irritation

Table 45.9 (continued)
The antipsychotics: Drug doses

Drug Generic name (Trade names)	Dosage	Nursing alert
A. Typical Antipsychotics		
1. Low-Potency Phenothiazines (cont'd)		
promazine (Sparine)	**Oral/IM:** Psychoses: *Adults:* 10–200 mg q4–6h up to 1000 mg/day. *Children > 12 years:* 10–25 mg q4–6h. Severe agitation: Adults: 50–150 mg initially; if required, additional doses may be given after 30 min up to a total dose of 300 mg, then maint. dose of 10–200 mg q4–6 h prn (not to exceed 1 g/24 h)	• **Oral:** Give with food or milk to reduce gastric irritation • **IM:** Give deep into large muscle mass. Avoid exposure to skin; can cause contact dermatitis
thioridazine (Mellaril)	Psychosis: **Oral:** *Adults/children > 12 years:* 50–100 mg tid initially; maintenance, 10–200 mg qid up to 800 mg/day. Depressive neuroses with anxiety, fears, depression; anxiety in the elderly: *Adults:* 25 mg tid (range, 20–200 mg/day). Behavioural problems in children: *Children > 2 years:* 0.25–3 mg/kg/day in 2–3 divided doses (10–25 mg bid or tid)	• Handle with care to prevent contact dermatitis • Give with food or fluid to reduce irritation. Dilute concentrate with water or juice just prior to administration. Shake suspension well before use
2. Mid/High-Potency Phenothiazine and Phenothiazine-like Drugs		
fluphenazine HCl (Moditen HCl, Permitil, Prolixin)	**Oral:** *Adults:* 0.5–10 mg/day in divided doses q6–8h initially; maint. dose, 1–5 mg/day. Initial dose in elderly or debilitated pts, 1–2.5 mg/day **IM:** *Adults:* 1.5–2.5 mg q6–8h. Initial dose in elderly or debilitated pts, 1–2.5 mg/day	• Handle with care to prevent contact dermatitis • Dilute concentrate into liquid (without caffeine) just prior to administration. Note that the concentrate form is 10x more concentrated than the elixir. Do not confuse with the decanoate or enanthate forms. Do not use solutions that contain precipitate. Drug should be protected from light
fluphenazine decanoate (Modecate)	**IM/SC:** *Adults:* 12.5–25 mg initially. May be slowly increased as needed (not to exceed 100 mg/dose). Some may require q4–6weeks dosing	• Handle with care to prevent contact dermatitis • See instructions for depot injections, Box 45.4 (page 517) • Do not use solutions that contain precipitate. Drug should be protected from light. Do not confuse with enanthate or hydrochloride forms
fluphenazine enanthate (Moditen Enanthate)	**IM/SC:** *Adults:* 25 mg q2weeks. May be slowly increased as needed (not to exceed 100 mg/dose). Some may require q1–3weeks dosing	• Handle with care to prevent contact dermatitis • Do not use solutions that contain precipitate. Drug should be protected from light. Do not confuse decanoate or hydrochloride forms • See instructions for depot injections, Box 45.4 (page 517)

(cont'd on next page)

Table 45.9 (continued)
The antipsychotics: Drug doses

Drug Generic name (Trade names)	Dosage	Nursing alert
2. Mid/High-Potency Phenothiazine and Phenothiazine-like Drugs (cont'd)		
fluspirilene (Imap, Imap Forte)	**IM:** Initially, 2–3 mg once a week. If akathisia does not develop after first dose, increase weekly by 1–2 mg prn. Optimal dose range, 2–10 mg once a week. Max., 15 mg/week	• Handle with care to prevent contact dermatitis • Do not use solutions that contain precipitate. Drug should be protected from light. Do not confuse decanoate or hydrochloride forms Give only IM, deep into muscle. Use 5-cm, 21-gauge needle for pts of normal weight; 6.5-cm needle for larger or obese pts. Injections given at least weekly
perphenazine (Trilafon)	**Oral** (tablets): Moderately disturbed, nonhospitalized pts: 4–8 mg tid, intially; reduce ASAP to minimum effective dosage. Max. in ambulatory pts, 24 mg. Severely disturbed, hospitalized pts and those with resistant mental or emotional disorders may require > 24 mg/day. **Oral** (liquid concentrate): In hospitalized pts, 8–16 mg bid–qid **IM:** Psychotic conditions: Usually, 5 mg; may repeat 1 6h. 10 mg initially may be required for control of symptoms in severe conditions. Total daily dosage should not exceed 15 mg in ambulatory pts or 30 mg in hospitalized pts	• **PO:** Dilute 5 mL oral concentrate into 60 mL liquid (water, milk, juice except apple) just prior to administration. Do not mix with beverages that contain caffeine (coffee or colas), tannics (tea) or pectinates (apple juice). Store in amber container to protect from light • **IM:** Give deep into large muscle mass. Avoid exposure to skin; can cause contact dermatitis
prochlorperazine (Stemetil)	Psychomotor agitation; psychoses: *Adults:* **Oral:** 5–10 mg 3–4x daily; increase prn (not to exceed 150 mg/day). **IM:** 10–20 mg q2–4h prn initially, then 10–20 mg q4–6h (may give up to q1h; not to exceed 150–200 mg/day. *Children:* **Oral, rectal:** *2–12 years* — 2.5 mg bid or tid (not to exceed 10 mg on first day; not to exceed 25 mg/day in children 6–12 years, or 20 mg/ day in children 2–5 years)	• Handle with care to avoid contact dermatitis • Do not crush or chew sustained-release forms. Give with food or fluids to reduce irritation • **IM:** Injections are administered deep into the buttocks. Pt should remain lying for 30 min due to risk for hypotension. Do not use solution that is deeply discoloured or contains a precipitate
pimozide (Orap)	**Oral:** Initially, 2–4 mg od, with weekly increments of 2–4 mg prn or until excessive adverse effects occur. Average maint. dose, 6 mg/day. Usual range, 2–12 mg/day. Max., 20 mg/day	• Give single dose in a.m.
trifluoperazine HCl (Stelazine)	Psychoses: *Adults:* **Oral:** 2–5 mg bid (up to 40 mg/day). **IM:** 1–2 mg q4–6h (up to 10 mg/day). *Children:* **Oral:** *6–12 years* — 1 mg 1–2x daily (up to 15 mg/day). **IM:** 1 mg 1–2x daily	• **IM:** Give deep into well-developed muscle (buttocks). Massage gently. Injection stings • **PO:** Dilute concentrate into any liquid just prior to administration • Handle with care to prevent contact dermatitis

Table 45.9 (continued)
The antipsychotics: Drug doses

Drug Generic name (Trade names)	Dosage	Nursing alert
3. Thioxanthenes thiothixene (Navane)	*Adults:* **Oral:** Initially, 5–10 mg daily. Gradually increase to optimally effective level (not to exceed 60 mg/day). Optimal range, 15–30 mg daily. Reduce dose for elderly	• Handle with care to avoid contact dermatitis • **PO:** Give with food or milk to reduce irritation. Dilute solution with any liquid prior to administration
4. Butyrophenones haloperidol (Haldol)	**Adults:** *Oral:* 0.5–5 mg bid or tid. Severe symptoms may require up to 100 mg/day. **IM:** 2–5 mg q1–8h, not to exceed 100 mg/day. **IV:** 0.5–50 mg; may be repeated in 30 min. Reduce dose for elderly. *Children:* **Oral:** Non-psychotic disorders and Tourette's syndrome: 50–75 µg/kg/day in 1–3 divided doses	• **IM:** Do not confuse with haloperidol decanoate (Haldol-LA®). Give deep into well-developed muscle • **PO:** Give with food or milk to reduce irritation. May give concentrate undiluted or diluted with liquid (without caffeine)
haloperidol decanoate (Haldol-LA)	**IM:** *Adults:* 10–15x previous daily oral dose, but not to exceed 100 mg initially. Given monthly (not to exceed 300 mg/month)	• Use depot injection technique (see Box 45.4, page 517) • Do not confuse with Haldol® injection
5. Dibenzoxazepine loxapine (Loxitane, Loxapac)	*Adults:* **Oral:** 10 mg bid; may be increased gradually over first 7–10 days prn. Usual maint. dose, 15–25 mg 2–4x daily. Severely ill may require up to 50 mg/day initially and maint. doses up to 250 mg/day. **IM:** 12.5–50 mg q4–6h prn (up to 250 mg/day)	• **PO:** Give with food or milk to reduce irritation. Dilute solution with juice prior to administration • **IM:** Inject deep into well-developed muscle
B. Atypical Antipsychotics clozapine (Clozaril)	*Adults:* **Oral:** Day 1: 12.5 mg od or bid. Day 2: 25 mg od or bid. If well tolerated, increase in increments of 25–50 mg/day, achieving a target dose of 300–450 mg/day by the end of 2 weeks. Subsequent increases should be made no more than 1–2x weekly, in increments not to exceed 100 mg. Dosage range, 300–600 mg/day in divided doses. Total daily dosage may be divided unevenly, with a larger portion hs	• Requires weekly hematological testing prior to delivery of the following week's supply of medication. Consult manufacturer's information
olanzapine (Zyprexa)	**Oral:** *Adults:* Initially, 5–10 mg od. Adjust prn in increments/decrements of 5 mg/day at intervals of not less than 1 week. 15 md/day or greater is recommended only after clinical assessment. Elderly or debilitated pts: Use with caution. Recommended initial dose is 5 mg in pts who have a predisposition to hypotensive reactions	• Give without regard to meals. Titrate dose to prevent severe hypotension

(cont'd on next page)

Table 45.9 (continued)
The antipsychotics: Drug doses

Drug Generic name (Trade names)	Dosage	Nursing alert
B. Atypical Antipsychotics (cont'd)		
risperidone (Risperdal)	*Adults:* **Oral:** Day 1: 1 mg bid. Day 2: 2 mg bid. Day 3: 3 mg bid. Further dosage adjustments, if indicated, should generally occur at intervals of not less than 1 week (increments/decrements of 1 mg bid are recommended). Max., 16 mg/day. *Geriatrics:* **Oral:** May require less drug, starting with 0.5 mg bid to a max. of 3 mg/day	• Titrate dose to prevent severe hypotension

Further Reading

Cohen LJ. Risperidone. *Pharmacotherapy* 1994;14:253–265.

Drugs for psychiatric disorders. *Medical Letter on Drugs and Therapeutics* 1994;36:89.

Ereshefsy L, Lacombe S. Pharmacological profile of risperidone. *Can J Psychiatry* 1993;38 (suppl 3):S80–S88.

Glod CA. Psychopharmacology and clinical practice. *Nurs Clin North Am* 1991;26(2):375–400.

Grant S, Fitton A. Risperidone. A review of pharmacology and therapeutic potential in the treatment of schizophrenia. *Drugs* 1994; 48:253–273.

Mellow A, et al. Sodium valproate in the treatment of behavioral disturbance in dementia. *J Geriatr Psychiatry Neurol* 1993;6:205–209.

Pollard A. Tranquilizing actions. *Nurs Times* 1994;11:34–46.

Risperidone for schizophrenia. *Medical Letter on Drugs and Therapeutics* 1994;36:33–44.

Staab W. Neuroleptic malignant syndrome: critical factors. *Crit Care Nurs* 1994;14(6):77–81.

Update on clozapine. *Medical Letter on Drugs and Therapeutics* 1994;35:16.

CHAPTER 46

Drugs for Mood Disorders

Topics Discussed
- Drug treatment of depression: TCAs, SSRIs, MAOIs
- Miscellaneous antidepressants
- Treatment of manic-depressive illness: Lithium
- For each drug discussed: Mechanism of action and pharmacologic effects, therapeutic uses, adverse effects
- Electroconvulsive therapy
- Treatment of depression in the older adult
- Nursing management

Drugs Discussed
Tricyclic Antidepressants (TCAs) and Analogues:
amitriptyline (am-ee-**trip**-tih-leen)
amoxapine (ah-**mox**-ah-peen)
clomipramine (kloe-**mip**-rah-meen)
desipramine (dez-**ip**-rah-meen)
doxepin (**dox**-eh-pin)
imipramine (im-**ip**-rah-meen)
maprotiline (mah-**proe**-ti-leen)
nortriptyline (nor-**trip**-tih-leen)
protriptyline (proe-**trip**-tih-leen)
trimipramine (try-**mip**-rah-meen)

Selective Serotonin Reuptake Inhibitors (SSRIs):
fluoxetine (flew-**ox**-eh-teen)
fluvoxamine (flew-**vox**-ah-meen)
nefazodone (nef-**az**-oh-done)
paroxetine (par-**ox**-eh-teen)
sertraline (**ser**-trah-leen)

Monoamine Oxidase Inhibitors (MAOIs):
moclobemide (moe-**kloe**-beh-myde)
phenelzine (**fenn**-ell-zeen)
tranylcypromine (tran-ill-**sip**-roe-meen)

Miscellaneous Antidepressants:
bupropion (byoo-**pro**-pee-on)
trazodone (**traz**-oh-done)
venlafaxine (ven-la-**fax**-een)

Drugs for the Treatment of Manic-Depressive Illness:
carbamazepine (kar-ba-**mazz**-eh-peen)
valproic acid (val-**proe**-ik)
lithium (**lith**-ee-um)

Drug Treatment of Depression

Depressive illness is the most common psychiatric condition, affecting as many as 10% to 15% of the population. The most serious outcome is suicide, which is a leading cause of death for many age groups in North America. Current treatment for depression includes drug therapy with the choice of a variety of classes of antidepressants, electroconvulsive therapy (ECT) and psychotherapy, alone or in combination.

Depression is characterized by feelings of sadness, despair or discouragement and loss of interest in one's usual daily activities. These alterations

Clinical Challenge

Consider this clinical challenge as you read through this chapter. The response to the challenge appears on page 542.

Clinical Challenge # 1

Mr. R., a 71-year-old man, is being discharged from the in-patient unit to a day hospital program. He has a 20-year history of depression and a variety of previous treatments including amitriptyline, lithium and ECT. He has been hospitalized on two occasions for suicidal ideation, and has admitted himself today through the Emergency Department.

Biophysical assessment: weight, 80 kg; height, 175 cm; no known allergies; lab values normal for age; borderline hypertension (135/90); pulse ranges from 74–90 and regular. Slight hypothyroidism.

Psychosocial assessment: lives in a seniors' lodge; no relatives in city; explains illness as "something that runs in the family." *Compliance:* has discontinued medications on his own in the past. States that drugs cause many problems such as difficulty voiding, lethargy and a very dry mouth. On admission, demonstrates inability to concentrate, lack of interest in environment and appearance, insomnia, poor appetite, and very slow speech. Good friend died recently.

Medication order: sertraline (Zoloft®) 50 mg/day.

1. What is the best administration schedule for the sertraline?
2. What are the most likely adverse effects? What actions would you take to reduce these?
3. What observations would indicate that the drug is effective?
4. You advise Mr. R. that he should notify staff at the day hospital if he develops symptoms of adverse reactions. What symptoms should he observe for?

---

in mood occur daily for a period of at least two weeks. Depression may not always be precipitated by stressful life events but can unexpectedly overwhelm a patient and his or her family. It is essential to differentiate depression from dementia (discussed in Chapter 45) and from normal grief reactions that occur in response to a major loss in life, such as the death of a loved one or a major illness.

Depressed people often report loss of appetite, insomnia, lack of interest, loss of concentration, weight loss or gain, intense feelings of guilt, worthlessness, hopelessness and thoughts of death. For some, suicidal ideation and behaviour may consume their waking moments. Immediate and effective treatment is not only important; it can be life-saving.

Drug treatment of depression has changed significantly in the past thirty years. Prior to 1957, amphetamine was often used. Although it produces central nervous system excitation and abolishes depression, its use created serious problems of drug dependence and profound depression upon drug withdrawal. The introduction of imipramine in 1957 provided the first of a new group of antidepressants called the *tricyclic antidepressants* (TCAs). These drugs revolutionized the treatment of depression. Now, for the first time, physicians could effectively treat depressed patients without fear of producing drug dependence. On the other side of the coin, TCAs have sedative, anticholinergic and hypotensive effects, and these actions frequently reduce patient compliance.

At the same time as TCAs were being introduced in the late 1950s and early 1960s, a group of drugs called *monoamine oxidase inhibitors* (MAOIs) were also being used. These frequently proved successful. However, they were often most toxic, particularly to patients who ate or drank foods containing tyramine (e.g., cheeses, wines and fish). Because of the need to constrain the diet of patients receiving MAOIs, many physicians restricted their use to people who failed to respond to treatment with TCAs.

Most recently, a new group of drugs, called selective serotonin reuptake inhibitors (SSRIs), has been introduced for the treatment of depression. Fluoxetine (Prozac®) was the first of this group to be approved for sale in North America. Several other drugs soon followed. The SSRIs have a different pharmacologic profile than either the TCAs or the MAOIs. Because they do not have significant sedative, anticholinergic or hypotensive effects, the SSRIs are often better accepted by patients.

This chapter reviews the basic pharmacologic effects, therapeutic uses and adverse effects of TCAs, SSRIs and MAOIs. These drugs have provided relief for millions of people plagued with depression. However, many of these drugs also have severe adverse effects and can even kill. Nurses should be aware of the benefits and risks of drug therapy. They should be able to recognize both improvement in patients as well as the appearance of drug-induced toxic reactions.

Tricyclic Antidepressants

Mechanism of action and pharmacologic effects. Tricyclic antidepressants (TCAs; these include amitriptyline, amoxapine, clomipramine, desipramine, doxepin, imipramine, nortriptyline and protriptyline) and maprotiline, a drug that is pharmacologically similar to the TCAs, elevate mood, increase physical activity and the activities of daily living, improve appetite and sleep patterns, and reduce morbid preoccupation in 60% to 70% of patients with major depression. The antidepressant response to these agents often is gradual (one to six weeks, or more).

Little is known about the cause(s) of depression or the means by which drugs relieve it. It has been speculated that depression is caused by a reduced release and action of norepinephrine and/or 5-hydroxytryptamine (5-HT, serotonin) in the brain. If that is the case, then increasing norepinephrine and/or 5-HT concentrations acting on brain receptors should reverse depression.

The best way to achieve this increase is to block neuronal reuptake of these substances (Figure 46.1). Neuronal reuptake refers to the abil-

Figure 46.1
Mechanism of action of tricyclic antidepressants

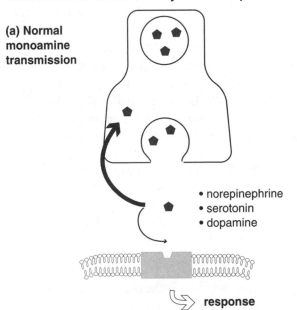

(a) Normal monoamine transmission

• norepinephrine
• serotonin
• dopamine

response

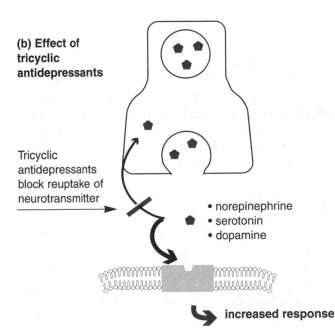

(b) Effect of tricyclic antidepressants

Tricyclic antidepressants block reuptake of neurotransmitter

• norepinephrine
• serotonin
• dopamine

increased response

Source: Harvey RA, Champe PC. *Lippincott's Illustrated Review: Pharmacology.* New York: J.P. Lippincott; 1992. Reproduced with permission.

Table 46.1
Properties of some tricyclic antidepressants

Generic name (trade name)	Usual oral dose[1]	Sedation[2]	Anticholinergic effects[2]
imipramine (Janimine®, Tofranil®)	Initially, 25 mg tid; incr. prn to 150 mg/day	++	++
clomipramine (Anafranil®)	Initially 25 mg tid; incr. prn to 150 mg/day	++	++
desipramine (Norpramin®, Pertofrane®)	Initially, 75–150 mg/day in divided doses. More severe cases may require up to 200 mg/day	+	+
amitriptyline (Elavil®, Endep®)	Initially, 25 mg tid; incr. prn to 150 mg/day	+++	+++
nortriptyline (Aventyl®, Pamelor®)	30–100 mg/day in divided doses	++	++
doxepin (Adapin®, Sinequan®)	Initially, 25 mg tid; incr. prn to 150 mg/day	+++	+++
protriptyline (Vivactil®, Triptil®)	15–30 mg/day in divided doses	0	++
maprotiline (Ludiomil®)	Initially, 75 mg/day in 2 or 3 divided doses, incr. prn gradually to 150 mg/day	+++	+/0

[1] Approximate doses for adult outpatients. Smaller doses are required for the young or elderly. Seriously ill, hospitalized patients may require higher doses. (For more detailed dosage schedules, see Table 46.15, pages 543–547.)

[2] 0 = none; + = slight; ++ = moderate; +++ = high

ity of nerve endings to reabsorb the neurotransmitter previously released. It is the major physiological mechanism for removing neurotransmitters from their receptors and terminating their actions. If the neurotransmitter — in this case either norepinephrine or 5-HT — is reabsorbed by the nerve, it cannot stimulate its receptors. If a drug blocks neuronal reuptake, it will raise the concentration of the neurotransmitter around receptors and increase the effect of the transmitter.

TCAs inhibit the neuronal reuptake of norepinephrine and serotonin, and this action plays a role in their effects. The story does not end here, however. TCAs inhibit neuronal reuptake from day 1 of treatment, but they require two to three weeks, or longer, to relieve depression. Obviously, because the time to treat depression does not correlate with onset of inhibition of neuronal reuptake, blocking reuptake is only the first step in the process of modifying mood. The changes in brain function that follow the block in neuronal reuptake are responsible for the time taken to produce relief. It is speculated that the block in neuronal

reuptake leads to a down-regulation or subsensitization of beta adrenergic receptors. This down-regulation of beta receptors requires two to three weeks to occur and correlates better with the relief of depression. Perhaps in another decade we can carry this story further and finally explain exactly how TCAs work.

TCAs also block alpha$_1$ adrenergic receptors, histamine (H$_1$) receptors and muscarinic receptors. These drugs sedate patients, and the sedative effects are attributed to their antihistaminic actions. Table 46.1 shows that the sedative and anticholinergic actions differ among the various TCAs.

It might seem unusual that antidepressant drugs sedate patients; one would expect them to have a stimulating effect. This is one of the paradoxes of some of these drugs. Doxepin and amitriptyline are the most potent antihistamines, as well as the best sedatives. Sedation is seen after the administration of the first dose or two.

The anticholinergic effects of TCAs include blurred vision, dry mouth, constipation and urinary retention. Amitriptyline and doxepin are the most potent anticholinergics; desipramine and protriptyline the weakest.

TCAs have marked effects on the cardiovascular system. Orthostatic hypotension is the most frequent and troublesome adverse effect seen with therapeutic doses. At normal doses, TCAs are antiarrhythmic. However, at high doses they block norepinephrine reuptake by cardiac sympathetic nerves and increase the risk for cardiac arrhythmias. Maprotiline has minimal or no effects on the cardiovascular system.

Therapeutic uses. Tricyclic antidepressants are used to treat major depression. They are most effective in patients suffering from more severe depression, particularly with greater vegetative disturbance and melancholia. A period of one to six weeks may be required before patients improve significantly. Little evidence can be found to demonstrate that one drug is more effective than the others. Usually, the more sedative drugs (amitriptyline and doxepin) are preferred for anxious or agitated depressives, while the less sedative drugs (protriptyline) are better for patients with psychomotor withdrawal.

Adverse effects. Autonomic effects constitute the majority of adverse reactions to tricyclic antidepressants. Orthostatic hypotension is the most common cardiovascular effect. Other effects seen with increasing doses are palpitation, tachycardia, cardiac arrhythmias and ECG abnormalities. Ventricular arrhythmias cause great concern. Ventricular tachyarrhythmias can be produced, and ventricular fibrillation is a cause of death in overdoses. As stated previously, maprotiline has minimal cardiovascular effects.

The anticholinergic actions of TCAs produce dry mouth and decreased sweating, constipation, urinary hesitancy and delayed ejaculation.

Confusion, seen most often in patients over the age of forty, is particularly likely to occur if the patient is receiving concomitant treatment with drugs that also possess anticholinergic effects, such as antipsychotics or antiparkinsonian agents. Tremors may also occur. The involvement of the sympathetic nervous system is suggested by the fact that propranolol, a beta adrenergic blocker, has been used with some success to reduce them.

Weight gain may be seen in patients receiving therapy with TCAs. Depending on the original status of the patient, this may or may not be an adverse effect. The reason for this effect may be partly due to the remission of depression. The drugs may also directly stimulate appetite.

Table 46.2 on the next page lists the clinically significant drug interactions with TCAs.

Selective Serotonin Reuptake Inhibitors

Mechanism of action and pharmacologic effects. The drugs fluoxetine (Prozac®), fluvoxamine (Luvox®), nefazodone (Serzone®), paroxetine (Paxil®), and sertraline (Zoloft®) inhibit selectively the neuronal reuptake of serotonin (5-hydroxytryptamine, 5-HT). They have little or no effect on the neuronal reuptake of norepinephrine.

The antidepressant action of selective serotonin uptake inhibitors (SSRIs) is presumed to be related to the inhibition of the neuronal uptake of serotonin (5-HT). Like the tricyclic drugs, SSRIs take one to six weeks to relieve depression.

Therapeutic uses. SSRIs are approved for the symptomatic relief of depressive illness. Their efficacy has been established primarily in moderately and severely depressed out-patients. The drugs may be particularly useful in patients with concurrent illness such as hypertension, coronary artery disease, prostatic enlargement or narrow-angle glaucoma; in those who can not tolerate the adverse effects of TCAs; and in the elderly.

Adverse effects. The most frequent adverse effects of SSRIs are headache, tremor, nausea, diarrhea, insomnia, agitation and nervousness. SSRIs may cause either agitation or sedation. These drugs do not have the anticholinergic, antihistaminic or alpha$_1$-receptor blocking activity of tricyclic antidepressants. As a result, they are less likely to cause orthostatic hypotension, tachycardia, delayed cardiac conduction, seizures, blurred vision or dry mouth (which may lead to serious dental problems). Although they generally do not cause weight gain in the short term, as the TCAs often do, with continued treatment patients taking SSRIs may also gain weight. Anorgasmia in both men and women and ejaculatory disturbances appear to be more common with these drugs than with tricyclic antidepressants.

Table 46.2
Tricyclic antidepressants: Drug interactions

Drug	Interaction
Alcohol	• Alcohol plus a TCA may produce greater than expected CNS depression and impairment in psychomotor skills
Amphetamines	• Amphetamines release norepinephrine and have enhanced effect in pts receiving a TCA
Anticholinergics	• Anticholinergics may show increased effects in the presence of a TCA (e.g., hyperpyrexia, paralytic ileus)
Antihistamines	• Antihistamines may show enhanced CNS depression in the presence of a TCA
Antipsychotics	• Antipsychotics may show enhanced CNS depression in the presence of a TCA
Barbiturates	• Barbiturates may potentiate the CNS depressant effects of TCAs. Chronic use of barbiturates, particularly phenobarbital, may stimulate the metabolism of TCAs
Benzodiazepines	• Benzodiazepines may show enhanced effects in the presence of TCAs with pronounced sedative properties, such as amitriptyline
Clonidine	• Clonidine plus desipramine may increase BP
Epinephrine and levarterenol	• Epinephrine and levarterenol given by IV infusions to subjects receiving imipramine can result in a 2- to 4-fold increase in the pressor response. These drugs should be used only with great caution in pts receiving TCAs
Guanethidine	• Guanethidine has a reduced antihypertensive effect in the presence of TCAs because TCAs inhibit the uptake of these drugs into adrenergic neurons
Lithium carbonate	• Lithium carbonate and a TCA can produce hyperpyrexia
MAOIs	• The use of MAOIs with TCAs is contraindicated. Pts may suffer hyperpyretic crises or severe convulsive seizures when such drugs are combined. Potentiation of adverse effects can be serious or even fatal
Narcotics	• TCAs with pronounced sedative effects may increase the CNS depression produced by narcotics

The possibility of overdosage is a serious concern in patients with depression. In this respect SSRIs appear to be much safer than the TCAs, which can cause lethal cardiac toxicity.

Table 46.3 lists the clinically significant drug interactions with SSRIs.

Monoamine Oxidase Inhibitors

Mechanism of action and pharmacologic effects. Monoamine oxidase (MAO) is a term used to refer to a group of enzymes widely distributed throughout the body that oxidatively deaminate and inactivate norepinephrine, dopamine and 5-hydroxytryptamine (5-HT; serotonin). Inhibition of monoamine oxidase increases brain levels of these neurotransmitters (Figure 46.2, page 530).

The monoamine oxidase inhibitors currently available for use in North America are phenelzine (Nardil®), tranylcypromine (Parnate®) and moclobemide (Manerix®). It is generally believed that these drugs relieve depression by increasing brain norepinephrine and/or 5-HT levels. This explanation is complicated, however, by the fact that enzyme inhibition appears after a few doses of the drug, but the antidepressant effects are seen only after two to four weeks of treatment.

Monoamine oxidase is currently subclassified into two types, A and B, which differ in their substrate specificity. Moclobemide is a reversible inhibitor of MAO-A. The estimated MAO-A inhibition is short-lasting (maximum, 24 h). Because of moclobemide's relatively short duration of action, it may be possible to control patients better with this drug than the other MAO inhibitors. Furthermore, the fact that moclobemide inhibits only MAO-A reduces its side effects and dangers in the presence of tyramine (see Interaction of Drugs and Foods with MAOIs, page 530).

Table 46.3
Selective serotonin reuptake inhibitors: Drug interactions

Drug	Interaction
Alprazolam	• Nefazodone can increase the plasma levels and effects of alprazolam. If alprazolam is coadministered with nefazodone, a reduction in the alprazolam dosage may be appropriate
Anticoagulants, oral	• Paroxetine should be administered with great caution to pts receiving oral anticoagulants because preliminary data suggest that combining paroxetine with warfarin may increase bleeding in the presence of unaltered prothrombin times
Anticonvulsants	• The coadministration of paroxetine with anticonvulsants may be associated with increased incidence of adverse experiences
Antidepressants, tricyclic	• There have been greater than 2-fold increases of previously stable plasma levels of other antidepressants when fluoxetine or fluvoxamine has been administered in combination with these drugs
Cimetidine	• Cimetidine, and other drugs that decrease drug metabolizing enzymes, can increase the plasma levels of paroxetine
Diazepam	• The half-life of concurrently administered diazepam may be prolonged in some pts taking fluoxetine
Drugs that are eliminated by metabolism	• Fluvoxamine may prolong the elimination of drugs that are metabolized by oxidation in the liver, and clinically significant interaction is more likely when the second agent, such as warfarin, phenytoin or theophylline, has a narrow therapeutic index
Lithium	• There have been reports of both increased and decreased lithium levels when lithium was used concomitantly with fluoxetine. Cases of lithium toxicity have been reported. Lithium levels should be monitored when these drugs are administered concomitantly. Lithium may enhance the serotonergic effects of fluvoxamine, thus these combinations should be used with caution
MAO inhibitors	• MAOIs are contraindicated in pts receiving SSRIs. SSRIs should not be administered within 14 days of discontinuing therapy with an MAOI
Triazolam	• Nefazodone can increase the plasma levels and effects of triazolam. The concomitant use of these two drugs should be avoided
Tryptophan	• Tryptophan should be used only with caution in conjunction with an SSRI because of the possibility of adverse reactions, such as agitation, restlessness and GI distress

In contrast to the sedative effects of TCAs, monoamine oxidase inhibitors (MAOIs) stimulate normal individuals. They also suppress REM sleep and are used to treat narcolepsy.

Therapeutic uses. MAOIs are usually used only after TCAs or SSRIs have failed to treat depression. Most physicians consider the latter two more effective and, with the exception of moclobemide, less toxic. For its part, moclobemide appears to be as effective and is well tolerated compared with TCAs such as imipramine and clomipramine. The good therapeutic control possible with moclobemide and the low incidence of drug interactions make it useful in the elderly.

Adverse effects. Phenelzine and tranylcypromine stimulate the central nervous system to produce tremors, insomnia and agitation. Convulsions have been reported occasionally, along with hallucinations and confusion.

Autonomic adverse effects caused by phenelzine and tranylcypromine include orthostatic hypotension. This can be treated immediately by having the patient lie down. If hypotension is severe, it may be necessary to reduce the dose of the drug or withdraw it entirely. Phenelzine and tranylcypromine can also decrease cholinergic stimulation, resulting in dry mouth, constipation, difficulty in urination, delayed ejaculation and impotence.

Figure 46.2
Mechanism of action of MAOIs

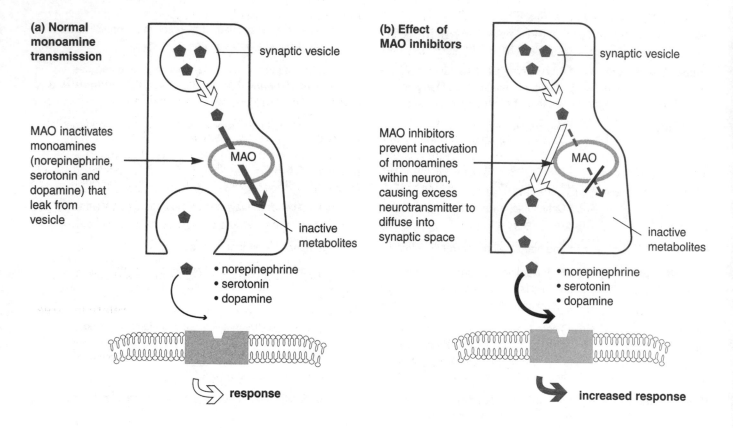

Source: Harvey RA, Champe PC. *Lippincott's Illustrated Review: Pharmacology.* New York: J.P. Lippincott; 1992. Reproduced with permission.

A low incidence of hepatotoxicity is reported with phenelzine and tranylcypromine. Its incidence does not appear to be related to duration of therapy or dose of the drug.

Acute overdose with either phenelzine or tranylcypromine presents very serious problems to both the patient and the medical team. Symptoms may be absent for several hours after ingestion of a large number of tablets and then proceed suddenly to severe fever, agitation, hyperexcitable reflexes, hallucination and increase or decrease in blood pressure. Treatment is largely symptomatic.

Moclobemide is generally well tolerated. The most common adverse effects seen are dry mouth, dizziness, headache, somnolence, nausea and insomnia. The incidence of anticholinergic side effects and orthostatic hypotension, common with TCAs, is less with moclobemide.

Interaction of drugs and foods with MAOIs. MAOIs that inhibit both MAO-A and MAO-B decrease the inactivation of sympathomimetic amines, leading to a potentiated adrenergic effect. The classical example of this type of interaction involves the ingestion of foods containing the chemical tyramine (e.g., cheese, beer, wine, pickled herring, snails, chicken liver and coffee in large quantities).

Tyramine is normally inactivated quickly by monoamine oxidase in the liver. When monoamine oxidase is inhibited, tyramine is not destroyed. Instead, it enters sympathetic nerves and releases norepinephrine, which produces a generalized vasoconstriction. The resulting hypertensive crisis may be characterized by a severe headache. Death can occur from an intracranial hemorrhage.

Moclobemide is less likely to block the metabolism of tyramine and the ingestion of tyramine, in amounts less than 100 mg, is highly unlikely to produce a clinically relevant elevation in blood pressure. Therefore, compared with the traditional MAOIs (phenelzine and tranylcypromine), there are no special dietary restrictions with moclobemide, and it may be taken with or without meals.

MAOIs should not be used with TCAs. By reducing both the reuptake of norepinephrine and, its enzymatic inactivation, the concomitant use of these drugs can produce a hyperpyretic crisis or severe convulsions.

MAOIs decrease the metabolism and increase the actions of a large number of drugs, such as narcotics, barbiturates, many anesthetics and anticholinergics. In the absence of an emergency, it is advisable to delay surgery for a few weeks to withdraw the patient from treatment with the MAOI.

Table 46.4 lists the clinically significant drug interactions with phenelzine and tranylcypromine, while Table 46.5 on the next page lists those with moclobemide.

Miscellaneous Antidepressants (Trazodone, Venlafaxine and Bupropion)

Trazodone, venlafaxine and bupropion share some properties with tricyclic antidepressants (TCAs) and selective serotonin reuptake inhibitors (SSRIs). However, each drug also differs significantly from the TCAs or SSRIs. As a result, we are discussing them under the general umbrella of miscellaneous antidepressants.

Trazodone (Desyrel®)

Mechanism of action and pharmacologic effects. In some respects, trazodone is similar to the SSRIs. Like these drugs, trazodone inhibits the neuronal reuptake of serotonin. However, trazodone has additional effects. It stimulates the neuronal release of norepinephrine and because of this action chronic trazodone treatment leads to a down-regulation (subsensitivity) of beta adrenergic receptors. This action may also play a role in the antidepressant effects of trazodone.

The down-regulation or subsensitivity of beta receptors produced by trazodone is similar to the effect proposed for TCAs. However, trazodone differs from TCAs in the fact that it is relatively free of antimuscarinic and cardiovascular adverse effects.

Therapeutic uses. Trazodone is approved for the symptomatic treatment of depressive illness.

Table 46.4
Phenelzine and tranylcypromine: Drug interactions

Drug	Interaction
Antidepressants, tricyclic	• The use of MAOIs with TCAs is contraindicated. Pts may suffer hyperpyretic crises or severe convulsive seizures when such drugs are combined. Potentiation of adverse effects can be serious or even fatal
Antidiabetic agents	• Antidiabetic drugs can have enhanced or prolonged hypoglycemic actions in the presence of an MAOI. This interaction applies to both insulin and oral hypoglycemics
Barbiturates	• Barbiturates may have their metabolism reduced by phenelzine or tranylcypromine
CNS depressants	• Morphine, meperidine, barbiturates and alcohol can have their effects potentiated by these MAOIs
Doxapram	• Doxapram can have its adverse CV effects (hypertension, arrhythmias) potentiated by these MAOIs
Meperidine	• Meperidine plus phenelzine or tranylcypromine may lead to excitation, sweating, rigidity and hypertension. Some pts develop hypotension and coma. Avoid concomitant use
Phenothiazines	• Phenothiazines may have additive hypotensive effects when administered with these MAOI
Reserpine	• Reserpine given subsequent to one of these MAOI can cause excitation and hypertension
Succinylcholine	• Succinylcholine may have prolonged effects in the presence of phenelzine because the MAOI may decrease plasma pseudocholinesterase, the enzyme responsible for inactivating succinylcholine
Sympathomimetics	• Amphetamines, ephedrine, levarterenol, levodopa, metaraminol, phenylephrine, phenylpropanolamine or pseudoephedrine must not be used concomitantly with phenelzine or tranylcypromine because combined use may cause severe hypertensive reactions

Table 46.5
Moclobemide: Drug interactions

Drug	Interaction
Alcohol	• The combination of alcohol and moclobemide should be avoided
Anesthetic agents	• Anesthetic agents should not be administered to pts receiving moclobemide for at least 2 days after moclobemide tx is stopped
Antidepressants, tricyclic	• TCAs should not be used concomitantly with moclobemide. Clinical interaction studies between moclobemide and a TCA (clomipramine) resulted in severe adverse reactions. Data involving other TCAs are limited
Antipsychotics	• In depressed pts with schizophrenic or schizoaffective disorder, psychotic symptoms may be exacerbated during tx with moclobemide. There is little experience regarding concomitant use of moclobemide and antipsychotic drugs. Thus, pts should be carefully monitored if concomitant tx is undertaken
Cimetidine	• Cimetidine, administered concomitantly with moclobemide, has led to a doubling of the area under the plasma concentration-time curve of moclobemide. Cimetidine tx is expected to double moclobemide's steady-state concentrations
SSRIs	• Clinical data are not available on the concomitant use of moclobemide, or other MAOIs, and SSRIs. Until such data become available, moclobemide should not be administered in combination with these agents
Sympathomimetics	• Sympathomimetics, plus moclobemide, may potentiate the increase in BP produced by the adrenergic drug. Pts should be advised to avoid concomitant use of all sympathomimetic amines until further studies have been conducted
Tyramine	• Tyramine, followed immediately by moclobemide, may increase BP. The potentiation of tyramine's effects may be minimized by administering moclobemide after, rather than before, a tyramine-rich meal

Controlled studies have demonstrated that trazodone is as effective as amitriptyline in patients with major depressive disorders and other subsets of depressive disorders. Because of its sedative effect, trazodone is generally more useful in depressive disorders associated with insomnia and anxiety.

Adverse effects. Trazodone is well tolerated. Drowsiness is the most common adverse effect (incidence, 15% to 20%). Nausea and vomiting occur less frequently and are mild. Dizziness and lightheadedness also may be noted. Dryness of the mouth, constipation and urinary retention are infrequent. Like the TCAs, trazodone can cause orthostatic hypotension. However, this effect generally lasts only four to six hours and can be lessened by administering each dose with food. Agitation is noted in less than one percent of patients.

Priapism has been associated with trazodone therapy (incidence 1:6000) and, if surgery is required, may lead to permanent impotence. Male patients should be alerted to the warning signs.

The neurotoxicity and respiratory depression commonly encountered after an overdose of a TCA are less severe with trazodone. Overdosage is relatively safe compared with the TCAs.

Table 46.6 lists the clinically significant drug interactions with trazodone.

Venlafaxine (Effexor®)

Mechanism of action and pharmacologic effects. Venlafaxine inhibits norepinephrine and serotonin reuptake and weakly inhibits dopamine reuptake. In this regard, its actions are similar to many of the TCAs. However, in contrast to TCAs, venlafaxine has no affinity for cholinergic, histaminergic or alpha$_1$-adrenergic receptors.

Therapeutic uses. Venlafaxine is approved for the symptomatic treatment of depressive illness. Its effectiveness has been demonstrated in

Table 46.6
Trazodone: Drug interactions

Drug	Interaction
Antihypertensives	• Because trazodone may cause hypotension, including orthostatic hypotension and syncope, caution is required if it is given to pts receiving antihypertensive drugs
CNS depressants	• Trazodone may enhance the CNS depression produced by alcohol, barbiturates, etc. Caution pts
Digoxin	• Trazodone may increase the plasma levels of digoxin
MAOIs	• Because it is not known whether an interaction will occur between trazodone and MAOIs, tx with trazodone should be initiated very cautiously if an MAOI is given concomitantly or has been discontinued shortly before trazodone is started
Phenytoin	• Trazodone may increase the plasma levels of phenytoin

controlled trials comparing it with placebo, imipramine and trazodone.

Adverse effects. The adverse effects of venlafaxine resemble those of SSRIs. Nausea, headache, anxiety, anorexia, nervousness, sweating, dizziness, insomnia and somnolence appear to be most common. Sexual dysfunction and weight loss have occurred. The weight gain and changes in cardiac conduction characteristic of the TCAs have not been reported, but dry mouth and constipation have occurred with the new drug more often than with placebo. Some patients have developed sustained increases in diastolic blood pressure during treatment with venlafaxine, particularly with dosages higher than 300 mg/day. For patients who experience a sustained increase in blood pressure during treatment with venlafaxine, either dosage reduction or discontinuation of venlafaxine should be considered.

Table 46.7 lists the clinically significant drug interactions with venlafaxine.

Bupropion (Wellbutrin®)

Mechanism of action and pharmacologic effects. Bupropion's mechanism of action is not known. Although bupropion blocks the reuptake of dopamine, this effect is seen only at doses that are higher than those needed for its antidepressant effects. Bupropion is a weak blocker of the neuronal reuptake of serotonin and norepinephrine, and it does not inhibit monoamine oxidase.

Bupropion is absorbed rapidly from the gastrointestinal tract, extensively metabolized in its first pass through the liver and eliminated primarily in the urine. With chronic use, the parent drug does not accumulate, but plasma concentrations of metabolites, which have longer half-lives, may increase.

Therapeutic uses. Bupropion is indicated for the treatment of major depression. The drug appears to be effective for the treatment of depression, without causing the sedation, orthostatic

Table 46.7
Venlafaxine: Drug interactions

Drug	Interaction
Inhibitors of drug metabolism by cytochrome P450IID6	• Drugs that inhibit cytochrome P450IID6, such as quinidine, may increase the serum concentrations and possibly the toxicity of venlafaxine in extensive metabolizers
MAOIs	• Because of its effect on adrenergic and serotonergic activity, venlafaxine should not be started until at least 14 days after an MAOI has been discontinued, and should be stopped at least 7 days before an MAOI is started

Table 46.8
Bupropion: Drug interactions

Drug	Interaction
Alcohol, clozapine, fluoxetine, haloperidol, lithium, loxapine, maprotiline, molindone, phenothiazines, TCAs, thioxanthenes, trazodone	• Concurrent use of these drugs with bupropion may lower the seizure threshold and increase the risk of major motor seizures
Benzodiazepines	• Abrupt discontinuation of a benzodiazepine may precipitate a seizure
Drugs that increase drug metabolism	• Since bupropion is extensively metabolized, drugs (e.g., cimetidine, carbamazepine, phenobarbital and others) that increase hepatic metabolism of drugs could cause adverse interactions
Levodopa	• Concurrent use of levodopa with bupropion may result in a greater incidence of adverse effects. Small initial doses of bupropion and small gradual dose increases are recommended during concurrent tx
Monoamine oxidase inhibitors	• Concurrent use of bupropion with MAOIs (including furazolidone, procarbazine and selegiline) may increase the risk of acute toxicity of bupropion and is contraindicated. A medication-free interval of at least 2 weeks should elapse between discontinuation of the MAOI and initiation of bupropion tx

hypotension, weight gain or sexual dysfunction associated with other antidepressants. The effects of the drug are seen in one to three weeks. Studies performed in patients sixty years of age and older have not demonstrated geriatic-specific problems that would limit the usefulness of bupropion in the elderly. However, older patients are known to be more sensitive to the anticholinergic, sedative and cardiovascular side effects of antidepressants. In addition, elderly patients are more likely to have age-related renal or hepatic function impairment, which may require dosage adjustment in patients receiving bupropion.

Adverse effects. Bupropion is generally well tolerated and causes fewer anticholinergic, sedative or adverse sexual effects than TCAs. It does not cause weight gain and does not affect cardiac conduction or cause orthostatic hypotension. Agitation has been the most frequent reason for stopping the drug. Dry mouth, headache, dizziness, insomnia, anorexia, weight loss, nausea and constipation have also occurred. Psychotic reactions have been reported, and symptoms have become worse in some depressed schizophrenic patients given bupropion.

The main concern in using bupropion is the risk for seizures. These occur more frequently at higher doses, the incidence being approximately 0.4% at doses up to 450 mg/day and increasing almost tenfold at doses between 450–600 mg/day. Equally divided doses taken three or four times a day at 4- to 6-hour intervals will avoid high peak concentrations of bupropion or its metabolites. Each single dose should not exceed 150 mg. The dosage should also be increased gradually to reduce the risk for seizures. Caution is used in patients with a history of seizures or cranial trauma, during concurrent use with other medications that may lower the seizure threshold, or when changes in treatment regimens occur.

Table 46.8 lists the clinically significant drug interactions with bupropion.

Nursing Management

Table 46.9 describes the nursing management of the patient receiving antidepressant drugs. Dosage details for individual drugs are given in Table 46.15, pages 543–547.

Table 46.9
Nursing management of the antidepressants

Assessment of risk vs. benefit	Patient data	• Assess to establish baseline VS, general state of health. Baseline lying and standing BP measures are important for those drugs with CV effects. Baseline lab tests will be completed by physician and/or nurse to determine any contraindications or precautions • Pts at high risk for suicide must be carefully assessed and monitored. Children should also be monitored carefully • *Pregnancy:* Risk category varies among drugs. Many are category C (animal studies show adverse effects to fetus but human data are unknown or insufficient); benefits may be acceptable despite risks. Others are category D (human fetal risk has been demonstrated). Always determine current status and future possibility of pregnancy prior to drug administration • *Children:* Despiramine has been reported in fatal cardia arrhythmias in children
	Drug data	• Select drugs based on symptoms (depression with/without agitation, anxiety) and side effect profile of the drug • *Some serious drug interactions:* Confer with pharmacist • Most serious adverse effects include CV effects on heart rate/rhythm and BP, urinary retention (with some drugs) and confusion. Overdose can be fatal. Rarely, agranulocytosis and allergic reactions have occurred • Photosensitivity occurs with some TCAs
Implementation	Rights of administration	• Using the "rights" helps prevent errors of administration
	Right route	• Give PO (most usual route); may occasionally be given IM (not preferred)
	Right time	• See Table 46.15. Note variation in dosage schedules among drugs in this class
	Nursing therapeutics	• Emotional support and therapeutic milieu are essential. Encourage expression of emotions and participation in group or individual tx • Implement measures to reduce adverse effects to promote compliance. Offer encouragement during initial phase of drug tx until effectiveness begins • Observe drug administration to ensure that pt is not "cheeking" pill. Ensure that pt does not have a supply of medications if suicidal ideation present
	Patient/family teaching	• Pt's need for information may be influenced by length of time required for tx or limited by serious illness • Compliance and follow-up are essential for successful tx. Review principles of pt education in Chapter 3 • Explain that successful tx of depression may require months • For MAOIs, give dietary information • Pts/families should know warning signs/symptoms of possible toxicities of drugs. Report immediately any signs of allergy, low BP or cardiac effects • Warn pts to avoid alcohol (increases risk for CNS depression) • *Discuss possibility of pregnancy:* Advise pt to notify physician; discuss birth control methods *(cont'd on next page)*

Table 46.9 (continued)
Nursing management of the antidepressants

Outcomes	Monitoring of progress	Continually monitor:
		• Clinical response indicating tx success (reduction in signs/ symptoms)
		• Observe or explore improvement in appetite, weekly weight, participation in daily living activities, improved concentration. Be particularly vigilant for changes in suicide ideation and behaviour
		• Signs/symptoms of adverse reactions: document and report immediately to physician

Treatment of Manic-Depressive Illness

Bipolar disorder, also referred to as manic-depressive illness, is a cyclic mood disorder characterized by alternating episodes of mania and depression. The manic phase is marked by euphoria, hyperactivity and flight of ideas, talkativeness, grandiosity, and irrational and high-risk activities (gambling, business ventures). Patients also have little need for sleep.

Clinical Challenge

Consider this clinical challenge as you read through this chapter. The response to the challenge appears on page 542.

Clinical Challenge #2

A 31-year-old woman is admitted to an acute psychiatric unit by her spouse. Her symptoms include increased energy (she has been sleeping only 2–3 h/night) and excessive talkativeness. Recently, she attempted to purchase a houseboat without having the necessary cash or credit. She has had no previous hospitalizations.

Biophysical assessment: weight and height normal for age; lab tests normal except slightly hypothyroid; CV status within normal limits.

Psychosocial assessment: unstable marriage, recently lost her job; relationship with her children, ages 10 and 13, has been good.

Medication order: includes chlorpromazine stat and lithium.

The patient asks the following questions:
1. Why do I have to take two drugs for my problem?
2. Why do I have to give so much blood? I'm always having blood tests.
3. The doctor said I'll have an ECG but I'm only 31 years old; there's nothing wrong with my heart.
4. I feel nauseated and my hands are shaky. Am I allergic to the drugs or is there too much in my system?

Lithium

Mechanism of action and pharmacologic effects. The mechanism of action of lithium is not known. Lithium is a positively charged ion, similar in this respect to sodium and potassium. It is unclear, however, whether its antimanic mechanism of action has any relationship to the actions of sodium or potassium. Lithium is known to affect a variety of neurohumoral signal transduction mechanisms and it may influence neurotransmitter systems by interfering with guanine nucleotide binding protein function.

Therapeutic concentrations of the drug have no noticeable effects in normal individuals. Lithium differs from other psychotropic drugs in that it is not a sedative, euphoriant or depressant. It corrects sleep patterns in the manic patient but has no primary action on sleep itself, other than perhaps a small decrease in REM phases.

Lithium carbonate is well absorbed from the intestine, producing sharp peaks in serum concentrations. The use of a sustained-release lithium carbonate preparation can reduce the frequency of absorption-related side effects in selected individuals who are particularly sensitive to rapid increases in serum lithium concentrations.

Lithium is excreted by the kidney, with a half-life of seventeen to thirty-six hours. In patients with renal impairment, the elimination of lithium is reduced. A reduction in sodium intake increases the renal reabsorption of lithium; therefore, patients taking lithium carbonate should not be given a low-sodium diet.

Lithium has a low therapeutic index and reaches toxic levels quickly. The serum concentration of lithium should be measured frequently during stabilization and routinely during the maintenance phase of treatment. Usually, blood is drawn prior to the morning dose. If serum concentrations are followed closely, lithium can be given safely. For long-term maintenance, serum concentrations between 0.8–1.0 mmol/L provide more protection against recurrent mood episodes than lower concentrations (0.4–0.6 mmol/L), but with a higher incidence of adverse effects. For many patients, serum concentrations of 0.6–0.7 mmol/L are effective and well tolerated. Mild to moderate toxic effects occur at 1.5–2.0 mmol/L and moderate to severe reactions above 2.) mmol/L. Table 46.10 on the next page describes the lithium dose-related toxic signs and symptoms.

Therapeutic uses. Manic and hypomanic patients are treated routinely with lithium carbonate. Lithium requires one to three weeks of treatment before it is fully effective. When mania is mild, lithium alone may suffice. In more severe cases, it is almost always necessary to give the lithium concurrently with an antipsychotic drug (usually haloperidol or chlorpromazine). After adequate serum levels of lithium have been reached, the antipsychotic may be withdrawn carefully. During the depressive phase, lithium may be combined with a TCA or bupropion.

Prophylactic lithium treatment is considered the therapy of choice to prevent recurrences of manic-depressive disorder. The drug is effective in 60% to 70% of patients treated. The decision to use lithium prophylactically is based on the number and severity of attacks suffered by a patient and the patient's ability to understand and comply with the treatment regimen.

Lithium is contraindicated in patients with significant CV or renal disease. It is also contraindicated in patients with evidence of severe debilitation or dehydration, sodium depletion, brain damage and in conditions requiring low sodium intake.

If lithium is either not effective, not tolerated or contraindicated, either carbamazepine or valproic acid may be used. Carbamazepine (Tegretol®) was the first drug to be widely studied as an alternative to lithium for patients with manic-depressive illness. Like lithium, carbamazepine reduces symptoms during both manic and depressed episodes. In addition, the drug appears to provide effective prophylaxis against recurrence of episodes. For patients with severe mania, and for those who cycle rapidly, carbamazepine may be superior to lithium. When given to manic patients who have failed to respond to lithium, carbamazepine has had a success rate of about 60%. For treatment of acute manic episodes, the dosage should be low initially (200–400 mg/day) and then gradually increased to as much as 1.6–2.2 g/day. Lower doses should be employed when carbamazepine is used together with lithium, valproic acid or an antipsychotic drug. The mechanism by which carbamazepine stabilizes mood is unknown.

Table 46.10
Lithium dose-related signs/symptoms

Lithium plasma level*	Signs/symptoms
At therapeutic blood levels < 1.5 mmol/L	• Polyuria, mild diarrhea, weight gain, edema, indigestion or nausea, drowsiness, headache, fine tremor of fingers (usually disappears after 2 weeks of tx)
1.5–2.0 mmol/L	• Persistent diarrhea, vomiting, muscle weakness, lack of coordination, sedation
2.0–2.5 mmol/L	• Ataxia, tinnitus, giddiness, blurred vision, high output of dilute urine, hypotension, ECG changes; may progress to seizures or coma
3.0 mmol/L	• Multiple organ systems involved, leading to coma and death

*In the United States, these values are usually expressed as mEq/L, where 1 mmol/L = 1 mEq/L

Valproic acid (Depakene®) is another promising alternative to lithium for manic-depressive patients who have failed to respond to lithium or who cannot tolerate its adverse effects. Clinical studies indicate that valproic acid can control symptoms in acute manic episodes and can provide prophylaxis against recurrent episodes of mania and depression. Like carbamazepine, valproic acid appears especially useful for patients with rapid-cycling bipolar disorder. Dosing should be initiated at 300–500 mg/day and then gradually increased to 750–3000 mg/day. Valproic acid alters GABA-mediated neurotransmission, and this action may underlie the drug's mood-stabilizing effects.

Adverse effects. Table 46.10 summarizes the toxic effects of lithium. Nausea, lethargy and fatigue may occur in the first weeks of treatment, even when serum concentrations are in the recommended range. Fine tremor of the hands is common, especially during initial treatment. If these pose a risk to patient compliance, it may be possible to reduce the dose of lithium or administer a small dose of propranolol. As the concentration of lithium increases, the fine tremor may become coarse and ataxia, dysarthria, loss of coordination, difficulty in concentration and mild disorientation are established. Other signs of neurological toxicity include muscle twitching and fasciculations in the limbs, hands and face, together with nystagmus, dizziness and visual disturbances. The signs of severe toxicity are restlessness, confusion, nystagmus, epileptic convulsions, delirium and eventually, coma and death.

Polyuria and polydipsia occur in 15% to 40% of patients treated with lithium. These effects do not bother most patients. Occasionally, severe polyuria may occur. Toxic renal effects, including tubular lesions, interstitial fibrosis and decreased creatinine clearance have been reported in patients treated chronically with lithium, but are uncommon. Nephrogenic diabetes insipidus (Chapter 40) is a renal complication that can persist for months or years in some patients.

Lithium can cause euthyroid goitre, hypothyroidism with or without goitre and abnormal endocrine test results. The incidence of lithium-induced goitres is about five percent. Hypothyroidism may begin weeks or years after starting therapy.

Lithium should be given with caution to elderly patients, those with dementia, cardiac disease, decreased sodium intake or increased sodium losses, and those taking nonsteroidal anti-inflammatory drugs. Lithium taken during pregnancy may cause a cardiac malformation in the fetus.

Table 46.11 lists the clinically significant drug interactions with lithium.

Nursing Management

Table 46.12 describes the nursing management of the patient receiving lithium. Drug doses are given in Table 46.15 (pages 543–547).

Table 46.11
Lithium: Drug interactions

Drug	Interaction
Diuretics	• Diuretics should be administered cautiously with lithium because lithium excretion decreases with sodium depletion
Potassium iodide	• Potassium iodide and lithium carbonate may have synergistic antithyroid activity
Sodium bicarbonate	• Sodium bicarbonate may increase the renal excretion of lithium
Sodium chloride	• Sodium chloride affects lithium excretion proportionally to the intake of NaCl. Pts on salt-free diets who receive lithium carbonate are prone to develop lithium toxicity. Increased sodium intake has been associated with reduced therapeutic response to lithium
Succinylcholine	• Succinylcholine may have its effects prolonged by lithium

Table 46.12
Nursing management of lithium

Assessment of risk vs. benefit	Patient data	• Assess to establish baseline VS, particularly renal and thyroid function and ECG • *Pregnancy:* Risk category D (human fetal risk has been demonstrated). Excreted in breast milk
	Drug data	• *Some serious drug interactions:* Confer with pharmacist • Most serious adverse effects are related to plasma levels. Levels of 3.5 mmol/L are life-threatening
Implementation	Rights of administration	• Using the "rights" helps prevent errors of administration
	Right route	• Give PO
	Right time	• Due to short half-life must be given 3–4x daily, except extended-release form, which may be given 2–3x/day • Best with meals to reduce gastric irritation
	Nursing therapeutics	• Emotional support and therapeutic relationship essential components of care. Depressive phase requires safety regarding suicidal ideation/behaviour. In the manic phase, pt and family require support to tolerate the risk-taking behaviours • Schedule lithium levels weekly during stabilization phase: should be drawn in a.m. prior to next dose, ideally 12 h after last dose • Ensure that pt swallows pill and does not "cheek" it • Provide diet adequate in sodium intake and encourage fluid intake of 2–3 L/daily
	Patient/family teaching	• Pt's need for information may be influenced by length of time required for tx or limited by serious illness. Pt may have difficulty comprehending information during manic or depressive crises • Compliance and follow-up are essential factors in successful tx. Review principles of pt education in Chapter 3

(cont'd on next page)

Table 46.12 (continued)
Nursing management of lithium

Implementation (cont'd)	Patient/family teaching (cont'd)	• Explain that successful tx of bipolar disorder may require months. Prevention of further occurrences requires continuing medication use • Pts/families should know warning signs/symptoms of possible toxicities of lithium; report immediately • Report occurrence of any flu-like illnesses that may cause dehydration, diarrhea or vomiting • *Discuss possibility of pregnancy:* Advise pt to notify physician; discuss birth control methods, breastfeeding risks. Pt may tolerate alternative drug tx for a planned pregnancy and breastfeeding
Outcome	Monitoring of progress	*Continually monitor:* • Clinical response indicating tx success (reduction in signs/symptoms) • Signs/symptoms of adverse reactions: Document and report immediately to physician • Plasma levels in association with clinical presentation of pt • P (rate/rhythm), daily fluid I/O, weekly weight and dietary intake of sodium

Electroconvulsive Therapy

Electroconvulsive therapy (ECT) is useful in the treatment of severe depression, particularly for those who have not responded to other treatments and those with suicidal ideation and behaviours. ECT is useful for the elderly patient who will tolerate this treatment better than the adverse effects of many of the antidepressants.

Modern ECT often involves treatment two or three times per week for a total of six to twelve treatments. An electrical current of 60–150 V is passed through the brain for a brief period (0.5–2 s). This results in a brain seizure that lasts 20–30 s which is manifested only by a brief twitching of muscles, if any observable signs occur.

Three drugs are important to ECT: pretreatment atropine (Chapter 28) reduces secretions and prevents aspiration; intravenous methohexital (Chapter 58) induces anesthesia and alleviates anxiety; and the skeletal muscle relaxant succinylcholine (Chapter 31) prevents a tonic-clonic seizure and the after-effects that would occur with such a total body seizure.

Treatment of Depression in the Older Patient

The incidence of mental illness, including depression and dementias, in the older population is 15%–25% and may be as high as 75%–90% for those residing in care facilities. Significant challenges in the treatment of this population arise from aging processes that may affect drug response, age-related diseases that may complicate drug therapy, and the risks associated with polypharmacy. As suggested above, ECT may be the treatment of choice for the older patient, particularly if the depression is severe or is accompanied by suicidal ideation.

When drugs are indicated, it is important to note the usual side-effect profile when choosing the best agent. For example, Table 46.13 illustrates the risks in treating older patients with tricyclic antidepressants. In choosing the correct antidepressant for a particular patient, it is important to consider the advantages and disadvantages of each drug, along with the particular needs of each individual. Table 46.14 summarizes the advantages and disadvantages of various drugs or drug groups for the older patient.

Table 46.13
Risks associated with use of TCAs in older patients

Adverse effect	Risk
Anticholinergic effects of dry mouth, constipation and urinary retention	• Exacerbation of existing problems of dehydration, poor diet, irregular bowel habits and prostatic hypertrophy. May cause dental problems, bowel impaction and admissions to hospital
Blurred vision	• Danger of falling, reduced quality of daily living through restriction of activities, risks associated with driving
Cardiovascular effects	• Increase risk r/t pre-existing heart disease; cerebral anoxia and confusion
Neurological effects	• Drowsiness or sedation could cause falls and injury

Table 46.14
Advantages and disadvantages of various drugs in the treatment of depression in the older adult

Drug class	Advantages	Disadvantages
TCAs	Effective Well known and researched Commonly used Effects are dose related; lower doses may minimize adverse reactions	Cardiotoxicity CNS toxicity
Trazadone	Effective Pharmacokinetics not substantially altered by age	Short-half life means multiple dosing, which may lead to compliance problems Risk for orthostatic hypotension (falls, injury, confusion)
Bupropion	Newer, not well studied in this population to date; metabolites may accumulate	Multiple daily doses (compliance issues)
SSRIs	Wide therapeutic index; no blood level monitoring required Few adverse effects; fewer cardiac, hypotensive and sedative actions Effective for several types of depression	Significant drug interactions Age-related dose adjustments required for some of this class (fluoxetine and paroxetine, but not sertraline) Long half-life requires substantial time to recover from adverse reactions

Response to Clinical Challenge #1

1. The best administration schedule for the sertraline is once daily in the morning or evening. May be best tolerated with food or milk.

2. The most likely adverse effects include headache, tremor, nausea, diarrhea, insomnia, agitation and nervousness. If effects are mild, Mr. R. may tolerate these as inconveniences. If they are more severe, he is likely to discontinue taking the drug.

Actions to reduce these adverse effects would include:

• for headache — reduce dosage if advised; use mild analgesic
• for nausea — take with food or milk
• for mild agitation — reduce dosage if advised; take in the morning if drug interferes with sleep or in evening if drug interferes with daytime activities
• for insomnia — take in morning.

If any of these are so severe that Mr. R. wants to discontinue the drug, another antidepressant should be tried.

3. Observations to indicate that the drug is effective would include improved appetite, increased concentration and interest in activities, expression of grief regarding the loss of his friend and a more hopeful attitude about the future.

4. Mr. R. should notify the staff at the day hospital if he develops symptoms of adverse reactions, particularly severe agitation and persistent headache. Generally, this drug is well tolerated.

Response to Clinical Challenge #2

1. The antipsychotic chlorpromazine (CPZ) has a quick onset of action; the lithium will require 1–3 weeks to control the symptoms. At that time, the CPZ will be withdrawn.

2. Lithium has a narrow therapeutic index. Frequent blood tests are taken during stabilization to determine the appropriate individual dose.

3. The ECG is to establish a baseline for comparison after drug therapy begins. Occasionally, lithium can cause changes in cardiac rhythms.

4. Nausea and fine tremors are common adverse effects even at therapeutic doses. Sometimes tolerance will develop. For other patients, these effects must be tolerated until the bipolar symptoms are controlled, at which time the drug dose can be reduced.

Further Reading

Choice of antidepressant drugs. *Medical Letter on Drugs and Therapeutics* 1993;35:25.
Drugs for psychiatric disorders. *Medical Letter on Drugs and Therapeutics* 1994;36:89.
Venlafaxine — a new antidepressant. *Medical Letter on Drugs and Therapeutics* 1994;36:49.

Table 46.15
Treatment of mood disorders: Drug doses

Drug Generic name (Trade names)	Dosage	Nursing alert
A. Tricyclic and Tricyclic-like Antidepressants		
amitriptyline (Elavil, Endep)	**Oral:** *Adults:* (Out-pts): Initially, 25 mg tid. May be increased to 150 mg/day. Increases should be made in late afternoon and/or hs. (Hospitalized, severely ill pts): Initially, 100 mg/day. May be increased to 200 mg/day. Some pts may need as much as 300 mg/day. *Adolescents/elderly:* Generally require lower doses, often 50 mg/day given as single or divided dose	•**PO:** Give without regard to meal schedule. If GI discomfort, dose may be given with food. Tablets can be crushed and added to food or mixed into liquid •Ensure that the pt swallows medication and does not "cheek" the tablet. Store in 4°C temperature in a well-closed container. The 10-mg tablets must be kept in a light-resistant container
amoxapine (Ascendin)	**Oral:** *Adults:* 100–150 mg daily initially, in divided doses; increase to 200–300 mg daily by end of first week (not to exceed 300 mg/day in out-pts, or 600 mg/day in divided doses in hospital). *Elderly:* 25 mg bid or tid; may be increased to 50 mg bid or tid (max., 300 mg/day)	•Ensure that pt swallows medication and does not "cheek" the tablet •Once optimal dose is achieved, may be given as a single hs dose; no single dose to exceed 300 mg
clomipramine HCl (Anafranil)	**Oral:** *Adults:* Initially, 25 mg/day, increased over 2-week period to 100 mg/day in divided doses. May be further increased over several weeks to max. of 250 mg/day in divided doses. *Children/adolescents:* Initially, 25 mg/day, increased over 2-week period to 3 mg/kg/day or 100 mg/day (whichever is less) in divided doses. May be further increased to 3 mg/kg/day or 200 mg/ day (whichever is less) in divided doses. Once stabilizing dose is reached, entire daily dose may be given hs	•Give with food to reduce gastric irritation •Once stabilizing dose is reached, entire daily dose may be given hs
desipramine HCl (Norpramin, Pertofrane)	**Oral:** *Adults:* Initially, 100–200 mg/day (in single or divided doses). For severely ill pts, increase gradually to 300 mg/day.	•Maintenance dose may be given as single dose hs or during the day if preferred; drug has low sedative action

(cont'd on next page)

Table 46.15 (continued)
Treatment of mood disorders: Drug doses

Drug Generic name (Trade names)	Dosage	Nursing alert

A. Tricyclic and Tricyclic-like Antidepressants (cont'd)

Drug Generic name (Trade names)	Dosage	Nursing alert
desipramine HCl (Norpramin, Pertofrane) (cont'd)		had a family hx of heart disease. Thus, obtain a family hx for heart disease or sudden death before starting tx. Then, get a 12-lead ECG. If significant arrhythmia is observed, run a 2-min rhythm strip to determine HR, P-R interval, QRS duration, and Q-T interval. Calculate the Q-Tc by dividing the measured Q-T by the square root of the R-R interval. Note the morphology of the ST segments and T waves. Repeat ECGs during the drug loading and maintenance phases. Monitor plasma drug levels at the same time ECGs are performed; ECG changes are more common at relatively high plasma concentrations. If there is a hx of heart disease or a significant baseline conduction delay, weigh the risks and benefits of TCA tx. Plasma desipramine levels should not exceed 300 ng/mL. P-R intervals should be <0.20 s and QRS duration <0.12 s. Max. Q-Tc should be 0.45 s
doxepin HCl (Adapin, Sinequan)	**Oral:** *Adults:* Initially, 25 mg tid. Increase by 25 mg at appropriate intervals until tx response is obtained. Optimum range, 100–150 mg/day. Max., 300 mg/day. *Elderly:* Total daily maint. dose up to 150 mg; may be given od. Proceed more cautiously with initial dose and increase more slowly	• The 150-mg capsule is intended for maintenance tx only and is not recommended for initiation of tx • Dilute concentrate with 120 mL liquid (water, milk or juice, but not carbonated drinks). Give with food to reduce gastric irritation
imipramine HCl (Janimine, Tofranil)	**Oral:** *Adults* (Out-pts): 25 mg tid. Increase gradually prn up to 150 mg/day. Max., 200 mg/day. (Hospitalized pts): Initially, 100 mg/day in divided doses. Increase prn to 200 mg/day. After 3 weeks of no significant response, dose may be increased to 250–300 mg/day. *Elderly/debilitated:* 30–40 mg/day in divided doses; increase gradually prn. Max., 100 mg/day	• Usually tolerated best in divided doses. Initiate with test dose and monitor BP. May give larger dose hs to minimize hypotension

Table 46.15 (continued)
Treatment of mood disorders: Drug doses

Drug Generic name (Trade names)	Dosage	Nursing alert
A. Tricyclic and Tricyclic-like Antidepressants (cont'd)		
maprotiline HCl (Ludiomil)	**Oral:** *Adults:* Initially, 75 mg/day; increase by 25 mg q2weeks to a max. of 150 mg/day. Some pts may require up to 225 mg/day. May be given in 3 divided doses or single daily dose. *Elderly:* Initially, 25 mg/day. Maintenance, 50–75 mg/day	• Give with food if nausea occurs. May give as single daily dose hs to reduce daytime sedation, if tolerated
nortriptyline HCl (Aventyl, Pamelor)	**Oral:** *Adults:* 25 mg tid or qid, up to 150 mg/day. *Elderly/adolescent:* 30–50 mg/day as a single dose or in divided doses	• Give with food if nausea occurs. May give as single daily dose hs to reduce daytime sedation, if tolerated
protriptyline HCl (Triptil, Vivactil)	**Oral:** *Adults* (out-pts): Initially, 15–30 mg/day. (Range, 20–60 mg/day divided into 2 or 4 doses.) When a satisfactory response is noted, reduce dose to smallest amount necessary to maintain relief. Hospitalized patients: 30–60 mg/day	• May be given at any time of day; least sedating of the TCAs
B. Selective Serotonin Reuptake Inhibitors (SSRIs)		
fluoxetine HCl (Prozac)	**Oral:** *Adults:* 20 mg/day in a.m. After several weeks, may increase by 20 mg/day at weekly intervals. Doses > 20 mg/day should be given in 2 divided doses, in a.m. and at noon (not to exceed 80 mg/day)	• Give early in day to avoid insomnia
fluvoxamine maleate (Luvox)	**Oral:** *Adults:* 50 mg/day hs. Increase after several days to 100 mg/day hs. Effective daily dose usually lies between 100–200 mg and should be adjusted gradually according to pt's response, up to a max. of 300 mg. Dosage increases should be made in 50-mg increments. Doses > 150 mg should be divided so that a max. of 150 mg is given hs	• Arrange dosing schedule for individual, depending on occurrence of somnolence or insomnia
nefazodone HCl (Serzone)	**Oral:** *Adults:* Initially, 200 mg/day (100 mg bid) with dose increases, after assessing response, following first week. Most pts respond to doses of 300–500 mg/day. Full antidepressant effect may be delayed for 4 weeks or longer. *Geriatrics, debilitated and hepatic impairment:* Initially, 100 mg/day (50 mg bid). Modify rate of subsequent dose titration as well as final target dose	• Give in divided doses for best results. Give with food if nausea occurs • May give as single daily dose hs to reduce daytime sedation, if tolerated

(cont'd on next page)

Table 46.15 (continued)
Treatment of mood disorders: Drug doses

Drug Generic name (Trade names)	Dosage	Nursing alert
B. Selective Serotonin Reuptake Inhibitors (SSRIs) (cont'd)		
paroxetine HCl (Paxil)	**Oral:** *Adults:* 20 mg as a single dose in a.m.; may be increased by 10 mg/day at weekly intervals (range, 20–50 mg). *Elderly or debilitated, severe hepatic or renal impairment:* Initially, 10 mg/day, not to exceed 40 mg/day	• Give in a.m. to reduce insomnia
sertraline (Zoloft)	**Oral:** *Adults:* Initially, 50 mg/day as single dose a.m. or p.m. May be increased at weekly intervals prn up to 200 mg/day	• May give as single daily dose hs to reduce daytime sedation, if tolerated
C. Monoamine Oxidase Inhibitors (MAOIs)		
moclobemide (Manerix)	**Oral:** *Adults:* Initially, 300 mg/day (in 2–3 divided doses); increase gradually to a max. of 600 mg/day, if needed. *Liver dysfunction:* Reduce daily dose to one-third or one-half the standard dose	• Give with or after food
phenelzine sulfate (Nardil)	**Oral:** *Adults:* Initially, 15 mg tid. Early-phase tx: Dose should be increased to at least 60 mg/day at a fairly rapid pace consistent with pt tolerance. May be necessary to increase dose up to 90 mg/day to obtain sufficient MAO inhibition. Many pts do not show a clinical response until tx at 60 mg has been continued for at least 4 weeks. Maint. dose: May be as low as 15 mg/day or qod, and should be continued for as long as is required	• Best given in divided doses • Significant food and drug interactions; instruct pt to consult physician prior to starting new drugs and before surgery
tranylcypromine sulfate (Parnate)	**Oral:** *Adults:* Initially, 10 mg bid. If no response after 2–3 weeks, increase to 30 mg/day (20 mg on arising and 10 mg in afternoon)	• Best given in divided doses • Significant food and drug interactions; instruct pt to consult physician prior to starting new drugs and before surgery
D. Miscellaneous Antidepressants		
trazodone HCl (Desyrel)	**Oral:** *Adults:* 150 mg/day in 3 divided doses; increase by 50 mg/day q3–4days until desired response (not to exceed 400 mg/day in out-pts or 600 mg/day in hospital). *Elderly:* Initially, 75 mg/day in divided doses. *Children 6–18 years:* 1.5–2 mg/kg/day in divided doses. May be increased q3–4days up to 6 mg/kg/day	• Best absorbed with food. May give larger portion of dose hs to minimize effects of dizziness

Table 46.15 (continued)
Treatment of mood disorders: Drug doses

Drug Generic name (Trade names)	Dosage	Nursing alert
D. Miscellaneous Antidepressants (cont'd)		
venlafaxine HCl (Effexor)	**Oral:** *Adults:* 75 mg/day in 2–3 divided doses. If no improvement after a few weeks, increase gradually to 150 mg/day. If needed, dose may be further increased up to 225 mg/day. Increments of up to 75 mg/day should be made at intervals of not less than 4 days. Max. for in-pts, 350–375 mg/day. *Hepatic impairment:* 50% of daily dose. *Renal impairment:* Decrease daily dose by 25–50%	• Best in divided doses. Monitor BP; may cause sustained hypertension
bupropion (Wellbutrin)	**Oral:** *Adults:* 100 bid (a.m. and p.m.) initially; after 3 days may be increased to 100 mg tid; after 4 weeks may increase to a max. daily dose of 450 mg daily in divided doses	• No single dose should exceed 150 mg. Wait at least 4–6 h between doses and divide qid if necessary to tolerate higher doses. Reduce hs dose if insomnia occurs.
E. Antimanic-Depressive Drug		
lithium carbonate (Carbolith, Duralith, Eskalith, Lithane, Lithotabs, Lithonane)	**Oral:** *Adults:* 900–1200 mg/day in 3–4 divided doses; usual dose, 300 mg tid or qid. Blood level monitoring necessary to determine proper dose. Extended-release forms (Duralith®, Eskalith-CR®, Lithizine®) may be given 2–3x daily. *Children:* 15–20 mg (0.4–0.5 mEq)/kg/day in 2–3 divided doses	• Do not interchange regular tabs with extended-release forms. Do not crush or chew extended-release forms • Advise pt not to change brands without advice • Give with food and water to reduce gastric irritation. Daily fluid intake should be 2500–3000 mL

Anxiolytics, Sedatives and Hypnotics

Topics Discussed
- The benzodiazepines
- Benzodiazepine antagonist: Flumazenil
- Nonbenzodiazepine anxiolytics
- For each drug discussed: Mechanism of action and pharmacologic effects, therapeutic uses, adverse effects
- Nursing management

Drugs Discussed

Benzodiazepines:
alprazolam (al-**praz**-zoe-lam)
bromazepam (broe-**maz**-eh-pam)
chlordiazepoxide (klor-dye-az-eh-**pox**-ide)
clorazepate (klor-**az**-eh-pate)
diazepam (dye-**az**-eh-pam)
flurazepam (flur-**az**-eh-pam)
ketazolam (ket-**az**-oh-lam)
lorazepam (lor-**az**-eh-pam)
nitrazepam (nye-**traz**-eh-pam)
oxazepam (ox-**az**-eh-pam)
temazepam (tem-**az**-eh-pam)
triazolam (trye-**az**-oh-lam)

Benzodiazepine antagonist:
flumazenil (flew-**maz**-eh-nil)

Nonbenzodiazepine Anxiolytics, Sedatives and Hypnotics:
amobarbital (am-oh-**bar**-bih-tal)
buspirone (byoo-**spee**-rone)
chloral hydrate (klo-ral **hye**-drate)
pentobarbital (pen-toe-**bar**-bih-tal)
secobarbital (see-koe-**bar**-bih-tal)
zopiclone (**zoe**-pih-klone)

Clinical Challenge

Consider the following clinical challenge as you read through this chapter. The response to the challenge appears on page 559.

A current debate in mental health care weighs the value of self-regulation against the benefits and risks of drug management. For each of the following situations, state (1) the goal of drug therapy, (2) whether the benefits outweigh the risks, and (3) whether a nondrug approach should be used.

A. A 47-year-old man is admitted to hospital for coronary surgery. The physician orders hs sedation.

B. A 48-year-old woman visits her family physician feeling depressed and lost since her husband died. She asks for something to make her feel better.

C. A teenager is being investigated for constant lower back pain. Should benzodiazepines be used?

D. A woman in her 80s is very lonely since her husband died. She is often tearful around her daughter, who asks the physician for something to calm her mother's nerves. When the physician discusses the possible risks, both mother and daughter reply, "What difference could it make at her age?"

Forty years ago the expression *anxiolytic,* or minor tranquilizer, was unknown. Brain depressants were called either sedatives or hypnotics. A *sedative* was generally agreed to be a drug that calmed the patient and allayed anxiety. A *hypnotic* produced greater depression and was used to induce sleep in the patient suffering from insomnia. However, there is nothing qualitatively different in the actions of sedatives and hypnotics: they differ only in the quantitative sense. Often, sedative drugs were given in large doses when a hypnotic effect was desirable.

In the late 1950s the so-called minor tranquilizers made their appearance in North America. However, the expression "minor tranquilizer" is a misnomer that should be avoided today, as there is nothing minor about their effects on the body and their therapeutic actions. Touted as capable of reducing our emotional reactions to stressful situations, these drugs became popular very quickly. Soon the term sedative began to slip into the background, and the expressions tranquilizer and anxiolytic became fashionable. It became most unpopular to consider giving a patient a drug that would "depress" the brain when one could use a tranquilizer that would, at least in the mind of the public, excommunicate that part of the brain responsible for emotion.

Over the years the fallacy in this thinking has become very evident. "Tranquilization" occurs only because brain function is depressed. Like the earlier sedative drugs, tranquilizers in higher doses can be used to produce sleep. When used this way, they are called hypnotics.

Anxiolytics, sedatives and hypnotics have frequently been misused by health professionals and abused by the lay public. However, they have also had a significant impact on the treatment of anxiety, tension, insomnia, alcohol withdrawal, convulsive disorders, preoperative sedation and agitated depression. This chapter will discuss the mechanism of action, therapeutic uses and adverse effects of these drugs, with particular emphasis on the nursing interventions in their appropriate use.

The Benzodiazepines

The introduction of chlordiazepoxide (Librium®) in 1960 heralded the arrival of the benzodiazepines. These drugs have virtually taken over the treatment of anxiety and insomnia, replacing the older, less effective and more toxic barbiturates that had been in use for decades.

The overuse of benzodiazepines is frequently criticized, and justifiably so. However, it is equally important to recognize the advantages these drugs brought to medicine over the previously prescribed barbiturates. Barbiturates had no selective antianxiety effects. For barbiturates to relieve anxiety, they had to sedate the patient. Lower doses of benzodiazepines appear to treat anxiety without producing marked CNS depression. Overdoses of barbiturates frequently killed patients, but even extreme doses of benzodiazepines are rarely lethal, so long as supportive therapy is carried out. Both barbiturates and benzodiazepines can, on chronic administration, produce psychological and physical dependence. However, dependence is greater, and the withdrawal effects far more severe, with barbiturate use.

Mechanism of Action and Pharmacologic Effects

Benzodiazepines modify behaviour. Regardless of what else is said to camouflage this point, nurses must never lose sight of the fact that the patient encased in a benzodiazepine bubble is not a normal individual — at least, not in the behavioural sense.

Benzodiazepines reduce anxiety by depressing the limbic system. The limbic system, composed of the septal region, the amygdala, the hippocampus and the hypothalamus, plays an important role in the emotional and autonomic responses to situations. The hypnotic effects of benzodiazepines can be attributed to depression of the limbic, neocortical and mesencephalic systems.

Diazepam is often used as a skeletal muscle relaxant in the injured athlete or the driver who has suffered whiplash. It has been contended that the relaxant action is due to an inhibition of brain stem and spinal cord function. However, it is also possible that patients fare better on the drug because they are sedated and do not move the damaged muscles.

The biochemical basis for the action of benzodiazepines has been the subject of intense investigation. It is now generally agreed that benzodiazepines work because they facilitate the action of γ-aminobutyric acid (GABA) in the central nervous system. Binding of GABA to its receptors in the CNS inhibits the formation of action potentials and depresses neuronal function. Benzodiazepines bind to specific, high-affinity sites on the cell membrane, which are separate from, but adjacent to, the receptors for GABA. The binding of benzodiazepines to their receptors enhances the affinity of GABA receptors for GABA. This results in a greater depression of neuronal function.

Pharmacokinetics

Benzodiazepines are absorbed rapidly. Their half-lives range from two to three hours for triazolam, to approximately fifty to one hundred hours for diazepam (Valium®) and flurazepam (Dalmane®) (Table 47.1). Chlordiazepoxide (Librium®), ketazolam (Loftran®) and diazepam are active in their own right and are also metabolized to active compounds. The half-lives given for these drugs take into account the durations of action of both the metabolites and the parent compounds. Flurazepam is rapidly converted to an active metabolite with a long half-life. Clorazepate is inactive. In stomach acid, it is converted to desmethyldiazepam, which is responsible for the effects produced by clorazepate.

Because benzodiazepines are often prescribed for long periods of time, their long-term pharmacokinetic characteristics are important. When a drug is taken chronically, approximately five half-lives are required from the time of the first dose for concentrations of the drug in the body to reach steady state. Therefore, drugs with long half-lives, such as diazepam, require two to three weeks before they reach plateau levels, and patients may not experience the full effects of these drugs until treatment has continued for two to three weeks. Benzodiazepines with shorter half-lives, such as oxazepam, reach plateau concentrations within one

Table 47.1
Properties of some benzodiazepines

Generic name (trade name)	Usual dose[1]	Peak time of effect (h)	Biologic half-life (h)	Therapeutic use(s)[3]
triazolam (Halcion®)	0.125–0.25 mg	2	2–3	Hypnotic
oxazepam (Serax®)	30–120 mg/day in divided doses	1–4	4–13	Anxiolytic
temazepam (Restoril®)	30 mg hs	0.8–1.4	8–10	Hypnotic
bromazepam (Lectopam®)	6–30 mg/day in divided doses	1–4	12	Anxiolytic
alprazolam (Xanax®)	0.25 mg bid–tid; incr. prn in 0.25-mg increments	1–2	6–20	Anxiolytic
lorazepam (Ativan®)	2 mg/day in 2–3 divided doses	1–6	12–15	Anxiolytic
chlordiazepoxide (Librium®)	10–40 mg/day in divided doses	2–4	20–24[2]	Anxiolytic
nitrazepam (Mogadon®)	5–10 mg hs	2	26	Hypnotic
clorazepate (Tranxene®)	30 mg/day in divided doses	1–2	48[2]	Anxiolytic
ketazolam (Loftran®)	15 mg od–bid; later, total daily dose can be given hs	?	50[2]	Anxiolytic
diazepam (Valium®)	4–40 mg/day in divided doses	1.5–2	50–100[2]	Anxiolytic
flurazepam (Dalmane®)	15 or 30 mg hs	1	50–100[2]	Hypnotic

[1] Refers to usual adult dosage. Dosage for elderly or debilitated pts should be halved. For detailed dosage schedules, see Table 47.9, pages 559–563.
[2] Refers to half-life of drug plus active metabolites.
[3] Refers to anxiolytic and hypnotic uses only.

to three days; for these agents, maximum effects are seen shortly after treatment is started.

Once a drug is stopped, it is eliminated from the body in relation to its half-life. Thus, the effects of chronic diazepam treatment last long after the drug is stopped. Lorazepam has a half-life of twelve to fifteen hours. Its effects disappear faster than those of diazepam once treatment is stopped. The rapid elimination of a benzodiazepine from the body following prolonged treatment can be a mixed blessing. Although the patient may not be bothered with the "hangover" effects of the drug, rapid elimination of the benzodiazepine often causes rebound excitation and a request for another prescription. Patients on shorter-acting benzodiazepines are thus more likely to become dependent on the drugs (see Tolerance and Dependence, below).

There is considerable misunderstanding of the importance of half-life in relation to duration of benzodiazepine action. The relationship of drug half-life to the termination of drug effects, following single or repeat doses, is best illustrated by referring to the two hypnotics triazolam and flurazepam. Triazolam has a much shorter half-life than the active metabolite of flurazepam. However, this does not mean that triazolam, given once or twice, has a shorter duration of action than flurazepam. During the initial nights of therapy with either drug, diffusion out of the brain and into other body tissues — not rate of elimination from the body — is the major factor responsible for terminating drug effect. As a result, flurazepam's duration of action is considerably shorter at this time than would be predicted on the basis of the long half-life of its active metabolite.

There is, however, a finite capacity for tissues to take up a drug like the active metabolite of flurazepam and remove it from the brain. The more frequently the drug is given, the less able are these tissues to take up more of subsequent doses. When this happens, diffusion out of the brain and into other body tissues stops being a major factor in terminating drug effect. At this point, the removal of flurazepam's active metabolite from the brain depends on its metabolism and elimination from the body. Now, if we compare flurazepam and triazolam, their respective rates of inactivation become progressively more important in determining duration of action. As a result, during chronic treatment, flurazepam has a long-term duration of action while triazolam has short-term effects. Patients taking flurazepam night after night may experience daytime hangover, as significant residual concentrations remain in the brain during waking hours. If triazolam is taken on a nightly basis, its concentration in the brain during the day should be low and hangover should not be a problem. The other side of the coin is that patients may awaken in the early hours of the morning when the concentration of triazolam in the brain falls below the hypnotic level.

Half-life should also be considered when benzodiazepines are used as antianxiety drugs. The advantage of a benzodiazepine such as oxazepam (Serax®), which has a relatively short half-life, is that hangover symptoms are minimal once the drug is stopped. However, drugs with shorter half-lives should be given several times a day to ensure adequate concentrations in the brain. Long-acting drugs, such as diazepam, produce more sustained blood levels. Although divided doses are recommended, diazepam can be taken once daily at bedtime. If patients follow this regimen, they should sleep well during the night and benefit from the antianxiety actions of the drug throughout the day. The disadvantage of longer-acting antianxiety drugs is a more prolonged hangover when they are stopped.

The decision to market a benzodiazepine either as an anxiolytic or a hypnotic is in many cases an arbitrary one. Obviously, it would make little sense to market a lower dose of triazolam as an anxiolytic. With a half-life of two to three hours, it would be necessary to take many doses each day. However, oxazepam and temazepam have similar half-lives. Oxazepam is sold mainly for the treatment of anxiety, and temazepam as a hypnotic. It would have made just as much sense to reverse the indications and use a lower dose of temazepam, three times daily, as an anxiolytic. Likewise, diazepam and flurazepam are very similar drugs. Either could be used in lower doses to relieve anxiety or in higher doses to produce sleep. Because diazepam was already on the market as an anxiolytic when flurazepam was introduced, the decision was made to sell relatively higher doses of flurazepam as a hypnotic.

Tolerance and Dependence

Tolerance is not uncommon with benzodiazepines, that is, the need for increased doses to obtain the same pharmacologic effect. In addition, concern is mounting about dependence liability, especially with benzodiazepines that have short half-lives. These drugs are more likely to leave the patient with rebound insomnia once the drug is discontinued. The danger of inducing drug dependence by yielding to requests for repeat prescriptions is obvious. It would be well to remember that under normal circumstances hypnotic drugs should not be used for more than fourteen to twenty-one nights consecutively. Patients also should be told to expect a few nights of relatively poor sleep once drug treatment is stopped. This is the price that must be paid for earlier drug-induced hypnosis.

Patients as well as professionals need to be aware of the acute withdrawal effects experienced by some people after taking triazolam. Awareness has resulted in a marked reduction in the use of this particular benzodiazepine as a hypnotic. Triazolam has the shortest half-life of any of the commonly used hypnotics, and it is thus not surprising that so many patients experience acute withdrawal effects when they cease to take this drug. Reducing the number of prescriptions written for triazolam should decrease the incidence of this complaint.

Dependence can also be a problem with antianxiety drugs, particularly those with shorter half-lives. Once therapy is discontinued, the patient may experience daytime anxiety and return to the physician for a repeat prescription.

Therapeutic Uses

Anxiety disorders, including panic and generalized anxiety, are the main indications for benzodiazepine use. These drugs may also be utilized for brief periods in stress-related conditions, but this must be done with some caution. A nonpharmacologic technique should be tried first (see Box 47.1).

Box 47.1
Patient teaching: Ten helpful hints to cope with anxiety

✔ When you feel your anxiety growing, SLOW DOWN. Take a few deep breaths and tell yourself to let go of the tension. Remember, "this too will pass."

✔ Try to meet your fears head on. At times it is natural to be afraid; just make sure that what you fear really does exist. You can overcome your fears once you understand the reasons behind them.

✔ Keep looking for different ways to deal with stress. Set aside some time each day and do something you enjoy. Physical activities like going for a walk or working around the house will help take your mind off your worries. You might try talking out your anxieties with a friend.

✔ Put yourself first, and learn to say no. How can people know how you feel unless you tell them? Stand up for your rights.

✔ Protect yourself. If you are not sure you are ready to handle a certain situation, put it off until you are ready.

✔ Don't be afraid to make decisions and stick to them.

✔ Concentrate on today. Yesterday is over, and what happens tomorrow depends on how you handle today.

✔ Take care of yourself physically. Stay in shape; work off excess tension by exercising several times a week. Regular exercise will also help you sleep better.

✔ Proper diet is just as important as exercise. Make sure you are eating regular, well-balanced meals, and avoid stimulating drinks such as coffee whenever possible. Remember, physical and emotional health go hand-in-hand.

✔ Your doctor might prescribe medication as a first step in helping you cope with your anxiety. This medication is beneficial because it does provide short-term relief, but it should not be used as a substitute for coping on your own. Talk to your doctor about the causes of your anxiety.

A "benzodiazepine crutch" to allay anxiety should be employed for short periods of time only.

Alprazolam (Xanax®) and bromazepam (Lectopam®) are second-generation benzodiazepines, claimed by some to provide better antianxiety effects with minimal sedation. Both drugs are used for short-term, symptomatic relief of excessive anxiety in patients with anxiety neurosis.

Insomnia is the second major use for benzodiazepines. The relative merits of short- and long-acting drugs have been discussed. Ideally, a hypnotic should produce sleep quickly and have no hangover effects the next day. The perfect hypnotic benzodiazepine has yet to be developed. Nitrazepam and flurazepam are long acting and may produce daytime hangover. Temazepam is an effective hypnotic with a half-life of eight to ten hours. Triazolam works quickly and is less likely to produce morning hangover, but with a half-life of two to three hours may allow the patient to awaken after just a few hours of sleep.

It is well to reiterate that hypnotics should not be used for more than fourteen to twenty-one days. To ignore this recommendation is to predispose the patient to the danger of drug dependence. Upon withdrawal, periods of rebound excitation and insomnia may be expected (especially with short-acting drugs) — a natural consequence of depressing the central nervous system night after night with any drug, then withdrawing it.

Rebound insomnia is less common when treatment with a long-acting hypnotic is stopped. For example, if flurazepam is administered on a regular basis, the body stores active metabolites. Once flurazepam treatment is stopped, the active metabolites leave their storage sites and enter the brain in ever-decreasing amounts over a period of several days or even weeks. In this way the patient is weaned off the medication and rebound insomnia is not so prevalent. On the other hand, daytime sedation may continue for a week or more.

Benzodiazepines can be used to reduce the CNS excitation that accompanies acute alcohol withdrawal. Once the patient is stabilized on the benzodiazepine, its dose can be reduced gradually and normal neuronal activity allowed to return slowly. Diazepam has been used for this purpose; other benzodiazepines may also be appropriate.

Adverse Effects

CNS depression is the major adverse reaction of benzodiazepines. Patients complain of fatigue, drowsiness and a feeling of detachment. Elderly patients are particularly prone to headache, dizziness, ataxia, confusion and disorientation.

Benzodiazepine use may also cause psychological impairment. This may be difficult to diagnose in the anxious patient because anxiety itself interferes with psychological performance. Relieving anxiety with a benzodiazepine may improve function and more than offset any direct action of the drug. Hostility has been reported after benzodiazepine use.

Although overdosage is common with benzodiazepines, few patients die. Unless consumed with another CNS depressant such as alcohol, a barbiturate, a tricyclic antidepressant or a narcotic, benzodiazepines rarely kill. The use of the benzodiazepine antagonist flumazenil (Anexate®, Mazicon®) to reverse the effects of a benzodiazepine is described later in this chapter.

The problems of benzodiazepine dependence have been described but warrant repeating. Psychological dependence is common, as evidenced by the continuing demand for repeat prescriptions. Physiological dependence is characterized by anxiety, agitation, restlessness, insomnia and tension following drug withdrawal. Although the symptoms of withdrawal are not as severe as those following cessation of alcohol or a barbiturate, one should not be deceived into believing that benzodiazepines do not produce physical dependence.

Table 47.2 on the next page lists the clinically significant drug interactions with benzodiazepines.

Benzodiazepine Antagonist: Flumazenil (Anexate®, Mazicon®)

Mechanism of Action and Pharmacologic Effects

Flumazenil is a benzodiazepine antagonist that blocks the effects of benzodiazepines on the brain by competitively inhibiting the benzodiazepine receptor. The antagonism is specific, since the

Table 47.2
Benzodiazepines: Drug interactions

Drug	Interaction
Antidepressants, tricyclic	• TCAs can potentiate the actions of benzodiazepines
CNS depressants	• Alcohol, antipsychotics, anesthetics, barbiturates, hypnotics, narcotics, and other CNS depressants have additive depressant effects on the CNS with benzodiazepines. They should be used together with caution. In particular, patients should be warned against the ingestion of moderate to large amounts of alcohol
Monoamine oxidase inhibitors	• MAOIs may potentiate the action of benzodiazepines and usually should not be given concurrently

effects of CNS depressants — such as nonbenzodiazepine sedatives, narcotics and anesthetics — are not blocked by flumazenil.

Therapeutic Uses

Flumazenil is approved for the complete or partial reversal of the central sedative effects of benzodiazepines. It may therefore be used in anesthesia and intensive care in the following situations: termination of general anesthesia induced and/or maintained with benzodiazepines, reversal of benzodiazepine sedation in short diagnostic and therapeutic procedures, and for the diagnosis and/or management of deliberate or accidental benzodiazepine overdosage.

Flumazenil has a shorter duration of action than most benzodiazepines. After intravenous administration, it is rapidly cleared by the liver, metabolized, and excreted in the urine, with a half-life of about one hour. Benzodiazepine antagonism begins within one to two minutes after intravenous injection, reaches a peak in six to ten minutes and lasts for about one hour, when the residual effect of the agonist may return, depending on the doses of the agonist and antagonist.

In view of the short duration of action of flumazenil and the possible need for repeat doses, the patient should remain closely monitored until all possible central benzodiazepine effects have subsided. Because of the possibility that resedation may occur, flumazenil should be administered only when the continued observation of patients for recurrence of sedation can be assured.

Adverse Effects

Flumazenil can cause nausea, dizziness, headache, blurred vision, increased sweating and anxiety, and may provoke a panic attack in some patients. The drug can cause convulsions in patients who are physically dependent on benzodiazepines or who are taking them to control epilepsy. In addition, patients who have taken overdoses of both the benzodiazepine and a tricyclic-type antidepressant have convulsed because flumazenil apparently antagonized the anticonvulsant effect of the benzodiazepine and unmasked the epileptogenic effects of the antidepressant. Cardiac arrhythmias apparently precipitated by flumazenil have also been reported.

Table 47.3 lists the clinically significant drug interactions with flumazenil.

Nonbenzodiazepine Anxiolytics, Sedatives and Hypnotics

Buspirone (Buspar®)

Mechanism of action and pharmacologic effects. Buspirone is a psychotropic drug with antianxiety properties. It belongs chemically to the class of compounds known as azaspirodecanediones. Buspirone shares some of the properties of the benzodiazepines and neuroleptics but is devoid of anticonvulsant and muscle relaxant properties. Its mechanism of action is not clear. Buspirone does not bind to the benzodiazepine GABA-receptor complex and thus its mechanism of action must differ from that of the benzodiazepines.

Table 47.3
Flumazenil: Drug interactions

Drug	Interaction
Multiple drug over-dosage	• Particular caution is necessary when using flumazenil in cases of multiple drug overdosage, since the toxic effects (cardiac arrhythmias and/or convulsions) of other psychotropic drugs, especially tricyclic anti-depressants, may increase as the effects of benzodiazepines subside

Therapeutic uses. Buspirone is indicated for the short-term symptomatic relief of excessive anxiety in patients with generalized anxiety disorder. Patients who have previously taken benzodiazepines may be less likely to respond to buspirone than those who have not. In controlled studies in healthy volunteers, single doses of buspirone up to 20 mg had little effect on most tests of cognitive and psychomotor function, although performance on a vigilance task was impaired in a dose-related manner.

Adverse effects. The most common adverse reactions encountered with buspirone are dizziness, headache, drowsiness and nausea. Approximately ten percent of patients discontinued buspirone because of their inability to tolerate the adverse effects of the drug.

Table 47.4 lists the clinically significant drug interactions with buspirone.

Zopiclone (Imovane®)

Mechanism of action and pharmacologic effects. Zopiclone is a short-acting hypnotic. It belongs to a novel chemical class, the cyclopyrrolones, which is structurally unrelated to existing hypnotics. Zopiclone is rapidly absorbed from the gastrointestinal tract. It is extensively metabolized and has an elimination half-life of approximately five hours. This is extended to over seven hours in elderly patients. Hepatic insufficiency also prolongs zopiclone's half-life to nearly twelve hours.

Therapeutic uses. Zopiclone is useful for the short-term management of insomnia characterized by difficulty in falling asleep, frequent nocturnal awakenings and/or early morning awakenings. As with all hypnotics, long-term continuous treatment is not recommended; a course of treatment should be no longer than four weeks in duration. Zopiclone is contraindicated in patients with myasthenia gravis or severe impairment of respiratory function, as well as those who have suffered acute cerebrovascular accidents.

Adverse effects. The most common adverse reaction seen with zopiclone is a bitter taste in the mouth. Severe drowsiness and impaired coordination are signs of drug intolerance or excessive doses. Patients may also experience somnolence, asthenia, dizziness, confusion, anterograde amnesia or memory impairment, feeling of drunkenness, euphoria, nightmares, agitation, anxiety or nervousness, hostility, depression, decreased libido, coordination abnormality, hypotonia, muscle spasms, paresthesias and speech disorder. These effects are completely consistent with a drug that depresses brain function, and can be expected with any of the medications discussed in this chapter.

Table 47.5 on the next page lists the clinically significant drug interactions with zopiclone.

Table 47.4
Buspirone: Drug interactions

Drug	Interaction
Food	• Food increases the bioavailability of buspirone
MAOIs	• Monoamine oxidase inhibitors and buspirone should not be used concomitantly because of reports of elevated BP in pts receiving both

Table 47.5
Zopiclone: Drug interactions

Drug	Interaction
Alcohol and other CNS depressants	• These have possible additive effects with zopiclone

Barbiturates

Barbiturates warrant only brief discussion. Many barbiturates remain on the market. However, with the exception of thiopental, used in anesthesia, and phenobarbital, administered for epilepsy, no justification can be found for their continued use. The availability of safer benzodiazepines, buspirone or zopiclone has made barbiturate use for sedation or hypnosis inappropriate. Barbiturates are more toxic on acute overdosage and can produce severe drug dependence.

Mechanism of action and pharmacologic effects. Barbiturates depress the central nervous system. By potentiating GABA-mediated inhibitory processes in the central nervous system, barbiturates exert muscle relaxant, anticonvulsant, sedative and hypnotic effects. Barbiturates also alter psychological functions. Psychomotor performance and complex tasks are most affected, especially those involving fine points of judgment. Increased doses lead to progressive impairment of brain function, culminating with respiratory failure.

Therapeutic uses. Although amobarbital (Amytal®), butabarbital sodium (Butisol®), pentobarbital sodium (Nembutal®) and secobarbital sodium (Seconal®) are still prescribed by a few physicians, the availability of the safer benzodiazepines has removed any need for the continued use of barbiturates as sedatives or hypnotics.

Adverse effects. Central nervous system depression is the major adverse effect of barbiturate use. Patients may experience drowsiness, confusion or even psychosis. Other signs of CNS depression include nystagmus, dysarthria and motor incoordination. The elderly are particularly at risk for ataxia and confusion. It is difficult to avoid many of these effects because satisfactory symptomatic control with barbiturates often requires oversedation.

Overdosage can cause respiratory failure. The concomitant use of a barbiturate with another CNS depressant, such as alcohol or a narcotic, compounds the problem.

Paradoxic excitation is difficult to explain. It is not known why certain patients become restless and excited — and may proceed to delirium —

Table 47.6
Barbiturates: Drug interactions

Drug	Interaction
Anticoagulants, oral	• Oral anticoagulants may interact with barbiturates, particularly phenobarbital, which can increase the liver metabolism of coumarin anticoagulants. As a result, the pharmacologic activity of the anticoagulants is reduced. Pts receiving coumarin anticoagulants should not have their barbiturate tx stopped or started without careful attention to possible dosage adjustment
Antidepressants, tricyclic	• TCAs may have their rates of metabolism increased by barbiturates, thereby decreasing their pharmacologic activities. On the other hand, when toxic doses of TCAs are used, barbiturates may potentiate the adverse effects
Contraceptives, oral	• Oral contraceptives may show reduced efficacy and increased incidence of breakthrough bleeding when used concomitantly with barbiturates
Monamine oxidase inhibitors	• MAOIs inhibit barbiturate metabolism. Give barbiturates with caution to pts receiving MAOIs

when given a barbiturate. This effect is particularly prevalent in the elderly.

Psychological and physical dependence is a very serious problem with barbiturates, and withdrawal effects can be particularly severe.

Microsomal enzyme induction can occur following chronic barbiturate use. This is more likely to occur if phenobarbital is used. Stimulation of microsomal enzymes may mean that the durations of action and therapeutic effects of many drugs are reduced.

Table 47.6 lists the clinically significant drug interactions with barbiturates.

Chloral Hydrate (Noctec®)

Chloral hydrate is available in capsule or elixir form. It works quickly and has a relatively short duration of action. Chloral hydrate is better suited for putting people to sleep rather than keeping them asleep. The drug is used often in pediatrics and geriatrics.

The adverse effects of chloral hydrate include gastric irritation. It should be given with milk or water to reduce the possibility of nausea or vomiting. The therapeutic ratio of chloral hydrate is similar to that of barbiturates. If large doses are taken, death can occur as a result of respiratory depression.

Table 47.7 lists the clinically significant drug interactions with chloral hydrate. Box 47.2 offers a sample patient teaching in nonpharmacological means of promoting sleep.

Nursing Management

The nursing management of patients receiving anxiolytic drugs is described in Table 47.8. Dosage details of individual drugs are given in Table 47.9 (pages 559–563)

Box 47.2
Patient teaching: Measures to promote sleep

Following this routine for 4–6 weeks can help to promote sleep.

✔ Establish a 24-h routine: arise and retire at the same time each day.

✔ Avoid daytime napping.

✔ Engage in physical activity throughout the day and avoid evening stimulation; e.g., read or listen to music rather than watch TV. Particularly, avoid stimulants such as caffeine.

✔ Have a warm bath and engage in a relaxation routine prior to bedtime.

✔ Use the bedroom for sleeping, not for other activities; maintain a comfortable bedroom environment.

✔ If not asleep in approximately 20 min, rise, leave the bedroom and engage in a quiet activity; then try again.

✔ Avoid worrying about sleeping!

Table 47.7
Chloral hydrate: Drug interactions

Drug	Interaction
Anticoagulants, oral	• Coumarin or indanedione-derivative oral anticoagulants may have their hypoprothrombinemic effects increased by the concomitant use of chloral hydrate, particularly during the first 2 weeks of concurrent tx. This effect is due to displacement of the anticoagulant from plasma protein binding sites. With continued concurrent use, anticoagulant activity may return to baseline level or be decreased. Frequent prothrombin-time determinations may be required, especially during initiation of chloral hydrate tx, to determine if dosage adjustment of the anticoagulant is necessary
CNS depressants	• The concurrent use of CNS depressants, including alcohol, with chloral hydrate will increase the depression of the central nervous system. Caution is recommended; the dosage of one or both agents should be reduced
Furosemide, IV	• Administration of chloral hydrate followed by IV furosemide within 24 h may result in diaphoresis, hot flashes, and variable blood pressure, including hypertension. This effect may be due to a hypermetabolic state caused by the displacement of thyroxin from its bound state

Table 47.8
Nursing management of the anxiolytics

Assessment of risk vs. benefit	Patient data	• Assess for hx of allergy (which may predispose to allergic reaction to benzodiazepines), signs/symptoms of presenting problem (i.e., anxiety, insomnia or panic disorder), hx of drug abuse or dependence and depression with suicidal ideation • Assess to establish baseline VS, general state of health • *Pregnancy:* Risk category D (human fetal risk has been demonstrated)
	Drug data	• Most serious drug interactions occur with other CNS depressants • Most serious adverse effects are CNS effects, both immediate (e.g., drowsiness, dizziness, fatigue, ataxia) and delayed (e.g., confusion, hangover, amnesia). Measures to prevent dependence and tolerance must be implemented
Implementation	Rights of administration	• Using the "rights" helps prevent errors of administration
	Right route	• Generally given PO, occasionally IV
	Right time	• See Table 47.9. NB variation in dosage schedules among drugs in this class
	Right technique	• IV administration requires knowledge of correct diluent and IV solution, correct dilution and rate of administration. Always refer to manufacturer's instructions for this route
	Nursing therapeutics	• Emotional support required for pts with panic or anxiety disorders. Encourage pt to use other approaches for control of anxiety and management of sleep disturbances, if possible (see Box 47.2 on previous page)
	Patient/family teaching	• Review principles of patient education (see Chapter 3) • Advise pts not to discontinue drug abruptly after prolonged use; can cause severe withdrawal symptoms. Advise pts of risks for dependence and tolerance. Encourage responsible self-medication • Pts/families should know warning signs/symptoms of possible toxicities of these drugs. Report immediately: excessive drowsiness, ataxia, slurred speech, skin rash, increased agitation • Warn pts to avoid alcohol (increased risk for CNS depression) • *Discuss possibility of pregnancy:* Advise pt to notify physician; discuss birth control methods
Outcomes	Monitoring of progress	*Continually monitor:* • Clinical response indicating tx success (reduction in signs/symptoms) • Signs/symptoms of adverse reactions; document and report immediately to physician • Signs/symptoms of developing dependence

Response to Clinical Challenge

A. An anxiolytic/hypnotic is useful in this situation because of its efficacy in alleviating the symptoms accompanying the expected anxiety associated with the preoperative period. An agent with a short half-life should be chosen to prevent any hangover effects and interaction with pre-op meds the following morning. This patient needs instructions regarding the risk of drowsiness if he awakens during the night (e.g., to go to the bathroom). The benefits outweigh the risks.

B. Relying on an anxiolytic or hypnotic in this situation may encourage dependence. The physician should (a) assess the patient's most troublesome symptoms and her available resources, (b) suggest others and (c) validate the normal grief reaction. The risks could outweigh the benefits.

C. Although some of the drugs in this class have muscle relaxant properties, their use during investigation may or may not be warranted. In this situation, the greatest risk is in the attitudes of professionals who tend to believe that if pain is relieved by a "tranquilizer," then it is not "real." Clearly, this prescribing a benzodiazepine would not serve this patient, and the use of these drugs may produce more negative than positive outcomes.

D. This is a common example of "ageism." The use of these drugs carries risks for older adults — to name only two, drowsiness or dizziness associated with falls, and memory impairment which could lead to misdiagnosis or loss of self-esteem. Normal grief reaction should be discussed, along with the patient's potential resources. Short-term hypnotic use may be indicated if sleep is seriously disturbed; however, the drug should be provided with information for responsible self-medication.

Table 47.9
The anxiolytics: Drug doses

Drug Generic name (Trade names)	Dosage	Nursing alert
A. Benzodiazepine Anxiolytics, Sedatives and Hypnotics		
alprazolam (Xanax)	**Oral:** For anxiety: *Adults:* 0.25–0.5 mg bid or tid prn (max., 4 mg/day). *Elderly, debilitated:* Initially, 0.25 mg bid or tid. For panic attacks: *Adults:* 0.5 mg tid; may be increased prn (max., 10 mg/day)	• **PO:** Can be given with food to minimize stomach upset. Ensure that pt swallows medication and does not attempt to "cheek" the tablet • Tablet may be crushed and mixed with food or liquid. Store medication between 15°C and 30°C
bromazepam (Lectopam)	**Oral:** *Adults:* Initially, 6–18 mg/day in equally divided doses, depending on severity of symptoms and response. Tx should be initiated by lower doses and adjusted prn. Optimal dosage may range from 6–30 mg/day, in divided doses. Doses up to 60 mg/day may be used in exceptional cases. *Elderly and debilitated:* Initially, not to exceed 3 mg/day in divided doses. Dosage can be carefully adjusted prn	• **PO:** Can be given with food to minimize stomach upset. Ensure that pt swallows medication and does not attempt to "cheek" the tablet • Tablet may be crushed and mixed with food or liquid. Store medication between 15°C and 30°C

(cont'd on next page)

Table 47.9 (continued)
The anxiolytics: Drug doses

Drug Generic name (Trade names)	Dosage	Nursing alert
A. Benzodiazepine Anxiolytics, Sedatives and Hypnotics (cont'd)		
chlordiazepoxide (Librium®)	**Oral:** For anxiety: *Adults:* 5–25 mg tid or qid. **IM/IV:** Initially, 50–100 mg, then 25–50 mg tid or qid prn. *Elderly:* Initially, 25–50 mg. *Children > 6 years:* 5 mg bid to qid prn, up to 10 mg bid or tid	• **PO:** Give with a full glass of water 1 h ac or 2 h pc. If stomach upset occurs, drug may be given with food • Ensure that pt swallows medication and does not attempt to "cheek" the tablet • **IV:** Inject slowly over 1 min. Do not administer cloudy solutions. Mix and use immediately; discard remainder. Protect powder from light and refrigerate • **IM:** Mix only with diluent provided by manufacturer. Diluent should be refrigerated. Administer only clear solution; discard any unused. Store medication between 15°C and 30°C
clorazepate dipotassium (Tranxene)	**Oral:** For anxiety: *Adults:* 15–60 mg/day in divided doses. *Elderly or debilitated:* 7.5–15 mg/day	• **PO:** Can be given with food to minimize stomach upset • Ensure that pt swallows medication and does not attempt to "cheek" the tablet • Do not administer antacids within 1 h of clorazepate administration. Store medication between 15°C and 30°C and protect it from light
diazepam (Valium)	**Oral:** For anxiety: *Adults:* 2–10 mg bid to qid. Extended-release form 15–30 mg od. **IM/IV:** 2–10 mg; may repeat in 3–4 h prn. *Children > 6 months:* 1–2.5 mg tid or qid	• **PO:** Can be given with food to minimize stomach upset. Sustained-released medication must be swallowed whole; however, short-acting tablets may be crushed and mixed with food or liquid • Ensure that pt swallows medication and does not attempt to "cheek" the tablet • **IM:** This route is rarely used; inject deeply into deltoid muscle • **IV:** Should not be mixed with other drugs. Direct IV push recommended; continuous infusion not recommended. Do not use a small vein to avoid venous irritation. Inject slowly, with pt in recumbent position. If direct injection is not possible, inject medication into tubing as close to site of vein insertion as possible

Table 47.9 (continued)
The anxiolytics: Drug doses

Drug Generic name (Trade names)	Dosage	Nursing alert
A. Benzodiazepine Anxiolytics, Sedatives and Hypnotics (cont'd)		
flurazepam HCl (Dalmane)	**Oral:** *Adults:* Usually, 30 mg hs. In some pts, 15 mg may suffice. *Elderly or debilitated:* Initially, 15 mg hs, until pt response is determined	• **PO:** May be crushed and added to food or liquid • Ensure that pt swallows medication and does not attempt to "cheek" the tablet • Store medication in a light-, heat- and moisture-resistant container, between 15°C and 30°C
ketazolam (Loftran)	**Oral:** *Adults:* 15 mg od or bid. Increases should be made in 15-mg increments according to pt response. Pts with sleep problems will benefit if most or all of daily dosage is given hs. *Elderly or debilitated:* One-half lowest adult dose	• Dosage may be divided or given as single dose according to pt's response
lorazepam (Ativan)	**Oral:** For anxiety: *Adults:* 1–3 mg bid or tid (up to 10 mg/day). *Elderly:* Initially, 0.5–2 mg/day in divided doses	• **PO:** Can be given with food to minimize stomach upset. Medication may be crushed and added to food or liquid. May be given sublingually • Ensure that pt swallows medication and does not attempt to "cheek" the tablet • Store medication between 15°C and 30°C • **IM:** Should be given at least 2 h before surgery and administered deep into muscle. Do not dilute medication • **IV:** Should be clear solution, mixed immediately prior to administration. Do not inject at a rate > 2 mg/min. Medication should be protected from light and refrigerated
nitrazepam (Mogadon)	**Oral:** For insomnia: *Adults:* Usually, 5–10 mg hs. *Elderly or debilitated:* Initially, 2.5 mg until pt response is determined (max., 5 mg/day)	• Give without regard to food
oxazepam (Serax)	**Oral:** *Adults:* 10–30 mg tid or qid. *Elderly:* Initially, 5 mg od or bid	• **PO:** Can be given with food to minimize stomach upset. Medication may be crushed and added to food or liquid • Ensure that pt swallows medication and does not attempt to "cheek" the tablet • Store medication between 15°C and 30°C in a tightly closed container

(cont'd on next page)

Table 47.9 (continued)
The anxiolytics: Drug doses

Drug Generic name (Trade names)	Dosage	Nursing alert
A. Benzodiazepine Anxiolytics, Sedatives and Hypnotics (cont'd)		
temazepam (Restoril)	**Oral:** *Adults:* 15 mg hs (max., 30 mg). *Elderly or debilitated:* Initially, 7.5 mg hs	• **PO:** Can be given with food to minimize stomach upset. • Ensure that pt swallows medication and does not attempt to "cheek" the tablet • Pt should remain in bed several hours after administration • Store medication in a light-, heat- and moisture-resistant container between 15°C and 30°C
triazolam (Halcion)	**Oral:** *Adults:* Initially, 0.125 mg hs (max., 0.25 mg). A dose of 0.5 mg should be used only for exceptional pts who do not respond adequately to a trial of the lower dose. *Elderly or debilitated and pts with disturbed liver/kidney function:* Should not exceed 0.125 mg hs	• **PO:** Can be given with food to minimize stomach upset • Ensure that pt swallows medication and does not attempt to "cheek" the tablet • Store medication in a heat- and moisture-resistant container between 15°C and 30°C
B. Benzodiazepine Antagonist		
flumazenil (Anexate, Mazicon)	Flumazenil should be administered IV by a physician with experience in anesthesiology. **IV:** For general anesthesia/sedation: *Adults:* Initially, 0.2 mg over 15 s. If desired level of consciousness is not obtained within 60 s, a further dose of 0.1 mg can be injected and repeated at 60-s intervals (max. total dose, 1 mg). Usual dose is between 0.3–0.6 mg. **IV:** For known or suspected benzodiazepine overdose: *Adults:* Initially, 0.3 mg over 30 s, followed by a series of 0.3-mg injections, each administered over a 30-s period, at 60-s intervals (max., 2.0 mg). If drowsiness recurs, an infusion of 0.1–0.4 mg/h may be useful. Rate of infusion should be individually adjusted to desired level of arousal	• **IV:** Should be given through free-flowing infusion. Use a large vein to avoid venous irritation. May be administered in diluted or undiluted form. Discard diluted solution after 24 h
C. Nonbenzodiazepine Anxiolytic		
buspirone HCl (Buspar)	**Oral:** *Adults:* Initially, 5 mg bid or tid. Dose may be increased by 5 mg q2–3 days (max., 45 mg/day in divided doses). Usual dose is 20–30 mg/day in 2–3 divided doses. *Elderly:* Max. daily dose should not exceed 30 mg for a duration not exceeding 4 weeks	• **PO:** Should be given with food to minimize stomach upset • Ensure that pt swallows medication and does not attempt to "cheek" the tablet • Store medication in a heat- and moisture-resistant container between 15°C and 30° C

Table 47.9 (continued)
The anxiolytics: Drug doses

Drug Generic Name (Trade Names)	Dosage	Nursing Alert
D. Nonbenzodiazepine Hypnotics		
zopiclone (Imovane)	**Oral:** *Adults:* Usual dose is 7.5 mg hs. This dose should not be exceeded. *Elderly/debilitated:* Initially, 3.75 mg hs. Up to 7.5 may be used with caution in appropriate cases	• Give without regard to food
chloral hydrate (Noctec)	**Oral:** Hypnotic: *Adults:* 500–1000 mg 15–30 min before bedtime. *Elderly:* Initially, 250 mg 15–30 min before bedtime. *Children:* 50 mg/kg (max., 1000 mg/single dose). Sedative: *Adults:* 250 mg tid pc (max., 2000 mg/day). *Children:* 25 mg/kg/day divided into 3–4 doses pc (max., 500 mg/dose). Premedicant: *Adults:* 500–1000 mg 30 min pre-procedure. *Children:* 25–50 mg/kg 30 min pre-procedure. May repeat in 30 min using half the dose (max., 1000 mg/single dose)	• **PO:** Should be given with food to minimize stomach upset. Administer drug with a full glass of water or juice • Ensure that pt swallows medication and does not attempt to "cheek" the tablet • Also available in suspension liquid and in two strengths; be certain of the dose you are giving. Shake well before administering • **IM:** Inject deeply; massage well. Reconstitute with 1.2 mL of bacteriostatic or sterile water for injection • **IV:** Sites should be changed q48–72h. Direct or intermittent infusion may be recommended • **Rectal:** Check for irritation; moisten suppository and gloved finger with water. Ensure that suppository is retained. Store suppositories in dark container in refrigerator

Further Reading

Cormack MA, Owens RG, Dewey ME. *Reducing Benzodiazepine Consumption. Psychological Contributions to General Practice.* New York: Springer-Verlag; 1989.

Drugs for psychiatric disorders. *Medical Letter on Drugs and Therapeutics* 1994;36:89.

CHAPTER 48

The Alcohols: Ethanol and Methanol

Topics Discussed
- Ethanol: Mechanism of action, immediate and chronic pharmacologic effects, pharmacokinetics, drug interactions
- Methanol
- Disulfiram
- Nursing management

Drugs Discussed
ethanol (**eth**-an-awl)
methanol (**meth**-an-awl)
disulfiram (dye-**sul**-fir-am)

Clinical Challenge

Consider this clinical challenge as you read through this chapter. The response to the challenge appears on page 568.

You are a case manager for clients who live in a senior citizens' apartment building. The seniors visit the clinic, and you also make home visits for follow-up.

You are working with Harold, a 76-year-old man who was widowed last year. You are concerned that his normal grief reaction has extended into depression. During a home visit, you discover that he is drinking beer daily to cope with his loneliness and loss. His son is concerned but does not know how to talk to his father, who used alcohol only socially prior to this year. His daughter thinks the family should not "nag" him ("If drinking eases his pain and helps him sleep, then what's the harm? Alcohol is no worse than some of the pills he could be taking!").

What is your response to this family?

Ethanol

Ethanol, or ethyl alcohol, is a simple aliphatic alcohol. It is found in varying concentrations in alcoholic beverages such as whisky, wine, beer and liqueurs. Ethanol has found great favour with the masses because it is a relatively cheap drug that can modify brain function. The effects of ethanol are dose dependent: small quantities may put a nice glow on the world, but larger amounts can produce unfortunate consequences.

Mechanism of Action and Pharmacologic Effects

Immediate effects. Ethanol depresses neuronal function in the central nervous system. It may be difficult to convince a drinker who feels larger than life that alcohol is depressing him. However, such is the case. Initially, as low concentrations of ethanol begin to wash over the brain, higher centres are depressed, and the mind is unfettered from its learned inhibitions. Confidence abounds, your boss's spouse looks better all the time, and life just couldn't be more enjoyable. At the same time, motor and intellectual functions that depend on polysynaptic pathways are impaired and finer grades of discrimination and concentration slip away.

As the concentration of ethanol in the brain increases, so does the degree of CNS depression, and the fortunes of our drinker decline. Operating a car becomes difficult, even illegal. An initial boisterous mood gives way to general depression as the effects of ethanol percolate farther down the brain stem. Mood swings, and perhaps even fist swings, become more prominent.

If our drinker continues to imbibe, profound brain depression ensues. Sleep is the usual and most benign result. However, if the concentration of ethanol is sufficiently high, respiratory failure and death can occur — and that really takes the fun out of a party.

The nice, warm glow produced by ethanol is due to moderate vasodilatation in the skin. This leads to an increase in heat loss. Ethanol also decreases heat production, so skiiers and snowmobilers should think twice before reaching for that hot toddy. Ethanol depresses the secretion of the antidiuretic hormone, producing a well-known renal response.

Anyone who has interviewed a toilet bowl at close range after a drinking bout will attest to the fact that ethanol can upset the stomach. Although it may be of only academic interest to drinkers at the time, concentrations of forty percent or more of ethanol cause congestive hyperemia and inflammation of the stomach. Food dilutes the concentration of ethanol in the stomach and reduces gastric irritation.

Chronic effects. Given the fact that some lost souls find ethanol appealing enough to return for more, we must consider the consequences of bathing the body tissues in it over long periods of time. Chronic excessive ethanol use produces serious neurological and mental disorders. These include brain damage, memory loss, sleep disturbances and psychoses. In addition, many alcoholics replace food with ethanol and as a result suffer from vitamin deficiencies. Evidence for this is found in the development of Wernicke's encephalopathy, polyneuritis, nicotinic acid deficiency encephalopathy and Korsakoff's psychosis.

The liver bears much of the brunt of long-term, high-dose ethanol consumption. Ethanol increases hepatic fat synthesis. Protein also collects in the liver. Eventually, the accumulation of both fat and protein leads to hepatic cirrhosis.

Ethanol may be the most common teratogen in North America. Fetal alcohol syndrome is well recognized and occurs with a frequency of four to seven per one thousand live births. Women should be advised to refrain from drinking even moderate amounts of ethanol during pregnancy. Fetal alcohol syndrome is characterized by low IQ and microcephaly, both reflections of CNS damage. Other characteristics are facial abnormalities that include a hypoplastic upper lip, a short nose, short palpebral fissures and slow growth.

Pharmacokinetics

Ethanol is absorbed from both the stomach and the duodenum, with absorption occurring faster from the latter site owing to its larger surface area. Often the rate-limiting factor in the absorption of ethanol is the speed with which it is passed to the duodenum. Suitably diluted and given to a person with an empty stomach, ethanol is passed quickly to the duodenum and absorbed within fifteen to thirty minutes. Food closes the pyloric sphincter. Ethanol taken with food is trapped in the stomach and absorbed more slowly.

Once absorbed, ethanol is distributed in the total body water before being metabolized to acetaldehyde by the enzyme alcohol dehydrogenase. Acetaldehyde is subsequently metabolized by acetaldehyde dehydrogenase. The inactivation of ethanol proceeds at a constant rate of 100 mg/kg of body mass/hour. Blood ethanol levels fall at the rate of approximately 0.015 g/100 mL/h. Under normal circumstances, about two percent of

Table 48.1
Ethanol: Drug interactions

Drug	Interaction
CNS depressants	• CNS depressant drugs, such as benzodiazepines, barbiturates, other hypnotics and sedatives, narcotics and tricyclic antidepressants, can produce profound brain depression and even death when taken with ethanol

ethanol is eliminated unchanged by the kidneys. The fact that ethanol can be expired has enabled scientists to develop the breathalyzer. Because the concentration of ethanol in alveolar air is in equilibrium with its level in blood and brain, it is possible to measure alveolar ethanol concentrations and calculate blood levels. In most parts of North America 0.08 g of ethanol per 100 mL of blood has been established as the legal limit for driving a motor vehicle.

Table 48.1 lists the clinically significant drug interactions with ethanol.

Nursing Management

A lengthy discussion of the nursing actions related to alcohol abuse and alcoholism is beyond the scope of this text. However, a brief overview of some of the responsibilities for nursing management will be provided.

All nurses have a responsibility to recognize the pharmacological as well as the social effects of ethanol and to develop a knowledge of referral sources. In the hospital setting, a drinking history should be obtained for all adults for three important reasons. First, ethanol is a drug and can interact with other drugs that may be prescribed in this treatment setting. Second, the effects of both short-term and chronic alcohol use should be understood in the context of the current presenting problem and in making an accurate diagnosis. Finally, alcohol abuse is an important factor in a substantial number of individuals seeking help at a hospital. Problem identification at this time can provide a valuable opportunity for appropriate services or referrals to be offered. Nurses can seek information in a non-judgmental way within the context of other lifestyle and treatment questions. Alcohol abuse is perhaps the most treatable of untreated disorders. With a positive approach and attitude, nurses can help many individuals to seek successful treatment.

Community health nurses can promote and protect population health and safety by offering educational sessions to increase public awareness of the importance of moderate use of alcohol. These sessions can also address the chronic effects of long-term abuse, the teratogenic effects of alcohol use during pregnancy, and the dangers of consumption concurrently with other medications.

Methanol

Methanol's actions on the brain are similar to those of ethanol. Concern over its acute toxicity results from the metabolism of methanol by alcohol dehydrogenase to formaldehyde, which in turn is converted to formic acid. Formaldehyde and formic acid are toxic to the retina and the optic nerve and can produce permanent blindness. In addition, formic acid produces metabolic acidosis which, if severe, can be fatal.

Treatment involves the administration of ethanol, which competes with methanol for the available alcohol dehydrogenase. This reduces the formation of formaldehyde and formic acid, and methanol is slowly eliminated unchanged in the urine. Methanol may also be eliminated by hemodialysis. It is also usual to treat the metabolic acidosis with intravenous sodium bicarbonate solutions.

Disulfiram (Antabuse®)

Disulfiram inhibits the enzyme acetaldehyde dehydrogenase. In the presence of disulfiram, ethanol ingestion causes large quantities of acetaldehyde to accumulate, producing intense flushing, tachycardia, nausea, vomiting and circulatory collapse.

Disulfiram is used as a deterrent to drinking. If the alcoholic knows that he is taking the drug, he is motivated to refrain from using ethanol lest he incur the unpleasant effects mentioned above. On the other hand, the individual must have the

Table 48.2
Disulfiram: Drug interactions

Drug	Interaction
Alfentanil	•Chronic preoperative administration or perioperative use of hepatic enzyme inhibitors, such as disulfiram, may decrease plasma clearance and prolong the duration of action of alfentanil
Anticoagulants, oral	•Anticoagulant effect may be increased during concurrent use with disulfiram because of the inhibition of the enzymatic metabolism of the anticoagulant. Also, disulfiram may act directly on the liver to increase the hypoprothrombinemia-inducing activity of coumarin derivatives. Anticoagulant dosage adjustments based on prothrombin-time determinations may be necessary during and following concurrent use
Anticonvulsants, hydantoin, especially phenytoin	•The concurrent use with disulfiram may increase the serum concentrations of hydantoins, possibly leading to hydantoin toxicity. Hydantoin serum concentrations should be obtained prior to and during concurrent therapy with disulfiram and dosage adjustments made accordingly
Isoniazid	•The concurrent use of disulfiram and isoniazid may result in an increased incidence of CNS effects, such as dizziness, incoordination, irritability or insomnia. A reduction of dosage or discontinuation of disulfiram may be necessary
Metronidazole	•The concurrent use of metronidazole with disulfiram may result in confusion and psychotic reactions because of combined toxicity. Metronidazole is not recommended concurrently with, and for 2 weeks following, disulfiram

will to stop drinking or he will not take disulfiram. The drug takes two to four hours to begin to act and reaches its maximum effect in twelve to twenty-four hours.

Disulfiram is not devoid of other toxicities. It blocks the enzyme dopamine-β-hydroxylase and thereby reduces catecholamine synthesis. This may explain the weakness, dizziness and cardiac arrhythmias seen in patients. Disulfiram may also produce a toxic psychosis or skin allergies on occasion.

Table 48.2 lists the clinically significant drug interactions with disulfiram.

Nursing Management

Table 48.3 describes the nursing management of patients receiving disulfiram. Dosage details are given in Table 48.4 (page 569).

Table 48.3
Nursing management of disulfiram

Assessment of risk vs. benefit	Patient data	•Assess to determine whether pt can understand the purpose and consequence of disulfiram use •Assess to establish baseline VS, general state of health and contraindications (e.g., hx of allergic response or heart disease) •*Pregnancy:* Risk category unknown; avoid during pregnancy
	Drug data	•Reaction will occur with any drugs that contain alcohol, e.g., cough remedies. Confer with pharmacist •Most serious adverse effects are cardiac dysrhythmias and psychosis

(cont'd on next page)

Table 48.3 (cont'd)
Nursing management of disulfiram

Implementation	Rights of administration	• Using the "rights" helps prevent errors of administration
	Right route	• Give PO. Must not be given within 12 h of last consumption of alcohol (preferably, 48 h of abstinence)
	Nursing therapeutics	• If drowsiness occurs with morning dose, may be given hs
	Patient/family teaching	• Compliance and follow-up are essential factors in successful tx; review principles of pt education in Chapter 3 • Explain that successful tx of alcohol abuse requires more than prevention of drinking with disulfiram • Emphasize importance of reading labels on all products that may contain alcohol and to determine use of wine or liqueurs in restaurants • Pts/families should know warning signs/symptoms of possible toxicities of drug. Report immediately: irregular pulse rate or psychotic symptoms • *Discuss possibility of pregnancy:* Advise pt to notify physician; discuss birth control methods
Outcomes	Monitoring of progress	*Continually monitor:* • Clinical response indicating tx success (reduction in signs/ symptoms) • Signs/symptoms of adverse reactions; document and report immediately to physician

Response to Clinical Challenge

Alcohol is a drug and should be treated with the general principle of weighing benefits against risks. The risks for Harold include: dizziness causing falls and injury; social isolation and withdrawal (solitary drinking); failure to seek more effective assistance for his loneliness and grief; physiological effects on liver, renal and gastric function.

Harold deserves more effective treatment than self-medicating with alcohol. Become familiar with community resources (programs and services, self-help groups, books and websites) that will help both Harold and his family. Explore grief counselling options for this man as well as for his son and daughter.

Further Reading

Adlaf EM, Smart RG. Drug use among adolescent students in Canada and Ontario: The past, present and future. *J Drug Issues* 1991;21(1):51–65.

Chaikelson J. Predictors of drinking among Canadian women and men. In: Adrian M, Lundy C, Eliany M, eds. *Women's Use of Alcohol, Tobacco and Other Drugs in Canada.* Toronto: Addiction Research Foundation; 1996.

Health and Welfare Canada *The National Alcohol and Other Drugs Survey.* Ottawa: Minister of Supply and Services Canada; 1990: cat. no. H39-175/ 1990E.

Robbins CA. Social roles and alcohol abuse among older men and women. *Family and Community Health* 1991;13:37–48.

Sobell LC, Sobell MB. Self-report issues in alcohol abuse: state of the art and future directions. *Behavioural Assessment* 1990;12:77–90.

Table 48.4
Disulfiram: Drug doses

Drug Generic Name (Trade Names)	Dosage	Nursing Alert
disulfiram (Antabuse)	**Oral:** *Adults:* A max. of 500 mg daily in a single dose should be given for 1–2 weeks, preferably taken in the morning. Pts experiencing a sedative effect may take the drug hs or, if necessary, dosage may be adjusted downward. Maintenance dose, 250 mg/day (range, 125–500 mg), not to exceed 500 mg/day	• Drug should not be administered until pt has abstained from alcohol for at least 12 h. Never give without pt's knowledge • May crush tablets and mix with food or fluid

Drugs for the Treatment of Neurologic and Neuromuscular Disorders

Recent years have seen major improvements in the treatment of neurologic and neuromuscular disorders. New drugs for the treatment of epilepsy and parkinsonism have afforded relief to many patients. These are discussed in Chapters 49 and 50, respectively.

Chapter 51 discusses drugs for the treatment of muscular skeletal disorders. Unfortunately, the advances seen in anticonvulsant and antiparkinsonian therapy have not been paralleled in the treatment of musculoskeletal disorders. The drugs used today are the same as those administered years ago. This does not mean that this area of pharmacotherapy should not be presented; to the contrary, if nurses are to play a major role in the management of clients with musculoskeletal disorders, they must understand the mechanisms of action, therapeutic uses, adverse effects and nursing actions related to the drugs that are currently available.

CHAPTER 49

Anticonvulsant Drugs

Topics Discussed
- Classification of epilepsy
- Antiepileptic drugs
- Drugs effective against generalized tonic-clonic seizures
- Newer adjuvant drugs for treatment of generalized tonic-clonic seizures
- Drugs effective against absence seizures
- Miscellaneous antiepileptics
- Nursing management

Drugs Discussed
carbamazepine (kar-ba-**maz**-eh-peen)
clobazam (**kloe**-baz-am)
clonazepam (kloe-**naz**-eh-pam)
diazepam (dye-**az**-eh-pam)
divalproex sodium (dye-val-**proe**-ex)
ethosuximide (eth-oh-**suck**-sim-ide)
gabapentin (gab-ah-**pen**-tin)
lamotrigine (lah-**moe**-trih-jeen)
lorazepam (lor-**az**-eh-pam)
phenobarbital (fee-noe-**bar**-bih-tal)
phenytoin (fen-ih-**toe**-in)
primidone (**prim**-ih-done)
valproic acid (val-**pro**-ik)
vigabatrin (vig-ah-**bay**-trin)

Clinical Challenge

Consider this clinical challenge as you read through this chapter. The response to the challenge appears on page 584.

You are the nurse in an elementary school. A 10-year-old pupil has recently been diagnosed with idiopathic epilepsy. He has a mixed seizure disorder with both tonic-clonic (grand mal) and occasional partial seizures. He is taking phenytoin daily.

What are the most important observations in your assessment visit with this boy? Outline the most significant points for a teaching plan for the child, including his teachers and family.

Classification of Epilepsy

Epilepsy is a group of disorders involving similar pathophysiological mechanisms occurring in different areas of the brain. (It is in fact more correct to refer to the condition as "the epilepsies.") It is estimated that 1% to 2% of the population experience one of the forms of epilepsy.

The various forms of epilepsy have different causes and present different clinical symptoms. Although it is always difficult to define a disorder precisely, the definition of epilepsy we favour is "a symptom of excessive temporary neuronal discharge, due to intracranial or extracranial causes ... characterized clinically by discrete episodes, which tend to be recurrent, in which there is a disturbance of movement, sensation, behaviour, perception and/or consciousness" (Sutherland JM, Eadie MJ, 1980).

This definition stresses the intermittent nature of epilepsy. Whereas it is true that patients may suffer attacks caused by abnormal neuronal firing, they can also experience long seizure-free periods. This is partly because epilepsy can result from many different causes affecting various parts of the brain. The symptoms of epilepsy depend on (1) the site of the epileptic focus and (2) the degree to which it spreads (Figure 49.1).

Etiologically, epilepsy can be classified as either primary or secondary.

Primary epilepsy. In primary epilepsy, the cause is not known; thus, it is also called idiopathic epilepsy. The condition is characterized by major (grand mal) or minor (petit mal; myoclonic and akinetic) seizures. This type of epilepsy usually manifests in childhood or adolescence.

Secondary epilepsy. Also called symptomatic epilepsy, this condition can result from either intracranial causes, such as cerebral tumours, cerebrovascular occlusive disease or head injury. Secondary epilepsy may also be caused by extracranial problems, such as anoxia, uremia or eclampsia. This type is more likely to occur in adulthood.

It is also popular to classify epilepsy on the basis of seizure patterns. Table 49.1 presents the classification suggested by the International League Against Epilepsy.

Figure 49.1
Manifestations of partial (symptomatic, cortical) epilepsy

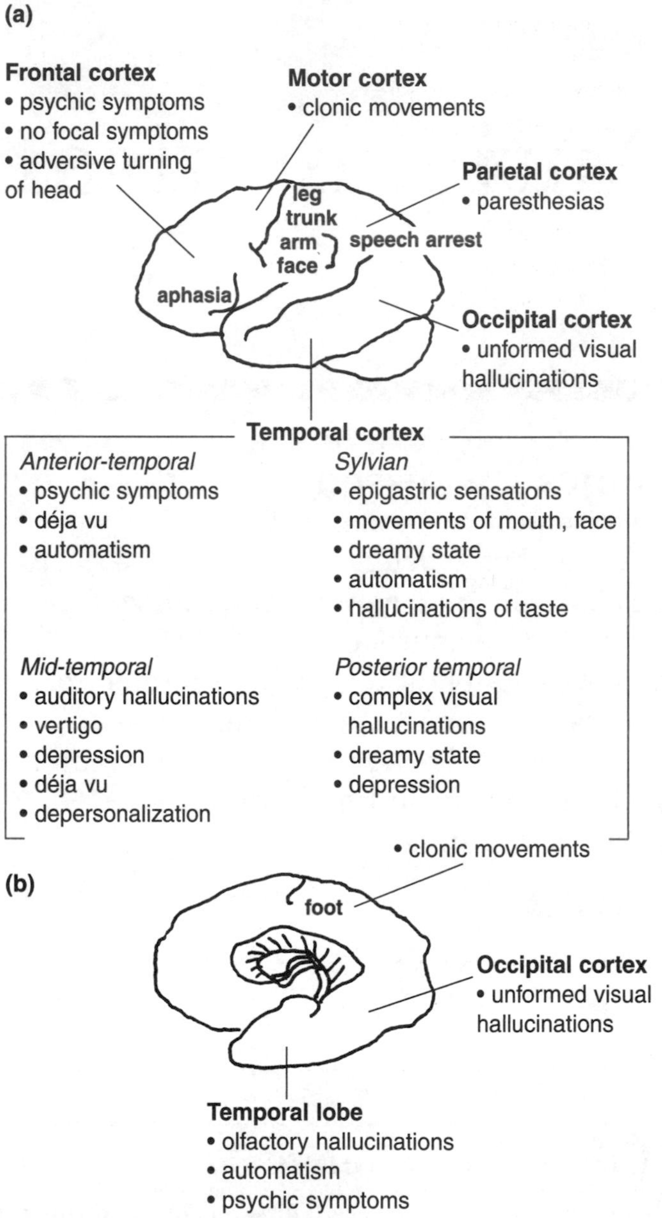

(a)

Frontal cortex
• psychic symptoms
• no focal symptoms
• adversive turning of head

Motor cortex
• clonic movements

Parietal cortex
• paresthesias

leg
trunk
arm
face
speech arrest

aphasia

Occipital cortex
• unformed visual hallucinations

Temporal cortex

Anterior-temporal
• psychic symptoms
• déja vu
• automatism

Sylvian
• epigastric sensations
• movements of mouth, face
• dreamy state
• automatism
• hallucinations of taste

Mid-temporal
• auditory hallucinations
• vertigo
• depression
• déja vu
• depersonalization

Posterior temporal
• complex visual hallucinations
• dreamy state
• depression

(b)

• clonic movements

foot

Occipital cortex
• unformed visual hallucinations

Temporal lobe
• olfactory hallucinations
• automatism
• psychic symptoms

Source: Sutherland JM, Eadie MJ. *The Epilepsies: Modern Diagnosis and Treatment.* 3rd ed. New York: Churchill and Livingstone; 1980: 27. Reproduced with permission.

Generalized seizures are characterized by an abnormal neuronal discharge that originates in the midbrain reticular formation. This part of the central nervous system acts much like a telephone system, connecting with all parts of the brain. Any neuronal discharge starting there or reaching there from another site may be transmitted to

Table 49.1
Characteristics of generalized, partial and unclassified epileptic seizures†

1. **Generalized seizures**
   Bilateral symmetrical seizures without local onset; clinically:
   (a) Absence seizures (petit mal)
   (b) Bilateral myoclonus
   (c) Infantile spasms
   (d) Clonic seizures
   (e) Tonic seizures
   (f) Tonic-clonic seizures (grand mal)
   (g) Akinetic seizures

2. **Partial seizures**
   Seizures beginning locally with:
   (a) Elementary symptomatology
   • motor
   • sensory
   • autonomic
   • compound forms

   (b) Complex symptomatology
   • impaired consciousness
   • complex hallucinations
   • affective symptoms
   • automatism (repetitive, purposeless behaviours)

   (c) Partial seizures becoming generalized tonic-clonic seizures

3. **Unclassified seizures**
   Seizures that cannot be classified because of incomplete data

† As suggested by International League Against Epilepsy, 1970.

other areas of the brain. The extent of its propagation and the areas of the brain to which it is transmitted determine the nature of the epileptic attack. As a result, generalized seizures may vary in severity. They always involve a loss of consciousness and bilateral motor events, but they can range from brief periods of unconsciousness (petit mal) to severe tonic-clonic (grand mal) seizures. Generalized seizures may be due to genetic factors that make the midbrain reticular formation unstable, or to structural abnormalities or chemical causes (such as uremia, eclampsia or anoxia).

Partial seizures result from an excessive neuronal discharge anywhere in the cerebral hemispheres. As Figure 49.1 shows, initial symptoms are determined by the anatomic site of the original discharge. The discharge may remain localized or it may spread to other anatomical areas of the brain. The farther it spreads, the greater will be its clinical effect. If the impulse reaches the midbrain reticular formation, it may be transmitted throughout the brain, producing a generalized seizure. If, for example, the neuronal discharge occurs in the motor cortex, unusual muscle movements will be seen. An illustration of this is the jacksonian (or cortical) march, which begins with involuntary movements in the fingers of one hand and then moves to include the hand, arm and leg of the same side, if the impulse spreads to other motor neurons on the same side of the cerebral cortex. If the impulse reaches the midbrain reticular formation, it may be carried to all areas of the brain, and a generalized seizure will occur. Etiologically, partial epilepsy is caused by pathology in a discrete area of the brain.

Antiepileptic Drugs

There is no ideal antiepileptic drug. Thus, patients can be treated with a variety of agents in an attempt to prevent seizures. In general, the drugs in use today control seizures in about 80% of patients. However, drug therapy must be individualized and, in some cases, only a combination of anticonvulsants can effectively achieve control.

Choice of drug therapy is determined by the kind(s) of seizures experienced:

Petit mal (absence) seizures are relatively uncommon and begin exclusively in childhood. Patients experience recurrent, brief, sudden interruptions of consciousness without falling and have minimal twitching around the face and eyes. The drugs of first choice are either valproic acid (Depakene®), divalproex sodium (Depakote®, Epival®) or ethosuximide (Zarontin®). Clonazepam (Klonopin®, Rivotril®) is an alternative drug.

Myoclonic seizures are characterized by bilateral myoclonic jerks of the limbs, face and trunk that, if severe, may throw the patient to the ground. There may be brief lapses of consciousness. Early treatment of myoclonic epilepsy in infancy (hypsarrhythmia) is imperative. Corticosteroids (e.g., prednisone, 10 mg three or four times daily) or corticotrophin (40 U daily) given for two weeks may stop these seizures and prevent mental deterioration. If these agents fail, clonazepam, valproic acid or nitrazepam may control the seizures but are less likely to prevent mental retardation. Myoclonic epilepsy in children, adolescents or adults is best treated with clonazepam or sodium valproate.

Generalized tonic-clonic seizures may be a manifestation of primary generalized epilepsy or may occur secondary to focal or myoclonic seizures. Carbamazepine (Tegretol®) or phenytoin (Dilantin®) are the drugs of first choice, with phenobarbital, primidone or valproic acid serving as second-line drugs. Phenobarbital is usually used for the prevention of febrile seizures in infants.

Partial or focal epilepsy may activate the deep central grey matter to produce a secondarily generalized tonic-clonic seizure. Phenytoin and carbamazepine are first-line drugs in the treatment of partial or focal epilepsy. Phenobarbital and primidone are second-line agents. Alternatives for refractory cases include acetazolamide, clorazepate and methsuximide.

Status epilepticus is the only situation in which urgent treatment of seizures is essential. It is usually treated with intravenous diazepam. Alternatively, phenobarbital or phenytoin can be administered intravenously.

Drugs Effective Against Generalized Tonic-Clonic Seizures

Phenytoin (Dilantin®)

Mechanism of action, pharmacokinetics and pharmacologic effects. Phenytoin is slowly absorbed from the gastrointestinal tract. Approximately ninety percent of the drug in the blood is bound to plasma proteins. Phenytoin appears to prevent the spread of seizure activity in the cerebrum by reducing sodium transport across cell membranes. Elimination of phenytoin depends on hepatic metabolism. At low doses the drug has a half-life of twenty-four hours. However, as the dosages of phenytoin increase, the metabolic pathways responsible for its inactivation become progressively more saturated, and the half-life of the drug increases. Relatively small increases in dose can produce significant increases in plasma concentrations and drug-related toxicity. Measuring phenytoin plasma levels is valuable in adjusting the dose. Plasma concentrations of phenytoin between 10–20 µg/mL (39.6–79.2 µmol/L) are often effective without causing undue toxicity.

Problems may be encountered if phenytoin is injected intramuscularly or intravenously. Phenytoin is soluble only in concentrated solutions at an alkaline pH. Dilantin injection solution has a pH of 12. If injected intramuscularly, body fluids rapidly change the pH of the drug solution to 7.35. Phenytoin is not soluble in a concentrated solution at this pH and precipitates in the muscle. Thereafter, its rate of absorption depends on slow dissolution in the muscle. Problems can also be encountered if phenytoin is placed in a glass intravenous bottle. In this environment the drug adheres to the glass. Using a glass container serves only to treat the inside of the bottle and not the inside of the patient.

Therapeutic uses. Phenytoin capsules are indicated for the control of generalized tonic-clonic and psychomotor (grand mal and temporal-lobe) seizures and prevention and treatment of seizures occurring during or following neurosurgery. The pediatric formulations (Infatabs® and suspension) are used for the control of generalized tonic-clonic (grand mal) and complex partial (psychomotor, temporal-lobe) seizures. When used parenterally, phenytoin is indicated for the treatment of status epilepticus of the grand mal type and the treatment of seizures occurring during or following neurosurgery.

Monotherapy is the preferred mode of therapy for most epileptic patients. If seizures continue and further increases in dosage appear inadvisable because of adverse effects or high serum concentrations of the drug, at least one and sometimes a second alternative drug should be tried before considering the use of two drugs at the same time. However, if multiple-drug therapy is required, phenytoin is often combined with phenobarbital, carbamazepine (Tegretol®) and/or primidone (Mysoline®) to manage difficult problems. Phenytoin may be combined with ethosuximide in the treatment of patients with both petit and grand mal.

Because of its effect on ventricular automaticity, intravenous phenytoin is contraindicated in sinus bradycardia, S-A block, second- and third-degree A-V block, and in patients with Adams-Stokes syndrome. Phenytoin should be used with caution in patients with hypotension and severe myocardial insufficiency.

Adverse effects. Phenytoin irritates the stomach, causing nausea and vomiting. Prolonged use can lead to gum hypertrophy, hirsutism, immunologic abnormalities, skin rashes and other hypersensitivity reactions. Gingival hyperplasia is the most common pediatric adverse effect, and can occur in up to twenty percent of children. Although gingival hyperplasia can be reduced by good oral hygiene, it remains an embarrassing problem.

Overdosage produces nystagmus, ataxia, diplopia and drowsiness. Generally, concentrations above 20 µg/mL (80 µmol/L) are associated with nystagmus, above 30 µg/mL (120 µmol/L) with ataxia and above 40 µg/mL (160 µmol/L) with lethargy.

Other adverse effects include hyperglycemia, osteomalacia (treated with high doses of vitamin D), lymphadenopathy, leukopenia, megaloblastic anemia (managed with folic acid) and aplastic anemia.

If given rapidly intravenously, phenytoin can produce hypotension. Cardiac arrhythmias, including ventricular fibrillation or arrest, can also occur.

The use of phenytoin has been associated with increased incidence of congenital malformations, such as cleft lip or palate and heart malformations in children of women receiving the drug. However, the great majority of mothers on antiepileptic medication deliver normal infants. *In any case, antiepileptic drugs should not be discontinued in*

Table 49.2
Phenytoin: Drug interactions

Drug	Interaction
Acute alcohol intake, chloramphenicol, chlordiazepoxide, cimetidine, diazepam, dicumarol, disulfiram, estrogens, ethosuximide, fluoxetine, halothane, isoniazid, methylphenidate, phenothiazines, phenylbutazone, salicylates, sulfonamides, trazodone	• These drugs may inhibit the metabolism of phenytoin, increasing its serum levels and effect
Alcohol	• Chronic use of ethanol can diminish the effect of phenytoin
Antidepressants, tricyclic	• High doses of TCAs may precipitate seizures and increase the required dose of phenytoin
Barbiturates	• Barbiturates may enhance metabolism of phenytoin. This effect is variable and unpredictable
Carbamazepine	• Carbamazepine may increase the metabolism and decrease the serum levels of phenytoin
Corticosteroids, coumarin anticoagulants, contraceptives (oral), digitoxin, doxycycline, estrogens, furosemide, quinidine, rifampin, vitamin D	• The efficacy of these drugs is reduced by phenytoin
Corticosteroids	• The metabolism of corticosteroids may be increased by phenytoin
Folic acid	• The replacement of folic acid in folate-deficient pts receiving phenytoin may increase the metabolism of phenytoin and decrease its serum level
Lidocaine IV	• IV lidocaine and IV phenytoin can cause excessive cardiac depression
Quinidine	• The metabolism of phenytoin can be increased by quinidine
Thyroid hormones	• Phenytoin may displace thyroid hormones from plasma proteins, thereby increasing free thyroxin levels

patients to whom the drug is administered to prevent major seizures, because of the strong possibility of precipitating status epilepticus.

Table 49.2 (page 576) lists the clinically significant drug interactions with phenytoin.

Carbamazepine (Tegretol®)

Pharmacokinetics and therapeutic uses. Carbamazepine's spectrum of activity is similar to that of phenytoin. It is considered a first-line drug for the treatment of generalized tonic-clonic seizures and partial seizures with complex symptomatology. Carbamazepine is ineffective in controlling petit mal, minor motor, myoclonic and predominantly unilateral seizures.

Carbamazepine is absorbed slowly from the gastrointestinal tract. Its half-life during chronic therapy may range from eight to over twenty-four hours. The drug's usual therapeutic range is 5–12 µg/mL (21.1–50.8 µmol/L); 15–17 µg/mL (63.3–71.7 µmol/L) may be necessary in some patients.

Adverse effects. At usual therapeutic doses, carbamazepine has a low incidence of adverse effects. The most common include gastric irritation, dizziness, diplopia and blurred vision. Carbamazepine can also produce oculomotor disturbances, tinnitus, abnormal involuntary movements, peripheral neuritis, rashes, congestive heart failure, hypotension, syncope, and cholestatic and hepatocellular jaundice. Agranulocytosis, thrombocytopenia and leukopenia are recognized adverse effects of the drug; fortunately, they are rare.

Table 49.3 lists the clinically significant drug interactions with carbamazepine.

Phenobarbital

Mechanism of action and therapeutic uses. Phenobarbital is a CNS depressant that may act as an antiepileptic by reducing sodium and potassium flux across cell membranes. It remains a popular drug for the treatment of tonic-clonic epilepsy, focal seizures and complex partial

---

Table 49.3
Carbamazepine: Drug interactions

Drug	Interaction
Acetazolamide, cimetidine, danazol, diltiazem, erythromycin, fluoxetine, isoniazid, propoxyphene, verapamil	• These drugs can increase plasma carbamazepine levels
Alcohol	• Tolerance to alcohol may be reduced in pts taking carbamazepine
Anticoagulants, oral	• Dosage of oral anticoagulants should be readjusted to clinical requirements whenever carbamazepine is started or stopped
Alprazolam, anticoagulants (oral), clobazam, clonazepam, contraceptives (oral), corticosteroids, cyclosporin, digoxin, doxycycline, ethosuximide, felodipine, haloperidol, imipramine, methadone, primidone, theophylline, thioridazine, valproic acid	• Induction of hepatic enzymes by carbamazepine may increase the metabolism and decrease the effects of these drugs
Contraceptives, oral	• Oral contraceptives may be less effective in the presence of chronic carbamazepine tx. Pts should be advised to use alternative, nonhormonal methods of contraception
Lithium	• Lithium and carbamazepine may increase the risk of neurotoxic side effects
Monoamine oxidase inhibitors	• MAOIs should not be administered immediately before, in conjunction with, or immediately after carbamazepine

Table 49.4
Phenobarbital: Drug interactions

Drug	Interaction
Anticoagulants (oral), anticonvulsants, antihistamines, contraceptives (oral), griseofulvin	• Phenobarbital may increase the metabolism of these drugs and decrease their effects
CNS depressants	• CNS depressants plus phenobarbital produce additive CNS depression
Methoxyflurane	• Methoxyflurane metabolism may be increased by chronic phenobarbital tx, resulting in the production of increased amounts of nephrotoxic metabolites
Vitamin D	• Vitamin D metabolism may be increased by phenobarbital

seizures. Phenobarbital is a long-acting barbiturate, with a half-life ranging from 60–120 h in adults. The plasma levels considered to be consistent with good therapeutic effect and minimal toxicity fall between 15–25 µg/mL (64.6–107.7 µmol/L). Phenobarbital is also employed prophylactically in young children when febrile seizures are feared.

Adverse effects. CNS depression is the major adverse effect of phenobarbital. This can be seen as either sedation or sleep and can be minimized by increasing the dose gradually. Fortunately, tolerance to the CNS-depressive effects of phenobarbital occurs when the drug is given chronically. Nevertheless, the first few weeks of treatment can be a problem.

Allergic rashes are reported in 1% to 2% of patients taking phenobarbital. Prolonged therapy may be associated with folate deficiency, hypocalcemia and osteomalacia. These effects will respond to folic acid treatment and high doses of vitamin D. Hypoprothrombinemia with hemorrhage has been reported in babies delivered from mothers given phenobarbital. This can be treated with vitamin K injections.

Table 49.4 lists the clinically significant drug interactions with phenobarbital.

Primidone (Mysoline®)

Mechanism of action, pharmacokinetics and pharmacologic effects. Primidone is structurally similar to phenobarbital and has a similar spectrum of antiepileptic activity. Primidone is quickly absorbed from the GI tract and metabolized to phenobarbital and phenylethylmalon-

amide, both having antiepileptic activity. The half-life of primidone is eight hours, and the half-lives of phenobarbital and phenylethylmalonamide are 60–120 h and 24–48 h, respectively. Therefore, patients treated with primidone accumulate its metabolites in their bodies. Effective plasma levels of primidone usually fall between 5–10 µg/mL (22.9–45.8 µmol/L). However, phenobarbital plasma levels frequently can be used to guide dosage.

Therapeutic uses. Primidone is useful in the prevention of grand mal and psychomotor seizures. It may be used alone or in combination with other anticonvulsants. To avoid undue CNS depression, primidone should be taken at night and the dose increased gradually.

Adverse effects. Primidone depresses the central nervous system and can cause sedation, vertigo, nystagmus, ataxia and diplopia. Other complaints include nausea and vomiting. Serious adverse effects are not common. However, leukopenia, thrombocytopenia, systemic lupus erythematosus and lymphadenopathy have been encountered. Similar to phenobarbital, primidone may cause maculopapular and morbilliform rashes, hemorrhage in the newborn, megaloblastic anemia and osteomalacia. The appearance of a rash is justification for stopping the drug. The other conditions may be treated as explained for phenobarbital. Because primidone is metabolized to phenobarbital, it has same drug interactions as phenobarbital (see Table 49.4).

Newer Adjuvant Drugs for Treatment of Generalized Tonic-Clonic Seizures

Between 50% and 70% of newly diagnosed patients with epilepsy will be seizure-free with initial antiepileptic drug monotherapy, regardless of the specific drug used. Switching to a second antiepileptic drug as monotherapy affords control in about one-third of the initially uncontrolled patients. Ultimately, however, even with different combinations of polytherapy, approximately 15% to 25% of epileptic patients have not been adequately controlled with the previously available epileptic drugs. There was, therefore, an urgent need for new, more effective antiepileptic drugs with less toxicity.

Gabapentin, lamotrigine and vigabatrin partly fill that need. These new drugs have been approved as add-on therapy, to be used with currently accepted antiepileptic drugs. Used in this manner, these drugs provide relief for many patients who previously had been uncontrolled.

Gabapentin (Neurontin®)

Mechanism of action and pharmacologic effects. The mechanism of action of gabapentin is not known. Its anticonvulsant action may result from altered transport or metabolism of brain amino acids. Gabapentin is rapidly absorbed after oral administration, with or without food, achieving maximum plasma concentrations within two to three hours. The fraction of the dose absorbed becomes smaller as the dose increases, apparently due to a saturable transport mechanism in the intestine. About sixty percent of a 300- to 600-mg dose is absorbed. Gabapentin is not metabolized and is almost completely excreted by the kidneys, with a relatively short half-life of five to seven hours.

Therapeutic uses. Gabapentin is effective as add-on therapy in some patients with drug-resistant partial epilepsy with or without generalization. In one double-blind, placebo-controlled trial, 1200 mg of gabapentin per day added to previous therapy decreased seizure frequency over three months by over fifty percent in twenty-nine percent of patients with partial epilepsy.

There is no interaction between gabapentin and phenytoin, valproic acid, carbamazepine or phenobarbital. Consequently, gabapentin may be used in combination with other commonly used antiepileptic drugs without concern for alteration of the plasma concentrations of gabapentin or the other antiepileptic drugs.

Adverse effects. Gabapentin appears to be well tolerated. Somnolence, dizziness, ataxia, fatigue and nystagmus have been the most common adverse effects when gabapentin was added to other antiepileptic drugs. These effects were usually mild to moderate in severity and often transient. Rash has occurred rarely. The absence of adverse reactions with other antiepileptic drugs is an advantage, particularly for adjunctive use.

Table 49.5 lists the clinically significant drug interactions with gabapentin.

Lamotrigine (Lamictal®)

Mechanism of action and pharmacologic effects. Lamotrigine is chemically unrelated to any other current antiepileptic drugs. It is thought to act by stabilizing neuronal voltage-dependent sodium channels, thus reducing the presynaptic release of excitatory amino acids, principally glutamate and aspartate, that are thought to play a role in the generation and spread of epileptic seizures.

Lamotrigine is almost completely absorbed from the GI tract, either with or without food. Plasma concentrations reach a peak in 1.5–5 h. The plasma half-life of a single dose is about 24 h.

Table 49.5
Gabapentin: Drug interactions

Drug	Interaction
Antacids	• Antacids decrease the bioavailability of gabapentin by about 20%. This interaction can be minimized by giving the anticonvulsant at least 2 h after the antacid

Table 49.6
Lamotrigine: Drug interactions

Drug	Interaction
Antiepileptic drugs	• The metabolism of lamotrigine is induced by antiepileptic drugs (e.g., phenytoin, carbamazepine, phenobarbital). This leads to a decrease in the half-life of lamotrigine to an average of 15 h. In pts withdrawn from enzyme-inducing antiepileptic drugs, plasma lamotrigine concentrations increased by > 100%
Valproic acid	• Valproic acid inhibits the elimination of lamotrigine and increases the half-life of lamotrigine up to 60 h. In pts receiving both valproic acid and enzyme-inducing agents (e.g., phenytoin, carbamazepine, phenobarbital), the half-life of lamotrigine is close to 24 h

Therapeutic uses. Lamotrigine is effective as add-on therapy in the treatment of drug-resistant partial epilepsy. In four randomized, placebo-controlled crossover trials in patients with drug-resistant partial epilepsy, lamotrigine produced a greater than fifty percent reduction in seizure frequency in twenty-two percent of patients.

Adverse effects. Dizziness, diplopia, ataxia, blurred vision, nausea, vomiting and rash have been the most common adverse effects when lamotrigine was added to other antiepileptic drugs. Rash has occurred in about ten percent of patients and caused about four percent to stop taking the drug. A few patients have developed rashes severe enough to require hospitalization, including Stevens-Johnson syndrome, and death has occurred rarely. Disseminated intravascular coagulation has been reported.

Table 49.6 lists the clinically significant drug interactions with lamotrigine.

Vigabatrin (Sabril®)

Mechanism of action and pharmacologic effects. Vigabatrin is an irreversible inhibitor of gamma-aminobutyric acid transferase (GABA-T), the enzyme responsible for the catabolism of the inhibitory neurotransmitter gamma-aminobutyric acid (GABA) in the brain. The mechanism of action of vigabatrin is attributed to the irreversible inhibition of GABA-T, and consequent increased levels of GABA.

The absorption of vigabatrin from the GI tract is rapid and almost complete. Food slightly reduces the rate, but not the extent, of vigabatrin absorption. Peak plasma concentrations are attained within 1–2 h after a single dose. Vigabatrin is neither protein bound nor metabolized. The drug is eliminated primarily by renal excretion, with renal clearance of unchanged drug accounting for about 60% to 70% of total clearance.

Therapeutic uses. Vigabatrin is approved for adjunctive management of epilepsy that is not satisfactorily controlled by conventional therapy. A meta-analysis of six studies found that vigabatrin produced a greater than fifty percent decrease in seizure frequency as add-on therapy in forty-six percent of adult patients with drug-refractory complex partial epilepsy. The antiepileptic efficacy and good clinical tolerability are generally maintained during treatment for up to seven years.

Adverse effects. Vigabatrin is generally well tolerated in epileptic patients. Adverse effects are mainly CNS related and probably a secondary consequence of increased GABA levels caused by vigabatrin. Somnolence was reported in 12.5% of patients. Dizziness, headache, nervousness, memory complaints, aggression, depression and diplopia have occurred in less than 4% of patients. The most frequent adverse event observed in children was "hyperactivity" (reported as hyperkinesia, 7.7%; agitation, 2.3%; excitation, 0.3%; or restlessness, 0.7%), which was reported in 11% of children.

Table 49.7 on the next page lists the clinically significant drug interactions with vigabatrin.

Table 49.7
Vigabatrin: Drug interactions

Drug	Interaction
Phenytoin	• A gradual reduction of about 20% in plasma phenytoin concentrations has been observed following add-on tx with vigabatrin. The mechanism whereby this occurs is unknown. Limited data from clinical trials suggest that increasing the phenytoin dose to compensate may not be necessary

Drugs Effective Against Absence Seizures

Ethosuximide (Zarontin®)

Pharmacokinetics and therapeutic uses.
Ethosuximide is a first-line drug for the treatment of petit mal epilepsy. With a half-life of thirty hours in children, ethosuximide requires five to seven days of regular treatment to reach steady-state levels. Therapeutic effects are usually obtained with serum levels of 50–100 µg/mL (354.2–708.3 µmol/L).

Adverse effects. Gastric irritation is the most common adverse reaction to ethosuximide. This can be minimized by giving the drug in divided daily doses. Other drug-related problems include CNS depression and rashes. Eosinophilia is seen in about ten percent of patients taking ethosuximide. Other blood problems that have occurred are pancytopenia and aplastic anemia. Systemic lupus erythematosus and Stevens-Johnson syndrome have also been noted rarely in patients given ethosuximide.

Valproic Acid (Depakene®)

Pharmacokinetics and therapeutic uses.
Valproic acid, or sodium valproate, is indicated as sole or adjunctive therapy in the treatment of simple or complex absence seizures, including petit mal, and is useful in primary generalized seizures with tonic-clonic manifestations. Valproic acid may also be used adjunctively in patients with multiple seizure types, which include either absence or tonic-clonic seizures.

Valproic acid is rapidly absorbed after oral administration. With a half-life of six to sixteen hours, the drug should be administered three or four times daily. Its therapeutic plasma window is 50–100 µg/mL (347–694 µmol/L).

Divalproex sodium (Depakote®, Epival®) is a derivative of valproic acid. Provided in enteric-coated tablets, it dissociates into valproic acid in the intestinal tract. The drug may produce less gastric distress than valproic acid.

Adverse effects. Anorexia, nausea and vomiting are major deterrents to the use of valproic acid. Taking the drug with food may help. Sedation, ataxia and incoordination occur very infrequently.

Minor elevations of transaminases (e.g., SGOT and SGPT) and LDH are frequent and appear to be dose related. Occasionally, laboratory tests also show increases in serum bilirubin and abnormal changes in other liver function tests. These results may reflect serious hepatotoxicity. Hepatic failure resulting in fatalities has occurred in patients receiving valproic acid. This has usually occurred during the first six months of treatment with valproic acid. Because children two years of age or younger have nearly a twenty-fold increase in risk of fatal hepatotoxicity, valproic acid should be used in this age group with extreme caution and as a sole agent. Liver function tests should be performed on patients receiving valproic acid prior to therapy and at frequent intervals thereafter, especially during the first six months. However, physicians should not rely totally on serum biochemistry, since these tests may not be abnormal in all instances, but should also consider the results of a careful interim medical history and physical examination. Care should be observed when administering valproic acid to patients with a prior history of hepatic disease.

Reports have appeared implicating valproic acid as a teratogen. The incidence of congenital malformations in the general population may be increased two- to threefold by valproic acid. The increase is largely associated with specific defects,

Table 49.8
Valproic acid: Drug interactions

Drug	Interaction
Alcohol	• Valproic acid can potentiate the CNS-depressant effects of ethanol
Clonazepam	• Clonazepam, used concomitantly with valproic acid, may produce absence status
Drugs affecting coagulation (e.g., ASA, warfarin)	• Anticoagulants (e.g., ASA, warfarin) should be used with caution with valproic acid because valproic acid affects the second stage of platelet aggregation
Phenobarbital	• Valproic acid can increase phenobarbital serum levels in pts taking phenobarbital or primidone

e.g., congenital malformations of the heart, cleft lip and/or palate, and neural tube defects. Nevertheless, the great majority of mothers receiving anticonvulsant medication deliver normal infants.

Table 49.8 lists the clinically significant drug interactions with valproic acid.

Clonazepam (Klonopin®, Rivotril®)

Therapeutic uses. Clonazepam is a benzodiazepine. It is indicated alone or as an adjunct in the management of myoclonic and akinetic seizures and petit mal variants. The drug may also be of some value in patients with absence spells (petit mal) who have failed to respond to succinimides.

Adverse effects. Sedation and drowsiness are the main complaints with clonazepam. In this regard it does not differ from other benzodiazepines (see Chapter 47). Ataxia may also be seen. Alterations in behaviour include aggressiveness, argumentativeness, hyperactivity, agitation, depression, euphoria, irritability, forgetfulness and confusion. These are particularly likely to occur in patients with a prior history of psychiatric disturbances and are known to occur in patients with chronic seizure disorders.

Table 49.9 lists the clinically significant drug interactions with clonazepam.

Miscellaneous Antiepileptics

Clobazam (Frisium®)

Clobazam is a benzodiazepine introduced for epilepsy refractory to standard therapy. In most studies, clobazam has been added to current antiepileptic therapy in patients with refractory seizures, and the drug appears to be a useful adjuvant medication in a variety of seizure types in adults and children. Clobazam has a rapid onset of action.

Clobazam appears to have a lower incidence of neurological adverse effects when compared with clonazepam. The adverse effects of clobazam are dose related. Most common are sedation, drowsiness, fatigue and dizziness. Ataxia, insomnia, depression, behavioural changes and weight gain have also been reported. As with other benzodiazepines, physical and psychological dependence have occurred. Clobazam must be discontinued slowly over several months to avoid withdrawal seizures.

Table 49.9
Clonazepam: Drug interactions

Drug	Interaction
CNS depressants, MAOIs, TCAs	• The action of benzodiazepines, such as clonazepam, may be potentiated by other CNS depressants, MAOIs and TCAs
Valproic acid	• Clonazepam, used concomitantly with valproic acid, may produce absence status

Diazepam (Valium®)

Intravenous diazepam is the recommended treatment for status epilepticus. Repeated injections are required to maintain the high brain levels necessary to terminate status epilepticus. Continued use of diazepam is not effective in the prevention of seizures. Detailed discussion of the pharmacology, adverse effects and drug interactions for benzodiazepines can be found in Chapter 47 and Table 47.2 (page 554).

Lorazepam (Ativan®)

Lorazepam is a benzodiazepine and is discussed in Chapter 47. It is effective for the initial treatment of status epilepticus and is regarded as a drug of choice for initial control of continuous generalized tonic-clonic or partial seizures. When lorazepam is administered intravenously for status epilepticus, the patient must be observed for signs of cardio-respiratory depression, especially when this drug is given with other antiepileptic agents. Seizure control after intravenous administration is usually achieved within three to five minutes; however, as long as ten minutes may be required in children, particularly if a lower dose (e.g., 0.05 mg/kg) is used.

Nursing Management

The nursing management of the patient receiving anticonvulsant drugs is described in Table 49.10. Dosage details of individual drugs are given in Table 49.11 (pages 585–587).

Table 49.10
Nursing management of the anticonvulsants

Assessment of risk vs. benefit	Patient data	• Assess to establish baseline VS, general state of health • *Pregnancy:* Risk category unknown for many of these drugs. Many women have had pregnancies while taking anticonvulsants without adverse effects to the baby. Risks of seizure must be weighed against potential risks to fetus. Valproic acid is classed as pregnancy risk category D (human fetus risk has been demonstrated)
	Drug data	• Physician should determine which drug is indicated, depending on type of seizure disorder and pt's risks for toxicity. Mixed disorders may require more than one drug for control • *Some serious drug interactions:* Confer with pharmacist • Most serious (but rare) adverse effects include blood cell abnormalities with carbamazepine, ethosuximide and primidone; hepatotoxicity with valproic acid • Most common adverse effects relate to CNS depression (sedation, drowsiness, lack of concentration, fatigue). Gingival hyperplasia with phenytoin can be embarrassing
Implementation	Rights of administration	• Using the "rights" helps prevent errors of administration
	Right route	• Generally given PO; IV may be used for status epilepticus
	Right time	• See Table 49.11. NB variation in dosage schedules among drugs in this class
	Right technique	• IV administration requires knowledge of correct diluent and IV solution, correct dilution and rate of administration. Always refer to manufacturer's instructions for this route. For direct IV, check agency policy regarding certification or education requirements. Specific precautions with this group because these drugs are very irritating to tissue: caution to prevent extravasation. Rate must not be exceeded. Resuscitation equipment must be readily available

Table 49.10 (continued)
Nursing management of the anticonvulsants

Implementation (cont'd)	Nursing therapeutics	• Epilepsy is still feared by many in society. Pt and family need accurate information, support and reassurance • Monitoring occurrence of seizures can help to identify triggers • Care during and following a seizure is important to provide safety and reassurance
	Patient/family teaching	• Pt/family require accurate information to promote successful drug tx. Compliance and follow-up are essential; review principles of pt education in Chapter 3 • With phenytoin, teach importance of good oral hygiene and regular dental check-ups • Alert pt that phenytoin can discolour urine (pink or reddish-brown) • Emphasize importance of routine schedule (no missed doses) and danger of sudden discontinuation. Same brand of drug should be used; not all brands are equivalent • For carbamazepine, sunscreen and protective clothing should be worn to prevent photosensitivity reactions to sunlight • Explain importance of routine blood work to determine plasma levels; adjust dosage prn • Pts/families should know warning signs/symptoms of possible toxicities of these drugs. Report immediately: rash, fever, sore throat, diarrhea, nausea, vomiting, unusual bleeding or bruising, weakness, dark urine, jaundice • Warn pts to avoid alcohol and OTCs that may cause drowsiness; will increase risk of CNS depression • Written instructions are helpful • *Discuss possibility of pregnancy:* Advise pt to notify physician; discuss birth control methods
Outcomes	Monitoring of progress	*Continually monitor:* • Clinical response indicating tx success (reduction in frequency/intensity of seizures) • Signs/symptoms of adverse reactions; document and report immediately to physician • Blood tests for plasma values may be ordered (weekly or periodically)

Response to Clinical Challenge

Important observations:
• Evaluate the effectiveness of the drug therapy: has he had any seizures? frequency? severity? improvements?
• Does he have any signs of gingival hyperplasia? other side effects?
• What are his emotional reactions to the disorder and to long-term drug therapy?
• What type of support does he receive from school, family and others?

Teaching points for the child:
• Assess his level of knowledge about his seizure disorder and his drug therapy. Determine what he has learned from others and reinforce or correct as necessary.
• Instruct in oral hygiene.
• Emphasize the importance of taking each dose as prescribed — not missing any doses and not discontinuing the drug.

Teaching points for the child's teachers:
• Explain the type of seizure disorder and the goals of drug treatment.
• Review the common side effects that might affect school work (e.g., drowsiness, lethargy, lack of concentration) and explain that dosage adjustments can help to reduce these effects. Encourage teachers to report their observations to family or to you.
• Reassure teachers regarding the boy's ability to live a healthy life.

Teaching points for the child's family:
• Determine their learning needs, and provide reinforcement or new information as required.
• Provide reassurance and encourage family to seek community support groups, if desired.

Further Reading

Drugs for epilepsy. *Medical Letter on Drugs and Therapeutics* 1995;37:37.
Gabapentin for epilepsy. *Medical Letter on Drugs and Therapeutics* 1994;39:36.
Kalviainen R, Keranen T, Riekkinen PJ Sr. Place of newer antiepileptic drugs in the treatment of epilepsy. *Drugs* 1993;46:1009–1024.
Lamotrigine for epilepsy. *Medical Letter on Drugs and Therapeutics* 1995;37:21.
Pugh CB, Garnett WR. Current issues in the treatment of epilepsy. *Clinical Pharmacy* 1991;10:335–358.
Sutherland JM, Eadie MA. *The Epilepsies: Modern Diagnosis and Treatment.* 3rd ed. Edinburgh, London, New York: Churchill Livingstone; 1980.

Table 49.11
The anticonvulsants: Drug doses

Drug Generic name (Trade names)	Dosage	Nursing alert
A. Drugs Effective Against Generalized Tonic-Clonic Seizures		
carbamazepine (Tegretol)	**Oral:** *Adults/children > 12:* Initially, 100–200 mg od–bid. Progressively increase in divided doses. Optimal dosage, 800–1200 mg/day. *Children 6–12 years:* Initially, 100 mg in divided doses on day 1. Increase gradually by adding 100 mg/day. Should generally not exceed 1000 mg/day	• Give with food to reduce gastric side effects. May crush tablets and mix with food. Must be taken in divided doses
phenobarbital	**Oral:** *Adults:* 120–250 mg; alternatively, 2–3 mg/kg daily. *Children:* 30–100 mg daily; alternatively, 3–5 mg/kg daily. These amounts are taken hs. Administration more than 1x/day is unnecessary Recurrent febrile seizures have been treated with an oral loading dose of 6–8 mg/kg, followed by a maint. dose of 3–4 mg/kg to maintain plasma concentrations of 15–30 µg/mL. **IV** (slow): For preventive management of status epilepticus: *Adults:* 15–20 mg/kg; alternatively, 10 mg/kg followed by another 10 mg/kg, if necessary. Usual rate should not exceed 100 mg/min; usual max. dose, 20 mg/kg. *Children:* 15–20 mg/kg; alternatively, 10 mg/kg followed by another 10 mg/kg, if necessary. Usual rate is 1–2 mg/kg/min; usual max. dose is 20 mg/kg	• **PO:** May crush tablets and mix with food • **IV:** For direct IV, follow agency policy. After reconstitution of powder following vial label, dilute further with 10 mL of sterile water and give each 50 mg over 1 min. Guard against extravasation. Use solution immediately. Follow with NS • Follow local policy with respect to controlled drugs
phenytoin (Dilantin)	**Oral:** *Adults:* Pts who have received no previous tx may be started on 100 mg tid, and the dose then adjusted. Maint. dose, 300–400 mg/day. *Children:* Initially, 5 mg/kg/day in 2 or 3 equally divided doses, with subsequent dosage individualized to a max. of 300 mg/day. Recommended daily maint. dosage is usually 4–8 mg/k **IV:** *Adults:* For status epilepticus: Loading dose of 10–15 mg/kg should be administered slowly at a rate not exceeding 50 mg/min. This should be followed by maint. doses of 100 mg PO or IV q6–8h	• **PO:** Give with meals to reduce gastric irritation. Mix liquid forms well and use calibrated device for accurate dosing. Advise pt to chew the chewable form thoroughly prior to swallowing. NB different brands of oral dosage forms may be equivalent • **IV:** Follow agency policy. Direct IV is recommended, or intermittent infusion followed by NS to prevent vein irritation. Watch carefully for extravasation. Do not add to large-volume infusion; will precipitate

(cont'd on next page)

Table 49.11 (continued)
The anticonvulsants: Drug doses

Drug Generic name (Trade names)	Dosage	Nursing alert
A. Drugs Effective Against Generalized Tonic-Clonic Seizures (cont'd)		
primidone (Mysoline)	**Oral:** *Adults/children > 8:* Initially, 100–125 mg hs for 3 days, then 100–125 bid for 3 days, then 100–125 mg tid for 3 days, then maint. dose of 250 mg 3–4x daily. Not to exceed 2 g/day. *Children < 8:* Initially, 50 mg hs for 3 days, then 50 mg bid for 3 days, then 100 mg bid for 3 days, then maint. dose of 125–250 mg tid (10–25 mg/kg/day)	• Give with food. Tabs may be crushed or mixed with food. Shake oral concentrate well and use calibrated measure to ensure accuracy
B. Adjuvant Drugs for Treatment of Generalized Tonic-Clonic Seizures		
gabapentin (Neurontin)	**Oral:** *Adults:* Initially, 300–400 mg/day; increase by increments of 300–400 mg/day to maint. dose of 900–1200 mg/day. Should be given in 3 equally divided doses	• May be taken without regard to food. May open capsule and mix with juice or food. Give immediately
lamotrigine (Lamictal)	**Oral:** *Adults* (without valproic acid): Weeks 1–2, 50 mg od; weeks 3–4, 50 mg bid. Maint. dose, 150–250 mg bid. Consult manufacturer's information for detailed dosage	• May be given without regard to food
vigabatrin (Sabril)	**Oral:** *Adults:* Initially, 1 g/day, although pts with severe seizures may require an initial dose of 2 g/day. Dose may be increased/decreased in increments of 0.5 g. Optimal range, 2–4 g/day. Children: Initially, 40 mg/kg/day; increase to 80–100 mg/kg/day prn	• May be given with or without food
C. Drugs Effective Against Absence Seizures		
ethosuximide (Zarontin)	**Oral:** *Adults/children > 6 years:* Initially, 500 mg/day in divided doses. Thereafter, dose must be individualized according to response and tolerance. Increase daily dose by 250 mg q4–7days. Daily dosage, 1–1.5 g in divided doses. *Children < 6 years:* 250 mg/day	• Give with food to reduce gastric distress. Ensure accuracy by using calibrated device to measure liquid form
valproic acid (Depakene)	**Oral:** *Adults:* Initially, 15 mg/kg/day, increased at 1-week intervals by 5–10 mg/kg/day. Max., 60 mg/kg/day. If dose exceeds 250 mg/day, give in divided doses. A 500-mg enteric-coated capsule may be substituted for 2 250-mg capsules	• Give with food to reduce GI effects

Table 49.11 (continued)
The anticonvulsants: Drug doses

Drug Generic name (Trade names)	Dosage	Nursing alert
C. Drugs Effective Against Absence Seizures (cont'd)		
divalproex sodium (Depakote, Epival)	**Oral:** *Adults/children:* Initially, 15 mg/kg/day, increasing at 1-week intervals by 5–10 mg/kg/day. Max., 60 mg/kg/day. When dose is ≥ 125 mg, give in divided doses	• For enteric-coated tablets, do not crush. May be given without regard to food
clonazepam (Klonopin, Rivotril)	**Oral:** *Adults:* Initially, not to exceed 1.5 mg/day, divided into 3 doses. May increase in increments of 0.5–1 mg q3days. Maint. dose, 8–10 mg/day in 3 divided doses. Max., 20 mg/day. *Children ≤ 10 years or 30 kg:* Initially, 10–30 µg/kg/day. Not to exceed 50 µg/kg/day, given in 2–3 divided doses. Dosage should be increased by no more than 250–500 µg q3days. Maint. dose, 100–200 µg/kg/day. Daily dose should be divided into 3 equal doses	• May be given with food if GI effects occur
D. Miscellaneous Antiepileptics		
clobazam (Frisium)	**Oral:** *Adults:* Initially, 5–15 mg/day; increase gradually to max. 80 mg/day, if necessary. *Children < 2 years:* Initially, 0.5–1 mg/kg/day. *Children 2–16 years:* Initially, 5 mg/day; may be increased q5days to max. 40 mg/day	• May be given without regard to food
diazepam (Valium)	(Anticonvulsant) **Oral:** *Adults:* 2–10 mg 2–4x daily or 15–30 mg of extended-release form od. **IV** (acute management of status epilepticus): *Adults:* 5–10 mg given at a usual rate of 2 mg/min. Usual max. dose, 20 mg. *Children:* 0.15–0.3 mg/kg, given over 2 min. Usual max. dose, 5–10 mg. **Rectal:** *Adults:* 0.15–0.5 mg/kg (up to 20 mg/dose). *Children:* 0.2–0.5 mg/kg	• **PO:** May be taken with food. May crush and mix with food. Do not crush extended-release form • **IV:** Follow agency policy for direct IV. Give at a rate of 5 mg over 1 min for adults; slower for children. Have resuscitation equipment available. Pt should remain supine; observe closely
lorazepam (Ativan)	**IV** (acute management of status epilepticus): *Adults:* 4 mg, given at a usual rate of 2 mg/min. Usual max. dose, 8 mg. *Children:* 0.05–0.1 mg/kg, given over 2 min. Usual max. dose, 0.2 mg/kg	• Follow agency policy regarding IV administration. Dilute immediately prior to administration and do not use if solution is discoloured or has precipitate. Patient should remain supine; observe closely

CHAPTER 50

Antiparkinsonian Drugs

Topics Discussed
- Parkinsonism
- Definition of akinesia, tremor, rigidity
- Etiology of parkinsonism
- Drugs for the treatment of parkinsonism: Dopaminergics and anticholinergics
- For all drugs discussed: Mechanism of action and pharmacologic effects, therapeutic uses, adverse effects
- Nursing management

Drugs Discussed

Dopaminergic Drugs:
amantadine (ah-**man**-tah-deen)
bromocriptine (broe-moe-**krip**-teen)
levodopa (lee-voe-**doe**-pah)
levodopa + benserazide (ben-**ser**-ah-zyde)
levodopa + carbidopa (kar-bih-**doe**-pa)
pergolide (**per**-goe-lyde)
selegiline (se-**lej**-ih-leen)

Central Anticholinergic Drugs:
benztropine (**benz**-troe-peen)
biperiden (bye-**per**-ih-den)
diphenhydramine (dye-fen-**hye**-drah-meen)
ethopropazine (ee-thoe-**proe**-pah-zeen)
orphenadrine (or-**fen**-ah-dreen)
procyclidine (proe-**cye**-klih-deen)
trihexyphenidyl (try-hex-ee-**fen**-ih-dill)

Clinical Challenge

Consider this clinical challenge as you read through this chapter. The response to the challenge appears on page 597.

Mr. T. is a 62-year-old man who was diagnosed with Parkinson's disease last year. For 10 months his symptoms were controlled with amantadine, and he continued to work. Recently, his symptoms have increased, and he has had to take early retirement, which was not his choice. He is attending the Parkinson Clinic for reassessment.

Your role at the clinic is to complete an assessment and history, review current drug therapy and discuss your recommendations with the neurologist. What assessment data will be important? What will be the likely next step in drug therapy?

Parkinsonism

Parkinsonism refers to two main disorders that present with similar clinical symptoms. The first is called *paralysis agitans* or *idiopathic Parkinson's disease.* It accounts for at least ninety percent of the cases of parkinsonism and, as the term idiopathic implies, its cause is unknown. The second condition is *secondary* or *symptomatic parkinsonism,* caused by a past infection with the virus of lethargic encephalitis.

Both Parkinson's disease and postencephalitic parkinsonism occur usually after the age of forty and are seen most often for the first time in patients between age fifty and sixty. The symptoms of parkinsonism can also be produced by drugs that either deplete dopamine stores in the brain or block dopaminergic receptors in the central nervous system. This side effect is of particular importance with antipsychotic drugs.

The most prominent symptoms of parkinsonism are akinesia, tremor and rigidity. *Akinesia* is difficulty in initiating movements or modifying ongoing motor activity. The patient may show slowness and loss of dexterity, as well as problems with speech, manual skills and gait. *Tremor* is seen at rest and usually disappears when the affected limb is moved. *Rigidity* is due to an abnormal increase in muscle tone, producing cogwheel resistance to passive movement of an extremity. In addition, the patient may suffer from a stoop when standing or walking and a characteristic posturing of the hands and feet. Perspiration, excessive salivation, seborrhea and difficulty in swallowing may also be seen. The occurrence and severity of the symptoms vary from patient to patient.

Etiology of Parkinsonism

A discussion of parkinsonism centres on the function of the basal ganglia. This area of the brain is responsible for the smooth control of skeletal muscle movement and contains high concentrations of the neurotransmitters dopamine and acetylcholine. The two appear to function as physiological antagonists, with dopamine acting as an inhibitory and acetylcholine as an excitatory neurotransmitter. Normal control of muscle movements depends on a delicate balance between these two. In patients with parkinsonism this balance is destroyed, as

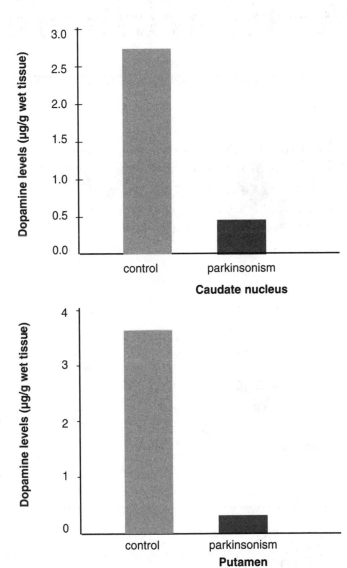

Figure 50.1
Concentrations of dopamine in the caudate nucleus and putamen at autopsy from control subjects and patients afflicted with parkinsonism

Source: Drawn from data provided in Hornykiewicz O. Parkinson's disease: from brain homogenates to treatment. *Fed Proc* 1973;32:183–190.

the levels of dopamine in the basal ganglia are reduced and acetylcholine acts unopposed (Figure 50.1).

This depletion of dopamine can be correlated with the degree of degeneration of substantia nigra. In the presence of dopamine deficiency, the normal balance between dopamine and acetylcholine is disturbed, and cholinergic activity predominates (see Figure 50.2, next page).

Figure 50.2
Balance between adrenergic and cholinergic mechanisms in the striatum

(a) Normal state

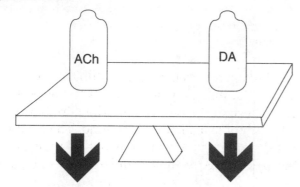

(b) Parkinsonism

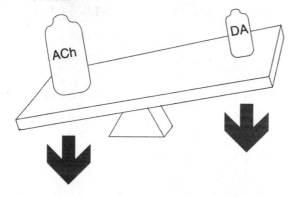

Ach = acetylcholine; DA = dopamine

Source: Yahr MD. The treatment of parkinsonism. *Med Clin North Am* 1972;56:1377–1382. Reproduced with permission.

Drugs for the Treatment of Parkinsonism

Drug treatment of parkinsonism is based on either stimulating dopamine receptors and/or blocking cholinergic receptors in the basal ganglia.

1. Dopaminergic Drugs

Levodopa (Dopar®, Larodopa®)

Mechanism of action and pharmacological effects. Levodopa is the immediate precursor of dopamine. When administered, a small portion of the dose enters the brain and is converted to

dopamine by the enzyme dopa decarboxylase. (If this statement needs further explanation, the reader is asked to review the biosynthesis of dopamine in Chapter 26.) Dopamine cannot be administered itself for the treatment of parkinsonism because, in contrast to levodopa, it will not cross the blood-brain barrier.

Levodopa is given orally. Despite the fact that attention is directed to its effects on the brain, only one percent of the administered dose reaches the central nervous system. Ninety-nine percent is converted to dopamine, norepinephrine and their metabolites in peripheral tissues. As a result, very large doses of levodopa must be given for the drug to produce significant changes in dopamine levels in the basal ganglia. The obvious consequence of administering very large doses is a high incidence of drug-related adverse effects.

Therapeutic uses. Levodopa, alone or combined with a dopa decarboxylase inhibitor (i.e., benserazide or carbidopa), is the most useful drug for the treatment of Parkinson's disease. Although treatment may be started with an anticholinergic or amantadine, the disease usually progresses to the point where levodopa is required within one year. Patients with postencephalic parkinsonism are also treated with levodopa. However, these individuals appear to tolerate only small doses of the drug and are more susceptible to its adverse effects.

The combination of levodopa and an anticholinergic may benefit patients who are not adequately treated by either drug alone. By increasing dopamine levels in the basal ganglia and blocking excessive cholinergic stimulation, these drugs, taken in combination, often afford greater relief than either used alone. Patients may also benefit from the combined use of amantadine and levodopa.

Levodopa is contraindicated in patients with parkinsonism secondary to the use of antipsychotic drugs because it will reverse the therapeutic benefits provided by phenothiazines and butyrophenones. Levodopa should not be administered to patients in whom sympathomimetic amines are contraindicated. Levodopa is contraindicated in patients with dementia accompanied by a significant degree of memory defect. It is also contraindicated in patients having episodic mental confusion, hallucinations or paranoid ideation. The drug should be used with caution in individuals with severe dizziness or fainting due to postural hypotension. It is contraindicated in patients with serious endocrine, renal, hepatic, cardiovascular or pulmonary disease. Patients with an existing or previously excised malignant melanoma must not be given levodopa because the drug can cause the disease to recur or lead to its progression or dissemination.

Adverse effects. Up to eighty percent of patients taking levodopa complain of anorexia, nausea, vomiting or epigastric pain. These effects can be reduced by taking the drug with food. About thirty percent of patients experience mild postural hypotension. An increase in cardiac arrhythmias is also a recognized adverse effect of levodopa.

Abnormal involuntary movements occur in about fifty percent of patients taking levodopa. Beginning approximately two to four months after starting therapy, they include faciolingual tics, grimacing, head bobbing and various rocking and rotating movements of the arms, legs or trunk.

Levodopa can also produce behavioural changes. Many patients with parkinsonism are elderly and may suffer from impairment of memory or dementia. Given to these individuals, levodopa can stimulate the central nervous system, resulting in hallucinations, paranoia, mania, insomnia and nightmares. It can also cause depression. Levodopa is perhaps best noted for its ability to stimulate the sexual interests of elderly patients, leading to additional behavioural changes.

Table 50.1 lists the clinically significant drug interactions with levodopa.

Levodopa plus Carbidopa (Sinemet®) and Levodopa plus Benserazide (Prolopa®)

Carbidopa and benserazide inhibit dopa decarboxylase. Because they do not cross the blood-brain barrier, these drugs reduce only the peripheral metabolism of levodopa to dopamine. The formation of dopamine in the brain is not affected. A higher percentage of the administered levodopa is converted to dopamine in the brain. By using either carbidopa or benserazide, it is possible to administer lower doses of levodopa, thereby reducing its peripheral adverse effects. As a result, the products Sinemet® and Prolopa® have replaced levodopa as the most useful agents for parkinsonism. The drug interactions for these products are the same as described for levodopa, except for the fact that pyridoxine does not interact with these compounds.

Bromocriptine (Parlodel®)

Bromocriptine stimulates dopaminergic D_2 receptors in the brain and has been found to be clinically useful as an adjunct to levodopa (usually with carbidopa or benserazide) in the symptomatic management of selected patients with Parkinson's

---

Table 50.1
Levodopa: Drug interactions

Drug	Interaction
Antidepressants, tricyclic	• If used with levodopa, TCAs can produce postural hypotension
Antihypertensive drugs	• Antihypertensive drugs can have their effects potentiated by levodopa
Antipsychotic drugs	• Antipsychotic drugs block dopamine receptors in the brain and reduce or abolish the effects of levodopa
Monoamine oxidase inhibitors	• MAOIs reduce dopamine and norepinephrine metabolism and increase their central and peripheral effects. Discontinue MAOIs
Pyridoxine	• Pyridoxine increases the extracerebral metabolism of levodopa, thus decreasing the amount available to the brain. Avoid pyridoxine unless a peripheral decarboxylase inhibitor (i.e., benserazide or carbidopa) is also given

disease who experience prominent dyskinesia or "wearing-off" reactions on long-term levodopa therapy. The best results with the drug have been seen early in the treatment of parkinsonism when it was given with Sinemet®. Doses of bromocriptine below 30 mg/day, combined with Sinemet®, can ameliorate the "on-off" and wearing-off effects encountered after long-term levodopa therapy.

The adverse effects of bromocriptine include nausea, vomiting, transient dizziness, abdominal pain, constipation and blurred vision, with or without diplopia. Digital vasospasm in response to cold, erythromelalgia, mental disturbances and dyskinesias may also be experienced. Bromocriptine, especially in higher doses, can produce mental disturbances. These include nightmares, mild agitation, hallucinations and paranoid delusions and are most common in elderly patients. The drug interactions for bromocriptine are the same as those previously described for levodopa with respect to tricyclic antidepressants, antihypertensives and antipsychotic drugs.

Pergolide (Permax®)

Pergolide is a long-acting dopamine agonist. Like bromocriptine, pergolide is effective when given with Sinemet®. Pergolide and bromocriptine appear similar in their therapeutic and adverse effects. However, some patients respond to one and not to the other.

Table 50.2 lists the clinically significant drug interactions with pergolide.

Selegiline (Eldepryl®)

Mechanism of action and therapeutic use. Selegiline, formerly known as l-deprenyl, acts indirectly to stimulate dopamine receptors. This drug is a selective monoamine oxidase type-B (MAO-B) inhibitor. It is a most interesting new compound,

and one that has stimulated a great deal of interest. Inhibition of MAO-B may block the metabolism of dopamine and increase the amount of dopamine available. Selegiline may also block dopamine neuronal reuptake, and this effect would also increase the amount of dopamine available to stimulate receptors.

Selegiline may be of value as an adjunct to levodopa (with or without a decarboxylase inhibitor) in the management of the signs and symptoms of Parkinson's disease. It may also be used in newly diagnosed patients before symptoms begin to affect the patient's social or professional life, at which time more efficacious treatment becomes necessary.

Adverse effects. Selegiline inhibits MAO-B, which is found in the brain, but not in the liver or intestine. It would not be expected, therefore, to interact with tyramine and sympathomimetics. In this sense, selegiline should not have the same adverse effects and drug interactions as the antidepressants phenelzine and tranylcypromine, which inhibit monoamine oxidase type A (MAO-A). These drugs interact with foods containing tyramine and sympathomimetics to produce significant, and sometimes dangerous, increases in blood pressure (see Chapter 46).

To date, clinical observations of selegiline appear to confirm its improved safety. It must be emphasized, however, that doses above 10 mg/day result in a loss of selectivity of selegiline towards MAO-B and an increase in the inhibition of MAO-A. At doses over 10 mg/day, patients are at increased risk for adverse reactions with tyramine-containing foods or sympathomimetics.

The adverse effects of selegiline are those usually associated with an excess of dopamine. The drug may potentiate the adverse effects of levodopa/carbidopa, and adjustments of drug dosages may be required. Hallucinations and confusion

---

Table 50.2
Pergolide: Drug interactions

Drug	Interaction
Dopamine antagonists	• Dopamine antagonists, such as the antipsychotics (phenothiazines, butyrophenones, thioxanthenes) or metoclopramide, ordinarily should not be administered concurrently with pergolide because these drugs may diminish pergolide's effectiveness

have been seen with the combined use of selegiline and levodopa/carbidopa. Other adverse effects include nausea, depression, loss of balance, insomnia, orthostatic hypotension, increased akinetic involuntary movements, arrhythmia, bradykinesia, chorea, delusions, hypertension, angina pectoris and syncope.

Amantadine (Symmetrel®)

Amantadine was first introduced as an antiviral agent for the prophylaxis of A_2 influenza. Because amantadine releases dopamine from the remaining intact dopaminergic nerves in the basal ganglia, it is also used to treat parkinsonism. Although less effective than levodopa, amantadine produces a more rapid response and fewer adverse effects, and its dosage is easier to adjust. Amantadine is indicated for the treatment of Parkinson's syndrome and in the short-term management of drug-induced extrapyramidal symptoms. Unfortunately, the initial clinical improvement may not be sustained. Performance deteriorates over three to six months. Therefore, amantadine is used most often with levodopa where it often improves the effects of the latter drug. However, amantadine usually has little effect in patients receiving near-maximal therapeutic benefits from levodopa.

The more important adverse effects with amantadine are orthostatic hypotensive episodes, congestive heart failure, depression, psychosis and urinary retention. Rarely, convulsion, reversible leukopenia and neutropenia, and abnormal liver function test results have been seen. Patients may also experience hallucinations, confusion or nightmares if high doses are used. These effects are more common if the patient is also receiving an anticholinergic.

In spite of the fact that the mechanism of action of amantadine is different from that of levodopa, its ultimate effect is the same. Amantadine increases the amount of endogenous dopamine available for use in the central nervous system. Therefore, the nursing process accompanying the use of amantadine is the same as that identified for levodopa.

Table 50.3 lists the clinically significant drug interactions with amantadine.

2. Central Anticholinergic Drugs

Trihexyphenidyl Hydrochloride (Artane®), Benztropine Mesylate (Cogentin®), Procyclidine Hydrochloride (Kemadrin®), Biperiden Hydrochloride (Akineton®)

Mechanism of action and pharmacologic effects. Anticholinergic drugs have been used for more than a century in the treatment of parkinsonism. As suggested earlier, the deficiency of dopamine in the basal ganglia exposes patients to excessive cholinergic stimulation. By administering an anticholinergic, it is possible to reduce the effects of acetylcholine and hopefully restore neurotransmitter balance.

Atropine and hyoscine, two classical anticholinergics, are no longer used because of their generalized effects on the body. In their place, newer agents have been synthesized with preferential effects on the brain. These include trihexyphenidyl hydrochloride (Artane®), benztropine mesylate (Cogentin®), procyclidine hydrochloride (Kemadrin®) and biperiden hydrochloride (Akineton®). The antihistamines diphenhydramine

---

Table 50.3
Amantadine: Drug interactions

Drug	Interaction
Amphetamine, dexamphetamine, methamphetamine, methylphenidate, pemoline	• These drugs should be used with caution with amantadine
Anticholinergics	• Anticholinergic effects are potentiated by amantadine. Confusion and hallucinations have been reported

Table 50.4
Anticholinergics: Drug interactions

Drug	Interaction
Amantadine	• Amantadine, given with a central anticholinergic, may potentiate the anticholinergic adverse effects of the latter drug

(Benadryl®) and orphenadrine (Disipal®) and the phenothiazine ethopropazine (Parsidol®) have antiparkinsonian activity because they, too, block cholinergic receptors in the basal ganglia.

Therapeutic uses. Anticholinergic drugs are used in patients at the early stage of disease, for those with minor symptoms, and in individuals who cannot tolerate levodopa. In addition, anticholinergic drugs are often used in conjunction with levodopa. Trihexyphenidyl, biperiden or benztropine are usually preferred for initial therapy. Levodopa, amantadine or an anticholinergic from another chemical class may be added if required. If therapy is started with levodopa, an anticholinergic may be added to achieve maximal response. Ethopropazine and diphenhydramine are often used in this situation. Patients often become refractive to anticholinergics during long-term therapy. This may be caused by progression of the disease.

Anticholinergics are also used to reduce drug-induced parkinsonism. This practice has been questioned, with the suggestion that anticholinergics may increase the probability of tardive dyskinesia caused by phenothiazines or butyrophenones.

Adverse effects. The adverse effects of these drugs can be attributed, in the main, to a reduction of peripheral cholinergic stimulation. Although more selective than atropine, the drugs can still produce cycloplegia, urinary retention and constipation. Because of their mydriatic effects, they can precipitate an attack of acute-angle glaucoma in patients predisposed to angle closure. The decrease in salivation that accompanies their use benefits the patient who experiences sialorrhea. Confusion and excitement can occur with large doses or in susceptible patients such as the elderly, patients with existing mental disorders, and those

taking other drugs with anticholinergic properties. Care must be taken in using anticholinergic therapy in patients over the age of seventy or any individual with dementia. Drowsiness and dizziness are common with the antihistamines diphenhydramine and orphenadrine and the phenothiazine ethopropazine.

Table 50.4 lists the clinically significant drug interactions with central anticholinergic drugs.

Nursing Management

Table 50.5 describes the nursing management of the patient receiving drugs for the treatment of Parkinson's disease. The nursing management for the use of drugs to manage the extrapyramidal symptoms associated with antipsychotic (neuroleptic) drug use is summarized in Table 50.6 (page 596). These drugs include benztropine, biperiden, procyclidine and trihexyphenidyl. (Further information on antipsychotic drugs is found in Chapter 45.)

Dosage details for individual drugs are given in Table 50.7 (pages 598–599).

Table 50.5
Nursing management of the antiparkinsonian drugs

Assessment of risk vs. benefit	Patient data	• Assess baseline lying and standing BP and P; s/s to determine drug response (akinesia, facial expression, rigidity, tremors, gait, general functional abilities with ADL) • *Pregnancy:* Risk category unknown; may not be of consequence, given the usual age of pts with the disorder
	Drug data	• Physician should determine which drug is warranted. Generally, drug tx for Parkinson's disease begins with amantadine or a similar agent. Levodopa should not be used for pts with drug-induced parkinson-like symptoms • *Several significant drug interactions:* Confer with pharmacist • Most serious adverse effects involve CNS (e.g., mild stimulation, hallucinations, delusions, confusion, nightmares and resulting disorganized behaviours). Older pts are more prone to these reactions
Implementation	Rights of administration	• Using the "rights" helps prevent errors of administration
	Right route	• Generally given PO
	Right time	• See Table 50.7. NB variation in dosage schedules among drugs in this class
	Nursing therapeutics	• Pts/families require emotional support. Parkinson's symptoms can cause significant disruption in daily life • Encourage pt to participate in activities and maintain level of self-dependence • Titrate drug doses carefully to achieve maximum symptom control with minimum side effects
	Patient/family teaching	• Pt's need for information may be influenced by presence of signs/symptoms • Compliance and follow-up are essential factors in successful tx; review principles of pt education in Chapter 3 • Explain that successful tx of Parkinson's disease requires careful titration of drug dosage to match individual response and that different drugs may achieve varying degrees of success • Advise pts/families that the appearance of troublesome CNS effects and behaviours will disappear with dosage reduction/discontinuation • Advise pt to monitor positive response to drugs, reduction of symptoms and occurrence of warning signs of toxicity
Outcomes	Monitoring of progress	*Continually monitor:* • Clinical response indicating tx success (reduction in signs/symptoms of Parkinson's and improvement in daily function) • Signs/symptoms of adverse reactions; document and report immediately to physician • Blood tests for renal, hepatic function and CBC may be ordered periodically

Table 50.6
Nursing management of drugs used to control EPS due to antipsychotics (neuroleptics)

Assessment of risk vs. benefit	Patient data	• Approximately one-third of pts receiving antipsychotic drugs will experience extrapyramidal symptoms (EPS) caused by the drugs' dopamine blockade on the extrapyramidal tracts in the CNS. The four common types of EPS include acute dystonia (severe muscle spasm which may involve the neck, mouth and tongue), akathisia (marked by pacing, restlessness, agitation); parkinsonism (drooling, cogwheel rigidity, tremors) and tardive dyskinesia (repetitive, involuntary bizarre movements of the tongue and mouth such as lip smacking, which occur after long-term tx) • Assess baseline lying and standing BP and P; s/s to determine drug response (akinesia, facial expression, rigidity, tremors, gait, general functional abilities with ADL) • *Pregnancy:* Risk category C (adverse effects demonstrated in animals; insufficient data in pregnant humans). Benefits of drug may outweigh risks. When used in the younger psychiatric pts, pregnancy counselling is essential. Often these drugs are used in conjunction with antipsychotic tx for dementia and may not be of consequence given the usual age of pts with this disorder
	Drug data	• Drug tx to prevent EPS caused by antipsychotic drugs is usually indicated for younger psychiatric pts on a short-term basis. Controversy exists regarding the possibility that this combination increases risks for tardive dyskinesia. Anticholinergic drugs are not effective in tx of tardive dyskinesia (see Chapter 45). When drugs are used for the older pt with psychotic symptoms accompanying dementia, careful consideration must be given to anticholinergic side effects. For this reason, higher-potency antipsychotics should be used with caution in this population • Most serious adverse effects relate to CNS (e.g., stimulation, hallucinations, delusions, confusion, nightmares and resulting disorganized behaviours). Older pts are more prone to these reactions
Implementation	Rights of administration	• Using the "rights" helps prevent errors of administration
	Right route	• Generally given PO
	Right time	• See Table 50.7. NB variation in dosage schedules among drugs in this class
	Nursing therapeutics	• Pts/families require emotional support; EPS can disrupt daily living and be very frightening. For the pt with dementia, CNS effects may be mistakenly attributed to the organic disorder. Although drug tx should be reduced or discontinued, this misinterpretation may lead to increased drug use
	Patient/family teaching	• Pt's need for information may be influenced by presence of signs/symptoms; during acute psychotic episodes, ability to comprehend information may be altered • Compliance and follow-up are essential factors in successful tx; review principles of pt education in Chapter 3 • Explain that use of antiparkinsonian drug is temporary to reduce side effects of antipsychotic medication. Advise actions to reduce dry mouth and constipation

Table 50.6 (continued)
Nursing management of drugs used to control EPS due to antipsychotics (neuroleptics)

Outcomes	Monitoring of progress	*Continually monitor:*
		• Clinical response indicating tx success (reduction in signs/symptoms of EPS and improvement in daily function)
		• Signs/symptoms of adverse reactions; document and report immediately to physician
		• Assess to determine whether drug or underlying disorder is the cause of altered behaviours

Response to Clinical Challenge

Important assessment data:
The assessment should focus on current symptoms, particularly muscle rigidity, tremor and ability to conduct ADL. A brief history describing improvement or worsening of symptoms is important. Exploration of any side effects caused by the amantadine, as well as daily compliance to the drug schedule, should be discussed.

Likely next step in drug therapy:
Amantadine is effective with few adverse effects and is often the first drug of choice. However, usually the individual with Parkinson's disease develops tolerance to the drug action of amantadine, or the disease progresses and a combination product of carbidopa + levodopa or benserazide + levodopa is required. This will be the likely next step — unless it is determined that the amantadine was not taken regularly, in which case instructions regarding measures to assist routine drug administration may be explored first.

Further Reading

Calne D. Diagnosis and treatment of Parkinson's disease. *Hospital Practice* 1995;30(1):83–86;90–92.

Sweeney P. Parkinson's disease: Managing symptoms and preserving function. *Geriatrics* 1995; 50(9):24–26;28–31.

Taira F. Facilitating self-care in clients with Parkinson's disease. *Home Healthcare Nursing* 1992;10(4):23–27.

Table 50.7
The antiparkinsonians: Drug doses

Drug Generic name (Trade names)	Dosage	Nursing alert
A. Dopaminergic Drugs		
levodopa (Dopar, Larodopa)	**Oral:** *Adults:* Initially, 500–1000 mg/day given in divided doses q6–12h. Increase by 100–750 mg/day q3–7days until response occurs or 8000 mg/day is reached. Usual maint. dose, 2000–8000 mg/day	• May be taken with food if gastric side effects occur. If pt has difficulty swallowing, may crush tablets and mix (e.g., with apple sauce or pure foods)
levodopa + benserazide (Prolopa)	**Oral:** For pts not on levodopa tx: Initially, 1 capsule of 100/25 mg 1–2x daily, increase by 1 capsule q3–4days until optimal tx effect is obtained. Optimal dosage for most pts is usually 4–8 capsules of 100/25 mg/day. For pts on levodopa tx, allow 12 h or more between last dose of levodopa and first dose of Prolopa®. A dosage of Prolopa® should be used that will provide approximately 15% of previous levodopa daily dosage	• Give with food or immediately pc. Capsules should be swallowed whole
levodopa + carbidopa (Sinemet)	**Oral:** *Adults:* For pts not on levodopa tx: Initially, 1 Sinemet® 100/25 tablet tid; increase by 1 tablet q3days until optimal effect is obtained or unacceptable adverse effects preclude further increases. For pts who previously received levodopa, levodopa should be discontinued at least 12 h before initiating tx with Sinemet®. Initial daily dose should provide approximately 20% of previous daily dose of levodopa	• Check dosage carefully (e.g., Sinemet® 10–100 indicates carbidopa 10 mg with levodopa 100 mg) • May be taken with food if GI upset occurs
bromocriptine mesylate (Parlodel)	**Oral:** *Adults:* 1.25 mg bid, increased by 2.5 mg/day in 2- to 4-week intervals. Usual dose range, 10–40 mg/day in 3 divided doses	• Give with milk or food to reduce gastric side effects. May crush tablets and mix with food
pergolide (Permax)	**Oral:** *Adults:* Initially, a single daily dose of 0.05 mg for the first 2 days. Gradually increase by 0.1–0.15 mg/day every third day over next 12 days of tx. Dosage may then be increased by 0.25 mg/day every third day until optimal dosage is achieved. In clinical studies, mean therapeutic dose of pergolide was 3 mg/day administered in 3 divided doses	• Pergolide is usually administered in divided doses 3x/day. During dosage titration, dosage of levodopa/carbidopa (Sinemet®) may be cautiously decreased • Give pergolide with food to reduce nausea. NB that this side effect usually reduces with continued use

Table 50.7 (continued)
The antiparkinsonians: Drug doses

Drug Generic name (Trade names)	Dosage	Nursing alert
A. Dopaminergic Drugs (cont'd)		
selegiline HCl (Eldepryl)	**Oral:** *Adults:* 5 mg bid	• Give doses with breakfast and lunch. When added to levodopa/carbidopa (Sinemet®) tx, dose of Sinemet® can be reduced gradually
amantadine HCl (Symmetrel)	**Oral:** *Adults:* 100 mg 1–2x daily	• Dividing dosage may reduce side effects. Give during daytime; avoid hs — may cause insomnia
B. Central Anticholinergic Drugs		
benztropine mesylate (Cogentin)	**Oral:** *Adults:* 0.5–6 mg/day in 1–2 divided doses	• Give with food to reduce gastric irritation. May crush tablets and mix with food
biperiden HCl (Akineton)	**Oral:** *Adults:* Initially, 2 mg tid–qid. Not to exceed 16 mg/day	• Give with food to reduce gastric side effects
diphenhydramine HCl (Benadryl)	**Oral:** *Adults:* For idiopathic and postencephalitic parkinsonism: Initially, 25 mg tid; increase gradually to 50 mg qid if required	• Give with meals or milk to reduce gastric side effect. May empty capsule and mix with food
ethopropazine HCl (Parsitan, Parsidol)	**Oral:** *Adults:* For idiopathic and postencephalitic parkinsonism: Initially, 50 mg tid; increase from 50–100 mg/day q2–3days until optimum effect is obtained or limit of tolerance is attained. For drug-induced extrapyramidal reactions: 100 mg bid	• Occasionally, nausea occurs. May take with food. Monitor s/s while increasing dose
orphenadrine HCl (Disipal)	**Oral:** *Adults:* Initially, 50 mg tid. Subsequent doses are adjusted to meet pt response and tolerance	• May be taken without regard to food
procyclidine HCl (Kemadrin)	**Oral:** *Adults:* For idiopathic and postencephalitic parkinsonism: Initially, 2.5 mg tid, pc; increase (if tolerated) to 5 mg tid, and occasionally 5 mg hs. For drug-induced extrapyramidal symptoms: Initially, 2.5 mg tid pc; may be increased by 2.5 mg/day until relief is obtained, usually with 10–20 mg/day	• Usually given pc. If insomnia occurs, hs dose may be omitted and higher doses given during the day
trihexyphenidyl HCl (Artane, Tremin)	**Oral:** *Adults:* For idiopathic and postencephalitic parkinsonism: 1 mg on day 1; increase by 2 mg daily q3–5days, up to 6–10 mg/day. Best tolerated in divided doses at mealtime. For drug-induced parkinsonism: Usually, 5–15 mg/day	• May give with or after meals. Establish effective dose before using extended-release form. If trouble swallowing, use elixir and accurate calibration device for administration

Drugs for the Treatment of Skeletal Muscle Disorders

Topics Discussed
- Spasticity
- Spasm
- Myasthenia gravis
- For each drug discussed: Mechanism of action and pharmacologic effects, therapeutic uses, adverse effects
- Nursing management

Drugs Discussed

Drugs for the Treatment of Spasticity:
baclofen (**bak**-loe-fen)
dantrolene (**dan**-troe-leen)
diazepam (dye-**az**-eh-pam)

Drugs for the Treatment of Spasm:
carisoprodol (kar-ih-soe-**proe**-dole)
chlorzoxazone (klor-**zocks**-ah-meen)
cyclobenzaprine (sye-klo-**ben**-zah-preen)
methocarbamol (meth-oh-**kar**-bah-mole)
orphenadrine (or-**fen**-ah-dreen)

Drugs for the Treatment of Myasthenia Gravis:
Cholinesterase inhibitors:
ambenonium (am-ben-**own**-ee-yum)
edrophonium (ed-roe-**fone**-ee-yum)
neostigmine (nee-oh-**stig**-meen)
pyridostigmine (peer-id-oh-**stig**-meen)

Adrenal corticosteroids:
prednisone (**pred**-nih-zone)

Clinical Challenge

Consider this clinical challenge as you read through this chapter. The response to the challenge appears on page 609.

Mildred is a 78-year-old woman who suffered a stroke, resulting in right-sided hemiparesis. She nows lives in a continuing care centre. Through her rehabilitation program she regained considerable physical function and speech. However, she continued to experience painful muscle spasticity, which has been successfully treated with dantrolene sodium.

During your monthly therapeutic monitoring, you notice the drug order for dantrolene. What assessment would you complete? What drug interactions warrant consideration? What concerns should you have regarding Mildred's drug therapy? What recommendations would you discuss with the physician and pharmacist?

Spasticity

Spasticity involves a velocity-dependent increase in tonic stretch reflexes that cause hyperactive reflexes, flexor or extensor spasms and loss of dexterity. The three major drugs used to treat spasticity are baclofen (Lioresal®), diazepam (Valium®) and dantrolene (Dantrium®).

Baclofen (Lioresal®)

Mechanism of action, pharmacologic effects and therapeutic uses. Baclofen inhibits mono- and polysynaptic pathways in the spinal cord and depresses the tonic stretch reflex. It has no peripheral muscle relaxant activity. Baclofen relieves involuntary flexor and extensor spasms and resistance to passive movements. The drug is indicated to alleviate the signs and symptoms of spasticity resulting from multiple sclerosis. It may also be of some value in the treatment of patients with spinal cord injuries and other spinal cord diseases.

Adverse effects. Baclofen is well tolerated by many patients. At full therapeutic doses, patients may initially experience drowsiness, dizziness, weakness and fatigue. Nausea, mild gastrointestinal upset, constipation or diarrhea, confusion, hypotension and urinary frequency are other reported adverse effects. Caution must be exercised if the drug is withdrawn. Abrupt withdrawal has, on occasion, led to severe reactions including visual and auditory hallucinations, status epilepticus, dyskinesia and confusion. Unless there are severe adverse effects, baclofen should be discontinued slowly over a period of one to two weeks. Baclofen has been known to disrupt blood glucose control in diabetic patients. Caution should be used and blood glucose levels monitored.

Table 51.1 lists the clinically significant drug interactions with baclofen.

Dantrolene Sodium (Dantrium®)

Mechanism of action, pharmacologic effects and therapeutic uses. Dantrolene inhibits muscle contraction by acting directly on skeletal muscles to suppress calcium release from the sarcoplasmic reticulum. It is valuable in the treatment of spasticity induced by spinal cord injury, cerebral palsy, multiple sclerosis and stroke, whenever such spasticity results in a decrease in the functional use of residual motor activity. The drug is not indicated in the relief of skeletal muscle spasms due to rheumatic disorders. Dantrolene is also used in the treatment of malignant hyperthermia.

Adverse effects. The most common adverse effects of dantrolene are muscle weakness, drowsiness, diarrhea, malaise and fatigue. Anorexia, nausea, vomiting and an acne-like rash are also caused by dantrolene. Dizziness, headache, nervousness, insomnia and depression may also be produced by the drug.

Dantrolene has the potential for hepatotoxicity and should not be used in conditions other than those recommended here. Idiosyncratic or hypersensitivity-mediated hepatocellular injury (which occurs rarely, but has been fatal) is the most serious adverse reaction. The risk appears to be greatest in patients over age thirty-five and in women, especially those receiving estrogen therapy. Hepatotoxicity occurs most frequently between three and twelve months after starting therapy. Therefore, routine baseline hepatic function studies should be performed prior to therapy, and alanine transaminase (ALT) or aspartate transaminase (AST) and alkaline phosphatase (AP) levels should be determined at appropriate intervals during therapy. The lowest effective dose (preferably no more than 400 mg daily) should be prescribed. Therapy should be continued for more than sixty days only if symptoms are relieved and there

---

Table 51.1
Baclofen: Drug interactions

Drug	Interaction
Alcohol and other CNS depressants	• These drugs may have additive CNS-depressant effects with baclofen

Table 51.2
Dantrolene: Drug interactions

Drug	Interaction
CNS depressants	• CNS depressants may increase the depressive effects of dantrolene
Estrogens	• Estrogens may increase the risk of dantrolene-induced liver damage

is no evidence of hepatic injury. Dantrolene is contraindicated in patients with active hepatic disease.

Table 51.2 lists the clinically significant drug interactions with dantrolene.

Diazepam (Valium®)

Mechanism of action, pharmacologic effects and therapeutic uses. Diazepam is a polysynaptic inhibitor in the brain stem and spinal cord. The drug also has secondary sedative effects. Diazepam assists patients with spasticity associated with spinal cord lesions, multiple sclerosis and other CNS lesions. It is also used adjunctively in acute, localized, severe traumatic disorders associated with painful muscle spasms.

Adverse effects. The adverse effects and drug interactions of diazepam are presented in Chapter 47 and Table 47.2 (page 554). The dose of the drug that relieves spasticity usually produces sedation and some incoordination.

Spasm

Spasm involves the involuntary contraction of a muscle or groups of muscles, usually accompanied by pain and limited function. Reflex spasm may be a protective mechanism in response to injury of a local nature. Most muscle strains and minor injuries respond rapidly to rest and physical therapy. Some, however, appear to benefit from additional use of a central skeletal muscle relaxant.

Central Skeletal Muscle Relaxants

Carisoprodol (Rela®, Soma®), Chlorzoxazone (Paraflex®), Cyclobenzaprine (Flexeril®), Methocarbamol (Delaxin®, Robaxin®), Orphenadrine (Disipal®, Norflex®)

Mechanism of action, pharmacologic effects and therapeutic uses. Central muscle relaxant drugs sedate patients and depress the facilitative and inhibitory neuronal activity affecting muscle stretch reflexes, primarily in the lateral reticular area of the brain stem. Most of them have been shown to be more effective than a placebo in treating localized muscle spasms. None has been demonstrated to be more effective than analgesic, anti-inflammatory drugs in relieving the pain of acute or chronic localized muscle spasm. There seems little reason to select one drug over the others. All are approximately equally effective and have similar adverse effects. Some are combined with analgesics. These include methocarbamol with ASA (Robaxisal®), chlorzoxazone plus acetaminophen (Parafon Forte®), acetaminophen plus codeine (Parafon C8®) and orphenadrine with ASA and caffeine (Norgesic®, Norgesic Forte®).

Table 51.3
Central skeletal muscle relaxants: Drug interactions

Drug	Interaction
CNS depressants	• CNS depressants may have additive CNS-depressant effects with central skeletal muscle relaxants
Monoamine oxidase inhibitors	• MAOIs interact with tricyclic antidepressants to produce hyperpyretic crises, severe convulsions and death. Cyclobenzaprine is similar in structure to TCAs, and the possibility of this interaction must be kept in mind

The U.S. Federal Drug Administration has classified these combinations as possibly effective. Central skeletal muscle relaxants are not recommended for the treatment of spastic disorders induced by cerebrospinal trauma, cerebral palsy or demyelinating disorders.

Adverse effects. All central skeletal muscle relaxants produce drowsiness, lightheadedness and dizziness. CNS depression is particularly pronounced for cyclobenzaprine, a drug that also causes dryness of the mouth.

Table 51.3 lists the clinically significant drug interactions with central skeletal muscle relaxants.

Nursing Management of Spasticity and Spasm

Table 51.4 describes the nursing management of the patient receiving drugs for the treatment of spasticity and muscle spasm. Dosage details for individual drugs are given in Table 51.7 (pages 607–609). The reader is also referred to Chapter 47 for further information on diazepam.

Table 51.4
Nursing management of drugs for spasticity and spasm

Assessment of risk vs. benefit	Patient data	• Baseline lab tests of liver function (e.g., AST, ALT, AP and bilirubin) • Assess to establish muscle rigidity, spasticity, pain, ROM. Determine risk for falls • *Pregnancy:* Risk category is unknown for some drugs in this category; check each drug. Some are category C (animal studies show adverse effects to fetus but human data are unknown or insufficient); benefits may be acceptable despite risks
	Drug data	• Select drugs based on underlying cause of spasticity (e.g., baclofen is not effective for spasticity caused by stroke, whereas dantrolene is not indicated for spasms caused by rheumatic disorders) • Most significant interaction is with other CNS depressants (e.g., alcohol). Dantrolene also interacts with estrogen • Most serious adverse effects are hepatic toxicity (dantrolene), withdrawal symptoms with sudden discontinuation (baclofen) and drowsiness with the risk of falls. Diazepam can also cause dependence, if used for prolonged duration
Implementation	Rights of administration	• Using the "rights" helps prevent errors of administration
	Right route	• Generally, give PO; check pt's ability to swallow pill
	Right time	• See Table 51.7. NB variation in dosage schedules among drugs in this class
	Nursing therapeutics	• Use measures to reduce spasticity and spasm (e.g., appropriate immobilization and exercise, cold compresses, physical tx) • Monitor initial reaction to drug (orthostatic hypotension, drowsiness) and supervise ambulation until response is known

(cont'd on next page)

Table 51.4 (continued)
Nursing management of drugs for spasticity and spasm

| Implementation (cont'd) | Patient/family teaching | • Pt's need for information may be influenced by length of time required for tx and underlying cause
• Review principles of pt education in Chapter 3
• Instruct pt/family that response to drug may not be immediate; generally, if adequate response is not achieved over several weeks, drug will be withdrawn and another tried
• Dantrolene may cause photosensitivity: instruct pt to use sunscreen and protective clothing when outdoors
• Instruct pt to monitor reaction to drug before engaging in activities such as driving and using power machinery
• Pts/families should know warning signs/symptoms of possible toxicities of these drugs. Report immediately: rash, itching, jaundice, abdominal pain and malaise
• Warn pts to avoid alcohol (increased risk for drowsiness; also hepatotoxicity with dantrolene)
• *Discuss possibility of pregnancy:* Advise pt to notify physician; discuss birth control methods |
| Outcomes | Monitoring of progress | *Continually monitor:*
• Clinical response indicating tx success (reduction in signs/symptoms)
• Blood glucose levels for diabetic pts receiving baclofen
• Signs/symptoms of adverse reactions; document and report immediately to physician
• Blood tests for hepatic function may be ordered (weekly or periodically) |

Myasthenia Gravis

Myasthenia gravis is an autoimmune disorder caused by a deficiency of skeletal muscle cholinergic (nicotinic) receptors as a result of antireceptor antibodies. Patients experience impaired neuromuscular transmission and demonstrate rapid fatiguability of skeletal muscles. Not all muscle fibres are equally involved, some being in a borderline condition and quickly paralyzed by activity, while others remain above threshold for some time. Myasthenic patients may be treated with reversible cholinesterase inhibitors and/or adrenal corticosteroids.

Cholinesterase Inhibitors

Ambenonium Chloride (Mytelase®), Edrophonium Chloride (Tensilon®), Neostigmine Bromide (Prostigmin®), Pyridostigmine Bromide (Mestinon®, Regonol®)

Mechanism of action and pharmacologic effects. By inhibiting acetylcholinesterase, these drugs prolong the survival of acetylcholine, permitting not only more receptor interactions but also a cooperative effect of several acetylcholine molecules on one receptor site. Unfortunately, cholinesterase inhibitors affect all cholinergic nerves, resulting in an increase in both nicotinic and muscarinic effects. (Nurses wishing to review the consequences of generalized cholinergic stimulation are referred to Chapter 27 in this book.)

Table 51.5
Cholinesterase inhibitors: Drug interactions

Drug	Interaction
Drugs that depress neuromuscular transmission	• These drugs are known to aggravate or unmask myasthenia gravis

Therapeutic uses. The primary indication for anticholinesterase therapy alone is to treat mild myasthenia, such as ocular myasthenia or mild residual involvement following thymectomy. More often, they are used with corticosteroids to treat patients with moderate to severe disease. Although anticholinesterase drugs improve many patients, muscle strength remains below normal in others. Pyridostigmine is usually the drug of choice because it produces fewer adverse effects than either neostigmine or ambenonium. Edrophonium has a more rapid onset and shorter duration of action. It is used exclusively for the diagnosis of myasthenia gravis and is given only under careful medical supervision.

Anticholinesterase drugs are contraindicated in patients with mechanical obstruction of the intestinal or urinary tracts and should be used with caution in people with bronchial asthma.

Adverse effects. Excessive cholinergic stimulation accounts for the majority of adverse effects. Muscarinic stimulation produces abdominal cramps, nausea, vomiting, diarrhea, hypersalivation, increased bronchial secretion, lacrimation, miosis and diaphoresis. Although these effects can be counteracted by atropine, neither this drug nor any other anticholinergic should be routinely incorporated into a patient's therapeutic regimen. Masking the signs of increased muscarinic stimulation may lead to cholinergic crisis. The effects of nicotinic stimulation include muscle cramps, fasciculations and weakness.

A cholinergic crisis may be difficult to differentiate from a myasthenic crisis. Both present with muscle weakness, the former as a result of an excessive accumulation of acetylcholine leading to a depolarizing skeletal muscle block, the latter because of the inability of acetylcholine to stimulate sufficient nicotinic receptors. Edrophonium may be used to differentiate between the two, but only after patients have first been intubated and controlled ventilation has been instituted. One to two milligrams of edrophonium given intravenously may improve strength in the patient with a myasthenic crisis but aggravate weakness in a cholinergic crisis.

Table 51.5 lists the clinically significant drug interactions with cholinesterase inhibitors used to treat myasthenia gravis.

Adrenal Corticosteroids

Mechanism of action and therapeutic uses. The pharmacology of adrenal corticosteroids is presented in detail in Chapter 66. With respect to the treatment of myasthenia gravis, adrenal corticosteroids suppress antireceptor antibody formation. They are used in patients not adequately managed with anticholinesterase therapy alone and, with increasing frequency, in place of cholinesterase inhibitors when one drug alone will suffice. The indications for corticosteroids also include older adults (usually over age forty) with moderate to severe involvement, whether or not they have undergone thymectomy. Corticosteroids may also be used for an interim period following thymectomy because of the delayed response often associated with this procedure. Other possible indications for the use of corticosteroids include preparation of patients for thymectomy and treatment of patients who refuse to undergo, or fail to respond to, thymectomy. These drugs can also be administered as maintenance therapy after surgical removal of an invasive thymoma.

Prednisone is the most frequently used corticosteroid. When given in a high-dose, alternate-day dose regimen, it usually improves muscular strength with reduced adverse effects. Treatment may be required indefinitely. Anticholinesterase therapy should be continued during the initial months of steroid treatment. Later, as the patient improves on corticosteroid treatment, the need for anticholinesterase therapy may decrease.

Adverse effects. The adverse effects and drug interactions of corticosteroids are presented in Chapter 66 and Table 66.3 (page 784).

Nursing Management

Table 51.6 describes the nursing management of the patient receiving drugs for treatment of myasthenia gravis. Dosage details of individual drugs are given in Table 51.7. The reader is also referred to Chapter 27 for further information on cholinesterase inhibitors and Chapter 66 for the nursing management related to corticosteroids.

Table 51.6
Nursing management of drugs for myasthenia gravis

Assessment of risk vs. benefit	Patient data	• Physician should determine any contraindications (e.g., mechanical obstruction of intestinal, urinary tracts; bronchial asthma) • Assess to establish baseline VS, general state of health • *Pregnancy and lactation:* Safety not established
	Drug data	• Duration of action varies from a few hours to several days/weeks
Implementation	Rights of administration	• Using the "rights" helps prevent errors of administration
	Right route	• Usually, PO; may also be given SC or IM
	Right dose	• Do not substitute oral and parenteral doses; higher doses are required PO
	Right time	• Give oral dose with food or milk to prevent nausea • Drug schedule must be individualized. Pt may wish to take drug 30 min ac, as drug action will promote ability to chew
	Nursing therapeutics	• Establish a careful dosage schedule and observe drug effects (e.g., improvement in ability to swallow or raise eyelids; reduced fatigue). Differentiate myasthenic crisis (extreme muscle weakness due to insufficient drug) from cholinergic crisis (extreme muscle weakness plus other s/s of cholinergic stimulation)
	Patient/family teaching	• Educate for general drug tx (see Chapter 3) • Pt/family need information and reassurance to manage drug tx. The constant challenge is to provide sufficient drug to enhance muscle function; excessive drug dose also causes muscle weakness. Help patient to develop a systematic approach to assessing muscle strength, and keep track of each drug dose and its effects • *Discuss possibility of pregnancy:* Advise pt to notify physician • Explain risks of lactation while on these drugs
Outcomes	Monitoring of progress	*Continually monitor:* • Muscle strength and daily function • Signs/symptoms of cholinergic crisis (hypersalivation, diaphoresis, hiccuping, nausea, vomiting, abdominal cramps, bronchoconstriction; possible CNS effects of slurred speech, respiratory arrest, seizures). Have respiratory support and atropine on hand; report immediately to physician

Table 51.7
Treatment of skeletal muscle disorders: Drug doses

Drug Generic name (Trade names)	Dosage	Nursing alert
A. Drugs for the Treatment of Spasticity		
baclofen (Lioresal)	**Oral:** *Adults:* 5 mg tid. May increase q3days by 5 mg/dose to max. of 80 mg/day (total daily dose may be given in divided doses qid)	• Instruct pts to discontinue drug slowly. Abrupt stoppage may cause severe reactions • May give with food or milk reduce gastric distress • **Safety alert:** Monitor initial response to prevent falls caused by hypotension
dantrolene sodium (Dantrium)	(For spasticity) **Oral:** *Adults:* Initially, 25 mg/day; increase to 25 mg bid–qid, then by increments of 25 mg up to 100 mg bid–qid if needed. Increments may be made q4–7days. Not to exceed 400 mg/day. *Children > 5 years:* 0.5 mg/kg bid; increase to 0.5 mg/kg tid–qid, then by increments of 0.5 mg/kg up to 3 mg/kg bid–qid. Not to exceed 100 mg qid	• **For spasticity:** May give with food to reduce gastric distress. Assess pt's ability to swallow capsule. If unable to swallow due to spasm, prepare oral suspension; open capsule, mix thoroughly with liquid and use immediately
	(For malignant hyperthermia) **IV push:** *Adults/children:* Begin with 2 mg/kg and continue until symptoms subside or a cumulative dose of 10 mg/kg has been reached. If the physiologic and metabolic abnormalities reappear, administration of dantrolene and other drugs (O_2, sodium bicarbonate) should be repeated. For prophylaxis: 2.5 mg/kg during induction of anesthesia. **Oral** (for prophylaxis): 4–8 mg/kg/day in 4 divided doses for 1–2 days prior to surgery, with the last dose given 3–5 h pre-op. The larger dose may cause considerable weakness	• **IV:** Follow agency policy regarding direct administration. Solution must be used within 6 h after reconstitution. Protect from light
diazepam (Valium®)	(Adjunctively for relief of skeletal muscle spasms) **Oral:** *Adults:* 2–10 mg tid–qid. (For muscle spasm associated with cerebral palsy, athetosis, stiff-man syndrome, or adjunctively in tetanus) **IV/IM:** 5–10 mg initially; then 5–10 mg in 3–4 h, if necessary. For tetanus, larger doses may be required	• **PO:** If pt is unable to swallow tablet, crush and mix with food, or use oral solution. Ensure that pt swallows medication and does not attempt to "cheek" tablet. (Also refer to Chapter 47) • **IM:** Inject deeply into deltoid muscle • **IV:** Should not be mixed with other drugs. Direct IV push recommended. Inject slowly into large vein with pt in recumbent position. If direct injection is not possible, inject medication into tubing as close to site of vein insertion as possible *(cont'd on next page)*

Table 51.7 (continued)
Treatment of skeletal muscle disorders: Drug doses

Drug Generic name (Trade names)	Dosage	Nursing alert
B. Central Skeletal Muscle Relaxants for the Treatment of Spasm		
carisoprodol (Rela, Soma)	**Oral:** *Adults:* 350 mg tid and hs. Not recommended for children < 12 years	•Give with food •**Safety:** Supervise ambulation to prevent falls until response to drug is known
chlorzoxazone (Paraflex)	**Oral:** *Adults:* 500 mg qid	•**Safety:** Supervise ambulation to prevent falls until response to drug is known
cyclobenzaprine HCl (Flexeril)	**Oral:** *Adults:* 10 mg tid, with a range of 20–40 mg/day in divided doses. Not to exceed 60 mg/day	•May give with food •**Safety:** Supervise ambulation to prevent falls until response to drug is known
methocarbamol (Delaxin, Robaxin)	**Oral:** *Adults:* 6 g/day for first 48–72 h of acute skeletal muscle spasm. Severe conditions: 8 g/day; reduce to 4 g/day. **IM:** *Adults:* 500 mg alternately in each gluteal region q8h. **IV:** *Adults:* 1–3 g/day at a rate not > 3 mL/min (100 mg/mL); some physicians substitute oral administration after 1–2 g have been administered. Do not give IV for more than 3 days	•**PO:** May give with food to reduce gastric distress. If difficulty swallowing, may crush tablets and mix with food or use IM or IV •**IM:** Limit each injection to 5 mL (500 mg) in each site •**IV:** Follow agency policy for direct IV. May be given at a rate of 300 mg (3 mL) over 1 min •**Safety:** Pt should remain lying 10–15 min after dose to prevent falls caused by orthostatic hypotension
orphenadrine HCl (Disipal, Norflex)	**Oral:** *Adults:* 100 mg bid	•May be taken without regard to food
C. Cholinesterase Inhibitors Used to Treat Myasthenia Gravis		
ambenonium chloride (Mytelase)	**Oral:** *Adults:* Initially, 5 mg tid or qid; increase prn. Adjust at intervals of 1–2 days to avoid accumulation. *Children:* Initially, 0.3 mg/kg/day in divided doses; increase if needed to 1.5 mg/kg/day in divided doses	•Give with milk or food. Dosage adjustments may be made according to pt's response (e.g., larger dose later in day if more fatigued)
neostigmine (Prostigmin)	**Oral:** *Adults:* Initially, 15 mg q3–4 h; increase at daily intervals until optimal response is achieved. Maint. dose, 150 mg/day (up to 375 mg/day, if needed). *Children:* 2 mg/kg/day in 3–4 divided doses. **SC/IM:** *Adults:* 0.5 mg. *Children:* 10–40 µg/kg; may give with 10 µg/kg atropine	•Give oral dose with food or milk to reduce GI effects •Pt may need to take 30 min ac for onset of drug action to assist with chewing •NB significant differences between oral and parenteral doses

Table 51.7 (continued)
Treatment of skeletal muscle disorders: Drug doses

Drug Generic name (Trade names)	Dosage	Nursing alert
C. Cholinesterase Inhibitors Used to Treat Myasthenia Gravis (cont'd)		
pyridostigmine bromide (Mestinon, Regonol)	**Oral:** *Adults:* 600 mg/day in divided doses. Range, 60–1500 mg. **Sustained-release:** 180–540 mg/day od or in 2 divided doses	• May be taken with food or milk to reduce gastric side effects • Pt may wish to take 30 min ac; drug action will assist in chewing
D. Adrenal Corticosteroid Used to Treat Myasthenia Gravis		
prednisone	**Oral:** *Adults:* Initially, 25 mg daily for 2 days; increase by 5 mg q2days until optimum response occurs. Usual dose, 50–60 mg/day. To begin a qod program, add 10 mg to the first day's dose (60 mg) and subtract 10 mg from the second day's dose (40 mg) each week until improvement reaches a plateau or until 100 mg is given qod. Reduce dosage if possible gradually over many months to establish minimum qod maintenance dose	• Do not confuse this medication with prednisolone; they are different medications • Give with food to reduce gastric irritation • Give in a.m. to coincide with normal circadian rhythm of cortisol secretion

Response to Clinical Challenge

Assessment:
Presence/absence of muscle spasticity or spasm, pain, range of motion, lab reports of liver function should also be checked.

Drug interactions to consider:
CNS depression can be enhanced by other depressants; is she receiving other CNS drugs? Hepatotoxicity risk is increased by concurrent use of estrogen. Is Mildred receiving any estrogen products?

Concerns regarding drug therapy:
The most serious adverse effect is liver damage. Are Mildred's lab tests normal? Does she have any signs/symptoms of liver toxicity?

Recommendations to discuss with physician/ pharmacist:
Depending on the assessment data, you might suggest slow reduction and discontinuation of the drug with increased use of physical therapy and comfort techniques for any spasticity or spasm.

Further Reading

Lepate G, Pestronk A. Autoimmune myasthenia gravis. *Hospital Practice* 1993;28(1):109–112; 115–117; 121–122.

Drugs to Alleviate Pain

More patients seek medical attention — or self-medicate — because of pain than for any other reason. Unit 11 deals with drug therapy for pain of various types.

Chapters 52 and 53 discuss narcotic and non-narcotic analgesics, respectively. Nurses must recognize the differences between these two groups of analgesics and understand the role of each in the treatment of pain.

Nurses should also familiarize themselves with the pharmacologic actions of drugs used to treat arthritis (Chapter 54), gout (Chapter 55) and migraine (Chapter 56). These drugs are most important and are frequently prescribed. Although they can provide welcome relief for many sufferers, they can also have profound adverse effects.

Chapters 57 and 58 present local and general anesthetics, respectively. Although these drugs are most frequently used by specialists in medicine, nurses must understand how they work and their possible adverse effects.

Narcotic Analgesics

Topics Discussed
● General properties of narcotics
● Definition of analgesic, acute pain, chronic pain, cross-tolerance
● Individual narcotic analgesics
● Agonist-antagonist narcotics
● Patient-controlled analgesia
● Narcotic antagonists
● For each drug discussed: Mechanism of action, pharmacologic effects, therapeutic uses, adverse effects
● Nursing management

Drugs Discussed

Narcotic Analgesics:
alfentanil (al-**fen**-tah-nil)
codeine (**koe**-deen)

fentanyl (**fen**-tah-nil)
hydrocodone (hye-droe-**koe**-done)
hydromorphone (hye-droe-**mor**-fone)
levorphanol (lee-**vor**-fan-ole)
meperidine (meh-**per**-ih-deen)
methadone (**meth**-ah-done)
morphine (**mor**-feen)
oxycodone (ox-ee-**koe**-done)
oxymorphone (ox-ee-**mor**-fone)
propoxyphene (pro-**pox**-ih-feen)

Mixed Agonist-Antagonist Analgesics:
butorphanol (byoo-**tor**-fah-nole)
nalbuphine (**nal**-byoo-feen)
pentazocine (pen-**taz**-oh-seen)

Narcotic Antagonist:
naloxone (**nal**-ox-one)

Clinical Challenge

Consider this clinical challenge as you read through this chapter. The response to the challenge appears on page 621.

You are working in a pediatric hospital. A 13-year-old boy, who was injured in a MVA, has had several surgeries. Prior to this surgery, one of the staff suggests that he use morphine PCA for self-management of postoperative pain.

Consider the advantages and disadvantages of this approach to pain management for this young patient. What arguments can you offer to support this suggestion, and what concerns should be addressed?

General Properties of Narcotics

Pain is a useful sensation when it protects the body from damage. Pushed to the extreme, however, or continued over long periods of time, pain is counterproductive, and steps must be taken to alleviate it. Drugs used to relieve pain are called *analgesics*. They are divided into *narcotic* and *non-narcotic* analgesics. (The latter group is also called the analgesic-antipyretics, and are discussed in Chapter 53.) This chapter discusses narcotic analgesics.

In 1680 the English physician Thomas Sydinham wrote, "Among the remedies which it has pleased Almighty God to give man to relieve his sufferings, none is so universal and so efficacious as opium." That statement is as true today as it was more than three hundred years ago. Morphine, the major narcotic contained in the opium plant, still serves as the ultimate standard of analgesic effectiveness. No other analgesic has proven so effective.

Narcotic analgesics may be further classified according to their source. These are:

- opium preparations;
- purified alkaloids of opium;
- semisynthetic modifications of morphine or codeine;
- synthetic compounds that resemble morphine in many of their actions.

Mechanism of Action and Pharmacologic Effects

All narcotics, regardless of their origin, reduce pain by stimulating opiate receptors in the central nervous system. In doing this they mimic the analgesic effects of naturally occurring brain opiates — the endorphins. Not all endogenous chemicals with opioid activity have been identified. However, two pentapeptides, leucine-enkephalin and methionine-enkephalin, have been found, which have properties similar to those of narcotics. By mimicking the actions of endogenous enkaphalins, opiates probably inhibit the release of excitatory transmitters from terminals of nerves that carry pain impulses.

At least four types of opioid receptors are found in the central nervous system. These are:

- *µ (mu) receptors,* which are thought to mediate supraspinal analgesia, respiratory depression, euphoria and physical dependence. These receptors are associated with morphine-like analgesia and euphoria.
- *K (kappa) receptors,* which mediate analgesia, miosis and sedation. These receptors are associated with pentazocine-like analgesia, sedation and miosis.
- *∂ (delta) receptors,* which are associated with alterations in affective behaviour.
- *Σ (sigma) receptors,* which are associated with dysphoria and psychotomimetic effects.

Pain is a universal experience, yet it is unique to each individual who experiences it. It can be classified in a variety of ways, but most commonly it is divided into *acute* and *chronic* pain. There are several differences between these types of pain, including the purpose and duration. For example, acute pain is usually short-lived and is often thought of as productive pain. Suppose you put your hand on a hot object. The pain you feel is productive because it alerts you to remove your hand from danger. In the same way, the pain of a myocardial infarct moves the sufferer to seek emergency medical treatment. The major goal of acute pain treatment is to alleviate the underlying cause, as well as to treat the pain.

In contrast, chronic pain is associated with long duration, from months to years. Often, the underlying cause of the pain cannot be alleviated. Thus, the major goal is to provide optimum relief with minimum sedation or long-term toxicities to enable the individual to function as independently and comfortably as possible. Managing chronic pain also requires flexibility in meeting changing needs. A third challenge is the long-term pain associated with terminal illness.

Narcotics can be useful in treating pain, irrespective of its duration. However, they are most useful for pain that emanates from the viscera.

Opiate receptors are found in high concentrations in the limbic system, the part of the brain that is responsible for emotion.

All narcotic analgesics have the same major pharmacologic properties. In addition to analgesia, their effects include *euphoria, drowsiness, depressed respiration, nausea and vomiting, miosis, altered gastrointestinal activity* and *dependence.* If narcotics are given chronically, *tolerance* occurs to many of these effects and larger doses must be given to provide satisfactory pain relief. Let's look at each of these effects in more detail.

Euphoria. This effect must not be minimized because the analgesia produced by narcotics depends, to a great degree, on their ability to induce euphoria. The emotional reaction to pain is very important. If a feeling of well-being can be produced in patients, the perception of, and reaction to, pain is reduced. Nurses have often heard patients state after receiving a narcotic that they can still feel pain but it no longer bothers them.

Drowsiness. This is a characteristic feature of stronger narcotics and plays a role in their analgesic effect. The word *narcosis* means a condition of stupour or insensitivity. Following the administration of a narcotic, patients may experience drowsiness, apathy and even sleep.

Respiratory depression. Narcotics depress respiration because they reduce the sensitivity of the brain-stem respiratory centres to increases in carbon dioxide tension. Therapeutic doses of morphine, for example, will depress the respiratory rate, minute volume and tidal exchange. As the dose is increased, respiratory depression deepens. Death from an overdose is due to respiratory failure.

Nausea and vomiting. Narcotics stimulate the chemoreceptor trigger zone in the medulla of the brain. Some patients never experience these effects; others are bothered with every dose. The more potent phenothiazine drugs (see Chapter 45) may block narcotic-induced nausea and vomiting.

Miosis. Miosis is a constriction of the pupil. Most narcotics produce this effect by stimulating the autonomic segment of the nucleus of the oculomotor nerve.

Constipation. This effect is prominent during chronic narcotic use. It is due to (1) a delayed emptying time of the stomach as a result of the constriction of the pyloric sphincter and increased tone of the antral portion of the stomach and duodenum, (2) a decrease in the propulsive contractions of the small intestine, together with an increase in nonpropulsive contractions and increased tone of the colon and (3) increased tone of the anal sphincter. The result of this triple-threat attack is constipation that can, when severe, proceed to obstipation (constipation severe enough to produce a serious obstruction).

Increased biliary tract pressure. Therapeutic doses of most narcotics increase biliary tract pressure. This can result in symptoms that vary from epigastric distress to typical biliary colic.

Physiological and psychological dependence. Both of these effects develop during chronic administration. They are one of the main reasons for caution in narcotic use. If a dependent subject is suddenly deprived of the narcotic, a withdrawal effect (absence syndrome) occurs quickly. Signs and symptoms of physiological withdrawal are autonomic hyperactivity, including diarrhea, vomiting, lacrimation, rhinorrhea, chills and fever. Patients may also suffer from abdominal cramps, pain and tremors.

Physiological dependence is an infrequent outcome when narcotics are taken to treat acute pain. Generally, the doses used and duration of treatment do not cause such dependence, and the narcotic can be stopped without withdrawal symptoms. Even if physiological dependence does occur, the withdrawal, while uncomfortable, is short-lived and is not life-threatening (as it is with barbiturates). Most significantly, physiological dependence does not lead to psychological dependence. Even in the management of long-term or chronic pain, narcotics may be indicated as the detrimental effects of living in chronic pain outweigh the risks of physiological dependence.

Psychological dependence is a far more vexing problem. It is difficult to explain why an individual who has been weaned off narcotics still feels a psychological compulsion to take the medication. Yet this does happen, and is the major reason why people return to old habits.

Tolerance. Tolerance occurs to the analgesic, euphoric and respiratory-depressant effects of narcotics. If a narcotic is used on a daily basis over a prolonged period of time, larger and larger doses must be given to maintain the same degree of analgesia. Once a patient develops tolerance to one narcotic, he or she will show tolerance to all other narcotics. This is known as *cross-tolerance*. Cross-tolerance does not extend to other groups of CNS depressants, such as alcohol or barbiturates. Tolerance does not develop to the GI or miotic effects of narcotics.

Pharmacokinetics

Narcotics are usually well absorbed from the gastrointestinal tract, but are often extensively inactivated during their first pass through the liver (first-pass effect). As a result, larger doses are usually required orally than parenterally. Most narcotics are effective for three to five hours.

Therapeutic Uses

Pain is the major reason for the use of narcotics. They should be used only when non-narcotic analgesics prove ineffective. On the other hand, narcotics should not be withheld from seriously ill patients because of fear of dependence, which matters little to the terminally ill patient. Further, it is important to use a narcotic in an effective dose. Often patients receive inadequate doses because of a caregiver's misplaced fear of dependency.

Narcotics are often used in severe pain resulting from trauma, surgery, obstetrics, renal and biliary colic, and carcinoma. Caution should be exercised in obstetrics because narcotics cross the placenta and can depress respiration in the newborn. Narcotics are not recommended while the cause of a patient's pain is being diagnosed, lest analgesia interfere with the diagnosis.

Dyspnea produced by acute left-ventricular failure and pulmonary edema may be treated with a narcotic. This effect is caused by a decrease in preload secondary to vasodilatation.

Diarrhea responds to narcotic treatment. (This topic is discussed in Chapters 60 and 61.) Diphenoxylate (Lomotil®) or loperamide (Imodium®) are the narcotics of choice because they are poorly absorbed and have minimal systemic effects.

Cough relief is afforded by some narcotics (see Chapter 71). By suppressing the cough centre in the medulla of the brain, many narcotics serve as excellent antitussives. The narcotics used most often are codeine and hydrocodone.

Narcotics are contraindicated in patients hypersensitive to the drugs. They are also contraindicated in those who have received monoamine oxidase inhibitors (MAOIs) within the previous fourteen days. Further, they are contraindicated in respiratory insufficiency or depression, in severe CNS depression, during an attack of bronchial asthma, in heart failure secondary to chronic lung disease, and in cardiac arrhythmias. Additional contraindications include increased intracranial or cerebrospinal fluid pressure, head injuries, brain tumour, acute alcoholism, delirium tremens, convulsive disorders, following biliary tract surgery, suspected surgical abdomen and surgical anastomosis.

Adverse Effects

The major adverse effects of narcotic analgesics are respiratory depression, dependence, constipation, nausea and vomiting. Concern over these effects has led to the use of non-narcotic analgesics in conditions in which they provide adequate relief of pain.

Although one must not minimize the danger of inducing narcotic dependence during chronic therapy, this concern should not serve as the basis for withholding treatment in the terminally ill. A more appropriate reason to show caution in the terminally ill patient is the ability of most narcotics to produce severe constipation, bordering on obstipation. Even the terminally ill must clear their intestines. If the narcotic binds the bowels, this can represent a serious medical/nursing problem.

The nausea and vomiting effects of narcotics can be minimized with antinauseant drugs, such as the phenothiazines or diphenhydramine.

Because of their ability to depress the respiratory centre, decrease ciliary activity, reduce the cough reflex and increase bronchomotor tone, narcotics must be used with caution in patients with excessive respiratory secretions or decreased ventilation.

Narcotics can cause hypoventilation and hypercapnia, resulting in cerebrovascular dilatation and increased intracranial pressure. Therefore, they must be used very cautiously, if at all, in patients with head injuries, delirium tremens and conditions in which intracranial pressure is increased.

Narcotics can produce hypotension and shock and should be given in reduced doses, if at all, to patients in shock or with decreased blood volume. If it is absolutely necessary to administer a narcotic to a patient in shock, it should be given intra-

Table 52.1
Narcotic analgesics: Drug interactions

Drug	Interaction
CNS depressants	• CNS depressants (e.g., alcohol, barbiturates, TCAs, antidepressants, MAOIs and phenothiazines) increase the central depressant effects of narcotics. Respiratory depression, hypotension and profound sedation or coma may result
Rifampin	• Rifampin stimulates the hepatic metabolism of methadone

venously to circumvent poor uptake following intramuscular or subcutaneous injection.

The spasmogenic effects of narcotics on the urinary bladder can lead to urinary retention in patients with prostatic hypertrophy or urethral stricture. Narcotics should be used in lower doses in patients with myxedema, hypothyroidism or hypoadrenalism.

Table 52.1 lists the clinically significant drug interactions with narcotic analgesics.

Individual Narcotic Analgesics

In view of the preceding discussion, a review of individual narcotic analgesics can be kept brief. Only particular aspects relating to the pharmacokinetics, relative potency and therapeutic uses for individual drugs will be discussed. The use of combination tablets, containing both a narcotic and a non-narcotic analgesic, is discussed in Chapter 53.

Opium Preparations (Pantopon®)

Pantopon® is a mixture of purified opium alkaloids in solution as hydrochloride salts. Pantopon® has the same indications as morphine and is used most commonly for postoperative pain. The analgesic effect of Pantopon® is the same as would be expected from its morphine content (50%). It has no proven advantage over an equivalent amount of morphine.

Purified Alkaloids of Opium

Morphine Sulfate

Morphine remains the standard against which all other narcotics must be compared. Although the drug is best administered parenterally, orally effective preparations are available. As for most narcotics, the half-life of morphine is about three to four hours. The major use of morphine is in the treatment of moderate to severe pain. In addition to the adverse effects of narcotics previously discussed, morphine can release histamine from mast cells, resulting in itching and skin rashes.

In the management of chronic or long-term pain, the accumulation of metabolites may be of concern. Hepatic metabolism of morphine gives rise to two glucuronides, morphine-6-glucuronide, which has analgesic activity, and morphine-3-glucuronide, which is inactive. A significant proportion of the analgesic action of morphine is in fact due to morphine-6-glucuronide, which can accumulate particularly in patients with renal dysfunction. This would include the aging patient, whose renal function may be reduced. As morphine-6-glucuonide builds up, it can cause sedation, increased respiratory depression, nausea and vomiting. For the older adult, reduced doses and longer intervals between doses may be important in preventing adverse effects.

Codeine Phosphate

Codeine is similar to morphine in its effects but much weaker. Administered orally in doses of 30–60 mg, codeine is effective in the treatment of mild to moderate pain. Sixty-five milligrams of the drug are equal in effectiveness to 650 mg of either ASA or acetaminophen. Codeine is often administered in combination with ASA or acetaminophen; the analgesia produced is usually greater than if either narcotic or non-narcotic is used alone.

Semisynthetic Modifications of Morphine or Codeine

Hydrocodone

Hydrocodone, a semisynthetic analogue of codeine, is an ingredient in some analgesic mixtures and has the same action as other opioids. It is more potent than codeine and its dependence liability is similar to that of other opioids given orally.

Hydromorphone (Dilaudid®)

Hydromorphone is a semisynthetic derivative of morphine. It is approximately eight times more potent than morphine and relatively more effective when given orally. Hydromorphone has the same actions and uses as morphine. It is indicated for the relief of moderate to severe pain.

Oxymorphone (Numorphan®)

Oxymorphone is another semisynthetic morphine derivative that is closely related to hydromorphone. The drug is indicated for the relief of moderate to severe pain. It is similar to both hydromorphone and morphine but is devoid of antitussive activity.

Oxycodone (Percodan®, Percocet®)

Oxycodone is available only in combination with ASA (Percodan®) or acetaminophen (Percocet®) for the treatment of pain. Oxycodone is effective orally and is more potent than codeine. As might be expected, its dependence liability is also greater than that of codeine. The doses for oxycodone in combination with either ASA or acetaminophen can be found in Chapter 53.

Synthetic Narcotics

Fentanyl (Sublimaze®, Duragesic®)

Fentanyl is a narcotic analgesic with actions similar to those of other narcotics. It produces analgesia, sedation, respiratory depression, constipation and physical dependence, but appears to have less emetic activity than other narcotic analgesics. Alfentanil, sufentanil and remifentanil are three similar narcotic analgesics. However, they are used exclusively in anesthesia and, accordingly, they are described in Chapter 58.

Fentanyl has been available for years in a parenteral formulation (Sublimaze®). Parenterally administered fentanyl is characterized by a relatively rapid onset and short duration of action. Its onset of action is almost immediate following intravenous administration; however, the maxi-

mum analgesic and respiratory depressant effect may not be noted for several minutes. The usual duration of the analgesic effect is 30–60 min after a single intravenous dose of up to 100 µg. Following intramuscular administration, the onset of action is from 7–8 min and the duration of action is 1–2 h. With epidural use, the onset of action is between 5–10 min following administration and the duration of action is generally 2–5 h.

Fentanyl is also marketed in a transdermal patch (Duragesic®) that provides continuous systemic delivery of the narcotic for up to seventy-two hours. This product is indicated in the management of chronic cancer pain in patients receiving opioid analgesia. It should provide significant convenience to patients requiring a continual cover of a narcotic. The disadvantages to Duragesic® are its long duration of action (and thus the difficulty of reversing drug-induced toxicities) and the lengthy interval until steady state is achieved.

Box 52.1 presents a sample patient teaching on the appropriate use of Duragesic®.

Meperidine HCl, Pethidine HCl (Demerol®)

Meperidine or pethidine is eight to ten times less potent than morphine (i.e., 10 mg morphine equals 80–100 mg meperidine). Oral meperidine is one-third to one-quarter as effective as the parenteral formulation. Meperidine's duration of action is two to four hours. A common mistake with this drug is to give it every six hours. Often this leaves the patient with two hours of pain before the next dose.

Meperidine is indicated for the relief of moderate to severe pain in many medical, surgical, obstetric and dental situations. It has less effect on the gastrointestinal tract than morphine and no antitussive properties. In obstetrics, meperidine does not antagonize the actions of an oxytocic. Therapeutic doses given during active labour do not delay birth; in fact, the frequency, duration and amplitude of uterine contractions sometimes may be increased. Meperidine does not interfere with normal postpartum contractions or involution of the uterus, and it does not increase the incidence of postpartum hemorrhage.

The pattern and overall incidence of adverse effects following the use of meperidine are similar to those observed after equianalgesic doses of mor-

---

Box 52.1
Patient teaching: Proper use of Duragesic®

✔ **Where to apply Duragesic®**

Select a dry, non-hairy area on your arms, chest or back. If the area you choose has body hair, clip (do not shave) the hair close to the skin with scissors.

    Do not put the patch on skin that is excessively oily, burned, broken out, cut, irritated or damaged in any way. If you need to clean the skin where the patch will be applied, use only clear water. Soaps, oils, lotions, alcohol or other products may irritate the skin under the patch.

✔ **How to apply Duragesic®**

• **Step 1.** Each patch is sealed in its own protective pouch. Do not remove the patch from the pouch until you are ready to use it. When you are ready, tear open the pouch along one of the edges or at one of the ends.

• **Step 2.** A stiff protective liner covers the sticky side of the patch — the side that will be put on your skin. Hold the liner at the edge and pull the patch from the liner. Try not to touch the sticky side of the patch. Throw away the liner.

• **Step 3.** Immediately after you have removed the liner, apply the sticky side of the patch to a dry area of your arms, chest or back. Press the patch firmly on your skin with the palm of your hand for about ten to twenty seconds. Make sure the patch sticks well to your skin, especially around the edges.

• **Step 4.** Wash your hands when you have finished applying the patch.

• **Step 5.** After wearing the patch for three days, or as directed by your doctor, remove it (see Disposing of Duragesic®). Then choose a different place on your skin to apply a new patch and repeat steps 1 to 4 in order.

✔ **Disposing of Duragesic®**

Before putting on a new Duragesic®, remove the patch you have been wearing. Fold the used patch in half so the sticky side sticks to itself, and flush down the toilet immediately.

Source: Canadian Pharmaceutical Association. *Compendium of Pharmaceuticals and Specialties.* 32nd ed. Ottawa: CPA; 1997. Reproduced with permission.

---

phine, except that constipation and urinary retention are less common. Meperidine differs from morphine in that toxic doses sometimes cause CNS excitation, characterized by tremors, muscle twitches and seizures; these effects are due largely to a metabolite, normeperidine. Since normeperidine is eliminated by both the kidney and the liver, decreased renal or hepatic function increases the likelihood of such toxicity. This can also pose a problem in patients over sixty years of age, who may have renal and/or hepatic insufficiency.

    Table 52.2 lists the clinically significant drug interactions with meperidine.

Table 52.2
Meperidine: Drug interactions

Drug	Interaction
CNS depressants	• CNS depressants (e.g., alcohol, barbiturates, TCAs, antidepressants, MAOIs and phenothiazines) increase the central depressant effects of narcotics. Respiratory depression, hypotension and profound sedation or coma may result
Monoamine oxidase inhibitors	• Meperidine should be avoided in pts receiving MAOIs, who may experience severe reactions, generally immediate, with excitation, sweating, rigidity and hypertension. Some pts develop hypertension and coma, and several deaths have been reported from this interaction. Other narcotics are not likely to cause such severe reactions

Levorphanol (Levo-Dromoran®)

Related both chemically and pharmacologically to morphine, levorphanol is four to five times more potent. Given orally, it is a more effective drug. Levorphanol may also be administered subcutaneously or by slow intravenous injection.

Methadone (Dolophine®)

Methadone is a synthetic narcotic with a half-life of twenty-five hours. Its long duration of action and excellent analgesic effects make it a good drug for the treatment of cancer. Methadone is also useful orally in narcotic detoxification programs. In this situation its long half-life is an advantage because patients may be treated once daily in a heroin clinic. Although methadone is similar to morphine and other potent narcotics, its long duration of action ensures less intense, but more prolonged, withdrawal symptoms.

Propoxyphene (Darvon®)

Propoxyphene HCl or napsylate (Darvon-N®) is effective for the relief of mild to moderate pain. Sixty-four milligrams of propoxyphene HCl and 100 mg propoxyphene napsylate contain equivalent amounts of propoxyphene and are as effective as 650 mg ASA. Propoxyphene owes its popularity over codeine and ASA to the fact that it does not irritate the stomach or constipate the patient. However, excessive doses have proven fatal, and for this reason, propoxyphene should not be prescribed to any patient with suicidal risk.

Agonist-Antagonist Narcotics

Most narcotics, such as morphine, codeine, meperidine and levorphanol, are agonists. They stimulate both μ (mu) and K (kappa) receptors. A few narcotics, such as pentazocine, butorphanol and nalbuphine, are called agonist-antagonist drugs. In the absence of agonists they produce analgesia. In the presence of pure agonists, they block many of the actions of the latter drugs. This action can be explained by the fact that they competitively block μ receptors, which are responsible for most of the analgesic effects of agonists such as morphine, while serving as agonists of K and Σ (sigma) receptors.

Individual Mixed Agonist-Antagonist Narcotics

Pentazocine (Talwin®)

Pentazocine is an agonist-antagonist drug, as described above. In the presence of other narcotics, it acts as a narcotic antagonist, blocking their actions on μ receptors. In the absence of other narcotics, its ability to stimulate K receptors becomes apparent and the drug produces analgesia. Pentazocine is claimed to cause less respiratory depression than morphine, but it is also less effective.

Pentazocine is indicated for relief of moderate to severe pain. It is also used as a preoperative or preanesthetic medication, and as a supplement to surgical anesthesia. The drug has the same adverse effects as other narcotics. Particular attention should be paid to the psychotomimetic effects of large doses. Pentazocine should not be given to patients who are dependent on narcotics because its antagonist properties on μ receptors may precipitate a withdrawal effect. In the United States, Talwin® tablets contain naloxone, an opioid antagonist (see below) to reduce the potential for abuse. Naloxone is not absorbed from the gastrointestinal tract and will not affect the analgesic effects of orally administered pentazocine. If, however, Talwin® tablets reach the street trade and are dissolved and injected, the naloxone will block the effects of the pentazocine.

Butorphanol Tartrate (Stadol®)

Butorphanol is more potent than either morphine or meperidine, with 2–3 mg parenterally producing analgesia equal to 10 mg morphine or 80 mg meperidine. It is ineffective if given by mouth. Butorphanol is indicated for relief of moderate to severe pain, including preoperative and postoperative pain and renal colic. The drug may also be used for analgesia during balanced anesthesia. Butorphanol is also prepared in a nasal spray (Stadol NS®) that is indicated for relief of moderate to severe acute pain. Box 52.2 gives a sample patient teaching in the proper use of Stadol® nasal spray.

Butorphanol is claimed to produce less respiratory depression than morphine. Its major side effects are drowsiness, weakness, sweating, nausea and a feeling of floating. Like pentazocine,

Box 52.2
Patient teaching: Use of Stadol NS® (nasal spray)

This medication is delivered by a nasal pump. Follow these steps to administer a dose.

✔ Gently blow your nose to clear nostrils.

✔ Remove the protective cap from the medication pump and prime the pump. To do this, hold the unit with tip between fingers and thumb on the bottom of the bottle, then press quickly and firmly until a spray is visible (this may require 4–7 strokes).

✔ While sitting up, insert the tip of the applicator about 1/2 inch into your nostril. Point the tip straight up your nose. Without inhaling, squeeze the pump once. This will deliver one dose of 1 mg. If a dose of 2 mg is ordered, repeat the procedure in the other nostril.

✔ Keep head still and sniff gently, with mouth closed, for several seconds. Do not blow nose.

✔ Cover the unit and store out of the reach of children. Follow the doctor's instructions regarding repeating the dose.

Source: Mead Johnson, Stadol NS® product insert sheet. Reproduced with permission.

butorphanol should not be given to patients who are dependent on narcotics because it will act as an antagonist and cause withdrawal effects.

Nalbuphine HCl (Nubain®)

Nalbuphine is about as potent as morphine and three times more active than pentazocine. Its adverse effects are similar to those of the stronger narcotics. Similar to pentazocine and butorphanol, nalbuphine should not be given to patients dependent on narcotics. Nalbuphine is indicated for relief of moderate to severe pain. It may also be used for preoperative analgesia, as a supplement to surgical anesthesia and for obstetrical analgesia during labour.

Patient-Controlled Analgesia

Patient-controlled analgesia (PCA) is a method of narcotics delivery via infusion pump that enables patients to self-administer the analgesic and thus control their own pain. Because the patients can administer small doses upon demand, plasma levels of drug are consistently maintained, resulting in more sustained pain relief.

The pumps have a timing control with a lockout mechanism that prevents overdosing. The patient is not dependent on the unit routine nor on the availability of staff for drug administration when pain returns. Many studies have shown that PCA results in earlier mobilization after surgery and reduced length of hospital stay. Most patients say they would use the approach again and would recommend it to others.

PCA requires nursing responsibility for supervision and monitoring of both therapeutic and nontherapeutic responses. Patient instruction is another role. Assessment prior to initiating the device is crucial: the nurse must ensure that the patient cannot self-administer a dose prematurely; that is, if a narcotic dose has been given by another route, such intravenously or orally, or in the postanesthetic recovery unit, the duration of action of this dose must pass before further doses can be self-administered.

Narcotic Antagonists

Narcotic antagonists competitively block opiate receptors and are used to treat narcotic overdoses. Naloxone (Narcan®) is the narcotic antagonist most frequently used in North America. When administered parenterally to a patient who has overdosed on a narcotic, it rapidly reverses the effect of the latter drug.

Nursing Management

Table 52.3 on the next page describes the nursing management of the patient receiving narcotic drugs. Table 52.4 (page 621) gives the titration of morphine and hydromorphone for oral and parenteral therapy. Dosage details of other drugs are given in Table 52.5 (pages 622–625).

Table 52.3
Nursing management of the narcotics

Assessment of risk vs. benefit	Patient data	• Physician should determine dosage, frequency and type of narcotic that is most effective for the type of pain • Assess to establish baseline VS, especially respiratory rate, and contraindications for use • Assess for pain: location, intensity, onset and pt reactions • *Pregnancy:* Risk category C (animal studies show adverse effects to fetus but human data are unknown or insufficient); benefits may be acceptable despite risks
	Drug data	• Select drugs based on pt age, presenting underlying problem, location and severity of pain and desired duration of action • Most serious adverse effects are CNS depression (including respiratory depression) and hypotension • Most common side effects are constipation and nausea
Implementation	Rights of administration	• Using the "rights" helps prevent errors of administration
	Right route	• Give by all routes: IV, IM, SC, PO, PCA, intrathecal, transdermal and nasal. Dosages are not interchangeable for different routes; usually, oral route requires higher doses • Rotate sites (e.g., morphine is irritating to SC tissues)
	Right dose	• See Table 52.5. Doses must be individualized. Generally, sharp, stabbing pain requires more analgesic than dull, constant pain. Aging pts often require lower doses • Dosage titration is important to ensure that pt's individual responses are considered. (See Table 52.4 for sample titration schedules for oral and parenteral routes)
	Right time	• Narcotics produce better analgesia when administered ATC before pain becomes severe, rather than prn
	Right technique	• IV administration requires knowledge of correct diluent and IV solution, correct dilution and rate of administration. Always refer to manufacturer's instructions for this route. For direct IV, refer to agency policy regarding certification. Rate must be carefully controlled; use infusion pump
	Nursing therapeutics	• Enhance comfort by such interventions as rest, fluids, positioning, massage, diversionary stimulation • *Emotional support:* Pain can produce anxiety • Prevent constipation by bowel protocol (e.g., dietary fibre, fluids, stool softeners and laxative, if required)
	Patient/family teaching	• Pt's need for information may be influenced by length of time required for tx or limited by serious illness. Pts/families should know warning signs/symptoms of possible toxicities of these drugs. Report immediately: excessive sedation, difficulty arousing • Warn pts to avoid dangerous activities (driving, operating heavy machinery) until response to drug is known • For PCA, instruct pt in use of device

Table 52.3 (continued)
Nursing management of the narcotics

Outcomes	Monitoring of progress	*Continually monitor:*
		• Clinical response indicating tx success (reduction in pain, increasing activity)
		• Assess pain 30–60 min after administration. Note duration of drug action
		• Signs/symptoms of adverse reactions; document and report immediately to physician

Response to Clinical Challenge

In considering the advantages and disadvantages of PCA for this young patient, you might have included the following:

Advantages:
• PCA has been found to be as or more effective than nurse-administered analgesia in many studies.
• Studies have shown a reduced length of stay with PCA.
• PCA allows for more steady plasma levels of the narcotic with more consistent pain relief.
• Patients do not have to wait for a nurse to be available to administer medication.

Disadvantages:
• Requires patient willingness and ability to learn to operate device.

• Initial implementation period is not without risk; caution must be taken to ensure that patient cannot activate device too soon after administration of narcotic by another route.
• PCA should not be used without appropriate supervision and monitoring of response.

Some arguments to support this suggestion:
• A 13-year-old boy is capable of learning to manage a PCA device and will probably have family members to assist.
• This route is preferable over the IM route for this young patient.
• The approach promotes self-care by involving the individual and family in the patient's recovery.

Some concerns that should be addressed:
• Effective teaching.
• Provision of adequate supervision and monitoring of response.

Table 52.4
Titration of morphine and hydromorphone for oral and parenteral therapy

Morphine (tabs or solution)			Hydromorphone		
Oral therapy					
Usual starting dose	If dosage is	Increase by	Usual starting dose	If dosage is	Increase by
5–10 mg q4h	5–30 mg q4h	5 mg/dose	1–2 mg q4h	1–6 mg q4h	1 mg/dose
	30–70 mg q4h	10 mg/dose		6–14 mg q4h	2 mg/dose
	70–100 mg q4h	20 mg/dose		14–20 mg q4h	4 mg/dose
	> 100 mg q4h	20–30 mg/dose		> 20 mg q4h	4–6 mg/dose
Continuous IV or SC therapy					
Usual starting dose	If dosage is	Increase by	Usual starting dose	If dosage is	Increase by
5–10 mg q4h	< 5 mg/h	1 mg/h	1–2 mg q4h	< 1 mg/h	0.25 mg/h
	5–20 mg/h	2 mg/h		1–4 mg/h	0.5 mg/h
	20–50 mg/h	5 mg/h		4–12.5 mg/h	1 mg/h
	> 50 mg/h	10–20 mg/h		> 12.5 mg/h	2–4 mg/h

Source: Calgary District Hospital Group Pharmacy. *TAP Newsletter.* Reproduced with permission.

Table 52.5
The narcotics: Drug doses

Drug Generic name (Trade names)	Dosage	Nursing alert
A. Opium Preparations		
purified opium alkaloids (Pantopon)	**IM/SC:** 5–20 mg	• 1 mL = 10 mg morphine. Observe for respiratory depression; treat with naloxone prn
B. Purified Alkaloids of Opium		
morphine sulfate	**Oral:** *Adults:* 10–30 mg q4h. Initially, as extended-release or sustained-release preparations, 30 mg q8h. **IM/SC:** 5–20 mg q4h prn. **IV:** 2.5–15 mg q4h or IV infusion initiated with a loading dose of 15 mg followed by infusion at 0.8–10 mg/h, rate increased prn. Doses of 20–150 mg/h have been used. **Rectal:** 10–30 mg q4h. **Epidural:** Initially, 2–10 mg/day, or 2–4 mg/day as a continuous infusion. **Intrathecal:** 0.2–1 mg as a single dose. *Children:* **SC:** 100–200 µg/kg q4h (not to exceed 15 mg/dose). **IM/IV:** 50–100 µg/kg (initially, not to exceed 10 mg/dose)	• **PO:** May be given with food. Do not crush, break or chew extended-release forms. Solutions may be diluted in fruit juice • **IV:** Do not use cloudy solution. Administer over 4–5 min or by continuous infusion. Have antidote available
codeine phosphate	**PO/IM/SC:** *Adults:* 15–60 mg q3–6h prn. *Children:* 0.5 mg/kg q4–6h (up to 4x daily) prn	• **PO:** May give with food or milk • **IM/SC:** Do not use solutions if discoloured or containing precipitate • ATC administration is more efficacious than prn. With long-term use, do not discontinue suddenly
C. Semisynthetic Modifications of Morphine or Codeine		
hydromorphone HCl (Dilaudid)	**Oral:** *Adults:* 2 mg q3–6h prn; may be increased to 4 mg q4–6h. **IM/SC:** 1–2 mg q3–6h, prn; may be increased to 3–4 mg q4–6h. **IV:** 0.5–1 mg q3h, prn. **Rectal:** 3 mg q4–8h, prn	• **PO:** May give with food or milk • **IV:** For direct IV, follow agency policy. Dilute with 5 mL NaCl or sterile water and give at a rate of 2 mg over 3–5 min. Check compatibility with other IV drugs/solutions
oxycodone HCl (Roxicodone)	**Oral:** *Adults:* 5–10 mg q4–6h	• May be given with food if GI upset occurs
oxymorphone HCl (Numorphan)	**SC/IM:** *Adults:* 1–1.5 mg q3–6h, prn. **IV:** 0.5 mg q3–6h, prn; increase prn. **Rectal:** 5 mg q4–6h, prn (Analgesia during labour) **IM:** 0.5–1 mg	• **Rectal:** Store suppositories in fridge and protect from light • **IV:** For direct IV, follow agency policy. Give dosage undiluted over 2–3 min. Check IV drug compatibility

Table 52.5 (continued)
The narcotics: Drug doses

Drug Generic name (Trade names)	Dosage	Nursing alert
D. Synthetic Narcotics		
fentanyl transdermal system (Duragesic)	Consult manufacturer's detailed information to convert opioid-tolerant pts from oral or parenteral opioids to Duragesic®	• Check dosage carefully. Available in systems supplying 25–100 µg/h. Supplementary doses may be required for breakthrough pain • For pt teaching, see Box 52.1 (page 617). Provide written instructions to pts re application, removal and disposal of patches. Wash hands with water only after applying patch and if any gel gets on the skin • Skin rash may occur at site. Rotate sites. Check site routinely to ensure that patch has not been accidentally removed
levorphanol tartrate (Levo-Dromoran)	**Oral:** *Adults:* Initially, 2 mg q4–5h; may be increased to 3–4 mg, prn. **SC/IV:** *Adults:* 2 mg q4–5h; may be increased to 3 mg if pain is severe	• **PO:** May give with food or milk • **IV:** Follow agency policy. Give slowly over 3–5 min • Pts should remain recumbent for 30–60 min after parenteral dose
meperidine HCl, pethidine HCl (Demerol)	**PO/IM/SC:** *Adults:* 50–150 mg q3–4h. *Children:* 1–1.8 mg/kg q3–4h (not to exceed 100 mg/dose). **IV:** *Adults:* 15–35 mg/h as continuous infusion (Analgesia during labour) **IM/SC:** 50–100 mg when contractions become regular; may repeat q1–3h	• Oral and parenteral doses are not interchangeable. The oral dose is approximately 50% as effective as the parenteral dose • **PO:** May give with food or milk • **IM:** Preferred over SC, which causes tissue irritation • **IV:** For direct IV, follow agency policy. Do not exceed rate of 25 mg/min. For continuous infusion, check drug compatibility; administer with infusion pump. Instruct pt re: use of PCA pump
methadone (Dolophine)	(Analgesia) **PO/IM/SC:** *Adults:* 2.5–10 mg q3–4h, up to 5–20 mg q6–12h. (Detoxification) **Oral:** *Adults:* 15–40 mg/day, initially, for 2–3 days, then decrease q2days.	• **PO:** May give with food or milk. Dilute liquid with 30 mL or more of water or juice
propoxyphene HCl (Darvon) propoxyphene napsylate (Darvon-N)	(Propoxyphene HCl) **Oral:** *Adults:* 65 mg q3–4h, prn (Propoxyphene napsylate) **Oral:** *Adults:* 100 mg q4h, prn	• **PO:** May give with food or milk *(cont'd on next page)*

Table 52.5 (continued)
The narcotics: Drug doses

Drug Generic name (Trade names)	Dosage	Nursing alert
E. Mixed Agonist-Antagonist Analgesics		
butorphanol (Stadol)	**IM:** *Adults:* 2 mg q3–4h, prn (range, 1–4 mg). **IV:** *Adults:* 1 mg push; an additional dose may be given immediately, prn. This dose can be repeated q3–4h	• **IM:** Administer deep into muscle; rotate sites • **IV:** For direct IV, follow agency instructions. Give slowly over 3–5 min
butorphanol tartrate (Stadol NS)	**Intranasal:** *Adults:* Initially, 1 spray (1 mg) in one nostril. If adequate pain relief is not achieved within 60–90 min, an additional 1-mg dose may be given. Repeat in 3–4 h as needed. Total daily doses of > 16 mg are not recommended. Depending on severity of pain, an initial dose of 2 mg (1 spray in each nostril) may be used in pts who will be able to remain recumbent in the event that drowsiness or dizziness occur. In such pts, additional doses should not be given for 3–4 h Use Stadol NS with caution in pts with hepatic impairment. Initial dosage interval should be increased to 6–12 h until response is well characterized. Subsequent dosings should be determined by pt response rather than scheduled at fixed intervals	• See Box 52.2 (page 619) for pt teaching
nalbuphine HCl (Nubain)	(For analgesia) **IM/SC/IV:** *Adults:* Usual dose, 10 mg q3–6h (single dose not to exceed 20 mg; total daily dose not to exceed 160 mg)	• **IM:** Give deep into muscle and rotate sites • **IV:** For direct IV, follow agency policy; do not exceed rate of 10 mg over 3–5 min. Store ampoules at room temperature and protect from excessive light
pentazocine HCl (tablets) (Talwin)	(For moderate to severe pain) **Oral:** *Adults:* 50–100 mg q3–4h (not to exceed 600 mg/day). **SC/IV/IM:** *Adults:* 30 mg q3–4h, prn (not to exceed 30 mg/dose IV or 60 mg/dose IM or SC; not to exceed 360 mg/day SC, IV or IM) (For obstetrics) **IM/IV:** *Adults:* 20 mg IV or 30 mg IM. When contractions become regular, may be repeated 2–3x at 2- to 3-h intervals	• **IM:** Give deep into muscle and rotate sites. Preferred parenteral route, as SC causes tissue irritation • **IV:** For direct IV, follow agency policy and do not exceed rate of 5 mg/min

Table 52.5 (continued)
The narcotics: Drug doses

Drug Generic name (Trade names)	Dosage	Nursing alert

F. Narcotic Antagonist

| naloxone HCl
(Narcan, Narcan Neonatal) | (Opioid-induced respiratory or CNS depression) **IV/IM/SC:** *Adults:* 0.4 mg; may repeat q2–3min (IV route is preferred). Some pts may require up to 2 mg. If pt is suspected of being opioid-dependent, initial dose should be decreased to 0.1–0.2 mg. May also be given by IV infusion at rate adjusted to pt's response. *Children:* 0.01 mg/kg q2–3min

(Postoperative respiratory depression) **IV:** *Adults:* 0.1–0.2 mg q2–3min until response obtained; may repeat q1–2h later if needed (0.5 µg/kg dose will not interfere with analgesia). *Children:* 5–10 µg; may repeat q2–3min until response obtained | •**IV:** Most rapid response with direct IV. Follow agency policy and administer at a rate of 0.1–0.4 mg in 15 s. Monitor clinical response carefully and titrate dose accordingly
•Check ampoule carefully; available in strengths of 0.02 mg/mL, 0.4 mg/mL and 1 mg/mL
•Continuous infusion may be required for tx of overdose with long-acting drugs |

Further Reading

Alcock N. Factors affecting the assessment of postoperative pain: A literature review. *J Adv Nurs* 1996;24(6):1144–1151.

Bedder M. Epidural opioid therapy for chronic non-malignant pain: critique of current experience. *J Pain Symptom Management* 1996;11(6):353–356.

Cokefair A, et al. An investigation of current literature on the effectiveness of PCA methods. *CRNA* 1996;7(3):126–134.

Drugs for pain. *Medical Letter on Drugs and Therapeutics* 1993;35:1–6.

Egbert A. Post-operative pain management in the frail elderly. *Clin Geriatric Med* 1996;12(3):583–599.

Haver M, et al. IV patient-controlled analgesia in critically ill post-op/trauma patients: research-based practice recommendations. *Dim Crit Care Nurs* 1995;14(3):144–153.

Lehmann K. New developments in patient-controlled post-operative analgesia. *Ann Med* 1995;27(2):271–282.

Lindaman C. Talking to physicians about pain control. *Am J Nurs* 1995;1:36–37.

Robison J, et al. Sublingual and oral morphine administration: review and new findings. *Nurs Clin North Am* 1995;30(4):725–743.

Skobel S. Epidural narcotic administration: what nursing should know. *Oncol Nurs Forum* 1996;23(10):1555–1562.

Vesely C. Pediatric patient-controlled analgesia enhancing the self-care construct. *Pediatr Nurs* 1995;21(2):124–128.

Williams C. PCA: a review of the literature. *J Clin Nurs* 1996;5(3):139–141.

Non-Narcotic Analgesics

Topics Discussed
- Single-ingredient products
- Analgesic products containing both a narcotic and a non-narcotic drug
- Co-analgesics
- For each drug discussed: Mechanism of action, pharmacologic effects, therapeutic uses, adverse effects
- Nursing process

Drugs Discussed
acetaminophen (ah-seat-ah-**min**-oh-fen)
acetylsalicylic acid (ah-see-til-sal-ih-**sill**-ik)
butalbital (byoo-**tal**-bih-tal)
diflunisal (dye-**floo**-nih-sal)
fenoprofen (fen-oh-**proe**-fen)
ibuprofen (eye-byoo-**proe**-fen)
ketorolac (kee-**toe**-role-ak)
naproxen (nah-**prox**-en)
paracetamol (par-ah-**see**-tah-mol)

Clinical Challenge

Consider this clinical challenge as you read through this chapter. The response to the challenge appears on page 633.

A mother brings her 3-year-old son to the local community health centre, concerned with his nausea, vomiting, diarrhea and abdominal pain, which started suddenly during the afternoon. The assessment reveals that he may have ingested several acetaminophen tablets last night but the mother assumed that they could not harm him because they are just an OTC painkiller. He did not complain of any symptoms prior to bedtime and slept well.

1. Are the child's symptoms consistent with acetaminophen overdose?
2. What is the major risk for this child?
3. What treatment should be commenced?

Non-narcotic analgesics are also called *analgesic-antipyretics* because they relieve pain and reduce fever. In contrast to narcotics, analgesic-antipyretics do not produce euphoria and drug dependence. Generally speaking, their analgesic activity is less than that of narcotics and they are used in pain of mild to moderate intensity. In progressive diseases, analgesic-antipyretics are often used first to treat pain and as the condition worsens, the patient is switched to a narcotic.

Non-narcotic analgesics are also used in the treatment of rheumatoid arthritis and osteo-arthritis (Chapter 54). Their use in these conditions will not be discussed in this chapter.

Single-Ingredient Products

Acetylsalicylic Acid, ASA (Aspirin®)

For years ASA has been the standard analgesic-antipyretic used in North America. In Canada, the full generic name for the drug is acetylsalicylic acid; Aspirin® is a trade name. In the United States, aspirin is a generic name, with many companies using it.

Mechanism of action and pharmacologic effects. ASA acts both peripherally and within the brain to produce analgesia. Peripherally, it interferes with the production of prostaglandins in various organs and tissues (Figure 53.1). Prostaglandin E_2 sensitizes pain receptors to noxious substances, such as histamine and bradykinin. By reducing the synthesis of prostaglandin E_2, ASA diminishes pain. Centrally, the drug acts in the hypothalamus to reduce pain perception.

ASA lowers elevated body temperatures. The antipyretic effects of the drug are due to its ability to interfere with production of prostaglandin E_1 in the brain. Prostaglandin E_1 is a powerful pyretic chemical, capable of increasing body temperature.

ASA also inhibits platelet aggregation (see Chapter 44). Doses of one to two grams per day reduce renal uric acid secretion. Five grams per day, or more, increase the elimination of uric acid from the body by reducing its reabsorption from the renal tubules. Large doses of ASA increase the renal reabsorption of sodium, chloride and water, producing edema.

Figure 53.1
Inhibition of prostaglandin synthesis by acetylsalicylic acid

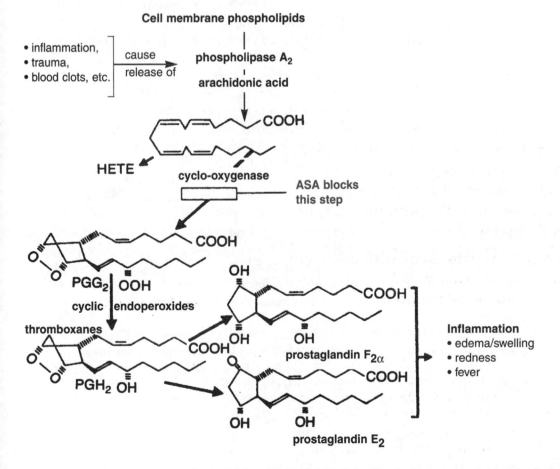

Source: Mazel P. Analgesics-antipyretics. In: Pradhan SN, Maickel RP, Dutta SN, eds. *Pharmacology in Medicine.* Bethesda, MD: SP Press International; 1986:224. Reproduced with permission.

Pharmacokinetics. ASA can be absorbed from both the stomach and the duodenum. However, its absorption proceeds faster from the latter site. Taking ASA with food slows absorption of the drug because food closes the pyloric sphincter, trapping ASA in the stomach.

Shortly after its absorption, ASA is metabolized to salicylate. Approximately ninety percent of the salicylate is metabolized in the liver. A glycine conjugate, called salicyluric acid, accounts for seventy-five percent of the metabolites. The capacity of the liver to furnish enough glycine to inactivate salicylate is limited. If the daily dose of ASA exceeds the capacity of the liver to provide glycine, serum salicylate levels rise sharply and the patient may become toxic. About ten percent of the salicylate in the body is eliminated unchanged by the kidney. If the urine is alkalinized, this can be increased three- to five-fold.

Therapeutic uses. ASA is an effective analgesic and antipyretic for the relief of mild to moderate pain. Six hundred fifty milligrams of ASA are as effective as 30 mg codeine or 100 mg propoxyphene napsylate. ASA is more effective in the relief of skeletal muscle pain than visceral pain and is often given to patients with headaches, neuralgias, myalgias or primary spasmodic dysmenorrhea. ASA is also a popular anti-inflammatory drug for the treatment of rheumatoid arthritis and osteoarthrosis. This aspect of its use is discussed in Chapter 54.

Concern over a possible correlation between the use of ASA as an antipyretic in children with varicella or influenza virus infection and the development of Reye's syndrome has led to the recommendation that the drug not be used in these conditions. ASA is also contraindicated in patients who are allergic to the drug, in those who have had a bronchospastic reaction, or in cases of generalized urticaria, angioedema, severe rhinitis, laryngeal edema or shock precipitated by ASA or nonsteroidal anti-inflammatory drugs (NSAIDs). Further, because of its irritant effects on the gastric mucosa, ASA is contraindicated in patients with active peptic ulcer.

Adverse effects. Gastric irritation, ranging from discomfort to gastric ulceration and hemorrhage, is a common adverse effect of ASA due to its direct irritant effects on the gastric mucosa, as well as its reduction of prostaglandin formation. Prostaglandin E_2 (PGE_2) promotes the secretion of protective gastric mucus. When its formation is blocked by ASA, gastric mucous secretion falls and the stomach is exposed to the digestive effects of its own secretion.

Enteric-coated ASA tablets do not dissolve until they reach the duodenum. They prevent the direct effect of ASA on the gastric mucosa, but have no effect on the action of the drug that is delivered to the stomach in the circulation after absorption.

ASA is rapidly metabolized in the body. Its primary product is salicylate, a vitamin K antagonist. Large doses of ASA taken for several days can cause hypoprothrombinemia. This effect is usually significant only in patients taking oral anticoagulants or suffering from liver disease.

ASA can cause serious allergic reactions, including acute asthmatic attacks, hives and hypotension. Patients allergic to ASA should not be given the drug nor any other nonsteroidal anti-inflammatory drug.

Mild toxicity is usually seen with serum salicylate levels of 500 μg/mL (3620 μmol/L). Hepatitis has been reported rarely in patients with systemic lupus erythematosus and juvenile rheumatoid arthritis with serum salicylate levels above 250 μg/mL (1810 μmol/L).

Large doses of ASA can be very toxic. Beginning with tinnitus and decreased hearing, the symptoms of acute poisoning can proceed to respiratory alkalosis. In response to the increased loss of CO_2, renal excretion of bicarbonate rises and systemic pH returns to normal — but at the cost of a reduced bicarbonate reserve. If sufficient ASA is consumed, metabolic rate increases and metabolic acidosis ensues. The final stage in salicylate intoxication is respiratory depression and death.

Box 53.1 summarizes the steps that can be taken to treat patients who have overdosed on ASA. Table 53.1 lists the drug's clinically significant interactions.

Box 53.1
ASA: Emergency treatment for overdose

Four steps can be taken to treat a patient who has overdosed on ASA.

✔ Gavage patient or induce vomiting to remove any unabsorbed drug
✔ Infuse Ringer's solution and isotonic sodium bicarbonate to restore normal electrolyte balance and pH
✔ Alkalinize urine with sodium bicarbonate to increase salicylate elimination
✔ Hemodialysis may also be tried to eliminate the drug

Table 53.1
ASA: Drug interactions

Drug	Interaction
ACE inhibitors	• NSAIDs, including ASA, reduce the ability of ACEIs to dilate renal blood vessels
Ammonium chloride and ascorbic acid	• Ammonium chloride and ascorbic acid acidify urine and increase the renal reabsorption of salicylates
Antacids	• Antacids, which alkalinize urine, reduce the renal reabsorption and lower the blood levels of salicylate
Anticoagulants, oral	• Oral anticoagulants may have increased effects with ASA. Large doses of ASA decrease prothrombin formation, displace oral anticoagulants from plasma proteins and produce GI bleeding
Antidiabetic agents	• Antidiabetic agents have increased effects with ASA, which decreases the hyperglycemia of diabetes and displaces tolbutamide and chlorpropamide from plasma protein binding
Corticosteroids	• Corticosteroids can enhance salicylate excretion
Dipyridamole	• Dipyridamole increases the risk of bleeding in pts taking ASA
Heparin	• The effect of heparin is increased by ASA
Methotrexate	• Salicylates reduce the renal excretion of methotrexate
Piroxicam	• Piroxicam and ASA should not be used together because of the danger of increased adverse effects
Spironolactone	• Salicylates reduce the diuretic effect of spironolactone
Uricosurics	• Small doses of salicylates may reduce the effects of uricosurics (e.g., probenecid, sulfinpyrazone)

Diflunisal (Dolobid®)

Diflunisal is a nonsteroidal, analgesic, anti-inflammatory, antipyretic drug that is administered twice daily. It appears to act peripherally by inhibiting prostaglandin synthesis. Diflunisal is indicated for relief of mild to moderate pain accompanied by inflammation in conditions such as musculoskeletal trauma, postdental extraction or postepisiotomy. It is also indicated for the symptomatic relief of osteoarthritis.

Diflunisal has a slow onset and long duration of action. The drug produces significant analgesia in one hour and maximum analgesia in two to four hours. Analgesic effects last eight to twelve hours.

Diflunisal is rapidly and completely absorbed following oral administration. Similar to ASA, diflunisal demonstrates concentration-dependent pharmacokinetics. Doubling the dose produces a greater than doubling of drug accumulation.

Table 53.2 on the next page lists the clinically significant drug interactions with diflunisal.

Table 53.2
Diflunisal: Drug interactions

Drug	Interaction
Acetaminophen	• Diflunisal may increase acetaminophen blood levels
Antacids	• Antacids can reduce the bioavailability of diflunisal
Anticoagulants, oral	• Diflunisal can increase the effects of dicumarol and warfarin
Furosemide	• Diflunisal can decrease the hyperuricemic effect of furosemide
Indomethacin	• Diflunisal may reduce the renal clearance and increase the plasma levels of indomethacin. Fatal GI hemorrhage has occurred
Thiazide diuretics	• Diflunisal can decrease the hyperuricemic effect of thiazide diuretics

Ketorolac Tromethamine (Toradol®)

Ketorolac is a nonsteroidal, anti-inflammatory drug (NSAID) that exhibits analgesic activity. It inhibits cyclo-oxygenase, thereby reducing prostaglandin synthesis. Ketorolac is considered to be a peripherally acting analgesic. At analgesic doses, it has minimal anti-inflammatory and antipyretic activity. When compared with other NSAIDs, ketorolac has the advantage of being available as an injectable product, as well as an oral drug.

Intramuscular injection of ketorolac is indicated for the short-term management of moderate to severe pain, including pain following major abdominal, orthopedic and gynecological operative procedures. Injectable ketorolac causes less pain at the injection site than morphine. Unfortunately, it is also about ten times more expensive than morphine.

Oral ketorolac is indicated for the short-term management of mild to moderately severe pain, including postsurgical pain (such as general, orthopedic and dental surgery), acute musculoskeletal trauma and postpartum uterine cramping.

The adverse effects of both oral and parenteral ketorolac are similar to those of other NSAIDs and include dyspepsia and GI pain. Patients taking the drug orally have also occasionally reported nausea, headache and dizziness. Parenteral ketorolac has been associated with drowsiness.

Table 53.3 lists the clinically significant drug interactions with ketorolac.

Other Nonsteroidal Anti-Inflammatory Drugs

Like ASA, nonsteroidal anti-inflammatory drugs inhibit the formation of the various prostaglandins and can be used as analgesic-antipyretics. Drugs such as ibuprofen (Advil®, Motrin®, Rufen®), naproxen sodium (Anaprox®) and fenoprofen (Nalfon®) are sold as analgesics. Their availability has decreased the need to use weaker narcotics.

Table 53.3
Ketorolac: Drug interactions

Drug	Interaction
Anticoagulants, oral	• Prothrombin time should be carefully monitored in all pts receiving oral anticoagulant tx concomitantly with ketorolac
Furosemide	• Ketorolac reduces the diuretic response to furosemide by about 20% in normovolemic subjects
Probenecid	• Concomitant administration of ketorolac and probenecid results in decreased clearance of ketorolac and an approximately 3-fold increase in ketorolac plasma levels and a twofold increase in terminal half-life. The concomitant use of ketorolac and probenecid is contraindicated

The pharmacology of these agents is discussed in detail in Chapter 54.

Acetaminophen, Paracetamol (Tylenol®)

Mechanism of action and pharmacologic effects. Acetaminophen is rapidly absorbed from the gastrointestinal tract and completely metabolized in the liver. Most of the drug is excreted in the urine as glucuronic acid, sulfuric acid and cysteine conjugates within twenty-four hours of administration.

The analgesic and antipyretic actions of acetaminophen are similar to those of ASA. Acetaminophen has no anti-inflammatory activity and does not affect platelet aggregation or irritate the stomach.

Therapeutic uses. Acetaminophen is indicated for the treatment of mild to moderate pain and the reduction of fever. The major use for the drug is as an analgesic-antipyretic in patients who cannot tolerate ASA. This applies to those who experience gastric discomfort with ASA or who are allergic to the drug. Acetaminophen should also be used in place of ASA in patients taking oral anticoagulants. The drug is valuable in relieving the pain of osteoarthritis. Because it is devoid of anti-inflammatory effects, it is less effective in rheumatoid arthritis.

Acetaminophen has proven popular in pediatrics because of its availability in liquid formulations. In addition, the previously mentioned concern over the connection between the use of ASA in children with varicella or influenza virus infection and the development of Reye's syndrome has led to the recommendation that acetaminophen be used in these conditions. Nurses should warn parents of the potentially lethal effects of the drug. It should be stored in a safe place in a childproof container.

Adverse effects. Taken in recommended doses, acetaminophen is well tolerated. Skin rash, drug fever and mucosal lesions have been reported occasionally. A few cases of neutropenia, pancytopenia and leukopenia have also been found.

Hepatic necrosis can occur if overdoses of acetaminophen are taken. Single doses of 10–15 g in adults may cause hepatotoxicity and 25 g or more can kill. The first signs of toxicity occur 12–24 h after acute overdose and include nausea, vomiting, diarrhea, diaphoresis, pallor and abdominal pain. Hepatic damage is seen 24–48 h after an overdose and is manifested by increased serum transaminases, lactic dehydrogenase, prothrombin time and serum bilirubin concentrations. Severe hepatic damage can subsequently proceed to liver failure, encephalopathy, coma and death. Acetaminophen, itself, is not responsible for the liver damage. The culprit is an acetaminophen metabolite that binds to the liver producing necrosis, primarily in the centrolobular region.

Box 53.2 on the next page describes the emergency treatment of the patient who has overdosed on acetaminophen; Table 53.4 lists the drug's clinically significant interactions.

Analgesic Products Containing Both a Narcotic and a Non-Narcotic Drug

Mechanism of Action and Pharmacologic Effects

Narcotic analgesics stimulate opiate receptors in the brain. Non-narcotic analgesics block the formation of prostaglandin E_2. Their different mechanisms of action make their combination rational. In addition, narcotics are effective for visceral pain, while most non-narcotics are effective for musculoskeletal pain and pain associated with inflammation. It is often possible to provide greater pain relief with a combination of a narcotic and a non-narcotic analgesic than with either drug alone.

There are, however, some disadvantages to using fixed-combination products containing a narcotic and a non-narcotic analgesic. These include the fact that the dosages of each ingredient are fixed, and this does not allow for individualization of the doses of each component. Further, the dose of the non-narcotic is frequently too low. For example, Percodan® tablets contain only 325 mg ASA, and a Tylenol #3® tablet has only 300 mg acetaminophen. The doses of each of these non-narcotic analgesics should be doubled to be effective. Finally, some analgesic products contain irrational combinations. Equagesic® tablets, for example,

Box 53.2
Acetaminophen: Emergency treatment for overdose

1. Activated charcoal is effective only when given within 1–2 h of the alleged overdose. Residual charcoal must be removed by gastric lavage with water prior to antidotal tx with acetyl-cystein (#3).

2. When serum determinations of acetaminophen are > 150 µg/mL (990 µmol/L) at 4 h, or > 40 µg/mL (260 µmol/L) at 12 h after the estimated time of ingestion, the pt is at risk for liver damage, and tx is required immediately. Ipecac-induced emesis or gastric lavage should, when possible, commence within 4 h of drug ingestion.

3. Acetylcysteine (Mucomyst®) is used as an antidote for severe acetaminophen poisoning. Because of the low inci-dence of adverse effects associated with acetylcysteine, tx should be initiated immediately without waiting for determina-tion of plasma acetaminophen levels. The decision to continue tx may then be guided by the lab results.

   Acetylcysteine is effective orally. A loading dose of 140 mg/kg is given as a single dose. A maintenance dose of 70 mg/kg is then given q4h for 17 doses. (Acetylcysteine, 20% solution, may be diluted to a 5% concentration with a soft drink to make it more palatable. This mixture should be con-sumed within 1 h of preparation.)

4. If nausea and vomiting occur within 1 h of the loading or maintenance dose of acetylcysteine, the entire dose should be repeated. If nausea and vomiting persist, a nonpheno-thiazine antiemetic (e.g., dimenhydrinate) may be adminis-tered.

5. The use of IV acetylcysteine is recommended when oral tx is not feasible or practical. A loading dose (150 mg/kg acetyl-cysteine) is infused in 200 mL of 5% dextrose in water (D5W) over 15 min, followed by an infusion of 50 mg/kg in 500 mL D5W over 4 h, and finally 100 mg/kg in 1000 mL D5W during the next 16 h. The total dose is 300 mg/kg, administered over 20 h.

Table 53.4
Acetaminophen: Drug interactions

Drug	Interaction
Anticoagulants, oral	• Chronic, high-dose acetaminophen may potentiate the anticoagulant effect of warfarin. Pts stabilized on oral anticoagulants should be advised to limit their intake of acetaminophen to not more than 2 g daily for no more than a few days at a time. ASA should not be used as an alternative

contain the tranquilizer meprobamate (Equanil®), which has no analgesic activity and is included to relieve anxiety. However, meprobamate can pro-duce severe CNS side effects and is rarely used today. Equagesic® tablets also contain ethohep-tazine, which does not have proven efficacy. Further, the dose of ASA in each Equagesic® tablet is 250 mg per tablet, an amount that is too low to have significant analgesic effect.

Mixtures Containing Codeine

ASA plus codeine preparations (e.g., Empirin/ Codeine®, 222®, 282®, 292®) or acetaminophen plus codeine products (e.g., Tylenol/Codeine®, Phenaphen/Codeine®) are most popular. (In the United States, these products also contain phenacetin.) The tablets contain either 15 mg, 30 mg or 60 mg codeine, together with 325 mg ASA or acetaminophen. Fifteen milligrams of codeine is, at best, minimally effective and it is not clear whether combinations containing this amount of narcotic are more effective than the analgesic-antipyretic alone. The preparations with 30 mg codeine in combination with either ASA or acetaminophen are most popular and more effec-tive than either ingredient used alone.

Mixtures Containing Propoxyphene

The rationale for combining propoxyphene with an analgesic-antipyretic is the same as that for similar combinations containing codeine. Control studies with propoxyphene combinations have been limited, but available results suggest that the analgesic effects of the individual components are additive. However, since propoxyphene is less effective than codeine, these combinations may be less effective than comparable codeine-containing preparations.

Mixtures Containing Oxycodone (Percodan®, Percocet®)

Oxycodone combined with non-narcotic analgesics is available as Percodan® and Percocet®. Each Percodan® tablet contains 5 mg oxycodone hydrochloride and 325 mg ASA. Percodan-Demi® tablets contain 2.5 mg oxycodone HCl and 325 mg ASA. Percocet® and Percocet-Demi® tablets contain acetaminophen in place of ASA. Oxycodone is more potent than codeine, and its dependence liability is also greater. Whereas the Percodan-Demi® and Percocet-Demi® tablets are indicated for the relief of mild to moderate pain, the full-strength Percodan® and Percocet® tablets are used in the treatment of moderate to moderately severe pain, including conditions accompanied by fever.

Mixtures Containing Codeine and Butalbital (Fiorinal-C®)

Fiorinal® preparations have been popular for many years. They contain ASA, caffeine and the barbiturate butalbital. Fiorinal-C® products also contain either 15 mg or 30 mg codeine. These products are indicated for relief of acute and chronic pain of mild, moderate or severe degree, which is accompanied by tension or anxiety, and in all cases in which a simultaneous sedative and analgesic action is required, such as tension headache, musculoskeletal pain, postoperative pain, dysmenorrhea and pain associated with dental procedures, neoplastic disease or trauma.

Butalbital has a longer half-life than the analgesics, and the chronic use of Fiorinal-C® will lead to barbiturate accumulation. In addition, there is the possibility that a preparation containing a barbiturate may induce dependence. Therefore, these products are not recommended for the routine or chronic management of pain.

Co-Analgesics

Several drugs having no direct analgesic actions of their own are used in concert with analgesics to relieve pain. These drugs act by reducing muscle spasm and tension, decreasing inflammation, alleviating edema, or treating the depression associated with chronic pain and the anxiety associated with acute pain. The most significant drug groups and their benefits in pain management are presented in Table 53.5 on the next page.

Nursing Management

Table 53.6 on the next page describes the nursing management of patients receiving non-narcotic analgesics. Dosage details of individual drugs are given in Table 53.7 (pages 635–636).

Response to Clinical Challenge

1. These are common symptoms of acetaminophen overdose that occur within 12–24 h after ingestion. The diagnosis can be confirmed by plasma levels. Owing to the elapsed time, the toxic level would be > 260 µmol/L.
2. The major risk for this child is hepatic damage caused by the metabolite that produces liver cell necrosis.
3. It is too late to use ipecac, gastric lavage or activated charcoal. Acetylcysteine should be administered immediately, even before plasma levels are determined.

Further Reading

Baker A, et al. Chronic pain management in cognitively impaired patients: a preliminary research project. *Perspectives* 1996;10(2):4–8.

Dellemya P. Do benzodiazepines have a role in chronic pain management? *Pain* 1994;57(2):137–152.

Drugs for pain. *Medical Letter on Drugs and Therapeutics* 1993;35:1–6.

MacMillian K. Pain corner: equivalent analgesic dose. *AARN Newsletter* 1990;46(3):25.

Stacey B. Effective management of chronic pain: the analgesic dilemma. *Postgraduate Medicine* 1996;100(3):281–284, 287–290, 293.

Table 53.5
Adjunctive drugs in pain management

Classification of co-analgesic (example)	Benefits in pain management
Anticonvulsants (carbamazepine)	• Inhibit nerve impulses; useful for trigeminal neuralgia superficial dyasthetic pain
Antidepressants (amitriptyline)	• Treat postherpetic neuralgia superficial dyasthenia; decrease mood disturbances of narcotics
Antipsychotics (haloperidol)	• Produce antiemetic, sedative actions; decrease agitation with pain (use cautiously because of possible adverse drug reactions)
Benzodiazepines (diazepam)	• Decrease anxiety, insomnia, muscle spasm
Corticosteroids (dexamethasone)	• Decrease inflammation, edema and intracranial pressure

Table 53.6
Nursing management of the non-narcotic analgesics

Assessment of risk vs. benefit	Patient data	• Most of these drugs are self-administered. The nurse may contribute to drug safety through pt and community education • *Pregnancy:* Risk category varies with drug. Benefits may be acceptable despite risks. The exception is diflunisal, which should not be taken during the 3rd trimester of pregnancy as it is known to cause premature closure of the ductus arteriosus in the fetus
	Drug data	• Although generally safe, these drugs can cause significant adverse reactions through immune reactions and with overdose • GI damage with ulceration and/or bleeding is of concern • A serious adverse effect is hepatotoxicity associated with acetaminophen overdose
Implementation	Rights of administration	• Using the "rights" helps prevent errors of administration
	Right route	• Most are PO; except ketorolac, which is available for IM injection
	Nursing therapeutics	• For management of chronic pain, comfort measures and emotional support can enhance effectiveness of drug tx, reduce required dose and provide a sense of individual control
	Patient/family teaching	• Pt's need for information may be influenced by indication for use (e.g., single-dose tx of headache or fever vs. long-term use for chronic pain) • Remind parents that ASA is not recommended for tx of viral illnesses in children/adolescents because of possibility of Reye's syndrome • Encourage pts to try nonpharmacological measures for control of pain (e.g., progressive muscle relaxation, visualization) • Pts/families should know warning signs/symptoms of possible toxicities of these drugs. Report immediately: signs of bleeding such as bruising, tarry stools; tinnitus (with ASA) • Warn pts to avoid/limit alcohol (increased risk for GI bleeding, hepatotoxicity) • *Discuss possibility of pregnancy:* Advise pt to discuss with MD

Table 53.6 (continued)
Nursing management of the non-narcotic analgesics

Outcomes	Monitoring of progress	*Continually monitor:* • Clinical response indicating tx success (reduction in signs/symptoms of fever, pain) • Signs/symptoms of adverse reactions; document and report immediately to physician

Table 53.7
The non-narcotic analgesics: Drug doses

Drug Generic name (Trade names)	Dosage	Nursing alert
A. Analgesics-Antipyretics		
acetylsalicylic acid, ASA (Aspirin)	**Oral/Rectal:** *Adults:* 325–1000 mg q4–6h prn (not to exceed 4 g/day).*Children 2-11 years:* 60–80 mg/ kg/day in 4–6 divided doses	• Give with meals, food or antacid to minimize direct gastric irritation. Do not crush or chew enteric-coated tablets or take enteric-coated tablets with antacids
acetaminophen, paracetamol (Tylenol)	(Analgesia) **Oral:** *Adults/children > 12 years:* 325–1000 mg q4–6h prn (not to exceed 4 g/day, or 2.6 g/day chronically). **Rectal:** 325–650 mg q4h prn (not to exceed 6 suppositories/24 h). *Children ≤ 12 years old should not receive more than 5 doses/24 h without notifying physician* **Oral/Rectal:** *Children 11–12 years:* 480 mg q4–6h prn; *9–11 years:* 400 mg q4–6h prn; *6–9 years:* 320 mg q4–6h prn; *4–6 years:* 240 mg q4–6h prn; *2–4 years:* 160 mg q4–6h prn. **Oral:** *Children 1–2 years:* 120 mg q4–6h prn; *4–12 months:* 80 mg q4–6h prn; *< 3 months:* 40 mg q4–6h prn	• Dose may be taken without regard to food. However, give with a full glass of liquid to enhance dissolution and absorption
diflunisal (Dolobid)	(Mild to moderate pain) **Oral:** 1000 mg initially, followed by 500 mg q12h	• Food slows absorption. For more rapid effect, take on empty stomach • If gastric upset occurs, give with food, milk or antacid
ibuprofen (Advil, Motrin, Rufen)	(Analgesia) **Oral:** *Adults:* 200–400 mg q4–6h (not to exceed 3200 mg/day)	• Food slows absorption. For more rapid effect, take on empty stomach • If gastric upset occurs, give with food, milk or antacid

(cont'd on next page)

Table 53.7 (continued)
The non-narcotic analgesics: Drug doses

Drug Generic Name (Trade Names)	Dosage	Nursing Alert
A. Analgesics-Antipyretics (cont'd)		
ketorolac tromethamine (Toradol)	**Oral:** 10 mg q4–6h. Doses > 40 mg/day are not recommended. Max. duration is 5 days for postsurgical pts and 7 days for pts with musculoskeletal pain	• **PO:** Give without regard to food
	IM: 10–30 mg initially, according to pain severity. Subsequent dosing may be 10–30 mg q4–6h prn to control pain. IM dosage should not exceed 2 days. Total daily IM dose should not exceed 120 mg. *For pts < 50 kg or > 65 years of age:* Initial IM dose should be 10 mg, and the total daily IM dose in elderly should not exceed 60 mg. Ketorolac is not recommended for pts with moderate to severe renal impairment	• **IM:** Store solution at room temperature with protection from light
naproxen sodium (Anaprox)	**Oral:** Initially, 550 mg followed by 275 mg q6–8h, prn. Total daily dose should not exceed 1375 mg. Alternatively, 1 550-mg DS (double-strength) tablet bid	• Food slows absorption. For more rapid effect, take on empty stomach • If gastric upset occurs, give with food, milk or antacid
B. Analgesic Products Containing Both a Narcotic and a Non-Narcotic Drug		
ASA/acetaminophen + caffeine + codeine	**Oral:** *Adults:* 1–2 tablets containing 15–30 mg codeine q4h, prn. One tablet containing 60 mg codeine q4h, prn	• May give with food, milk or antacid to minimize direct gastric irritation of ASA
ASA + oxycodone HCl (Percodan) acetaminophen + oxycodone (Percocet)	**Oral:** *Adults:* 1 tablet q6h, prn. Percodan-Demi® and Percocet-Demi® tablets: *Adults:* 1–2 tablets q6h. *Children > 12 years:* 1/2 tablet q6h; *6–12 years:* 1/4 tablet q6h. (Not indicated for children < 6 years)	• May give with food, milk or antacid to minimize direct gastric irritation of ASA
ASA + caffeine + propoxyphene HCl (Darvon Compound 65) acetaminophen + propoxyphene napsylate (Darvocet-N)	**Oral:** *Adults:* 1 capsule 3–4x daily	• May give with food, milk or antacid to minimize direct gastric irritation of ASA
ASA + caffeine + codeine + butalbital (Fiorinal-C)	**Oral:** *Adults:* 1–2 capsules containing 15 or 30 mg codeine stat, then 1 capsule q3–4h, prn	• May give with food, milk or antacid to minimize direct gastric irritation of ASA

Antiarthritic Drugs

Topics Discussed

● First-line therapy: Nonsteroidal anti-inflammatories
● Second-line therapy: Antimalarials, gold compounds, pencillamine, azathioprinc, methotrexate, adrenal corticosteroids
● For each drug discussed: Mechanism of action and pharmacologic effects, therapeutic uses, adverse effects
● Nursing management

Drugs Discussed

Viscosupplementation:
hylan G-F 20 (**hye**-lan)

First-Line Drugs: Nonsteroidal Anti-Inflammatories:
acetylsalicylic acid (ah-see-til-sal-ih-**sill**-ik)
diclofenac (dye-**kloe**-fen-ak)
etodolac (ee-**toe**-doe-lak)
fenoprofen (fen-oh-**proe**-fen)
flurbiprofen (flyoor-bih-**proe**-fen)
ibuprofen (eye-byoo-**proe**-fen)

indomethacin (in-doe-**meth**-ah-sin)
ketoprofen (kee-toe-**proe**-fen)
meclofenamate (mek-loe-**fen**-am-ate)
nabumetone (nah-**byoo**-meh-tone)
naproxen (nah-**prox**-en)
phenylbutazone (feen-il-**byoo**-tah-zone)
piroxicam (peer-**ox**-ih-kam)
sulindac (**soo**-lin-dak)
tiaprofenic acid (tye-ah-proe-**feen**-ik)
tolmetin (**tole**-met-in)

Second-Line Drugs:
adrenal corticosteroids (a-**dreen**-al kor-ti-koe-**steer**-oids)
auranofin (oh-**rane**-oh-fin)
aurothioglucose (or-oh-thye-oh-**glue**-kose)
azathioprine (az-ah-**thye**-oh-preen)
chloroquine (**klor**-oh-kwin)
gold sodium thiomalate (thye-oh-**may**-late)
hydroxychloroquine (hye-drox-ee-**klor**-oh-kwin)
methotrexate (meth-oh-**trex**-ate)
penicillamine (pen-ih-**sill**-ah-meen)

In recent years many new drugs have been introduced for the treatment of arthritis. Before discussing the pharmacotherapy of arthritis, it is important to separate first-line nonsteroidal anti-inflammatory, or symptomatic, drugs from second-line agents, such as the antimalarials, gold and penicillamine. The latter are remittive, slow acting and potentially much more toxic than the nonsteroidal anti-inflammatory drugs (NSAIDs). As a result, they are used only after NSAIDs have proven unsatisfactory.

Clinical Challenge

Consider this clinical challenge as you read through this chapter. The response to the challenge appears on page 646.

Mrs. C., age 75, has recently moved into the assisted-living apartment that you visit weekly in your role as community health nurse. She enjoyed good health until age 70, when she developed mild COPD and degenerative joint disease (osteoarthritis) of both hands, which has affected her ability to prepare meals and clean house. The distal joints of both hands are enlarged, and Mrs. C.'s ROM is limited. Currently she is taking sulindac (Clinoril®) 150 mg PO bid. Sometimes she augments her drug therapy with acetaminophen prn for joint pain and the occasional dose of ASA for headache. She was using alcohol — a daily drink before supper — for poor appetite, pain and to help her relax. She continues to have pain; on a recent visit to a local walk-in clinic, she received an order for diclofenac (Voltaren®).

What teaching/monitoring is indicated in this situation?

Before we consider the anti-inflammatory drugs, it is worth pointing out that acetaminophen — which has no anti-inflammatory action at all — is often the drug of choice for the treatment of osteoarthritis, a chronic degenerative disease characterized by variable (but often minor) degrees of inflammation. The significant analgesic relief and relative lack of serious adverse effects of acetaminophen have made it the first-line therapy for many osteoarthritic patients. The pharmacology of acetaminophen is described in Chapter 53.

Also noteworthy is a relatively new treatment for osteoarthritis of the knee, involving the intra-articular injection of hylan G-F 20 (Synvisc®). This drug is a sterile, nonpyrogenic, elastoviscous fluid containing hylans, which are derivatives of hyaluronan (the sodium salt of hyaluronic acid). Hyaluronan is the component of the synovial fluid that provides elastoviscosity. In most patients with osteoarthritis, hyaluronan is less concentrated and has a lower molecular weight. Decreasing hylauronan's molecular weight and lowering its concentration drastically reduces the elastoviscosity of the synovial fluid. Hylan G-F 20 treatment involves three injections, one week apart. This regimen, called *viscosupplementation,* replenishes hyaluronan and augments the elastoviscosity of the synovial fluid and the intercellular matrix of the tissues of the joint. For many patients with

osteoarthritis of the knee, three injections of hylan G-F 20 provide relief for several months, with minimal risk of systemic adverse effects.

First-Line Therapy: Non-Steroidal Anti-Inflammatory Drugs

The number of nonsteroidal anti-inflammatory drugs (NSAIDs) has increased dramatically in the past twenty-five years and continues to grow as researchers seek agents with increased efficacy and minimal side effects. This need is driven, in part, by an aging population. Currently, ten percent of our population is over age sixty-five, and many experience musculoskeletal disorders. As many as one in three visits to the family doctor are for complaints of acute or chronic musculoskeletal pain. Many agents, such as naproxen, tolmetin, fenoprofen, ketoprofen, flurbiprofen, diclofenac, sulindac and piroxicam, have been added to the inventory of drugs that help arthritic patients with their pain and discomfort. The term nonsteroidal is used differentiate these drugs from the corticosteroids, which are also used to alleviate inflammation in arthritis.

NSAIDs are used to treat rheumatoid arthritis,

osteoarthritis and ankylosing spondylitis, conditions marked, to a greater or lesser degree, by pain and inflammation. Drug therapy is aimed at reducing both pain and inflammation. NSAIDs are better agents for the treatment of inflammatory arthritic conditions than standard analgesics, such as acetaminophen and narcotics, which are devoid of anti-inflammatory effects.

Mechanism of Action

NSAIDs inhibit prostaglandin synthesis. To understand the significance of this action, it is essential first to discuss the role played by prostaglandins in inflammation.

Inflammation is a reaction of both blood vessels and cells to a stimulus from infecting microorganisms, physical trauma or immunological attack. In the first century CE the Roman writer Cornelius Celsus described the major signs of inflammation as *rubor et tumor cum calore et dolore* (redness and swelling with heat and pain). To these four signs Rudolph Virchow added a fifth in 1858: disturbed function. Although these signs apply to all forms of inflammation, and not solely to rheumatoid arthritis, they describe the agonies of the arthritic patient, and the processes against which therapy is aimed.

Rheumatoid arthritis is a chronic inflammatory disease of connective tissue, especially within the joints. About three percent of women and one percent of men are affected. Rheumatoid arthritis can also occur in children. It is generally believed to be caused by an antigen-antibody reaction. Whether the antigen is introduced directly into the body or formed within the body is not known. It is clear, however, that the body reacts to the presence of the antigen by producing antibodies specific to the antigen. The initial, or acute, response to the antigen-antibody reaction is vasodilatation (*rubor*), increased blood flow (*calore*) and increased vascular permeability. As a result of the increase in vascular permeability, plasma water, protein and blood cells, notably neutrophilic leukocytes and monocytes, escape into the tissues to produce a swelling (*tumor*).

How, then, are prostaglandins involved in acute inflammation? Shortly after the antigen-antibody interaction and the attempts by neutrophils to phagocytose the immune complex, two important endogenous mediators of inflammation are released into the affected tissues. These are bradykinin, formed in blood, and histamine, released from mast cells. Both chemicals dilate blood vessels, increase vascular permeability and produce pain (*dolore*). Prostaglandin E_2 (PGE_2) and prostaglandin $F_{2\alpha}$ ($PGF_{2\alpha}$) are formed from arachadonic acid in neutrophils by the enzyme cyclo-oxygenase. Released into tissues when neutrophils are destroyed in their attempt to digest the antigen-antibody complex, PGE_2 and $PGF_{2\alpha}$ increase the biological activities of both bradykinin and histamine. In the absence of normal quantities of PGE_2 and $PGF_{2\alpha}$, the abilities of histamine and bradykinin to dilate blood vessels, increase vascular permeability and produce pain are reduced.

If not resolved, the acute phase of arthritic inflammation may proceed to a chronic stage as the synovial membrane changes into a granulomatous tissue called *pannus*. The invasion of joint cartilage and subchondrial bone at the synovial attachment by pannus results in the destruction of cartilage and erosion of bone. Over time, pannus may be gradually transformed into fibrous or even osseous tissue, leading to *ankylosis* (stiffening). Because of this, it is important to reduce acute inflammation to minimize the development of chronic inflammation.

Although much will be said here of the beneficial effects of NSAIDs, it is important to recognize their limitations. They do not block all manifestations of inflammation. They neither block antibody production, nor diminish the roles played by the complement and clotting systems in inflammation. NSAIDs fail to modify the chemotactic actions of T-lymphocytes, which attract neutrophils from blood and reduce the migration of macrophages away from inflamed tissues. Finally, NSAIDs neither reduce the release of destructive lysosomal enzymes by neutrophils nor diminish the production of hydrogen peroxide (or any other toxic oxygen products) by leukocytes. Thus, it is not surprising that these drugs fail to arrest the disease process of rheumatoid arthritis or, in some cases, even to provide adequate relief of pain.

As for osteoarthritis, little is known of its etiology. It is characterized by deterioration of articular cartilage and bony outgrowths at joint margins. About five percent of people past age fifty are affected. If inflammation is present, it is usually less severe than is seen with rheumatoid arthritis. Although acetaminophen is often used to treat osteoarthritis, NSAIDs are also used.

Pharmacologic Effects

Pharmaceutical companies are quick to point out the differences between their NSAIDs and those of their competitors. However, it would be more appropriate to describe these drugs' similarities because they share most of their effects. In addition to their anti-inflammatory actions, other effects of NSAIDs that depend on their ability to block prostaglandin synthesis include:

• *analgesia:* PGE_2 and $PGF_{2\alpha}$ sensitize nerve endings to pain.
• *antipyresis:* NSAIDs lower body temperatures in a febrile patient by dilating the small vessels in the skin. This action may depend on the inhibition of PGE_2 and PGI_2 formation in the hypothalamus. Prostaglandins are necessary for pyrogen-induced fever.
• *gastric irritation:* NSAIDs can irritate the stomach locally. Following absorption, they can also damage the stomach. The latter effect is due to an inhibition of PGE_2 and PGI_2 synthesis in the gastric mucosa. PGE_2 and PGI_2 inhibit gastric acid secretion and promote the secretion of cytoprotective mucus in the intestine.
• *reduced platelet aggregation:* Some NSAIDs inhibit platelet aggregation. Thromboxane A_2, which is similar in structure to prostaglandins, is formed in platelets from arachadonic acid and promotes platelet aggregation. The inhibition of cyclooxygenase by NSAIDs reduces thromboxane A_2 synthesis.
• *decreased renal function:* PGE_2 increases the renal excretion of sodium, chloride and water. Inhibition of its formation results in salt and water reabsorption. Renal prostaglandins reduce the vasoconstriction produced by norepinephrine and angiotensin II. In patients with reduced renal function, prostaglandins are important in maintaining renal blood flow. In these patients, NSAIDs can significantly affect renal function (see Adverse Effects, below).

Therapeutic Uses

NSAIDs are first-line therapy for the treatment of rheumatoid arthritis, osteoarthritis and ankylosing spondylitis. (They can also be used to treat acute attacks of gout; see Chapter 55.) However, acetylsalicylic acid (ASA) is still the drug of first choice for many clinicians. If ASA fails to achieve the desired therapeutic effects, or produces an unacceptable degree of gastric distress, an NSAID may be given.

The newer NSAIDs constitute a major advance. These include ibuprofen (Motrin®, Rufen®), fenoprofen (Nalfon®), ketoprofen (Orudis®), naproxen (Naprosyn®), flurbiprofen (Ansaid®), tolmetin (Tolectin®), sulindac (Clinoril®), diclofenac (Voltaren®), piroxicam (Feldene®) and tiaprofenic acid (Surgam®). Many patients who were not treated effectively with the older drugs ASA, indomethacin or phenylbutazone — or who demonstrated untoward effects with these agents — have been helped by the newer compounds.

There is considerable patient-to-patient variability in response to any drug. The appropriate NSAID for any patient is the one that works on that patient at that particular time. Evidence also suggests that patients who initially respond favourably to a drug may become tolerant to it later. The variability in patient response, together with the often-encountered development of tolerance, provides some justification for the large number of drugs currently on the market. Nursing evaluation helps to establish drug efficacy and tolerance for individual patients.

NSAIDs should not be used in patients who have previously exhibited a hypersensitivity reaction (e.g., angioedema, bronchospasm) to ASA or other NSAIDS. Anaphylactoid reactions have occurred in patients with known ASA hypersensitivity. NSAIDs are also contraindicated in patients with nasal polyps.

Adverse Effects

PGE_2 synthesis in the stomach protects the gastric mucosa. Because of their ability to inhibit PGE_2 synthesis, all NSAIDs can irritate the stomach and produce peptic ulceration and gastric bleeding. This is one of the two major reasons, along with lack of effect, for switching from one drug to another. On an individual basis, one drug may cause considerable distress while another produces little discomfort.

NSAIDs can cause marked CNS toxicity, including headache, dizziness, nervousness, confusion, insomnia and drowsiness. These effects are particularly prevalent with indomethacin.

Most NSAIDs reduce platelet aggregation and adhesiveness. Their use with oral anticoagulants or heparin may cause bleeding and should be approached with caution. This interaction is definite with ASA, meclofenamate and phenylbutazone, and possible with fenoprofen, indomethacin, ketoprofen, piroxicam and choline magnesium salicylate. It is unlikely with ibuprofen, naproxen, sulindac and tolmetin.

All NSAIDs should be administered cautiously to patients at risk for reduced renal function (e.g., patients with advanced age, renal dysfunction, atherosclerosis, hepatic cirrhosis, concomitant diuretic treatment, low serum sodium, hyperkalemia and acute gouty arthritis). Prostaglandins are important in maintaining renal blood flow in these individuals. The adverse effects of NSAIDs include renal insufficiency, nephrotic syndrome with interstitial nephritis, hyperkalemia, hyponatremia and papillary necrosis.

Most NSAIDs precipitate bronchoconstriction in patients who have demonstrated ASA-induced asthma; thus, all NSAIDs are contraindicated in these patients.

NSAIDs frequently cause dermatologic reactions. Urticaria, exanthema, photosensitivity and pruritus are the most often reported reactions.

Acetylsalicylic Acid, ASA (Aspirin®)

ASA remains a first-line drug for treatment of arthritis. The direct irritation of ASA on the gastric mucosa can be reduced by the use of enteric-coated tablets or by taking the drug with meals. However, enteric-coated tablets may not completely prevent this adverse effect: once the drug is absorbed and carried back to the stomach via the bloodstream, ASA can prevent prostaglandin synthesis, thereby damaging the gastric mucosa.

High doses of ASA can saturate the capacity of the body to eliminate salicylate. When this happens, small increases in dose produce an abrupt increase in blood and tissue salicylate levels. Patients may suddenly experience salicylate poisoning. Determinations of serum salicylate levels can assist in titrating the proper dose. Anti-inflammatory therapeutic serum levels are 15–30 mg of salicylate/dL (1.1–2.2 mmol/L).

Choline magnesium trisalicylate (Trilisate®) and choline salicylate (Arthropan®) are two nonacetylated salicylates that are claimed to produce less gastric irritation than ASA. As they have not compared well against enteric-coated ASA tablets, their place in therapy should be reserved for patients who cannot tolerate ASA.

The clinically significant drug interactions for ASA are presented in Table 53.1 (page 629).

Propionic Acid Derivatives (Profens): Ibuprofen (Motrin®, Rufen®), Fenoprofen (Nalfon®), Flurbiprofen (Ansaid®), Ketoprofen (Orudis®), Naproxen (Naprosyn®), Tiaprofenic Acid (Surgam®)

The propionic acid derivatives (*profens*) differ little from one another. Naproxen has a half-life of ten to seventeen hours and may be given twice daily. All profens are appropriate for the treatment of rheumatoid arthritis and osteoarthritis. Because of interpatient variability, there appears to be little basis for arbitrarily selecting one over the others.

Among the profens, fenoprofen is most likely to produce dizziness, lightheadedness, drowsiness, headache and confusion. This drug is also more commonly associated with renal adverse effects than the other profens.

Table 54.1 lists the clinically significant drug interactions with the profens.

Table 54.1
Propionic acid derivatives (profens): Drug interactions

Drug	Interaction
ACE inhibitors	• NSAIDs can reduce the vasodilator actions of ACEIs
Anticoagulants	• Because most NSAIDs (e.g., ASA, meclofenamate, phenylbutazone) reduce platelet aggregation, they should be used only with great caution in conjunction with oral anticoagulants or heparin

Indolacetic Acids: Indomethacin (Indocid®, Indocin®), Tolmetin (Tolectin®), Sulindac (Clinoril®)

Indomethacin is an effective anti-inflammatory drug for the treatment of rheumatoid arthritis, osteoarthritis of the hip, ankylosing spondylitis, psoriatic arthritis and arthritis associated with enteropathic disease. Unfortunately, the drug often produces severe gastric distress. Indomethacin use is also associated with a high incidence of headaches, dizziness and lightheadedness, particularly in the elderly. Indomethacin capsules should be administered two to three times daily. The sustained-release product (Indocid-SR®) may be given twice daily. Indocid suppositories are usually inserted prior to retiring.

Tolmetin is indicated for the treatment of rheumatoid arthritis. Although less effective than indomethacin, tolmetin is also less irritating to the stomach. Nevertheless, it causes GI adverse effects in about thirty percent of patients.

Sulindac is an effective NSAID, indicated for the treatment of rheumatoid and osteoarthritis. It is also approved in some countries for the treatment of ankylosing spondylitis, acute painful shoulder and acute gouty arthritis. Inactive in its own right, sulindac is converted to its active sulfide metabolite within the body. The half-life of the sulfide is eighteen hours, and sulindac may be given twice daily. GI adverse effects (constipation, epigastric pain, nausea) occur in about twenty-five percent of patients.

Table 54.2 lists the clinically significant drug interactions with indomethacin.

Fenamates: Diclofenac (Voltaren®) and Meclofenamate Sodium Monohydrate (Meclomen®)

Both diclofenac and meclofenamate are effective NSAIDs for the treatment of rheumatoid arthritis and osteoarthritis. GI effects are the most frequent adverse reactions of either drug. The drug interactions for these drugs are the same as those previously described for the profens.

Piroxicam (Feldene®)

Piroxicam owes its popularity to its half-life of thirty-eight hours, enabling once-daily dosing. Some patients who previously had not been adequately treated have responded to piroxicam. However, the same statement can be made for any NSAID. Gastric distress can be severe with piroxicam, particularly if more than the recommended dose of 10–20 mg/day is used. Peptic ulceration, perforation and GI bleeding — sometimes severe, and in some instances fatal — have been reported with piroxicam therapy.

Table 54.3 lists the clinically significant drug interactions with piroxicam.

Etodolac (Lodine®, Utradol®)

Etodolac, like other NSAIDs, inhibits prostaglandin synthesis. However, the drug differs structurally from all other NSAIDs and belongs to none of the classes previously described. Etodolac is approved for acute or long-term use in the relief of signs and symptoms of rheumatoid arthritis and osteoarthritis. It is well absorbed following oral administration. The systemic availability of

---

Table 54.2
Indomethacin: Drug interactions

Drug	Interaction
ACE inhibitors	• NSAIDs can reduce the vasodilator actions of ACEIs
Diflunisal	• Diflunisal may decrease the renal clearance of indomethacin. Fatal GI hemorrhage has been associated with the combined use of these drugs
Diuretics, potassium-sparing	• Potassium-sparing diuretics, together with indomethacin, may result in hyperkalemia and nephrotoxicity
Lithium	• Indomethacin may reduce the elimination and increase the serum levels of lithium
Probenecid	• Probenecid inhibits the renal transport of indomethacin, thereby increasing its plasma levels

Table 54.3
Piroxicam: Drug interactions

Drug	Interaction
Acetylsalicylic acid	• ASA can reduce plasma concentrations of piroxicam to 80% of normal levels. Further, there is no evidence to suggest that the combination of these drugs produces greater improvement than either drug alone. Concurrent use increases likelihood of adverse effects and is not recommended
Anticoagulants, oral; sulfonylurea anti-diabetics; phenytoin	• These drugs may be displaced from their plasma protein binding sites and their effects increased by piroxicam
Lithium	• Piroxicam can decrease the elimination and increase the serum levels of lithium
NSAIDs	• Concurrent use of another NSAID with piroxicam is not recommended: there is no evidence that combined tx is better than using a single agent, and potential for adverse effects is increased

etodolac is at least eighty percent. Its contraindications, precautions, warnings, adverse effects and drug interactions are similar to those for the other NSAIDs.

Nabumetone (Relafen®)

Nabumetone is the only nonacidic NSAID and, as a result, does not directly irritate the gastric mucosa. Further, once the drug is absorbed, its active metabolite is a less potent inhibitor of prostaglandin synthesis in the stomach than other NSAIDs. For these reasons, nabumetone has fewer gastric adverse effects. Besides its anti-inflammatory action, nabumetone is also an effective analgesic and antipyretic, and is approved for acute and chronic relief of the signs and symptoms of rheumatoid arthritis and osteoarthritis.

Table 54.4 lists the clinically significant drug interactions with nabumetone.

Phenylbutazone (Butazolidin®)

Phenylbutazone is a very effective anti-inflammatory and may be used for the symptomatic treatment of acute superficial thrombophlebitis, acute attacks of gout, rheumatoid arthritis and ankylosing spondylitis. However, its toxicities include nausea, vomiting, peptic ulceration (sometimes with hemorrhage and perforation), agranulocytosis and aplastic anemia. Thus, this drug should be held in reserve until other NSAIDs have been tried unsuccessfully. Agranulocytosis occurs soon after the onset of therapy in young patients and is rarely fatal. Aplastic anemia may appear after months of therapy in older patients and has a very high mortality rate.

Table 54.5 on the next page lists the clinically significant drug interactions with phenylbutazone.

Table 54.4
Nabumetone: Drug interactions

Drug	Interaction
Chlorpropamide, sulfonylureas, tolbutamide, warfarin	• In vitro studies have shown that, because of its affinity for protein, the active metabolite of nabumetone may displace these and other plasma protein bound drugs from plasma protein binding sites. Use these drugs together with caution
Digoxin	• Monitor digoxin levels and, if necessary, adjust dosage of digoxin when administered concomitantly with nabumetone
Lithium	• NSAIDs have been reported to increase steady-state plasma lithium concentrations. Monitor lithium levels when initiating, adjusting, or discontinuing nabumetone tx

Table 54.5
Phenylbutazone: Drug interactions

Drug	Interaction
Anticoagulants, oral	• Oral anticoagulants should not be used with phenylbutazone because phenylbutazone may prolong prothrombin time
Hypoglycemic agents	• Phenylbutazone may increase the actions of insulin and oral hypoglycemics

Second-Line Drugs

Antimalarials

Chloroquine Phosphate (Aralen®) and Hydroxychloroquine Sulfate (Plaquenil Sulfate®)

Therapeutic uses. Although their mechanism of action is not understood, both chloroquine phosphate and hydroxychloroquine sulfate are used in rheumatoid arthritis, in juvenile arthritis, and for the arthritic and skin manifestations of systemic lupus erythematosus. About seventy percent of patients with rheumatoid arthritis obtain moderate relief.

Adverse effects. Although gastric intolerance may occur with either drug, the most common adverse effect is eye damage. This may involve either (1) corneal infiltration, which is reversible on discontinuation of the drug or (2) retinopathy, which can cause irreversible visual loss. The risk of retinopathy is small if doses less than 400 mg chloroquine or 250 mg hydroxychloroquine are taken daily. The importance of regular ophthalmologic monitoring must be stressed. Chloroquine or hydroxychloroquine should not be administered in the presence of retinal or visual field changes.

Gold Compounds

Aurothioglucose (Solganol®) and Sodium Aurothiomalate (Myochrysine®)

Therapeutic uses. Both the oil-based aurothioglucose and the water-based sodium aurothiomalate are injected intramuscularly. Although the mechanism of action of gold is not known, it is useful and may even alter the disease course in patients with active adult or juvenile rheumatoid arthritis or psoriatic arthritis. It may be used in patients who have failed to respond to treatment with NSAIDs, rest and physical therapy. Because of its slow onset of action (up to three or four months before possible benefit), gold should be added to a background of maintenance NSAID therapy. Treatment with gold should be instituted before irreversible changes occur in the affected joints. Unfortunately, there is no convincing evidence that gold prevents joint damage.

Adverse effects. Approximately thirty percent of patients discontinue gold therapy because of its adverse effects, the most common being skin rashes and mucous membrane lesions. Gold can also cause irreversible aplastic anemia, agranulocytosis and thrombocytopenia. Proteinuria, resulting from a membranous glomerulonephritis, is seen in 2% to 10% of patients receiving gold therapy. Patients receiving gold should undergo regular laboratory monitoring.

Gold preparations are contraindicated in the presence of renal or hepatic disease, history or presence of pernicious anemia, thrombocytopenia or other blood dyscrasias, or acute disseminated lupus erythematosus. They should also not be used in pregnancy, during lactation or in cases of diabetes mellitus, eczema, chronic dermatitis, advanced cardiovascular disease or hemorrhagic diathesis.

Auranofin (Ridaura®)

Auranofin is an oral gold preparation that appears to be as effective, and is perhaps better tolerated, than gold sodium thiomalate. Patients with rheumatoid arthritis improve within three to four months of starting therapy. The most frequent adverse effects of auranofin are GI disturbances (changes in bowel habits, loose stools, diarrhea). Like parenteral gold, auranofin can cause skin reactions. Patients may demonstrate proteinuria.

Table 54.6
Penicillamine: Drug interactions

Drug	Interaction
Antimalarial or cyto- toxic drugs, gold, oxyphenbutazone, phenylbutazone	• These drugs should not be given concomitantly with penicillamine because they are associated with similar serious hematologic and renal adverse effects

Auranofin has the same contraindications and precautions as parenteral gold. Blood dyscrasias (including leukopenia, granulocytopenia and thrombocytopenia) have all been reported with injectable gold and auranofin. These reactions may occur separately or in combination at any time during treatment. Because they have potentially serious consequences, blood dyscrasias should be constantly watched for, through monitoring of the formed elements of the blood, every two weeks for the first three months of treatment and at least monthly thereafter.

Penicillamine (Cuprimine®, Depen®)

Mechanism of action and therapeutic uses. Penicillamine may have an immunosuppressive action on T-cells. It is as effective as gold or azathioprine in the treatment of rheumatoid arthritis but of little value in ankylosing spondylitis or psoriatic arthritis. Penicillamine should be reserved for patients who have not responded adequately to treatment with NSAIDs.

Adverse effects. Skin rashes and GI disturbances are the most common adverse effects, but renal damage or bone marrow depression are the major reasons for stopping the drug. Other toxicities of penicillamine include autoimmune diseases such as systemic lupus erythematosus, myasthenia gravis, polymyositis and a syndrome similar to Goodpasture's. It can also cause painful breast engorgement in females and congenital abnormalities in infants born to patients taking the drug. Because of its potential for causing renal damage, penicillamine should not be administered to rheumatoid arthritis patients with a history or other evidence of renal insufficiency.

Table 54.6 lists the clinically significant drug interactions with penicillamine.

Azathioprine (Imuran®)

The immunosuppressant azathioprine should be used only in severe, active, progressive rheumatoid arthritis that has failed to respond to conventional treatment. It should be given together with NSAIDs; gold, antimalarials and penicillamine should be discontinued. Azathioprine can cause nausea and vomiting, leukopenia, thrombocytopenia and anemia. Complete blood counts, including platelet counts, should be performed periodically.

Table 54.7 lists the clinically significant drug interactions with azathioprine.

Methotrexate (Rheumatrex®)

Methotrexate is a competitive inhibitor of the enzyme folic acid reductase. In rheumatoid arthritis, the mechanism of action of methotrexate is

Table 54.7
Azathioprine: Drug interactions

Drug	Interaction
Allopurinol	• Allopurinol, administered concomitantly in a dose of 300–600 mg/day, will require a reduction in the dose of azathioprine to 25% to 30% of the usual dose
Bone marrow suppressants	• Use these drugs with caution together with azathioprine

unknown, but it may affect immune function. Usually, the effects of methotrexate on articular swelling tenderness in rheumatoid arthritis can be seen as early as three to six weeks.

Although the drug clearly ameliorates symptoms of inflammation, there is no evidence that it induces remission of rheumatoid arthritis. No beneficial effect has been demonstrated on bone erosions and other radiologic changes that result in impaired joint use, functional disability and deformity. Most studies of methotrexate in patients with rheumatoid arthritis are relatively short term (three to six months). Data from long-term studies indicate that an initial clinical improvement is maintained for at least two years with continued therapy.

Methotrexate should be used only by physicians whose knowledge and experience includes the use of antimetabolite therapy. The drug is indicated in the management of selected adults with severe, active or definite rheumatoid arthritis who have had an insufficient therapeutic response to, or were intolerant of, an adequate trial of first-line therapy, including full-dose NSAIDs and, usually, a trial of a least one or more disease-modifying antirheumatic drugs.

Methotrexate is contraindicated in pregnancy, blood dyscrasias, liver disease and active infectious disease; during immunization procedures; in nursing mothers; and when there is overt or laboratory evidence of immunodeficiency syndromes. The most common adverse reactions include nausea, stomatitis, GI discomfort, diarrhea, vomiting and anorexia. Clinical laboratory findings include elevation of liver enzymes and occasionally, decreased white blood cell counts. In general, the incidence and severity of side effects are considered to be dose related.

Adrenal Corticosteroids

Therapeutic uses. The pharmacology of adrenal corticosteroids and their drug dosages are presented in detail in Chapter 66. Corticosteroids may be administered systemically when more conservative measures have failed, or during the hiatus between the initiation of second-line therapy and its onset of action in a patient whose condition cannot be controlled by rest, physical measures, analgesics and NSAIDs.

Prednisone is the steroid used most frequently. Long-acting corticosteroids, such as prednisolone tebutate (Hydeltra TBA®), betamethasone sodium phosphate and acetate (Celestone Soluspan®), triamcinolone acetonide (Kenalog®), triamcinolone hexacetonide (Aristospan®) and methylprednisolone (Depo-Medrol®) may be used intra-articularly. The indications for intra-articular therapy include (1) the patient with otherwise well-controlled arthritis in whom a single joint is particularly resistant, (2) the individual in whom one or two particularly active joints are impeding ambulation or physiotherapy, or (3) the patient with one active joint, in whom NSAIDs are contraindicated.

Adverse effects. The adverse effects and drug interactions of corticosteroids are presented in Chapter 66 and Table 66.3 (page 785).

Nursing Management

Table 54.8 describes the nursing management of the patient receiving antiarthritis drugs. Dosage details of individual drugs are given in Table 54.9 (pages 648–654).

Response to Clinical Challenge

Mrs. C. may benefit from an explanation of the desired actions of each of the drugs she is using (ASA, acetaminophen and sulindac) as well as the potential interaction with alcohol. In particular, the variability in response by individuals to antiarthritic drugs and the possibility that tolerance can develop over time may explain why she is not receiving the desired pain control from her current drug therapy. The risks of polypharmacy and visiting various doctors should be reviewed. There is no research evidence to suggest that combining these agents achieves more desirable outcomes. Determining which drug is causing side effects may be difficult.

Mrs. C.'s drug therapy will be more successful if one prescriber assesses the presenting problems, orders drugs in adequate doses for a reasonable trial and discontinues drugs that are not helpful.

Table 54.8
Nursing management of the antiarthritics

Assessment of risk vs. benefit	Patient data	• These drugs are often self-administered. The nurse may contribute to drug safety through pt and community education • Drugs are also commonly used in long-term care. Older pts are at greater risk for nephrotoxicity and gastric bleeding, with a significant risk for death • *Pregnancy:* Risk category varies with drug or is unknown. Benefits may be acceptable despite risks. Given that most frequent use is in the older population, pregnancy risk may not be relevant
	Drug data	• Although generally safe, these drugs can cause significant adverse reactions. GI damage with ulceration and/or bleeding is of concern; renal toxicity can occur with long-term or high dosage
Implementation	Rights of administration	• Using the "rights" helps prevent errors of administration
	Right route	• Most drugs are given PO; except gold products, which are given IM
	Nursing therapeutics	• Approaches will depend on indication for drug use (e.g., rheumatoid arthritis occurs in young adults or children and is lifelong, vs. acute musculoskeletal injury requiring short-term use) • For management of chronic pain, comfort measures and emotional support can enhance effectiveness of drug tx, reduce required dose and provide a sense of individual control
	Patient/family teaching	• Pt's need for information may be influenced by age and indications for use (e.g., single-dose tx vs. long-term use for chronic pain) • Advise that anti-inflammatory response may require 1–4 weeks for maximum effect; thus, a reasonable trial period must be used to determine drug efficacy • Encourage pts to try nonpharmacological measures for control of pain (e.g., massage, relaxation/visualization techniques) • Pts/families should know warning signs/symptoms of possible toxicities of drugs. Report immediately: bleeding such as bruising, tarry stools; gastric distress; renal effects such as edema, elevated BP • Warn pts to avoid/limit alcohol to decrease risk of GI bleeding, hepatotoxicity • *Discuss possibility of pregnancy:* Advise pt to consult MD
Outcomes	Monitoring of progress	*Continually monitor:* • Clinical response indicating tx success (reduction in signs/ symptoms of pain, inflammation) • Signs/symptoms of adverse reactions; document and report immediately to physician • Given the use of these drugs in residential care, implement a surveillance plan for pts taking them who are unable to report side effects (e.g., those with dementia or speech impairment) • Periodic checks of hemoglobin, serum urea nitrogen, creatinine and electrolyte levels may be useful

Table 54.9
The antiarthritics: Drug doses

Drug Generic name (Trade names)	Dosage	Nursing alert
A. First-Line Therapy: Nonsteroidal Anti-Inflammatory Drugs		
acetylsalicylic acid, ASA (Aspirin)	**Oral:** *Adults:* 3.6–5.4 g/day. *Children weighing ≤ 25 kg:* Up to 120 mg/kg/day; *weighing > 25 kg:* 2.4–3.6 g/day	• Take with adequate water to ensure dissolution and absorption. Take with food, milk or antacid to reduce direct GI irritation. Do not crush/chew enteric-coated tablets; do not take enteric-coated tablets with antacids (separate by 1–2 h)
diclofenac sodium (Voltaren, Voltaren SR)	**Oral/enteric-coated tablets** (for rheumatoid arthritis): Initially, 75–150 mg/day in 3 divided doses. Dose should be reduced in maint. tx to usually 75–100 mg/day in 3 divided doses. (For osteoarthritis): Initially, 75 mg/day in 3 divided doses. Max. daily dose, 150 mg **Oral/sustained-release tablets:** Tx should be initiated and individual titration carried out using enteric-coated tabs. Pts on maint. dose of 75 mg/day can be changed to od dosage of sustained-release tabs of 75 mg, administered a.m. or p.m. Pts on maint. dose of 100 mg/day of enteric-coated tabs may be changed to od dosage of sustained-release 100-mg tabs, administered a.m. or p.m. Pts on maint. dose of 150 mg/day may be changed to bid dosage of 1 sustained-release 75-mg tab, administered a.m. and p.m. **Rectal:** 50 or 100 mg may be given as substitute for the last of the 3 oral daily doses, to a total daily dose not > 150 mg	• Take with adequate water to ensure dissolution and absorption. Take with food, milk or antacid to reduce direct GI irritation. Instruct pt not to crush enteric-coated or extended-release tablets
etodolac (Lodine, Ultradol)	**Oral:** *Adults:* 200–300 mg bid. Pts may also respond to od dose (400- or 600-mg) administered in evening	• Food may slow absorption. For rapid onset, take on empty stomach. However, if GI upset occurs, take with food, milk or antacids. Take with adequate water to ensure dissolution and absorption

Table 54.9 (continued)
The antiarthritics: Drug doses

Drug Generic name (Trade names)	Dosage	Nursing alert
A. First-Line Therapy: Nonsteroidal Anti-Inflammatory Drugs (cont'd)		
fenoprofen calcium (Nalfon)	**Oral** (rheumatoid arthritis): Initially, 600 mg 3–4x/day. Once a satisfactory response has been obtained, decrease daily dose in increments of 300 mg until minimum effective dose has been established. Max. daily dose should not exceed 3.0 g **Oral** (osteoarthritis): 300–600 mg 3–4x/day to alleviate pain and increase mobility. Adjust dose to pt's need. Only infrequently will it be necessary to increase daily dose to 2.4 g	• Food may slow absorption. For rapid onset, take on empty stomach. However, if GI upset occurs, take with food, milk or antacids. Take with adequate water to ensure dissolution and absorption
flurbiprofen (Ansaid, Froben)	**Oral:** 200 mg/day given in divided doses. Some pts may require up to 300 mg/day. Adjust dose until the min. effective maint. dose is established	• Food may slow absorption. For rapid onset, take on empty stomach. However, if GI upset occurs, take with food, milk or antacids. Take with adequate water to ensure dissolution and absorption
ibuprofen (Motrin)	**Oral:** *Adults:* Initially, 1200 mg divided into 3–4 equal doses. Depending on response, adjust dose upward or downward. Daily dosage should not exceed 2400 mg. Maint. dose will range from 800–1200 mg/day	• Food may slow absorption. For rapid onset, take on empty stomach. However, if GI upset occurs, take with food, milk or antacids. Take with adequate water to ensure dissolution and absorption
indomethacin (Indocid)	**Oral** (rheumatoid arthritis, ankylosing spondylitis): *Adults:* Initially, 25 mg bid or tid; increase by 25 or 50 mg/day at weekly intervals until a max. of 200 mg/day is reached. **Sustained-release capsules** (containing 75 mg indomethacin): 1–2x/day **Oral** (severe osteoarthritis and degenerative joint disease of the hip): *Adults:* Initially, 25 mg bid or tid. If response is not adequate, increase daily dosage by 25 mg at weekly intervals until satisfactory response is obtained or dosage of 150–200 mg/day is reached. **Rectal:** 100–200 mg (i.e., 100 mg hs and another 100 mg the following a.m.)	• Give with food, milk or antacid to reduce GI irritation. Instruct pt not to crush or chew extended-release tablets. Shake oral suspension well prior to administration

(cont'd on next page)

Table 54.9 (continued)
The antiarthritics: Drug doses

Drug Generic name (Trade names)	Dosage	Nursing alert
A. First-Line Therapy: Nonsteroidal Anti-Inflammatory Drugs (cont'd)		
ketoprofen (Orudis, Orudis SR, Oruvail)	**Oral:** 150–200 mg daily in 3–4 divided doses. Usual maint. dose, 100 mg bid. Pts on maint. dose of 200 mg/day may be changed to od dosing of Orudis SR® tablets (200 mg), given in a.m. or p.m. *Pts with impaired renal function or elderly:* Initial dose should be reduced by 1/2–1/3. Oruvail® capsules: 150 or 200 mg od, taken in a.m. or p.m. *Pts with impaired renal function or elderly:* Dosage should be reduced. Lower strength (150-mg capsule) should be used **Rectal:** One 50- or 100-mg suppository a.m. and p.m. or 1 suppository hs, supplemented as needed by divided oral doses	• Food may slow absorption. For rapid onset, take on empty stomach. However, if GI upset occurs, take with food, milk or antacids. Take with adequate water to ensure dissolution and absorption
meclofenamate (Meclomen)	**Oral** (rheumatoid arthritis and osteoarthritis): *Adults:* 200–400 mg daily in 3–4 equal doses	• Drug may be taken with meals or milk. Chewable tablets may be chewed or swallowed whole
nabumetone (Relafen)	**Oral:** *Adults:* Initially, 1000 mg daily taken as a single dose with or without food. Dosage may be increased to 1500 mg or 2000 mg/day, given either as a single dose or in 2 divided doses. Dosage adjustments should not be made more frequently than at 1-week intervals	• Give with meals or antacid to reduce direct GI irritation
naproxen (Naprosyn)	**Oral:** *Adults:* Usual total daily dose, 500 mg in divided doses. May be increased gradually to 750 or 1000 mg or decreased, depending on pt's response	• Food may slow absorption. For rapid onset, take on empty stomach. However, if GI upset occurs, take with food, milk or antacids. Take with adequate water to ensure dissolution and absorption
phenylbutazone (Butazolidin)	**Oral** (ankylosing spondylitis): *Adults:* Initially, 300–600 mg/day in 3–4 divided doses. Maint. dose should not exceed 400 mg/day. If a favourable response is not obtained, discontinue drug. If a dose of 100 or 200 mg/day controls symptoms, drug may be given for longer periods of time under careful observation. *Elderly (> 60 years):* Restrict phenylbutazone to short-term tx (max. 1 week, if possible), or avoid using	• Because of higher incidence of toxicities, use only when other drugs fail. Take with food

Table 54.9 (continued)
The antiarthritics: Drug doses

Drug Generic name (Trade names)	Dosage	Nursing alert
A. First-Line Therapy: Nonsteroidal Anti-Inflammatory Drugs (cont'd)		
piroxicam (Feldene)	**Oral** (rheumatoid arthritis and ankylosing spondylitis): Initially, 20 mg od. If desired, this dose may be given as 10 mg bid. Most pts will be maintained on 20 mg/day **Oral** (osteoarthritis): Initially, 20 mg od. If desired, this dose may be given as 10 mg bid. Usual maint. dose, 10–20 mg/day. *Elderly and debilitated pts:* Consider using lower starting dose and increasing dose only if symptoms remain uncontrolled **Rectal:** Dosage of piroxicam suppositories, when used alone, is identical with the dosage of piroxicam capsules	• **PO:** Take with food or antacids to reduce direct gastric irritation • **Rectal:** Store suppositories at room temperature. Instruct pts on correct use
sulindac (Clinoril)	**Oral** (osteoarthritis, rheumatoid arthritis, ankylosing spondylitis): 150 mg bid, with food. Dosage may be lowered or raised depending on response. Doses > 400 mg/day are not recommended **Oral** (acute painful shoulder/subacromial bursitis/supraspinatus tendinitis; acute gouty arthritis): 200 mg bid. After satisfactory response has been achieved, dosage may be reduced according to response. In acute painful shoulder, tx for 7–14 days is usually adequate. In acute gouty arthritis, tx for 7 days is usually adequate	• Food may slow absorption. For rapid onset, take on empty stomach. However, if GI upset occurs, take with food, milk or antacids. Take with adequate water to ensure dissolution and absorption
tiaprofenic acid (Surgam, Surgam SR)	**Oral/standard-release tablets** (rheumatoid arthritis): Usual initial and maint. dose, 600 mg/day in 3 divided doses. Some pts may do well on 300 mg bid. Max. daily dose, 600 mg. (Osteoarthritis): Usual initial and maint. dose, 600 mg/day in 2–3 divided doses. Max. daily dose, 600 mg **Oral/sustained-release capsules** (Surgam SR®) (rheumatoid arthritis and osteoarthritis): Initial and maint. dose, 2 sustained-release capsules of 300 mg od	• Effects of food on absorption unknown. Do not crush or chew sustained-release tablets

(cont'd on next page)

Table 54.9 (continued)
The antiarthritics: Drug doses

Drug Generic name (Trade names)	Dosage	Nursing alert
A. First-Line Therapy: Nonsteroidal Anti-Inflammatory Drugs (cont'd)		
tolmetin sodium (Tolectin)	**Oral** (rheumatoid arthritis, ankylosing spondylitis): *Adults:* Initially, 1200 mg/day in 3 doses. Individualize maint. dose to obtain min. effective dose, i.e., between 600–1800 mg/day, given tid or qid. Doses > 2000 mg/day are not recommended. (Osteoarthritis): Initially, 800–1200 mg/day, given tid or qid. Adjust upwards or downwards to achieve min. effective dose. Maint. dose usually lies between 600–1600 mg/day, given tid or qid. Doses > 1600 mg/day are not recommended *Children ≥ 2 years* (juvenile rheumatoid arthritis): Initially, 20 mg/kg/day in divided doses (tid or qid). When control has been achieved, usual doses range from 15–30 mg/kg/day. Doses > 30 mg/kg/day are not recommended	• Food may slow absorption. For rapid onset, take on empty stomach. However, if GI upset occurs, take with food, milk or antacids. Take with adequate water to ensure dissolution and absorption
B. Second-Line Antiarthritic Drugs		
1. Antimalarials		
chloroquine phosphate (Aralen)	**Oral:** *Adults:* 250 mg od with p.m. meal or hs	• Take with food
hydroxychloroquine sulfate (Plaquenil Sulfate)	**Oral:** *Adults:* 200 mg od or bid with meals (max., 6.4 mg/kg/day)	• Take with food
2. Gold Compounds		
auranofin (Ridaura)	**Oral:** Usual starting dose, 6 mg/day. This dose may be given bid (1 3-mg capsule with breakfast and 1 with evening meal) or od (2 3-mg capsules with breakfast or 2 3-mg capsules with evening meal)	• Give with food

Table 54.9 (continued)
The antiarthritics: Drug doses

Drug Generic Name (Trade Names)	Dosage	Nursing Alert

B. Second-Line Antiarthritic Drugs (cont'd)

2. Gold Compounds (cont'd)

Drug Generic Name (Trade Names)	Dosage	Nursing Alert
aurothioglucose (Solganol) sodium aurothiomalate (Myochrysine)	**IM:** *Adults* (single weekly injections): 10 mg, week 1; 25 mg, week 2; 25 or 50 mg, week 3 and each week thereafter until total dose of 800 mg to 1 g has been given. In the face of no improvement, drug may either be discontinued or increased in increments of 10 mg q1–4weeks; max. single injection, 100 mg. If pt has responded and there is no evidence of toxic effects, 25–50 mg may be given q2–3weeks, and then monthly **IM:** *Children:* 1 mg/kg weekly for 20 weeks. Continue same dose at 2- to 4-week intervals after initial 20 weeks for as long as tx appears successful and there are no signs of toxicity. No single dose should exceed 50 mg (except for the largest of adolescents)	• To facilitate withdrawal of suspension from vial, immerse in warm water bath and then shake well. Administer deep into gluteal muscle, using larger-gauge needle. Pt should remain lying for 10 min after injection
3. Penicillamine penicillamine (Cuprimine, Depen)	**Oral:** *Adults:* Initially, 125 mg–250 mg od; increase prn by 125–250 mg/day at 1- or 3-month intervals. If there is no improvement and no signs of potentially serious toxicity are seen after 2–3 months of tx with doses of 500–750 mg/day, increases of 125–250 mg/day at 2- to 3-month intervals may be continued until satisfactory remission occurs or signs of toxicity develop. If there is no discernible improvement after 3–4 months of tx with 1000–1500 mg penicillamine daily, it may be assumed pt will not respond and drug should be stopped **Oral:** *Children:* Initially, 5 mg/kg/day; increase to 10–15 mg/kg/day after 2 months if response to lower dose fails to produce desired effect	• Administer penicillamine on an empty stomach, at least 1 h ac or 2 h pc, and at least 1 h apart from any other drug, food or milk, to permit maximum absorption
4. Immunosuppressant azathioprine (Imuran)	**Oral:** *Adults:* Initially, 1 mg/kg/day (50–100 mg) as single dose or in 2 divided doses; increase prn after 6–8 weeks by 0.5 mg/kg/day at 4-week intervals to a max. of 2.5 mg/kg/day	• Give with food

(cont'd on next page)

Table 54.9 (continued)
The antiarthritics: Drug doses

Drug Generic name (Trade names)	Dosage	Nursing alert

B. Second-Line Antiarthritic Drugs (cont'd)

5. Folic Acid Reductase Inhibitor

Drug	Dosage	Nursing alert
methotrexate sodium (Rheumatrex)	**Oral:** Initially, 7.5 mg 1x/week, or divided oral doses of 2.5 mg at 12-h intervals for 3 doses given as a course 1x/week. Dose may be increased to 15 mg/week after 6 weeks in nonresponsive pts. If necessary, dosage may be gradually increased further to achieve optimal response, but ordinarily not to exceed total weekly dosage of 20 mg. Once response has been achieved, each schedule should be reduced, if possible, to lowest possible amount of drug and with longest possible rest period. Although rare, some pts may be maintained on a dose of 2.5 mg/week	• Best absorbed on empty stomach (1 h ac or 2 h pc). Remind pt that dose is weekly and not daily

6. Adrenal Corticosteroids

Refer to Table 66.5 (pages 789–792) for dosage information and nursing alerts

Further Reading

Al-Arfag A, Davis P. Osteoarthritis: current drug treatment regimens. *Drugs* 1991;41:193–201.

Drugs for pain. *Medical Letter on Drugs and Therapeutics* 1993;35:1–6.

Furst DE. Rational use of disease-modifying antirheumatic drugs. *Drugs* 1990;36:19–37.

Manson J, et al. A prospective study of aspirin use and primary prevention of cardiovascular disease in women. *JAMA* 1991;266, 521–527.

McCormack K, Brune K. Dissociation between the antinociceptive and anti-inflammatory effects of the nonsteroidal anti-inflammatory drugs: a survey of their analgesic efficacy. *Drugs* 1991;41:533–547.

Panayi SG, Roth SH. Symposium on NSAIDs: reducing the risk. *Drugs* 1990;40(suppl 5).

Strom B, et al (1993). Nonsteroidal anti-inflammatory drugs and neutropenin. *Arch Int Med* 1993; 153:2119–2124.

Antigout Drugs

Topics Discussed
- Drugs that act in the joint
- Drugs that reduce uric acid synthesis
- Drugs that increase renal excretion of uric acid (uricosurics)
- For each drug discussed: Mechanism of action, pharmacological effects, therapeutic uses, adverse effects
- Nursing management

Drugs Discussed
allopurinol (al-oh-**pure**-ih-nole)
colchicine (**kol**-chih-seen)
probenecid (proe-**ben**-eh-sid)
sulfinpyrazone (sul-fin-**peer**-ah-zone)

Clinical Challenge

Consider this clinical challenge as you read through this chapter. The response to the challenge appears on page 660.

You are a nurse practitioner in a small rural community. Brian, a 15-year-old high school student, visits the health office complaining of extreme pain in his right knee. The joint is red, swollen and extremely tender to touch; he cannot stand on the affected leg without considerable pain. Brian indicates that he injured his knee last week playing football and assumed that these sudden symptoms were related to that event. His family history reveals that his father had several attacks of gout in the foot. You take a blood sample and advise immediate rest for the joint.

1. What blood work will confirm your suspicions of gout?
2. What drugs can be ordered?
3. What major points should be included in teaching Brian about this disorder and the drug therapy?

Gout is a disorder in uric acid metabolism. The normal range for serum urate concentrations is 3–8 mg/100 mL (190–490 mmol/L). People with serum urate concentration in this range have little risk for gout. Individuals at high risk have serum urate levels of 10–11 mg/100 mL (610–675 mmol/L). In the latter group, the concentration of urate exceeds the capacity of the body fluids to hold it in solution, and sodium urate crystals may deposit in a joint. When neutrophils attempt to phagocytose the crystals, inflammation ensues and the patient experiences gout (see Figure 55.1 on the next page).

Figure 55.1
Role of monosodium urate crystals and neutrophils in gout

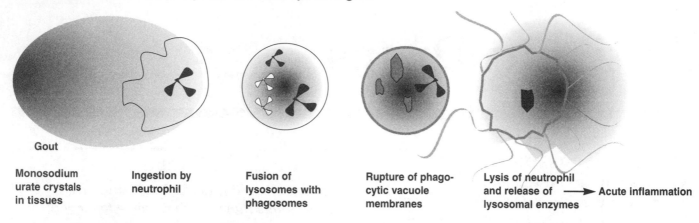

| Gout | | | | |
| Monosodium urate crystals in tissues | Ingestion by neutrophil | Fusion of lysosomes with phagosomes | Rupture of phago-cytic vacuole membranes | Lysis of neutrophil and release of lysosomal enzymes ⟶ Acute inflammation |

Source: Ryan GB, Majno G. *Inflammation, Scope Productions.* The Upjohn Company, MI, USA; 1974:54. Reproduced with permission.

Drugs for the treatment of gout can act (l) in the joint to reduce inflammation, (2) in the tissues to decrease the production of uric acid or (3) in the kidneys to increase uric acid excretion.

Drugs That Act in the Joint

Colchicine

Mechanism of action and pharmacologic effects. Sodium urate deposits in joints if its concentration in joint fluids exceeds its solubility. When neutrophils attempt to phagocytose urate crystals they are destroyed, freeing chemicals that not only cause inflammation but also attract more neutrophils from the blood. The newly arrived neutrophils in turn attempt to phagocytose the sodium urate crystals and they, too, are destroyed, freeing additional inflammatory and chemotactic chemicals. This process can repeat itself many times.

Colchicine is not an analgesic. Its ability to reduce pain is restricted to gout. Following absorption from the gastrointestinal tract, colchicine concentrates in the liver, spleen, GI tract and neutrophils. Its ability to concentrate in neutrophils may be most important because colchicine reduces inflammation by decreasing the release of chemotactic factors from neutrophils, with the result that

fewer neutrophils are subsequently attracted to the affected joint.

Therapeutic uses. In patients with gout, colchicine reduces inflammation in the affected joint(s) and can terminate an acute attack. Prompt oral treatment usually provides relief of pain and inflammation within twenty-four to forty-eight hours. Colchicine can also be given in reduced doses to prevent attacks or diminish their severity. It should be administered until all visible or radiographically demonstrated tophi are dissolved. Colchicine has an important value as an aid in the diagnosis of acute gout, since response to the drug is very specific.

During initial treatment with allopurinol or uricosurics (discussed later in this chapter), patients often experience more attacks. Colchicine can be given at this time to reduce the number of attacks.

Colchicine may not be effective in pseudogout, a condition that results from the deposition of calcium pyrophosphate dehydrate or calcium hydroxyapatite (as opposed to the deposition or urate crystals in gout) and which may present as acute chronic arthritis, particularly in elderly people. The acute inflammatory response of pseudogout

Table 55.1
Colchicine: Drug interactions

Drug	Interaction
Vitamin B$_{12}$	• Colchicine can reduce absorption of vitamin B$_{12}$

resembles gout, but usually involves the knee joint rather than the big toe. Although colchicine may not be effective in pseudogout, NSAIDs or intra-articular corticosteroid injection can resolve attacks of pseudogout.

Colchicine is contraindicated in patients with serious gastrointestinal, renal or cardiac disease. It has also produced teratogenic effects in some species of animals. Thus, if prescribed during pregnancy, or if a patient becomes pregnant while taking the drug, the woman should be told of the potential hazard to the fetus.

Adverse effects. Diarrhea, nausea, vomiting and abdominal pain often occur with the use of colchicine. If these effects occur the drug should be stopped, regardless of the condition of the joint(s). Large doses of colchicine cause a burning sensation in the throat, bloody diarrhea, hematuria, oliguria, CNS depression and death. Extravasation of intravenous colchicine results in inflammation and necrosis of the skin and soft tissues.

Table 55.1 lists the clinically significant drug interactions with colchicine.

Nonsteroidal Anti-Inflammatory Drugs

The pharmacology of nonsteroidal anti-inflammatory drugs (NSAIDs) is presented in Chapter 54. Indomethacin, phenylbutazone and oxyphenbutazone have been used for years to provide short-term treatment of acute attacks of gout. More recently, the newer NSAIDs have largely supplanted colchicine for acute attacks because of the latter's invariable tendency to produce gastrointestinal upset. To be effective for gout, however, NSAIDs should be used promptly and in optimal doses. NSAIDs are also frequently effective in treatment of pseudogout (see Therapeutic Uses under Colchicine, above).

The adverse effects, drug interactions and nursing process for these drugs are presented in Chapter 54.

Drugs That Reduce Uric Acid Synthesis
Allopurinol (Lopurin®, Zyloprim®)

Mechanism of action and pharmacologic effects. Allopurinol is rapidly absorbed from the gastrointestinal tract. Peak plasma concentrations are obtained thirty to sixty minutes after drug ingestion. Allopurinol and its major metabolite, oxypurinol, inhibit xanthine oxidase, the enzyme responsible for the synthesis of uric acid. Both plasma and urine uric acid levels fall within a few days to two weeks of starting treatment.

Therapeutic uses. Allopurinol is used to treat chronic tophaceous gout. Administered chronically, the drug inhibits the formation of tophi, mobilizes stored urates and decreases the size of tophi already formed. Because it does not depend on the kidney for its effects, allopurinol benefits patients who have already developed renal obstructions as a result of uric acid stones, or individuals with excessively high urate excretion who have not responded to uricosuric drugs. Allopurinol is contraindicated in nursing mothers and in children (except in those with hyperuricemia secondary to a malignancy).

Adverse effects. Skin rashes, gastrointestinal upset, hepatotoxicity and fever are the most common adverse effects of allopurinol. Attacks of acute gout may occur more frequently during the first months of treatment with allopurinol. The number of attacks can be kept to a minimum by administering colchicine and increasing fluid consumption to ensure adequate diuresis.

Table 55.2 on the next page lists the clinically significant drug interactions with allopurinol.

Drugs That Increase Renal Excretion of Uric Acid (Uricosurics)

Probenecid (Benemid®)

Mechanism of action and pharmacologic effects. Uric acid undergoes filtration, reabsorption and secretion in the nephron as follows:

1. Uric acid is filtered through the renal glomeruli.
2. Next, some of the filtered uric acid is reabsorbed back into the blood from the proximal convoluted tubules.
3. Finally, uric acid is secreted from the blood into the renal tubules.

Table 55.2
Allopurinol: Drug interactions

Drug	Interaction
Anticoagulants, oral	• Oral anticoagulants may have their metabolism inhibited by allopurinol
Azathioprine	• Allopurinol reduces the inactivation of azathioprine
Chlorpropamide	• Allopurinol can decrease the renal excretion and increase the hypoglycemic effects of chlorpropamide
Cyclophosphamide	• Cyclophosphamide may produce increased incidence of bone marrow depression in the presence of allopurinol
Mercaptopurine (6-MP)	• Allopurinol reduces the inactivation of mercaptopurine
Uricosurics	• Uricosurics may decrease oxypurinol excretion

Stated simply, the amount of uric acid cleared in the urine is a result of filtration + secretion − reabsorption, or (1 + 3) − 2.

Probenecid decreases uric acid reabsorption (see item 2, above). The resulting increase in uric acid excretion causes a substantial fall in plasma uric acid levels. However, even high doses of probenecid fail to prevent more than fifty percent of the filtered uric acid from being reabsorbed.

Therapeutic uses. Probenecid is indicated for the treatment of hyperuricemia in all stages of gout and gouty arthritis, except a presenting acute attack. It prevents or reduces joint changes and tophi that occur in chronic gout. Because acute attacks of gout may occur during the first months of therapy, treatment should include colchicine and an increase in fluid consumption.

Adverse effects. Probenecid's adverse effects include headache, anorexia, nausea, vomiting, urinary frequency, hypersensitivity reactions (dermatitis, pruritus and fever), sore gums, flushing, dizziness, anemia and anaphylactoid reactions. Hemolytic anemia has been reported. This may be related to a genetic glucose-6-phosphate dehydrogenase deficiency in red blood cells. Probenecid is contraindicated in patients with uric acid kidney stones. It is also contraindicated in persons with blood dyscrasias and in children under age two.

Table 55.3 lists the clinically significant drug interactions with probenecid.

Sulfinpyrazone (Anturan®)

Sulfinpyrazone is a potent uricosuric with the same mechanism of action and clinical uses as

Table 55.3
Probenecid: Drug interactions

Drug	Interaction
Acetaminophen	• Probenecid may increase peak plasma concentrations of acetaminophen
Cephalosporins	• The renal excretion of cephalosporins is inhibited by probenecid
Dapsone	• The renal excretion of dapsone may be inhibited by probenecid
Indomethacin	• The renal excretion of indomethacin may be inhibited and its plasma levels increased by probenecid
Methotrexate	• The renal excretion of methotrexate may be reduced and its plasma levels increased by probenecid.
Para-aminosalicylic acid (PAS)	• Probenecid may inhibit the renal excretion of PAS
Penicillins	• Probenecid inhibits the renal excretion of penicillins
Salicylates	• Salicylates are contraindicated because they antagonize the uricosuric action of probenecid

Table 55.4
Sulfinpyrazone: Drug interactions

Drug	Interaction
Insulin and oral hypoglycemics	• Sulfinpyrazone may potentiate the actions of insulin and oral hypoglycemics
Salicylates	• Salicylates may cause unpredictable, and at times serious, prolongation of bleeding times. In combination with sulfinpyrazone, salicylates may cause bleeding episodes
Sulfonamides	• Sulfinpyrazone may potentiate the actions of sulfonamides
Warfarin	• Sulfinpyrazone can increase the actions of warfarin

probenecid. It may be given to patients receiving maximally effective doses of probenecid for enhanced uricosuric effect. Gastric irritation is its most common adverse event.

Table 55.4 lists the clinically significant drug interactions with sulfinpyrazone.

Nursing Management

Table 55.5 describes the nursing management of the patient receiving drugs for treatment of gout. Dosage details of individual drugs are given in Table 55.6 (pages 660–661).

Table 55.5
Nursing management of antigout drugs

Assessment of risk vs. benefit	Patient data	• Assess for baseline joint involvement, signs/symptoms, mobility • *Pregnancy:* Risk category varies with drug or is unknown. Benefits may be acceptable despite risks
	Drug data	• Although generally safe, these drugs can cause allergic reactions and/or GI distress (in which cases drug must be discontinued). Action requires 24–48 h
Implementation	Rights of administration	• Using the "rights" helps prevent errors of administration
	Right route	• Usually, give PO, except colchicine, which can be given IV. NB that extravasation causes severe tissue necrosis
	Nursing therapeutics	• Comfort measures to promote pain relief in affected joint should accompany drug tx • Promote increased fluid intake (2 L/day) for better excretion of uric acid crystals
	Patient/family teaching	• Pt's need for information may be influenced by age and indications for drug use (e.g., tx for acute episode vs. long-term prophylaxis) • Advise that response may require 24–48 h • Warn pts to avoid/limit alcohol; may increase occurrence of gout. For chronic or recurrent gout, pt should try low-purine diet • *Discuss possibility of pregnancy:* Advise pt to consult physician

(cont'd on next page)

Table 55.5 (continued)
Nursing management of antigout drugs

Outcomes	Monitoring of progress	*Continually monitor:*
		• Clinical response indicating tx success (reduction in signs/symptoms of pain, inflammation)
		• Signs/symptoms of adverse reactions; document and report immediately to physician
		• Given the use of these drugs in residential care centres, implement a surveillance plan for pts who are unable to report side effects (e.g., those with dementia or impaired speech)
		• Periodic checks of hemoglobin, serum urea nitrogen, creatinine and electrolyte levels may be useful

---

Response to Clinical Challenge

1. A high serum level of uric acid suggests a diagnosis of gout.
2. Colchicine has been the drug of choice in the past; however, NSAIDs are increasingly being prescribed.
3. Brian should know that colchicine is specific for gout and will relieve the inflammation in 24–48 h. Colchicine will not immediately relieve the pain. If he has a recurrent episode, Brain should consider reducing purine in his diet. His possible use of alcohol should be explored.

Further Reading

Gout and hyperuricemia. *AMA Drug Evaluations Subscriptions* 1993; III. Immunology:1:37–1:45.

Table 55.6
The antigout drugs: Drug doses

Drug Generic name (Trade names)	Dosage	Nursing alert
A. Antigout Drugs That Act in the Joint		
colchicine	**Oral:** Start at the first warning of an acute attack. Give 1 or 1.2 mg initially, followed by subsequent 0.5- or 0.6-mg doses q2h until pain is relieved or toxic symptoms appear. Total amount usually required in course of tx may range from 4–8 mg. As interval tx, 0.5 or 0.6 mg may be taken 1–4x/week for mild or moderate case, 1–2x/day in severe cases. Dosage reduction is indicated if weakness, anorexia, nausea, vomiting or diarrhea occurs	• Give with food to reduce gastric irritation • NB dosage schedule may not be daily

Table 55.6 (continued)
The antigout drugs: Drug doses

Drug Generic name (Trade names)	Dosage	Nursing alert
B. Drugs That Reduce Uric Acid Synthesis		
allopurinol (Zyloprim)	**Oral:** Dose varies with severity of disease. Min. effective dose is 100–200 mg; average doses are 200–300 mg/day for mild gout, 400–600 mg/day for moderately severe tophaceous gout and 700–800 mg/day for severe conditions. Max. dose in pts with normal renal function is 800 mg/day. Divide total daily requirements into 1–3 doses. For daily doses ≤ 300 mg, take od pc (allopurinol is generally better tolerated if taken with food). Divided doses should not exceed 300 mg Reduce dose for pts with renal insufficiency. If CrCl = 10–20 mL/min, a daily dose of 200 mg is suitable. When CrCl < 10 mL/min, daily dosage should not exceed 100 mg. With extreme renal impairment (CrCl < 3 mL/min), interval between doses may also need to be lengthened	• Give pc. May crush tablets and mix with food
C. Uricosuric Drugs		
probenecid (Benemid)	**Oral:** *Adults:* 250 mg bid for 1 week, followed by 500 mg bid thereafter. If necessary, dose may be increased by 500-mg increments q4weeks within tolerance (and usually not > 2 g/day) if s/s of gouty arthritis are not controlled or the 24-urate excretion is not > 700 mg. Dose should be adjusted in pts with renal impairment. Probenecid may not be effective in chronic renal insufficiency, particularly when the GFR is ≤ 30 mL/min	• Take with food or antacid
sulfinpyrazone (Anturan)	**Oral:** Days 1 and 2, 100 mg bid or 200 mg od; days 3 and 4, 200 mg bid; days 5 and 6, 200 mg tid; from day 7 onward, 200 mg qid	• Take with food or antacid • Follow dosage schedule; use calendar or chart to record varying daily dose regime

Antimigraine Drugs

Topics Discussed
- Drugs to prevent migraine attacks
- Drugs to treat migraine attacks
- For each drug discussed: Mechanism of action, pharmacologic effect, therapeutic uses and adverse effects
- Nursing management

Drugs Discussed
amitriptyline (am-ee-**trip**-til-leen)
dihydroergotamine (dye-hye-droh-er-**got**-am-een)
ergotamine (er-**got**-am-een)
flunarizine (flew-**nar**-eh-zeen)
methysergide (meth-ih-**ser**-jide)
pizotyline (pih-**zot**-ih-leen)
propranolol (proe-**pran**-oh-lole)
sumatriptan (soo-ma-**trip**-tan)

Migraine headaches are associated with a dilatation of the arteries of the scalp and face. However, although migraine attacks are characterized by an abnormal reactivity of blood vessels to stimuli, vasodilatation alone cannot entirely explain the pain. Exercise and heat exposure will dilate scalp arteries without producing pain. Other factors must be involved in migraine headaches.

It is now recognized that migraine headaches are caused by dilatation of the arteries of the scalp, together with the release of 5-hydroxytryptamine (5-HT, serotonin), histamine, bradykinin, substance P and prostaglandins that sensitize pain receptors in the scalp vessel wall and adjoining tissue. Pulsation in scalp arteries, together with sensitization of pain receptors, leads to the pain of migraine.

Migraine headaches may be divided into two major groups — common migraine and classic migraine. Both types tend to be severe, characterized by a throbbing, sharp pain that is made worse by movement. *Common migraine* has a high incidence, reputedly affecting 10% to 20% of the population. In common migraine the patient may experience a prodromal period before an attack. The prodromal symptoms involve changes in mood, activity, appetite or fluid balance. The patient may experience depression, lethargy or elation, a craving for unusual food, or edema. These symptoms give way to headache pain as blood vessels in the scalp and face dilate.

Classic migraine is much rarer, occurring about one-tenth as often as common migraine. It is characterized by the presence of an aura, lasting for periods of five to thirty minutes, between the prodromal period and the headache. The aura causes visual disturbances, often characterized by the presence of bright or coloured lights, or holes in the visual field. Complex visual disturbances or hemiparesis may occur. The aura is due to pronounced vasoconstriction, with an accompanying cerebral ischemia.

Drugs are used either to prevent attacks (by inhibiting vasodilatation) or to terminate an attack (by producing analgesia or by constricting the already dilated vessels).

Clinical Challenge

Consider this clinical challenge as you read through this chapter. The response to the challenge appears on page 671.

Colleen, a 21-year-old college student, experiences frequent migraine headaches, exacerbated by certain environmental conditions. While away at school, Colleen does not have a regular family physician. She has made several trips to the Emergency Department of a nearby hospital where she has received several different treatments, including an injection of sumatriptan. Although these various drugs have produced some relief, none has been completely successful.

One evening Colleen is struck with a severe attack and a friend takes her to the city's urgent-care health centre. The nurse there notices that Colleen is wearing dark glasses, is very pale and appears stressed. She quickly moves her into a darkened room and completes an assessment. The physician orders an intranasal dose of dihydroergotamine, which is effective within 15 min.

1. Why have previous drug treatments not been successful?
2. What is the mechanism of action of dihydroergotamine?
3. What information should Colleen have before leaving the health centre?

Drugs to Prevent Migraine Attacks

Beta blockers, antidepressants, 5-HT (5-hydroxy-tryptamine, serotonin) antagonists and calcium channel blockers are used to prevent migraine headaches. The disparity in their mechanisms of action reflects our lack of understanding of the multifactorial etiology of migraine headaches and our willingness to try many types of drugs in an attempt to prevent attacks. In addition, non-steroidal anti-inflammatory drugs (NSAIDs) have been used to prevent migraine attacks.

Beta Blockers

Propranolol is the beta blocker most commonly used for migraine prevention. Other beta blockers that have shown antimigraine effectiveness include timolol (Blocadren®), atenolol (Tenormin®), nadolol (Corgard®) and metoprolol (Betaloc®, Lopresor®, Lopressor®). Because propranolol is the only beta blocker officially recommended for migraine prophylaxis in North America, it will be the only agent presented here.

Propranolol reduces the number of moderately severe migraine attacks in more than fifty percent of cases. Its clinical effectiveness does not differ markedly from that of the 5-HT antagonist pizotyline (see below). Like pizotyline, propranolol is often ineffective in patients with severe migraine.

The adverse effects of propranolol, its drug interactions and related nursing management are described in Chapters 30, 34 and 36. It is less toxic than the 5-HT antagonist methysergide (described below) and warrants a trial before patients are prescribed the latter compound.

Tricyclic Antidepressants

Tricyclic antidepressants (TCAs) can prevent migraine in some patients and may be given concurrently with other prophylactic agents. Amitriptyline (Elavil®) has been used most frequently. Its pharmacology, drug interactions and related nursing management are discussed in Chapter 46. The mechanism of amitriptyline's antimigraine action is not clear. Amitriptyline appears to be an effective prophylactic in approximately 55% to 60% of migraine patients.

5-Hydroxytryptamine Antagonists

Pizotyline, Pizotifen (Sandomigran®)

Pizotyline blocks 5-HT receptors but it is not clear whether this mechanism explains the drug's ability to prevent migraine attacks. Approximately 33% to 66% of patients respond to the drug after three to four weeks of treatment. Compared with methysergide (see below), pizotyline has fewer adverse effects. The adverse effects of pizotyline include CNS depression, which may disappear after a few days of treatment, and an increase in appetite with weight gain. Other adverse effects that occur less frequently include fatigue, nausea, dizziness, headache, confusion, edema, hypotension, depression, weakness, epigastric distress, dry mouth, nervousness, impotence and muscle pain. In normal doses pizotyline has minimal anticholinergic effects. Nevertheless, because of its anticholinergic potential, pizotyline is contraindicated in patients taking monoamine oxidase inhibitors, as well as in patients with pyloroduodenal obstruction or stenosing pyloric ulcers.

Table 56.1 lists the clinically significant drug interactions with pizotyline.

Methysergide (Sansert®)

Mechanism of action, pharmacologic effects and therapeutic uses. Like pizotyline, methysergide is also a 5-HT antagonist. It is not clear whether this action explains or is just coincidental to its ability to prevent migraine attacks.

With a 70% to 80% success rate, methysergide is more effective than most other drugs, but also more toxic. Its adverse effects have limited its use to patients who do not respond to other drugs. The useful effects of methysergide may begin within a few days or may take two to three weeks to occur. The drug is indicated in the prophylactic treatment of severe recurring vascular headaches that occur one or more times weekly, or vascular headaches that are so severe or uncontrollable that preventative therapy is indicated regardless of frequency. Methysergide has proven effective in reducing or eliminating the pain and frequency of attacks of classical migraine, common migraine and cluster headache (histaminic cephalgia).

Adverse effects. Methysergide may produce retroperitoneal fibrosis, as well as fibrosis in the pleura and heart valves. Because the risk of these adverse effects increases with the length of treatment, methysergide should not be taken continuously for longer than six months. Methysergide should be discontinued for at least one month before beginning treatment again. Other adverse effects include insomnia, nausea, vomiting, heartburn, abdominal discomfort and diarrhea. These occur more frequently than the serious adverse effects described above and can be avoided by giving the drug with food or minimized by starting treatment with small doses.

Methysergide is contraindicated in a wide range of conditions. These include peripheral vascular disease (because on rare occasions, methysergide can produce pronounced vasoconstriction), coronary artery disease, severe arteriosclerosis, moderate to severe hypertension, and valvular heart disease. The drug is also contraindicated in pulmonary or collagen disease, impaired liver or renal function, urinary tract disease, and cachectic or septic states.

Flunarizine (Sibelium®)

Mechanism of action and pharmacologic effects. Flunarizine is a calcium channel blocker. Structurally different from other commercially available calcium channel blockers, flunarizine has no direct effects on the heart. The drug selectively blocks the entry of calcium into cells when calcium is stimulated to enter cells in excess, thereby preventing cell damage caused by calcium overload in various tissues. It inhibits the contraction of

---

Table 56.1
Pizotyline: Drug interactions

Drug	Interaction
CNS depressants	•CNS depressants may potentiate the depressant effects of pizotyline on the brain

vascular smooth muscle mediated by the entry of extravascular calcium, and it protects endothelial cells against damage from calcium overload and brain cells from the effects of hypoxia.

It has been postulated that migraine pathogenesis involves an initial decrease in cerebral blood flow, leading to ischemia and hypoxia. Hypoxia causes an excessive influx of calcium into cells, resulting in cerebral cellular dysfunction. The involvement of calcium in these processes, together with the action of flunarizine to block calcium entry channels, explains the clinical effectiveness of the flunarizine.

Therapeutic effects. Flunarizine is at least as effective in preventing migraine attacks as the other drugs discussed in this chapter (i.e., beta blockers, antidepressants and 5-HT antagonists). Furthermore, it is at least as well tolerated as the other drugs, and better tolerated than methysergide. Flunarizine is most beneficial for reducing migraine frequency. It appears to have less effect on the severity and duration of attacks.

Adverse effects. Flunarizine is usually well tolerated. Its adverse effects include drowsiness, weight gain, headache, insomnia, nausea, gastric pain and dry mouth. The most serious adverse effect reported during clinical trials was depression. Long-term therapy in the elderly has produced extrapyramidal effects, which are usually reversible when the drug is stopped. Flunarizine is contraindicated in patients with a history of depression or pre-existing extrapyramidal disorders.

Nonsteroidal Anti-Inflammatory Drugs

The pharmacology of NSAIDs, together with their associated nursing process, is presented in Chapter 54. These drugs are effective both in terminating attacks (see below) and in preventing them. In one trial, naproxen (Naprosyn®) was found effective in preventing attacks in fifty-one percent of patients, compared with nineteen percent for placebo.

Drugs to Treat Migraine Attacks

Analgesics

Analgesics, such as ASA with codeine, may relieve migraine pain. They are best taken early in the attack before the pain has had an opportunity to become established. Narcotics stronger than codeine are not recommended because of the danger of dependence. NSAIDs can be quite effective in the treatment of migraine attacks. Naproxen (Naprosyn®; 825 mg at the onset and 275 mg 30 min later, prn) has been shown to be as effective as ergotamine (2 mg at the onset, with 1 mg 30 min later, prn) in relieving the pain of migraine attacks, and more effective in relieving nausea and motor symptoms.

There has been a tendency to couple analgesic use with the administration of barbiturates. The products Fiorinal® (which contains ASA and a barbiturate) and Fiorinal-C® (which also contains codeine) are popular. There is little evidence to support the contention that barbiturates increase the analgesic effects of these products. Nurses should be aware of the danger of dependence if they are used chronically. The patient's consumption of the medication should be monitored closely.

Ergotamine and Dihydroergotamine (Ergomar®, Ergostat®, Gynergen®, Medihaler-Ergotamine®, Migranal®)

Mechanism of action and pharmacologic effects. Ergotamine is a vasoconstrictor that reduces migraine-induced vasodilatation. The drug should not be used in patients with pre-existing vascular disease, such as atherosclerosis, hypertension, Raynaud's phenomenon and Buerger's disease, because its vasoconstrictor properties can lead to ischemia.

Therapeutic uses. Ergotamine is an effective drug to abort a migraine attack, and should be taken (orally or sublingually) as soon as the patient feels an attack starting. As the drug itself is not well absorbed, caffeine is often incorporated into ergotamine products to improve absorption. Since ergotamine can produce nausea, and migraine headaches also produce nausea,

Table 56.2
Ergotamine and dihydroergotamine: Drug interactions

Drug	Interaction
Alpha adrenergic drugs	• An alpha adrenergic and ergotamine should not be used together because the concomitant use of two vasoconstrictors may result in excessive peripheral vasoconstriction and hypertension
Dopamine	• Dopamine and ergotamine should not be used together because the concomitant use of two vasoconstrictors may result in excessive peripheral vasoconstriction and hypertension
Erythromycin	• If erythromycin is used concomitantly with ergotamine, it may lead to an elevated concentration of ergotamine in the plasma, thereby leading to untoward peripheral vasoconstriction

antinauseant drugs are also combined with ergotamine.

Ergotamine can be given rectally as suppositories, and this route is indicated for the nauseated or vomiting patient. The drug can also be given by inhalation from a pressurized nebulizer. Administered this way, ergotamine may be rapidly and completely absorbed. This route of administration is useful to treat patients whose severe headaches occur without warning. However, many patients have difficulty mastering the technique of inhaling the drug. Further, the opportunity to administer an overdose is great. One can sympathize with the patient who feels that if one puff is good, two will be better. However, this philosophy can lead to ergotamine toxicity because larger than recommended amounts of the drug may be taken.

Ergotamine, or its analogue dihydroergotamine, may be given by injection. This is a procedure used only in emergency departments of hospitals or physicians' offices. It is the most effective means to terminate an attack, but caution should be taken to ensure that an overdose is not given. It is anticipated that a new intranasal formulation of dihydroergotamine (Migranal®) will provide good relief, with fewer adverse effects than ergotamine. Its availability should also reduce the need for trips to emergency departments.

Adverse effects. Ergotamine's major adverse effects are generalized vasoconstriction and stimulation of the vomiting centre in the brain. Patients may experience nausea and vomiting, weakness in the legs, muscle pains in the extremities, numbness and tingling of fingers and toes, precordial distress and pain, and transient tachycardia or bradycardia.

Ergotamine is metabolized in the liver and also eliminated unchanged by the kidneys. It is contraindicated in patients with hepatic or renal disease because it may accumulate to toxic levels. Ergotamine is also contraindicated in the presence of sepsis, occlusive vascular tissues, hypertension, peptic ulcer, infectious states, malnutrition, severe pruritus, pregnancy or lactation.

Table 56.2 lists the clinically significant drug interactions with ergotamine and dihydroergotamine.

Sumatriptan Succinate (Imitrex®)

Mechanism of action and pharmacologic effects. Sumatriptan is a selective 5-hydroxytryptamine$_1$-like (5-HT$_1$-like) receptor agonist. This activity is responsible for a selective vasoconstriction within the carotid arterial circulation supplying the intracranial and extracranial tissues, such as the brain and meninges. The activation of the 5-HT$_1$-like receptors by sumatriptan suggests the possibility that the mechanism of the antimigraine action of sumatriptan could involve vasoconstriction of the dural blood vessels.

Therapeutic uses. Sumatriptan is indicated for the relief of migraine attacks with or without aura. The drug is contraindicated in patients with ischemic heart disease, angina pectoris, previous myocardial infarction and uncontrolled hypertension. Sumatriptan is also contraindicated in patients taking ergotamine-containing preparations. Until further data are available, the use of sumatriptan is contraindicated in patients with hemiplegic migraine, basilar migraine, and in patients receiving treatment with MAO inhibitors, selective 5-HT reuptake inhibitors and lithium.

Adverse effects. The most common adverse reaction associated with sumatriptan administered subcutaneously is transient pain at the site of injection. Other side effects that have been reported for both the oral and subcutaneous routes, but were more common for subcutaneous treatment, include sensations of tingling, heat, heaviness, pressure or tightness in any part of the body, chest symptoms, flushing, dizziness and feelings of weakness. Fatigue and drowsiness have been reported at slightly higher rates for the oral route, as were nausea and vomiting; the relationship of the latter adverse reactions to sumatriptan is not clear.

Nursing Management

Table 56.3 describes the nursing management of the patient receiving antimigraine drugs. Dosage details of individual drugs are given in Table 56.4 (pages 668–671).

Table 56.3
Nursing management of the antimigraine drugs

Assessment of risk vs. benefit	Patient data	• Physician should assess type and frequency of migraine attacks and determine which drug tx is recommended • *Pregnancy:* Risk varies from drug to drug; risk for each drug should be balanced against benefit
	Drug data	• Some drugs prevent migraine attacks, while others treat them. Drugs have different side effects; methysergide is probably the most toxic, particularly when used for prolonged, continuous tx
Implementation	Rights of administration	• Using the "rights" helps prevent errors of administration
	Right route	• Give IV, PO, intranasally and by inhalation
	Right technique	• Consult product information for proper administration by intranasal and inhalation routes • IV administration requires knowledge of correct diluent and IV solution, correct dilution and rate of administration. Always refer to manufacturer's instructions for this route
	Nursing therapeutics	• At least 10% of the population experience migraines, which may occur infrequently or daily. Sufferers appreciate emotional support and understanding of the disruption and disability that may be caused
	Patient/family teaching	• Differentiate between drugs to stop/treat attacks from those that are used for prophylaxis • Self-care strategies, such as keeping a diary to detect triggers for attacks, can be helpful • Instruct pt regarding techniques for intranasal or inhalation use • *Discuss possibility of pregnancy:* Advise patient to notify physician; discuss birth control methods
Outcomes	Monitoring of progress	*Continually monitor:* • Frequency and severity of migraines • Occurrence of adverse effects

Table 56.4
The antimigraine drugs: Drug doses

Drug Generic name (Trade names)	Dosage	Nursing alert
A. Drugs Used to Prevent Migraine Attacks		
1. Beta Blocker		
propranolol HCl (Inderal)	**Oral:** Initially, 40 mg bid; increase gradually prn. Usual range, 80–160 mg/day	• Take with food. Do not crush or chew extended-release preparations
2. Tricyclic Antidepressant		
amitriptyline HCl (Endep, Elavil)	**Oral:** Initially, 25 mg hs; increase prn by 25 mg q1–2weeks to 100–200 mg/day	• Take with a snack hs
3. 5-Hydroxytryptamine Antagonists		
pizotyline hydrogen maleate (Sandomigran)	**Oral:** Initially, 0.5 mg hs; increase gradually to 0.5 mg tid. Range, 1–6 mg/day	• Take with food. Store in airtight, light-resistant container
methysergide maleate (Sansert)	**Oral:** 2 mg at night; increase gradually to 2 mg tid with meals. There must be a medication-free interval of 3–4 weeks after every 6-month course of tx	• Take with food or milk. Use chart or calendar to track required drug-free interval
4. Calcium Channel Blocker		
flunarizine HCl (Sibelium)	**Oral:** *Adults:* Usual dosage, 10 mg/day administered in the evening. Pts who experience side effects may be maintained on 5 mg hs. Clinical experience indicates that onset of effect is gradual and max. benefits may not be seen before pt has completed several weeks of continuous tx. Tx therefore should not be discontinued for lack of response before adequate time has elapsed (e.g., 6–8 weeks)	• Take hs without regard to food
B. Drugs Used to Treat Migraine Attacks		
1. Ergot Alkaloids		
ergotamine tartrate (Ergomar, Ergostat, Gynergen)	**Oral** (Gynergen®): 2 mg at first sign of an attack and 1 mg q30min, prn, to a max. of 6 mg/day, 10 mg/week	• Instruct pt to use at first warning signs of headache and show how to self-administer the medication • **PO:** May give with food

Table 56.4 (continued)
The antimigraine drugs: Drug doses

Drug Generic name (Trade names)	Dosage	Nursing alert
B. Drugs Used to Treat Migraine Attacks (cont'd)		
1. Ergot Alkaloids (cont'd)		
ergotamine tartrate (Ergomar, Ergostat, Gynergen) (cont'd)	**Sublingual** (Ergomar®): Begin tx at first sign of an attack with 2 mg. Continue with 2 mg at 30-min intervals, prn. Total 24-h dosage should not exceed 6 mg, or 10 mg/weekly **Inhalation** (Medihaler-Ergotamine®): A single inhalation (0.36 mg) at the first sign of an attack, repeated in 5 min if relief is not obtained. Any additional inhalations should be spaced at intervals of not < 5 min. Not > 6 inhalations should be taken in any 24-h period, and drug is not to be used more frequently than 5 consecutive days in a 7-day period	• **Sublingual:** Do not eat, drink or smoke while holding drug in mouth
dihydroergotamine mesylate (Migranal)	**IM** (for acute migraine attack): 1 mg at first warning sign of headache, repeated at 30-min to 1-h intervals, prn, to a total of 3 mg/attack **IV** (for cluster headache [Horton's syndrome]): 0.5 mg by slow injection. Max. weekly dose, 6 mg **Intranasal** (Migranal®): At first s/s of an attack, 1 spray (0.5 mg) should be administered to each nostril; if necessary, 15 min later, an additional spray (0.5 mg) should be administered to each nostril, for a total dosage of 4 sprays (2.0 mg). Clinical response begins approximately 30 min following administration. No more than 4 sprays (2.0 mg) should be administered for any single migraine headache. No more than 8 sprays (4.0 mg) should be administered during any 24-h period. Max. weekly dosage, 24 sprays (12.0 mg)	• **IV:** Follow agency policy • **Intranasal:** Prior to administration, pump must be primed (squeeze 4 times). Once applicator has been prepared, it should be discarded, with any remaining drug, after 24 h
ergotamine + caffeine (Cafergot)	**Oral:** *Adults:* 2 tablets initially; if necessary, 1 tablet q30min. Max., 6 tablets/day, 10 tablets/week. *Children 6 to 12 years:* Initially, 1 tablet; additional doses of 1 tablet may be given 2x only. Max., 3 tablets/day, 5 tablets/week. Must not be administered prophylactically to adults or to children	• May be taken with food, if pt is not experiencing nausea due to migraine

(cont'd on next page)

Table 56.4 (continued)
The antimigraine drugs: Drug doses

Drug Generic name (Trade names)	Dosage	Nursing alert
B. Drugs Used to Treat Migraine Attacks (cont'd)		
1. Ergot Alkaloids (cont'd)		
ergotamine + caffeine + belladonna + pentobarbital (Cafergot-PB, Bellergal Spacetabs)	**Oral** (Cafergot-PB® tablets): *Adults:* As for Cafergot® tablets.(Bellergal® tablets): *Adults:* 3 or 4 tablets daily; in more resistant cases, dosage may be increased to 6 tablets daily (max. dose), reducing dosage gradually after some days to lowest effective dose. Max., 33 tablets/week. (Bellergal Spacetabs®): 1 in a.m., 1 in p.m. Max., 16 tablets/week **Rectal** (Cafergot-PB® suppositories): *Adults:* 1 suppository initially; repeat in 1 h, prn. Max., 3/day; 5/week. *Children 6–12 years:* Initially, 1/2 suppository; additional doses of 1/2 suppository may be given 2x only, prn, in the course of an attack. Max., 1.5 suppositories/ attack or per day; 2.5 suppositories/week	• Do not substitute different formulations (e.g., Cafergot-PB® contains a barbiturate, while Cafergot® does not)
ergotamine + caffeine + belladonna (Wigraine)	**Oral/Rectal:** 1–2 tablets or suppositories at first sign of an attack, followed by 1–2 tablets or suppositories q20–30min until pain subsides. Max., 6 tablets or suppositories per attack (12 tablets or suppositories per week)	• Do not substitute different formulations (e.g., Cafergot® or Cafergot-PB® for Wigraine)
2. 5-Hydroxytryptamine$_1$ Agonist		
sumatriptan succinate (Imitrex)	Indicated only for intermittent tx of migraine headache with or without aura; should not be used prophylactically. Sumatriptan may be given PO or SC. Clinical response begins 10–15 min following SC injection and 30 min following oral administration. Further doses should not be taken if pt shows no response to initial tx of single attack. Should not be taken within 24 h following administration of any ergotamine-containing preparation. Conversely, ergotamine-containing preparations should not be taken < 6 h following sumatriptan administration	

Table 56.4 (continued)
The antimigraine drugs: Drug doses

Drug Generic name (Trade names)	Dosage	Nursing alert

B. Drugs Used to Treat Migraine Attacks (cont'd)

2. 5-Hydroxytryptamine₁ Agonist (cont'd)

sumatriptan succinate (Imitrex) (cont'd)	**Oral:** *Adults:* 100 mg. Pts who have had a successful response (i.e., no pain or mild pain) may treat a later recurrence of headache with an additional 100-mg dose. Not > 300 mg should be taken in any 24-h period. *Hepatic impairment:* A 50-mg dose (single tablet) may be considered since plasma sumatriptan concentrations up to 2x those seen in healthy subjects have been observed in pts with mild to moderate impairment following a 50-mg oral dose	
	SC: *Adults:* A single 6-mg injection. Pts who have had a successful response (i.e., no pain or mild pain) may treat a later recurrence of headache with one additional 6-mg dose, provided 1 h has elapsed since first dose. Max. dose in 24 h: 2 6-mg injections	• Instruct pt in use of auto injector (prefilled syringe for SC self-administration)

Response to Clinical Challenge

1. Treatment and prevention of migraine headaches are achieved through the use of several different agents: response to both the therapeutic actions and the occurrence of side effects varies among individuals. Successful treatment may depend on trial of different drugs.
2. Dihydroegotamine produces vasoconstriction, which is thought to relieve the migraine-related vasodilation.
3. Colleen should know:
• how to administer the drug intranasally
• the drug's expected actions and side effects
• how often she can repeat a dose
• the importance of taking the drug early in the course of the migraine to stop the attack.

Further Reading

Andersson KE, Vinge E. β-Adrenoreceptor blockers and calcium antagonists in the prophylaxis and treatment of migraine. *Drugs* 1990;39:355–373.
Jacob B. Emergent neurologic events. *Crit Care Clin North Am* 1995;7(3):427–444.
Lipton R, et al. Headaches in the elderly. *J Pain Symptom Management* 1993;8(2):87–97.
Silberstein S. Migraine and women: the link between headache and hormones. *Postgraduate Medicine* 1995;97(4):147–153.

Local Anesthetics

Topics Discussed
● Local anesthetics (esters and amides):
Mechanism of action and pharmacologic
effects, pharmacokinetics, therapeutic
uses, adverse effects
● Common local anesthetics
● Nursing management

Drugs Discussed
bupivacaine (byoo-**piv**-eh-kane)
cocaine (koe-**kane**)
lidocaine (**lye**-doe-kane)
mepivacaine (meh-**piv**-eh-kane)
procaine (**proe**-kane)
tetracaine (**tet**-rah-kane)

Clinical Challenge

*Consider this clinical challenge as you read through this chapter. The response to the challenge
appears on page 676.*

You are working on an obstetrics unit where epidural anesthetics are used.
What observations should be made during administration?

Local anesthetics are used to block pain sensation from discrete areas of the body. They either anesthetize nerve endings or prevent the subsequent conduction of impulses in the peripheral nerves leading to the brain. Local anesthetics prevent the nerve action potential from reaching the threshold necessary for the electrical transmission of impulses.

Mechanism of Action and Pharmacologic Effects

To understand how local anesthetics work, we must briefly review how nerves carry impulses.

Impulses are transmitted by successive depolarizations of the neuronal membrane. Depolarization depends on the flux of potassium and sodium across the membrane. In the resting state, the neuronal membrane is largely impermeable to sodium. As a result, sodium concentrations outside the nerve are much higher than inside. By way of

contrast, potassium is concentrated inside the nerve. When a nerve is stimulated and a wave of depolarization sweeps along it, the neuronal membrane becomes permeable to sodium and sodium enters the nerve. At the same time, potassium leaves. These ion changes are essential if a nerve is to transmit an impulse. Subsequently, the nerve repolarizes by pumping sodium out, allowing potassium to re-enter. It is then ready to accept the next impulse.

Local anesthetics exist in solution in the body in both the ionized and nonionized forms. The latter, being more lipid soluble, penetrate the nerve membrane. Once inside the nerve some of the molecules ionize, attach to the nerve membrane, and interfere with neuronal ion transport. They block nerve conduction by decreasing or preventing the large transient increase in the permeability of the membrane to sodium ions.

Figure 57.1 shows the effects of a local anesthetic on the intracellular nerve action potential.

Figure 57.1
Intracellular nerve action potential prior to and following exposure to lidocaine

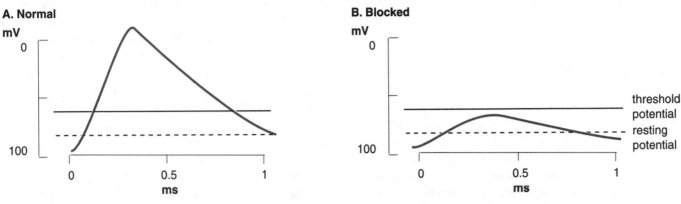

Source: Attia RR, Grogono AW. *Practical Anesthetic Pharmacology.* New York: Appleton-Century-Crofts; 1978. Reproduced with permission.

Pharmacokinetics

Local anesthetics are either applied to the surface of a mucous membrane or injected in the vicinity of the nerve(s) to be blocked. The extent of the nerve block produced depends on the drug's ability to penetrate the nerve and to block the transmission of impulses along the cell membrane. The duration of activity of a local anesthetic is determined by the speed at which it diffuses away from the nerve and is absorbed by the blood.

Most local anesthetic solutions are prepared in at least two concentrations. They are also supplied with and without epinephrine. For example, procaine hydrochloride can be found in 1% and 2% solutions, with and without epinephrine. The higher concentration produces neuronal blockade for a longer period of time. It may also block more neurons. In light of these comments, it might seem reasonable to use the higher concentration each time. However, this is not true. The higher concentration is more likely to produce adverse effects and may not be required. For example, smaller nerves have larger surface areas relative to their size and may be blocked by lower concentrations of a local anesthetic. Furthermore, nonmyelinated nerves are more readily paralyzed than myelinated neurons. Finally, nerves lying near the outside of a nerve bundle are blocked more easily than those inside. In each of these situations in which a block of a small nerve, a nonmyelinated neuron or nerves near the outside of a bundle may be required, it may be possible to use the lower concentration of the anesthetic.

Epinephrine is added to ensure that the local anesthetic stays local. Once the anesthetic leaves the site of administration, it loses its value to the patient. Large quantities of a local anesthetic entering the general circulation can produce systemic toxicity. Therefore, epinephrine is often added as a vasoconstrictor to prevent rapid absorption and ensure a longer duration of action.

There are situations when epinephrine is contraindicated. It can prove catastrophic if injected into a finger, toe, ear or nose, as the reduction in blood flow to these areas can produce gangrene. Imagine the consequences of using a local anesthetic containing epinephrine to produce a ring block prior to performing a circumcision.

Once absorbed, epinephrine may produce systemic effects. For example, the cardiac palpitations encountered in a dentist's chair are not always due to the stark terror of the moment. They can also result from absorption of the epinephrine in the local anesthetic solution.

Following their absorption, local anesthetics are metabolized. The local anesthetic esters procaine, chloroprocaine, tetracaine and cocaine are rapidly destroyed by cholinesterase in plasma. Ten to twelve percent of a cocaine dose is excreted unchanged.

The local anesthetic amides bupivacaine, etidocaine, lidocaine, mepivacaine and prilocaine are inactivated by hepatic mixed-function oxidases. They have considerably longer half-lives than the esters, ranging from 96 min for lidocaine to 210 min for bupivacaine. The longer half-lives of the amides is a problem only if, as a result of an overdose or inadvertent intravenous administration, significant amounts reach the systemic circulation. Used properly, local anesthetics are absorbed slowly, and differences in rates of metabolism have no clinical significance.

Therapeutic Uses

Topical anesthesia involves the application of a local anesthetic to mucous membranes for the purpose of anesthetizing the surface areas of the nose, mouth, throat, esophagus, tracheobronchial tree and genitourinary tree. Cocaine, tetracaine and lidocaine are used most often. Procaine and mepivacaine are not effective because they do not penetrate mucous membranes. The choice of drug depends on the site to be anesthetized. Cocaine can be used for the ear, nose and throat, but not the urethra, rectum or skin. Tetracaine is recommended for all sites except the urethra. Benzocaine can be used for the ear, nose, throat, urethra, rectum and skin, but not the eye.

Infiltration anesthesia is the injection of a local anesthetic directly into the tissues concerned. Epinephrine approximately doubles the duration of anesthesia. Lidocaine is used most frequently. Infiltration anesthesia offers the advantage of good anesthesia while maintaining normal physiological function. Unfortunately, it requires relatively large amounts of anesthetic and is appropriate only for minor surgery.

Nerve block anesthesia is used for larger areas of the body and is produced when a local anesthetic is injected in the vicinity of peripheral nerves or nerve plexuses. Nonmyelinated nerve pain fibres are blocked before myelinated motor neurons, making it possible to block pain without decreasing movement.

Intravenous regional anesthesia involves the injection of a local anesthetic, without a vasoconstrictor or preservatives, into a vein of a previously exsanguinated limb for operations of the elbow or areas distal to it. It may also be used to anesthetize the foot, but is not suitable for the entire leg because of the large amount of local anesthetic required. When the operation is finished, the tourniquet is released. If the tourniquet has been inflated for at least fifteen minutes, only 15% to 30% of the original local anesthetic flows into the general circulation.

Spinal anesthesia is a safe and effective method for operations on the lower abdomen, extremities and perineum. It is produced when a local anesthetic is injected into the subarachnoid space usually between the second and fifth lumbar vertebrae. The major factors controlling the level of anesthesia are (1) site of injection, (2) specific gravity and volume of solution, (3) position of the patient and (4) volume of the spinal subarachnoid space. Isobaric, hyperbaric or hypobaric solutions may be injected, depending largely on the administrator's personal preference. The level of block can be kept low in the distal subarachnoid space by making the solution hypertonic with glucose and sitting the patient in a head-up position. Duration of anesthesia depends on the rate of drug absorption into blood. This can be reduced by adding epinephrine to the solution. Spinal anesthesia produces sympathetic denervation, causing a fall in peripheral resistance, venous return, cardiac output and blood pressure. Venous return can be guaranteed if sympathetically blocked areas are elevated above the level of the right atrium.

The uses for spinal anesthesia include caesarean sections, where it is a frequent choice. Onset of action is rapid and hypotension is common, if measures are not taken to prevent this (i.e., prophylactic volume loading and use of a vasopressor).

Epidural anesthesia is accomplished when a local anesthetic is injected into the epidural space. The anesthetic diffuses into the subarachnoid space, where it acts like a spinal anesthetic, and outside the spinal cord into the paravertebral area, where it produces multiple paravertebral blocks. Epidural anesthesia is usually subdivided into thoracic epidural, lumbar epidural and caudal epidural. Thoracic epidural anesthesia is useful in surgical procedures involving the thorax or upper abdomen. Lumbar epidural anesthesia is the most frequently employed and is useful in obstetrics and for surgical procedures involving the lower abdomen. Caudal anesthesia is usually reserved for interventions on the pelvis and perineum and for vaginal deliveries.

Epidural anesthesia is frequently used for women in labour, and it now sets the standard for pain relief. It requires skilled and experienced personnel for safe institution and management, with the aim of blocking T11 and T12 during the first stage of labour, and in addition S2 to S4 in the second stage. Epidural analgesia is particularly indicated in patients with preeclampsia.

Adverse Effects

Local anesthetics can stimulate the central nervous system. Generally, the more potent local anesthetics are more likely to produce restlessness, tremors and, if the concentration is sufficiently high, clonic convulsions. The sequel to central stimulation is depression and death as a result of respiratory failure.

Local anesthetics are potent myocardial depressants. If present in adequate concentrations they decrease electrical excitability, conduction rate and force of contraction. In the case of lidocaine, these properties are used to make the drug a very valuable agent for the treatment of ventricular arrhythmias (see Chapter 33). However, one should not confuse the deliberate, controlled use of lidocaine for this purpose with the consequences of inadvertently confronting the heart with large amounts of the drug. In the latter situation, patients experience bradycardia, hypotension and heart block, which can progress to cardiac and respiratory arrest. The cardiovascular symptoms usually begin after the signs of CNS intoxication.

Hypersensitivity reactions may occur following the use of local anesthetics. They appear as allergic dermatitis, asthma or fatal anaphylaxis. Hypersensitivity is seen mainly with the esters benzocaine, cocaine, procaine and tetracaine. Individuals allergic to one ester are usually allergic to the others. These patients should receive one of the amides.

Common Local Anesthetics

Cocaine is too toxic to be injected but provides excellent surface anesthesia when applied topically. It has good vasoconstrictor potency and promotes the shrinking of mucous membranes. Cocaine should not be used in the genitourinary areas because it is absorbed too quickly. Solutions range from 1% to 10%.

Procaine (Novocain®) was the standard local anesthetic against which all others were compared. It has been replaced by lidocaine in this regard. Procaine penetrates mucous membranes poorly and should not be used for topical anesthesia. When procaine is injected, anesthesia begins quickly. Depending on the concentration used or the presence of a vasoconstrictor, the duration of anesthesia can last for an hour or longer.

Tetracaine (Pontocaine®) is also a local anesthetic ester. Its onset of action (ten minutes or more) and duration of action are longer than procaine's. For injection purposes, the drug is available in 0.3% solution. Topically, it works well in concentrations of 0.5% to 2%.

Lidocaine (Xylocaine®) is more potent and versatile than procaine and can be used for infiltration and nerve block anesthesia, as well as topical anesthesia. It is prepared in concentrations ranging from 0.5% to 2%. Lidocaine is an amide and may be used in patients who are hypersensitive to local anesthetic esters.

Mepivacaine (Carbocaine®) is an amide with essentially the same properties as lidocaine, with the exception that it has poor activity when used topically, and a longer duration of action when injected.

Bupivacaine (Marcaine®) is another amide. Its properties are similar to those of the other drugs. Bupivacaine is used for infiltration, nerve block and peridural anesthesia. It is more potent and longer acting than mepivicaine. Bupivacaine is available in injection solutions of 0.25%, 0.5% and 0.75%.

Dibucaine (Nupercaine®) is a very potent amide with a long duration of action. The concentrations available for injection usually range from 0.05% to 0.1%. Dibucaine is also used often for topical anesthesia.

Table 57.1 on the next page lists the clinically significant drug interactions with local anesthetic esters while Table 57.2 lists those with local anesthetic amides.

Nursing Management

Table 57.3 (page 677) describes the nursing management of the patient receiving local anesthetic drugs. Dosage details of individual drugs are given in Table 57.4 (pages 677–678).

Table 57.1
Local anesthetic esters: Drug interactions

Drug	Interaction
Beta blockers	• Propranolol, and possibly other beta blockers, potentiates cocaine-induced coronary vasoconstriction (potentiation of alpha adrenergic effects of cocaine). Avoid concurrent use
Echothiophate iodide	• When used for prolonged periods in the eye, echothiophate iodide reduces pseudocholinesterase activity, resulting in reduced rate of inactivation of local anesthetic esters, e.g., procaine and tetracaine
Guanethidine, MAOIs, TCAs	• All these drugs potentiate the vasoconstrictor effects of cocaine. In addition, TCAs and MAOIs increase the activity of epinephrine. Local anesthetic solutions containing epinephrine should be used with caution, if at all, in pts receiving TCAs or MAOIs

Table 57.2
Local anesthetic amides: Drug interactions

Drug	Interaction
Beta blockers	• Propranolol, metoprolol and possibly other beta blockers decrease the metabolism and increase the toxicity of lidocaine. Monitor lidocaine concentrations
Cimetidine	• Cimetidine can possibly decrease the metabolism and increase the toxicity of IV or epidural lidocaine. Decrease infusion rate and monitor lidocaine concentrations
Phenytoin	• IV administration of phenytoin, together with IV lidocaine, can produce excessive cardiac depression
Ranitidine	• Ranitidine may decrease bupivacaine metabolism and increase its toxicity. Monitor clinical status
TCAs and MAOIs	• TCAs and MAOIs increase the activity of epinephrine. Local anesthetic solutions containing epinephrine should be used with caution, if at all, in pts receiving TCAs or MAOIs
Verapamil	• Verapamil and epidural bupivacaine can produce severe hypotension and bradycardia

Response to Clinical Challenge

The main observations of the woman in labour would include:
• vital signs, including pulse rate and rhythm
• symptoms such as nervousness, dizziness, blurred vision
• signs such as tremors or drowsiness, which suggest CNS effects that can progress to respiratory distress or convulsions.

Routine assessment of the baby would also be important (heart rate and rhythm). At birth, observation of respiratory rate and depth are essential.

Further Reading

Sectish T. Use of sedation and local anesthetic to prepare children for procedures. *Am Fam Phys* 1997;55(3):909–916.

Sklar D. Local anesthetics. *Ann Emerg Med* 1996; 27(4):464–465.

Thorp J, Breedlove G. Epidural analgesia in labor: an evaluation of risks and benefits. *Birth Issues in Perinatal Care and Education* 1996;23(2):63–83.

Table 57.3
Nursing management of the local anesthetics

Assessment of risk vs. benefit	Patient data	• Usually, selection and administration of local anesthetics is the responsibility of the physician, dentist or anesthetist • Assess to establish baseline VS, general state of health. Monitor fetal heart tones when drug is used in delivery • *Pregnancy:* Risk category B (animal studies may or may not show risk; if risk has been shown in animals, none has been shown in human studies)
	Drug data	• Select drugs based on desired onset and duration of action, site of action and pt hx
Implementation	Rights of administration	• Using the "rights" helps prevent errors of administration
	Right route	• May be applied topically or by injection
	Right time	• See Table 57.4. NB variation in dosage schedules among drugs in this class
	Right technique	• Check agency policy regarding certification program
Outcomes	Monitoring of progress	*Continually monitor:* • Clinical response indicating tx success • Signs/symptoms of adverse reactions; esp. monitor central nervous and cardiovascular systems. Report immediately to physician • Local tissue irritation and generalized allergic reactions (rash, urticaria, edema or anaphylaxis)

Table 57.4
The local anesthetics: Drug doses

Drug Generic name (Trade names)	Dosage	Nursing alert
A. Local Anesthetic Esters		
cocaine HCl	**Topical:** For ENT/bronchoscopy, 4% cocaine HCl. For corneal anesthesia, 0.25-0.5% solution	• Follow agency policy re: certification for administration of local anesthesia
procaine HCl (Novocain)	**Infiltration:** Up to 100 mL of 0.25% or 0.5% solution with or without epinephrine. **Nerve block:** Up to 50 mL of 1% or 25 mL of 2% solution with or without epinephrine	• Ensure that correct solution is chosen (with or without epinephrine). Do not substitute

(cont'd on next page)

Table 57.4 (continued)
The local anesthetics: Drug doses

Drug Generic name (Trade names)	Dosage	Nursing alert
A. Local Anesthetic Esters (cont'd)		
tetracaine HCl (Pontocaine)	**Subarachnoid:** Dilute 1% solution with equal volume of 10% dextrose. For obstetric saddle block, 2–4 mg. For lower extremities and perineal operations, 3–6 mg. For most caesareans and lower abdominal surgery, 9–12 mg. For upper abdominal surgery, 12–15 mg	• Follow agency policy re: certification for administration. Calculate and prepare solution carefully; supplied in 20-mg ampoule
B. Local Anesthetic Amides		
bupivacaine HCl (Marcaine, Sensorcaine)	**Solution** (caudal/epidural/peripheral nerve block): For incomplete motor block, 0.25%. Motor block but incomplete muscular relaxation, 0.5%. Complete motor block, 0.75%. For detailed dosage, consult product literature	• Read label carefully. Supplied in varying strengths (0.25%, 0.5%, 0.75%) with or without epinephrine • Follow agency policy re: certification for administration
lidocaine HCl (Xylocaine)	**Infiltration/IV** (regional nerve block, epidural, spinal and topical anesthesia): See product literature for various formulations available and recommended dosages	• Follow agency policy re: certification for drug administration. Use infusion pump to ensure accuracy
mepivacaine HCl (Carbocaine)	**Nerve block:** 5–20 mL of 1% or 1.5%. **Epidural block:** 15–25 mL of 1%. **Infiltration:** Up to 40 mL of 1% solution.	• Follow agency policy re: certification for drug administration. Read label carefully; may or may not contain preservative

General Anesthetics

Topics Discussed
- Inhalation Anesthetics
- Intravenous Anesthetics
- For each drug discussed: Mechanism of action, pharmacologic effects, therapeutic uses, adverse effects
- Nursing management

Drugs Discussed

Inhalation Anesthetics:
enflurane (**en**-flyoor-ayne)
ether (**ee**-thur)
halothane (**hal**-oh-thayne)
isoflurane (eye-soe-**flyoor**-ayne)
methoxyflurane (meth-ox-ee-**flyoor**-ayne)
nitrous oxide (**nye**-truss **ox**-eyed)

Intravenous Anesthetics:
alfentanil (al-**fen**-tah-nil)
diazepam (dye-**az**-eh-pam)
droperidol (droe-**per**-ih-dole)
fentanyl (**fen**-tah-nil)
ketamine (**ket**-ah-meen)
methohexital (meth-oh-**hex**-ih-tal)
midazolam (mid-**ay**-zoe-lam)
propofol (**proe**-poe-fol)
remifentanil (rem-ee-**fen**-tah-nil)
sufentanil (soo-**fen**-tah-nil)
thiamylal (thye-**am**-il-lawl)
thiopental (thye-oh-**pen**-tal)

Clinical Challenge

Consider this clinical challenge as you read through this chapter. The response to the challenge appears on page 690.

You are working in an operating room where many patients receive inhalation anesthetics. Consider the occupational health risks related to exposure to these agents. You might ask:

1. Does the site have a scavenging system to remove the gas?
2. What is the mean exposure of gas for those working in the operating theatres?
3. What reproductive health risks might be related to continued exposure to nitrous oxide?

Anesthesia is the loss of sensation. General anesthesia is a state of unconsciousness with the absence of pain. General anesthetics produce, in varying degrees, the following effects:

• amnesia;
• loss of consciousness;
• analgesia;
• loss of reflexes; and
• muscle relaxation.

General anesthesia is usually produced by the inhalation or intravenous administration of drugs. This chapter discusses these drugs.

Inhalation Anesthetics

Mechanism of Action and Pharmacologic Effects

Inhalation anesthetics depress CNS function, beginning with the cerebral cortex and moving down the central nervous system (with increasing concentrations) to inhibit the basal ganglia, cerebellum, spinal cord and medulla oblongata, in that order. It is fortunate that spinal function is affected before medullary activity because this allows the anesthetic to paralyze both the sensory and motor functions of the cord before it stops respiration. Complete CNS paralysis is apparent when the respiratory and cardiovascular centres in the medulla oblongata are completely depressed. Although many theories have been advanced to explain the means by which inhalation anesthetics work, their exact mechanism of action is not known.

Two factors control the degree of CNS depression: the concentration of the drug and its intrinsic activity. The latter is expressed as the *minimal alveolar concentration* (MAC) necessary to prevent movement in fifty percent of individuals subjected to a painful stimulus.

Pharmacokinetics

The pharmacokinetics of inhalation anesthetics is complex. The induction of anesthesia involves the following steps:

1. inhalation of the anesthetic and mixing it with gas already present in alveoli;
2. diffusion of the anesthetic into the pulmonary circulation;
3. transport of the anesthetic in blood throughout the body; and
4. diffusion of the anesthetic from blood into brain.

Inhalation anesthetics are administered as gases. They exist under pressure in the gas machine, lungs and blood. Although these points may seem obvious, they bear mentioning because this chapter is the first to discuss gaseous drugs.

Once absorbed through alveoli, anesthetics are held in solution in the blood under pressure. The partial pressure of an anesthetic determines the rate at which it leaves the blood and enters the brain. The higher the partial pressure of the gas in blood, the greater the force pushing it into the brain. For its part, the partial pressure of the gas is determined by its concentration and solubility in blood. Gases with poor solubility in blood attain high partial pressures rapidly and are forced into the brain quickly.

From the preceding discussion, it is logical to conclude that anesthetic gases differ in their blood solubility. This is true. The importance of blood solubility to the onset and duration of action of an anesthetic can be illustrated by referring to two agents that differ markedly in this regard. Nitrous oxide is poorly soluble in blood. As a result, when nitrous oxide is inhaled and passes from alveoli into blood, its partial pressure increases rapidly, reflecting the inability of blood to dissolve and hold large amounts of the gas. The high partial pressure of the gas in blood quickly drives the anesthetic into the brain, giving the drug a rapid onset of action.

By contrast, ether is very soluble in blood. When ether is inhaled, its partial pressure rises very slowly. Keeping in mind that it is the partial pressure of the gas in blood that drives the anesthetic into the brain, the reader can readily understand why ether enters the brain slowly. Thus, induction of anesthesia with ether proceeds over a longer period of time. Most gaseous anesthetics have blood solubilities and partial pressures between the extremes of ether and nitrous oxide.

Once the operation is complete and the anesthetist turns off the gas machine, the rates of recovery from nitrous oxide and ether differ markedly. In the case of nitrous oxide, recovery is very rapid. The high partial pressure of this gas in blood rapidly drives the drug back into the alveoli, from whence it is expired. The resulting fall in nitrous oxide levels in blood quickly draws the gas out of the brain. The capacity of blood to dissolve and hold ether is much greater. As a result, the drug is not cleared as quickly by the lungs. Because it continues to circulate through the body, perfusing the brain, ether's recovery time is longer. From this discussion we can derive a principle:

Anesthetic gases with low solubility in blood accumulate quicker in the brain during inhalation and leave more rapidly once administration of the anesthetic is stopped.

Other factors that influence the onset of anesthesia are (1) the inspired concentration, (2) the alveolar ventilation and (3) the cardiac output.

Inspired concentration is important in determining the uptake of gas by blood and brain. Here the principle is:

The higher the inspired concentration, the more rapid will be the rate of increase of the partial pressure of the anesthetic in blood.

This is particularly true for gases readily soluble in blood. If the initial inspired anesthetic tension is set higher than required for the maintenance of anesthesia, the concentration and partial pressure of the gas in blood will rise more rapidly and the drug will enter the brain more quickly. This technique is called *overpressure.*

If the patient breathes more rapidly, increased quantities of anesthetic enter the blood, saturating it quickly and raising the partial pressure of the gas. The principle here is:

Improving alveolar ventilation increases the rate of anesthetic uptake by blood.

Again, the effect is greater for agents readily soluble in blood.

Increasing cardiac output improves blood flow through the lungs. Because a greater volume of blood is exposed to the gas in the alveoli per unit of time, it becomes more difficult to saturate it with anesthetic. Thus, the principle is:

Increasing cardiac output reduces the rate at which partial pressure increases, thereby delaying induction of anesthesia.

Here too, the effect is greatest with those anesthetics possessing good blood solubility. Excitement, fever and other hypermetabolic states, all conditions that increase cardiac output, delay anesthetic induction. Conversely, shock reduces cardiac output. As a result, anesthetic induction occurs very quickly in a patient in shock.

Stages of Anesthesia

Over sixty years ago, anesthetists recognized four stages of anesthesia as they related to the effects of ether. These reflect increasing concentrations of the anesthetic in the central nervous system and the progressive deterioration of neuronal function. The stages are still used today to describe the depth of anesthesia, even though they may be somewhat obscured in the newer anesthetics.

Stage I. Also known as the stage of analgesia, stage I begins at the time of drug administration and lasts until the patient loses consciousness. The patient starts this stage with normal memory and sensation and leaves with amnesia and analgesia.

Stage II. The second stage (delirium or excitement) starts with loss of consciousness and continues to the point where the patient is ready for surgery. Excitement and involuntary activity may be present. At this time the patient may shout, sing, laugh or attempt to fight. Sympathetic nervous system activity is high. The pupils may be dilated, the heart rate fast, and the blood pressure raised. These effects are due to the release of lower and more primitive areas of the brain from the overriding influence of higher inhibitory centres, which have just been depressed. As a result, basic emotional reactions appear unfettered by learned inhibitions. Anesthetists try to pass patients through stage II as quickly as possible.

Stage III. The third stage (surgical anesthesia) starts when the patient leaves stage II and continues until the cessation of spontaneous respiration. At one time, stage III was divided into four planes to delineate the extent of muscular relaxation and respiratory depression. Today, this has little meaning, as drugs such as tubocurarine or succinylcholine (see Chapter 31) are used for the specific purpose of relaxing muscles. As the name indicates, this is the stage during which surgery is performed.

Stage IV. The fourth stage (respiratory paralysis) begins with respiratory failure and concludes with complete circulatory collapse.

Specific Inhalation Anesthetics

Ether

Ether, or diethyl ether to be correct, is a colourless, highly volatile liquid with a pungent odour. In contrast to most inhalation anesthetics, it has significant solubility in water. With the exception of nitrous oxide, ether is the oldest inhalation anesthetic in use. It was first used in 1842 and, although its popularity has dropped greatly over the past thirty years, ether is still used occasionally. Our interest in it, however, is largely historical.

Anesthesia with ether is characterized by prolonged induction and emergence. Patients suffer from a high incidence of postanesthetic nausea and vomiting. Ether is also very irritating; its use results in increased salivary, bronchial and gastric secretions. Laryngeal spasm is not uncommon with the drug. In addition, ether is flammable, thus all possibility of sparks in the operating room must be eliminated.

Nitrous Oxide

Nitrous oxide, with a low solubility in blood, has a rapid onset of action and a quick recovery. It is an excellent baseline anesthetic and is often used in conjunction with other anesthetics to allow for lower concentrations of the latter drugs. The main limitation to nitrous oxide use is its weak potency. The minimal alveolar concentration (MAC) for nitrous oxide is 100%. Obviously, it is impossible to give a patient 100% nitrous oxide, unless you want him to asphyxiate. Nitrous oxide should be administered with at least 30% oxygen during induction and maintenance.

Halothane (Fluothane®)

Halothane was introduced in the mid 1950s. Since that time it has become one of the most popular inhalation anesthetics in North America. It is a potent anesthetic with a MAC of 0.76%, compared with 100% for nitrous oxide. Halothane induces anesthesia rapidly with little or no excitement but does not provide good muscular relaxation. As a result, neuromuscular blockers are often required. Nitrous oxide is often used concomitantly to reduce the concentration of halothane required. Controlled ventilation may be required, particularly if deep anesthesia is indicated. Halothane can lower blood pressure and sensitize the myocardium to catecholamines.

Hepatitis, occurring three to ten days after operation and preceded by fever, is a rare complication. It is believed to be a hypersensitivity reaction and is unpredictable in its occurrence. A portion of the administered halothane is metabolized in the liver, and it is believed that one of the metabolites is responsible for the hepatitis.

Enflurane (Enthrane®)

Enflurane has a MAC of 1.68%. Its action is characterized by rapid onset and quick recovery. Enflurane produces better muscle relaxation and less myocardial sensitization to catecholamines than halothane. It also causes profound respiratory depression. Nitrous oxide is often used to enable the anesthetist to administer a lower concentration of enflurane. Episodes of tonic-clonic or twitching movements or grand mal seizures, particularly in children, have occurred with enflurane. Liver damage has also been reported, but no cause-and-effect relationship with enflurane has been established.

Methoxyflurane (Penthrane®)

With a MAC of 0.16%, methoxyflurane is the most potent anesthetic available. Because of its high solubility in blood, methoxyflurane is rarely used for induction. Nitrous oxide or barbiturates are administered for induction. Awakening from methoxyflurane is slow because of its high solubility in blood. Methoxyflurane produces good muscle relaxation and minimal sensitization of the myocardium to catecholamines. The drug is also a good analgesic, and patients often awake free of pain. The major deterrent to its use is the high risk for renal failure. Methoxyflurane is metabolized, in part, giving rise to inorganic fluoride that can damage the kidneys. Although its nephrotoxicity is usually reversible, many anesthetists feel this is too high a price to pay for use of the drug.

Isoflurane (Forane®)

A potent anesthetic with a MAC of 1.2%, isoflurane has a pungent odour that limits the concentration patients will accept without coughing or holding the breath. Induction is usually smooth if patients are premedicated and given nitrous oxide or intravenous agents. Isoflurane does not sensitize the myocardium to catecholamines.

Table 58.1 lists the clinically significant drug interactions with inhalation anesthetics.

Intravenous Anesthetics

Total intravenous anesthesia can be an effective alternative to inhalation anesthesia. The ideal intravenous anesthetic should provide smooth induction, have a predictable dosage and a large therapeutic index (high margin of safety), produce minimal cardiovascular and respiratory depression, allow rapid and complete recovery, provide absence of pain or injury from injection and be stable in solution.

Barbiturates

Thiopental (Pentothal®) is a potent intravenous anesthetic used to provide rapid induction. Emergence, usually quick, may be delayed if large doses are given by continuous intravenous drip. Laryngospasm may occur during induction. Thiopental depresses both respiration and circulation. High doses are required to relax skeletal muscles. Thiopental decreases urine output by reducing perfusion pressure, constricting renal arteries and releasing the antidiuretic hormone (ADH).

Methohexital sodium (Brevital Sodium®) is a short-acting barbiturate used for induction and in

---

Table 58.1
Inhalation anesthetics: Drug interactions

Drug	Interaction
Amiodarone	• Amiodarone plus halothane, isoflurane or enflurane can result in increased CV toxicity. Monitor CV status
Aminoglycoside antibiotics	• Aminoglycoside antibiotics, plus enflurane or methoxyflurane, can produce increased renal toxicity. Avoid concurrent use, especially in pts with renal damage
ACE inhibitors	• Captopril has been reported to produce additive hypotension with nitrous oxide, enflurane, halothane and isoflurane. Monitor BP
Antihypertensive drugs	• Guanethidine, methyldopa, reserpine or spirolactone, together with enflurane, halothane, isoflurane or nitrous oxide, can produce additive hypotension. Monitor BP
Beta blockers	• Beta blockers and halothane can produce additive hypotension. Monitor BP
Fentanyl	• Enflurane or halothane may decrease the metabolism and increase the toxicity of fentanyl. Monitor closely
Epinephrine	• Epinephrine plus halothane may result in fatal arrhythmias. Avoid concurrent use
Isoniazid	• Isoniazid and enflurane may be nephrotoxic. Avoid concurrent use
Sympathomimetic amines	• Sympathomimetic amines, plus enflurane or isoflurane, may produce cardiac arrhythmias. Monitor cardiac rhythm
Sympathomimetic bronchodilators	• Halothane and sympathomimetic bronchodilators can produce cardiac arrhythmias. Avoid concurrent use
Tetracyclines	• Tetracyclines and methoxyflurane may result in fatal renal toxicity
Theophyllines	• Halothane and a theophylline product can increase ventricular arrhythmias. Use with caution

conditions such as electroconvulsive therapy, when loss of consciousness is required.

Thiamylal sodium (Surital®) is similar to thiopental and has the same uses and adverse effects.

The drug interactions for barbiturates are provided in Table 47.6 (page 556).

Benzodiazepines

Diazepam (Valium®) can be used intravenously to induce anesthesia. However, it has a slower onset than thiopental and, except in patients with cardiovascular disease, is usually less satisfactory. Its therapeutic applications include basal sedation during regional analgesia, cardioversion, and endoscopic and dental procedures. Intravenous diazepam can produce superficial, painless venous thrombosis at the injection site and is associated with a high incidence of phlebitis.

Midazolam (Versed®) is a short-acting, water-soluble benzodiazepine. Depending on the route of administration and dose used, midazolam can produce sedative-hypnotic effects or induce anesthesia. The administration of midazolam may often be followed by anterograde amnesia. Onset of sedative effects after intramuscular administration is about fifteen minutes, with peak sedation occurring thirty to sixty minutes following injection. Sedation after intravenous injection is usually achieved within three to six minutes. When midazolam is used intravenously, induction of anesthesia can usually be achieved in 1.5 min when narcotic premedication has been administered and in 2–2.5 min without narcotic premedication.

Midazolam is indicated as an intramuscular premedication prior to diagnostic procedures. As an intravenous agent, it can be used for patients requiring conscious sedation prior to and during short endoscopic diagnostic procedures and direct-current cardioversion. Midazolam can also be used intravenously as an induction anesthetic.

Table 47.2 (page 554) lists the drug interactions of benzodiazepines, including diazepam and midazolam.

Propofol (Diprivan®)

Propofol is an intravenous hypnotic agent that can be used for both induction and maintenance of anesthesia as part of a balanced anesthesia technique for inpatient and outpatient surgery. The drug is formulated in an oil-in-water emulsion. Intravenous injection of a therapeutic dose of propofol produces hypnosis rapidly and smoothly, usually within forty seconds from the start of an injection, although induction times of greater than sixty seconds have been observed.

Fentanyl (Sublimaze®), Sufentanil (Sufenta®), Alfentanil (Alfenta®) and Remifentanil (Ultiva®)

These four drugs belong to a general class of injectable anesthetic/analgesic opioid compounds known as 4-anilidopiperidines. As a class of drugs, these agents have been of great value as analgesics/anesthetics.

Fentanyl was first introduced in the early 1960s, and it demonstrated distinct advantages over morphine in surgical procedures. Its principal advantages were a shorter duration of action and greater cardiac stability. Fentanyl is often combined with the drug droperidol, a butyrophenone, with properties similar to those of the antipsychotic haloperidol (see Chapter 45). The two are often used together to produce neuroleptanalgesia, a state in which consciousness is not lost but the anxiety of the patient is allayed and the ability to perceive pain reduced or abolished. Neuroleptanalgesia may be valuable for diagnostic and therapeutic procedures. Innovar® is a fixed-ratio combination of fentanyl and droperidol. It is often used to premedicate patients or as an adjunct to inhalation anesthesia.

The subsequent introduction of sufentanil, and later alfentanil, provided drugs with shorter durations of action than fentanyl and thus some clinical advantage. Over the past decade or two, attention has focused primarily on alfentanil. Anesthesia with alfentanil is characterized by a more rapid onset and shorter duration of action than fentanyl or sufentanil.

Despite the improvement that alfentanil and sufentanil offer over fentanyl, both are far from ideal. Their shortcomings include the facts that:

• their pharmacokinetic and pharmacodynamic half-lives are too long to allow exact intraoperative control of blood levels and, consequently, drug effects;

• their reduced clearance on prolonged or repeated administration leads to accumulation and delayed recovery; and

• they depend on hepatic metabolism for elimination. This is slower than the metabolism of remifentanil by plasma and tissue esterases (see below). As a consequence of the fact that alfentanil and sufentanil are metabolized in the liver, increasing their dosage or prolonging their duration of administration leads to drug accumulation and delayed recovery.

Remifentanil appears to have overcome these problems. It is rapidly inactivated by plasma and tissue esterases. As a result, its dosage can be titrated easily to meet the needs of each patient. Because remifentanil is rapidly inactivated, its dosage can be increased or prolonged, without fear of accumulation or delayed recovery. Remifentanil can also be given over prolonged periods without fear of drug accumulation, and it does not depend on hepatic metabolism for elimination.

Ketamine (Ketalar®)

Ketamine is a nonbarbiturate anesthetic that can be administered intravenously or intramuscularly. It is sometimes called a dissociative anesthetic because patients become unresponsive to pain and to the environment. Duration of anesthesia is short. Ketamine is useful for repeated anesthesia in burn patients, for diagnostic studies, for sedating uncontrollable patients and for minor surgical procedures. An anticholinergic should be administered concomitantly to reduce salivary secretion.

The use of ketamine is limited because of its ability to produce elevated blood pressure, vivid dreams, hallucinations and other psychic disturbances after recovery. These effects may be reduced by oral premedication with 4 mg lorazepam or 10 mg diazepam. Alternatively, intravenous diazepam (0.15–0.30 mg/kg) can be administered at the end of anesthesia.

Nursing Management

Table 58.2 describes the nursing management of the patient receiving general anesthetic drugs. Dosage details of individual drugs are given in Table 58.3 (pages 686–689).

Table 58.2
Nursing management of the general anesthetics

Assessment of risk vs. benefit	Patient data	• Usually, selection and administration of general anesthetics is the responsibility of the physician, dentist or anesthetist • Assess to establish baseline VS, general state of health • *Pregnancy:* Risk category varies
	Drug data	• Select drugs based on desired onset, duration of action and pt hx
Implementation	Rights of administration	• These drugs are usually administered by a physician or other certified personnel
Outcomes	Monitoring of progress	*Continually monitor:* • Clinical response indicating tx success. Monitor the following VS for deviations from norm: T, P (rate, rhythm, quality), BP (compared with baseline), R (rate, depth, equality of bilateral chest expansion, regularity), colour (nailbeds, lips) • Emergence from anesthetic (this usually occurs in a specialized unit) • *Signs/symptoms of adverse reactions:* Monitor central nervous and CV systems; report immediately to physician

Table 58.3
The general anesthetics: Drug doses

Drug Generic name (Trade names)	Dosage	Nursing alert
A. Inhalation Anesthetics		
nitrous oxide	**Inhalation** (low anesthetic potency): For sedation, 25%; for analgesia, 25% to 50% with O_2; for induction, 70% N_2O with 30% O_2 for 2–3 min	• Used in dentistry for its analgesic properties
enflurane (Enthrane)	Surgical anesthesia in 7–10 min: 2% to 4.5%. Maintenance: 0.5% to 3%	• Observe pt for seizures
halothane (Fluothane)	**For induction:** 1% to 4%. Maintenance: 0.5% to 2%	• Observe for respiratory depression. Have resuscitation equipment on hand
isoflurane (Forane)	**For induction:** 3% to 3.5% in O_2 or in N_2O/O_2. Maintenance: 0.5% to 3%	• Observe for respiratory depression; have resuscitation emergency equipment on hand
methoxyflurane (Penthrane)	**Inhalation:** For analgesia, 0.3% to 0.8%. Maintenance: Together with at least 50% N_2O	• Useful in labour, in low doses; does not suppress uterine contractions
B. Intravenous Anesthetics		
thiopental sodium (Pentothal Sodium)	**IV:** *Adults:* 50–100 mg intermittently q30–40s prn. Alternatively, a single injection of 3–5 mg/kg. Maintenance: 50–100 mg of 2.5% solution prn. *Children 5–15 years:* 2.5% solution injected slowly and intermittently at 30-s intervals. Total dose, 4–5 mg/kg. Maintenance: *Children 30–50 kg:* 25–50 mg intermittently. **Rectal** (basal anesthesia): *Children:* 30 mg/kg in 40% suspension	• Follow agency policy re: certification for drug administration. Use infusion pump to ensure accuracy. Check IV compatibility
diazepam (Valium)	**IV:** For induction: 0.1–1.5 mg/kg. Basal sedation: 2–5 mg q30s	• Resuscitation equipment must be on hand for IV administration. Follow agency policy re: certification for drug administration

Table 58.3 (continued)
The general anesthetics: Drug doses

Drug Generic name (Trade names)	Dosage	Nursing alert
B. Intravenous Anesthetics (cont'd)		
midazolam (Versed)	**IM** (preoperative sedation/memory impairment): *Adults:* 70–80 µg/kg 1 h before surgery (usual dose, 5 mg). **IV** (conscious sedation for short procedure): *Adults:* 1–2.5 mg initially; dosage may be increased further prn. Doses > 5 mg are rarely needed. *Elderly (> 60 years) or debilitated patients:* Initial dose should not exceed 1.5 mg, with doses > 3.5 mg rarely needed. (Induction of anesthesia): *Adults:* 200–350 µg/kg initially. May give additional dose of 25% of initial dose if needed, up to 600 µg/kg total. If > 55 years, initial dose should be 150–300 µg/kg. For seriously ill or debilitated pts, initial dose may be 150–250 µg/kg. If pt is premedicated, initial dose should be further reduced	• Resuscitation equipment must be on hand for IV administration. Follow agency policy re: certification for drug administration
propofol (Diprivan)	**IV:** *Adults* (induction): 2–2.5 mg/kg. *Elderly and debilitated:* 1–1.5 mg/kg. (Maintenance) *Adults:* 0.1–0.2 mg/kg/min. For detailed information, consult manufacturer's dosage recommendations	• Dose is titrated to pt's response; monitor continuously • Follow agency policy re: direct IV. For preparation of infusion, shake well, dilute only with D5W (concentration, 2 mg/mL). No preservatives; use strict aseptic technique. Discard unused solution within 6 h. Choose large vein; drug is irritating. Lidocaine may be given to reduce local pain
droperidol (Inapsine)	**IM:** *Adults* (premedication): 2.5–10 mg, administered 30–60 min pre-op. Diagnostic (without general anesthetic): 2.5–10 mg 30–60 min preprocedure. Additional IV: 1.25–2.5 mg may be given. **IV** (induction): 2.5 mg/9–11 kg	• Follow agency policy re: direct IV. Administer slowly and monitor site to avoid extravasation. Resuscitation equipment must be at hand
fentanyl citrate (Sublimaze)	**IM** (for premedication): *Adults:* 0.05–0.1 mg (1–2 mL) 30–60 min prior to surgery. This dose should be decreased in the elderly or poor-risk pt	
	IV (for induction): *Adults:* 0.05–0.1 mg (1–2 mL) initially, repeated at 2- to 3-min intervals until satisfactory induction is achieved. If attenuation of sympathetic activity is desired (e.g., coronary artery disease), a total dose of 50–120 µg/kg is required.	• Follow agency policy re: direct IV. Use infusion pump for intermittent infusion. Resuscitation equipment must be available

(cont'd on next page)

Table 58.3 (continued)
The general anesthetics: Drug doses

Drug Generic name (Trade names)	Dosage	Nursing alert
B. Intravenous Anesthetics (cont'd)		
fentanyl citrate (Sublimaze) (cont'd)	**IV** (cont'd): The dose should be reduced to 0.025–0.05 mg (0.5–1 mL) in elderly or poor-risk patients. For maintenance: 0.025 mg to one-half the loading dose may be administered if lightening of anesthesia is manifested by movement. Change in VS may or may not occur. *Children* (for induction and maintenance): 2–3 µg/kg	
droperidol + fentanyl (Innovar)	**IV:** Neuroleptanesthesia can be induced with 1 mL/9–12 kg (smaller does may be adequate), administered slowly (1 mL q1–2min), followed by N_2O and O_2 when drowsiness develops. Thiopental 100 mg also may be used to hasten induction. Anesthesia can be maintained with N_2O or with fentanyl alone (usual dose, 0.05–0.1 mg q30–60min) when clinical sig**ns** indicate that anesthesia may be too light	• Follow agency policy for direct IV. Rate not to exceed 1 mL q1–2min. Use infusion pump for intermittent infusion. Monitor continuously
alfentanil HCl (Alfenta)	**IV:** *Adults* (for short procedures in pts breathing spontaneously or with assisted ventilation with N_2O/O_2): A slow (20-min) bolus injection of 8–20 µg/kg administered prior to induction with a barbiturate: a maint. dose of 3–5 µg/kg is then given. (For long procedures): Loading dose may be increased to 50–75 µg/kg. A variable-rate, continuous infusion (approximately 0.5–3 µg/kg/min) is recommended for maintenance. In the absence of signs of lightening anesthesia, infusion rates always should be decreased. If additional opioid is required during the final 15 min of surgery, bolus doses of 7 µg/kg are preferred to continuing or increasing the infusion rate	• Follow agency policy re: direct IV. Use tuberculin syringe to ensure accuracy with small dosages. Rate should not exceed 1–1.5 µg/kg/min. Use infusion pump for continuous infusion
remifentanil (Ultiva)	**IV:** *Adults* (induction of anesthesia): 0.5–1 µg/kg/min (through intubation). Maintenance of anesthesia with N_2O (66%): 0.4 µg/kg/min (dosage range, 0.1–2 µg/kg/min). Maintenance of anesthesia with isoflurane (0.4–1.5 MAC): 0.25 µg/kg/min (dosage range, 0.05–2 µg/kg/min). Maintenance of anesthesia with propofol (100–200 µg/kg/min.): 0.25 µg/kg/min (dosage range, 0.05–2 µg/kg/min)	• Follow agency policy re: direct IV. Use tuberculin syringe to ensure accuracy with small dosages. Monitor continuously. Use infusion pump for continuous infusion (cont'd on next page)

Table 58.3 (continued)
The general anesthetics: Drug doses

Drug Generic name (Trade names)	Dosage	Nursing alert
B. Intravenous Anesthetics (cont'd)		
remifentanil (Ultiva) (cont'd)	**IV** (cont'd): Spontaneous ventilation anesthesia: 0.04 μg/kg/min (dosage range, 0.025–0.1 μg/kg/min). Continuation as an analgesic into the immediate postoperative period: 0.1 μg/kg/min (dosage range, 0.025–0.2 μg/kg/min)	
sufentanil citrate (Sufenta)	**IV** (for general surgery requiring intubation and mechanical ventilation): *Adults:* 1–2 μg/kg with N_2O/O_2. For maintenance, 10–25 μg (0.2–0.5 mL) prn or by continuous infusion (For major surgical procedures requiring some attenuation of sympathetic response to surgical stimuli) *Adults:* 2–8 μg/kg with N_2O/O_2. For maintenance, 25–50 μg (0.5–1 mL) prn, or by continuous infusion of 0.3–1 μg/kg/min (For induction in pts undergoing CV procedures) *Adults:* 8–30 μg/kg or more with O_2 and nondepolarizing muscle relaxant; for maintenance, 25–50 μg (0.5 to 1 mL) prn, or continuous infusion at the higher dose range. Postoperative mechanical ventilation will be required with these doses *Children 2–12 years undergoing CV surgery:* 10 μg/kg or more with O_2 only (For induction for neurosurgical procedures) *Adults:* 1–2 μg/kg with a benzodiazepine or small doses of thiopental and O_2 and a nondepolarizing muscle relaxant; for maintenance, incremental doses not exceeding 1 μg/kg/h or a continuous infusion not exceeding that rate	• Follow agency policy re: direct IV. Use tuberculin syringe to ensure accuracy with small dosages. Suggested IV rate is 250–300 μg/min. Use infusion pump for continuous infusion
ketamine HCl (Ketalar)	**IV:** For induction, 1.0–4.5 mg/kg administered over 60 s. Maintenance, 50% induction dose prn **IM:** For induction, 6.5–13 mg/kg. Maintenance, 50% induction dose prn. For analgesia, 2 mg/kg	• For direct IV follow agency policy. Rate, 1–2 mg/min. For continuous infusion, prepare solution with NS or D5W at a concentration of 1 mg/mL. Use infusion pump

> **Response to Clinical Challenge**
>
> 1. A scavenging system to remove gas is an important occupational protection.
> 2. The recommended level of nitrous oxide should not exceed 22 ppm.
> 3. Reduced fertility is one potential risk of continued exposure to nitrous oxide. (For more information, refer to the readings listed at the end of this chapter.)

Further Reading

Austin PR, Austin PJ (1996). Measurement of nitrous oxide concentration in a simulated postanesthetic care unit environment. *J Perianesth Nurs* 1996; 11(4):259–266.

Curley M, Molengraft J. Providing comfort to critically ill pediatric patients. Isoflurone. *Crit Care Nurs Clin North Am* 1995;7(2):267–274.

Dougherty J. Same day surgery: the nurse's role. *Orthoped Nurs* 1996;15(4):15–18.

Dunnihoo M, et al. The effects of total intra-venous anesthesia using propofol, ketamine and vancuronium on cardiovascular response and wake-up time. *AANA Journal* 1994;62(3):261–264.

Hawks S. Clinical aspects of nurse anesthesia practice. *Nurs Clin North Am* 1996;31(3):591–605.

Keating H. Patient controlled analgesia with nitrous oxide in cancer pain. *J Pain Symptom Management* 1996;11(2):126–130.

McAuliffe M, Hartshorn E. Anesthetic drug inter-actions. *CRNA* 1994;5(3):124–129.

Phillips M. Into the land of nod. Drugs used during anesthesia in day surgery. *Can Operating Room Nurs J* 1994;12(4):4–9.

Rowland A, et al. Reduced fertility among women employed as dental assistants exposed to high levels of nitrous oxide. *New Engl J Med* 1992; 32(327):993–997.

Shortridge-McCauley L. Reproductive hazards: an overview of exposure to health care workers. *AAOHN Journal* 1995;43(12):614–621.

Vessering T. Narcotics and the implications of post-anesthetic recovery unit. *Nurs Clin North Am* 1993;28(3):573–580.

Walker J. What's new with inhaled anesthetics. *J Perianesth Nurs* 1996;11(5):330–333.

Drugs and the Gastrointestinal Tract

Stretching approximately twelve metres in the adult, the gastrointestinal (GI) tract plays an important role in our general well-being. Similar to other organ systems, the gastrointestinal tract, too, is subject to disease, and the importance of placating it cannot be overemphasized. Failure to restore peace and harmony within the entrails can divert attention from almost all other activities and make a normal lifestyle virtually impossible.

Unit 12 addresses the problems of the gastrointestinal tract with a discussion of antiulcer therapy (Chapter 59), drugs for the treatment of chronic inflammatory bowel disease (Chapter 60), agents for the treatment of diarrhea and constipation (Chapter 61) and antiemetic and antinauseant drugs (Chapter 62).

Antiulcer Drugs

Topics Discussed
- Peptic ulcer disease
- Drug therapy of peptic ulcers: Antibacterials, drugs that block the secretion of gastric acid, drugs that reduce the effects of secreted gastric acid and pepsin
- For each drug discussed: Mechanism of action and pharmacologic effects, therapeutic uses, adverse effects
- Nursing management

Drugs Discussed
aluminum hydroxide (ah-**lyoo**-min-num hye-**drok**-side)
amoxicillin (ah-mox-ee-**sill**-in)
bismuth subsalicylate (**biss**-muth sub-sal-**iss**-il-late

cimetidine (sim-**met**-ih-deen)
clarithromycin (klar-ith-roe-**mye**-sin)
famotidine (fah-**moe**-tih-deen)
lansoprazole (lanz-**op**-rah-zole)
magnesium hydroxide (mag-**nee**-zee-um hye-**drok**-side)
metronidazole (me-troe-**nye**-dah-zole)
misoprostol (mye-soe-**prost**-ole)
nizatidine (niz-**zat**-ih-deen)
omeprazole (oh-**mep**-rah-zole)
pirenzepine (peer-**enz**-ah-peen)
ranitidine (rah-**nit**-id-een)
sucralfate (soo-**kral**-fate)
tetracycline (tet-rah-**sye**-kleen)

Clinical Challenge

Consider this clinical challenge as you read through this chapter. The response to the challenge appears on page 698.

You are an occupational health nurse working for a large urban employer. A 38-year-old woman attends the clinic for advice regarding peptic ulcer disease. She had a peptic ulcer about 10 years ago and is currently undergoing diagnostic testing for the possibility of a recurrence. Previously she was treated with a special diet, prescribed antacids and instructed to stop smoking and reduce her caffeine intake. As the sole supporter for two children, she is worried that her current job stress is the cause of the ulcer; friends have suggested that she may have to quit work if this is so.

1. What other information would you ask?
2. What general education would you provide to this woman?

An ulcer is a hole in the tissue covering one of the surfaces of the body. Ulcers may be found in the skin, the cornea of the eye and the lining of the gastrointestinal (GI) tract. Peptic ulcers appear in those parts of the GI tract that are exposed to gastric juice containing acid and pepsin and extend at least through the entire thickness of the esophageal, gastric or duodenal mucosa. Duodenal ulcers are most common.

The consequences of an ulcer vary depending on its site and extent. For example, if an ulcer occurs close to a large artery it may erode the wall of the vessel and cause a severe hemorrhage. Although most ulcers do not penetrate deeper than the esophageal, gastric or duodenal muscle layers, a few, called penetrating ulcers, may perforate through the entire wall, allowing for the flow of fluid from the GI tract into the peritoneal cavity. This can be a life-threatening situation. If the site of the penetrating ulcer occurs adjacent to another organ, such as the liver or pancreas, the escape of gastric secretions may damage these tissues.

Peptic Ulcer Disease

Our understanding of peptic ulcer disease was significantly changed in 1983 when it was discovered that a spiral gram-negative bacterium covered the gastric mucosa in many patients. The bacteria was called *Campylobacter pylori*. It would later be renamed *Helicobacter pylori*. Research has shown *H. pylori* to be an important factor in the pathogenesis of gastritis, peptic ulcer disease and possibly other diseases of the stomach. *H. pylori* is associated with about 70% of the cases of gastric ulcers and 85% to nearly 100% of duodenal ulcers.

The discovery of *Helicobacter pylori* provided a new insight into the pathogenesis of ulcers and the treatment of peptic ulcer disease. Since the 1950s, attention has been paid to reducing gastric acid secretion, or neutralizing stomach acid, in an attempt to prevent peptic ulcers. This view led to the introduction of antacids, followed by H_2 blockers, sucralfate, the synthetic prostaglandin misoprostol and finally, the proton pump inhibitors. Despite the effectiveness of these medications, ulcers recurred in up to eighty percent of patients within one year of stopping the drugs.

Attention is now focused directly at treating the *H. pylori* infection. This has improved ulcer healing and reduced relapses dramatically.

Epidemiology of *Helicobacter pylori*

Helicobacter pylori is very common. The infection is acquired early in life and persists unless treated. The most important risk factor for developing it appears to be one's socioeconomic conditions in childhood. In developing nations, the rates of infection can reach 80% to nearly 100% by age twenty. In industrialized countries such as Canada, prevalence is low in childhood but increasing numbers are infected with advancing age. By the age of fifty, nearly fifty percent of the population may be infected.

H. pylori infection is usually asymptomatic. It is spread from person to person. More evidence supports fecal–oral transmission rather than oral–oral spread.

H. pylori typically infects the antrum of the stomach rather than the duodenum. Patients with duodenal ulcers have a characteristic triad of chronic antral gastritis, elevated gastric acid secretion (secondary to increased serum gastrin levels) and gastric metaplasia in the duodenum. Under these conditions *H. pylori* can migrate from the surface of the antrum to colonize foci of duodenal gastric metaplasia resulting in duodenitis, which facilitates development of ulcers.

H. pylori is thought to induce ulceration through one of two mechanisms. The "leaky roof" hypothesis holds that *H. pylori* produces toxins and induces inflammation by stimulating the immune system. This leads to destruction of the intact mucosal barrier, resulting in ulcers. The alternative hypothesis holds that *H. pylori* infection leads to increased levels of gastrin, which in turn stimulates excess acid production from parietal cells, ultimately resulting in peptic ulceration.

Drug Therapy of Peptic Ulcers

Our discussion of drug therapy for peptic ulcers will begin with the antibacterial treatment of *H. pylori*. This will then be followed by a discussion of drugs that block the secretion of gastric acid and drugs that reduce the effects of secreted gastric acid and pepsin. Together, all these groups play a role in the management of peptic ulcer disease.

Antibacterial Drugs

The antibacterial drugs used to treat *Helicobacter pylori* infections are discussed in detail in Unit 3 of this book. As a result, they can be presented briefly in this chapter.

The ideal therapy for *H. pylori* infection has yet to be defined. Many dual (two-drug) or triple (three-drug) therapies have been used. However, the current accepted standard appears to be triple therapy with bismuth subsalicylate (Pepto-Bismol®), tetracycline and metronidazole. This regime is given for two weeks and results in cure in up to ninety percent of patients. The treatment is generally well tolerated. Patients taking metronidazole may experience a metallic taste. Metronidazole also produces an disulfiram-like effect when combined with alcohol, and this can decrease compliance. Where metronidazole resistance is suspected (especially where the drug is frequently used to treat other infections), adding omeprazole, in a dose of 20 mg twice daily, virtually eliminates the problem of drug resistance. This quadruple-therapy regime provides the best overall cure rates.

Dual therapies using omeprazole and antibiotics, such as amoxicillin, have improved compliance but are less effective and are not currently recommended. A new therapy, known as MOC (metronidazole, omeprazole, clarithromycin), is gaining popularity because it has a good success rate and the twice-daily dosing may improve compliance. This involves administering metronidazole 500 mg twice daily, omeprazole 20 mg twice daily and clarithromycin 250 mg twice daily.

Drugs That Block the Secretion of Gastric Acid

The fasting stomach continuously secretes acid. Peak amounts are released near midnight and lowest quantities shortly before awakening.

Gastric acid is secreted by parietal cells in the stomach. The formation and secretion of gastric acid occurs in two stages. First, histamine, acetylcholine or gastrin stimulate the parietal cells to begin the process of acid formation. Subsequently, the enzyme H^+,K^+-ATPase (often called the proton pump) completes the formation and secretion of gastric acid. The proton pump is the final common pathway for the secretion of gastric acid.

Figure 59.1 illustrates the parietal cell and the role of acetylcholine, gastrin and histamine, and their relationship to the H^+,K^+-ATPase pump, in the secretion of gastric acid.

Histamine$_2$ (H$_2$) Blockers

Cimetidine (Tagamet®)

Mechanism of action and pharmacologic effects. Histamine receptors in the stomach are called H_2 receptors to distinguish them from the H_1 receptors found elsewhere in the body that are responsible for histamine's effects on bronchioles, skin, nasal mucosa and conjunctiva.

Cimetidine is a reversible, competitive antagonist of the actions of histamine on H_2 receptors. It inhibits, in a dose-dependent manner, histamine-

Figure 59.1

Conceptual model of the parietal cell and some mechanisms believed to be involved in the control and inhibition of gastric acid secretion

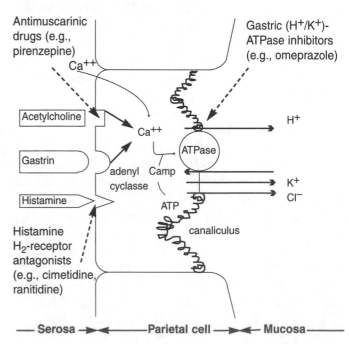

Source: Clissold SP, Campoli-Richards DM. Omeprazole. A preliminary review of its pharmacodynamic and pharmacokinetic properties, and therapeutic potential in peptic ulcer disease and Zollinger-Ellison syndrome. *Drugs* 1986;32:15–47. Reproduced with permission.

evoked gastric acid secretion. It also inhibits secretion induced by gastrin and partially blocks acetylcholine-stimulated gastric acid secretion. Cimetidine reduces both the volume of gastric juice secreted and its hydrogen ion concentration. The output of pepsin generally falls in parallel with the diminished volume of gastric secretion.

Therapeutic uses. Cimetidine is indicated for primary therapy for conditions where the inhibition of gastric acid secretion is likely to be beneficial, such as: duodenal ulcer; nonmalignant gastric ulcer; gastroesophageal reflux disease; management of upper GI hemorrhage; pathological hypersecretion associated with Zollinger-Ellison syndrome, systemic mastocytosis and multiple endocrine adenomas. The drug is also approved for prophylaxis of recurrent duodenal or gastric ulcer, stress ulceration and aspiration pneumonitis.

Cimetidine promotes both duodenal and gastric healing. Many patients relapse when cimetidine is stopped. This should come as no surprise if *H. pylori* is involved.

Adverse effects. Cimetidine's adverse effects include diarrhea, muscular pain, skin rash, dizziness and mental confusion. It also blocks androgen receptors and can cause gynecomastia and breast tenderness. Rarely, cimetidine can cause hepatitis, bone marrow depression and elevation of serum creatinine levels.

Table 59.1 lists the clinically significant drug interactions with cimetidine.

Ranitidine (Zantac®)

Ranitidine is four to nine times more potent than cimetidine. Maximal inhibition of gastric acid secretion is obtained with a dose of 150 mg of the drug. Ranitidine does not interfere with drug metabolism. It is indicated in the treatment of duodenal ulcer, benign gastric ulcer, reflux esophagitis, postoperative peptic ulcer, Zollinger-Ellison syndrome and other conditions where reduction of gastric secretion and acid output is desirable. Ranitidine is generally well tolerated.

Famotidine (Pepcid®)

Famotidine is a competitive inhibitor of H_2 receptors, and its effects are very similar to those of ranitidine. It is indicated in the treatment of acute duodenal ulcer, acute benign gastric ulcer and the Zollinger-Ellison syndrome. Famotidine is also used prophylactically in duodenal ulcer patients. It usually is well tolerated; most adverse reactions have been mild and transient. These include headache, dizziness, constipation and diarrhea.

Nizatidine (Axid®)

Nizatidine is another competitive, reversible antagonist of H_2 receptors. Its properties are similar to those of ranitidine and famotidine. Nizatidine is indicated in the treatment of acute duodenal ulcer and acute benign gastric ulcer and for the prevention of duodenal ulcer.

Anticholinergic Drugs

Mechanism of action and pharmacologic effects. The pharmacology of anticholinergics and their implications for nursing care have been presented in detail in Chapter 28. Anticholinergics block muscarinic receptors in the stomach, thereby preventing acetylcholine, released by the vagus, from stimulating gastric acid secretion.

Table 59.1
Cimetidine: Drug interactions

Drug	Interaction
Anticoagulants (oral), chlordiazepoxide, diazepam, lidocaine, phenytoin, propranolol, theophylline	• These drugs may have their hepatic metabolism reduced by cimetidine. As a result, their elimination is reduced and their blood levels are increased. The dosages of these drugs may require adjustment when starting or stopping cimetidine

Unfortunately, high doses of most anticholinergics are usually required, with the result that a general parasympathetic block often is produced throughout the body.

Therapeutic uses. The value of most anticholinergics is limited by relatively poor efficacy and unacceptable adverse effects. Pirenzepine (Gastrozepin®) is more effective than its predecessors. It also has little CNS toxicity and minimal peripheral adverse effects.

Combination products are available containing both an anticholinergic and a CNS depressant. These products are used as adjunctive therapy in the treatment of peptic ulcers, the irritable bowel syndrome and acute enterocolitis. The therapeutic rationale for combining a CNS depressant with an anticholinergic must be questioned.

Anticholinergic drugs, including pirenzepine, are contraindicated in glaucoma, obstructive uropathy due to prostatism and obstructive diseases of the GI tract.

Adverse effects. A major drawback to the use of anticholinergics for the treatment of peptic ulcers is the variety of adverse effects seen. With the exception of pirenzepine, anticholinergic treatment often blocks all cholinergic innervation, and the patient experiences dry mouth, mydriasis, cycloplegia, anhidrosis, tachycardia, urinary retention and decreased intestinal motility.

Prostaglandin Analogues

Misoprostol (Cytotec®)

Mechanism of action and pharmacologic effects. Misoprostol is a synthetic analogue of PGE_1. The drug has both gastric antisecretory and cytoprotective effects. The antisecretory effect occurs through direct action on the parietal cells. Misoprostol exerts its cytoprotective effect by enhancing natural mucosal defence mechanisms. It can protect the gastric mucosa against various irritants such as alcohol, acetylsalicylic acid and some nonsteroidal anti-inflammatory drugs (NSAIDs).

Therapeutic uses. Misoprostol is indicated for treatment of duodenal ulcer and also for treatment and prevention of NSAID-induced gastric ulcers (≥ 0.3 cm in diameter). *The drug is contraindicated in pregnancy, and women should be advised to use strict contraceptive measures while taking it.* If pregnancy is suspected, the use of misoprostol should be discontinued, and the pregnancy followed very closely (weekly) for the next four weeks.

Adverse effects. Diarrhea and abdominal pain are the most common adverse effects of misoprostol. Other adverse effects include nausea, headache and dizziness.

H^+,K^+-ATPase (Proton Pump) Inhibitors

Omeprazole (Losec®, Prilosec®) and Lansoprazole (Prevacid®)

Mechanism of action and pharmacologic effects. Omeprazole and lansoprazole inhibit the gastric enzyme H^+,K^+-ATPase (the proton pump), which is responsible for secretion of H^+ by the parietal cells of the stomach. These drugs produce a dose-dependent inhibition of both basal acid secretion and stimulated acid secretion. Omeprazole also has antimicrobial activity both in vitro and in vivo against *Helicobacter pylori,* the gramnegative bacilli now strongly associated with peptic ulcers (see discussion at the beginning of this chapter). Daily oral doses of omeprazole or lansoprazole reduce 24-h intragastric acidity by approximately eighty percent. Neither food nor antacids have any effect on omeprazole's bioavailability.

Therapeutic uses. Omeprazole and lansoprazole are very effective in treating duodenal ulcer, gastric ulcer and reflux esophagitis. However, the fact that they are more costly than H_2 blockers has reduced their use in these conditions. Because of cost considerations, these drugs should be reserved for patients with ulcers shown to be resistant to H_2-antagonist therapy and patients with reflux esophagitis who have not responded to treatment with an H_2 blocker. Proton pump inhibitors are also used to reduce gastric acid secretion in patients with Zollinger-Ellison syndrome.

Adverse effects. Omeprazole is well tolerated, and incidence of adverse reactions is low. When they have occurred, most adverse effects have been

Table 59.2
Omeprazole and lansoprazole: Drug interactions

Drug	Interaction
Diazepam	• Repeated doses of omeprazole can increase the half life of diazepam
Phenytoin	• Repeated doses of omeprazole can increase the half-life of phenytoin

mild and transient, and there has been no consistent relationship with treatment. The adverse reactions experienced with omeprazole include nausea, headache, diarrhea, constipation, abdominal pain, dyspepsia, flatulence and vomiting. Omeprazole is metabolized in the liver via the cytochrome P_{450} system.

Lansoprazole is also well tolerated. Abdominal pain, nausea and diarrhea have been reported. Like omeprazole, lansoprazole is metabolized by the cytochrome P_{450} system. Both drugs can interact with other drugs that are metabolized by the same system.

Table 59.2 lists the clinically significant drug interactions with omeprazole and lasoprazole.

Drugs That Reduce the Effects of Secreted Gastric Acid and Pepsin

Antacids

Mechanism of action and pharmacologic effects. Antacids neutralize gastric acid. Prior to the introduction of cimetidine, antacids were the standard treatment for peptic ulcers because they relieved pain and promoted healing. As the pH of the stomach increases, the action of pepsin decreases. At pH values between 4 and 5, the proteolytic action of pepsin is completely inhibited.

Therapeutic uses. Antacids are helpful in treating peptic ulcer disease, particularly duodenal ulcers. They are less effective in gastric ulcers.

It is important to select an antacid that is not absorbed (i.e., a nonsystemic antacid). Sodium bicarbonate is rapidly absorbed. Although it will increase the pH of the stomach, it will, if enough is taken, also raise the systemic pH of the body. Calcium carbonate is partially absorbed and also is not recommended for chronic use. Aluminum and magnesium salts are not absorbed and are preferred for chronic therapy.

Adverse effects. If systemic antacids are used chronically, they can increase the systemic pH of the patient. Nonsystemic antacids are salts of aluminum and magnesium. Both affect the bowel, but in different directions. Aluminum produces constipation; magnesium causes diarrhea. In an attempt to counterbalance the constipating effects of one with the laxative properties of the other, many antacid products contain both aluminum and magnesium salts.

Table 59.3 lists some of the clinically significant drug interactions with antacids; see Table 59.5 for further information.

Table 59.3
Antacids: Drug interactions

Drug	Interaction
Iron preparations	• Iron preparations may have decreased absorption when taken shortly before, with, or within a few hours after aluminum-containing antacids
Isoniazid	• Isoniazid may not be absorbed if taken before, with, or within a few hours after aluminum hydroxide or magaldrate
Phenothiazines	• Phenothiazines may not be absorbed if taken shortly before, with, or within a few hours of an antacid
Tetracyclines	• Tetracyclines may have reduced absorption if taken shortly before, with, or within a few hours of an antacid

Sucralfate (Carafate®, Sulcrate®)

Mechanism of action and pharmacologic effects. Sucralfate is not absorbed from the GI tract. It exerts a generalized gastric cytoprotective effect by enhancing natural mucosal defence mechanisms. In addition, sucralfate has greater affinity for ulcerated gastric or duodenal mucosa. The drug produces an adherent and cytoprotective barrier at the ulcer site. This barrier protects the site from the potential ulcerogenic properties of acid, pepsin and bile.

Therapeutic uses. Sucralfate is indicated for treatment of duodenal and nonmalignant gastric ulcers and for prophylaxis of duodenal ulcer recurrence.

Adverse effects. Sucralfate's adverse effects are mild and rarely lead to discontinuing the drug. Constipation, seen in about two percent of patients, is the main complaint. Other adverse effects reported include diarrhea, nausea, gastric discomfort, indigestion, dry mouth, skin rash, pruritus, back pain, dizziness, sleepiness and vertigo.

Nursing Management

Table 59.4 describes the nursing management of the patient receiving antiulcer drugs. Dosage details of individual drugs are given in Table 59.5 (pages 700–704).

Response to Clinical Challenge

1. You should explore other causative factors, such as use of NSAIDs. For example, does the client use ASA regularly?
2. Myths regarding the causes of ulcers are common; stress is often considered the major factor. Although it can be a mediating factor in healing, stress per se does not cause peptic ulcers. You should explain the role of *H. pylori* and the types of treatment currently available. Instructions on coping mechanisms to reduce the typical responses to stress can be helpful in promoting healing and in the client's general well-being.

Further Reading

Burak K, Worobetz L. *Helicobacter pylori:* are stomach problems 'bugging' your patients? *Sask Med J* 1996;7:1–5.

Drugs for treatment of peptic ulcers. *Medical Letter on Drugs and Therapeutics* 1994;36:65–69.

Keithley JK. Histamine H$_2$ receptor antagonists. *Nurs Clin North Am* 1991;26(2):361–374.

Table 59.4
Nursing management of the antiulcer drugs

Assessment of risk vs. benefit	Patient data	• Physician should determine type and probable cause of ulcers • Assess to establish baseline VS, general state of health, particularly nutritional status • Cautious use for elderly pts and those with renal impairment • *Pregnancy:* Risk category varies among drugs in this class. For many, benefits may be acceptable despite risks; advise pt to consult with physician/pharmacist. NB: Misoprostol, metronidazole and tetracycline are contraindicated in pregnancy
	Drug data	• Generally, drugs are well tolerated, but some histamine blockers can cause hematologic adverse effects such as agranulocytosis, neutropenia
Implementation	Rights of administration	• Using the "rights" helps prevent errors of administration
	Right route	• Given mainly PO; sometimes IV
	Right time	• Many of these drugs should be given at a separate time from antacids; instruct pt accordingly
	Right technique	• IV administration requires knowledge of correct diluent and IV solution, correct dilution and rate of administration. Always refer to manufacturer's instructions or agency handbook for this route
	Nursing therapeutics	• Although stress does not produce ulcers, it does play a role in delaying healing. Explore adaptive and coping behaviours with pt; introduce relaxation approaches
	Patient/family teaching	• Pt's need for information may be influenced by hx of ulcers. Explore use of caffeine, dietary irritants and smoking, as all can produce gastric acid secretion • Triple and quadruple therapy require up to 2 weeks for effectiveness; explain reasons for combinations and assess pt understanding of regimen • Pts/families should know warning signs/symptoms of possible toxicities of these drugs. Report immediately: rash, fever, sore throat, diarrhea, nausea, vomiting, unusual bleeding or bruising • Warn pts to avoid alcohol; can increase risk of gastric irritation • *Discuss possibility of pregnancy:* Advise pt to notify physician; discuss birth control methods
Outcomes	Monitoring of progress	*Continually monitor:* • Clinical response indicating tx success (reduction in signs/symptoms) • Signs/symptoms of adverse reactions; document and report immediately to physician • With long-term tx, periodic blood tests for bone marrow function may be ordered

Table 59.5
The antiulcer drugs: Drug doses

Drug Generic name (Trade names)	Dosage	Nursing alert
A. Drugs to Combat *Helicobacter pylori*		
1. Triple Therapy		
bismuth subsalicylate (Pepto-Bismol) + metronidazole (Flagyl) + tetracycline	**Oral:** 2 Pepto-Bismol® tablets qid plus tetracycline 250 mg qid and metronidazole 250 mg tid for 2 weeks	• *Bismuth subsalicylate:* Shake liquid thoroughly before using. *Metronidazole:* Take with food or milk. May crush tabs and mix with food (NB: contraindicated in pregnancy). *Tetracycline:* Not recommended in pregnancy or for children < 8 years. Take on empty stomach (1 h ac or 2 h pc). Note drug–food interactions: do not give within 1 h of milk, antacids or iron supplements
2. Dual Therapy		
omeprazole magnesium (Losec, Prilosec) + amoxicillin (Amoxil)	**Oral:** Omeprazole 20 mg bid or 40 mg od plus amoxicillin 750 mg bid for 14 days	• *Omeprazole:* May be taken with antacids. Do not crush or chew capsules. Best if taken before meals, preferably in am. *Amoxicillin:* Take without regard to food; capsules may be emptied and mixed with liquid or food. Chewable tabs should be chewed or crushed not swallowed whole. Ensure that suspension is mixed prior to use
omeprazole magnesium (Losec, Prilosec) + clarithromycin (Biaxin)	**Oral:** Omeprazole 40 mg od plus clarithromycin 500 mg tid for 14 days, followed by omeprazole 20 mg od for 14 days	• *Omeprazole:* As above. *Clarithromycin:* Give without regard to food
3. MOC (Metronidazole + Omeprazole + Clarithromycin) Therapy		
metronidazole (Flagyl) + omeprazole magnesium (Losec) + clarithromycin (Biaxin)	**Oral:** Metronidazole 500 mg bid plus omeprazole 20 mg bid and clarithromycin 250 mg bid	• *Metronidazole:* As above. *Omeprazole:* As above. *Clarithromycin:* As above

Table 59.5 (continued)
The antiulcer drugs: Drug doses

Drug Generic name (Trade names)	Dosage	Nursing alert
B. Drugs That Decrease Acid Secretion		
1. Histamine$_2$ (H$_2$) Blockers		
cimetidine (Tagamet)	**Oral** (duodenal ulcer and nonmalignant gastric ulcer): *Adults:* 800 mg hs; or 600 mg bid at breakfast and hs; or 300 mg qid, with meals and hs. (Prophylaxis of recurrent duodenal or gastric ulcer): 400 mg hs or 300 mg bid at breakfast and hs. (NSAID-induced lesions and symptoms): 800 mg hs or 400 mg bid at breakfast and hs, for 8 weeks. (Gastroesophageal reflux disease): 800 mg hs or 600 mg bid at breakfast and hs, or 300 mg qid, with meals and hs, for 8–12 weeks. (Zollinger-Ellison syndrome): 300 mg qid with meals and hs. Adjust dosage to meet needs of pt (usually not > 2400 mg/day). *Children 1–12 years:* 20–25 mg/kg/day in divided doses q4–6 h	• **PO:** Do not give within 1 h of antacids. Give with meals
	IV (management of upper GI hemorrhage): Injection or intermittent infusion of 300 mg q6h until 48 h after active bleeding has stopped. At this time an oral dosage regimen of 600 mg bid, at breakfast and hs, or 300 mg q6h may be instituted. Recommended dosage for intermittent IV infusion: 300 mg q6h. For impaired renal or hepatic function: Consult manufacturer's information	• **IV:** For direct IV, follow agency policy re: certification. For intermittent infusion, mix with compatible solution (see product information) and infuse over 15–20 min. May also be given by continuous infusion
ranitidine HCl (Zantac)	**Oral** (for duodenal ulcer and benign gastric ulcer): 300 mg od hs or 150 mg bid in a.m. and hs. (For maintenance tx for duodenal ulcer and benign gastric ulcer): 150 mg hs. (For reflux esophagitis): Acute tx: 300 mg hs, or 150 mg bid, taken a.m. and hs for up to 8 weeks. In pts with moderate to severe esophagitis, increase to 150 mg qid for up to 12 weeks. Long-term management: 150 mg bid. (Tx of NSAID-induced lesion and GI symptoms and prevention of recurrence): 150 mg bid for 8–12 weeks. (Zollinger-Ellison syndrome): 150 mg tid, initially; adjust dosage to needs of pt. Doses up to 6 g/day have been well tolerated	• **PO:** Give without regard to meals. Do not give antacids within 1 h • **IV:** For direct IV, follow agency policy re: certification. Rate: Administer over at least 5 min. For intermittent infusion, dilute according to product information and give over 15–20 min. May also be given by continuous infusion
	IM: 50 mg q6–8h. **IV:** Injection, 50 mg q6–8h; intermittent infusion, 50 mg q6–8h	*(cont'd on next page)*

Table 59.5 (continued)
The antiulcer drugs: Drug doses

Drug Generic name (Trade names)	Dosage	Nursing alert
B. Drugs That Decrease Acid Secretion (cont'd)		
1. Histamine$_2$ (H$_2$) Blockers (cont'd)		
famotidine (Pepcid)	**Oral** (duodenal ulcer/acute tx): 40 mg hs for 4–8 weeks. Maintenance tx: 20 mg hs for up to 6–12 months. (Benign gastric ulcer): 50 mg hs for 9–12 weeks. (Zollinger-Ellison syndrome): 20 mg q6h. Adjust to needs of pt. Doses up to 800 mg/day have been administered. (Gastro-esophageal reflux disease): **Oral:** 20 mg bid **IV:** 20 mg q12h For renal insufficiency, consult manufacturer's information	• **PO:** May be given with food and/or antacids. Shake suspension well prior to use. Instruct pt to use calibrated device (not household spoon) to measure dose • **IV:** For direct IV, follow agency policy re: certification. Rate: Administer over 2 min. For intermittent infusion, dilute according to product information and give over 15–20 min
nizatidine (Axid)	**Oral** (duodenal or gastric ulcer): 300 mg hs, or 150 mg bid. Maintenance: 150 mg hs for 6–12 months. (Gastroesophageal reflux disease): 150 mg bid For renal insufficiency, consult manufacturer's information	• Ideal dosage schedule is hs, but dose may be divided bid. Do not give within 1 h of antacids • Instruct pt to use calibrated device (not household spoon) to measure dose
2. Anticholinergic Drug		
pirenzepine (Gastrozepin)	**Oral** (duodenal ulcer and nonmalignant gastric ulcer): 50 mg bid, a.m. and p.m. In pts with more pronounced symptoms, 50 mg tid can be given. In pts requiring long-term tx, pirenzepine can be given continuously for up to 3 months	• Best taken 30 min ac
3. Prostaglandin Analogue		
misoprostol (Cytotec)	**Oral** (tx and prevention of NSAID-induced gastroduodenal ulcers): 400–800 µg/day in divided doses. (Tx of duodenal ulcer): 800 µg/day for 4 weeks in 2 or 4 equally divided doses (i.e., 200 µg qid or 400 µg bid). Last dose should be taken hs with food. Tx should be continued for a total of 4 weeks unless healing in less time has been documented by endoscopic examination For geriatric or renally impaired pts, consult manufacturer's information	• Best taken with food; may reduce incidence of diarrhea and abdominal cramping. Do not take with antacids containing magnesium

Table 59.5 (continued)
The antiulcer drugs: Drug doses

Drug Generic name (Trade names)	Dosage	Nursing alert

B. Drugs That Decrease Acid Secretion (cont'd)

4. Proton Pump Inhibitors

Drug	Dosage	Nursing alert
omeprazole magnesium (Losec, Prilosec)	**Oral** (duodenal ulcer/acute tx): 20 mg od. Healing usually occurs within 2 weeks. For pts not healed after this initial course, an additional 2 weeks of tx is recommended. Refractory pts: 20–40 mg od. Healing usually achieved within 4 weeks. (Gastric ulcer/acute tx): 20 mg od. Healing usually occurs within 4 weeks. Refractory pts: 40 mg od. Healing usually achieved within 8 weeks. (Reflux esophagitis/acute tx): 20 mg od; 40 mg od for refractory pts. Maintenance: 20 mg od. (Zollinger-Ellison syndrome): Initially, 60 mg od; titrate to needs of pt. Doses up to 120 mg tid have been administered *H. pylori*-associated peptic ulcer disease: Consult information at the top of this Table	• May be taken with antacids. Do not crush or chew capsules. Best if taken ac, preferably in a.m. With doses > 80 mg, divide for bid dosing
lansoprazole (Prevacid)	**Oral** (duodenal/gastric ulcer): 15 mg/day before breakfast. (Reflux esophagitis): 30 mg/day before breakfast for 4–8 weeks	• Give 30 min ac. Capsules should be swallowed whole

C. Drugs That Reduce the Effects of Secreted Gastric Acid and Pepsin

1. Antacids

Drug	Dosage	Nursing alert
aluminum hydroxide (Amphogel)	**Oral** (gastric and duodenal ulcers to relieve pain): Liquid containing 320 mg/5 mL, 10 mL 5–6x/day between meals and hs. Tablets containing 600 mg, 1 tablet 5–6x/day	• Shake liquid preparation well prior to use. Instruct pt to use calibrated measure (not household spoon) to measure dose. Tablets should be chewed thoroughly, followed by water • Usual schedule, 1 h ac/3 h pc and hs • May be combined with magnesium antacid to reduce constipation. May contain sodium; check label if sodium-restricted diet
magnesium hydroxide, milk of magnesia	**Oral** (gastric and duodenal ulcers to relieve pain): 5–10 mL qid	• Tablets should be chewed thoroughly, followed by water. Shake liquid preparations well prior to use. Instruct pt to use calibrated measure (not household spoon) to measure dose • NB: Used as laxative with higher doses (i.e., 30–60 mL). May be combined with aluminum to prevent diarrhea

(cont'd on next page)

Table 59.5 (continued)
The antiulcer drugs: Drug doses

Drug Generic name (Trade names)	Dosage	Nursing alert
C. Drugs That Reduce the Effects of Secreted Gastric Acid and Pepsin (cont'd)		
1. Antacids (cont'd)		
aluminum and magnesium hydroxide (Maalox, Mylanta, Gelusil, Riopan)	**Oral** (gastric and duodenal ulcers to relieve pain): 10–20 mL ac and hs, or more often prn	• Tablets should be chewed thoroughly, followed by water. Shake liquid preparations well prior to use. Instruct pt to use calibrated measure (not household spoon) to measure dose • NB: Used as laxative with higher doses (i.e., 30–60 mL). May be combined with aluminum to prevent diarrhea
2. Gastroduodenal Cytoprotective Agent		
sucralfate (Carafate, Sulcrate)	**Oral** (duodenal and gastric ulcers): *Adults:* 1 g qid, 1 h ac and hs, on an empty stomach. For duodenal ulcer, may give 2 g bid, on waking and hs on an empty stomach. (Prophylaxis of GI hemorrhage due to stress ulceration): 1 g orally or via N/G tube 4–6x/day	• Best on empty stomach, 1 h ac. Do not give with antacid; separate by 30 min prior to or 1 h after drug dosage • Do not crush or chew tablets. Shake suspension well prior to use. Flush N/G tube with water to prevent clogging

CHAPTER 60

Drugs for the Treatment of Chronic Inflammatory Bowel Disease

Topics Discussed
● Chronic inflammatory bowel disease (CIBD): Ulcerative colitis and Crohn's disease
● Drug treatment of CIBD: Anti-inflammatories, immunosuppressants, antibiotics, histamine-release inhibitors
● Drugs to assist in the normalization of bowel habits: Narcotics, anticholinergics, bile acid sequestrants
● Nursing management

Drugs Discussed
5-aminosalicylic acid (ah-meen-oh-sal-ih-**sill**-ik)
amoxicillin (ah-mox-ee-**sill**-in)
azathioprine (az-ah-**thye**-oh-preen)
betamethasone (bay-tah-**meth**-ah-sone)

chloramphenicol (klor-am-**fen**-ih-kole)
cholestyramine (kole-es-**teer**-ah-meen)
cotrimoxazole (koe-trim-**ox**-ah-zole)
cromolyn (**kroe**-moe-lin)
diphenoxylate—atropine (dye-fen-**ox**-ee-late **at**-troe-peen)
hydrocortisone (hye-droe-**kor**-tih-sone)
loperamide (loe-**per**-ah-myde)
mercaptopurine (mer-kap-toe-**pyoor**-een)
mesalamine (mee-**sal**-ah-meen)
methylprednisolone (meth-il-pred-**niss**-oh-lone)
metronidazole (met-roe-**nye**-dah-zole)
olsalazine (ole-**sal**-ah-zeen)
prednisone (**pred**-nih-sone)
sulfasalazine (sul-fah-**sal**-ah-zeen)
tetracycline (tet-rah-**sye**-kleen)

Chronic Inflammatory Bowel Disease

Chronic inflammatory bowel disease (CIBD) may be divided into ulcerative colitis and Crohn's disease. With an annual incidence in North America and Europe of between five and ten new cases per 100 000 population for ulcerative colitis and three to five new cases per 100 000 for Crohn's disease, these conditions are not among the most common medical disorders. However, for those patients afflicted, CIBD can be devastating, not only alter-

ing lifestyle but also presenting the prospect of death. Nursing these individuals presents special problems. It is important that nurses understand the nature of the two diseases and the drugs used to treat them if they are to provide appropriate nursing care.

Ulcerative colitis and Crohn's disease have many similarities. They are both ulcerating inflammatory diseases of the intestine that often present with diarrhea, rectal bleeding, abdominal pain, fever or weight loss. The two conditions have identical extracolonic manifestations that include arthritis, ankylosing spondylitis, eye damage,

Clinical Challenge

Consider this clinical challenge as you read through this chapter. The response to the challenge appears on page 712.

Denise is a 27-year-old woman who has recently attended your wellness clinic and joined the chronicity support group. Two years ago she was diagnosed with Crohn's disease: she experienced severe abdominal pain, anorexia, diarrhea, fever and weight loss.

Initially, Denise was treated with sulfasalazine but developed a severe skin reaction. Prednisone was tried with some success, but she became increasingly concerned with the adverse effects she was experiencing and the potential long-term effects of steroid therapy. She has had surgery, with a temporary colostomy. During one of the group sessions, Denise makes the following statements: "I failed at drug therapy so I guess there is no hope for me to be cured"; "I'm tired of people blaming me for my disease; whenever I have a flare-up of symptoms, my friends and family ask me what I did wrong. They think I don't handle stress well."

1. What information about Crohn's disease and drug treatment would you use to address Denise's statements?
2. What is the relationship between stress and inflammatory bowel disease?

venous thromboses, skin problems and kidney, liver and pancreas deterioration. Ulcerative colitis differs from Crohn's disease in that it involves only the mucosa of the large intestine. In contrast, Crohn's disease affects the entire gastrointestinal (GI) wall. Furthermore, although the ileum and colon are its most common sites, Crohn's disease can also be found in the stomach, duodenum, jejunum and rectum.

Current research indicates that genetic factors may play an important role in the incidence of these two diseases. Although stress increases the symptoms of both and may inhibit healing, it is not the cause.

Drug Treatment of Chronic Inflammatory Bowel Disease

Drug therapy of ulcerative colitis or Crohn's disease involves the use of anti-inflammatory agents, immunosuppressants and antibiotics or antibacterials. No drug is curative, and there is some doubt

whether treatment even alters the course of these diseases, especially Crohn's disease. The use of these drugs, alone or in combination, is based on the assumption that ulcerative colitis and Crohn's disease are inflammatory disorders that may have an immunological or infectious basis, or both. Other forms of drug treatment include the use of cromolyn to reduce the release of histamine from mast cells in the GI tract and narcotics to treat diarrhea symptomatically.

It is not the place of this book to discuss other forms of therapy. Readers should refer to a medical-surgical nursing text to familiarize themselves with the use of elemental diets and parenteral hyperalimentation, since they may form an important component of complete therapeutic regimen for patients with CIBD. Readers are also encouraged to seek information on ostomy procedures, as temporary or permanent ileostomy and colostomy may be required if drug treatment is not successful. Knowledge of local community support groups is helpful. Living with unpredictable chronic illness can tax both the patient and the family.

Anti-Inflammatory Agents

Sulfasalazine (Azulfidine®, Salazopyrin®, SAS-500®)

Mechanism of action and pharmacologic effects. Sulfasalazine is split by bacteria in the lower colon into sulfapyridine, a sulfonamide antibacterial, and mesalamine (5-aminosalicylic acid, or 5-ASA), an anti-inflammatory chemical. It is believed that sulfasalazine owes its therapeutic value to the actions of the mesalamine component.

Therapeutic uses. Sulfasalazine is indicated for adjunctive therapy in the treatment of severe ulcerative colitis, proctitis or distal ulcerative colitis, and Crohn's disease. It is especially used for chronic administration. Sulfasalazine is contraindicated in patients who are hypersensitive to sulfonamides or salicylates. It should also not be used in infants under age two.

Adverse effects. The common adverse effects of sulfasalazine are nausea and vomiting, anorexia, arthralgia, skin rashes, erythema, pruritus, urticaria, fever, headache and apparently reversible oligospermia. Sulfasalazine may also cause methemoglobinemia, hemolytic anemia, megaloblastic anemia, leukopenia and cyanosis.

Table 60.1 lists the clinically significant drug interactions with sulfasalazine.

Olsalazine (Dipentum®)

Mechanism of action and pharmacologic effects. The conversion of olsalazine to 5-aminosalicylic acid (5-ASA) in the colon is similar to that of sulfasalazine. On a weight basis, olsalazine delivers twice the amount of 5-ASA to the colon, compared with sulfasalazine. There is no residual carrier molecule (sulfapyridine) following olsalazine administration.

Therapeutic uses. Olsalazine has been approved for the long-term maintenance of patients with ulcerative colitis in remission. It is also used in the treatment of acute ulcerative colitis of mild to moderate severity, with or without the concomitant use of steroids. Olsalazine is contraindicated in patients who are hypersensitive to salicylates.

Adverse effects. In general, olsalazine is well tolerated. Its adverse effects appear to be mild and transient. The drug appears to induce loose stools in approximately fifteen percent of patients. This incidence may be reduced if the dose is increased slowly and taken with food.

Mesalamine, 5-Aminosalicylic Acid (Asacol®, Pentasa®, Salofalk®)

Mechanism of action and pharmacologic effects. As previously noted, sulfasalazine is a combination of sulfapyridine linked to mesalamine (5-ASA). Intestinal bacteria in the ileum and colon break sulfasalazine down to these two components. Sulfapyridine is absorbed and metabolized in the liver, whereas mesalamine is excreted in the feces. Mesalamine is responsible for the anti-inflammatory effects and sulfapyridine for many of the adverse effects of sulfasalazine. It is therefore reasonable to expect that 5-ASA should be as effective as sulfasalazine, but with a reduced incidence of adverse effects.

For 5-ASA to work, however, it must be delivered in high concentration to the site of inflammation. This means the use of controlled-release formulations that protect the drug from dissolution until it reaches the inflamed section of the intestine. Plain 5-ASA tablets are not effective because they dissolve quickly and the drug is rapidly and completely absorbed from the upper GI tract. If, on the other hand, 5-ASA is released in the colon from a controlled-release product, it is poorly absorbed

---

Table 60.1
Sulfasalazine Drug interactions

Drug	Interaction
Digoxin	• Sulfasalazine may decrease the absorption of digoxin. Pts receiving both drugs should be observed carefully for evidence of reduced digoxin effect

and able to treat inflammation in this part of the intestine.

To provide the concentrations of 5-ASA required for effective anti-inflammatory activity, pharmaceutical companies developed oral formulations that release the drug close to the site of inflammation. Several manufacturers have developed different galenic preparations of mesalamine, designed to release the drug slowly as it progresses through the intestine, or quickly at specific sites, such as the colon.

For example, Asacol® is formulated to withstand pH values below 7 and to release its drug in the distal part of the ileum and colon. Salofalk®, on the other hand, begins to release its drug higher in the intestine because its coating starts to dissolve at pH values above 5.5. Pentasa® tablets disintegrate in the stomach to liberate individually coated microgranules which release 5-ASA throughout the GI tract. The release of 5-ASA from Pentasa® is relatively slow in the acidic conditions of the proximal small intestine and more rapid at the high pH found in the distal ileum and colon. Consistent with its ability to release 5-ASA slowly through the entire intestinal tract, Pentasa® is the only mesalamine product specifically indicated as an adjunct in the management of mild-to-moderate Crohn's disease.

Because each of these products has its own unique drug delivery system, they are not interchangeable. Each product has a place in therapeutics and each meets the needs of a different group of patients, depending on the sites of intestinal inflammation.

Therapeutic uses. Mesalamine is indicated as adjunctive therapy in the treatment of ulcerative colitis. As indicated above, each product is specifically designed to release its active ingredient in different portions of the intestinal tract to treat varying areas of inflammation.

Rectal suppositories and a rectal suspension are also available. The suppositories are indicated in the management of ulcerative proctitis and as adjunctive therapy in more extensive distal ulcerative colitis. The rectal suspension is used in the management of distal ulcerative colitis extending to the splenic flexure including refractory distal ulcerative colitis. In addition, the rectal suspension is approved as adjunctive therapy in more exten-

sive disease as well as for the prevention of relapse in distal ulcerative colitis. Long-term mesalamine therapy may be necessary to prevent recurrent relapses of active colitis.

These products are contraindicated in patients with a history of sensitivity to salicylates and in patients under the age of two years.

Adverse effects. Because mesalamine does not contain the sulfonamide sulfapyridine, its unwanted effects are less frequent and less severe than those of sulfasalazine. Occasionally patients may have mild nausea, colic or headache.

Corticosteroids

Mechanism of action and pharmacologic effects. The pharmacology of corticosteroids and the nursing actions related to their use are presented in Chapter 66. The anti-inflammatory effects of glucocorticoids account, at least in part, for their effectiveness in CIBD. Their immunosuppressive actions may also play a role in their ability to placate the irritated intestine.

Therapeutic uses. Corticosteroids are indicated in ulcerative colitis to reduce acute inflammation. Their value in preventing recurrence is still debatable. Once a decision is made to use corticosteroid treatment, the initial dose should be sufficient to produce remission, and therapy should be maintained for a period of time to ensure success. Thereafter, an attempt should be made to withdraw the drug.

Corticosteroid enemas may be effective if the condition is restricted to the left side of the colon. Their use greatly reduces the risk of systemic adverse effects. Hydrocortisone (Cortenema®), methylprednisolone (Medrol Enpak®) and betamethasone (Betnesol®) are available in enema form. The enema can be attempted once nightly for two to four weeks. If this treatment does not prove successful, oral steroid therapy should be introduced. On the other hand, success within this time may be followed by enema treatment every other night for seven days and then every third night for an additional week. The intermittent use of corticosteroid enemas may be successful in the management of many patients with mild chronic ulcerative colitis.

Moderate inflammatory bowel disease may need oral corticosteroid treatment. Although many steroids could be used, prednisone is most often prescribed because it is effective and usually cheap. Triamcinolone is not recommended because effective doses produce profound nitrogen loss.

If the patient presents for the first time in acute distress and requires hospitalization, intravenous corticosteroid treatment, such as hydrocortisone sodium succinate, may be required.

Adverse effects. Caution should be used in prescribing corticosteroids, which are double-edged swords. Although they can provide dramatic relief for patients, these drugs also produce many adverse effects, including pituitary-adrenal suppression, increased susceptibility to infection, osteoporosis, hyperglycemia, "buffalo hump," "moon face" and the possibility of psychotic disturbances. Their systemic use is justified only after other treatments have failed. The adverse effects and drug interactions of corticosteroids are presented in greater detail in Chapter 66.

Immunosuppressants

Azathioprine (Imuran®) and Mercaptopurine (Purinethol®)

Azathioprine and mercaptopurine are immunosuppressants and reduce the proliferation of B-lymphocytes, T-lymphocytes and macrophages. Their use is based on the belief that CIBD may be the result, at least in part, of an immunological disorder. Azathioprine and mercaptopurine are used most often with corticosteroids in Crohn's disease because they reduce the dose of steroid required.

The adverse effects of these drugs are attributable to their ability to impair cell multiplication.

In addition to their immunosuppressant effects, azathioprine and mercaptopurine can depress bone marrow and produce pancreatitis, alopecia and rashes. These effects are rarely seen with the low dosages of the drugs used to treat Crohn's disease.

Table 60.2 lists the clinically significant drug interactions with immunosuppressants.

Antibiotics

The use of antibiotics or antibacterials in the treatment of chronic inflammatory bowel disease is based on the premise that an infectious agent may be the cause of the disorder. The evidence to support this view is, at best, tenuous. Ampicillin, the tetracyclines, trimethoprim plus sulfamethoxazole (Bactrim®, Septra®) and chloramphenicol have been tried, with questionable success. Metronidazole (Flagyl®) is indicated in the treatment of Crohn's disease not responsive to sulfasalazine.

Nurses should identify and be familiar with the specific drugs used in the various sites and the adverse effects of each. The pharmacology and the related nursing responsibilities of each drug are presented in Unit 3.

Histamine-Release Inhibitor

Cromolyn/Sodium Cromoglycate (Nalcrom®)

Cromolyn, or sodium cromoglycate, reduces the release of histamine from mast cells. It is marketed in an oral dosage form (Nalcrom®) for the treatment of food allergies and CIBD. The initial dose for adults is 200 mg four times daily before meals.

Cromolyn produces few adverse effects. Unfortunately, it is often ineffective; comparative studies have shown cromolyn to be less effective

Table 60.2
Immunosuppressants: Drug interactions

Drug	Interaction
Allopurinol	• Allopurinol interacts with both azathioprine and 6-mercaptopurine (6-MP). Azathioprine is metabolized first to 6-MP, which is then converted to inactive products. Allopurinol increases 6-MP blood levels by reducing its metabolism. If allopurinol is given, the dose of azathioprine or 6-MP should be reduced to approximately 25%–33% of the usual amount administered

than sulfasalazine. Some patients respond to cromolyn, but more improve on sulfasalazine. Cromolyn must be used more extensively before we can establish its place in the treatment of CIBD. It now appears justified only in those patients who either have not responded to, or are allergic to, sulfasalazine.

Drugs to Assist in the Normalization of Bowel Habits

Drugs can be used to treat the diarrhea of CIBD. However, this form of treatment is secondary to the more specific therapy outlined earlier. In addition, antidiarrheal drugs should not be used in acute colitis because they can precipitate toxic dilatation of the colon under these circumstances.

Narcotics

Mechanism of action and pharmacologic effects. Narcotics have a constipating action because they decrease the propulsive motility of the colon. Diphenoxylate (Lomotil®) and loperamide (Imodium®) stimulate narcotic receptors in the intestine. These drugs are preferred over other narcotics because their effects are largely restricted to the intestinal tract. Diphenoxylate is poorly absorbed, and this results in minimal systemic effects. Loperamide is also poorly absorbed from the GI tract and does not cross the blood-brain barrier. As a result, it has few systemic effects and does not cause drug dependence. For this reason, many countries do not classify loperamide as a narcotic.

Therapeutic uses. Diphenoxylate has been on the market for many years and is the favourite of many physicians. Loperamide was introduced later; it is at least as effective as diphenoxylate. These drugs should be used as adjuncts to rehydration therapy for the symptomatic control of chronic diarrhea associated with CIBD. Diphenoxylate must be kept out of the reach of children because accidental overdosage may cause severe or even fatal respiratory depression. The use of diphenoxylate or loperamide is not recommended in children under two years of age.

Adverse effects. The systemic adverse effects of diphenoxylate include nausea, drowsiness, lethargy, sedation, respiratory depression, dizziness, vomiting, anorexia, pruritus and skin eruptions. These reactions are characteristic of most narcotics. They are less likely to occur when a poorly absorbed drug like diphenoxylate is administered. However, abdominal bloating and cramps, paralytic ileus and toxic megacolon can also occur if care is not taken to monitor the patient. The most frequent effect of loperamide is constipation, a sign of overdosage. Loperamide can also produce toxic megacolon.

Table 60.3 lists the clinically significant drug interactions with diphenoxylate.

Anticholinergics

Anticholinergic drugs can also be used to reduce diarrhea. Their actions and the nursing management related to their use are discussed in detail in Chapter 28. Propantheline, marketed as Pro-Banthine®, is an example of an anticholinergic. A dose of 15 mg or more of this drug has been used to decrease the incidence and degree of diarrhea. However, all anticholinergics produce a variety of adverse effects that include dry mouth, absence of saliva, lack of sweat, mydriasis, cycloplegia and tachycardia. Under these circumstances, it might be hard for patients to remember why they took the drug in the first place.

Table 60.3
Diphenoxylate: Drug interactions

Drug	Interaction
CNS depressants	• Diphenoxylate may potentiate the actions of CNS depressants (e.g., barbiturates, benzodiazepines, phenothiazines, narcotics, ethanol)
Monoamine oxidase inhibitors	• MAOIs can precipitate a hypertensive crisis in pts receiving diphenoxylate

Bile Acid Sequestrants

Cholestyramine (Questran®)

Cholestyramine is a nonabsorbed resin that sequesters bile acids and may be of considerable assistance to the patient after ileal resection. The pharmacology of this drug, together with its drug interactions and doses, is discussed in Chapter 42.

Nursing Management

Table 60.4 describes the nursing management of the patient receiving drugs for the treatment of chronic inflammatory bowel disease. Dosage details for individual drugs are given in Table 60.5 (pages 713–714).

Table 60.4
Nursing management of drugs for chronic inflammatory bowel disease

Assessment of risk vs. benefit	Patient data	• Physician should determine whether severity of disease warrants use of drugs in this class • *Allergy:* Assess for allergy to sulfonamides or salicylates (contraindicates use of sulfasalazine, mesalamine and olsalazine) • Assess to establish baseline VS, general state of health, liver and renal function • *Pregnancy:* Risk category varies with class. For category C (animal studies show adverse effects to fetus but human data are unknown or insufficient), benefits may be acceptable despite risks. This may change near term
	Drug data	• Select drugs based on severity of symptoms and hx of related allergies • *Some serious drug interactions:* Confer with pharmacist • Most serious adverse effects are allergic and/or photosensitivity reactions and hematologic effects of bone marrow depression. Steroids have significant long-term adverse effects
Implementation	Rights of administration	• Using the "rights" helps prevent errors of administration
	Right route	• Give by oral and rectal routes
	Nursing therapeutics	• *Emotional support:* Chronic illness with unpredictable flare-ups challenge both pt and family. Drugs may not be successful and pt may have to adapt to temporary or permanent ileostomy or colostomy. Explore possibility of community support group for education and social support
	Patient/family teaching	• Pt's need for information may be influenced by length of time required for tx or limited by serious illness • Compliance and follow-up are essential for successful tx of CIBD; review principles of pt education in Chapter 3 • Explain that success may require trials with various drugs • Teach pt to avoid exposure to sun and to use clothing or sun-blocking agents • Pts/families should know warning signs/symptoms of possible toxicities of these drugs. Report immediately: rash, fever, sore throat, diarrhea, nausea, vomiting, unusual bleeding or bruising • *Discuss possibility of pregnancy:* Advise pt to notify physician; discuss birth control methods *(cont'd on next page)*

Table 60.4 (continued)
Nursing management of drugs for chronic inflammatory bowel disease

Outcomes	Monitoring of progress	*Continually monitor:*
		• Clinical response indicating tx success (reduction in signs/symptoms)
		• Signs/symptoms of adverse reactions; document and report immediately to physician
		• With long-term tx, periodic blood tests to monitor bone marrow function may be ordered

---

Response to Clinical Challenge

1. The etiology of Crohn's disease is not known, but genetic factors are associated with it. Drug treatment is based on the severity and type of symptoms. For some patients who can tolerate the drugs' actions, including the nontherapeutic effects, drugs may be successful. Others require surgery, including temporary ostomies while the bowel heals and permanent ostomies when significant portions of the bowel are removed.

2. Although the stress response can increase symptoms and delay healing, stress alone is not the cause of inflammatory bowel disorders.

Further Reading

Doughty D. What you need to know about inflammatory bowel disease. *Am J Nurs* 1994(7):24–31.

Phillips S, Warren J. Supporting the patient with inflammatory bowel disease. *Nurs Times* 1995;91(27):38–39.

Rhodes J, et al. Inflammatory bowel disease management. Some thoughts on future drug developments. *Drugs* 1997;53(2):189–194.

Table 60.5
Treatment of chronic inflammatory bowel disease: Drug doses

Drug Generic name (Trade names)	Dosage	Nursing alert
A. Anti-Inflammatory Agents		
sulfasalazine (Azulfidine, Salazopyrin, SAS-500)	**Oral:** *Adults* (severe, acute attacks): 1–2 g tid–qid. (Prophylaxis): 1 g bid–tid. *Children 25–35 kg:* 500 mg tid; *35–50 kg:* 1 g bid–tid. (Prophylaxis): *25–35 kg:* 500 mg ibid–tid; *35–50 kg:* 500 mg bid **Rectal:** *Adults* (proctitis and distal ulcerative colitis): 1 enema (3 g) daily, preferably hs	•**PO:** Ensure adequate fluid intake (1–1.5 L/day) to prevent crystalluria. Shake suspension well prior to use. Give uncoated tabs with food to minimize gastric irritation. Do not crush or chew enteric-coated form. Slowly increase dose during first weeks of tx to reduce side effects. Promote fluid intake to reduce side effects •**Rectal:** Review self-administration of enema with pt. Solution should be retained
olsalazine sodium (Dipentum)	**Oral:** *Adults:* Increase gradually over 1 week starting with 500 mg/day. If no response is achieved with 2 g and drug is well tolerated, dose may be increased to 3 g daily. A single dose should not exceed 1 g. Usual adult dose (including elderly): Acute, 500 mg qid; prophylaxis, 500 mg bid. *Children:* No specific dose has been defined. Adjust dosage to pt's weight, age	•Take drug at regular intervals with meals
mesalamine, 5-aminosalicylic acid (Asacol)	**Oral:** *Adults:* 2–8 tablets (800–3200 mg) per day in divided doses. Severe active disease: Dose may be increased to 12 tablets (4800 mg) daily	•Do not substitute for other mesalamine products. Do not crush or chew enteric-coated tabs
mesalamine, 5-aminosalicylic acid (Pentasa)	**Oral** (ulcerative colitis): Initially, 0.5 g qid (daily dose, 2 g); increase prn to 1 g qid. (Crohn's disease): 1 g qid for mild to moderate disease	•Take before meals and hs with fluids. Do not chew, break or crush before swallowing. Do not substitute for other mesalamine products
mesalamine, 5-aminosalicylic acid (Salofalk)	**Oral** (acute ulcerative colitis): 1000 mg tid–qid **Rectal:** Two 250-mg or one 500-mg suppository bid or tid. Rectal suspension (acute episodes): *Adults:* 1 unit-dose (4 g/60 g 5-ASA) hs, retained during entire rest period. (Prevention of relapse): 2 g/60 g administered hs and retained during entire rest period	•Do not substitute for other mesalamine products •Instruct pt in self-administration of suppositories and enema

(cont'd on next page)

Table 60.5 (continued)
Treatment of chronic inflammatory bowel disease: Drug doses

Drug Generic name (Trade names)	Dosage	Nursing alert
B. Corticosteroids		
prednisone	**Oral:** Adults: Usually, 40 mg/day in 4 equal doses for 4–6 days. Reduce by 5 mg/week to 20 mg/day. Maintain for 1 month, then withdraw at rate of 5 mg/week	• Give with food to reduce gastric irritation. Shake oral solution prior to use. Instruct pt to use calibrated device (not household spoon) to measure dose
hydrocortisone enema (Cortenema)	**Rectal:** 1 retention enema, containing 100 mg hydrocortisone in 60 mL, hs for 2–3 weeks, and every second day thereafter	• Instruct pt in self-administration of enema. Solution should be retained for up to 8 h, if possible
methylprednisolone retention enema (Medrol Enpak)	**Rectal:** 1 retention enema containing 40 mg methylprednisolone acetate, od–bid	• As above
betamethasone disodium phosphate (Betnesol)	**Rectal:** 1 retention enema containing 5 mg betamethasone/100 mL, nightly for 2–4 weeks	• As above
C. Immunosuppressant Drug		
azathioprine (Imuran)	**Oral/parenteral:** Adults: 2 mg/kg/day or 100–200 mg/day	• Give with meals. Dose may be divided to reduce nausea
D. Narcotic Antidiarrheal Drugs		
diphenoxylate HCl + atropine sulfate(Lomotil)	**Oral:** Adults: Usually, 5 mg tid–qid. Max. recommended dose, 20 mg/24 h in divided doses. Adjust dose downward as soon as initial control of symptoms is accomplished	• May be taken with food. May crush tabs. Shake liquid preparations prior to use. Instruct pt to use calibrated measure (not household spoon) to ensure accuracy
loperamide HCl (Imodium)	**Oral:** Adults (acute diarrhea): 4 mg initially, followed by 2 mg after each unformed stool. Daily dosage should not exceed 16 mg. (Chronic diarrhea): 4 mg initially, followed by 2 mg after each unformed stool until diarrhea is controlled; thereafter, dosage should be reduced to meet individual requirements. Children (acute or chronic diarrhea): Use only with the advice of a physician. 2–5 years old (10–20 kg): 1 mg tid; 5–8 years (20–30 kg): 2 mg bid; 8–12 years (> 30 kg): 2 mg tid	• Shake solution well prior to use. Instruct pt to use calibrated measure (not household spoon) to ensure accuracy. NB: Solution contains alcohol

Laxatives and Antidiarrheal Drugs

Topics Discussed

- The bowels
- Drugs that act within the intestinal lumen
- Antibiotics/antibacterials
- Drugs that act on the gut wall
- Drug treatment of constipation: Bulk laxatives, osmotic laxatives, stool softeners, chemical stimulants
- Nursing management

Drugs Discussed

agar (**ag**-ahr)
ampicillin (am-pih-**sill**-in)
bisacodyl (bis-ah-**koe**-dill)
bismuth subsalicylate (**biss**-muth sub-sal-**iss**-ih-late)
cholestyramine (kole-es-**teer**-ah-meen)
cotrimoxazole (koe-trim-**ox**-ah-zole)
diphenoxylate–atropine (dye-fen-**ox**-ee-late **at**-troe-peen)
docusate (**dok**-yoo-sate)
doxycycline (dox-ee-**sye**-kleen)
kaolin (**kay**-oh-lin)
karaya (kah-**ray**-ah)
loperamide (loe-**per**-ah-myde)
magnesium hydroxide (mag-**nee**-zee-um hye-**drok**-side)
magnesium sulfate (mag-**nee**-zee-um **sul**-fate)
pectin (**peck**-tin)
phenolphthalein (fee-nole-**thal**-een)
psyllium (**sill**-ee-yum)
trimethoprim–sulfamethoxazole (try-**meth**-oh-prim sul-fah-meth-**ox**-ah-zole)

Clinical Challenge

Consider this clinical challenge as you read through this chapter. The response to the challenge appears on page 726.

You are planning to travel to a foreign country and are concerned that you may experience constipation due to changes in daily activity, and/or diarrhea related to changes in your diet.

Conduct personal research at a pharmacy and decide which laxative and antidiarrheal drug you would take with you.

The Bowels

The actions of the bowels have weighed heavily on the collective mind of humankind since the beginning of time. No organ system has been the subject of so much introspection as the lower regions of the intestines. They have been coddled and cursed, irrigated and irritated, placated and purged — all in the interest of ensuring the daily bowel movement.

Our fascination with colonic function is understandable. Despite their distance from the brain, the bowels can be real attention-getters. Everyone has had the experience of enduring several feces-free days. The profound sense of relief that follows that first bowel movement is an experience to be treasured.

Today's frenetic lifestyle presents the colon with ever greater challenges. People travel more now than ever before, and travel often upsets the colonic humours, presenting problems of economic and social significance. Many an executive has flown half-way around the world to chair a meeting, only to be rendered nonoperational by a seemingly continuous flow of stools. Others have experienced just the opposite effect: in these individuals, travel pulls tight the strings of the anal sphincter. Still others suffer alternately the bullet of constipation and the torrent of diarrhea. There is nothing quite like flying from Los Angeles to New York on a Monday, only to have one's bowels arrive with a clap of thunder on Friday evening, just in time for your after-dinner speech at the wind-up banquet. Experienced travellers cannot be blamed if they are unsure whether to buy a bit of internal dynamite to break the logjam on days three to four, or a medicated cork to stem the tide on day five.

Frequency of bowel movements and consistency of stools have also been discussed for centuries. Folklore holds that one, and only one, bowel movement per day is essential for good health. Fortunately, this is not true, or many of us would be quite ill. In one study of 1100 post office employees, it was found that only 53 had regular daily bowel movements. Obviously, other explanations must be sought for the failure of the mail to arrive on time! Lest we snicker unfairly at the posties, a survey of 440 nurses yielded essentially the same results. Other studies have shown that 99% of people have between three movements per week and three per day. It is the nurse's responsibility to explain this fact to patients. If this is understood, much of the perceived need for laxatives or antidiarrheal preparations will disappear.

It is easier to count stools than to measure their consistency. Yet it is just as important to know something of their nature. Forcing a cardiac patient to strain in producing a hard torpedo can be just as dangerous as neglecting the patient with liquid diarrhea as he quickly dehydrates. Although it may be convenient simply to ask the patient about the physical nature of his stools, it may also be unreliable. Most patients are not experienced stool gazers and may have little to compare against their own efforts. Thus an individual may claim, incorrectly, that his movements are not hard if he has been used to clearing cannon balls. Nurses should be well-experienced stool watchers and, unpleasant as this may be, are often in the best position to study their consistency.

It must be apparent to even the casual observer that laxatives and antidiarrheal preparations are overused. Patients must be advised that the daily bowel movement is not sacred. Deviations from this pattern may be normal. There are, however, indications for the use of drugs that modify the bowels. The means by which these agents produce their effects, and their appropriate uses, form the basis for the rest of this chapter.

Functional Diarrhea

It is important to differentiate between functional and organic diarrhea. The former condition requires minimal investigation; the latter an extensive workup. The use of an antidiarrheal preparation to treat organic disease may initially alleviate the patient's symptoms, but delay more appropriate treatment.

The causes of diarrhea may vary from patient to patient. They include: (1) increased water arriving at the colon, (2) decreased colonic water reabsorption, (3) increased pressure gradient from cecum to anus, or (4) decreased sigmoid segmentation. The last-named cause is best understood when it is recognized that the sigmoid section of the colon acts as a sphincter or valve, regulating the passage of material to the rectum. Decreased sigmoid segmentation reduces the valve effect and increases the volume of material presented to the rectum. Drugs given to treat diarrhea act to reduce either the volume of material arriving at the rectum or the peristaltic activity of the intestine. In either case, the urge to defecate is reduced.

Drugs That Act Within the Intestinal Lumen

Psyllium (Hydrocil®, Metamucil®)

Psyllium is capable of treating constipation or diarrhea. In the latter situation it absorbs water from the developing feces in the intestine to form a gel, thereby reducing the possibility of a watery diarrhea. Psyllium also absorbs bile acids. This may be important for its antidiarrheal action because bile acids can stimulate the colon. Nursing evaluation of patients following administration of psyllium must document the number of stools per day and describe the characteristics of the fecal material. This information is essential in order to establish the effectiveness of the drug.

Pectin

Pectin is a dietary fibre obtained from citrus rind. The mechanism by which it reduces diarrhea is not clear, as it is destroyed within the intestine. Pectin is usually used in conjunction with kaolin in products such as Kaopectate®.

Kaolin

Kaolin is hydrated aluminum citrate. Combined with pectin as attapulgite, it has been a time-honoured treatment for diarrhea. Although its mechanism of action is not clear, explanations for its effects include an ability to bind bacteria, toxins, bile acids and other material in the gut. It has also been claimed that the astringent effect of aluminum contributes to the action of kaolin. An astringent is an agent that contracts body tissue

and blood vessels. For example, a styptic pencil, used to stem the flow of blood after shaving, is an astringent. In that sense one could think of kaolin ingestion as swallowing a styptic pencil. That should be enough to pucker anyone's intestines and reduce diarrhea!

Table 61.1 lists the clinically significant drug interactions with kaolin–pectin formulations.

Bismuth Subsalicylate

Pepto-Bismol®, containing bismuth subsalicylate, has been used for years to treat diarrhea. It has found favour with North Americans visiting Mexico. Pepto-Bismol® has reduced complaints of diarrhea, nausea and abdominal cramping caused by toxigenic *Escherichia coli* and shigella. At the present time it is not clear if the beneficial results are due to the bismuth or the subsalicylate — undoubtedly a purely academic point to the unfortunate soul watching his or her intestines being flushed away by Mexico's finest water. Obviously, much work remains to be done before the actions of this old remedy are completely understood.

A note of caution about Pepto-Bismol®: the use of 240 mL daily has been suggested for prevention of travellers' diarrhea. This contains the equivalent salicylate content to 2.6 g of ASA or, put another way, eight 325-mg (5-grain) tablets. If this dose of Pepto-Bismol® is given to patients taking large doses of ASA for arthritis, toxic concentrations of salicylate can accumulate in the body. In addition, patients taking oral anticoagulants, uricosurics or methotrexate may experience adverse drug interactions if they consume the recommended dose of Pepto-Bismol®.

Table 61.2 on the next page lists the clinically significant drug interactions with bismuth subsalicylate.

Table 61.1
Kaolin + pectin: Drug interactions

Drug	Interaction
Digitalis glycosides	• Digitalis glycosides undergo reduced absorption in the presence of kaolin–pectin preparations

Table 61.2
Bismuth subsalicylate: Drug interactions

Drug	Interaction
Anticoagulants, oral; ASA and other salicylates; hypoglycemics, oral	• The activities of these drugs may increase in the presence of bismuth subsalicylate because the latter compound can displace these drugs from plasma proteins
Uricosurics	• Uricosurics (probenecid or sulfinpyrazone) may have reduced activity in the presence of bismuth subsalicylate because the latter drug can decrease the tubular secretion of uricosurics

Cholestyramine (Questran®)

Cholestyramine binds bile salts. Its use in the treatment of hyperlipidemia and the nursing processes related to its use are discussed in Chapter 42. The drug has been reported to be effective in the treatment of patients with irritable bowel problems secondary to bile salt malabsorption. Although cholestyramine has varyingly been described as tasting like plastic or dehydrated horse manure, relatively small amounts are used to treat diarrhea, thereby reducing the taste problem. Four to six grams per day of the drug have been recommended in this situation.

Antibiotics/Antibacterials

Travellers' diarrhea is caused by an infection and, as a result, would not normally be discussed in a unit dealing with chronic functional diarrhea. However, this is the most appropriate location in the book for this topic.

Bacterial infection from enterotoxigenic *Escherichia coli* is the most common cause of travellers' diarrhea. Other pathogens include shigella, salmonella and viruses. Any tourist who has undergone the three-dimensional experience (nausea, vomiting and diarrhea) of travellers' diarrhea must have wondered if there was not something that he or she could have taken to prevent such a plague.

Some studies have suggested that the tetracycline antibiotic doxycycline (Vibramycin®) is effective as a prophylactic. Although a definitive dose has not been established, it would appear that 100–200 mg daily of doxycycline will suffice for most individuals. To the purist, this use of a "therapeutic umbrella" might not seem justified. It is often pointed out by such people that travellers' diarrhea is a self-limited illness of several days' duration. Presumably, all one has to do is to wait out the storm. However, after passing more than ten loose stools per day, the storm may overtake the patient. Sulfonamides and trimethoprim–sulfamethoxazole (Bactrim®, Septra®) have also been reported to prevent travellers' diarrhea.

It is one thing to try to protect a patient from the scourge of the "Aztec two-step" and quite another to cure the problem once it has settled in. Antimicrobial treatment begun after the symptoms have started probably does not reduce the number of days the patient is incapacitated if the diarrhea is due to enterotoxigenic *E. coli*. Obviously, stool cultures should be taken from patients experiencing severe diarrhea (more than ten loose stools per day) with blood and mucus in the stools. Between the time of taking the cultures and obtaining the results, cotrimoxazole (Bactrim® or Septra®, one tablet every twelve hours) or ampicillin (500 mg four times daily) could be given. The pharmacology of cotrimoxazole is discussed in detail in Chapter 15; doxycycline is presented in Chapter 13.

Drugs That Act on the Gut Wall

Narcotics

Narcotics decrease the propulsive action of the colon and increase distal segmentation, improving the valve action of the sigmoid section of the colon. Although these drugs are effective, caution should be exercised in their use to treat diarrhea. In particular, narcotics should not be used in any bacterial infection causing diarrhea, including travellers' diarrhea, because they can worsen the condition by reducing or preventing the clearance of pathogens

Table 61.3
Diphenoxylate: Drug interactions

Drug	Interaction
CNS depressants	• Barbiturates, benzodiazepines, ethanol and other CNS depressants may have their actions potentiated by diphenoxylate
Monoamine oxidase inhibitors	• MAOIs, together with diphenoxylate, may precipitate a hypertensive crisis

from the intestines. Narcotics can worsen antibiotic-induced colitis or precipitate toxic megacolon in severe ulcerative colitis. These drugs are also contraindicated in pseudomembranous enterocolitis.

Although most narcotics could be selected for their actions on the bowels, a few have been chosen for the treatment of diarrhea. Tincture of opium or camphorated tincture of opium (paregoric) are the historical favourites of many physicians.

Codeine has also been used on many occasions for the treatment of functional diarrhea. It is effective and considerably cheaper than diphenoxylate or loperamide. The constipating action of codeine is obvious to anyone who has taken the drug for the relief of pain. Thirty milligrams of codeine three times daily will cement the bowels of most mortals.

Diphenoxylate plus atropine (Lomotil®) is a popularly prescribed narcotic for the treatment of diarrhea. It is less well absorbed than codeine but is still capable of producing systemic effects. Many nurses and mothers have come to depend on this drug for the treatment of diarrhea and colic in children. Lomotil® is formulated in a palatable cherry-flavoured liquid containing 2.5 mg of diphenoxylate per 5 mL. The use of this product in the treatment of chronic inflammatory bowel disease (CIBD) is discussed in Chapter 60.

Loperamide (Imodium®) is a very popular antidiarrheal narcotic. It is very poorly absorbed, does not cross the blood-brain barrier and has few systemic effects. Loperamide is more potent and longer-acting than diphenoxylate. Its use in CIBD is presented in Chapter 60.

Nurses should caution parents to keep narcotics away from children because accidental poisoning is common. With the exception of loperamide, narcotics can produce nausea, sedation and dizziness.

The nursing process for narcotics in the use

of CIBD is discussed in detail in Chapter 60. Table 61.3 lists the clinically significant drug interactions with diphenoxylate.

Nursing Management

Table 61.4 on the next page describes the nursing management of the patient receiving antidiarrheal drugs. Dosage details for individual drugs are given in Table 61.7 (pages 724–726).

Drug Treatment of Constipation

A cathartic is an agent that causes the evacuation of the bowels. A laxative can also be defined this way, but is usually considered to be milder in action than a cathartic. In this book, the terms laxative and cathartic will be used interchangeably.

Regardless of the name used, these drugs are often abused. Many in our society equate purging with purifying. In the United States alone, over $100 million per year is spent on laxatives, and much of this money is wasted. At least one study has shown that most patients, previously taking laxatives daily, continued to be "regular fellows" when switched to identical-looking placebos.

The above statements notwithstanding, laxatives do have a small place in health care. First, however, it must be emphasized that all laxatives are contraindicated in patients with cramps, colic, nausea, vomiting, fever or undiagnosed abdominal pain. Also, since some laxatives can be shared by a nursing mother with her infant, nurses should teach lactating mothers to use diet and exercise as well as other nondrug remedies to prevent constipation or to treat it. The role of laxatives in the treatment of functional constipation is always secondary to a fibre-rich diet and other nondrug alter-

Table 61.4
Nursing management of antidiarrheal drugs

Assessment of risk vs. benefit	Patient data	• These drugs are often used for self-medication. Pts should consult with a health provider for advice in choosing a suitable product • For antibiotic prophylaxis, physicians should determine any allergies or contraindications • *Pregnancy:* In general, these drugs are risk category C (animal studies show adverse effects to fetus but human data are unknown or insufficient); benefits may be acceptable despite risks. Exceptions include the antibiotics (see Unit 3 for more details on these drugs)
	Drug data	• Select drugs based on underlying cause of diarrhea • Generally well tolerated; however, overuse can cause constipation
Implementation	Nursing therapeutics	• Enhance general health status (nutrition, fluids, hygiene)
	Patient/family teaching	• Instruct pt regarding dietary and fluid intake. Increase fluids to prevent dehydration (esp. for children and older pts). Advise not to use for prolonged periods of time without medical diagnosis • If using antibiotics prophylactically, avoid sun exposure by protective clothing and use of sun-blocking agents
Outcomes	Monitoring of progress	• Instruct pt to monitor clinical response indicating tx success (reduction in signs/symptoms). Be alert for signs/symptoms of dehydration or electrolyte imbalance related to diarrhea

natives. Laxatives may be indicated for the maintenance of soft feces, to prevent straining, especially in patients with cardiovascular problems or anorectal disorders. They can also be used to evacuate the bowels prior to diagnostic procedures or surgery.

Laxatives act by (1) retaining water in the intestine, thereby liquefying the feces (bulk laxatives and osmotic laxatives), (2) softening the stools to facilitate their evacuation (stool softeners) or (3) irritating the colon to increase peristalsis (chemical stimulants). Regardless of the means by which these drugs work, all three groups fall under the general category of laxatives.

Although we may not agree with much of the use of laxatives, it is essential to review how they produce their effects.

Bulk Laxatives

Bran

Bran has been known as a laxative for at least 2500 years. Found in cereals such as All-Bran®

and Fine Bran®, it mixes with food where its hydrophilic action enables it to retain water in the intestine and increase stool volume.

A major disadvantage to the use of bran is its taste. Many users claim that it tastes like a mixture of sawdust and cardboard. This can make it difficult for the constipated patient to ingest sufficient quantities of bran for it to work. About 20 g of bran daily are required; this can be obtained from two to three heaping tablespoonsful of Fine Bran® or All-Bran®, respectively. If the patient prefers, bran alone may be purchased and incorporated into other foods.

Psyllium

Psyllium is obtained from the seed coat of an Indian plant. It is found in several products including Metamucil®, Hydrocil®, Effersyllium® and Serutan®.

Psyllium has the capacity to hold water in the intestinal lumen and swell to many times its original volume. Given in a dose of 2–6 g three times daily, psyllium may soften hard stools. The drug is best taken in juice at mealtimes and accompanied by an additional 200 mL (8 oz) of water. Psyllium has been known to cause allergic reactions, both in patients and in nurses mixing the granules.

Agar and Karaya

The gums agar and karaya attract water. They are incorporated in several laxative products. Many patients feel that they have derived benefit from products containing these substances. Nurses should evaluate patients receiving karaya for allergic reactions such as urticaria, rhinitis, dermatitis and asthma.

Osmotic Laxatives

Osmotic laxatives are not well absorbed from the intestinal tract. As a result of the osmotic pressure created by the nonabsorbed solute, water is also retained in the intestinal lumen. The increased volume of water liquefies feces as they develop and promotes easy defecation.

Magnesium Sulfate and Magnesium Hydroxide

The expression "a dose of salts" was common some years ago. The introduction and extensive marketing of newer laxatives has reduced both the use of this expression and the drugs to which it referred. Saline laxatives are poorly absorbed from the gastrointestinal tract and retain water in the intestine by their osmotic action.

Magnesium sulfate (Epsom salts) is commonly used, in spite of the fact that it has a bitter, unpleasant taste. When taken in 5- to 15-g doses it produces a semifluid catharsis within three hours. Low doses of magnesium hydroxide (milk of magnesia) neutralize stomach acid. Larger amounts produce catharsis. It is important for the user to understand this dose-dependent response. Otherwise, the overzealous use of magnesium hydroxide by the patient seeking antacid relief may yield an entirely unexpected effect with a well-defined endpoint.

If absorbed, magnesium is eliminated from the body by renal excretion. Although the absorption of magnesium from these salts is not more than twenty-five percent of the dose, they should not be administered to patients with renal impairment because the concentration of magnesium can climb into the toxic range (see Chapter 38).

Lactulose (Cephalac®, Chronulac®)

Lactulose is a disaccharide, composed of galactose and fructose. It is not hydrolyzed in the small intestine and therefore not absorbed. The osmotic pressure caused by the retention of lactulose in the intestinal lumen results in the retention of water and electrolytes.

Prior to administration, nursing assessment of the patient should be undertaken to establish any previous history of diabetes or the presence of an existing pregnancy. In both cases, lactulose administration is contraindicated.

Although lactulose may be effective in relieving constipation, quantities up to 8 g daily may be required. Some patients find these quantities difficult to take because the drug has a sweet, syrupy taste. For this reason administration often includes diluting the drug in water or other juices, given with the patient's dessert at mealtime.

Lactulose is also marketed under the trade name Cephalac®. This product provides symptomatic improvement and some normalization of the electroencephalogram in about three-fourths of patients with portal systemic encephalopathy associated with chronic liver disease. Concentrations of ammonia in the blood are reduced by 25% to 50% because of the ability of lactulose to reduce the absorption of ammonia and possibly other toxic amines from the intestinal tract.

Stool Softeners

Mineral Oil

The very name stool softeners conjures up an image of their mechanism of action. Obviously, soft stools are easier for those tender tissues down below to clear than hard stools. The oldest stool softener in use is mineral oil. This substance is also marketed as liquid petrolateum or liquid paraffin. It is used to lubricate stools, for stools, like pistons, run easier and faster when they are oiled.

In spite of its place in history, mineral oil is not a good laxative. When aspirated it produces acute pneumonitis, chronic diffuse pneumonitis or localized granulomas. This occurs most often in young and elderly patients who take the product chronically. Mineral oil will also block absorption of the fat-soluble vitamins A, D, E and K. Finally, oil may leak through the anal sphincter. In addition to being unpleasant itself, the leakage of oil can cause pruritus. The primary nursing responsibility related to the use of mineral oil is patient teaching to inform the patient of these adverse effects.

Dioctyl Sodium Sulfosuccinate, Docusate Sodium (Colace®)

Docusate is a detergent, and although it is tempting to state that it cleans patients out, we will not yield to the impulse. It is incorporated into too many products for all to be listed here. Probably the most commonly used is Colace®; the one with the most intriguing name is Afko-Lube®. Other common trade names include Comofax® and Modane Soft®.

Docusate is claimed to soften the stool by the accumulation of water in the intestine. It can disrupt the gastric mucosal barrier and is best reserved for situations in which a stool softener is required for a short period.

Table 61.5 lists the clinically significant drug interactions with docusate sodium.

Chemical Stimulants

Chemical stimulants are taken for the purpose of irritating the intestine and thereby increasing its motility. Once irritated, the intestine can be a difficult beast to tame. Many a sorry soul has taken a drug in this category only to wish later that he could restrain the tiger in his tank. After all, enough is enough. All chemical stimulants produce griping, increased mucus secretion, and in some people, excessive evacuation of fluid.

Phenolphthalein

Phenolphthalein is the active ingredient in many products, including such household remedies as Ex-Lax®, Feen-A-Mint® and Phenolax®. The drug produces its irritant effect on the colon. As a result, a period of several hours is required before the effects of phenolphthalein are seen. For this reason, it is best taken at night before retiring. Recently, concern has been expressed over the possible carcinogenic potential of phenolphthalein, and regulatory agencies have moved to restrict the distribution of products containing this drug.

Bisacodyl (Dulcolax®, Theralax®)

Bisacodyl is similar to phenolphthalein in its effects on the colon. It is given orally or rectally. In the colon it initiates repetitive peristalsis. A soft, formed stool is usually produced six to ten hours after oral administration and fifteen to sixty minutes after insertion into the rectum. The usual oral dose should be administered from an airtight container that has been stored in a cool place (at temperatures below 30°C or 86°F). Patient teaching should include instructions to swallow the tablets whole. Chewing destroys the enteric coating and results in gastric irritation. Taking the tablets within one hour of ingesting either milk or an antacid may also destroy the enteric coating and produce gastric irritation.

Castor Oil

Castor oil — the very name used to strike fear in the hearts of children. Untold numbers grew to adulthood despite a weekly purgation with castor oil. Derived from the *Ricinus communis* seed and containing the active ingredient ricinoleic acid, castor oil acts on the small intestine. It is usually prescribed only when prompt, thorough evacuation of the bowel is desired.

Table 61.5
Docusate sodium: Drug interactions

Drug	Interaction
Mineral oil	• The absorption and hepatotoxicity of mineral oil may increase with the concomitant administration of docusate

Castor oil will produce abdominal cramps and loose bowel movements within two hours. It is usually administered on an empty stomach. The drug is not given during pregnancy because it has been associated with the onset of labour. Castor oil's unpleasant taste can be made more palatable if it is offered in a large glass to which is added 125 mL (4–5 oz) of citrus juice and 2 mL (1/2 teaspoon) of baking soda. This mixture is stirred rapidly and consumed quickly.

Nursing Management

Table 61.6 describes the nursing management of the patient receiving laxatives. Dosage details of individual drugs are given in Table 61.7 (pages 724–726).

Table 61.6
Nursing management of laxatives

Assessment of risk vs. benefit	Patient data	• These drugs are often used for self-medication. Pts should consult a health provider for advice on choosing a suitable the product • Oils should not be used by anyone who has difficulty swallowing or is immobile in bed • *Pregnancy:* In general, these drugs are risk category C (animal studies show adverse effects to fetus but human data are unknown or insufficient). Benefits may be acceptable despite risks. One exception is castor oil, which is contraindicated in pregnancy
	Drug data	• Select drugs based on underlying cause of constipation • Some agents are used prophylactically to prevent constipation in certain chronic conditions, including heart disease where straining during a bowel movement may cause the Valsalva manoeuvre (pt holds breath and tightens muscles) • Generally well tolerated; however, overuse can cause cramping, diarrhea, electrolyte imbalance and functional bowel dependence (bowel lose peristalsis). Overuse of oils can reduce absorption of nutrients, especially fat-soluble vitamins
Implementation	Nursing therapeutics	• Plan time of administration according to expected onset of action. Provide privacy and promote regular bowel pattern • Enhance general health status (nutritional fibre intake, fluids, daily exercise/activity) • Ensure that bulk-forming agents are taken with adequate fluids; can cause obstruction in the GI tract
	Patient/family teaching	• Instruct pt regarding dietary and fluid intake; increase daily exercise/activity and promote regular bowel habits
Outcomes	Monitoring of progress	*Continually monitor:* • Clinical response indicating tx success (regular, formed bowel movements without straining) • Signs/symptoms of diarrhea and functional dependence with overuse or electrolyte imbalance related to diarrhea

Table 61.7

Laxatives and antidiarrheals: Drug doses

Drug Generic name (Trade names)	Dosage	Nursing alert
A. Antidiarrheal Drugs		
1. Drugs Acting in the Intestinal Lumen		
psyllium hydrophilic mucilloid (Hydrocil, Metamucil)	**Oral:** 7 g mixed with glass of water or other suitable fluid 1–3x/day. Second glass of water enhances drug's effects	• Give with full glass of liquid to ensure granules are dissolved and do not lodge in esophagus. Administer immediately after mixing
kaolin–pectin mixture; attapulgite (Kaopectate)	**Oral** (after each movement): *Adults:* 60–120 mL. *Children > 12 years:* 60 mL; *6–12 years:* 30–60 mL; *3–6 years:* 15–30 mL; *< 3 years:* 5 mL or more prn	• Shake suspension well prior to administration. Instruct pt to use calibrated device (not household spoon) to ensure accuracy
bismuth subsalicylate (Pepto-Bismol)	**Oral/suspension:** *Adults:* 30 mL. *Children 10–14 years:* 20 mL; *6–10 years:* 10 mL; *3–6 years:* 5 mL. Repeat q30–60min prn to 7–8 doses. **Tablets:** *Adults:* 2 tablets. *Children 10–14 years:* 1 tablet; *6–10 years:* 2/3 tablet; *3–6 years:* 1/3 tablet; repeat q30min, not to exceed 8 doses	• Shake liquid well prior to use. Tablets should be chewed or dissolved before swallowing. Instruct pt to use calibrated device (not household spoon) to ensure accuracy
2. Narcotic + Anticholinergic diphenoxylate HCl + atropine sulfate (Lomotil)	**Oral:** *Adults:* Initially, 5 mg diphenoxylate (2 tablets) tid or qid (max., 20 mg diphenoxylate/24 h in divided doses). Reduce dose as soon as initial symptom control is accomplished. Maint. dose may be as low as 1/4 initial dose. *Children:* Not for use in children < 2 years of age. Initially, 0.3–0.4 mg diphenoxylate per kg daily in divided doses. Reduce dose as soon as initial symptom control is accomplished	• May be taken with food. May crush tablets. Shake liquid preparations prior to use. Instruct pt to use calibrated measure (not household spoon) to ensure accuracy
3. Narcotic loperamide HCl (Imodium)	**Oral:** *Adults* (acute diarrhea): 4 mg initially, followed by 2 mg after each unformed stool. Daily dose should not exceed 16 mg. (Chronic diarrhea): 4 mg initially, followed by 2 mg after each unformed stool until diarrhea is controlled; thereafter, dose should be reduced to meet pt's requirements. *Children* (acute or chronic diarrhea): *2–5 years (10–20 kg):* 1 mg tid; *5–8 years (20–30 kg):* 2 mg bid; *8–12 years (> 30 kg):* 2 mg tid. Use only on advice of MD	• Shake solution well prior to use. Instruct pt to use calibrated measure (not household spoon) to ensure accuracy • Note: Solution contains alcohol

Table 61.7 (continued)
Laxatives and antidiarrheals: Drug doses

Drug Generic name (Trade names)	Dosage	Nursing alert
B. Laxatives		
1. Osmotic Laxative		
magnesium citrate (Citro-Mag)	**Oral** (for use in diagnostics): 200 mL magnesium citrate solution (1.55 g–1.9 g/100 mL magnesium oxide with citric acid anhydrous and potassium bicarbonate for effervescence)	• Chill prior to use to make more palatable. Push fluids prior to and following administration
magnesium sulfate, Epsom salts	**Oral:** *Adults:* 5–15 g prn	• More effective if taken on empty stomach. Dissolve in full glass of water and following another glass of any liquid. Administer early in day. Acts in 3–6 h
magnesium hydroxide, milk of magnesia	**Oral:** *Adults:* 15–30 mL prn	• Faster onset if taken on empty stomach. Usual onset of action: 3–6 h. Give early in day • Instruct pt to use calibrated measure (not household spoon) to ensure accuracy
lactulose (Chronulac)	**Oral:** 15–60 mL (10–40 g of lactulose) daily, prn	• Usual action within 24–48 h. Mix with liquid (juice, water, milk)
2. Stool Softeners mineral oil	**Oral:** *Adults:* 15–45 mL daily	• Do not administer if pt has difficult swallowing or is immobile. Administer hs with pt sitting (not reclining) • Do not give within 2 h of food; interferes with absorption of fat-soluble vitamins
docusate sodium, dioctyl sodium sulfosuccinate (Colace)	**Oral:** *Adults/older children:* 100–200 mg; *0–3 years:* 10–40 mg; *3–6 years:* 20–60 mg; *6–12 years:* 40–120 mg. May be given in divided dosage with water **Rectal:** Retention enema: 5 mL of drops (50 mg) to 90 mL enema fluid. Flushing enema: 1 mL of drops (10 mg) to 100 mL of enema fluid. To counteract barium constipation: Add 10–20 mL (100–200 mg) to barium mixture before administration	• Usual action within 1–3 days. May dilute oral solution in milk or juice

Table 61.7 (continued)
Laxatives and antidiarrheals: Drug doses

Drug Generic name (Trade names)	Dosage	Nursing alert
B. Laxatives (cont'd)		
3. Chemical Stimulants		
phenolphthalein (Ex-Lax, Feen-A-Mint, Phenolax, many others)	**Oral:** *Adults:* 60 mg. *Children:* 15–30 mg	• **PO:** Give tablets with full glass of water hs. Onset of action, 6–12 h. Instruct pt to chew the chewable tablets; do not swallow whole • Advise pt that drug may discolour urine
bisacodyl (Dulcolax, Therolax)	**Oral:** *Adults* (acute and chronic constipation): 5–15 mg in the evening or before breakfast. (Proctoscopic, radiographic or preoperative preparation): 10–15 mg the evening before, supplemented by administration of a 10-mg suppository or the contents of 1 Micro-Enema® rectally 1–2 h prior to scheduled procedure **Rectal:** *Children 6–12 years:* 5-mg suppository or approximately one-half the contents of 1 Micro-Enema®	• **PO:** Do not crush or chew enteric-coated tablets; take separate from antacids by 1 h • **Rectal:** Insert suppositories as high as possible against rectal wall, but avoid feces. Encourage pt to retain suppository until onset of action (within 15–30 min)

Response to Clinical Challenge

In choosing the proper drug, you should consider such factors as your age, your general health status, other medical conditions and drugs that you may be taking. This research will be useful to you personally as well in counselling others.

Further Reading

Cohen M. Medication errors. Lactulose versus Kayexalate: Unlikely bedfellows. *Nursing* 1996; 26(5):18.

Hall G, et al. Managing constipation using a research-based protocol. *Medsburg Nursing* 1995;4(1):11–20.

Steward E, et al. A strategy to reduce laxative use among older people. *Nurs Times* 1997;93(4):35–36.

C H A P T E R   6 2

Antiemetic Drugs

Topics Discussed
- Nausea, vomiting and motion sickness
- Anticholinergic drugs
- Antihistamines
- Antidopaminergic drugs
- Antipsychotic drugs
- 5-Hydroxytryptamine$_3$ (5-HT$_3$) antagonists
- Miscellaneous drugs
- For each drug discussed: Mechanism of action and pharmacologic effects, therapeutic uses, adverse effects
- Nursing management

Drugs Discussed
cisapride (**siss**-ah-pride)
cyclizine (**cye**-kleh-zeen)
dimenhydrinate (dye-men-**hye**-drin-ate)
domperidone (dome-**pair**-ih-done)
granisetron (gran-**iss**-eh-tron)
hydroxyzine (hye-**drok**-sih-zeen)
hyoscine (**hye**-oh-seen)
meclizine (**meck**-liz-een)
metoclopramide (met-oh-**kloe**-pram-ide)
nabilone (**nab**-ih-loan)
ondansetron (on-**dan**-seh-tron)
perphenazine (per-**fen**-ah-zeen)
prochlorperazine (proe-klor-**pair**-ah-zeen)
promethazine (proe-**meth**-ah-zeen)
scopolamine (scoe-**pole**-ah-meen)
thiethylperazine (thye-eth-il-**pair**-ah-zeen)

Clinical Challenge

Consider this clinical challenge as you read through this chapter. The response to the challenge appears on page 733.

Helen, a 23-year-old woman pregnant with her first child, is experiencing morning sickness. She visits the Women's Health Centre to read information on nausea in pregnancy and to determine her options for alleviating this troublesome symptom.
   What is she likely to discover about the use of antiemetics during pregnancy?

Nausea, Vomiting and Motion Sickness

This chapter reviews the treatment of nausea, vomiting and motion sickness. Drugs used to treat these conditions may be classified as (1) anticholinergics, (2) antihistamines, (3) antidopaminergics, (4) 5-hydroxytryptamine$_3$ antagonists and (5) miscellaneous drugs. For the first three groups, only their use to reduce nausea, vomiting or motion sickness will be discussed here, as the detailed pharmacology of these agents can be found in Chapters 28, 72 and 45, respectively.

As suggested by the Clinical Challenge, nausea and vomiting in the first trimester of pregnancy are common. However, these are due to physiological changes in most cases and usually do not require drug therapy. Although drug therapy may seem appealing to the nauseated patient, it must be remembered that all drugs can cross the placenta. During the first trimester, the fetus is developing rapidly and is particularly susceptible to the actions of drugs. Administering some drugs during this period can produce significant damage to growing tissues and organs. The effects of drug on the unborn are not restricted to the first trimester and potentially can cause harm at any time during pregnancy. Nurses should be aware that some antiemetics are contraindicated in pregnancy, while others may be used if the benefits outweigh the risks. For example, if a woman is losing weight due to nausea, or is unable to function in her daily life, the cautious use of an antiemetic may be justified. However, prior to embarking on drug treatment, patients should be instructed in nonpharmacological alternatives. These include eating dry foods, such as crackers, immediately upon awaking, sipping carbonated beverages or juices or water, eating small, frequent meals and avoiding any foods or smells that cause nausea.

Anticholinergic Drugs

Scopolamine

Mechanism or action and pharmacologic effects. Anticholinergic drugs block muscarinic receptors competitively throughout the body (Chapter 28). They also reduce the excitability of the labyrinth receptors, depressing conduction in vestibular pathways or preventing recruitment of impulses at the chemoreceptor trigger zone. Stimulation of the chemoreceptor trigger zone in the brain activates the vomiting centre. Anticholinergic drugs, such as scopolamine (hyoscine), which reduce the sensitivity of the chemoreceptor trigger zone are often effective in the treatment of nausea and vomiting.

Therapeutic uses. Scopolamine (hyoscine) is the anticholinergic used most frequently. Its value as an antinauseant is counterbalanced by its

adverse effects resulting from a generalized cholinergic block. The introduction of the transdermal therapeutic system (Transderm-SCOP®, Transderm-V®) has been a significant advance. These flat, circular units continuously release scopolamine over thirty-six to forty-eight hours. Applying one disc behind the ear often provides effective protection against nausea and vomiting associated with motion sickness, without producing undue systemic adverse effects. An anticholinergic should not be used by persons suffering from glaucoma or when it causes pressure pain behind the eye.

Adverse effects. Dryness of the mouth, cycloplegia and drowsiness are the most common adverse effects of scopolamine. They are experienced less frequently if the transdermal delivery system is used. Infrequently, patients may experience disorientation, memory disturbances, restlessness, giddiness, hallucinations and confusion when scopolamine is administered systemically. Because of the CNS depression that scopolamine can produce, patients should be cautioned about engaging in activities that require mental alertness, such as driving a car or operating dangerous machinery. The drug interactions for anticholinergic agents are found in Table 28.1 (page 275).

Antihistamines
Cyclizine, Dimenhydrinate, Hydroxyzine, Meclizine, Promethazine

Mechanism of action and pharmacologic effects. Several antihistamines are used to prevent vertigo, motion sickness and the nausea of pregnancy. These include cyclizine (Marezine®, Marzine®), dimenhydrinate (Dramamine®, Gravol®), hydroxyzine (Atarax®, Orgatrax®, Vistaril®), meclizine (Antivert®, Bonamine®, Bonine®) and promethazine (Phenergan®, Remsed®). Their mechanism of action is not completely understood. They may affect neural pathways originating in the labyrinth.

Therapeutic uses. The therapeutic indications differ slightly from product to product, but all are indicated for the prevention and relief of the nausea or vomiting of motion sickness. The drugs are also recommended for the treatment of vertigo. With the exception of hydroxyzine, all antihistamines are effective in treating the nausea of pregnancy. However, antiemetics are generally not recommended during pregnancy. Hydroxyzine and promethazine are indicated for the treatment of postoperative emesis. Finally, dimenhydrinate, meclizine and promethazine may be used in the treatment or prophylaxis of the nausea and vomiting of radiation sickness.

Adverse effects. Drowsiness is the most common adverse effect of antihistamines. Dizziness may also occur. All antihistamines possess appreciable anticholinergic activity. Patients may experience dry mouth, nose and throat; blurred vision; difficult or painful urination; thickening of bronchial secretions; and tachycardia. Depending on the drug used, patients may also complain of headache, loss of appetite, nervousness, restlessness, skin rash, upset stomach or stomach pain, excitement and nausea. The drug interactions for antihistamines are presented in Table 72.1 (page 847).

Antidopaminergic Drugs

Antipsychotic Drugs

Mechanism of action and pharmacologic effects. Dopamine is the neurotransmitter in the chemoreceptor trigger zone. Antipsychotic drugs block dopamine receptors. Phenothiazines, such as perphenazine and prochlorperazine, reduce nausea or vomiting, or both. Only thioridazine (Mellaril®), of the commonly used phenothiazines, appears devoid of antinauseant activity. These drugs also block alpha$_1$ and dopaminergic receptors throughout the body, accounting for many of the peripheral effects (see Chapters 30 and 45).

Therapeutic uses. Dopaminergic blocking drugs reduce the sensitivity of the chemoreceptor trigger zone to numerous emetic stimuli, such as antineoplastics, radiation, uremia, estrogens, tetracyclines and narcotics. They do not appear to be effective in controlling motion sickness or treating vertigo. The contraindications to their use are described in Chapter 45.

Adverse effects. The adverse effects of phenothiazines are discussed in detail in Chapter 45. Drowsiness is the most common adverse reaction when these drugs are used as antinauseants. Other commonly encountered effects are orthostatic hypotension, dryness of the mouth and nasal congestion. Extrapyramidal reactions resulting from inhibition of dopaminergic receptors in the basal ganglia are well-recognized adverse effects of phenothiazines. The drugs are also capable of producing cholestatic jaundice, granulocytopenia, urticaria, dermatitis, thrombocytopenia, leukopenia, agranulocytosis, purpura, pancytopenia, gastroenteritis, photosensitivity, galactorrhea and edema of the extremities.

Patients with a hypersensitivity to one phenothiazine should not be treated with any of these drugs. They are contraindicated in patients with bone marrow depression and in pregnant women with a history of preeclampsia. Care should be taken if the patient is already receiving another CNS depressant or antihypertensive agents. The drug interactions for these compounds are presented in Table 45.2 (page 511).

Metoclopramide (Maxeran®, Reglan®) and Domperidone (Motilium®)

Mechanism of action and pharmacologic effects. Metoclopramide blocks dopaminergic receptors at the chemoreceptor trigger zone. It also increases gastrointestinal (GI) motility. Metoclopramide increases the strength of contractions of the gastric antrum and speeds gastric emptying. The drug relaxes the duodenal bulb and accelerates upper GI tract transit, there alleviating gastric stasis. Because of these actions, metoclopramide can be used to treat delayed gastric emptying.

Domperidone blocks peripheral dopamine receptors. Its antiemetic activity is similar to metoclopramide's, but the incidence of extrapyramidal side effects is lower with domperidone because it does not easily cross the blood-brain barrier. Domperidone increases lower esophageal sphincter pressure, the duration of antral and duodenal contractions, and the gastric emptying of liquids and semisolids.

Therapeutic uses. Metoclopramide injection is useful in preventing the nausea and vomiting associated with cancer chemotherapy. When used preoperatively, oral metoclopramide may reduce narcotic-induced postoperative vomiting. Metoclopramide is also indicated as an adjunct in the management of delayed gastric emptying associated with subacute and chronic gastritis or following vagotomy and pylorplasty and other surgical procedures.

Domperidone is indicated in the symptomatic management of upper GI motility disorders associated with chronic and subacute gastritis and diabetic gastroparesis. The drug may also be used to prevent GI symptoms associated with the use of dopamine-agonist antiparkinsonian agents (see Chapter 50).

Neither metoclopramide nor domperidone should be used whenever stimulation of GI motility might be dangerous, e.g., in the presence of GI hemorrhage, mechanical obstruction or perforation.

Adverse effects. Drowsiness, fatigue and lassitude occur in about ten percent of patients receiving metoclopramide. Less frequent adverse reactions are insomnia, headache, dizziness and bowel disturbances. Parkinsonism or extrapyramidal symptoms (see Chapter 45), or both, have been reported in about one percent of patients.

The overall incidence of side effects with domperidone was less than seven percent. The more serious or troublesome adverse effects (galactorrhea, gynecomastia, menstrual irregularities) are dose related and gradually resolve after lowering the dose or discontinuing therapy.

Table 62.1 lists the clinically significant drug interactions with metoclopramide, while Table 62.2 lists those with domperidone.

Thiethylperazine (Torecan®)

Thiethylperazine is a phenothiazine that is particularly useful to treat nausea and vomiting associated with anesthesia. It also relieves nausea and vomiting caused by mildly emetic chemotherapeutic agents, radiation therapy and toxins. This drug does not prevent vertigo or motion sickness.

Untoward effects are infrequent, mild, and transitory with usual doses. Adverse reactions noted occasionally include drowsiness, dizziness, dryness of the mouth and nose, tachycardia, and anorexia. Like other phenothiazines, thiethylperazine may produce extrapyramidal reactions.

5-Hydroxytryptamine$_3$ (5-HT$_3$) Antagonists

Ondansetron (Zofran®)

Mechanism of action and pharmacologic effects. Ondansetron is a selective antagonist of the serotonin receptor subtype 5-HT$_3$. The antiemetic effect of ondansetron is probably due to the selective antagonism of 5-HT$_3$ receptors on neurons located in either the peripheral or central nervous systems, or both.

Therapeutic uses. Ondansetron is approved for the management of nausea and vomiting associated with emetogenic chemotherapy and radiotherapy. It is also indicated for the prevention and treatment of postoperative nausea and vomiting. Ondansetron is not effective in preventing motion-induced nausea and vomiting.

Table 62.1
Metoclopramide: Drug interactions

Drug	Interaction
Anticholinergics	• Anticholinergics antagonize the GI effects of metoclopramide
Antipsychotic drugs	• Antipsychotic drugs have potentiated effects in the presence of metoclopramide
Cholinergics	• Cholinergics may increase the effects of metoclopramide
CNS depressants	• CNS depressants may produce additive sedative effects with metoclopramide
Digoxin	• Metoclopramide may decrease the absorption of digoxin

Table 62.2
Domperidone: Drug interactions

Drug	Interaction
Antacids and H$_2$ blockers	• Antacids and H$_2$ blockers should be avoided because domperidone requires gastric acid for absorption
Anticholinergics	• Anticholinergics may compromise the beneficial effects of domperidone
Monoamine oxidase inhibitors	• MAOIs should be administered with care when pts are taking domperidone

Adverse effects. Ondansetron is well tolerated. The most frequent adverse events reported in controlled clinical trials were headache (11%) and constipation (4%).

Granisetron HCl (Kytril®)

The actions, indications, and efficacy of this 5-HT$_3$ receptor antagonist are similar to those of ondansetron. Like the latter drug, granisetron alone is superior to metoclopramide/dexamethasone combinations for prevention and control of acute nausea and vomiting associated with cisplatin and other highly emetogenic cancer chemotherapeutic regimens.

Granisetron is well tolerated, though constipation, diarrhea, headache and transient hypotension have occurred in some patients. Extrapyramidal adverse reactions have not been reported.

Miscellaneous Drugs

Cannabinoid Drug: Nabilone (Cesamet®)

Nabilone is a synthetic cannabinoid with antiemetic properties which have been found to be of value in the management of some patients with nausea and vomiting associated with cancer chemotherapy. It also has sedative and psychotropic effects.

Nabilone is used in the management of severe nausea and vomiting associated with cancer chemotherapy. The most frequently observed adverse reactions are drowsiness, vertigo, psychological high, dry mouth, depression, ataxia, blurred vision, sensation disturbance, anorexia, asthenia, headache, orthostatic hypotension, euphoria and hallucinations, in that order.

Gastrokinetic Drug: Cisapride (Prepulsid®)

Mechanism of action and pharmacologic effects. The inclusion of cisapride in this chapter is open to criticism because cisapride is not indicated in the treatment of nausea. However, because of this drug's similarity to metoclopramide and domperidone, this chapter is the most appropriate place to present this interesting compound.

Cisapride's activity is considered to be due to enhancement of the physiological release of acetylcholine at the myenteric plexus. The drug increases esophageal peristaltic activity and lowers esophageal sphincter tone, thereby decreasing reflux of gastric contents into the esophagus and improving esophageal clearance. Gastric and duodenal emptying are also enhanced by cisapride as a consequence of increased gastric and duodenal contractility and antroduodenal coordination. Cisapride decreases duodenogastric reflux. The drug also enhances intestinal propulsive activity and improves both small and large bowel transit. Cisapride is free of dopamine-receptor blocking activity. Because it is not a cholinomimetic, cisapride does not increase basal or pentagastrin-induced gastric acid secretion.

Therapeutic uses. Cisapride is indicated in the symptomatic management of GI motility disorders, including gastroesophageal reflux disease; gastroparesis, whether idiopathic or associated with diabetic neuropathy; and intestinal pseudo-obstruction. Like metoclopramide and domperidone, cisapride is contraindicated whenever GI stimulation might be dangerous.

Adverse effects. The most frequent adverse effects of cisapride involve the GI tract — diarrhea and abdominal discomfort. Most adverse effects are transient and rarely necessitate discontinuation of therapy.

Nursing Management

Table 62.3 describes the nursing management of the patient receiving antiemetic drugs. Dosage details are given in Table 62.4 (pages 733–737).

Table 62.3
Nursing management of the antiemetic drugs

Assessment of risk vs. benefit	Patient data	• *Pregnancy:* Risk category for most of these drugs is B or C; however, many have not been sufficiently studied in pregnant women. Caution is thus advised
	Drug data	• Physician should determine underlying cause of nausea and vomiting and which drug action is warranted • Most drugs in this class are well tolerated but do cause CNS effects, such as drowsiness (which can be dangerous if pt drives or engages in hazardous work). Some drugs cause extrapyramidal and other CNS adverse reactions
Implementation	Nursing therapeutics	• Enhance general health status (nutrition, rest, fluids, hygiene) • Ensure adequate fluid intake to prevent dehydration and electrolyte imbalance • Instruct pt in supportive measures that alleviate nausea
	Patient/family teaching	• As these drugs are often used for self-medication, teach regarding proper use of drug • Pts/families should know warning sings/symptoms of possible adverse reactions of these drugs. Report immediately: extrapyramidal symptoms, excessive drowsiness • Warn pts to avoid alcohol (increased risk of CNS depression) • *Discuss possibility of pregnancy:* Advise pt to discuss with physician
Outcomes	Monitoring of progress	*Continually monitor:* • Clinical response indicating tx success • Adverse effects, esp. signs/symptoms of dehydration and electrolyte imbalance

Response to Clinical Challenge

Your response could include the following points:

• Most drugs can cross the placenta into fetal circulation and may cause harm at any point during pregnancy.
• During the first trimester the fetus is developing rapidly; drug effects at this time can produce significant damage to growing tissues and organs.
• Some antiemetics are contraindicated in pregnancy while others may be used if the benefits outweigh the risks. Nonpharmacologic measures (e.g., eating dry crackers; sipping carbonated beverages; eating small, frequent meals) should be tried before drug therapy is considered.

Box 62.1 lists the pregnancy categories of some commonly prescribed antiemetic drugs.

Further Reading

Bruera E, et al. Chronic nausea in advanced cancer patients: a retrospective assessment of metoclopramide-based antiemetic regimen. *J Pain and Symptom Management* 1996;11(3):147-153.

Box 62.1
Pregnancy risk categories of antiemetic drugs

Generic name (Trade name)	Risk category
cisapride (Prepulsid)	C
cyclizine (Marezine, Marzine)	B
dimenhydrinate (Dramamine, Gravol)	B
domperidone (Motilium)	Unknown
granisetron (Kytril)	Unknown
hydroxyzine (Atarax, Orgatrax, Vistaril)	Unknown
meclizine (Antivert, Bonamine, Bonine)	B
metoclopramide (Maxeran, Reglan)	B
ondansetron (Zofran)	B
perphenazine (Trilafon)	Unknown
prochlorperazine (Compazine, Stemetil)	C
promethazine (Phenergan, Remsed)	Unknown
scopolamine, hyoscine	C

Category B: Animal studies have not shown a risk to the fetus, but controlled studies have not been conducted in pregnant women; or, animal studies have shown an adverse effect on the fetus, but adequate studies in pregnant women have not shown a risk to the fetus during the first trimester or in later trimesters.

Category C: Animal studies show adverse effects to fetus but human data are unknown or insufficient; benefits may be acceptable despite risks.

Table 62.4
The antiemetics: Drug doses

Drug Generic name (Trade names)	Dosage	Nursing alert
A. Anticholinergic Drugs		
scopolamine, hyoscine	**IM/IV/SC:** *Adults:* 0.3–0.65 mg. *Children:* 6 μg/kg or 0.2 mg per m²	• For direct IV, follow agency policy re: certification
transdermal scopolamine (Transderm-SCOP, Transderm-V)	**Topical:** Apply 1 disc to postauricular skin approx. 12 h before antiemetic effect is required	• Apply only one disc at any one time

Table 62.4 (continued)
The antiemetics: Drug doses

Drug Generic name (Trade names)	Dosage	Nursing alert
B. Antihistamines		
cyclizine (Marezine, Marzine)	For postoperative vomiting: **IM:** *Adults:* 50 mg 15–30 min before end of operation; may be repeated tid during the first few postoperative days prn. *Children ≤ 6 years:* 25% of adult dose; *6–10 years:* 50% of adult dose **IV:** Injection may be given IV if diluted to at least 10 mL with sterile water or normal saline and administered slowly. To prevent postoperative vomiting, give slow IV 20 min before expected end of surgery	• For direct IV, follow agency policy re: certification
dimenhydrinate (Dramamine, Gravol)	**Oral:** *Adults* (motion sickness nausea, vomiting, dizziness and vertigo): 50–100 mg q4h prn to a max. of 400 mg in 24 h. For extended relief: 1–2 long-acting 75-mg capsules q8h to a max. of 5 capsules in 24 h. *Children < 2 years:* As directed by a physician; *2–6 years:* 15–25 mg q6–8h prn to a max. of 75 mg in 24 h; *6–8 years:* 25–50 mg q6–8h prn to a max. of 150 mg in 24 h; *8–12 years:* 25–50 mg q6–8h prn to a max. of 150 mg in 24 h; *≥ 12 years:* 50 mg q4–6h prn to a max. of 300 mg in 24 h **Rectal:** *Adults:* 50–100 mg suppository q6–8h prn. *Children 2–6 years:* 12.5–25 mg, not to be repeated except on the advice of a physician; *6–8 years:* 12.5–25 mg q8–12h prn; *8–12 years:* 25–50 mg q8–12h, prn: *≥ 12 years:* 50 mg q8–12h prn Postoperative nausea: *Adults:* 50–100 mg orally or 50 mg IM as a preoperative dose, to be followed postoperatively by similar doses prn to a max. of 400 mg in 24 h Radiation sickness: 50–100 mg, administered rectally or parenterally 30–60 min before tx. Repeat prn to a max. of 400 mg in 24 h	• For motion sickness, initial dose should be taken at least 30 min and preferably 1–2 h before departure • Do not crush or chew long-acting capsules • Instruct pt in self-administration of rectal suppository • Store in cool place

Table 62.4 (continued)
The antiemetics: Drug doses

Drug Generic name (Trade names)	Dosage	Nursing alert
B. Antihistamines (cont'd)		
meclizine HCl–nicotinic acid (Antivert, Bonamine, Bonine)	**Oral:** *Adults* (motion sickness): 25–50 mg taken at least 1 h prior to travelling. (Labyrinthine and vestibular disturbances): 25–100 mg daily in divided doses. (Radiation sickness): 50 mg 2–12 h prior to radiation tx. *Children:* One-half the adult dose	• Give with food or milk to reduce gastric irritation. Available in chewable form
promethazine (Phenergan)	(Antiemetic) **Oral/Rectal/IM/IV:** *Adults:* 10–25 mg q4h prn. *Children > 2 years:* 0.25–0.5 mg/kg 4–6x daily (Motion sickness) **Oral:** *Adults:* 25 mg 30–60 min prior to departure; may be repeated in 8–12 h. *Children > 2 years:* 12.5–25 mg or 0.5 mg/kg 30–60 min prior to departure; may be given bid	• **PO:** Give with food or milk, if possible, to reduce gastric irritation. Tabs may be crushed and mixed with food • **IV:** For direct IV, follow agency policy re: certification • **IM:** Inject deep into muscle mass • **Rectal:** Instruct pt re: self-administration of suppository
C. Antipsychotic Drugs		
perphenazine (Trilafon)	**IM** (severe nausea and vomiting): *Adults:* Usual dose for rapid control of vomiting is 5 mg. Rarely, a 10-mg dose is necessary. Do not exceed 15–30 mg/day **Oral** (severe nausea and vomiting): *Adults:* 8–16 mg daily in divided doses; 24 mg occasionally may be necessary; early dosage reduction is desirable	• Oral concentrate and injection solution may cause contact dermatitis; avoid contact with skin and wash thoroughly if this occurs • To prepare oral solution, add 5 mL of concentrate to 60 mL of diluent; do not use any solutions containing caffeine, tannins (e.g., tea) or pectinates (e.g., apple juice). May use water, milk, other juices or pop • Do not confuse syrup (2 mg/5 mL) with concentrate (16 mg/5 mL)
prochlorperazine (Compazine, Stemetil)	(To control nausea or vomiting) **Oral/Rectal:** *Adults:* 5–10 mg tid or qid. In mild cases, a single dose of 5–10 mg is often adequate. *Children 9–13 kg:* 2.5 mg 1–2x/day, max. 7.5 mg/day; *14–17 kg:* 2.5 mg bid or tid, max. 10 mg/day; *18–39 kg:* 2.5 mg tid or 5 mg bid, max. 15 mg/day **IM:** *Adults:* 5–10 mg bid or tid. **IV:** *Adults:* 2.5–10 mg; rate not to exceed 5 mg/min. May be repeated in 30 min. Single dose not to exceed 10 mg (or 40 mg/day)	• **PO:** Give with food or milk, if possible, to reduce gastric irritation. Do not crush or chew sustained-release caps, and do not substitute for tabs • Oral and injectable solutions may cause contact dermatitis; avoid contact with skin and wash thoroughly if this occurs. • **IM:** Inject deep into muscle mass. Do not use solution that is discoloured or contains precipitate • **IV:** For direct IV, follow agency policy re: certification

(cont'd on next page)

Table 62.4 (continued)
The antiemetics: Drug doses

Drug Generic name (Trade names)	Dosage	Nursing alert
D. Antidopaminergic Drugs metoclopramide HCl (Maxeran, Reglan)	**Oral** (delayed gastric emptying): *Adults:* 5–10 mg tid or qid ac. *Children:* 2.5–5 mg tid ac. (Diagnostic radiology): *Adults:* 20 mg 5–10 min before barium swallow. (Reduction of post-operative vomiting induced by narcotics): *Adults:* 20 mg 2 h before anesthesia **IV** (prevention of chemotherapy-induced vomiting): *Adults:* 1–2 mg/kg 30 min prior to chemotherapy; 1–2 mg/kg may be given additionally q2h for 2 doses, then q3h for 3 additional doses. **IM** (postoperative nausea/vomiting): *Adults:* 10–20 mg	• **PO:** If possible, give with food or milk to reduce gastric irritation • **IM:** Give deep into muscle mass • **IV:** Follow product instructions for dilution and rate, and agency policy re: certification
domperidone maleate (Motilium)	**Oral** (upper GI motility disorders): *Adults:* 10 mg tid or qid, 15–30 min ac and hs, prn. In severe or resistant cases, dose may be increased to a max. of 20 mg tid or qid. (Nausea and vomiting associated with dopamine-agonist antiparkinsonian agents): 20 mg tid or qid	• Indication for use determines appropriate time of administration
thiethylperazine (Torecan)	**Oral/IM/Rectal:** *Adults:* 10 mg 1–3x daily	• Inject deep into muscle mass. Pt should remain lying down for 1 h to prevent hypotension
E. 5-HT₃ Antagonists ondansetron HCl dihydrate (Zofran)	(Highly emetogenic chemotherapy — e.g., regimens containing cisplatin) **IV:** Initially, 8 mg infused over 15 min given 30 min prior to chemotherapy, followed by 1 mg/h by continuous infusion for up to 24 h; or, 32 mg diluted in 50–100 mL of saline or other compatible infusion fluid and infused over not less than 15 min, given 30 min prior to chemotherapy. Post-chemotherapy: After first 24 h, 8 mg PO q8h for up to 5 days (Less emetogenic chemotherapy — e.g., regimens containing cyclophosphamide, doxorubicin, epirubicin, fluorouracil and carboplatin) **IV:** Initially, 8 mg infused IV over 15 min, given 30 min prior to chemotherapy; or, 8-mg tablet PO 1–2 h prior to chemotherapy. Post-chemotherapy: 8-mg tablet PO bid for up to 5 days	• **IV:** Check product information or agency handbook for dilution and rate of administration. Compatible with D5W and NS; stable for up to 48 h

Table 62.4 (continued)
The antiemetics: Drug doses

Drug Generic name (Trade names)	Dosage	Nursing alert
E. 5-HT₃ Antagonists (cont'd)		
ondansetron (Zofran) (cont'd)	*Children:* 3–5 mg/m² IV over 15 min immediately before chemotherapy. After therapy, 4 mg PO q8h for up to 5 days (Radiotherapy-induced nausea and vomiting): *Adults:* Initially, 8 mg PO 1–2 h before radiotherapy.(Post-radiotherapy): 8 mg PO q8h for up to 5 days after course of tx. (Postoperative nausea and vomiting): *Adults:* For prevention, 16 mg PO 1 h prior to anesthesia. Alternatively, a single dose of 4 mg may be given by slow IV injection	
granisetron HCl (Kytril)	**IV:** *Adults:* 10 µg/kg infused over 5 min within 30 min before initiation of chemotherapy **Oral:** 2 mg on day of chemotherapy. This may be administered either as a single dose (2 x 1 mg) 1 h before chemotherapy, or as divided dose of 1 mg 1 h before chemotherapy followed by second 1-mg dose 12 h postchemotherapy	• Taken only on days that chemotherapy is administered • **IV:** For direct IV, check agency policy for certification. Prepared solution is stable for 24 h at room temperature
F. Miscellaneous Drugs		
1. Cannabinoid nabilone (Cesamet)	**Oral:** *Adults:* 1 mg or 2 mg bid. If required, administration of nabilone can be continued up to 24 h after chemotherapeutic agent is given. Max. recommended daily dose is 6 mg, in divided doses	• First dose should be given the night before initiating administration of chemotherapeutic medication. Second dose is usually administered 1–3 h before chemotherapy
2. Gastrokinetic Drug cisapride monohydrate (Prepulsid)	**Oral** (gastroesophageal reflux disease): *Adults:* Symptomatic management: 5–10 mg tid or qid, 15 min ac and hs; or, 20 mg bid, before breakfast and hs. Prophylaxis: 10 mg bid, before breakfast and hs, or 20 mg od, hs. In pts with severe disease, it may be necessary to increase dose to a max. of 20 mg bid. (Gastroparesis and pseudo-obstruction):	• Ensure that drug is taken 15 min ac • Should be taken with a liquid to ensure dissolution and absorption of tab

Endocrine Pharmacology

By definition, an endocrine gland produces one or more internal secretions that are introduced directly into the bloodstream and carried to other parts of the body whose functions they regulate or control. The endocrine glands are the thyroid, parathyroid, pancreas, adrenal cortex and gonads.

Unit 13 discusses the use of drugs as replacement therapy in cases of endocrine deficiency, as well as their use to reduce endocrine function in situations of hypersecretion. In the case of the adrenal cortex, we also discuss in detail the anti-inflammatory actions of the glucocorticoids and their importance in health care.

CHAPTER 63

Drugs and the Thyroid

Topics Discussed
- Drugs for hypothyroidism
- Drugs for hyperthyroidism
- For each drug discussed: Mechanism of action and pharmacologic effects, therapeutic uses, adverse effects
- Nursing management

Drugs Discussed
levothyroxine (lee-voe-thye-**rox**-in)

liothyronine (lye-oh-**thye**-roe-neen)

methimazole (meth-**im**-ah-zole)

potassium iodide (poe-**tass**-ee-yum **eye**-oh-dyed)

propylthiouracil (proe-pil-thye-oh-**yoor**-ah-sill)

sodium iodide (**so**-dee-yum **eye**-oh-dyed)

thyroglobulin (thye-roe-**glob**-yoo-lin)

thyroid (**thye**-royd)

Clinical Challenge

Consider this clinical challenge as you read through this chapter. The response to the challenge appears on page 745.

Ellen, a 36-year-old woman, has experienced significant weight loss in spite of increasing appetite. She has also had episodes of palpitations and fatigue. She is very concerned about these symptoms and mentions them to you at her visit to the Wellness Clinic. Consider the following questions:

1. What might account for Ellen's symptoms?
2. What tests will she require to confirm the diagnosis?
3. What options will she have for treatment?

The thyroid is the largest endocrine gland. Normally weighing about twenty grams, it can increase its size twenty- to thirty-fold if a goitre develops. The major function of the thyroid gland is the synthesis, storage and secretion of the iodinated chemicals L-triiodothyronine (T_3) and L-thyroxine (T_4). To accomplish this task, the thyroid actively extracts iodide from the plasma, oxidizes it to iodine before coupling the iodine to the amino acid tyrosine, forming either monoiodotyrosine or diiodotyrosine. T_3 is formed from one molecule each of monoiodotyrosine and diiodotyrosine. T_4 is produced from two molecules of diiodotyrosine. Once synthesized, both T_3 and T_4 are stored within the thyroid as thyroglobulin and released into the circulation following stimulation of the gland by the thyroid-stimulating hormone (TSH). Some of the T_4 released is subsequently converted to T_3.

Thyroid activity is controlled by TSH, released from the pituitary. For its part, TSH release is triggered by the secretion of the thyrotrophic-releasing hormone from the hypothalamus. TSH increases both the synthesis and secretion of T_3 and T_4. Removal of the anterior pituitary leads to a diminished thyroid mass as well as decreased production and secretion of thyroid hormones. The administration of pituitary extracts to hypophysectomized patients restores normal TSH levels and returns thyroid structure and function to normal.

A balance exists between the secretion of TSH and the thyroid hormones. An increase in circulating levels of T_3 and T_4 decreases TSH secretion. The reverse is also true: a decrease in circulating T_3 and T_4 increases TSH secretion.

Once secreted, T_3 and T_4 are highly bound to specific plasma proteins called thyroid-binding globulin and thyroid-binding prealbumin. T_3 and T_4 are also bound nonspecifically to albumin. A smaller percentage of T_3 is bound, and as a result more of this hormone is found free in blood. Only T_3 and T_4 molecules free in plasma water can enter body cells and exert an effect. Thus, T_3 produces a more rapid effect than T_4.

T_3 and T_4 increase tissue metabolic rate. In addition to activating mitochondrial protein synthesis, they stimulate the cell membrane sodium pump, causing an expenditure of energy. Thyroid hormones are also necessary for general growth and for maturation and development of the central nervous and skeletal systems. Thyroid deficiency in childhood results in cretinism, a condition characterized by growth failure and mental retardation.

Diseases of the thyroid can be divided into those that involve only a change in gland size (adenamatous goitre, thyroid cancer or nontoxic diffuse goitre) and those that involve an alteration in its secretion (hypothyroidism or hyperthyroidism). In hypothyroidism or hyperthyroidism, drug therapy plays an important role in restoring health.

Drugs for Hypothyroidism

Nursing assessment of patients with hypothyroidism reveals fatigue, decreased heart rate, swelling of the hands and the area around the eyes, constipation, dry skin, brittle hair and menstrual irregularities. These symptoms can range from mild to severe. If mild, they may be inapparent to the patient and detectable only by laboratory examination. When severe, they can extend to a characteristic guttural voice, thickened boggy skin (myxedema), slow mental processes, loss of body hair, intolerance to cold, ascites, pericardial effusion, frank myxedema, coma and death.

Hypothyroidism can be primary or secondary. If primary, the disorder lies within the gland itself. This may occur as a result of radioiodine therapy, partial or total surgical removal of the gland, or treatment with antithyroid drugs. Primary hypothyroidism is also caused by the autoimmune destruction of the gland (Hashimoto's thyroiditis). Secondary hypothyroidism results from the failure of the pituitary to secrete adequate amounts of TSH.

Regardless of the cause, thyroid hormone therapy is essential to reverse the clinical abnormalities and restore euthyroidism. Several products are available that provide T_3 or T_4, or both. Their pharmacologic actions, therapeutic uses and adverse effects are identical. They differ only in their actual content of T_3 and T_4, the speed with which they produce their effects, the absolute doses used and their cost. Table 63.1 summarizes the differences between these products.

Table 63.1
Preparations containing thyroxine (T_4) and/or liothyronine (T_3)

	Thyroid	Thyroglobulin	Sodium levothyroxine	Sodium liothyronine
Source	animal thyroids	animal thyroids	synthetic	synthetic
Content	$T_3 + T_4$	$T_3 + T_4$	T_4	T_3
Standardization	organic I content	organic I content	analysis of T_4 content	analysis of T_3 content
Approx. equiv. doses	60 mg	60 mg	0.1 mg	25 µg
Approx. peak action	2 weeks	2 weeks	2 weeks	0.5 week
Approx. duration of action	3 weeks	3 weeks	3 weeks	1 week

Desiccated Thyroid Tablets (Thyrar®)

Desiccated thyroid tablets are prepared by removing fat and water from hog or beef thyroids. They are the cheapest form of therapy but have several drawbacks. The tablets are standardized on the basis of their iodine content rather than on the amounts of T_3 and T_4 present. Because the major portion of iodine in the gland is in the form of inert iodotyrosines, the iodine assay does not reflect the biologic potency of the tablets. In addition, the ratio of T_4 to T_3 can vary from 2:1 to 3:1, depending on the particular batch of tablets. The iodine assay will not measure the actual levels of each hormone or the relative ratios of one to the other.

L-Thyroxine, Levothyroxine (Eltroxin®, Levothyroid®, Synthroid®)

Oral and injectable forms of l-thyroxine (T_4) are the preferred treatment. The advantages of these preparations over desiccated thyroid include reliable potency and the absence of wide swings in serum T_3 and T_4 levels. Converted in part to T_3 in the body, T_4 provides a reliable source of both thyroid hormones. The amount of T_4 usually considered equivalent to 60 mg of desiccated thyroid or 25 µg of liothyronine sodium (T_3) is 0.1 mg.

Liothyronine: L-Triiodothyronine (Cytomel®)

Liothyronine (T_3) is 2.5 to 3.3 times more potent than l-thyroxine (T_4). Its effects are seen sooner, and at first glance liothyronine may seem more attractive than T_4. However, stabilization of a patient on T_3 may be more difficult because it is cleared from the body faster than T_4. Furthermore, treatment with T_4 provides a reliable source of both T_3 and T_4.

Combinations of Liothyronine and L-Thyroxine, Liotrix (Euthroid®, Thyrolar®)

These preparations contain the sodium salts of T_4 and T_3 in a 4:1 ratio and are designed to mimic normal thyroid secretion. However, the patient-to-patient variations in normal serum T_3 levels make it difficult to achieve this goal. It is difficult to see how these products provide any advantage over the cheaper T_4-containing tablets which are converted, at least in part, to T_3 in the body.

Thyroglobulin (Proloid®)

Obtained from frozen hog thyroid, thyroglobulin meets USP standards for iodine, as assayed biologically. Its indications, adverse effects, precautions and doses are the same as those for thyroid tablets, with which it is equipotent.

Special Treatment Problems

The treatment of the hypothyroid neonate or child presents a special problem. Children, particularly neonates, are at risk if thyroid activity is low. If hypothyroidism is suspected in the neonate or child, serum should be drawn for thyroid function tests and therapy begun immediately without waiting for the results. The risk of giving thyroid hormone to a neonate who does not require it is minimal compared to the danger of withholding the drug if the baby is hypothyroid. One protocol calls for 10–12 µg of T_4 to be given for every kilogram of body weight, initially. This can be reduced to 8 –10 µg/kg after three months. Thereafter, the dose may be reduced according to the manufacturer's directions.

Although myxedema coma is rare, it can have a fifty percent mortality rate. To handle this situation, an initial intravenous dose of 300–500 µg of T_4 can be given, followed by 50–100 µg intravenously daily.

Table 63.2 on the next page lists the clinically significant drug interactions with thyroid replacement drugs.

Nursing Management

Table 63.3 on the next page describes the nursing management of the patient receiving thyroid preparations. Dosage details of individual drugs are given in Table 63.6 (pages 747–748).

Table 63.2
Thyroid replacement: Drug interactions

Drug	Interaction
Anticoagulants, oral	• Oral anticoagulants may have their effects increased by all forms of thyroid replacement. Reduce anticoagulant dose by one-third when thyroid replacement is started. Thereafter, adjust anticoagulant doses on the basis of prothrombin times
Cholestyramine and colestipol	• Cholestyramine and colestipol bind thyroxine and liothyronine in the intestine, thus impairing their absorption. Four to 5 h should elapse between the administration of cholestyramine or colestipol and thyroid hormones
Estrogens and progestins	• Estrogens and progestins may increase serum thyroxine-binding globulin, possibly increasing the dose of thyroxine replacement tx required
Hypoglycemics, oral	• Oral hypoglycemics may have their effects reduced by thyroid replacement. It may be necessary to increase the dose of the antidiabetic drug if thyroid replacement tx is started. Conversely, decreasing the dose of the thyroid preparation may cause hypoglycemic reactions if the dosage of the oral hypoglycemic drug is not adjusted
Insulin	• Insulin may require an increase in dosage if thyroid replacement tx is used
Phenytoin	• Phenytoin may displace thyroxine from plasma protein binding sites, thereby temporarily increasing free or active levels of thyroxine. As a result, phenytoin may increase the activity of thyroxine

Table 63.3
Nursing management of thyroid replacement drugs

Assessment of risk vs. benefit	Patient data	• Assess to establish baseline VS, general state of health, clinical indicators of present condition • *Pregnancy:* Risk category varies with drug but is generally category A (no risk to the fetus has been shown in studies that are adequate and well controlled)
	Drug data	• *Some serious drug interactions:* Confer with pharmacist • May alter effectiveness of oral anticoagulants. Vigilant monitoring required
Implementation	Rights of administration	• Using the "rights" helps prevent errors of administration
	Right route	• Give PO
	Right time	• Best administered as a single dose prior to, or with, breakfast; helps to maintain regular hormone blood levels, promotes ease of drug regime for pt, and may prevent drug-related insomnia
	Nursing therapeutics	• Both apical P and BP should be monitored prior to and during tx • *Emotional support:* Provide reassurance regarding drug tx; Explain that thyroid hormone tx does not cure hypothyroidism; it is replacement tx only and may be lifelong

Table 63.3 (continued)
Nursing management of thyroid replacement drugs

| Implementation (cont'd) | Patient/family teaching | • Instruct pt to take medication exactly as directed, at same time each day. If a dose is missed, take as soon as remembered unless it is almost time for the next dose
• If 2–3 doses are missed, pt should contact physician. Pts should not discontinue medication without physician's knowledge and approval
• Instruct family and pt to check pulse correctly. Dose should be withheld if resting pulse is > 100 beats/min. If this should occur, notify physician
• Pts should also be advised that changing brands of medication should be avoided. Changing brands once a stable response is achieved may result in problems with bioequivalence
• Inform pts who take anticoagulant medication in combination with this drug to report unusual bruising or bleeding to their physician at once
• Advise pt to notify physician if any of the following occur: headache, nervousness, diarrhea, excessive sweating, heat intolerance, chest pain, increased pulse rate, palpitations. Instruct older pts to watch for s/s of aggravated CV disease (chest pain, dyspnea, tachycardia)
• Instruct pt to avoid taking other medications (Rx or OTCs) concurrently without advising physician or pharmacist
• Instruct pts to inform physician or dentist that they are taking this medication prior to tx or surgery |
| Outcomes | Monitoring of progress | *Continually monitor:*
• Follow-up exams: thyroid function tests should be performed yearly
• Signs/symptoms of adverse reactions; document and report immediately to physician
• Signs/symptoms of hyperthyroidism: tachycardia, chest pain, nervousness, insomnia, diaphoresis, tremors, weight loss
• Signs of myocardial ischemia and tachyarrhythmias |

Drugs for Hyperthyroidism

The major signs and symptoms of hyperthyroidism are well known. They include heat intolerance, loss of weight, bruit over the thyroid, a hyperkinetic circulatory state (including a rapid heart rate and dysrhythmias) and dyspnea. Unusual muscle fatigue, irritability and the presence of eye signs, such as lid lag, weakness of the extraocular muscles and proptosis may also be seen. The great majority of North American patients with hyperthyroidism suffer from either Graves's disease or toxic adenoma of the thyroid. The distinction between the two is important. Graves's disease is an autoimmune disorder caused by the existence in the blood of thyroid-stimulating antibody (TSAb). It may be treated surgically, with iodine-131 (^{131}I), or with antithyroid drugs. A toxic adenoma of the thyroid is a benign neoplasm that requires removal to produce a cure.

Propylthiouracil (Propacil®, Propyl-Thyracil®) and Methimazole (Tapazole®)

Mechanism of action and pharmacologic effects. Propylthiouracil and methimazole block the oxidative iodination of tyrosine, thereby preventing the formation of T_3 and T_4. Propylthiouracil also impairs the peripheral conversion of T_4 to T_3. Methimazole does not affect the conversion of T_4 to T_3.

Table 63.4
Propylthiouracil and methimazole: Drug interactions

Drug	Interaction
Anticoagulants	• The activity of anticoagulants may be potentiated by the antivitamin-K activity attributed to methimazole. Propylthiouracil has occasionally been reported to cause hypoprothrombinemia which would increase the effect of anticoagulants. Doses of oral anticoagulants, administered concurrently with propylthiouracil, should be adjusted accordingly
Sulfonamides	• Sulfonamides should not be administered concomitantly with propylthiouracil as both can cause agranulocytosis

Therapeutic uses. Propylthiouracil and methimazole are used to prepare patients for surgery, to assist in the management of patients in thyrotoxic crisis and for chronic treatment of hyperthyroidism. Titrating the dose according to the response should make the patient euthyroid in three to six weeks. Thereafter, the dose should be reduced gradually, with the ultimate maintenance dose being achieved in a few months. Generally, antithyroid drugs are administered for one to two years and are then tapered or discontinued to establish whether remission has occurred.

Remissions occur in 30% to 40% of patients with Graves's disease after long-term antithyroid therapy, and in these individuals propylthiouracil or methimazole can be successfully stopped. Remission occurs only in patients with relatively small goitres. Patients with larger goitres (> 45 g) invariably require further treatment. Combining propylthiouracil or methimazole in doses designed to make the patient slightly hypothyroid, with sufficient T_4 to maintain euthyroidism, has been claimed to increase the chance of disease remission. One dosage regimen calls for T_4 to be administered in a dose of 100 µg/day, together with methimazole, 10 mg/day.

Both propylthiouracil and methimazole are contraindicated in nursing mothers. Concerns over the use of either drug in pregnancy are expressed later in this chapter (see Special Treatment Problems). It goes without saying that in the treatment of thyrotoxicosis during pregnancy, propylthiouracil or methimazole should be used in the smallest possible doses. Rare cases of scalp defects have occurred in infants born to mothers who have used methimazole during pregnancy. Because scalp defects have not been reported in offspring of patients treated with propylthiouracil, this drug may be preferable to methimazole in pregnant women requiring treatment with antithyroid drugs.

Adverse effects. Propylthiouracil produces numerous adverse effects, including skin rash, urticaria, fever, granulocytopenia, agranulocytosis, pancytopenia, hepatitis, myalgia and headache. Methimazole's adverse effects include nausea, vomiting, epigastric distress, headache, fever, arthralgia, pruritus, edema and pancytopenia. Overtreatment with either propylthiouracil or methimazole can result in goitre. The decrease in serum T_3 and T_4 increases TSH secretion, producing hyperplasia of the thyroid.

The effects of propylthiouracil on the fetus have been presented above. Both drugs can produce hypothyroidism in the fetus. Methimazole can also produce rare scalp defects in the fetus. As result, propylthiouracil is preferred in pregnant women. Both propylthiouracil and methimazole are contraindicated in the nursing mother.

Table 63.4 lists the clinically significant drug interactions with propylthiouracil and methimazole.

Potassium Iodide, Sodium Iodide, Strong Iodine Solutions

Mechanism of action and pharmacologic effects. Large doses of iodide or iodine inhibit, at least temporarily, organic iodine formation and thyroid hormone release. High doses may also prevent the effects of TSH on the thyroid gland.

Therapeutic uses. Iodine or iodide is given after treatment with an antithyroid drug such as propylthiouracil, to prepare hyperthyroid patients for thyroidectomy. Iodide is also given intravenously approximately two to three hours after an antithyroid drug to treat thyrotoxic crisis or neonatal thyrotoxicosis.

Adverse effects. These drugs produce an unpleasant taste of iodine and a burning in the mouth. Patients may experience a sore mouth and throat, as well as hypersalivation, painful salivary glands, acne and other rashes. Diarrhea and a productive cough may also be seen. Sensitive individuals may experience angioedema with swelling of the larynx and dyspnea.

Special Treatment Problems

Hyperthyroidism in pregnancy is a special treatment problem. In the nongravid state, hyperthyroidism may be treated by surgically removing the thyroid, destroying it with ^{131}I, or administering propylthiouracil or methimazole. In pregnancy, however, most physicians prefer not to subject the patient to the stress of surgery. Radioactive iodine is also not appropriate because it crosses the placenta and can damage the fetal thyroid. Therefore, the only treatment remaining is propylthiouracil or methimazole. As stated earlier, because methimazole administration during pregnancy has been associated with rare cases of scalp defects, many physicians prefer to use propylthiouracil. In using either of these drugs, however, it is important to titrate the dose carefully to guard against producing a hypothyroid goitre in the fetus.

Thyroid storm is a rare, life-threatening disorder that occurs during the course of untreated hyperthyroidism that may be precipitated by infection, trauma, or surgery. It is associated with heightened manifestations of hyperthyroidism with hyperpyrexia, dehydration and even congestive heart failure. Thyroid storm must be treated quickly because it represents a danger to life. Treatment includes propylthiouracil 300 mg every six hours, sodium iodide 50 mg intravenously (one dose given at least one hour after propylthiouracil), propranolol 40 mg orally every six hours, and restoration and maintenance of adequate hydration. Prednisone 60 mg daily is often administered, although there is no clear evidence of its value.

Adjunctive Drugs

Many of the effects of hyperthyroidism resemble excessive sympathetic nervous system stimulation. These include tachycardia, palpitations, sweating, tremor and nervousness. The use of beta blockers has been mentioned in the treatment of thyroid storm. Their administration should not be restricted to the acute needs of patients with severe hyperthyroidism. Drugs such as propranolol (Inderal®) can benefit many hyperthyroid patients by reducing or abolishing some or all of the effects mentioned earlier. It should be recognized, however, that a beta blocker provides only symptomatic treatment. The activity of the thyroid gland and the concentrations of serum T_3 and T_4 still remain elevated. More specific treatment, such as surgery, ^{131}I or antithyroid drugs, is still required to reduce thyroid function.

Benzodiazepines may also play a role in the treatment of hyperthyroidism to reduce the anxiety of patients. The drug of choice is probably one with a relatively long half-life, such as diazepam.

Nursing Management

Table 63.5 on the next page describes the nursing management of the patient receiving thyroid antagonists. Dosage details of individual drugs are given in Table 63.6 (pages 747–748).

Response to Clinical Challenge

1. Ellen's symptoms are consistent with hyperthyroidism. Due to excessive thyroid hormones, metabolic rate is accelerated with resulting hunger, weight loss and heat intolerance.
2. The diagnosis can be confirmed by examinations and thyroid lab tests.
3. Besides drug therapy, other treatment options include surgical removal or radioactive iodine therapy.

Further Reading

Medication use in hypothyroid patient. *Home Care Provider* 1996;1(2):97–99.

Table 63.5
Nursing management of thyroid antagonists

Assessment of risk vs. benefit	Patient data	• Assess to establish baseline VS, general state of health, clinical indicators of present condition • *Pregnancy:* Risk category D (human fetal risk has been demonstrated but benefits might outweigh possible risks). Baby might develop thyroid problems; monitor carefully at birth. Drug passes into breast milk and thus should be not used during lactation
	Drug data	• *Some serious drug interactions:* Confer with pharmacist • May alter effectiveness of oral anticoagulants; vigilant monitoring and dosage adjustment are required
Implementation	Rights of administration	• Using the "rights" helps prevent errors of administration
	Right route	• Give PO
	Right time	• May be given without regard to food (which may increase or decrease absorption), but should be given at same time with respect to meals each day
	Nursing therapeutics	• Review hyperthyroidism with pt/family. Explain that remissions can occur with long-term antithyroid tx (i.e., 1–2 years) and drugs may be discontinued. Other options for tx include surgical removal or radioactive iodine tx
	Patient/family teaching	• Advise pt to report suspected pregnancy to physician prior to tx • Missed doses may precipitate hyperthyroidism. Instruct pt to take medication exactly as directed. If a dose is missed, it should be taken as soon as it is remembered, unless it is almost time for next dose. If more than one dose is missed, pt should contact physician • Discontinuing medication should be initiated only after consultation with physician • Pt should monitor weight, checking it 2–3x/week. If any significant change occurs, contact physician • Medication may cause drowsiness; pts should avoid driving and other activities that require alertness until response is known • Pts should be advised to report sore throat, fever, chills, headache, malaise, weakness, yellowing of eyes or skin, unusual bleeding or bruising, rash or any symptoms of hypothyroidism or hyperthyroidism. • Instruct pt to avoid taking other medications (Rx or OTCs) containing iodine concurrently without advising physician or pharmacist • Instruct pts to carry ID that describes the medication and their regimen with them at all times • Advise pts to consult dietitian regarding dietary sources of iodine (food with high concentrations should be avoided) • Some cold medications contain iodine as an expectorant. Advise pt to consult with pharmacist prior to using OTC cold remedies • Instruct pts to inform physician or dentist that they are taking this medication prior to tx or surgery • Remind pts of importance of routine lab testing and exams

Table 63.3 (continued)
Nursing management of thyroid antagonists

Outcomes	Monitoring of progress	*Continually monitor:*
		• Signs/symptoms of hyperthyroidism or thyrotoxicosis (tachycardia, palpitations, nervousness, insomnia, fever, diaphoresis, heat intolerance, tremors, weight loss, diarrhea) • Signs/symptoms of hypothyroidism (intolerance to cold, constipation, dry skin, headache, listlessness, fatigue, weakness • Skin rash or swelling of cervical lymph nodes. If these signs appear, tx should be discontinued • Signs/symptoms of iodism (metallic taste, stomatitis, skin lesions, cold symptoms, severe GI upset). Should these be observed, contact physician immediately

Table 63.6
Treatment of thyroid disorders: Drug doses

Drug Generic name (Trade names)	Dosage	Nursing alert
A. Thyroid Preparations		
thyroid USP (Armour Thyroid®, S-P-T, Thyrar)	**Oral** (for myxedema): Initially, 30–180 mg daily. (Other hypothyroid states): 60–300 mg daily. Usual maint. dose, 30–125 mg/day	• Administer as a single dose, preferably before or with breakfast (promotes stable hormone blood levels and prevents drug-related insomnia). Monitor apical P and BP prior to and during tx
l-thyroxine, levothyroxine sodium (Eltroxin, Levothyroid, Synthroid)	**Oral** (primary hypothyroidism): Approximately 1.6 µg/kg/day **IV** (for myxedema coma): *Adults:* 2–4 mL of a solution containing 100 µg/mL, infused slowly; 1–3 mL may be given on 2nd day if necessary, then 1 mL/day until oral administration is possible	• Check tablet dosage carefully; drug is available in many strengths • Monitor apical P and BP prior to and periodically during tx
liothyronine sodium, l-triiodothyronine (Cytomel, Tertroxin)	**Oral:** *Young and middle-aged adults* (mild hypothyroidism): Initially, 25 µg daily; increase by 12.5 or 25 µg at intervals of 1–2 weeks prn. (Severe hypothyroidism) Initially, 5 µg daily; increase by 5–10 µg at intervals of 1–2 weeks until a daily dose of 25 µg is reached; thereafter, increase amount by 12.5–25 µg at 1- to 2-week intervals prn. Usual maint. dose, up to 75 µg/day. *Older adults:* Initially, 2.5–5 µg daily for 3–6 weeks; amount is then doubled q6weeks	• Administer as a single dose, preferably before or with breakfast (promotes stable hormone blood levels and prevents drug-related insomnia) • Monitor apical P and BP prior to and during tx • Because of rapid onset of action, initial dose should be low and gradually increased, especially for elderly pts

Table 63.6 (continued)
Treatment of thyroid disorders: Drug doses

Drug Generic name (Trade names)	Dosage	Nursing alert
B. Antithyroid Drugs propylthiouracil (Propacil, Propyl Thyracil)	**Oral:** *Adults:* Initially, 50–100 mg q8h, with increases prn to a max. of 500 mg/day. Initial doses as high as 900 mg/day may be required. When doses > 300 mg/day are needed, drug should be administered q4–6 h. Pt should be examined regularly by a physician and dose adjusted until pt is euthyroid (usually after 6–8 weeks). At this stage, dosage should be reduced by 33% q4–6weeks to maint. dose of 50 mg bid or tid *Children* (initial dose guideline): 150 mg/m^2/24 h. *Children ≥ 10 years:* 150–300 mg/day in divided doses, at regular intervals; *6–10 years:* 50–150 mg/day in divided doses, at regular intervals. General maint. dose: 50 mg bid when euthyroid	• Give with or without food but administer at same time each day. Food may increase or decrease absorption • Store in light-resistant container
methimazole (Tapazole)	**Oral:** *Adults:* Initially, 15 mg for mild hyperthyroidism, 30–40 mg for moderately severe hyperthyroidism, and 60 mg for severe hyperthyroidism, divided into 3 doses at 8-h intervals. Maint. dosage, 5–15 mg daily. *Children:* Initially, 0.4 mg/kg/day, divided into 3 doses and given at 8-h intervals. Maint. dosage is approximately 1/2 initial dose	• Give with or without food, but administer at same time each day. Food may increase or decrease absorption • Store in light-resistant container
potassium iodide, sodium iodide, strong iodine solution	**Oral:** *Adults/children* (to prepare pts for thyroidectomy): 2–6 drops strong iodine solution USP tid or 1 or 2 drops tid of potassium iodide solution USP for 10 days before surgery. (For thyroid storm): 1 h after antithyroid drugs and as part of the medical emergency tx, at least 2 drops strong iodide solution or 50–100 mg potassium iodide solution USP, q6–12 h **IV** (for thyroid storm): 50–100 mg sodium iodide USP daily, beginning 1 h after initial doses of propylthiouracil and propranolol have been administered	• **PO:** Syrup and tablets available. Tabs should be stored in light-resistant container. Oral solution is usually colourless but may darken on standing; this does not affect potency • Dissolve tabs in 200 mL (8 oz) fruit juice, milk or water. Administer pc to decrease GI irritation. Pts should be hydrated to mask salty taste of solution. Administer liquid through a straw to prevent discoloration of teeth • Avoid enteric-coated tablets, which have been linked to bowel lesions and other serious complications including perforation, hemorrhage and obstruction • If medication is prescribed as radiation protectant, it should be administered exactly when ordered. In case of nuclear emergency, medication will provide 90–99% protection when given immediately after exposure. Potassium iodide offers 50% protection when administered within 3–4 h of exposure

Drugs and the Parathyroid Gland

Topics Discussed
- Plasma calcium
- Drugs for hypoparathyroidism
- Treatment of hyperparathyroidism
- Nursing management

Drugs Discussed
calciferol (kal-**siff**-eh-role)

calcitonin (kal-sih-**toe**-nin)

calcitriol (kal-sih-**trye**-ole)

calcium (**kal**-see-um)

cholecalciferol (kole-eh-kal-**siff**-eh-role)

dihydrotachysterol (dye-hye-droe-tak-**iss**-ter-ole)

ergocalciferol (er-goe-kal-**siff**-eh-role)

prednisone (**pred**-nih-zone)

vitamin D_2

vitamin D_3

Clinical Challenge

Consider this clinical challenge as you read through this chapter. The response to the challenge appears on page 752.

Ellen, age 36, has recently been diagnosed with hyperthyroidism. She relied on drug therapy for several months without signs of remission and, unfortunately, experienced agranulocytosis. This was diagnosed immediately when she reported sore throat, fever and malaise, and drug therapy was discontinued. Ellen decided on surgical removal of the thyroid gland. Following this, she may be at risk for hypoparathyroidism.

Explain this risk to Ellen and possible symptoms related to the condition. What treatment plan can avoid the associated symptoms?

Plasma Calcium

The parathyroid hormone (PTH), vitamin D and calcitonin regulate calcium and phosphate metabolism. Calcium serves both mechanical and metabolic functions in the body. Mechanically, it is the main constituent in bone, where the great majority of body calcium is found. Metabolically, calcium is essential for nerve and muscle function, cardiac activity, the actions of cell membranes and the clotting of blood.

It is because of calcium's metabolic functions that we focus attention on its plasma concentration. Plasma levels of calcium depend on its absorption from the intestine, the quantity stored in bone, and the amount eliminated by the kidneys. Forty percent of plasma calcium is bound to albumin and not able to diffuse into tissues. Another ten percent is present as citrate or phosphate salts. The remainder of plasma calcium is present in its ionic form, and it is this fraction that leaves the vascular bed to influence metabolic functions.

Normal plasma calcium levels range from 9–10.5 mg/100 mL (2.2–2.56 mmol/L). PTH is secreted in response to a fall in the levels of ionized plasma calcium. It increases the intestinal absorption of calcium, mediates the transfer of calcium from bone to blood, and decreases the renal excretion of calcium. If it can be stated that a fall in ionized calcium concentration in plasma triggers the release of PTH, the converse is also true: high levels of ionized calcium in plasma decrease PTH secretion.

For its part, vitamin D stimulates the absorption of calcium and phosphate. Vitamin D is not active itself. Rather, it is a prohormone, converted to 25-hydroxy vitamin D in the liver. Its subsequent metabolism in the kidney to the active 1,25-dihydroxy vitamin D (calcitriol) stimulates calcium absorption.

Calcitonin is a hormone secreted by the thyroid gland. Released in response to an increase in plasma-ionized calcium, it decreases bone resorption and increases calcium excretion.

Drugs for Hypoparathyroidism

In the past this condition often resulted from total, or partial, surgical thyroidectomy. Located behind both the upper and lower poles of the thyroid gland, the parathyroids are "sitting ducks" to be removed inadvertently during thyroidectomy. The use of radioactive iodine, propylthiouracil or methimazole to reduce thyroid function has decreased the incidence of hypoparathyroidism. In idiopathic hypoparathyroidism, the gland ceases to function for unknown reasons.

Vitamin D and Calcium Supplements

Mechanism of action and pharmacologic effects. Hypoparathyroidism is characterized by hypocalcemia and hyperphosphatemia with a history of symptoms that include paresthesias and muscle spasms that may proceed to tetany and convulsions. Preparations of PTH are not available for therapeutic use. Patients may be treated by giving vitamin D_2 or vitamin D_3 plus elemental calcium. The goal of therapy is to stabilize plasma calcium levels at no higher than 9 mg/100 mL (2.2 mmol/L) to prevent hypercalciuria.

Adverse effects. The primary adverse effects resulting from the use of vitamin D or calcium, or both, is hypercalcemia manifesting as muscle weakness, increased myocardial irritability, polyuria with accompanying thirst, anorexia, nausea, vomiting, bone pain, either constipation or diarrhea, lethargy, exhaustion, mental confusion and irritability.

Table 64.1 lists the clinically significant drug interactions for calcium.

Treatment of Hyperparathyroidism

More than eighty-five percent of cases of primary hyperparathyroidism are due to a chief cell adenoma of the parathyroid gland. Patients often present with symptoms of hypercalcemia, bone disease and renal calculi. The diagnosis of hyperparathyroidism is usually made in the clinical laboratory. Serum calcium levels are usually in the range of 2.69–3.42 mmol/L (11–14 mg/100 mL). In some cases, they may be higher.

Hyperparathyroidism is usually treated by surgical removal of the hyperfunctioning tissue. If this is not possible, medical treatment may ameliorate the symptoms caused by the hypercalcemia. An attempt is often made to restore body fluids, electrolytes and renal function to normal. This involves the administration of fluids, with or

Table 64.1
Calcium: Drug interactions

Drug	Interaction
Corticosteroids	• The administration of a corticosteroid may interfere with calcium absorption
Digoxin and other digitalis glycosides	• Digitalis products and calcium ions have similar effects on the myocardium. The injection of calcium preparations is strictly contraindicated in digitalized pts
Tetracyclines	• Tetracycline absorption is reduced by oral calcium preparations

without saline, and large doses of loop diuretics, such as furosemide or ethacrynic acid, to increase calcium excretion. Nursing responsibilities related to the use of these medications were discussed in depth in Chapter 38. Readers are advised to refer to that material. Neutral phosphate solutions, given either orally or intravenously, will also lower plasma calcium levels as the element moves into bone.

Corticosteroids, such as prednisone, which decrease calcium absorption, and calcitonin may be tried in the treatment of hyperparathyroidism. The nursing activities initiated as the result of the prescription of corticosteroids are presented in detail in Chapter 66.

Nursing Management

Table 64.2 describes the nursing management of the patient receiving drugs for hypoparathyroidism. Dosage details of individual drugs are given in Table 64.3 (pages 752–754).

Table 64.2
Nursing management of hypoparathyroidism

Assessment of risk vs. benefit	Patient data	• For tx of hypoparathyroidism with vitamin D, calcium and diet, complete a nutritional assessment with particular emphasis on dietary calcium and vitamin D • Assess signs/symptoms including VS, calcium levels and fluid I/O ratio. Check pt's hx for previous incidence of renal calculi • *Pregnancy:* Risk category C (animal studies show adverse effects to fetus but human data are unknown or insufficient); benefits may be acceptable despite risks
	Drug data	• *Some serious drug interactions:* Confer with pharmacist • Most serious adverse effects are caused by hypercalcemia
Implementation	Rights of administration	• Using the "rights" helps prevent errors of administration
	Right route	• Give PO
	Nursing therapeutics	• Complete nutritional assessment or refer to dietitian for counselling • Emphasize importance of self-management of hypoparathyroidism • Dry mouth, nausea, vomiting, metallic taste and constipation may be early symptoms of toxicity. Therefore, monitor pt's eating as well as bowel habits
	Patient/family teaching	• Emphasize necessity for lifelong tx and provide suggestions to assist with following a regular regimen (e.g., dosette, calendar with medication schedule) • Instruct pt to adhere to dietary and supplemental requirements (calcium, 1000 mg) • Pts should avoid OTC drugs unless approved by physician • Pts should avoid magnesium-containing antacids • Instruct pt/family in s/s of drug efficacy and also of drug overdose, esp. hypercalcemia as manifested by muscle weakness, bone pain, polyuria without thirst, anorexia, nausea, vomiting • Instruct pts to report any s/s of vitamin D intoxication (weakness, nausea, vomiting, dry mouth, constipation, muscle or bone pain, metallic taste)

(cont'd on next page)

Table 64.2 (continued)
Nursing management of hypoparathyroidism

Outcomes	Monitoring of progress	*Continually monitor:*
		• Clinical response indicating tx success (reduction in signs/symptoms)
		• When high doses are used, monitor the following frequently: serum and urine calcium, potassium and urea levels
		• Signs/symptoms of adverse reactions; document and report immediately to physician. Most serious adverse reactions occur with hypercalcemia and include myocardial irritability, mental confusion as well as symptoms described earlier
		• Serum calcium level (serum Ca level x serum PO_4 level should not exceed 70). During titration, determine serum calcium 2x/week
		• Periodic monitoring of plasma calcium levels may be ordered to assess drug tx

---

Response to Clinical Challenge

During surgery to remove the thyroid gland, the parathyroids may also be removed, resulting in hypoparathyroidism. The common symptoms are paresthesias, muscle spasms (which may produce tetany) and convulsions, if not treated. To avoid the symptoms caused by hypocalcemia, treatment with vitamin D, calcium supplements and dietary regulation is usually successful.

Table 64.3
Treatment of parathyroid disorders: Drug doses

Drug Generic name (Trade names)	Dosage	Nursing alert
A. Vitamin D and Vitamin D-like Preparations		
vitamin D_2, ergocalciferol, calciferol (Deltalin, Drisdol)	**Oral** (for hypoparathyroidism): *Adults:* Initially, 50 000–200 000 IU daily after acute tetany is controlled with IV calcium. Maint. dose, 25 000–1 000 000 IU/day. *Children:* 10 000–25 000 IU daily	• **PO:** Given in tablet, capsule and liquid form. If pt is unable to absorb oral form, then give IM injection of vitamin D dispersed in oil • Proceed with caution if administered to cardiac pts, especially those receiving digitalis glycosides. Dosages of 60 000 IU/day can cause hypercalcemia

Table 64.3 (continued)
Treatment of parathyroid disorders: Drug doses

Drug Generic name (Trade names)	Dosage	Nursing alert
A. Vitamin D and Vitamin D-like Preparations (cont'd)		
vitamin D$_3$, cholecalciferol, dihydro-tachysterol (Hytakerol)	**Oral:** Tx must be strictly individualized and maintained under careful control of the calcium levels of the blood and urine. *For acute cases:* 0.75–2.5 mg daily for several days. Maint. dose is from 0.25–1.75 mg weekly, depending on blood and urine calcium levels	• **PO:** Supplied in tablets, capsules or oral solution. Medication should be stored in light-resistant, tightly closed container. Do not refrigerate
calcitriol (Rocaltrol)	*Effectiveness of tx is predicated on adequate daily calcium intake, i.e., 800 mg for adults and 350 mg for infants during the first 6 months of life* (Hypocalcemia in chronic renal failure) **Oral:** *Adults:* 0.25 µg calcitriol initially; increase by 0.25 µg calcitriol/day at 4- to 8-week intervals. Usual dose, 0.5–1.0 µg/day. *Children:* 0.25–2 µg/day **IV:** *Adults:* 0.5 µg (0.01 µg/kg) 3x/week. May increase by 0.25–0.5 µg/dose at 2- to 4-week intervals. Usual dose, 0.5–3.0 µg 3x/week (0.01–0.05 µg/kg 3x/week) (Hypoparathyroidism or pseudohypoparathyroidism) **Oral:** *Adults:* 0.25 µg/day; may increase at 2- to 4-week intervals (usual range, 0.5–2 µg/day). *Children 1–5 years:* 0.25–0.75 µg/day (0.04–0.08 µg/kg/day)	• **PO:** Supplied in capsule form. Protect from heat and light • This is the most potent form of vitamin D available. Anyone taking it without a prescription is at serious risk for toxicity. Instruct pts never to permit anyone else to take their medication
B. Mineral		
calcium (available in various salt forms)	(Tx of calcium deficiency, including hypoparathyroidism) **Oral:** *Adults:* Approx. 2 g elemental calcium/day in divided doses **IV:** *Adults:* Initially, 20 mL of 10% solution of calcium gluconate, injected slowly, followed by slow infusion of 0.3–0.8% solution (30–40 mL of 10% solution in 500–1000 mL of isotonic NaCl or D5W injection) over 3–12 h. *Infants:* 2 mL/ kg of 10% solution	• **PO:** Check tabs; available in many forms and strengths • **IV:** For direct IV, check agency policy. For intermittent infusion, dilute according to manufacturer's instructions

(cont'd on next page)

Table 64.3
Treatment of parathyroid disorders: Drug doses

Drug Generic name (Trade names)	Dosage	Nursing alert
C. Hormonal Therapy		
calcitonin salmon (Calcimar, Miacalcin)	(Paget's disease) **IM/SC:** *Adults:* 100 IU/day initially; maint. dose, 50 IU/day or 50–100 IU every 1–3 days. (Hypercalcemia) **IM/SC:** *Adults:* Initially, 4 IU/ kg q12h; can increase up to 8 IU/kg q6h. (Osteoporosis) **IM/SC:** 100 IU q1–3days	• **IM/SC:** If dose to be administered exceeds 2 mL, use IM route. Supplied in ampoules; refrigerate between 2°C to 8°C. Once reconstituted, solution should be used within 2 h • Administer hs to minimize nausea and vomiting • This hormone is a protein; therefore, systemic allergic reaction is possible. A skin test should be performed prior to tx; epinephrine should be kept handy • For 20–30% of pts, facial flushing and warmth after injection will occur. Reassure them that this is a transient effect (usually lasting 1 h)
prednisone	**Oral:** (Hyperparathyroidism): Initially, 5–60 mg/day, divided into 4 equal doses. Maint. dose, 5–10 mg/day	• Do not confuse this medication with prednisolone; they are different medications • Give oral dose with food to reduce gastric irritation. For replacement tx, give 2/3 dose in a.m., 1/3 in afternoon • Intermediate-acting; may be used for qod tx. For inflammatory conditions, administer in a.m. to mimic body's normal diurnal secretion

CHAPTER 65

Drugs for the Treatment of Diabetes Mellitus

Topics Discussed
- Diabetes mellitus: Types I and II
- Drugs used to treat diabetes mellitus
- For all drugs: Mechanism of action and pharmacologic effects, therapeutic uses, adverse effects
- Nursing management for drugs
- Management of diabetes mellitus

Drugs Discussed

Hormones:
glucagon (**glew**-kah-gon)
insulin (**in**-syoo-lin)

Alpha-Glucosidase Inhibitor:
acarbose (**ack**-ar-bose)

Sulfonylureas:
acetohexamide (ah-seet-oh-**hex**-ah-myde)
chlorpropamide (klor-**proe**-pah-myde)
gliclazide (**glye**-klah-zide)
glyburide (**glye**-byoo-ryde)
tolbutamide (tole-**byoo**-tah-mide)

Biguanide:
metformin (met-**for**-min)

Insulin Resistance Improving Agent:
troglitazone (troe-**glit**-ah-zone)

Clinical Challenge

Consider this clinical challenge as you read through this chapter. The response to the challenge appears on page 777.

As a community health nurse, you provide health promotion services to students, teachers and families through the Wellness Clinic at the high school in a small town. You have been working with a 15-year-old student and his family since his recent diagnosis of diabetes mellitus.

Brian has learned to inject insulin and monitor his blood glucose. Today, you are urgently called by a teacher to assess Brian who is in the gym. You find that his pulse is rapid, he is very pale and diaphoretic. He appears frightened and has difficulty answering your questions.

1. What information do you need immediately to diagnose the situation?
2. What is the most likely diagnosis?
3. What immediate treatment will you initiate?

Diabetes Mellitus

Diabetes mellitus is a major medical and economic problem. The World Health Organization estimated that there were six million people with insulin-dependent diabetes mellitus (IDDM, or type I diabetes mellitus) worldwide in 1992. It is also estimated that the worldwide population of individuals with non–insulin-dependent diabetes mellitus (NIDDM, or type II diabetes mellitus) is increasing and may reach 100 million by the year 2000.

Diabetes is associated with increased mortality and a high risk for vascular, renal, retinal and neuropathic complications. These can be prevented if blood glucose levels are kept in the normal range. However, this is easier said than done. Despite significant advances in the treatment of diabetes over the past twenty years (new oral hypoglycemics and human insulin), many patients are still not well controlled.

In this light, it is of great interest to note several new products that offer alternative forms of drug therapy for diabetes — specifically, acarbose, troglitazone, and insulin lispro, all of which are discussed later in this chapter.

Role of Insulin

Before discussing the treatment of diabetes, we must reflect on the effects of insulin and its relationship to glucose metabolism, for these are interwoven. A 70-kg human has only 350–400 g of glucose and glycogen. Despite this, glucose plays a vital role in body metabolism. It is the major source of energy for all cells and the only source for brain and nerve tissue. Glucose is also readily converted to fats and may supply carbon atoms for the synthesis of some amino acids.

Insulin is synthesized in the islets of the pancreas. In non-diabetic individuals, glucose absorption from the gastrointestinal tract stimulates insulin release from the pancreas. However, insulin-dependent (type I) diabetics have little or no insulin in the pancreas and cannot respond to glucose absorption with the release of insulin. Non-insulin-dependent (type II) diabetics release insulin in response to glucose absorption, but because of tissue resistance to the actions of insulin, the hormone has reduced effect.

Insulin regulates the entry of glucose into many tissues. Under its influence, glucose enters skeletal and cardiac muscle and fat to act as a source of energy. In the absence of insulin, glucose cannot enter these tissues. Not all tissues depend on insulin for the entry of glucose. Glucose can enter nerve tissue, kidney tubules, liver and intestinal mucosa cells even in the absence of insulin.

Insulin can also influence glucose metabolism. In its presence, glucose is converted in the liver to its storage form, glycogen. The absence of insulin, and the consequent inability of the body to use glucose as an energy source, forces the body to move to other food stores. Triglycerides are broken down to fatty acids, which are then metabolized in the liver and elsewhere to provide energy. The increased utilization of fat results in the accumulation of its metabolic byproducts, ketone bodies. Betahydroxybutyric acid and acetoacetate are the two main ketone bodies that accumulate. Insulin deficiency causes muscles to waste because protein is converted to amino acids, which are then metabolized to provide energy.

Diagnosis of Diabetes Mellitus

The medical diagnosis of diabetes mellitus can be based on the unequivocal elevation of plasma glucose concentration, together with the classic symptoms of polyuria, ketonuria, polydipsia and weight loss. Patients whose nursing assessment reveals these symptoms should be referred to a physician immediately for further assessment and diagnosis. The physician may also diagnose diabetes mellitus on the basis of elevated fasting plasma glucose (FPG) concentrations on more than one occasion, or elevated plasma glucose concentrations after an oral glucose tolerance test (OGTT) on more than one occasion.

Table 65.1 sets out the diagnostic criteria for diabetes mellitus in nonpregnant adults and children; it also establishes the criteria for impaired glucose tolerance in these subpopulations. These patients occupy a grey area between normals and diabetics. They should be monitored by a physician to determine whether diabetes mellitus will ensue.

Classes of Diabetes Mellitus

Type I. Type I or insulin-dependent diabetes mellitus (IDDM) patients have little or no insulin in the pancreas. These people usually experience

Table 65.1
Diagnostic criteria for diabetes mellitus

Diabetes mellitus in nonpregnant adults

Any of the following are considered diagnostic of diabetes:

A. Presence of classic symptoms of diabetes, such as polyuria, polydipsia, ketonuria and rapid weight loss, together with gross and unequivocal elevation of plasma glucose.

B. Elevated fasting glucose concentration on more than one occasion:

venous plasma	$\leq$	140 mg/dL (7.8 mmol/L)
venous whole blood	$\geq$	120 mg/dL (6.7 mmol/L)
capillary whole blood	$\geq$	120 mg/dL (6.7 mmol/L)

If the fasting glucose concentration meets these criteria, the oral glucose tolerance test (OGTT) is *not required*. Indeed, virtually all persons with fasting plasma glucose (FPG) > 140 mg/dL will exhibit an OGTT that meets or exceeds the criteria in C, below.

C. Fasting glucose concentration less than that which is diagnostic of diabetes (B, above) but sustained elevated glucose concentration during the OGTT on more than one occasion. *Both* the 120-min sample *and* some other sample taken between administration of the 75-g glucose dose and 120 min later must meet the following criteria:

venous plasma	$\geq$	200 mg/dL (11.1 mmol/L)
venous whole blood	$\geq$	180 mg/dL (10.0 mmol/L)
capillary whole blood	$\geq$	200 mg/dL (11.1 mmol/L)

Impaired glucose tolerance (IGT) in nonpregnant adults

Three criteria must be met: the fasting glucose concentration must be below the value that is diagnostic for diabetes; the glucose concentration 120 min after a 75-g oral glucose challenge must be between normal and diabetic values; and a value between 30-min, 60-min or 90-min OGTT value later must be unequivocally elevated.

Fasting value:

venous plasma	$<$	140 mg/dL (7.8 mmol/L)
venous whole blood	$<$	120 mg/dL (6.7 mmol/L)
capillary whole blood	$<$	120 mg/dL (6.7 mmol/L)

30-min, 60-min or 90-min OGTT value:

venous plasma	$\geq$	200 mg/dL (11.1 mmol/L)
venous whole blood	$\geq$	180 mg/dL (10.0 mmol/L)
capillary whole blood	$\geq$	200 mg/dL (11.1 mmol/L)

120-min OGTT value:

venous plasma of between	140–200 mg/dL (7.8–11.1 mmol/L)
venous whole blood of between	120–180 mg/dL (6.7–10.0 mmol/L)
capillary whole blood of between	140–200 mg/dL (7.8–11.1 mmol/L)

Normal glucose levels in nonpregnant adults

Fasting value:

venous plasma	$<$	115 mg/dL (6.4 mmol/L)
venous whole blood	$<$	100 mg/dL (5.6 mmol/L)
capillary whole blood	$<$	100 mg/dL (5.6 mmol/L)

120-min OGTT value:

venous plasma	$<$	140 mg/dL (7.8 mmol/L)
venous whole blood	$<$	120 mg/dL (6.7 mmol/L)
capillary whole blood	$<$	140 mg/dL (7.8 mmol/L)

OGTT values between 30-min, 60-min or 90-min OGTT value later:

venous plasma	$<$	200 mg/dL (11.1 mmol/L)
venous whole blood	$<$	180 mg/dL (10.0 mmol/L)
capillary whole blood	$<$	200 mg/dL (11.1 mmol/L)

Glucose values above these concentrations but below the criteria for diabetes or IGT should be considered nondiagnostic for these conditions.

Diabetes mellitus in children

Either of the following are considered diagnostic of diabetes:

A. Presence of classic symptoms of diabetes, such as polyuria, polydipsia, ketonuria and rapid weight loss, together with a random plasma glucose greater than 200 mg/dL.

B. In asymptomatic individuals, both an elevated fasting glucose concentration and a sustained elevated glucose concentration during the OGTT on more than one occasion *Both* the 120-min sample *and* some other sample taken between administration of the glucose dose (1.75 g/kg ideal body weight, up to a maximum of 75 g) and 120 min later must meet the criteria below:

Fasting value:

venous plasma	$\geq$	140 mg/dL (7.8 mmol/L)
venous whole blood	$\geq$	120 mg/dL (6.7 mmol/L)
capillary whole blood	$\geq$	120 mg/dL (6.7 mmol/L)

120-min OGTT value and an intervening value:

venous plasma	$\geq$	200 mg/dL (11.1 mmol/L)
venous whole blood	$\geq$	180 mg/dL (10.0 mmol/L)
capillary whole blood	$\geq$	200 mg/dL (11.1 mmol/L)

Impaired glucose tolerance (IGT) in children

Two criteria must be met: the fasting glucose concentration must be below the value that is diagnostic of diabetes, and the glucose concentration 120 min after an oral glucose challenge must be elevated.

Fasting value:

venous plasma	$<$	140 mg/dL (7.8 mmol/L)
venous whole blood	$<$	120 mg/dL (6.7 mmol/L)
capillary whole blood	$<$	120 mg/dL (6.7 mmol/L)

120-min OGTT value:

venous plasma	$>$	140 mg/dL (7.8 mmol/L)
venous whole blood	$>$	120 mg/dL (6.7 mmol/L)
capillary whole blood	$>$	120 mg/dL (6.7 mmol/L)

Normal glucose levels in children

Fasting value:

venous plasma	$<$	130 mg/dL (7.2 mmol/L)
venous whole blood	$<$	115 mg/dL (6.4 mmol/L)
capillary whole blood	$<$	115 mg/dL (6.4 mmol/L)

120-min OGTT value:

venous plasma	$<$	140 mg/dL (7.8 mmol/L)
venous whole blood	$<$	120 mg/dL (6.7 mmol/L)
capillary whole blood	$<$	140 mg/dL (7.8 mmol/L)

an abrupt onset of symptoms, insulin deficiency and dependency on injected insulin to sustain life. They are prone to ketosis. In the past this condition was called juvenile or growth-onset diabetes because it occurred most often in juveniles; however, it can occur at any age. Thus, it is inappropriate to classify it by age.

Type II. Type II, or non–insulin-dependent diabetes mellitus (NIDDM), results from a combination of environmental and complex genetic factors. Approximately ninety percent of diabetics have type II diabetes, and seventy percent of these individuals are obese. NIDDM tends to occur in later life, and for this reason it was formerly called adult-onset diabetes mellitus. Type II diabetics may be asymptomatic for years with only a slow progression of the disease. Despite this, NIDDM patients demonstrate the typical chronic associations and complications of diabetes. These are atherosclerosis, microangiopathy, neuropathy, retinopathy and cataracts.

Maturity-onset diabetes of the young (MODY) is a subset of type II diabetes with characteristics of both types I and II.

The exact cause (or causes) of type II diabetes is still unclear. However, it appears that the development of tissue resistance to the actions of insulin occurs initially in the disease in most type II patients. As a result of insulin resistance, glucose is not taken up into skeletal muscle and glycogen synthesis in the liver is impaired. Most patients with NIDDM are initially hyperinsulinemic because the beta cells of the pancreas respond to peripheral insulin resistance by increasing basal and postprandial insulin secretion. As the diabetes progresses with the further aggravation of insulin resistance, the increased secretory load placed on the pancreas results in pancreatic failure and a decrease in the secretion of insulin.

Several factors play a role in the pathology of NIDDM. These include hyperglycemia, hyperinsulinemia and insulin resistance. Hyperglycemia leads to the formation of advanced glycation end products and sugar alcohols. These accumulate in a variety of tissues and disrupt normal organ function, producing retinopathy, neuropathy, cataracts and pancreatic beta-cell dysfunction.

Two important developments have recently occurred in the treatment of NIDDM. Because insulin resistance appears to be a primary defect in type II diabetes, attention has been directed recently into developing drugs that can restore the sensitivity of tissues to insulin. For example, the drug troglitazone (Rezulin®), described later in this chapter, enhances insulin action by increasing insulin-stimulated glucose uptake in skeletal muscle and adipose tissue, and decreasing hepatic glucose output. The attenuation of hyperglycemia and hyperinsulinemia leads to regranulation of the pancreatic beta cells and re-establishment of pancreatic insulin secretion.

A second new drug, acarbose (Prandase®, Precose®; see discussion later in this chapter) inhibits intestinal alpha-glucosidase, the enzyme responsible for the hydrolysis of sucrose into absorbable monosaccharides. By inhibiting this enzyme, acarbose reduces the rate at which glucose is absorbed following a meal and decreases postprandial hyperglycemia. More than just a drug, acarbose acts as an adjunct to dietary therapy in patients requiring additional help in managing postprandial peaks in blood sugar. It may also forestall, or even prevent, the institution of conventional antihyperglycemic therapy, with all its problems.

Gestational diabetes. Gestational diabetes (Table 65.2) refers to the onset of glucose intolerance in women during pregnancy. By definition it

Table 65.2
Gestational diabetes

Two or more of the following values after a 100-g oral glucose challenge must be met or exceeded:

	Venous plasma	Venous whole blood	Capillary whole blood
Fasting	105 mg/dL (5.8 mmol/L)	90 mg/dL (5.0 mmol/L)	90 mg/dL (5.0 mmol/L)
1 h	190 mg/dL (10.6 mmol/L)	170 mg/dL (9.5 mmol/L)	170 mg/dL (9.5 mmol/L)
2 h	165 mg/dL (9.2 mmol/L)	145 mg/dL (8.1 mmol/L)	145 mg/dL (8.1 mmol/L)
3 h	145 mg/dL (8.1 mmol/L)	125 mg/dL (7.0 mmol/L)	125 mg/dL (7.0 mmol/L)

excludes women who were diabetic before pregnancy. If patients remain diabetic after delivery, they must be reclassified as type I (insulin-dependent) or type II (non–insulin-dependent) diabetics.

Drugs Used in the Treatment of Diabetes Mellitus

The treatment of patients with diabetes mellitus has two goals. The initial or short-term objective of treatment is to relieve the symptoms of the disease, to overcome ketoacidosis and to restore normal growth, weight gain and resistance to infections by achieving normal blood sugar levels. This goal has been achieved with more success than the long-term objective, which is to avoid the complications of diabetes mellitus, particularly those affecting the vascular and nervous systems that often appear after fifteen to twenty years of the disease.

Insulin-dependent diabetics obviously require treatment with that hormone. Non-insulin-dependent patients may respond to changes in diet, together with drug therapy using alpha-glucosidase inhibitors, oral hypoglycemics, insulin or insulin plus troglitazone.

Hormones

Insulin

Pharmacokinetics. Preparations are available that contain beef plus pork, or only pork, insulin. These are formulated to provide rapid, intermediate or prolonged effects. The pharmacokinetic characteristics of these insulins are summarized in Table 65.3 on the next page. These values should not be taken to indicate specific times in hours for the onset and duration of action because of the great intra- and interpatient variability observed. They do, however, provide an approximate comparison of the pharmacokinetics of the various insulin preparations.

Regular crystalline insulin is clear in appearance. Its peak activity can be seen in 2–4 h, and its duration of action is 6–8 h. Longer-acting insulins are complexed with large protein molecules (NPH, PZI) or formulated as large crystals (lente series) to reduce their rates of absorption. Semilente insulin is turbid and has a rapid onset of action.

However, its actions are more prolonged than those of regular crystalline insulin.

NPH and lente insulins are intermediate-acting products. Peak activity occurs 6–12 h after injection. Durations of action last from 24–28 h. Protamine zinc insulin and ultralente insulin are prolonged-acting products. Peak activity is seen 14–24 h after injection. Durations of action extend to 36 h or more.

The *Iletin II® insulins* are highly purified insulins. They are particularly suitable for patients now taking beef–pork insulin who have persistent local or systemic allergy, or those currently taking beef–pork insulin or beef insulin who have developed insulin lipodystrophy.

Human biosynthetic insulin (Humulin®, Novolin®) is a highly purified insulin formed by recombinant DNA. Identical to human insulin and free of animal pancreatic impurities, it is less likely to induce immunoglobulin E and G (IgE and IgG) production. Its use should result in reduced incidence of allergies and resistance. Human insulin may be recommended for (1) newly diagnosed insulin-dependent patients, (2) newly diagnosed insulin-requiring patients with maturity-onset diabetes, (3) patients with existing maturity-onset diabetes who are new to insulin therapy and (4) patients who have developed lipoatrophy from injections of beef or pork insulin.

Humulin® is formulated as a rapidly acting preparation with a short duration (6–8 h) of action (Humulin R®). It is also produced in the form of two intermediate-acting products: Humulin N® is an NPH insulin and Humulin L® is a lente insulin. Both have durations of action of up to 24 h. Humulin U® is an ultralente insulin with a slower onset of action than regular insulin and a longer duration of action (at least 24 h).

Most recently, human insulin has been provided in a very rapidly acting, short-duration product called *insulin lispro* (Humalog®). At physiologic concentrations, insulin lispro exists in solution as a monomer. As such, its rate of absorption from subcutaneous sites of injection is faster than that of regular human insulin.

Subcutaneously injected regular insulin typically results in serum insulin concentrations that peak later and remain elevated for a longer time than those following normal pancreatic insulin secretion in non-diabetics. As a result, patients

Table 65.3
Characteristics of insulins

Trade name (Route)	Source	Action (h)		
		Onset	Peak effect	Duration
Regular Iletin I (IV, SC)	beef/pork	0.5	2–4	5–7
Regular Iletin II (IV, SC)	pork	0.5	2–4	5–7
Semilente II (SC)	pork	1–2	2–4	12–16
NPH Iletin I (SC)	beef/pork	1–2	6–12	24–28
NPH Iletin II (SC)	pork	1–2	6–12	24–28
Lente Iletin I (SC)	beef/pork	1–3	6–12	24–28
Lente Iletin II (SC)	pork	1–3	6–12	24–28
Ultralente Iletin I (SC)	beef/pork	4–6	18–24	36 or more
Protamine Zinc Iletin I (SC)	beef/pork	4–6	14–24	36 or more
Protamine Zinc Iletin II (SC)	pork	4–6	14–24	36 or more
Human insulins				
Humalog (SC)	recombinant DNA	0.3–0.5	0.5–2.5	3–4.3
Humulin R (IV, SC)	recombinant DNA	0.5–1.0	1–5	6–8
Humulin N (SC, IM)	recombinant DNA	1–2	6–12	18–24
Humulin 30/70 (SC, IM)	recombinant DNA 30% regular insulin 70% NPH insulin			up to 24
Humulin L (SC, IM)	recombinant DNA	4–6	14–24	up to 24
Humulin U (SC, IM)	recombinant DNA			24 or more

Iletin II = Highly purified insulins containing < 1/1 000 000 parts proinsulin, compared with < 20 parts proinsulin in normal insulin. Human insulin formed by recombinant DNA is less likely to induce IgE and IgG.

IV = intravenous; SC = subcutaneous; IM = intramuscular

Source: Yesterday, Tomorrow — Total Commitment to Total Diabetes Care. Indianapolis: Eli Lilly. Reproduced with permission.

using intensive insulin regimens with regular insulin to decrease postprandial hyperglycemia often do not achieve adequate control, because regular insulin is absorbed more slowly than blood glucose levels rise. Larger doses of regular insulin could be injected to produce concentrations sufficient to control postprandial hyperglycemia. However, this would subsequently lead to late hypoglycemia due to the relatively long duration of activity of regular insulin. Since insulin lispro is absorbed more quickly than regular insulin, it is more effective at reducing postprandial blood glucose levels. Furthermore, because it has a shorter duration of action, insulin lispro is less likely to produce subsequent hypoglycemia after the absorption of food has finished. For this reason, it can also be taken closer to meals.

Table 65.3 lists the characteristics of currently available insulins.

Therapeutic uses. Insulin must be used in patients with insulin-dependent diabetes and should be considered for individuals afflicted with diabetes mellitus before thirty years of age. Any patient with ketosis, persistent ketonuria or ketoacidosis should be treated with insulin. Insulin should be administered to diabetics with severe infections and gangrene. It is also indicated in non–insulin-dependent diabetics in whom diet or oral hypoglycemics, or both, have failed. Insulin should also be used in non–insulin-dependent diabetics who are taking corticosteroids or suffering from reduced kidney or liver function, or during surgery or pregnancy.

Gestational diabetes should be treated with insulin, if diet alone is unsuccessful. Oral hypoglycemics are not indicated because they will cross the placenta and stimulate fetal insulin production abnormally.

The choice of the appropriate insulin preparation(s) depends on the unique needs of each patient. Insulin lispro provides the most rapid absorption and shortest duration of action for insulin. In future, it may replace the previously available rapidly acting insulins, which heretofore have been the preparations of choice when immediate effect is required.

Several doses of a rapidly acting insulin per day could also be used as maintenance therapy. However, many patients find several daily injections unacceptable. In these situations, the intermediate- or prolonged-acting formulations may be selected to meet the requirements of each patient.

Insulin resistance. Insulin resistance has already been discussed as it relates to non–insulin-dependent (type II) diabetics. This form of insulin resistance is due to peripheral resistance to the action of the hormone. Insulin resistance can also be caused by the presence of large amounts of IgG insulin-binding antibodies. Most patients require less than 50–60 U/day of insulin. This is slightly more than the 30–40 U that a normal human secretes daily. Doses in excess of 100 U/day are uncommon. If the dosage requirements reach 200 U/day, insulin resistance is said to have occurred.

Insulin resistance due to antibody binding is rare with human-type insulin. True resistance to animal-source insulin (> 200 U/day) should prompt a switch to human-type insulin (usually allowing a gradually decreasing dose.)

Obesity reduces target organ sensitivity as a result of the previously described peripheral resistance to the action of the hormone seen in type II patients. A reduction in weight or food intake will usually restore normal insulin sensitivity. Cushing's disease and hyperthyroidism will increase the dosage of insulin required.

Acute insulin resistance can occur during stress. Surgery, trauma, emotional upheaval or infections are common causes. Large doses of insulin, water and electrolytes may be required while the precipitating cause is addressed.

Adverse effects. Hypoglycemic reactions are of the greatest concern. The signs of hypoglycemia depend on the rate of fall of blood sugar. If blood sugar levels decrease rapidly, sympathetic nervous system stimulation increases and patients experience hunger, anxiety, warmth and sweating, tremor, weakness, confusion, emotional instability, palpitations, pallor, fatigue, paresthesias and hyperesthesias of the lips, nose or fingers. If blood glucose levels fall slowly, these effects may not be seen. Severe hypoglycemia produces profound CNS dysfunction, resulting in convulsions, coma and sometimes death.

Allergic reactions, both local and systemic, are also a potential problem. Drug sensitivity, usually beginning several weeks after starting therapy and characterized by an erythematous, indurated area around the injection site, is the most common reaction. Generalized reactions usually start with urticaria and may rarely proceed through angioedema and anaphylaxis. Patients who are allergic to standard insulin preparations may be tried on either the highly purified insulins (Iletin II®) or human insulin (Humulin®, Novolin®).

Lipodystrophies, involving either atrophy or hypertrophy of fat, can occur at sites in which insulin is injected repeatedly.

Table 65.4 on the next page lists the clinically significant drug interactions with insulin.

Glucagon

Mechanism of action and pharmacologic effects. Glucagon is a hormone synthesized and stored in the alpha cells of the pancreatic islets. The contrasts between it and insulin are striking, despite the fact that the two are stored in adjacent pancreatic cells. Insulin secretion is increased when glucose is absorbed from the GI tract. The release of glucagon is depressed by glucose absorption. Once released, insulin facilitates the storage of food energy. Glucagon, released when blood sugar levels fall, acts to mobilize glucose to provide energy. Accordingly, insulin secretion is increased and glucagon release decreased following a meal. During a fast, the reverse is true: glucagon secretion is increased and insulin decreased.

Therapeutic uses. Glucagon is useful in counteracting severe hypoglycemic reactions in

Table 65.4
Insulin: Drug interactions

Drug	Interaction
Beta blockers, non-selective	• Nonselective beta blockers enhance the hypoglycemia produced by insulin by interfering with catecholamine-induced glycogenolysis. In addition, the warning sign of tachycardia that may accompany hypoglycemia is usually not seen in pts treated with beta blockers. Concomitant use of a beta blocker and insulin should be avoided, if possible. When this is not possible, pts should be monitored carefully
Contraceptives, oral	• Oral contraceptives may increase daily insulin requirements
Diuretics	• Diuretics may increase, decrease or not affect insulin requirements
Epinephrine	• Epinephrine increases blood sugar and reduces the effects of insulin
Ethanol	• Ethanol can increase insulin's hypoglycemic actions
Guanethidine	• Guanethedine can increase insulin's hypoglycemic actions
Hormones	• Hormones such as growth hormone, corticotrophin, glucocorticoids, thyroid hormone and glucagon reduce the hypoglycemic actions of insulin
MAOIs	• MAOIs can increase the hypoglycemic actions of insulin
Phenytoin	• Phenytoin may antagonize the hypoglycemic effects of insulin
Salicylates	• Salicylates, in daily doses of 1.5–6 g, can increase insulin's hypoglycemic effects in some pts
Steroids, anabolic	• Anabolic steroids can increase insulin's hypoglycemic effects in some pts

diabetics, but only if liver glycogen is available. Glucagon is of little or no value in states of starvation, adrenal insufficiency or chronic hypoglycemia. The patient with insulin-dependent diabetes may not respond as well to glucagon as the non–insulin-dependent stable diabetic. Both should be given supplementary carbohydrate as soon as possible.

A dose of 0.5–1 mg glucagon given subcutaneously, intramuscularly or intravenously usually awakens the unconscious hypoglycemic patient in 5–20 min. If response is delayed, there is no contraindication to the administration of one or two additional doses of glucagon; however, the use of parenteral glucose must be considered. Intravenous glucose should be given if the patient fails to respond to glucagon.

Adverse effects. Glucagon is largely free of untoward effects. Nausea and vomiting may occur with large doses. Since glucagon is a protein, the possibility of hypersensitivity reactions remains.

Nursing Management

Table 65.5 describes the nursing management of the patient receiving insulin. Dosage details of individual drugs are given in Table 65.12 (pages 773–776).

Alpha-Glucosidase Inhibitor

Acarbose (Prandase®, Precose®)

Mechanism of action and pharmacologic effects. Acarbose inhibits the enzyme alpha-glucosidase in the brush border membrane of the small intestine. Alpha-glucosidase is responsible for the hydrolysis of sucrose into absorbable monosaccharides. By inhibiting this enzyme, acarbose delays glucose absorption, reduces postprandial hyperglycemia and decreases glycosylated hemoglobin (HbA_{1c}) in type II diabetes mellitus patients. Acarbose can be used as an adjunct to prescribed diet for the management of blood glucose levels in NIDDM patients who are inadequately controlled by diet alone.

Acarbose differs significantly from the oral hypoglycemics (see below). Although oral hypoglycemics (i.e., sulfonylureas and metformin) diminish postprandial hyperglycemia, neither of these groups of drugs affects the rate at which glucose is absorbed. In both cases, the body is exposed to high levels of absorbed glucose, thereby stress-

Table 65.5
Nursing management of insulin

Assessment of risk vs. benefit	Patient data	• Physician should determine which insulin protocol is required. Baseline lab tests include FPG, postprandial glucose, glycosylated hemoglobin (HbA$_{1c}$, also known as diabetic control index; this is a long-term indicator of the average blood glucose levels over a period of time) • Assess for baseline VS, general state of health, nutritional status • *Pregnancy:* Risk category B (studies in animals may or may not have shown risk; if risk has been shown in animals, no risk has been shown in human studies; if risk has not been shown in animals, there are insufficient data in pregnant women)
	Drug data	• Select insulin product based on individual pt factors • Most serious adverse effect is caused by insulin reaction (hypoglycemia)
Implementation	Rights of administration	• Using the "rights" helps prevent errors of administration
	Right route	• Give SC through intermittent injection or by newer methods of continuous infusion • In emergencies, give regular insulin IV (preferred) or IM, if necessary
	Right time	• See Table 65.12. NB variation in dosage schedules among insulins due to onset and duration of action
	Right technique	• **SC:** See Box 65.1 (page 765) • **IV:** Administration requires knowledge of correct diluent and IV solution, correct dilution and rate of administration. Always refer to manufacturer's instructions for this route. Rate must be carefully controlled. Due to reaction with containers and tubing, insulin loses most of its potency when given by continuous infusion; direct injection preferred. Check agency policy regarding certification for this procedure
	Nursing therapeutics	• Encourage self-management (nutrition, exercise/activity, hygiene) • Ensure pt understands that this medication does not cure the condition, but does control symptoms and may prevent complications associated with the disease • *Emotional support:* Diabetes is a lifelong condition with many serious complications • Provide nutritional counselling or refer to dietitian • Be prepared to treat hypoglycemic (insulin) reactions immediately. If pt is able to swallow, provide fast-acting source of carbohydrates such as fruit juice, sugar cubes, hard candies; if unable to swallow, IV glucose is the preferred tx, although parenteral glucagon may be used initially

(cont'd on next page)

Table 65.5 (continued)
Nursing management of insulin

Implementation (cont'd)	Patient/family teaching	• Pt's need for information is influenced by many individual factors including beliefs regarding the condition, previous experience with diabetes, education, culture and age. Compliance and follow-up are essential factors in successful tx: review principles of pt education in Chapter 3 • Pts/families should know warning signs/symptoms of insulin reaction caused by hypoglycemia (see Monitoring, below). Treat immediately; if untreated, can progress to coma, sometimes quickly • Instruct pts on proper use of equipment for monitoring capillary blood glucose levels • Pts/families should know that stress and illness can alter insulin requirements: medical attention may be required • Advise pts to wear a medical ID bracelet at all times. They should also carry insulin, a syringe and carbohydrates (e.g., sugar cubes, hard candies) with them • As cigarette smoking decreases insulin absorption, pts who continue to smoke should be advised to refrain from smoking within 30 min of injecting insulin • Emphasize importance of tx regimen, including diet, exercise, avoiding infection, regular examinations, timing of eating and injections
Outcomes	Monitoring of progress	*Continually monitor:* • Clinical response indicating tx success (reduction in signs/ symptoms) • Signs/symptoms of adverse reactions; document and report immediately to physician • Be especially alert for s/s of hypoglycemia (blood glucose level < 3.8 mmol/L) and treat immediately. Symptoms may occur rapidly due to sympathetic response, e.g., pallor, sweating, nervousness, trembling, tachycardia, weakness and hunger. Symptoms may also occur slowly, e.g., headache, blurred or double vision, incoherent speech, mental confusion, coma and convulsions. These signs generally appear when blood glucose is < 3 mmol/L • Signs/symptoms of hyperglycemia or ketosis: dry, flushed skin, dry mouth and excessive thirst; anorexia; dyspnea; acetone breath odour; hypotension; weak, rapid pulse • Blood tests to monitor glucose levels, including regular blood glucose levels through self-monitoring and periodic lab tests and HbA$_{1c}$

ing the capacity of pancreatic beta cells to deal with sudden peaks in blood sugar. This may play a role in the progressive deterioration of beta-cell function seen in NIDDM patients receiving a sulfonylurea or metformin.

Compared with sulfonylurea treatment (see discussion below), acarbose decreases both postprandial and fasting plasma insulin levels. The significance of this point must not be minimized. Hyperinsulinemia that results from sulfonylurea therapy may accelerate the progression of macrovascular disease.

When administered over several years, the sulfonylureas and metformin gradually lose their effect. This is likely due to deterioration in pancreatic beta-cell function. Acarbose, on the other

---

Box 65.1
Insulin: Technique for SC injection

✔ The usual administration route for insulin is SC. This route reduces the rate of absorption and the amount of pain. Use only insulin syringes to ensure accurate dosage

✔ Do not use insulin that changes colour or becomes clumped and/or granular in appearance. Always check the expiration date on vials of insulin prior to use

✔ Rotate vial between palms to ensure homogeneous suspension prior to withdrawing

✔ When mixing two insulins, always withdraw regular insulin before modified insulin. This step prevents accidental contamination of the regular insulin

✔ Pinch a fold of skin with three fingers at least 3 in apart; insert needle at a 45°–90° angle. Aspirate to insure medication is not inadvertently administered IV or IM

✔ Store insulin in a cool area. Refrigeration is desirable, but not essential; vial can be kept at room temperature for 1 month. Prevent exposure to direct heat and sunlight and do not freeze

✔ Prefilled syringes may be stored in refrigerator for one week: store with needle pointing up to prevent clogging. Prior to use, gently rotate syringe to mix suspension

---

hand, does not depend on the pancreas for its primary effect. In the face of decreased pancreatic function, acarbose should continue to reduce the rate of glucose absorption, putting less stress on the already compromised pancreas.

Acarbose does not produce hypoglycemia, and this gives it a unique margin of safety compared with the oral hypoglycemics.

Finally, acarbose does not increase body weight, whereas sulfonylureas have been shown to increase the weight of NIDDM patients.

Therapeutic uses. Acarbose can be used as adjunctive therapy for the management of blood glucose levels in non–insulin-dependent diabetic patients who are inadequately controlled by diet alone. If a program of diet and regular exercise fails to result in adequate glycemic control, the use of acarbose should be considered before resorting to other treatments, such as oral hypoglycemics.

Adverse effects. Only 1% to 2% of an oral dose of acarbose is absorbed from the gastrointestinal (GI) tract as unchanged drug, and this limits its systemic adverse effects. The majority of adverse experiences with acarbose involve GI symptoms. Most are of mild or moderate intensity and are dose dependent. Acarbose can produce flatulence, diarrhea and abdominal pain. These effects can be minimized by starting with a low dose and slowly titrating upwards.

Because of these effects, acarbose is contraindicated in patients with inflammatory bowel disease, colonic ulceration, partial intestinal obstruction or in patients predisposed to intestinal obstruction. In addition, acarbose should not be used in patients who have chronic intestinal diseases associated with marked disorders of digestion or absorption and in patients who suffer from states that may deteriorate as a result of increased gas formation in the intestine, e.g., larger hernias.

Table 65.6 on the next page lists the clinically significant drug interactions with acarbose.

Oral Hypoglycemic Drugs

Oral hypoglycemic drugs can be divided into sulfonylureas and biguanides. Table 65.7 on the next page lists some of the oral hypoglycemics available in North America. The second-generation sulfonylureas are more potent than the first-generation agents, but are no more effective. As metformin is the only biguanide available in Canada, it is the only one we will discuss here.

Sulfonylureas and Metformin

Mechanism of action and pharmacologic effects. Sulfonylureas require the presence of insulin to be effective. Their mechanism of action is depicted in Figure 65.1 on the next page. These drugs (1) stimulate the release of insulin from the pancreas, (2) increase the action of insulin on the liver to decrease hepatic glucogenesis and (3) increase the action of insulin on muscle to increase glucose utilization.

Table 65.6
Acarbose: Drug interactions

Drug	Interaction
Cholestyramine	• The concomitant administration of cholestyramine may enhance the effects of acarbose, particularly with respect to reducing postprandial insulin levels
Drugs that produce hyperglycemia	• Certain drugs tend to produce hyperglycemia and may lead to loss of blood glucose control. These include diuretics (thiazides, furosemide), corticosteroids, phenothiazines, thyroid products, estrogens, oral contraceptives, phenytoin, nicotinic acid, sympathomimetics and isoniazid. When such drugs are administered to a pt receiving acarbose, the pt should be closely observed for loss of blood glucose control
Intestinal absorbents/ digestive enzyme preparations	• Intestinal absorbents (e.g., charcoal) and digestive enzyme preparations containing carbohydrate-splitting enzymes (e.g., amylase, pancreatin) may reduce the effect of acarbose and should not be taken concomitantly

Table 65.7
Some oral hypoglycemic drugs used in North America

Drug and class	Duration of action (h)
Sulfonylureas	
First generation	
Acetohexamide (Dimelor®)	12–24
Chlorpropamide (Chloronase®, Diabinese®)	24–72
Tolazamide (Diabewas®, Tolinase®)	12–24
Tolbutamide (Mobenol®, Orinase®)	6–12
Second generation	
Gliclazide	10–16
Glyburide	24–24
Biguanide	
Metformin (Glucophage®)	5–6

Figure 65.1
Actions of sulfonylureas

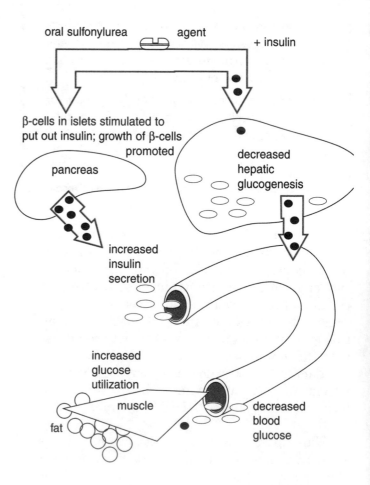

Source: Waife SO. Oral hypoglycemic agents. In: *Diabetes Mellitus.* Indianapolis: Eli Lilly; 1980:123. Reproduced with permission.

Sulfonylureas are well absorbed when taken orally. They differ mainly in their respective durations of action. With the exception of chlorpropamide, all sulfonylureas are extensively metabolized in the body. Chlorpropamide is not significantly metabolized. It is cleared largely unchanged by the kidneys. This drug has the longest half-life of the sulfonylureas and can be given on a once-daily basis.

Metformin also requires the presence of insulin to lower blood sugar. Its mechanism of action is not clear. Metformin may decrease the absorption of glucose from the intestinal tract or increase its utilization in the body by stimulating anaerobic glycolysis, or both.

Therapeutic uses. Oral hypoglycemics are used only in patients with non–insulin-dependent diabetes mellitus. Contraindications to their use include ketoacidosis; coma; stress conditions such as severe infection, trauma or surgery; and the presence of frank jaundice or liver/renal disease or impairment. Oral hypoglycemics should not be administered during pregnancy or lactation. It should be noted that these drugs do not prevent the cardiovascular complications of diabetes mellitus.

Over time, patients may become progressively less responsive to therapy with oral hypoglycemics. Therefore, patients should be monitored with regular clinical and laboratory evaluations, including blood glucose and glycosylated hemoglobin (HbA$_{1c}$) determinations, to determine the minimum effective dosage and to detect primary failure (inadequate lowering of blood glucose concentrations at the maximum recommended dosage) or secondary failure (progressive deterioration in blood sugar control following an initial period of effectiveness).

The rate of primary failure will vary greatly depending upon patient selection and adherence to diet and exercise. The etiology of secondary failure is multifactorial and may involve progressive beta-cell failure as well as exogenous diabetogenic factors such as obesity, illness or drugs, or tachyphylaxis to the sulfonylureas. If a loss of adequate blood glucose-lowering response to a sulfonylurea is detected, the addition of a different type of oral antidiabetic may be considered, although insulin is often required.

Adverse effects. The majority of adverse effects associated with sulfonylureas have been dose related, transient and have responded to dose reduction or withdrawal of the drug. Severe hypoglycemia, which mimics acute CNS disorders, may occur with a sufonylurea. Hepatic and/or renal disease, malnutrition, debility, advanced age, alcoholism, adrenal or pituitary insufficiency may be predisposing factors. Nausea, epigastric fullness and heartburn are common reactions to sulfonylureas. These tend to be dose related and may disappear when dosage is reduced or the total daily dose is administered in divided doses. Sulfonylureas can also cause allergic skin reactions, such as pruritus, erythema, urticaria and morbiliform or maculopapular eruptions.

The most frequently reported adverse reactions to metformin are a metallic taste in the mouth, epigastric discomfort, nausea and vomiting. Diarrhea and anorexia are reported rarely. Most of these reactions are transient and can be controlled by reducing the dosage or discontinuing therapy.

Table 65.8 on the next page lists the clinically significant drug interactions with sulfonylureas, while Table 65.9 lists those with metformin.

Table 65.8
Sulfonylureas: Drug interactions

Drug	Interaction
Allopurinol, anabolic steroids, fluconazole, H_2-antagonists, NSAIDs, MAOIs, salicylates, sulfonamides	• Hypoglycemia may be potentiated when a sufonylurea is used with any of these drugs
Anticoagulants, oral	• Coumarin derivatives, when administered with sulfonylureas, may initially result in increased plasma concentrations of both drugs. With continued tx, decreased anticoagulant concentrations and increased hepatic metabolism of sulfonylureas may occur. Adjustment in dosage for both drugs may be required
Beta blockers	• Beta blockers may delay recovery from hypoglycemia and suppress hypoglycemic symptoms (with the exception of sweating). They may also inhibit insulin secretion. Cardioselective beta blockers in low doses may be safer than nonselective beta blockers
Corticosteroids, oral contraceptives, estrogens, rifampin, thiazide diuretics	• These drugs may cause hyperglycemia when used with a sulfonylurea
Ethanol	• Intolerance to alcohol (disulfiram-like reaction: flushing, sensation of warmth, giddiness, nausea and occasionally tachycardia) may occur in pts treated with sulfonylureas. This reaction occurs more frequently with chlorpropamide. Unpredictable fluctuations in serum glucose levels, most commonly hypoglycemia, may also occur following alcohol ingestion

Table 65.9
Metformin: Drug interactions

Drug	Interaction
Beta blockers, clofibrate, MAOIs, phenylbutazone, probenecid, salicylates, long-acting sulfonamides, tuberculostatics	• Administering any of these drugs with metformin can produce a hypoglycemic reaction
Oral contraceptives (estrogen plus progestins), corticosteroids, diuretics (thiazides, furosemide), nicotinic acid	• These drugs produce hyperglycemia and may lead to loss of blood sugar control
Phenprocoumon	• The elimination rate of this anticoagulant has been reported to be increased by 20% when used concurrently with metformin. Therefore, pts receiving phenprocoumon or other antivitamin-K anticoagulants, together with metformin, should be watched carefully. In such cases, an important increase in prothrombin time may occur upon cessation of metformin tx, with increased risk for hemorrhage

Insulin Resistance Improving Agent

Troglitazone (Rezulin®)

Mechanism of action and pharmacologic effects. Troglitazone acts primarily by treating insulin resistance. Troglitazone specifically improves sensitivity to insulin in muscle and adipose tissue and inhibits gluconeogenesis. The drug decreases hepatic glucose output and increases insulin-dependent glucose disposal in skeletal muscle. It is not chemically or functionally related to either the sulfonylureas, the biguanides or the alpha-glucosidase inhibitors. Unlike sulfonylureas, troglitazone does not cause an increase in the secretion of insulin.

Therapeutic uses. Troglitazone is indicated for the treatment of patients with type II diabetes inadequately controlled with insulin therapy. By decreasing insulin resistance, concomitant therapy with troglitazone and insulin improves glucose control. As glycemic control is improved, it may be possible to reduce the dose of insulin or even completely eliminate insulin for some patients. *However, a reduction in insulin dosage should not come at the expense of optimal diabetes control.*

Troglitazone would appear to provide an easy-to-implement intervention that simplifies attempts to improve glucose control by not requiring massive insulin dosage with the concomitant weight gain that usually occurs with insulin. Adding troglitazone to insulin treatment in resistant patients will lower glucose levels, and at the same time decrease insulin dosage, lower HbA_{1c} and improve lipid parameters. Troglitazone performs these functions without exposing the patient to undue risks for hypoglycemia.

The possibility of reducing insulin dosage has another important implication. There is some evidence that very high insulin doses may promote atherogenesis and hasten cardiovascular disease. By enabling physicians to reduce the dosage of insulin, where possible without compromising glycemic control, it may be possible to prevent or reduce the CV complications of hyperinsulinemia.

The future role of troglitazone in the treatment of type II patients should not be minimized. Thirty to fifty percent of all NIDDM patients take insulin to control their blood glucose, even though sulfonylureas and metformin have been available for years. In this large subpopulation of patients, the use of insulin is not as straightforward as many believe, as many patients (including the elderly) do not readily adapt to insulin use. This is particularly a problem with the more obese patients with insulin resistance who frequently require ever-increasing doses of insulin to control blood glucose and steadily gain weight from the insulin, without necessarily achieving improved glucose control. It is in these individuals that troglitazone may provide its most significant therapeutic contribution.

Adverse effects. In general, troglitazone is well tolerated. The overall incidence and types of adverse reactions in controlled clinical trials was comparable in troglitazone-treated patients and those receiving placebo. In these studies, 2.2% of troglitazone-treated and 0.6% of placebo-treated patients had reversible elevations of AST or ALT greater than three times the upper limit of normal. It is recommended that liver function tests be done at the start of therapy, monthly for the first six months, bimonthly for the fremainder of the first year of therapy and periodically thereafter. Troglitazone is not recommended in the presence of acute liver disease. In the presence of previous hepatic disease, caution should be observed and liver function tests monitored, as above.

Table 65.10 lists the clinically significant interactions with troglitazone.

Nursing Management

Table 65.11 on the next page describes the nursing management of the patient receiving oral hypoglycemic agents. Dosage details of individual drugs are given in Table 65.12 (pages 773–776).

Box 65.2 (pages 771–772) provides an overview of management of diabetes mellitus, including nonpharmacologic and pharmacologic measures.

Table 65.10
Troglitazone: Drug interactions

Drug	Interaction
Cholestyramine	• The concomitant administration of cholestyramine with troglitazone reduces the absorption of troglitazone by 70%. Coadministration is not recommended

Table 65.11
Nursing management of the oral hypoglycemics

Assessment of risk vs. benefit	Patient data	• Assess for baseline VS, general state of health, nutritional status • *Pregnancy:* Risk category varies with drug. Generally, these drugs are not recommended during pregnancy and lactation
	Drug data	• Most serious adverse effects are related to drug-induced hypoglycemia and allergic reactions
Implementation	Rights of administration	• Using the "rights" helps prevent errors of administration
	Right route	• Give PO
	Nursing therapeutics	• Encourage self-management (nutrition, exercise/activity, hygiene) • Ensure pt understands that this medication does not cure the condition, but does control symptoms and may prevent complications associated with the disease • *Emotional support:* Diabetes is a lifelong condition with many serious complications • Provide nutritional counselling or refer to dietitian • Treat hypoglycemic reactions immediately: If pt is able to swallow, provide fast-acting source of carbohydrates such as fruit juice, sugar cubes, hard candies; if unable to swallow, IV glucose is preferred tx, although parenteral glucagon may be used initially
	Patient/family teaching	• Pt's need for information is influenced by many individual factors including beliefs regarding the condition, previous experience with diabetes, education, culture and age. Compliance and follow-up are essential factors in successful tx; review principles of pt education in Chapter 3 • Pts/families should know warning signs/symptoms of hypoglycemic reaction and how to treat immediately • Pts should be advised to avoid large amounts of alcohol because of possible disulfiram-like reaction • Pt should be instructed to report any abnormal blood or urine glucose tests • Advise pt to consult with pharmacist or physician prior to using OTC medications • Advise pts to wear a medical ID bracelet at all times. They should also carry a supply of carbohydrates in case of mild hypoglycemic episodes • *Discuss possibility of pregnancy:* Advise pt to notify physician and discuss transferring to insulin
Outcomes	Monitoring of progress	*Continually monitor:* • Clinical response indicating tx success (reduction in signs/symptoms) • Signs/symptoms of adverse reactions; document and report immediately to physician. Observe for hypoglycemia, hyperglycemia and allergic reactions • Blood tests to monitor glucose levels, including regular blood glucose levels through self-monitoring and periodic lab tests and HbA$_{1c}$

Box 65.2
Management of diabetes mellitus

A. Nonpharmacological approaches

Patients must be educated about diabetes. At the same time, a multidisciplinary health care team must work together to optimize management of the condition. Dietary advice should be given to all patients. In type I diabetes, along with insulin therapy, a meal plan designed by a dietitian forms the basis for all other therapies. Regular exercise is also part of optimal management; it reduces weight, lowers blood glucose and lipid levels, decreases insulin resistance, reduces cardiovascular disease, lowers blood pressure and promotes general well-being.

Patients must also be taught to recognize and treat hypoglycemic reactions (e.g., by never missing meals or snacks; anticipating exercise with extra carbohydrate; taking oral sugar prn). Patients who can reliably monitor their own blood glucose can make appropriate adjustments to their treatment programs.

B. Type I diabetes mellitus (insulin-dependent diabetes mellitus; IDDM)

Nonpharmacological approaches to the treatment of type I diabetes are not enough. Insulin must be started immediately. Patients with type I who are more than moderately ketotic, dehydrated, vomiting or severely nauseated or who live far from a treatment centre are usually admitted to hospital for acute treatment and education. Others can be treated as outpatients if a dietitian, nurse educator and physician are available and patients have been taught a diet, insulin injection and self-monitored blood glucose techniques.

Patients with type I diabetes should receive human insulin at the time of diagnosis to reduce symptoms and to emphasize the importance of prompt blood glucose reduction. Patients who are in good control on nonhuman insulin need not be switched to human insulin.

Type I patients who are not ketoacidotic are treated with an initial insulin total daily dosage of 0.5 U/kg ideal body weight. Short- and intermediate-acting insulin should be started immediately. The goal in the first week is to achieve modestly elevated blood glucose levels (8–10 mmol/L) to avoid hypoglycemia when the patient resumes activity. A long-term blood glucose level of 5–8 mmol/L should be the goal in most patients.

C. Diabetic ketoacidosis

Diabetic ketoacidosis occurs with severe insulin deficiency and may be apparent at diagnosis or in patients with established diabetes (types I and II) associated with acute infections, myocardial infarction, surgery and omission of insulin.

It is characterized by dehydration, acidotic breathing, obtundation to the point of coma, marked ketonuria and ketonemia, metabolic acidosis with electrolyte abnormalities (hyponatremia, normal or elevated serum potassium despite net potassium depletion, depressed serum bicarbonate), prerenal azotemia and markedly elevated glucose (sometimes only a modest increase in glucose, despite serious ketoacidosis).

Treatment includes hospitalization and immediate administration of rapid-acting insulin, 5–10 U/h by continuous IV infusion. IV fluids and electrolytes should be administered (commonly, 0.45% saline with the addition of potassium 20–40 mmol/L). Frequently, 1–2 L 0.9% saline should be given in the first 2 h, depending on the extent of dehydration, before switching to 0.45% saline. Bicarbonate is administered if serum bicarbonate is < 6 mmol or pH ≤ 7.1.

Hourly monitoring of glucose and electrolytes guides the gradual reduction of insulin dosage and modification of fluid and electrolyte administration. When glucose levels fall below 11 mmol/L (rate of fall, usually 5 mmol/h), physicians frequently start 5% glucose IV 100 mL/h to provide calories and prevent hypoglycemia.

Supportive measures (nasogastric tube, antibiotics, cardiac monitoring prn) should be continued until the patient is fully conscious and cooperative. Once the patient is able to begin oral feeding, a switch is made to subcutaneous insulin.

D. Type II diabetes mellitus (non–insulin-dependent diabetes mellitus; NIDDM)

Nonpharmacological approaches to the treatment of type II diabetes (see above) should be tried before drug therapy is instituted. If dietary management proves insufficient to restore normal blood sugar levels, acarbose should be considered.

If dietary management plus an alpha-glucosidase inhibitor fails to restore normal blood sugar, oral hypoglycemics may be used. A two-week trial is likely sufficient to determine response and adequacy of dose.

If either a sulfonylurea or metformin alone fails to control blood sugar and HbA_{1c} values, the two may be combined. There is no advantage to combining two sulfonylureas.

If oral agents fail to control NIDDM patients, insulin is used. It is also preferred as initial therapy by many physicians in patients younger than 40, women contemplating pregnancy (tight control 1–2 months preconception and in early pregnancy prevents malformations), nonobese patients and those with maturity-onset diabetes of the young (MODY), nonketotic severely hyperglycemic patients,

(cont'd on next page)

Box 65.2 (continued)
Management of diabetes mellitus

D. Type II diabetes mellitus (non–insulin-dependent diabetes mellitus; NIDDM) (cont'd)

alcoholic patients and those with pre-existing complications. The decision to switch to insulin therapy should not be delayed if other measures fail to control blood glucose.

In patients who have not responded adequately to insulin, troglitazone can be added to insulin therapy. This novel drug increases tissue sensitivity to insulin and has been approved for the treatment of patients with type II diabetes inadequately controlled with insulin therapy. As glycemic control improves, it may be possible to reduce the dose of insulin or even completely eliminate it in some patients. However, reduction in insulin dosage should not come at the expense of optimal diabetes control.

E. Hypoglycemic emergency (insulin reaction)

Hypoglycemia occurs more frequently when tight control is pursued. Except in a small number of patients, this does not justify undertreating. Hypoglycemic reactions can be classified as mild, severe or dangerous.

Mild reactions present with sweating, shaking, hunger, weakness and tachycardia. These symptoms are easily recognized and treated by the patient.

Severe reactions start as mild but if not treated, progress to additional neurologic symptoms (e.g., confusion, aggressiveness, disorientation, coma) that prevent the patient from taking appropriate measures.

In dangerous reactions, the patient cannot recognize early signs (hypoglycemic unawareness) in order to take corrective action; the level of control must be reconsidered to avoid recurrence.

The conscious patient requires immediate ingestion of 10–15 g glucose (e.g., 125–250 mL unsweetened juice, 3–5 Life Savers® or 2–3 sugar cubes). For compromised patients, one packet of Monogel® or 15 mL (1 tablespoon) of corn syrup or honey in the cheek should suffice; these are viscous and less likely to be aspirated. Glucose, 25 g IV], is a reliable treatment if the patient is unconscious. Alternatively, glucagon 1 mg IM or SC (repeated prn) will increase blood glucose for 20–30 min, allowing the patient to swallow carbohydrate. Glucagon enhances glycogenolysis and may not be effective in malnourished patients. Once blood glucose returns to normal, the reasons for the hypoglycemia should be explored to avoid recurrences.

F. Intensive insulin therapy

In intensive insulin therapy, patients are required to have at least 4 injections of insulin daily or use an insulin infusion pump (see below). The expense associated with an insulin pump and its sometimes imperfect biotechnology have meant that most patients use the daily injection technique.

In this treatment, patients must monitor their blood glucose frequently, usually at least 4–7 times daily. They need to learn from theoretical knowledge and practical experience how their blood glucose concentrations can fluctuate in response to changes in physical activity and food consumption. Then, the patient makes frequent adjustments to the insulin dosage as necessary. The aim is to keep blood glucose concentrations as near normal as possible. This management method requires a great deal of patient education and is most easily conducted where there is close involvement between patients and a multidisciplinary health care team.

In the Diabetes Control and Complications Trial (DCCT) (see Further Reading), intensive treatment reduced HbA_{1c} by about 2% and reduced both the development and progression of diabetic complications by 35% to 76%. However, it was also associated with a threefold higher incidence of severe hypoglycemic episodes. Thus, intensive insulin therapy should be used with caution in patients prone to hypoglycemia. Many patients also find the demand of managing diabetes on an hour-to-hour basis too much of a psychological burden. Thus, counselling and selection of patients for intensive treatment must be conducted carefully by experienced health care professionals.

G. Continuous subcutaneous infusion of insulin

Continuous subcutaneous insulin infusion (CSII) is accomplished using a portable infusion pump connected to an indwelling SC catheter. The only form of insulin employed for CSII is regular insulin. To provide a basal level of insulin, the pump is set to infuse the hormone continuously at a slow but steady rate. To accommodate insulin needs created by eating, the pump is triggered manually to provide a bolus dose of insulin matched in size to the caloric content of each meal. Thus, CSII can adapt to changes in insulin needs. Home monitoring of blood glucose is an essential component of CSII.

The most troubling problem with CSII is severe hypoglycemia, which has occurred when pump malfunction caused the infusion of excessive doses of insulin. CSII has also produced local allergic reactions and infections at the site of needle insertion. The final drawback is that CSII is expensive.

Table 65.12
Treatment of diabetes: Drug doses

Drug Generic name (Trade names)	Dosage	Nursing alert
A. Hormones **1. Very Rapidly Acting Insulin** insulin lispro (Humalog)	**SC:** Quicker onset of action and shorter duration of activity than animal-source or other DNA recombinant-source insulins. Dosage depends on pt requirements and should be based on amount and frequency of administration to maintain near-normal blood glucose concentrations. Pts receiving insulin for the first time can be started on insulin lispro in the same manner as they would on animal-source or human insulin. Some pts transferring to insulin lispro may require a change in dosage from that used with their previous insulin. If adjustment is needed, it may be made with the first dose or over a period of several weeks	• Store in a cool area. Refrigeration is desirable, but not essential; vial can be kept at room temperature for 1 month. Prevent exposure to direct heat and sunlight and do not freeze • Do not use insulin that changes colour or becomes clumped and/or granular in appearance. Always check expiration date on vials prior to use • Advise pt to keep to the same brand of syringe or needle • Remind pt, when mixing two insulins, always to draw up into syringe in the same order • Follow correct technique for SC injection (see Box 65.1, page 765). Administer 15–30 min prior to meal • Do not use for IV administration
2. Rapidly Acting Insulins regular insulin (Insulin Toronto, Insulin-Toronto [Beef], Insulin-Toronto [Pork], Iletin I) highly purified insulin (Velosin, Regular Iletin II Pork) human biosynthetic insulin (Humulin R)	**SC:** Individualize according to blood or urine glucose. As adjunct to intermediate-acting preparations, commonly 5–10 U regular insulin is given in same syringe before breakfast or evening meal. Dose of regular insulin must be adjusted according to blood glucose measurements at appropriate time (e.g., after breakfast and before lunch for a.m. dose; after evening meal and before bedtime snack for before-evening meal dose of regular insulin) **IV** (for ketoacidosis): *Adults:* 5–10 U/h by infusion. More may be required in some insulin-resistant pts. *Children:* Range, 0.1 U/kg/h to the adult dose, given by continuous infusion	• Store in a cool area. Refrigeration is desirable, but not essential; vial can be kept at room temperature for 1 month. Prevent exposure to direct heat and sunlight and do not freeze • Do not use insulin that changes colour or becomes clumped and/or granular in appearance. Always check expiration date on vials prior to use • Advise pt to keep to the same brand of syringe or needle • Remind pt, when mixing two insulins, always to draw up into syringe in the same order • Follow correct technique for SC injection (see Box 65.1, page 765). Administer 15–30 min prior to meal • **IV:** This is the only form of insulin that can be used. Give by direct injection at a rate of 50 U over 1 min. Check agency policy regarding certification. For continuous infusion, use infusion pump and check compatibility with other medications. This is not preferred route, as 20%–80% of drug potency is lost due to reaction with tubing and container. Monitor blood glucose levels frequently during infusion • Peak effect occurs 2–4 h after administration. Monitor for hypoglycemia at this time

(cont"d on next page)

Table 65.12 (continued)
Treatment of diabetes: Drug doses

Drug Generic name (Trade names)	Dosage	Nursing alert
A. Hormones (cont'd) **2. Rapidly Acting Insulins (cont'd)**		
semilente insulin (Semilente Insulin, Semilente Iletin I)	**SC** (for newly diagnosed mild diabetics): Initially, 10–20 U 30 min before breakfast. At least 2 daily doses may be necessary. No standard dose can be cited for this drug	• Store in a cool area. Refrigeration is desirable, but not essential; vial can be kept at room temperature for 1 month. Prevent exposure to direct heat and sunlight and do not freeze • Do not use insulin that changes colour or becomes clumped and/or granular in appearance. Always check expiration date on vials prior to use • Advise pt to keep to the same brand of syringe or needle • Remind pt, when mixing two insulins, always to draw up into syringe in the same order • Follow correct technique for SC injection (see Box 65.1, page 765). Administer 15–30 min prior to meal • Do not use for IV administration • Peak effect occurs 2–4 h after administration. Monitor for hypoglycemia at this time
3. Intermediate-Acting Insulins NPH insulin, isophane insulin (NPH Insulin, NPH Iletin, NPH Insulin [Beef], NPH Insulin [Pork], NPH Insulin [Isophane]) highly purified insulin (Insulatard NPH, Iletin II Pork) human biosynthetic insulin (Humulin N) lente insulin (Lente Insulin, Lente Iletin I, Lente Insulin Pork) lente insulin highly purified (Lente Iletin II Pork)	**SC:** Individualize dosage. Initially, 10–20 U or more 30–60 min before breakfast, often combined with regular insulin. If needed, NPH and regular insulin may be given in divided doses to provide approximately 1/3 daily requirement 30 min before evening meal	• As above, except peak effect occurs 6–12 h after administration. Monitor for hypoglycemia at this time
4. Long-Acting Insulins protamine zinc insulin (Protamine Zinc Insulin, Protamine Zinc Iletin, Protamine Zinc [Beef], Protamine Zinc [Pork]) ultralente insulin (Ultra Lente Insulin, Ultra Lente Iletin) human biosynthetic insulin (Human L Lente)	**SC:** Individualize on basis on pt response	• As above, except peak effect occurs 14–24 h after administration. Monitor for hypoglycemia at this time

Table 65.12 (continued)
Treatment of diabetes: Drug doses

Drug Generic name (Trade names)	Dosage	Nursing alert
A. Hormones (cont'd) **5. Polypeptide Hormone**		
glucagon HCl (Glucagon Injection)	**SC/IM/IV** (for hypoglycemia): *Adults/children > 20 kg:* 1 mg (1 U). *Children < 20 kg:* 0.5 mg (0.5 U) or dose equivalent to 20–30 µg/kg. Pt will usually awaken within 15 min. If response is delayed, there is no contraindication to administration of 1–2 additional doses of glucagon. IV glucose must be given if pt fails to respond to glucagon	•Diluent is provided for use only in the preparation of glucagon for intermittent parenteral injection and for no other use. Directions: 1. Dissolve lyophilized glucagon in the accompanying diluent. If glucagon is to be given in doses > 2 mg, it should be reconstituted with sterile water for injection instead of the supplied diluting solution and used stat 2. Glucagon should not be used in concentrations > 1 mg/mL (1 U/mL) 3. Solutions should not be used unless they are clear and of a watery consistency
B. Alpha-Glucosidase Inhibitors acarbose (Prandase, Precose)	**Oral:** Individualize dosage on the basis of both effectiveness and tolerance while not exceeding 100 mg tid. Usual starting dosage is 25 mg tid. Maint. dosage: After the initial dosage of 25 mg tid, increase to 50 mg tid. Some pts may benefit from further increasing dosage to 100 mg tid	•Take 3x daily with first bite of each meal •Dosage of acarbose should be adjusted at 4- to 8-week intervals based on 2-h postprandial glucose levels and tolerance
C. Sulfonylurea Oral Hypoglyemics acetohexamide (Dimelor, Dymelor)	**Oral** (pts not previously receiving insulin or drug tx): In mild, stable diabetes (after dietary regulation), initially, 250 mg daily before breakfast; increase by increments of 250–500 mg q5–7days, prn. Pts who require 1.5 g daily usually benefit from bid dosage, given before the a.m. and evening meals. Pts who do not respond to 1.5 g daily will usually not respond to a higher dose (Transfer from tolbutamide) Initial dose of acetohexamide should be about 1/2 tolbutamide dose, up to a max. of 1.5 g acetohexamide (Transfer from chlorpropamide) Initial acetohexamide dose should be about double the dose of chlorpropamide	•Take single daily dose before breakfast. If multiple doses required, take with a.m. and evening meals. If pt is transferring from another oral agent, no transition period is required. If pt is transferring from insulin to an oral antidiabetic, then pt should monitor blood glucose levels at least 3x/day ac
chlorpropamide (Chloronase, Diabinese)	**Oral:** Initially, 250 mg daily. Older pts should be started on 100–125 mg daily. Dosage may be adjusted upward or downward by 50–125 mg at intervals of 3–5 days prn. Usual range, 100–500 mg daily. Maint. doses > 500 mg daily should be avoided	•No transition period is required if pt is transferring from another oral antidiabetic. Give total daily dose with breakfast unless gastric upset occurs, then divide dose and give with a.m. and evening meals

(cont'd on next page)

Table 65.12 (continued)
Treatment of diabetes: Drug doses

Drug Generic name (Trade names)	Dosage	Nursing alert
C. Sulfonylurea Oral Hypoglycemics		
gliclazide (Diamicron)	**Oral:** Initially, 160 mg/day, taken as 1 80-mg tablet bid with meals. Rec. daily dose, 80–320 mg. Total daily dose should not exceed 320 mg	• Dosages of ≥ 160 mg should be divided into 2 equal doses and given bid
glyburide (Diabeta, Euglucon)	**Oral:** Newly diagnosed diabetics: Initially, 5 mg daily (2.5 mg in pts > 60 years), continued for 5–7 days. Increase or decrease by steps of 2.5 mg prn. Max. daily dose, 20 mg. Majority of pts can be controlled by 5–10 mg/day	• Give daily dose during or immediately after breakfast, or at lunch if pt usually has a light breakfast. If dosage > 10 mg, take 10 mg in a.m. and remaining dose with evening meal • Do not substitute different brands; may not be bioequivalent
tolbutamide (Mobenol, Orinase)	**Oral** (newly diagnosed diabetics): 1–2 g daily as single dose in a.m. or in divided doses, for 4 weeks or until pt responds; then adjust maint. dose (usually, 0.5–2 g) to smallest daily dose required to maintain optimum control	• May be taken as single dose in a.m. or divided into 2 doses and taken with a.m. and evening meals
D. Biguanide Oral Hypoglycemic		
metformin HCl (Glucophage)	**Oral:** Usually, 500 mg tid or qid, or 850 mg bid or tid. Max. dose should not exceed 2.5 g/day	• To minimize gastric reactions such as nausea and vomiting, take with food
E. Insulin Resistance Improving Agent		
troglitazone (Rezulin)	**Oral:** Usually, 400 mg od. Initially, 200 mg od; increase prn in 2–4 weeks to 400 mg od. Max. rec. dose, 600 mg daily. It is recommended that insulin dose be reduced by 10%–25% when fasting plasma glucose concentrations decrease to < 6.7 mmol/L (120 mg/dL). Further adjustments should be individualized based on glucose-lowering response. Therefore, dose increases should be done gradually. Use of troglitazone in pts with liver disease should be done only with caution. Monitor long-term use of troglitazone in pts with renal impairment	• Take with a meal • Remind pt that maximum effectiveness may not be achieved for 6–12 weeks

Response to Clinical Challenge

1. The most helpful information for immediate diagnosis includes: capillary blood glucose level, time of last insulin injection, time/amount of last meal.

2. The most likely explanation for these symptoms is hypoglycemia caused either by excessive insulin or inadequate food intake. Symptoms could also be related to a change in Brian's daily exercise patterns. For example, he may have expended more energy in the gym than usual at this time of day.

3. Immediate treatment should be to provide oral, rapid-acting carbohydrates, such as fruit juice, a sugar cube or hard candy very quickly. This should be followed by longer-acting carbohydrates (starches) to maintain the blood sugar level. You should also be familiar with agency policy regarding the protocol for treatment of hypoglycemic episodes. This may include parenteral administration of glucose or glucagon.

Further Reading

American Diabetes Association. Position statement: continuous SC insulin infusion. *Diabetes Care* 1997;20(suppl 1):S50.

Anderson J, et al. Reduction of postprandial hyperglycemia and frequency of hypoglycemia in IDDM patients on insulin-analog treatment. *Diabetes* 1997;46(2):265–270.

Diabetes Control and Complications Trial (DCCT) Research Group. The effect of intensive treatment of diabetes on the development and progression of long-term complications in insulin-dependent diabetes mellitus. *New Engl J Med* 1993;329:977.

DCCT Research Group. Epidemiology of severe hypoglycaemia in the Diabetes Complications and Control Trial. *Am J Med* 1991;90:450.

Hirsch IB, Farkas-Hirsch R. Type I diabetes and insulin therapy. *Nurs Clin North Am* 1993;28(1):9–23.

Palmer DG, Inturrisi M. Insulin infusion therapy in the intrapartum period. *J Perinatal Neonatal Nurs* 1992;6(1):25–36.

Savinette-Rose B, Balmer L. Understanding continuous subcutaneous insulin infusion therapy. *Am J Nurs* 1997;97(3):42–49.

U.K. Prospective Diabetes Study Group. Perspectives in diabetes. Study 16: Overview of 6 years' therapy of type II diabetes: a progressive disease. *Diabetes* 1995;44:1249–1258.

U.K. Prospective Diabetes Study Group. Study 13: Relative efficacy of randomly allocated diet, sulfonylurea, insulin, or metformin in patients with newly diagnosed non–insulin-dependent diabetes followed for three years. *Brit Med J* 1995; 310:83–88.

CHAPTER 66

Adrenal Corticosteroids

Topics Discussed
- Physiological control of adrenal cortical hormone release
- Actions of glucocorticoids
- Synthetic corticosteroids
- Systemic corticosteroid therapy
- Topical corticosteroid therapy
- Nursing management

Clinical Challenge

Consider this clinical challenge as you read through this chapter. The response to the challenge appears on page 788.

Jay is a 27-year-old man admitted to Emergency by his wife, who states that he is receiving corticosteroid therapy. He presents with severe muscle weakness, low blood pressure, extreme fatigue, dyspnea and dizziness.

What do you suspect? What treatment is indicated?

Drugs Discussed
amcinonide (am-**sin**-oh-nyde)
beclomethasone (beck-loe-**meth**-ah-zone)
betamethasone (bay-tah-**meth**-ah-zone)
clobetasol (kloe-**bay**-tah-sole)
clobetasone (kloe-**bay**-tah-zone)
cortisol (**kor**-tih-sole)
cortisone (**kor**-tih-zone)
desonide (**dess**-oh-nyde)
desoximetasone (dess-ox-ee-**met**-ah-zone)
dexamethasone (dex-ah-**meth**-ah-zone)
diflurasone (dye-**flyoor**-ah-zone)
fludrocortisone (flew-droe-**kor**-tih-zone)
fluocinolone (flew-oh-**sin**-oh-lone)
fluocinonide (flew-oh-**sin**-oh-nyde)
halcinonide (hal-**sin**-oh-nyde)
hydrocortisone (hye-droe-**kor**-tih-zone)
methylprednisolone (meth-il-pred-**niss**-oh-lone)
paramethasone (pair-ah-**meth**-ah-zone)
prednisolone (pred-**niss**-oh-lone)
prednisone (**pred**-nih-zone)
triamcinolone (trye-am-**sin**-oh-lone)

Physiological Control of Adrenal Cortical Hormone Release

The adrenal cortex secretes glucocorticoids, mineralocorticoids and sex hormones. This chapter focuses on the pharmacologic properties of glucocorticoids and the general principles and nursing management underlying their systemic use. The actions of the major mineralocorticoid hormone, aldosterone, are here mentioned only briefly, as they are covered in greater detail in Chapter 39. Sex hormones are discussed in Chapter 67.

Glucocorticoids are so named because they have important actions on glucose metabolism. However, their effects are not limited to glucose. These hormones exert major actions on all aspects of carbohydrate, fat and protein metabolism. They also modify cardiovascular function and reduce the response to inflammatory stimuli.

Mineralocorticoids increase the renal reabsorption of sodium, chloride and water, while promoting the excretion of potassium and hydrogen ions. If plasma sodium falls or plasma potassium increases, or if blood pressure drops, the adrenal cortex releases aldosterone, resulting in an increase in sodium and a drop in potassium levels.

Although the expression corticosteroid can be taken to mean any chemical, natural or synthetic, that possesses glucocorticoid and/or mineralocorticoid properties, it is usually used to refer to drugs with predominantly glucocorticoid effects. In this chapter the words glucocorticoid and corticosteroid are used interchangeably.

Many drugs have been synthesized to mimic, in part or in whole, the effects of the glucocorticoids. These drugs are used to treat many diseases. Their uses in bronchial asthma, rheumatoid arthritis, chronic inflammatory bowel disease and skin disorders, to mention but four areas, are discussed in separate chapters. Glucocorticoids owe their therapeutic usefulness to their marked metabolic, anti-inflammatory and immunosuppressive actions.

Regulation of Glucocorticoid Release

Hydrocortisone, also called cortisol, is synthesized in the adrenal cortex and released in response to stimulation from the hypothalamus and pituitary. The hypothalamus releases a chemical called the corticotrophin-releasing factor (CRF), which stimulates secretion of the adrenocorticotrophic hormone (ACTH) from the pituitary. ACTH, in turn, stimulates the adrenal cortex to synthesize and release cortisol. A major factor controlling the release of CRF and ACTH is the circulating level of glucocorticoids. In the face of low plasma cortisol concentrations, CRF and ACTH secretion increase. By way of contrast, high levels of cortisol or synthetic glucocorticoids depress CRF and ACTH release. The influence of CRF, ACTH and circulating cortisol levels on the secretion of cortisol is depicted in Figure 66.1.

Stress increases the release of corticosteroids. In response to stress, blood levels of ACTH increase rapidly. Shortly thereafter, cortisol secretion is increased.

Cortisol secretion is subject to diurnal variation. High blood levels of cortisol are found in the

Figure 66.1
Hypothalamic–pituitary–adrenal axis

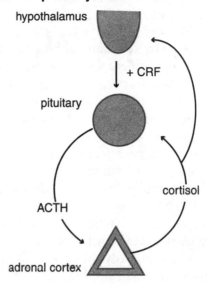

Pituitary ACTH secretion is regulated by negative-feedback effects of cortisol on the pituitary. Hypothalamic drive of ACTH release is mediated by corticotrophin-releasing factor (CRF). Cortisol inhibits pituitary response to CRF and may inhibit the secretion of CRF also.

Source: Baxter JD, Forsham PH. Tissue effects of glucocorticoids. *Am J Med* 1972;53:573–589. Reproduced with permission.

early morning hours around 06:00 (a stressful time for most of us), and low levels in the late evening. Individuals who work from midnight to 08:00 and sleep throughout the day show peak plasma cortisol levels just after arising, around 16:00, and low levels just prior to retiring.

Actions of Glucocorticoids

Metabolic Effects

Glucocorticoids produce a variety of effects. They influence the intermediary metabolism of carbohydrates, fats and proteins and modify salt and water balance. In supraphysiological doses, glucocorticoids have marked anti-inflammatory and immunosuppressive effects.

The metabolic actions of glucocorticoids are complex and involve both anabolic and catabolic effects. They increase glucose synthesis and impair its utilization. As a result, blood sugar levels rise. Glucocorticoids have a catabolic action on fat and muscle, releasing free fatty acids, glycerol and amino acids from these tissues and increasing their levels in the blood. Gluconeogenesis — the formation of glucose from fatty acids and amino acids — increases. In addition to their catabolic actions on muscle, glucocorticoids reduce amino acid uptake into this tissue, resulting in muscle wasting. In response to the increase in blood amino acids, glucagon is secreted, further accelerating hepatic glucose output.

The effects of glucocorticoid therapy on fat tissue are apparent to any nurse who has participated in the clinical management of patients receiving these drugs. As suggested above, the direct effects of glucocorticoids on fat tissue are antianabolic (a decrease in glucose uptake into fat) and catabolic (a breakdown of fat already formed, with an increase in free fatty acid production). These actions are counterbalanced, at least in part, by insulin released in response to the increase in blood glucose levels. Insulin has opposite effects to those of glucocorticoids: it stimulates lipogenesis and inhibits lipolysis. The consequence of the antagonism between a glucocorticoid and insulin is a redistribution of fat in the body. At sites in which the actions of the corticosteroid predominate, fat is lost; in areas in which insulin dominates, fat accumulates. Nurses will notice a characteristic "moon face" and "buffalo hump" in patients on high-dose glucocorticoid therapy as fat accumulates around the face and in the supraclavicular area following prolonged treatment.

The metabolic effects of glucocorticoids on liver, muscle, lymphoid, skin and adipose tissue are summarized in Figure 66.2.

Glucocorticoids interfere with the metabolic actions of vitamin D, causing a reduction in calcium absorption and an increase in its renal clearance. These actions account for the osteoporosis induced by glucocorticoids.

Anti-inflammatory and Immunosuppressive Effects

Glucocorticoids owe much of their therapeutic usefulness to their marked anti-inflammatory effects. These actions are nonspecific and can be directed against inflammatory responses to immunologically mediated disorders as well as to mechanical or chemical injury, or infection. The anti-

Figure 66.2
Glucocorticoid action on carbohydrate, lipid and protein metabolism

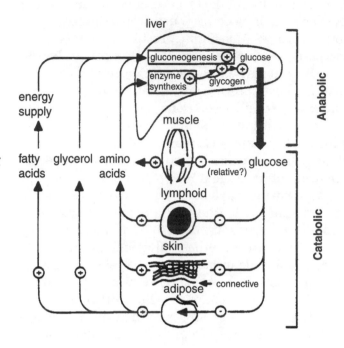

Arrows indicate the general flow of substrate in response to the catabolic and anabolic actions of the glucocorticoid when unopposed by secondary secretions of other hormones. The + and – signs indicate stimulation and inhibition, respectively.

Source: Baxter JD, Forsham PH. Tissue effects of glucocorticoids. *Am J Med* 1972;53:573–589. Reproduced with permission.

inflammatory and immunosuppressive responses to corticosteroids correlate with their glucocorticoid potency. In developing new corticosteroids for the treatment of inflammatory disorders, efforts are made to design drugs with marked glucocorticoid and minimal mineralocorticoid effects.

Inflammation was described nearly 1900 years ago as *rubor et tumor cum calore et dolore* (redness and swelling with heat and pain). Glucocorticoids treat each symptom. First, they potentiate the vasoconstrictor effects of circulating epinephrine and norepinephrine, thereby reducing blood flow and redness. The reduced blood flow to the inflamed area also diminishes heat at the affected site. Swelling is a result of increased capillary permeability and the leakage of fluid from blood vessels. Glucocorticoids decrease capillary permeability and reduce the loss of plasma into inflamed tissues. Finally, much of the pain is due to the release of two endogenous mediators of inflammation — histamine and bradykinin. Mast cells synthesize, store and release histamine. Glucocorticoids reduce histamine release by diminishing the accumulation of mast cells at the site of inflammation. The chemical prostaglandin E_2 is synthesized within neutrophils. It serves to increase the pain-producing activities of both histamine and bradykinin. Glucocorticoids reduce neutrophil migration to the site(s) of inflammation and decrease prostaglandin E_2 synthesis and release. Glucocorticoids also diminish T-lymphocyte levels in blood, thereby reducing the cell-mediated immunity response to an inflammatory stimulus.

To the description of inflammation as redness, swelling, heat and pain, may be added one more facet — disturbed function. As a result of fibrin deposition, capillary and fibroblast proliferation and the deposition of collagen and cicatrization (scarring), the ability of a joint to move normally is disturbed. Glucocorticoids reduce fibrin deposition and minimize both capillary and fibroblast proliferation. They also decrease the deposition of collagen and cicatrization.

The use of glucocorticoids to treat inflammatory conditions is a double-edged sword. Although the suppression of inflammation may afford considerable relief or even prove life saving, glucocorticoids can also suppress signs of infection. Furthermore, patients on long-term, high-dose corticosteroid treatment regimens have reduced immunologic capability and are at greater risk for infections.

Synthetic Corticosteroids

The introduction of hydrocortisone (cortisol) as a drug provided a major therapeutic advance. However, because cortisol possesses both significant glucocorticoid and mineralocorticoid actions, newer steroids have been synthesized with the aim of accentuating glucocorticoid activity and reducing or abolishing mineralocorticoid properties. These include prednisone, prednisolone, methylprednisolone, triamcinolone, betamethasone, beclomethasone and dexamethasone.

In addition to having greater glucocorticoid activity, with diminished mineralocorticoid effects,

Table 66.1
Durations of action and equivalent doses of commonly used corticosteroids

Compound	Duration of action*	Equivalent dose**
Hydrocortisone	S	20 mg
Cortisol	S	25 mg
Prednisone	I	5 mg
Prednisolone	I	5 mg
Methylprednisolone	I	4 mg
Triamcinolone	I	4 mg
Betamethasone	L	0.6 mg
Dexamethasone	L	0.75 mg

* S, short (8- to 12-h biological half-life); I, intermediate (12- to 36-h biological half-life); L, long (36- to 72-h biological half-life)
** These dose relationships apply only to oral or IV administration.

the newer steroids have longer half-lives than hydrocortisone. Their biological half-lives are considerably longer than their chemical half-lives because the consequences of steroid action outlast by many hours the presence of the drug in tissues. Glucocorticoids are classified as short-acting, intermediate-acting and long-acting on the basis of their biological half-lives (Table 66.1). Cortisone and prednisone are inactive; they are converted to cortisol and prednisolone, respectively, in the liver. The latter chemicals are responsible for the pharmacological effects of cortisone and prednisone.

Systemic Glucocorticoid Therapy

Replacement Therapy

Corticosteroids may be administered as replacement therapy in primary or secondary adrenal insufficiency.

Primary adrenal insufficiency is characterized by inadequate cortisol production, despite the presence of large quantities of ACTH. The most frequent cause of primary adrenal insufficiency, or Addison's disease, is idiopathic atrophy of the adrenal glands, which results in a deficiency of both cortisol and aldosterone. Treatment for this condition involves the use of both a glucocorticoid and a mineralocorticoid. An appropriate dosage regimen for the treatment of Addison's disease is 20 mg/day of cortisol and 0.1 mg/day of the mineralocorticoid fludrocortisone (Florinef®).

Adrenal insufficiency secondary to pituitary insufficiency is characterized by low levels of both ACTH and cortisol and normal levels of aldosterone. Treatment involves replacement of the missing cortisol. Thirty-five to 40 mg of cortisone or 20–25 mg of cortisol can be given daily. The normal diurnal secretion of cortisol will be simulated if approximately two-thirds of the daily dose is given on arising in the morning and the remaining one-third around 16:00.

Congenital adrenal hyperplasia (adrenogenital syndrome) results from enzyme deficiencies in the synthesis of cortisol. As a result of low cortisol levels, ACTH secretion is increased, elevating the synthesis and secretion of adrenal androgens. Evidence of the condition in the female is often seen at birth as masculinization of the external genitalia. Diagnosis of the adrenal genital syndrome in males may not be made until later in infancy or in childhood. Treatment involves administration of a glucocorticoid to suppress ACTH secretion. It may also be necessary to administer a mineralocorticoid if a reduction in both glucocorticoid and mineralocorticoid synthesis occurs.

Suppressive Therapy

Corticosteroids may be given either on a short-term, high-dose; long-term, low-dose; or long-term, high-dose basis for their anti-inflammatory or immunosuppressive effects. The short-term, high-dose regimen, as used for the treatment of emergencies such as status asthmaticus and anaphylactic shock, does not produce pituitary–adrenal suppression. Long-term, low-dose corticosteroid therapy is used in the treatment of chronic conditions such as rheumatoid arthritis. Serious adverse effects can occur, but they are not as severe as when long-term, high-dose therapy is employed for conditions such as autoimmune hemolytic anemia and temporal arteritis, which require this regimen.

Alternate-day steroid therapy is intended to minimize the consequences of chronic high-dose glucocorticoid treatment. Patients are usually started on a daily corticosteroid regimen until

relief is obtained. Thereafter, it may be possible to convert them gradually to alternate-day treatment by doubling the daily glucocorticoid dose and administering it as a single dose on alternate mornings. Intermediate-acting steroids, such as prednisone (with a biologic half-life of 1.5 days), are most appropriate for alternate-day treatment. They provide protection for most of each forty-eight-hour period but still allow enough drug-free time for pituitary–adrenal responsiveness to return before the next dose. Unfortunately, conditions requiring high-dose, long-term treatment often require daily therapy to respond. Short-acting steroids such as cortisol are inadequate for most patients, because the length of time between the cessation of their action and the next dose is usually too long to provide significant protection. On the other hand, long-acting steroids are also inappropriate when used on an alternate-day basis. Because their durations of action exceed forty-eight hours, the patient's pituitary–adrenal function cannot recover before the next dose is given.

The use of supraphysiological doses of a glucocorticoid (75 mg cortisol or equivalent doses of a synthetic steroid) for longer than two weeks results in suppression of the pituitary–adrenal axis, which may persist for as long as nine to twelve months following withdrawal of treatment. As a result, to avoid an acute adrenal crisis, glucocorticoid therapy should not be withdrawn abruptly. The first step is to administer the total daily dose on a once-daily basis. Thereafter, the dose can be decreased gradually to physiological levels.

Therapeutic uses. Glucocorticoids are used nonspecifically in the treatment of inflammatory diseases of the intestine, bronchioles, nose, eyes, ears, skin and joints. Their uses in the treatment of arthritis, chronic inflammatory bowel disease and asthma are described in Chapters 54, 60 and 69, respectively, and need not be repeated here. The use of topical corticosteroids to treat dermatological conditions is outlined below. It should be pointed out that fear of their adverse effects has relegated glucocorticoids to a position behind other less effective, but also less toxic, drugs for the treatment of many systemic problems.

Corticosteroids are used to treat allergic diseases. However, they are indicated only in situations not controlled adequately by less dangerous agents, such as antihistamines. Since glucocorticoids do not act immediately, life-threatening situations, such as anaphylaxis and angioneurotic edema of the glottis, should be treated with subcutaneous epinephrine. Glucocorticoids are then used in short-term, high doses as second-line treatment.

Corticosteroids may be used in the treatment of rheumatic carditis, collagen vascular diseases, renal diseases, cerebral edema, malignant hematological diseases, liver diseases and shock. None of these will be presented in detail in this book. Nurses are encouraged to seek out relevant reference texts if they wish to understand the therapeutic value of steroids in the above conditions.

Adverse effects. Box 66.1 lists some of the more important complications of long-term, suppressive corticosteroid therapy. The adverse effects are, in most cases, a direct consequence of the major pharmacologic properties of corticosteroids and are more often seen when higher doses are used. Following chronic steroid therapy, myopathy presents as a proximal muscle weakness; marked wasting of the musculature is seen in the extremities.

Peptic ulceration is a commonly accepted adverse effect of glucocorticoid therapy. Some authorities dispute the view that glucocorticoids predispose patients to ulcers.

The CNS disturbances produced by corticosteroids vary from insomnia, nervousness and slight mood changes, to schizophrenia and suicide attempts. Reactions of this nature are generally more frequent and more severe in patients with known psychological difficulties.

As a result of their mineralocorticoid activity, many steroids can create problems in patients with pre-existing hypertension or cardiovascular disease. In these individuals, dexamethasone or triamcinolone (corticosteroids with minimal mineralocorticoid activity) may be preferred, together with a restriction of dietary salt and/or the use of diuretics with supplementary potassium.

The ability of glucocorticoids to induce osteoporosis has already been explained. Patients who are more likely to develop osteoporosis, such as postmenopausal women and elderly, immobilized and diabetic patients, suffer greater risk for compression fractures of the vertebral column. For

---

Box 66.1
Complications of corticosteroid therapy

Musculoskeletal
Myopathy
Osteoporosis/vertebral compression
Fractures
Aseptic necrosis of bone

Gastrointestinal
Peptic ulceration (often gastric)
Gastric hemorrhage
Intestinal perforation
Pancreatitis

Ophthalmologic
Glaucoma
Posterior subcapsular cataracts

Cardiovascular and renal
Hypertension
Sodium and water retention, edema
Hypokalemic alkalosis

Metabolic
Precipitation of clinical manifestations of genetic diabetes
   mellitus, including ketoacidosis
Hyperosmolar nonketotic coma
Hyperlipidemia
Induction of centripetal obesity

Endocrine
Growth failure
Secondary amenorrhea
Suppression of hypothalamic–pituitary–adrenal system

Central nervous system
Psychiatric disorders
Pseudocerebral tumour

Inhibition of fibroblasts
Impaired wound healing
Subcutaneous tissue atrophy

Suppression of the immune response
Superimposition of a variety of bacterial, fungal, viral and
   parasitic infections in steroid-treated pts

Source: Melby JC. Clinical pharmacology of systemic steroids. *Ann Rev Pharmacol Toxicol* 1977;17:511–527. Reproduced with permission.

these individuals, supplementary therapy with vitamin D and calcium is recommended.

Glucocorticoids stimulate the formation and diminish the utilization of glucose. Thus, latent diabetes mellitus may be unmasked by prolonged steroid therapy and pre-existing disease is often aggravated. Secondary to an alteration in adipose tissue metabolism, patients may accumulate fat in the supraclavicular area ("buffalo hump") and acquire a "moon face."

Corticosteroids can reduce significantly the host defence mechanism. Attention should be given to the possibility of a pre-existing infection before starting steroid therapy, not only for the systemic administration of drugs, but also for their topical use.

Table 66.2 lists the clinically significant drug interactions with systemic corticosteroids.

Topical Corticosteroids

Mechanism of Action and Pharmacologic Effects

Corticosteroids reduce inflammation by causing vasoconstriction, impairing chemotaxis, reducing prostaglandin formation, stabilizing lysosomal membranes in neutrophils and diminishing the lymphocytic response to allergic stimuli. Because of these actions, corticosteroids are incorporated into lotions, gels, creams, and ointments for the treatment of a variety of dermatologic conditions. Corticosteroids also suppress mitosis and are used in the treatment of psoriasis.

Potency of Different Corticosteroids

In using topical steroid therapy safely, it is important for nurses to recognize the differences in potency among the various products on the market. Corticosteroids range in potency from low potency through moderately potent, very potent to most potent. Representatives of each group are presented in Table 66.3 on page 786.

Table 66.2
Systemic corticosteroids: Drug interactions

Drug	Interaction
Amphotericin B	• Amphotericin B may have its potassium-depleting effects increased by glucocorticoids
Anticoagulants, oral	• Oral anticoagulants can have their effects antagonized by corticosteroids, which increase blood coagulability. Conversely, corticosteroids can increase the danger of hemorrhage because of their effects on vascular integrity. Because of the risk of GI ulceration as well as the possible risk of hemorrhage, pts who receive both corticosteroids and oral anticoagulants should be monitored carefully
Antidiabetic agents	• Antidiabetic agents may have their effects reduced by glucocorticoids, which increase blood sugar. Closely monitor pts receiving both drugs
Barbiturates	• Barbiturates, particularly phenobarbital, may increase the metabolism of corticosteroids, necessitating an increase in steroid dosage
Diuretics	• Diuretics (thiazides, chlorthalidone, ethacrynic acid, furosemide) may cause excessive loss of potassium in pts also receiving a glucocorticoid
Estrogen products	• Estrogen-containing products (such as oral contraceptives) can increase serum cortisol-binding globulin
Indomethacin	• Indomethacin is ulcerogenic. Combined effects of this drug and corticosteroids may result in increased incidence and/or severity of GI ulceration. If possible, avoid concomitant use
Phenytoin	• Phenytoin may increase the rate of corticosteroid metabolism
Rifampin	• Rifampin may increase the rate of metabolism of corticosteroids, thereby decreasing their pharmacologic effects
Salicylates	• Salicylates may have their serum concentrations reduced by corticosteroids, although the concomitant use of both drugs is not contraindicated. Salicylism may occur if the dose of the corticosteroid is reduced

Although the more potent steroids will usually provide a rapid and profound response, the temptation to use these products should be resisted because they are also capable of causing severe local adverse effects. Drugs in the very potent and most potent categories should be used only when the less potent products fail.

Role of the Vehicle

The choice of a vehicle is important in determining steroid absorption. To exert an anti-inflammatory effect, a corticosteroid must penetrate the stratum corneum of the epidermis to reach the dermis. Occlusion of pores with dressings (e.g., plastic wrap) has long been recognized as an effective way of increasing topical corticosteroid activity. The increased hydration of the stratum corneum, which accompanies occlusion, facilitates transport of a corticosteroid to deeper skin tissues. Ointments are the most occlusive vehicles and are most effective in promoting steroid penetration. Creams are less occlusive and generally less effective in guaranteeing penetration. Lotions are least occlusive. Gels usually contain alcohol and a jelling agent, such as propylene glycol. They are most suitable for hairy areas of the body and should not be used on mucous membranes because the alcohol may be severely irritating.

These comments must be weighed with the knowledge that creams, being oil-in-water vehicles, are more miscible with, and suitable for, wet or weepy dermatoses. Fortunately, wet or weepy skin problems offer less of a barrier, and thus creams provide adequate steroid penetration. Dry dermatoses offer greater impediment and usually require treatment with ointments. Lotions, like gels, are often used on hairy areas of the body.

Regional differences exist with respect to the ease with which drugs penetrate the skin. The back, scalp, axillae, forehead, jaw angle and scrotum present little impediment to drug absorption. They are best treated with weaker steroids (e.g., hydrocortisone). Only hydrocortisone should be used on the face and in the groin and axillae. If diaper rash requires steroid use, only hydrocortisone should be applied. The plantar surface of the foot and the ankle present greater barriers to absorption and may require stronger corticosteroids.

Therapeutic Uses

Allergic contact dermatitis, primary irritant dermatitis, endogenous eczema (e.g. atopic, neurodermatitis, cheiropompholyx), psoriasis (especially of the face and flexures), seborrheic eczema and varicose eczema usually respond well to topical corticosteroids. Alopecia areata, discoid lupus erythematosus, granuloma annulare, hypertrophic scars and keloids may respond to topical steroids but are treated faster with intralesional corticosteroids. The same statement can be made for necrobiosis lipoidica, nodular prurigo, pretibial myxedema and sarcoidosis.

Topical corticosteroids should not be used alone in skin infections; they reduce the host's defence mechanisms and permit the spread of infection. In addition, by reducing inflammation, they lull the patient, the physician and the nurse into the belief that the condition is on the wane. In cases of impetiginized eczema, which are usually colonized by *Staphylococcus aureus,* corticosteroids should be combined with antimicrobials. Other indications for combination products include seborrheic eczema, diaper rash, otitis externa, and intertriginous eruptions. However, the use of a combination preparation can also produce problems, such as the emergence of resistant strains, contact sensitization (particularly to neomycin) and skin staining (with iodochlorhydroxyquin [Vioform®]).

Adverse Effects

The major complications occurring after prolonged topical corticosteroid treatment involve the dermis. Dermal atrophy is a common adverse effect; dermal collagen is damaged and striae appear. This is more likely to occur in children and adolescents. The more potent steroids cause thinning of the epidermis. Rebound pustulation can also be seen when a strong corticosteroid is discontinued.

Consistent with the effects of corticosteroids on the host defence mechanisms, their topical application may both mask and encourage skin infections. Thus, it is important to determine if a topical inflammatory condition is secondary to an infection. When it is impossible to differentiate between an inflammatory condition and inflammation secondary to an infection, the patient should be treated with a combination of a steroid and appropriate antibacterials and antifungals.

Table 66.3
Classification of topical corticosteroids

Generic name	Trade name
Low-potency	
Hydrocortisone 1%	Aeroseb-HC, Alphaderm, Cetacort, Cort-Dome, Cortef, Cortril, Emo-Cort, Hydro-Cortilean, Hytone, Nutracort, Synacort, Unicort
Methylprednisolone 0.25%	Medrol
Moderately potent to potent	
Betamethasone valerate 0.05%	Betnovate, Celestoderm-V/2, Valisone
Clobetasone butyrate 0.05%	Eumovate
Desoximetasone 0.05%	Topicort Mild, Topicort LP
Fluocinolone acetonide 0.01%	Fluoderm, Fluonid, Synalar, Synamol
Fluocinonide 0.01%	Lidemol, Lidex, Topsyn
Halcinonide 0.025%	Halog
Hydrocortisone valerate 0.2%	Westcort
Triamcinolone acetonide 0.025%	Aristocort, Aristocort "D", Kenalog, Triacet, Triaderm
Potent to very potent	
Amcinonide 0.1%	Cyclocort
Beclomethasone dipropionate 0.025%	Propaderm
Betamethasone benzoate 0.025%	Beben, Betnisone, Uticort
Betamethasone valerate 0.1%	Betaderm, Betnovate, Celestoderm-V, Valisone
Desonide 0.05%	Tridesilon
Desoximethasone 0.25%	Topicort
Diflurasone diacetate 0.05%	Fluoderm, Fluonide, Synalar, Synamol
Fluocinonide 0.05%	Lidemol, Lidex, Topsyn
Flurandrenolide 0.05%	Cordran, Drenison
Halcinonide 0.1%	Halciderm, Halog
Triamcinolone acetonide 0.1%	Aristocort, Aristocort "R", Kenalog, Triacet, Triaderm
Very potent	
Betamethasone dipropionate 0.05%	Diprosone
Most potent	
Clobetasol propionate 0.05%	Dermovate
Fluocinolone acetonide 0.2%	Synalar HP
Triamcinolone acetonide 0.5%	Aristocort, Aristocort A, Aristocort C, Kenalog, Triacet

Nursing Management

Table 66.4 describes the nursing management of the patient receiving corticosteroids. Dosage details of individual drugs are given in Table 66.5 (pages 789–792).

**Table 66.4
Nursing management of the corticosteroids**

Assessment of risk vs. benefit	Patient data	• Because of the many adverse effects of the corticosteroids, the physician should determine whether severity of condition warrants use of the drug. Goal of drug tx influences choice of drug, dosage and route • Assess to establish baseline VS, general state of health • Assess conditions that require cautious drug use or enhanced monitoring such as diabetes, hypertension, peptic ulcer • Assess for clinical indicators of present infection, which contra-indicates drug use • *Pregnancy:* Most drugs in class are risk category C (animal studies show adverse effects to fetus but human data are unknown or insufficient); benefits may be acceptable despite risks
	Drug data	• *Some serious drug interactions:* Confer with pharmacist • Many serious adverse effects related to dosage and duration of drug tx (see Box 66.1, page 783) • Steroids are available in many dosage forms and preparations. Always check drug names and strengths carefully
Implementation	Rights of administration	• Using the "rights" helps prevent errors of administration
	Right route	• Give PO, IV, IM, topically and by local injection (intra-articular and intralesional), inhalation or nasal spray. NB that injection preparations may be available as various esters, including acetate and sodium phosphate. The acetate form must never be used IV
	Right time	• To reduce adrenal suppression, these drugs may be given on a qod cycle. Document carefully and instruct pt to use calendars or other memory devices to ensure accurate administration • Oral steroids are best given in the a.m. with food to reduce gastric irritation, to mimic the body's normal circadian production of natural cortisol. If divided doses are required, give 2/3 the dose in the a.m. and 1/3 prior to 16:00 h
	Right technique	• IV administration requires knowledge of correct diluent and IV solution, correct dilution and rate of administration. Always refer to manufacturer's instructions for this route. Specific precautions with this group because acetate form must not be given IV. Rate must be carefully controlled • Topical application also requires correct technique to ensure absorption for the pt without subjecting the nurse to a dose as well. Apply sparingly to clean skin. Wear gloves or finger cot to prevent absorbing drug. Apply occlusive dressing only if ordered. Do not substitute products, as potency varies
	Nursing therapeutics	• Some complications of corticosteroid tx can be minimized through nursing interventions, i.e.: *Osteoporosis* — dietary counselling to ensure adequate intake of calcium, vitamin D and daily activity/exercise; *peptic ulceration* — administration of drug with food;

(cont'd on next page)

Table 66.4 (cont'd)
Nursing management of the corticosteroids

Implementation (cont'd)	Nursing therapeutics (cont'd)	*CV effects* — prevention of sodium and water retention through dietary restrictions; *suppression of immune response* — aseptic precautions and improved host defences through hygiene, nutrition, rest and lifestyle to minimize exposure to infections; *psychological effects* — observe for signs of depression or emotional changes, provide reassurance and support to pt and family, discuss pt/family reactions to body image changes; *ophthalmic changes* — with long-term tx, instruct pt to have periodic eye examinations for glaucoma and cataracts
	Patient/family teaching	• Teach proper technique for nasal spray administration, i.e., blow nose before administration; hold head upright, breathe through nose during administration; sniff hard after for several minutes. If nasal passages are blocked, nasal decongestant should be used prior to administration to ensure penetration of spray • Instruct pt to report early warning signs/symptoms of adrenal suppression, e.g., muscle weakness, fatigue, joint pain, dyspnea, dizziness, fainting • Emphasize importance of maintaining drug tx and danger of sudden withdrawal • Pt should provide emergency information (i.e., wear medical-alert ID) and carry adequate supply of medication at all times • Pts should not receive vaccinations during steroid tx • Discuss pregnancy and potential risks to baby if high-dose tx is required. Baby may be born with adrenal insufficiency and require replacement tx. Lactation is not recommended during high-dose tx
Outcomes	Monitoring of progress	*Continually monitor:* • Clinical response indicating tx success (reduction in signs/symptoms) • Signs/symptoms of adverse reactions; document and report immediately to physician • Periodic monitoring of electrolytes and blood glucose may be indicated

Response to Clinical Challenge

Given Jay's symptoms, you should suspect adrenal insufficiency. Long-term or high-dose corticosteroid therapy produces adrenal suppression. If Jay has missed doses of his drug, he could be in adrenal crisis. The most important questions would centre on his drug therapy: the current drug, dosage, time of last dose.

If Jay is experiencing adrenal crisis, treatment would include emergency administration of a steroid by IV route for immediate onset of action. Careful monitoring is essential.

Further Reading

Armstrong R, Bolding F. Septic arthritis after arthroscopy: the contributing roles of intra-articular steroids and environmental factors. *Am J Inf Control* 1994(1):16–18.

Handerhan B. Recognizing adrenal crisis: how to respond to severe steroid withdrawal. *Nursing* 1992;22(4):33.

Table 66.5
The corticosteroids: Drug doses

Drug Generic name (Trade names)	Dosage	Nursing alert
A. Short-Acting Glucocorticoids		
hydrocortisone, cortisol (Cortef, Solu-Cortef)	**Oral** (for chronic adrenocortical insufficiency): 12–18 mg/m²/day, 2/3 in a.m. on rising, 1/3 in afternoon. (For congenital adrenal hyperplasia): 10–25 mg/m²/24 h [1/3 q8h], or 1/3 in a.m. and 2/3 in evening **IV** (for emergencies): Initially, 100–500 mg, delivered over 30 s (if 100 mg) to 10 min (if 500 mg) and repeated, if necessary. (For salt-losing crisis in congenital adrenal hyperplasia): 50–100 mg with IV fluids for 1–2 days until crisis is controlled **IM** (for emergencies when IV route is not possible): 100–500 mg, repeated at intervals of 2, 4 or 6 h, prn	• Give PO, IV and IM • **PO:** Give with meals in a.m. to mimic circadian rhythm. If doses are divided, last dose should be given by 16:00. Drug should be stored in light-proof containers • **IM:** Administer deeply into large muscle mass; use 19-gauge needle. Site of injection should be rotated. Avoid deltoid muscle • **IV:** Follow agency policy. Reconstitute drug with solution provided. For a dose of 100 mg, rate of infusion should be at least 30 s. If dose is ≥ 500 mg, be certain infusion occurs over at least 10 min. Diluted solutions should be used within 24 h. Observe BP and serum electrolyte levels
cortisone acetate (Cortone Acetate)	**Oral** (for chronic adrenal insufficiency): 12–20 mg/m²/day. (For congenital adrenal hyperplasia): 10–30 mg/m²/day **IM** (for chronic adrenocortical insufficiency): Initially, 20–30 mg daily. Larger doses (up to 300 mg) are indicated in shock unresponsive to conventional tx if adrenocortical insufficiency exists or is suspected. Maint. dosage is determined by gradually decreasing initial dose to the lowest amount that maintains adequate clinical response. In general, cortisone should not be given IM for acute adrenal insufficiency because absorption may be erratic and inadequate *Infants and young children with congenital adrenal hyperplasia:* Administration only q3–4days may be adequate for maintenance. Drug withdrawal should be done gradually	• Give PO, IM or SC • **PO:** Divide dose, giving 2/3 in a.m. and 1/3 in afternoon. Give with meals to reduce gastric irritation. When oral tx is not feasible, then IM injection is used
B. Intermediate-Acting Glucocorticoids		
prednisolone (Delta-Cortef, Dua-Pred, Hydeltra-TBA, Hydeltrasol, Predaline RP, Meticortolone, Saracort, Sterane)	**Oral** (for replacement): 4 mg/m²/day. (For anti-inflammatory effects): 5–60 mg/day	• **PO:** Given in a.m. to mimic the body's normal secretion. Oral dose may also be given 2/3 in a.m. and 1/3 in afternoon. Give with food to prevent gastric irritation

(cont'd on next page)

Table 66.5 (continued)
The corticosteroids: Drug doses

Drug Generic name (Trade names)	Dosage	Nursing alert
B. Intermediate-Acting Glucocorticoids (cont'd)		
prednisolone (Delta-Cortef, Dua-Pred, Hydeltra-TBA, Hydeltrasol, Predaline RP, Meticortolone, Saracort, Sterane) (cont'd)	**IV** (for emergencies): 25–50 mg prednisolone sodium phosphate. **Intra-articular/intrabursal injection** (for arthritis or bursitis): 25 mg for larger joints; 10–15 mg for smaller joints	• **IV:** For IV infusion, be certain to use prednisolone sodium phosphate; never give acetate form IV • **IM:** Shake solution before drawing up • Do not confuse this medication with prednisone; they are different medications
prednisone (Deltasone, Meticorten, Orasone)	**Oral** (for replacement tx): 4 mg/m^2/day, 2/3 in a.m., 1/3 in afternoon. (Inflammatory conditions): 5–60 mg/day	• Do not confuse this medication with prednisolone • **PO:** Give with food to reduce gastric irritation. For replacement tx, give 2/3 dose in a.m., 1/3 in afternoon. Intermediate-acting drug may be used for qod tx • For inflammatory conditions, administer in a.m. to mimic the body's natural secretion
methylprednisolone (Medrol, Depo-Medrol, Solu-Medrol)	**Oral:** *Adults:* Initially, 4–48 mg/day, in single dose or divided doses. If used chronically, when dose is stabilized, daily dose may be doubled and given qod. *Children* (adrenal insufficiency): 117 µg/kg/day in 3 divided doses. (Other uses): 4.7 µg/kg to 1.67 mg/kg/ day in 3–4 divided doses **IM/IV:** *Adults* (methylprednisolone sodium succinate): 10–40 mg. High-dose tx of 30 mg/ kg may be given IV q4–6h for up to 72 h. (For multiple sclerosis): 160 mg/day for 7 days, then 64 mg qod for 1 month. *Infants and children* (methylprednisolone sodium succinate; for adrenal insufficiency): 117 µg/kg/day in 3 divided doses. (Other uses): 139–835 µg/kg q12–24h. **IM:** *Adults* (methylprednisolone acetate): 40–120 mg daily, weekly or q2weeks. **Intra-articular/intralesional:** *Adults* (methylprednisolone acetate): 4–80 mg q1–5 weeks	• **PO:** Give with food to prevent gastric irritation • **IV:** Be sure to use methylprednisolone sodium succinate; do not use acetate form for IV. When direct injection is ordered, inject diluted drug into a vein, or into an IV-compatible solution at a rate of at least 1 min (regardless of dose). If drug is ordered to treat shock, administer massive doses over at least 10 min. This rate will prevent arrhythmias and circulatory collapse • **IM:** Give deep into gluteal muscle. With large doses of acetate, salt dermal atrophy may occur. Thus, give large doses in several small injections and rotate injection site • Avoid SC route as it may result in atrophy or sterile abscesses • When immediate onset of action is required, do not use acetate salt. Do not confuse Solu-Medrol® with Solu-Cortef®

Table 66.5 (continued)
The corticosteroids: Drug doses

Drug Generic name (Trade names)	Dosage	Nursing alert
B. Intermediate-Acting Glucocorticoids (cont'd)		
triamcinolone (Aristocort, Aristospan, Kenacort, Kenalog)	**Oral** (for adrenocortical insufficiency): *Adults:* 4–12 mg/day as single dose or 2–4 divided doses. *Children:* 117 µg/kg/day (3.3 mg/m^2/day) as single dose or divided doses. (For other uses): *Adults:* 4–48 mg/day as single dose or 2–4 divided doses (up to 60 mg/day). *Children:* 416 µg to 1.7 mg/kg/day (12.5–50 mg/m^2/day) as single dose or divided doses **IM:** *Adults:* 40–80 mg q4weeks as acetonide suspension or 40 mg weekly as diacetate suspension. *Children:* 40 mg q4weeks or 30–200 µg/kg (1–6.25 mg/m^2) given q1–7days as acetonide suspension or 40 mg weekly as diacetate suspension **Intra-articular:** *Adults:* 2.5–15 mg as acetonide suspension or 3–48 mg q1–8weeks as diacetate suspension or 2–20 mg q3–4weeks as hexacetonide suspension. **Intralesional:** *Adults:* 1 mg q7days or longer as acetonide suspension or 3–48 mg q1–8weeks as diacetate suspension or 0.5 mg/2.5 cm^2 of affected skin as hexacetonide suspension	• **PO:** May give with food to reduce gastric irritation • **IM:** Inject deep into gluteal muscle. To prevent muscle atrophy, rotate injection sites • Parenteral formulation is not for IV use. Do not interchange injection products. Dosages and duration of action vary
C. Long-Acting Glucocorticoids		
betamethasone (Celestone, Celestone Phosphate, Celestone Soluspan)	**Oral** (for adrenocortical insufficiency): *Children:* 17.5 µg/kg (500 µg/m^2) daily in 3 divided doses. (For other uses): *Adults:* 0.6–7.2 mg/day as single daily dose or in divided doses. *Children:* 17.5–250 µg/kg (1.875–7.5 mg/m^2) daily in 3 divided doses **IM** (for adrenocortical insufficiency): *Children:* 17.5 µg/kg (500 µg/m^2) daily in 3 divided doses every third day, or 5.8–8.75 µg/kg (166–250 µg/m^2) daily as single dose (Betamethasone sodium phosphate) **IM/IV:** *Adults:* Up to 9 mg betamethasone base (12 mg betamethasone phosphate), prn. **IM:** *Children:* 17.5–125 µg/kg (0.625–3.75 mg/m^2) of the base q12–24h. **Intra-articular/ Intralesional:** *Adults:* Up to 9 mg betamethasone base (12 mg betamethasone phosphate), prn	• **PO:** Give with food to prevent gastric irritation and in a.m. to mimic normal circadian production • **IM:** Administer deep into muscle mass and rotate sites to prevent muscle atrophy • **IV:** Use only sodium phosphate; do not use acetate suspension. Follow agency policy regarding direct IV and administer over at least 1 min (regardless of dose). For intermittent infusion, consult manufacturer's information for compatibility • Avoid SC route (risk of abscess formation)

(cont'd on next page)

Table 66.5 (continued)
The corticosteroids: Drug doses

Drug Generic name (Trade names)	Dosage	Nursing alert
C. Long-Acting Glucocorticoids (cont'd)		
betamethasone (Celestone, Celestone Phosphate, Celestone Soluspan) (cont'd)	(Betamethasone sodium phosphate/ betamethasone acetate suspension) **IM:** *Adults:* 0.5–9 mg/day. **Intra-articular:** *Adults:* 1.5–12 mg (dose depends on joint); may be repeated prn. **Intralesional:** *Adults:* 1.2 mg/m^2 of affected skin (not to exceed 6 mg); may be repeated weekly	
dexamethasone (Decadron, Delalone, Dexone, Hexadrole)	**Oral** (for adrenal insufficiency): *Children:* 23.3 µg/kg or 670 µg/m^2/day in 3 divided doses. (For anti-inflammatory and most other uses): *Adults:* 0.5–9 mg/day in single dose or 3–4 divided doses. *Children:* 83.3–333.3 µg/kg or 2.5–10 mg/m^2/day in 3–4 divided doses **IM/IV** (for anti-inflammatory and most other uses): *Adults:* 0.5–24 mg/day (phosphate). **IM:** *Adults:* 8–16 mg/day (acetate). **Intra-articular:** *Adults:* 4–16 mg (acetate) as single dose; may be repeated q1–3weeks	• **PO:** Give with food to prevent gastric irrita- tion and in a.m. to mimic normal circadian production • **IV:** Use only sodium phosphate; do not use acetate suspension. Follow agency policy regarding direct IV and administer over at least 1 min (regardless of dose). For intermit- tent infusion, consult manufacturer's informa- tion for compatibility. Use solution within 24 h • **IM:** Administer deep into muscle mass and rotate sites to prevent muscle atrophy • Avoid SC route (risk of abscess formation) • For dexamethasone suppression test as diagnosis for depression: Follow protocol precisely
paramethasone (Haldrone)	**Oral** (for anti-inflammatory effects): 2–24 mg/ day	• **PO:** Give with food to prevent gastric irrita- tion and in a.m. to mimic normal circadian production
D. Mineralocorticoids		
fludrocortisone acetate (Florinef Acetate)	**Oral** (for chronic primary adrenocortical insuf- ficiency): Initially, 0.05–0.1 mg fludrocortisone acetate/day; increase up to 0.2 mg daily. (For salt-losing forms of congenital adrenal hyper- plasia) Initially, doses up to 0.2 mg/day. This can be reduced gradually over several months to 0.05–0.1 mg/day	• **PO:** Give with food to prevent gastric irrita- tion and in a.m. to mimic normal circadian production

The Sex Hormones

Topics Discussed
- Physiological secretion
- Pharmacologic preparations
- For each drug: Mechanism of action and pharmacologic effects, therapeutic uses, adverse effects
- Nursing management

Drugs Discussed

Estrogens:
estradiol (ess-trah-**dye**-ole)
estrone (**ess**-trone)
conjugated estrogens (**ess**-troe-jenz)
diethylstilbestrol (dye-eth-il-stil-**bess**-trole)
ethinyl estradiol (**eth**-in-il ess-trah-dye-ole)

Antiestrogen:
clomiphene (**kloe**-mih-feen)

FSH Inhibitor:
danazol (**dan**-ah-zole)

Selective Estrogen Receptor Modulator:
raloxifene (ral-**ox**-ih-feen)

Bisphosphonates:
alendronate (ah-**len**-droe-nate)
etidronate (eh-tih-**droe**-nate)

Progestins:
progesterone (proe-**jess**-ter-own)
hydroxyprogesterone caproate (hye-drox-ee-proe-**jess**-ter-own)
levonorgestrel (lee-voe-nor-**jess**-trel)
medroxyprogesterone acetate (med-rox-ee-proe-**jess**-ter-own)
megestrol (meh-**jess**-trole)
norethindrone (nor-**eth**-in-drone)
norethynodrel (nor-eth-**thin**-oh-drel)

Androgens:
fluoxymesterone (flew-ox-ee-**mess**-ter-own)
methyltestosterone (meth-ill-tess-**toss**-ter-own)
testosterone enanthate (eh-**nan**-thayt)

Antiandrogen:
finasteride (fin-**ass**-ter-eyed)

Clinical Challenge

Consider this clinical challenge as you read through this chapter. The response to the challenge appears on page 803.

Consider the following questions, which are commonly asked of nurses in many clinical settings. Prepare a brief teaching summary for each:

1. Should I take estrogen or hormone replacement therapy at menopause?
2. What are the benefits and risks of using oral contraceptives?
3. What might happen if a young athlete (male or female) uses androgenic agents to enhance growth and performance?

Physiological Secretion and Action of the Sex Hormones

No organs are the subject of so much social commentary as the ovaries and testes. Never content to carry on their work quietly, these organs occupy centre stage as they promote both the reproductive and recreational activities of men and women.

Students of gonadal function readily recognize the exocrine and endocrine importance of the ovaries and testes. The exocrine activities are manifest in the synthesis and release of ova or sperm, and their endocrine prowess is demonstrated by the formation and secretion of estrogens, progesterone and androgens.

Role of the Pituitary

Behind every successful gonad stands a good pituitary. Follicle-stimulating hormone (FSH) and luteinizing hormone (LH), secreted by the anterior pituitary, control both the exocrine and endocrine functions of the ovaries and testes (Figure 67.1). In females, FSH stimulates the ovaries to produce ova and estrogens. LH acts first in concert with FSH in females to promote ovulation, and later alone to stimulate progesterone and estrogen synthesis by the corpus luteum. In males, FSH increases growth of the seminiferous tubules and LH stimulates production of testosterone by Leydig cells in the testes. FSH, LH and testosterone act together to stimulate spermatogenesis. Without FSH and LH, humans would find this world much less crowded and a lot less interesting.

Estrogens and Progesterone

The word estrogen is used to describe a chemical that possesses female sex hormone properties. The human ovary secretes two estrogens, estradiol, sometimes called estradiol-17-beta, and estrone. A third estrogen, estriol, is a metabolic product of both estradiol and estrone. Estradiol is the estrogen of greatest biological significance in humans.

Once secreted, estrogens have pronounced effects on the body. Among other things, their presence or absence determines an individual's sex. Few tissues in the body are not affected by estrogens. In the female, estrogens are responsible for the physiologic changes that occur at puberty and are essential for the development of the reproduc-

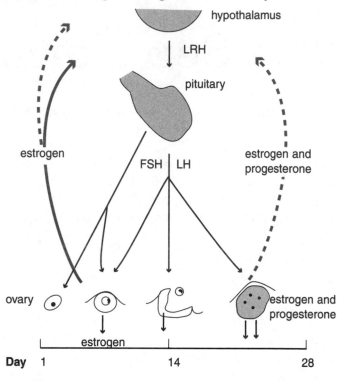

Figure 67.1
Endocrine changes during the menstrual cycle

Dashed arrows indicate inhibitor effects; solid lines, stimulatory effects.

Source: Ganong WF. The gonads: development and function of the reproductive system. In: *Review of Medical Physiology.* 11th ed. Los Altos: Lange; 1983:336. Reproduced with permission.

tive organs. They increase the mitotic activity and stratification of the cells of the vaginal epithelium and cause a proliferation of the uterine cervical mucosa. Estrogens produce endometrial mitoses, increase the height of the epithelium and improve the blood supply and capillary permeability of uterine vessels. In response to estrogen stimulation, uterine water and electrolyte content increase. In contrast, ovariectomy produces atrophic changes in all uterine tissues. Estrogens also stimulate stromal development and ductal growth in the breasts.

Estrogens are responsible for the accelerated growth phase in maturing females and for closing the epiphyses of the long bones at puberty. The other metabolic actions of the estrogens include at least a partial responsibility for the maintenance of normal skin and blood vessel structure in females. Although estrogens do not stimulate bone formation, they decrease the rate of bone resorption in ovariectomized women.

Progesterone is also secreted by females. It is synthesized and secreted by the corpus luteum and placenta. Progesterone's effects are usually seen only when tissues have been stimulated previously by estrogens. Both hormones are important in establishing the proper uterine environment for the fertilized egg. Whereas estrogens act to stimulate the growth of sensitive tissues, progesterone, released later in the menstrual cycle, converts the newly formed cells into secretory tissue. For example, estrogens increase stromal and ductal development in the breasts, and progesterone subsequently prepares the mammary glands for lactation. Progesterone reduces uterine motility and prepares the estrogen-stimulated endometrium for egg implantation and gestation.

In view of their importance to ovulation, fertilization and implantation, it is not surprising that FSH, LH, estrogens and progesterone show cyclic surges in secretion. FSH and LH secretions peak shortly before ovulation occurs (Figure 67.2). Plasma estradiol levels (E2) rise quickly before FSH and LH release occurs. Thereafter, plasma estradiol falls, only to rise again six to eight days after ovulation, before decreasing once more prior to menstruation. In contrast to the biphasic pattern of estrogen release, progesterone secretion remains low during the first half of the cycle and increases markedly after ovulation and corpus luteum formation. 17-Hydroxyprogesterone (17-OHP) is a progesterone metabolite. Its levels reflect progesterone release. This secretory pattern (Figure 67.2) is understood when it is remembered that a function of progesterone is to prepare the estrogen-stimulated endometrium for the implantation of the fertilized egg and gestation. If fertilization does not occur, progesterone secretion falls and menstruation ensues.

Androgens

Male sex hormones are collectively called androgens. Testosterone is the major androgen secreted by males. The secretion of androgens begins in earnest at the time of puberty and is responsible for the conversion of the boy to the man. The testes are the main source of androgens in males, and they secrete large amounts of testosterone. Many other organs, such as the skin, salivary and adrenal glands, can also secrete androgens. Under normal conditions, however, their contribution to

Figure 67.2
Plasma levels of gonadotropins and gonadal steroids during the human menstrual cycle

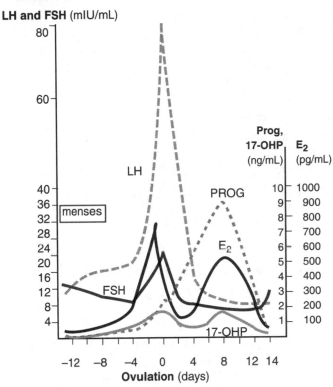

The cycle is centered on day 0, the day of midcycle LH peak. LH = leuteinizing hormone; FSH = follicle-stimulating hormone; PROG = progesterone; E2 = plasma estradiol; 17-OHP = 17-hydroxyprogesterone.

Source: Speroff L, Vande Wiele RL.(1971), Regulation of the human menstrual cycle. *Amer J Obstet Gynec* 1971;109:234–247. Reproduced with permission.

the total androgen pool in the male is small. Androstenedione is secreted by female adrenals, and accounts for most of the androgens found in women. Under normal conditions, androgen secretion in women is much lower than the quantities of estrogens released.

Testosterone is responsible for the full morphological and functional development of the male reproductive tract, including the accessory glands and external genitalia. Castration removes the major source of androgens from the body, and it is impossible for the skin, salivary glands or adrenals to pick up the slack. In the face of such a calamity the seminal vesicles and prostate suffer a marked reduction in size and secretory capacity.

Androgens are also responsible for many of the other characteristics that distinguish males from females. They initiate recession of the male hairline (setting up the rumour that bald men are more virile) and determine distribution and growth of hair on the face, body and pubes. Androgens can also take credit for the bass section in the church choir because they enlarge the larynx and thicken the vocal chords.

The effects of androgens on sexual development in the male are more obvious than their actions on body metabolism, but these should not be forgotten. The secretion of testosterone increases protein anabolism and decreases protein catabolism. Androgens increase the ability of muscles to work by stimulating the number, thickness and tensile strength of muscle fibres. Following the separation of a male from his testicles, most skeletal muscles either stop accumulating protein or accumulate it at a reduced rate.

Pharmacologic Preparations of the Sex Hormones

Estrogens

Pharmacokinetics. The naturally occurring estrogens are estradiol, estrone and estriol. Only estradiol is used as a drug, and its action is greatly reduced by significant metabolism as it passes through the liver in the portal circulation (the first-pass effect). Several approaches may be used to overcome this problem. It may be injected as estradiol benzoate, estradiol cypionate (Depo-Estradiol®, E-Ionate PA®) and estradiol valerate (Delestrogen®). In these forms estradiol is absorbed slowly, misses the portal circulation and has a long duration of action.

Another approach that facilitates oral administration and still circumvents first-pass metabolism is to administer synthetic estrogenic drugs that are not rapidly inactivated by the liver. These include ethinyl estradiol (Estinyl®, Feminone®), diethylstilbestrol (Honvol®, Stibilium®, Stilphosterol®) and quinestrol (Estrovis®). A popular oral product, Premarin®, is obtained from pregnant mares' urine. Premarin® contains the sodium salts of conjugated estrogen sulfates.

A more recent development in estrogen therapy is the development of a transdermal therapeutic system (Estraderm®). The 17-β-estradiol is held in a reservoir between an occlusive backing and microporous membrane that controls the rate of release of the drug. A contact adhesive holds the system to the skin through which the estradiol then passes, entering the blood of the dermis. In appropriately selected postmenopausal women, Estraderm® is both effective and well tolerated.

Estrogen preparations are also available as gels, vaginal creams and implants.

Therapeutic uses. Estrogens are used for several therapeutic indications. Their most common use is in oral contraceptives. As this involves the concomitant administration of a progestin, the subject of oral contraceptives is discussed later in this chapter.

Estrogen use is contraindicated in patients with active hepatic dysfunction or disease, especially of the obstructive type. They are also contraindicated in women having a personal history of breast or endometrial cancer. Endometrial hyperplasia also contraindicates estrogen therapy without accompanying progestagen. Other contraindications for estrogen use include undiagnosed vaginal bleeding, history of cerebrovascular accident, coronary thrombosis, presence or history of classical migraine, history of thrombophlebitis or thromboembolic disease, partial or complete loss of vision or diplopia arising from ophthalmic vascular disease, and suspected pregnancy.

Estrogens can be used as replacement therapy. This is most commonly seen in treating the symptoms of menopause. The decline in ovarian function often produces characteristic hot flashes that may alternate with chills. Inappropriate sweating and paresthesias can also occur. Other symptoms of menopause are muscle cramps, myalgias, arthralgias, overbreathing, palpitations, anxiety, faintness and syncope. Estrogen treatment relieves the hot flashes and other vasomotor effects, as well as atrophic vaginitis.

Estrogens are also effective in preventing postmenopausal osteoporosis. However, concern that estrogen treatment may increase the risk of breast and uterine carcinoma has stopped many women from taking these drugs. Further, estrogen treatment can cause uterine bleeding, increase the risk for venous thromboembolic events, produce cholelithiasis, cause headaches and result in pain and enlargement of the breast. These effects, too, have limited the use of estrogens to prevent postmenopausal osteoporosis.

It is most interesting, therefore, to look at the

recent development of newer products designed to prevent postmenopausal osteoporosis, such as the bisphosphonates etidronate (Didronel®) and alendronate (Fosamax®). These drugs inhibit osteoclast-mediated bone resorption and are not encumbered by the toxicities of estrogens or the concerns that estrogen therapy may increase the risk of breast or uterine cancer. The product Didrocal® contains both etidronate and calcium, and has proven to be most popular in the treatment of postmenopausal osteoporosis.

Interest is particularly strong in raloxifene HCl (Evista®), a drug that is in the final stages of development in Canada. Raloxifene behaves as an estrogen agonist in the skeleton and on cholesterol metabolism, but as an estrogen antagonist in both the uterus and breast. In postmenopausal women, the estrogen-agonist properties of raloxifene allow the drug to increase bone mineral density, thereby reducing the risk of postmenopausal osteoporosis. Raloxifene also acts like an estrogen by lowering LDL cholesterol. At the same time, the drug's estrogen-antagonist effects on breast and uterus provide a significant advantage over estrogens. In contrast to estrogens, there is no evidence to date that raloxifene increases the risk of uterine or breast cancer. Furthermore, in well women, raloxifene has not been associated with an increase in benign breast-related adverse events, such as breast pain, breast enlargement and fibrocystic disease, in contrast to the observed increase with estrogen therapy. To date, no evidence has been found that raloxifene increases the risk of cardiovascular death, myocardial infarction, stroke or any other major arterial cardiovascular event. Raloxifene may increase the risk of venous thrombolytic events in women with risk factors such as increasing age, obesity or prior MI.

Replacement estrogen therapy is indicated when the ovaries fail to develop. In Turner's syndrome, ovarian dysgenesis with dwarfism occurs. Treatment with an estrogen produces breast enlargement and menses but does not cause the normal growth spurt or ovarian maturation. Hypopituitarism causes ovarian, thyroidal and adrenal cortical failure. Replacement therapy in girls involves treatment with thyroxine, adrenal cortical hormones and an estrogen.

Estrogens can provide relief from dysmenorrhea by inhibiting ovulation. Cyclic therapy with oral contraceptives is often successful. However, the current trend is to treat primary dysmenorrhea with inhibitors of prostaglandin $E_{2\alpha}$ synthesis. Prostaglandin $E_{2\alpha}$ accumulates in the uterus immediately before menstruation and provokes uterine contractions. Drugs such as ASA (Aspirin®), ibuprofen (Motrin®, Rufen®), naproxen (Naprosyn®), naproxen sodium (Anaprox®) and mefenamic acid (Ponstan®, Ponstel®) block prostaglandin synthesis. They are given for three to four days each month, just before and during the first one or two days of menstruation.

Estrogens are often used to suppress postpartum lactation because they inhibit prolactin secretion.

An estrogen, often combined with a progestin in an oral contraceptive tablet, can be used to treat endometriosis by reducing FSH secretion. Although some patients can be withdrawn from this treatment after four to six months and remain symptom free, most relapse and require additional estrogen therapy or surgery. The drug danazol (Cyclomen®, Danocrine®) also prevents FSH secretion. It appears more effective in endometriosis treatment with a lower rate of relapse once withdrawn. Danazol is also used in the treatment of benign fibrocystic breast disease.

Adverse effects. Nausea is the most frequent adverse effect of estrogen treatment. This can be compared with the morning sickness experienced during the early months of pregnancy. If large doses of an estrogen are used, patients may suffer anorexia, mild diarrhea and/or vomiting. The effects of estrogens on blood coagulation are discussed later in this chapter (see Contraceptives). Other common adverse effects of estrogen therapy are breast tenderness, weight gain due to edema and hypertension.

Table 67.1 lists the clinically significant drug interactions with estrogens, while Table 67.2 lists those of some alternatives to estrogen replacement therapy — alendronate, etidronate and danazol.

Antiestrogens: Clomiphene (Clomid®, Serophene®)

Mechanism of action and pharmacologic effects. Stimulation of the estrogenic receptors by estradiol, estrone and estriol reduces FSH and LH secretion. Clomiphene competes with estrogens for

Table 67.1
Estrogens: Drug interactions

Drug	Interaction
Anticoagulants, oral	• Estrogens may increase the activity of certain clotting factors in the blood, thereby requiring an increase in oral anticoagulant dosage. If a pt is taking an estrogen for contraception, it would probably be preferable to use another birth control method
Corticosteroids	• Estrogens can raise the level of cortisone-binding globulin in plasma and increase the binding corticosteroids. Estrogens may also slow the normal metabolism of hydrocortisone
Rifampin	• Rifampin may increase the rate of metabolism of estrogens, thereby reducing their effectiveness. If the pt is taking the estrogen product for contraception, it is probably best to use another birth control method

Table 67.2
Alternatives to estrogen replacement therapy: Drug interactions

Drug	Interaction
	A. With alendronate sodium (Fosamax®)
Calcium supplements, antacids and other oral medications	• It is likely that calcium supplements, antacids and some other oral medications will interfere with the absorption of alendronate. Thus, pts must wait at least 30 min after taking alendronate before taking any other drug
Ranitidine, IV	• IV ranitidine has been shown to double the bioavailability of oral alendronate. The clinical significance of this increased bioavailability, and whether similar increases will occur in pts given oral H$_2$-antagonists, is unknown
	B. With etidronate disodium + calcium carbonate (Didrocal®)
Antacids	• Antacids containing calcium or aluminum should not be taken within 2 h before or after ingesting etidronate disodium, since these may reduce the absorption of etidronate disodium and could lead to tx failure
Food	• Food in the stomach or upper portions of the small intestine, particularly materials with a high calcium content such as milk, may reduce the absorption of etidronate disodium
Laxatives	• Laxatives containing magnesium should not be taken within 2 h before or after ingesting etidronate disodium, since these may reduce the absorption of etidronate disodium and could lead to tx failure
Vitamins	• Vitamins with mineral supplements (such as iron or calcium) should not be taken within 2 h before or after ingesting etidronate disodium, since these may reduce the absorption of etidronate disodium and could lead to tx failure
	C. With danazol (Cyclomen®, Danocrine®)
Anticoagulants, oral	• Danazol may potentiate the effects of oral anticoagulants. In cases in which oral anticoagulants are given concurrently with danazol, careful attention to and, if necessary, readjustment of their dosages is recommended

their receptor sites in the body. By blocking the actions of endogenous estrogens, clomiphene prevents the normal "feedback inhibition" of FSH and LH secretion. Increased quantities of the gonadotropins are secreted, leading to ovarian stimulation, ovulation and sustained corpus luteum formation.

Therapeutic uses. Clomiphene is effective in the treatment of infertility due to anovulation. It is used in cases of female infertility when anatomical causes have been ruled out. Clomiphene is ineffective in women who have ovarian or pituitary failure or who suffer from undeveloped ovaries. Animal studies have demonstrated teratogenicity at doses twenty to thirty times the dose recommended for humans. As a result, clomiphene should not be administered during pregnancy. In addition, clomiphene is contraindicated in patients with liver disease or a history of liver dysfunction, and in patients with bleeding of undetermined origin.

Adverse effects. The adverse effects of clomiphene result from hyperstimulation of the ovaries. Hot flashes and flushing occur commonly. Multiple cysts are formed, resulting in a higher incidence of multiple births. However, the 6% to 8% incidence of multiple births produced by clomiphene is not as high as the 15% to 25% seen after Pergonal® (FSH, LH) gonadotrophin administration. Approximately three-quarters of the multiple births resulting from clomiphene treatment are twins.

Progestins

Pharmacokinetics. Progesterone is rapidly inactivated by the liver and has little activity if given orally. The hormone may be administered intramuscularly to circumvent first-pass liver metabolism.

A progestin is a drug that mimics some properties of progesterone. Although some progestins have properties that resemble progesterone very closely, others have inherent estrogenic and androgenic effects. It is beyond the scope of this text to detail the properties of each progestin. Instead, we will describe the therapeutic uses of some of the more commonly used chemicals.

Medroxyprogesterone acetate (Depo-Provera®) and hydroxyprogesterone caproate (Delalutin®) are two progestins designed for intramuscular injection. Several progestins are available for oral administration. These drugs are not rapidly inactivated when they pass through the liver in the portal circulation. They include megestrol acetate (Megace®, Pallace®), norethindrone (Micronor®, Norlutin®), norethindrone acetate (Norlutate®) and norethynodrel.

Therapeutic uses. The major therapeutic use of progestins is in oral contraceptive tablets. This application is discussed later in this chapter.

Dysfunctional uterine bleeding often results from the continuous action of estradiol, causing endometrial hyperplasia, with insufficient progesterone secreted to maintain the endometrium.

Progestin therapy often assists the patient. It can be given orally or intramuscularly in the last half of the cycle for six months. After discontinuation, regular spontaneous menstruation may return.

The concomitant use of progestin and estrogen therapy for the treatment of dysmenorrhea, endometriosis and postpartum lactation has been discussed previously in this chapter. Other indications for progestin therapy are endometrial carcinoma and early pregnancy (threatened abortion and habitual abortion). The use of a progestin for the prevention of abortion must be weighed against the fact that the drug may cause virilization and genital deformities in the fetus.

Premenstrual syndrome (PMS) is the cyclical occurrence of mild to severe symptoms in relation to the menstrual cycle. Although the cause is not known, it is hypothesized that hormonal fluctuations play an important role in the symptoms. Many strategies for self-management of the syndrome are successful; however, for those women whose symptoms are severe, drug therapy is sometimes warranted. One approach has been the use progesterone suppositories, specifically prepared by the pharmacist. Although the research is unclear, anecdotal reports indicate success for some women.

Progestin therapy is contraindicated in the presence of thrombophlebitis, thromboembolic disorders and cerebral apoplexy. These drugs are also contraindicated in patients with a past history of undiagnosed vaginal bleeding, breast pathology and urinary tract bleeding.

Adverse effects. Inferential evidence suggests an association between progestin administration early in pregnancy and the occurrence of congenital malformations. Other adverse effects in women taking progestins include breakthrough bleeding, intercyclic spotting, changes in menstrual flow, amenorrhea, changes in cervical erosion and cervical secretion, and breast tenderness. Patients may experience edema and weight gain. Skin sensitivity reactions consisting of urticaria, pruritus, edema and generalized rash have occasionally occurred.

Contraceptives

Oral contraceptive tablets became widely available in the early 1960s. Their use expanded rapidly: by

1965 approximately 15% of all married women 15 to 44 years of age in the United States were taking them. By 1973 this had increased to 25%, or about 6.6 million women. In 1977 it was estimated that 54 million women in the world were consuming oral contraceptive tablets.

These figures should not come as a surprise. For centuries, humankind has sought a truly efficient method of birth control. Oral contraceptives meet that need, providing efficacy so near to 100% that closer estimates are not possible. More recently, injectable contraceptives have been placed on the market and these, too, provide effective, safe contraception.

Types of products and patterns of administration. Oral contraceptives contain either a combination of an estrogen plus a progestin, or a progestin alone. Box 67.1 presents a list of oral contraceptives on the market. Combination estrogen–progestin tablets are most popular. These products can be classified as *monophasic, biphasic* or *triphasic*.

For the monophasic products, the ratio of estrogen to progestin is the same in each pill, which is taken daily for twenty-one days, followed by a seven-day "pill-free" period. The biphasic and triphasic preparations provide two or three different pills, respectively, containing varying amounts of estrogen and progestin. When taken as directed, these pills deliver different doses of progestin and estrogen on different days of the twenty-one-day cycle. For example, Triphasil 21® provides 50 µg levonorgestrel plus 30 µg ethinyl estradiol on days 1 through 6, 75 µg levonorgestrel plus 40 µg ethinyl estradiol on days 7 through 11 and 125 µg levo-norgestrel plus 30 µg ethinyl estradiol on days 12 through 21. This dosage pattern more closely approximates the estrogen-to-progestin ratios that occur during the menstrual cycle. The purpose of introducing the biphasic and triphasic oral contraceptive products was to decrease the incidence and severity of drug-induced adverse effects, such as breakthrough bleeding.

Oral contraceptives prevent ovulation if taken the same time each day from the fifth to the twenty-sixth day of the cycle. Day 1 is the first day of menstruation. Bleeding occurs three or four days after stopping the tablets and the cycle is repeated, beginning on day 5. Concern over the possible

---

Box 67.1
Oral contraceptive products

Monophasic oral contraceptives
50 µg estrogen
Ethinyl estradiol/ethynodiol diacetate (Demulen 50®)
Mestranol/norethindrone (Norinyl 1/50®, Ortho-Novum 1/50®)
Ethinyl estradiol/norgestrel (Ovral®)

< 50 µg estrogen
Ethinyl estradiol/desogrestrel (Marvelon®, Ortho-Cept®)
Ethinyl estradiol/ethynodiol acetate (Demulen 30®)
Ethinyl estradiol/levonorgestrel (Mini-Ovral®)
Ethinyl estradiol/norethindrone (Brevicon 1/35®, Brevicon 0.5/35®, Ortho 0.5/35®, Ortho 1/35®)
Ethinyl estradiol/norethindrone acetate (Loestrin 1.5/30®, Minestrin 1/20®)
Ethinyl estradiol/norgestimate (Cyclen®)

Biphasic oral contraceptives
Ethinyl estradiol/norethindrone (Ortho 10/11®, Synphasic®)

Triphasic oral contraceptives
Ethinyl estradiol/norethindrone (Ortho 7/7/7®, Triphasil®, Triquilar®)
Ethinyl estradiol/norgestimate (Tri-Cyclen®)

Progestin-only oral contraceptive
Norethindrone (Micronor®)

---

toxicity of estrogens has led to the introduction of products containing as little as 20 µg of estrogen.

Progestin-only tablets are available as oral contraceptives. Containing either 0.35 mg norethindrone (Micronor®, Nor QD®) or 0.075 mg norgestrel (Ovrette®), these products must be taken every day of the cycle at the same time each day. They inhibit the secretion of pituitary gonadotropins, thereby preventing follicular maturation and ovulation, as well as causing changes in the cervical mucus and endometrium. The contraceptive efficacy of progestin tablets is 97% to 98%, somewhat lower than conventional estrogen–progestin tablets. Progestin tablets may cause troublesome irregular bleeding. Contraindications to the use of oral contraceptives have been described earlier in this chapter (see the sections "Estrogens" and "Progestins").

Injectable contraceptives have been used worldwide for many years. Medroxyprogesterone acetate (Depo-Provera®), administered intramuscularly in a dose of 150 mg every three months, is safe and effective. An injection schedule of four times a year simplifies compliance. Medroxyprogesterone acetate produces amenorrhea in the majority of women, but there are some who have irregular bleeding and progestational side effects, such as bloating, weight gain/loss and mood swings. This drug is an excellent product for those women who must avoid high doses of estrogen, such as migraine sufferers. It can be used in the postabortal state (five days postpartum) and during lactation (six weeks postpartum).

Levonorgestrel (Norplant®) is administered in the form of progestin-containing rods that are implanted in the subcutaneous tissue of the upper, inner arm. When given this way, levonorgestrel provides a long-term (up to five years) reversible contraceptive product that has efficacy close to that of tubal ligation. Norplant rods should be removed at the end of five years. This product may cause dysfunctional or breakthrough bleeding. Occasionally, it can be difficult to remove the rods. Levonorgestrel rods have similar side effects and benefits as Depo-Provera®. The major drawback to Norplant is the expensive up-front costs.

Despite the ready availability of numerous contraceptive products, there will always remain the need for a "morning after" pill to provide emergency contraception. This need is frequently met by administering ethinyl estradiol and levonorgestrel (two tablets of Ovral®), together with an antinauseant, followed by a second identical dose twelve hours later. These drugs prevent pregnancy up to seventy-two hours after a single episode of unprotected intercourse. This is followed by menstrual bleeding twenty-one days after treatment when it is successful. This method is claimed to have a ninety-eight percent success rate when used correctly.

Contraception during breastfeeding presents another problem. An IUD can be inserted four to six weeks postpartum, once involution has occurred and the uterus is firm enough to decrease the risk of insertional perforation. Alternatively, progestin-only pills can be used during lactation, without increasing thromboembolic rates in the puerperium. These pills must be taken the same time each day, and patients must not miss a dose. Low-dose combination oral contraceptives can be used once milk supply is well established. However, there is some decrease in milk quantity.

Adverse effects. Concern has been expressed about the safety of oral contraceptives. This concern has centred in the past on the effects of the estrogen component in the tablets. The greatest attention has been given to the cardiovascular complications of oral contraceptive use. In particular, concern has been expressed that these drugs increase the likelihood of venous thromboembolic disorders, myocardial infarction (MI) and stroke. Oral contraceptives do increase the incidence of venous thromboembolism, and this risk increases about threefold during the first month of treatment. Thereafter, the risk remains constant, falling to control levels within a month of stopping treatment. Obesity or moderate cigarette smoking increases the risk of oral contraceptive-induced venous thromboembolism in women over age thirty-five.

The risk of thromboembolism may be reduced significantly by using low-dose estrogen preparations. Tablets containing 50–80 μg of either ethinyl estradiol or mestranol are only one-third to one-half as likely to produce venous thromboses as preparations with 100–150 μg of these estrogens.

The increased risk of MI in women over thirty-five appears to be related to the amount of estrogen in the tablet, the age of the patient and the woman's smoking habits. Decreasing the estrogen component from 100–150 μg of ethinyl estradiol or mestranol per pill to 30 μg significantly diminishes the risk for MI.

Risk for MI is higher in women over the age of thirty-five who smoke. Low-dose oral products may be considered for contraception in nonsmoking women over thirty-five.

Risk for MI in users of oral contraceptives is also increased in patients with a history of preeclamptic toxemia, hypertension, type II hyperlipoproteinemia or diabetes. Hypertension increases the likelihood of oral contraceptive users' experiencing a thrombotic stroke. Both cigarette smoking and hypertension increase the risk for hemorrhagic stroke in women taking the pill.

Androgens

Pharmacokinetics. Testosterone is the major androgen secreted by the testes. Similar to estradiol and progesterone, testosterone cannot be given orally because it is rapidly inactivated during its first pass through the liver in the portal circulation. To circumvent first-pass metabolism, testosterone may be injected intramuscularly as the propionate, enanthate or cypionate ester. Methyltestosterone (Metandren®) can be taken either orally or sublingually. Other orally effective androgens are fluoxymesterone (Halotestin®), oxandrolone (Anavar®) and stanozolol (Winstrol®).

Therapeutic uses. Androgens are used for replacement therapy. Patients suffering from hypogonadism, associated with testicular failure, respond well to long-acting androgens, such as testosterone cypionate (Andro-Cyp®, Depo-Testosterone®, T-Ionate-PA®) or testosterone enanthate (Delatestryl®), with the development of secondary sex characteristics and increased potency. Androgens are also given at the age of puberty to males with hypopituitarism.

In view of the widespread use of estrogen therapy in postmenopausal women, it seems fair and reasonable to offer equal opportunity to men in the form of androgen treatment. It is well known that testicular function decreases gradually with advancing years. Signs of this include decreased libido, decreased sexual activity and reduced muscle mass and strength. Plasma testosterone levels decrease around the age of fifty. In cases where plasma testosterone levels are well below those expected, androgen replacement therapy may increase libido, keep the peace at home and maintain secondary sex characteristics.

Androgens are known to stimulate erythropoiesis. Use has been made of this effect to treat patients with hypoplastic anemia, the anemia of cancer, aplastic anemia, red cell aplasia, hemolytic anemias and those related to renal failure, lymphomas, leukemias and myeloid metaplasias.

Androgens are used for the treatment of recurrent and metastatic carcinoma of the breast; the response is much better in tumours containing estrogen or progesterone receptors, or both.

Several androgens — ethylestrenol (Maxibolin®), methylandrostenolone (Dianobol®) and stanozolol (Winstrol®) — are used for their anabolic effects. They are employed to help postoperative recovery and to treat chronic debilitating diseases. Although possibly beneficial on a short-term basis, they do not alter the outcome of the underlying disease. Their use to accelerate growth is the subject of great controversy. Some children undergo a growth spurt when treated with an anabolic androgen, but the epiphyses may close, compromising future growth.

Athletes may use anabolic androgens in an attempt to gain weight quickly. Although this effect may take place, much of the initial increase in weight results from the retention of sodium, chloride and water by the kidney. Androgens may increase muscle mass, weight and strength and can appeal to individuals with strong backs and weak brains. However, one cannot condone hormonal therapy in otherwise healthy young men and women. Long-term androgen therapy decreases FSH and LH secretion, leading to testicular atrophy. From the coach's point of view, this might not be a bad idea. It certainly will tend to reduce the desire for extracurricular activity and keep the athlete's mind only on sports.

Androgens are contraindicated in carcinoma of the male breast; known or suspected carcinoma of the prostate; and cardiac, hepatic or renal decompensation. Use is also contraindicated in patients with hypercalcemia or impaired liver function, prepubertal males, patients easily stimulated sexually and pregnant or lactating women.

Adverse effects. Women taking androgens experience menstrual irregularities. Masculinization can also occur. This is seen first as acne, growth of facial hair and deepening of the voice. Later, male-pattern baldness and excessive body hair may become evident. Marked development of the skeletal muscles and veins, together with hypertrophy of the clitoris, may later ensue.

Androgens increase salt and water reabsorption by the kidneys. Edema can be a problem for patients receiving large doses for cancer. It is also undesirable in patients with congestive heart failure, kidney disease or hypoproteinemia.

Other adverse effects of androgens include biliary stasis leading to jaundice, and hepatic

Table 67.3
Androgens: Drug interactions

Drug	Interaction
Anticoagulants, oral	• Oral anticoagulants should be avoided if possible in pts receiving anabolic steroids because the steroids may decrease clotting factor formation, increase clotting factor degradation and increase the affinity of receptor sites for the anticoagulant. If it is essential to treat pts with both drugs, they should be monitored carefully for excessive anticoagulant response
Antidiabetic drugs	• Anabolic steroids may decrease blood sugar in some diabetic pts. Further, they may reduce the rate of metabolism of oral hypoglycemics. Therefore, pts should be monitored closely for signs of hypoglycemia if anabolic steroids are added to an antidiabetic drug regimen. Particular attention should be paid to possible alterations in antidiabetic dosage requirements

adenocarcinoma. Impotence and azoospermia are adverse effects of chronic androgen treatment. This may seem strange, given the fact that testosterone is required, together with FSH and LH, for spermatogenesis. However, as discussed above, daily use of androgens leads to a decrease in FSH and LH secretion, with the consequent ill effects.

Table 67.3 lists the clinically significant drug interactions with androgens.

Antiandrogen: Finasteride (Proscar®)

Mechanism of action and pharmacologic effects. Finasteride is a competitive and specific inhibitor of 5-alpha-reductase, an intracellular enzyme that metabolizes testosterone into the more potent androgen dihydrotestosterone. Within twenty-four hours after the oral administration of a single dose of finasteride, circulating dihydrotestosterone levels are reduced by approximately sixty percent.

Therapeutic uses. Finasteride is indicated for the treatment of symptomatic benign prostatic hyperplasia, to cause regression of the enlarged prostate, improve urine flow and improve the symptoms associated with benign prostatic hyperplasia.

Adverse effects. Finasteride is well tolerated. In clinical studies, 1.4% of patients were withdrawn because of adverse reactions attributable to finasteride. The most frequent reactions were impotence (3.7%), decreased libido (3.3%) and decreased volume of ejaculate (2.8%).

Nursing Management

Table 67.4 describes the nursing management of the patient receiving hormone replacement drugs. Dosage details of individual drugs are given in Table 67.5 (pages 805–809).

Response to Clinical Challenge

Your responses are probably appropriate for the situations described. It is important that you prepare your own teaching summary; you will use the information often in both professional and personal settings.

Further Reading

Boroditsky R, Fisher W, Sand M. The 1995 Canadian Contraceptive Study. *J SOGC* 1996;1(December; suppl):31.

Collins JA, Gunby J. Oral contraceptive use and the cardiovascular health of Canadian women. *J SOGC* 1997;19:125–137.

Pill scares and public responsibility. Editorial. *Lancet* 1996;347:1707.

WHO Collaborative Study of Neoplasia and Steroid Contraceptives. Breast Cancer and depot-medroxyprogesterone acetate: a multinational study. *Lancet* 1991;33:833–838.

Table 67.4
Nursing management of hormone replacement drugs

Assessment of risk vs. benefit	Patient data	• Assess to establish baseline VS, general state of health, hx of malignancies and CV disease; rule out pregnancy prior to drug tx. Hx of smoking is relevant as it increases risks of estrogen use • *Pregnancy:* Risk category X (human fetal risk clearly documented; avoid use during pregnancy)
	Drug data	• Choice of drug and dosage varies with indication for use and pt tolerance. Goal is to use lowest effective dose • *Some serious drug interactions:* Confer with pharmacist. Most significant interaction occurs with anticoagulants • Most serious adverse effects are risks associated with embolism (with estrogens) and unacceptable virilization (with androgens)
Implementation	Rights of administration	• Using the "rights" helps prevent errors of administration
	Right route	• Give PO, most commonly; but also IV, IM, topically (vaginal cream) and transdermally (patch)
	Right technique	• IV administration requires knowledge of correct diluent and IV solution, correct dilution and rate of administration. Always refer to manufacturer's instructions for this route
	Nursing therapeutics	• Education for informed choice in the use of these drugs is essential, including information that promotes compliance and effective application by the various routes • *Emotional support:* Drugs are sometimes used to treat infertility or some malignancies
	Patient/family teaching	• Patient's need for information may be influenced by indication for tx: e.g., oral contraceptive or replacement therapy vs. tx of cancers • Compliance with drug schedule and follow-up are essential factors in successful use of oral contraceptives. Review principles of pt education in Chapter 3 • Pts/families should know warning signs/symptoms of possible toxicities of these drugs • For estrogens, report immediately: sudden shortness of breath or sharp chest pain; calf pain; sudden disturbance in speech, vision or severe headache; unusual vaginal bleeding; jaundice, unusual swelling of extremities. Warn pts to avoid smoking; increases risk of CV adverse effects, such as embolism • For androgens, report immediately: muscle cramps or spasms (caused by hypercalcemia); virilization in women (acne, hirsuitism, hoarseness, changes in libido, baldness); excessive hormonal effects in men (impotence, oligospermia, priapism), altered blood glucose levels in diabetics • Explain photosensitivity with some of these drugs, i.e., importance of using sunblock and protective clothing if exposed to sun • *Discuss possibility of pregnancy:* Advise pt to notify physician; discuss birth control methods. Essential to avoid pregnancy while taking these hormones

Table 67.4 (continued)
Nursing management of hormone replacement drugs

Outcomes	Monitoring of progress	*Continually monitor:* •Clinical response indicating tx success (reduction in signs/symptoms) •Signs/symptoms of adverse reactions; document and report immediately to physician. Observe for: thrombophlebitis (redness, swelling, unilateral calf pain with Homan's sign), pulmonary embolism (sudden chest pain, unexplained cough or dyspnea), cerebrovascular complications (sudden headache, dizziness, blurred vision, speech impairments), electrolyte and blood glucose imbalance •Virilization in males may not be undesirable unless accompanied by priapism, impotence or premature closure of epiphysis with resulting retardation of growth; however, in females it may be intolerable unless drug is required to control metastatic disease

Table 67.5
The sex hormones: Drug doses

Drug Generic name (Trade names)	Dosage	Nursing alert
A. Estrogens		
estradiol 17-β (Estrace, Estraderm)	**Oral** (for menopausal symptoms): Initially, 1–2 mg/day. Maintenance, 0.5–2 mg/day, usually for 21 days, followed by 7-day rest. **Estraderm® patches:** Apply twice weekly	•Instruct pt in self-administration of oral tabs or patch application. Take oral tabs with food to reduce nausea
estradiol cypionate (Depo-Estradiol) estradiol valerate (Delestrogen)	**IM** (for replacement): Estradiol cypionate: 1–5 mg q3–4weeks. Estradiol valerate: 10–20 mg q4weeks	•Ensure solution is well mixed prior to administration (e.g., roll vial between palms; do not shake). Inject deep into large muscle mass and rotate sites •Do not substitute cypionate for valerate; dosage not equivalent
estrone piperazine (Ogen)	**Oral** (cyclically, for replacement): 0.75–1.5 mg/day. A progestin may be added on last 10–13 days or continuously. **Vaginal** (for atrophic vaginitis or kraurosis vulvae): 2–4 g/day, cyclically	•Follow manufacturer's instructions for insertion of vaginal cream. Pt should wash vaginal area prior to instillation and lie flat for at least 30 min after. Avoid tampons. Wash applicator after each use

Table 67.5 (continued)
The sex hormones: Drug doses

Drug Generic name (Trade names)	Dosage	Nursing alert
A. Estrogens (cont'd)		
conjugated estrogens (Premarin)	**Oral** (menopausal symptoms): 0.625–1.25 mg/day, cyclically or continuously; a progestin may be added during last 10–13 days per month or continuously in women with an intact uterus. (Replacement in hypogonadism): 0.625–1.25 mg/day. (Dysfunctional uterine bleeding due to atrophic endometrium): 5 mg/day in divided doses for 1 week with a progestin (e.g., MPA 10 mg) added to regimen on last 5 days; alternatively, 2.5–3.75 mg plus MPA 10 mg daily for 7–10 days. (Breast carcinoma in women > 5 years postmenopause): 10 mg tid for at least 3 months. (Prostatic carcinoma): 1.25–2.5 mg tid	• **PO:** Give with food to reduce nausea
	IV (for emergency of dysfunctional uterine bleeding in presence of denuded endometrium): 25 mg q4h for 3 doses, followed by an estrogen–progestin preparation orally **Vaginal** (for atrophic vaginitis/kraurosis vulvae): 2–4 g/day	• **IV:** Store powder in refrigerator. Reconstitute by adding 5 mL sterile water for injection slowly into vial, letting it flow against the side; gently rotate to dissolve — do not shake. Follow agency policy re: direct IV administration. Inject slowly (rate, 5 mg/min) • **Vaginal:** Instruct pt re: instillation
ethinyl estradiol (Estinyl, Feminone)	**Oral** (menopausal symptoms): 5 or 10 μg/day for 21 days. A progestin may be added for last 10 days. This is followed by a 7-day period without medication. (Functional uterine bleeding): 0.5 mg od or bid until hemostasis is secured; then cyclic administration of 0.05 mg od–tid during first 2 weeks of menstrual cycle; followed by progesterone for 5 days. Three cycles may be given. (Carcinoma of breast in postmenopausal women): 0.10 mg tid. (Prostatic carcinoma): 0.15–3 mg/day hs	• Check dosage carefully; available in variable strengths. Calculate carefully; dose may be ordered in mg and tabs available in μg
diethylstilbestrol diphosphate (Honvol, Stilphosterol)	**Oral:** *Adults* (hypogonadism or replacement): 0.2–0.5 mg/day and cyclically. A progestin may be added during last 10–13 days. (Postmenopausal breast cancer): 15 mg/day. (Prostatic carcinoma): 1–3 mg/day	• **PO:** Give with food to reduce nausea. Do not crush or chew enteric-coated tabs
	IV (prostatic carcinoma): *Adults:* Initially, 500–1000 mg/day until response is obtained (5 or more days); then 250–500 mg 1–2x	• **IV:** Dilute in 250–500 mL NS or D5W. Initiate infusion slowly to test tolerance (1–2 mL/min x 15 min). If no reaction, infuse dosage over 1 h

Table 67.5 (continued)
The sex hormones: Drug doses

Drug Generic name (Trade names)	Dosage	Nursing alert
B. Progestins		
progesterone (PMS: Progesterone)	**IM** (secondary amenorrhea): *Adults:* 50–100 mg (single dose) or 5–10 mg daily for 6–8 days, given 8–10 days prior to expected menstrual period. (Abnormal uterine bleeding) 50–100 mg (single dose) or 5–10 mg daily for 6 days. (Corpus luteum insufficiency): 12.5 mg/ day at onset of ovulation for 2 weeks (may continue until 11th week of gestation)	• **IM:** Shake vial prior to withdrawing dose. Give oily solution (in peanut or sesame oil base) deep into muscle mass. Rotate sites. Check for allergies to peanuts or sesame before administration
hydroxyprogesterone caproate (Delalutin)	**IM** (for menstrual disorders): 125–250 mg/ cycle	• **IM:** Give oily solution (in sesame or castor oil base) deep into muscle mass. Rotate sites
medroxyprogesterone acetate (Oral: Provera; IM: Depo-Provera)	**Oral** (for amenorrhea and dysfunctional uterine bleeding): 5–10 mg/day for 10 days. (Endometriosis) 10–30 mg/day. (Menopausal replacement) 10 mg for last 10–13 days of estrogen administration or 2.5 mg daily with estrogen for continuous tx **IM** (endometriosis): 150 mg q3months. (Endometrial carcinoma) Initially, 400–1000 mg weekly	• **PO:** Take at same time each day to promote compliance • **IM:** Give deep into muscle mass; rotate sites. Shake vial prior to administration
norethindrone (Norlutin)	**Oral** (amenorrhea and dysfunctional uterine bleeding): 5–20 mg/day, starting on day 5 of cycle and ending on day 25. (Endometriosis) Initially, 10 mg/day for 2 weeks; incr. by 5 mg/ day q2weeks until dose of 30 mg/day is reached. May be held at this level for 6–9 months or until breakthrough bleeding demands temporary termination	
norethindrone acetate (Norlutate)	**Oral** (amenorrhea and dysfunctional uterine bleeding): 2.5–10 mg/day, starting on day 5 of cycle and ending on day 25. (Endometriosis) Initially, 5 mg/day for 2 weeks; incr. by 2.5 mg/ day q2weeks until 15 mg/day is reached. May be held at this level for 6–9 months or until breakthrough bleeding demands temporary termination. (Menopausal replacement tx) 1 mg for 10 to 13 days of each month of estrogen administration	• Do not substitute for norethindrone acetate; doses not equivalent

Table 67.5 (continued)
The sex hormones: Drug doses

Drug Generic name (Trade names)	Dosage	Nursing alert
C. Androgens		
fluoxymesterone (Halotestin)	**Oral: (**Androgen deficiency): 5–20 mg/day. (Malignant breast carcinoma in women): 10–40 mg/day in divided doses	• May take with food to reduce nausea
methyltestosterone (Metandren, Testred)	**Oral:** (Male hypogonadism): 10–40 mg/day [tablets]. (Eunuchoidism): 10–40 mg/day [tablets]. (Female carcinoma of breast): 100 mg [tablets] bid for 2–4 weeks; then halved, if response is evident	• Do not substitute buccal tablets for oral tablets. The dosage of the buccal tablets is usually 1/2 that of the oral tablets. Dosage expressed here is for oral tablets. Instruct pt re: use of buccal tabs: Place between cheek and gum until tab dissolves (30–60 min). Do not eat, drink or smoke while buccal tablet is in place. Rinse mouth after tab is absorbed
testosterone enanthate (Delatestryl)	**IM** (in women, to enhance libido): 100 mg q4weeks; use only if uterus is normal size. (For mammary cancer in premenopausal women): 200–400 mg q2weeks or more; dosage adjusted depending on clinical response **IM** (For hypogonadism in men): 200–400 mg q4weeks. (For cryptorchidism): 100–200 mg q4weeks. Chorionic gonadotropin usually should be tried first. Use only when no obstructive anatomic lesion exists. If descent has not occurred after 3–4 months, surgical transplantation should be considered. (For oligospermia): 100–200 mg q4–6weeks for development and maintenance of testicular tubular function; 200 mg every week for 6–12 weeks for suppression of spermatogenesis and rebound stimulation	• Inject deep into muscle mass; rotate sites. Mix solution thoroughly prior to administration
D. Bisphosphonates to Treat Osteoporosis in Postmenopausal Women		
alendronate sodium (Fosamax)	**Oral** (osteoporosis in postmenopausal women): 10 mg od. (Paget's disease of bone): 40 mg od for 6 months	• Take at least 30 min before first food, beverage or medication of the day with a full glass of plain water only. Waiting longer than 30 min before eating will improve absorption of alendronate

Table 67.5 (continued)
The sex hormones: Drug doses

Drug Generic name (Trade names)	Dosage	Nursing alert
D. Bisphosphonates to Treat Osteoporosis in Postmenopausal Women (cont'd)		
etidronate disodium + calcium carbonate (Didrocal)	**Oral:** Didrocal tx is a cyclical regimen administered in 90-day cycles. Each cycle provides 14 white 400-mg etidronate disodium tablets to be taken od for 14 days, followed by 76 blue calcium carbonate tablets to be taken od for next 76 days	• Didrocal® tx should be administered on an empty stomach, 1 tablet/day with full glass of water. To aid compliance, pt should take hs, at least 2 h before or after eating. To maximize absorption of etidronate disodium, pt should not take the following within 2 h of dosing: food, especially food high in calcium, such as milk or milk products; antacids; vitamins with mineral supplements such as iron; calcium supplements; laxative containing magnesium. Use calendar to assist compliance to regimen
E. Antiestrogenic: Ovulatory Drug		
clomiphene citrate (Clomid, Serophene)	**Oral:** 50 mg daily for 5 days, started at any time in pt who has had no recent uterine bleeding. If progestin-induced bleeding is planned or if spontaneous uterine bleeding occurs before tx, start 5-day regimen on or about 5th day of cycle. In absence of ovulation, give 100 mg/day for 5 days as early as 30 days after previous tx. Never give more than 100 mg for 5 days. If ovulatory menses have not occurred after 3 courses, diagnosis should be re-evaluated	• Verify when to start tx, i.e., on 5th day of cycle. First day of menstrual flow is day 1 of menstruation cycle • NB: If dose is missed, take as soon as remembered, even if this requires doubling the dose. Notify physician if more than 1 dose is missed • Take at same time each day. Instruct pt in self-measurement of basal temperature to detect ovulation
F. Inhibitor of FSH Secretion		
danazol (Cyclomen, Danocrine)	**Oral: (Endometriosis):** 200–800 mg/day in 2–4 divided doses, administered without interruption for 3–6 months. (Fibrocystic breast disease): 100–400 mg/day in 2 divided doses. Should be continued uninterrupted until complete disappearance of symptoms or for 6 months, whichever occurs first	• May take with food. Begin during menstruation or do pregnancy test prior to starting drug
finasteride (Proscar)	**Oral** (symptomatic benign prostatic hypertrophy): One 5-mg tablet daily	• May be taken without regard to food

CHAPTER 68

Drugs That Stimulate or Relax the Uterus

Topics Discussed
- Uterine stimulants
- Uterine relaxants
- For each drug: Mechanism of action and pharmacologic effects, therapeutic uses, adverse effects
- Nursing management

Drugs Discussed

Uterine Stimulants:
dinoprostone (dye-noe-**prost**-own)
ergonovine (er-goe-**noe**-veen)
methylergonovine (meth-ill-er-goe-**noe**-veen)
oxytocin (ox-ee-**toe**-sin)

Uterine Relaxant:
ritodrine (**rit**-oh-dreen)

Clinical Challenge

Consider this clinical challenge as you read through this chapter. The response to the challenge appears on page 814.

You are a midwife working in a large research birthing centre. A 31-year-old woman, Beth, is admitted in labour with her second child. The membranes have ruptured and her contractions have reduced significantly. An oxytocin drip is considered.

Following vaginal delivery, Beth experiences excessive bleeding. Oxytocin is ordered IM.

1. During Beth's labour, what examinations/assessment should be completed prior to initiating this drug? What questions regarding Beth's history are most relevant?
2. If the drip is commenced during labour, what monitoring should occur?
3. What is the rationale for use of this drug after delivery? What dose would be used? What is the optimal site for administration?

Uterine Stimulants

Although many drugs can stimulate the uterus, only oxytocin, the ergot alkaloids ergonovine and methylergonovine, and some prostaglandins have the selectivity and predictability of action required for this purpose.

Oxytocin (Pitocin®, Syntocinon®)

Mechanism of action and pharmacologic effects. Specific oxytocin receptors are present in the uterus during pregnancy, particularly during the latter phases. At this time the uterus is highly responsive to oxytocin, which stimulates both the

Table 68.1
Oxytocin: Drug interactions

Drug	Interaction
Vasopressors	• Severe hypertension may occur if oxytocin follows administration of a vasopressor

frequency and force of uterine contractions. These effects of oxytocin are estrogen dependent.

Specific receptor sites for oxytocin are also present in the mammary gland during lactation. At this time oxytocin stimulates myoepithelial cell contractions, forcing milk from the alveoli of the breast.

Oxytocin relaxes vascular smooth muscle, decreasing both systolic and diastolic blood pressure, as well as producing flushing and an increase in peripheral circulation.

Therapeutic uses. Intravenous oxytocin is used to induce and augment labour. Oxytocin may be used in inevitable or incomplete abortion. Intramuscular oxytocin is used after delivery to prevent or control hemorrhage, restoring normal tone to the hypotonic uterus. Used as an intravenous bolus, it may cause transient hypotension. Intranasal oxytocin is used to stimulate milk letdown.

Adverse effects. Oxytocin, given in labour, can cause uterine rupture. It rarely causes anaphylactoid or allergic reactions. Some studies indicate that neonates delivered from oxytocin-treated mothers have shown an increased incidence of jaundice. Prolonged use of high-dose oxytocin combined with dextrose and water can cause water intoxication.

Table 68.1 lists the clinically significant drug interactions with oxytocin.

Ergonovine Maleate (Ergotrate Maleate) and Methylergonovine Maleate (Methergine)

Mechanism of action and pharmacologic effects. Ergonovine and methylergonovine are potent uterine stimulants. Although uterine sensitivity increases as pregnancy proceeds, even the immature uterus responds to these drugs. Ergot alkaloids can constrict blood vessels and should not be given to patients with chronic or pregnancy-induced hypertension.

Therapeutic uses. These drugs are used after delivery of the placenta and following suction curettage or instillation abortion to produce firm uterine contractions and decrease uterine bleeding. Both drugs have a rapid onset of action, which varies according to the route of administration (IV, 40 s; IM, 7–8 min; PO, 10 min). Their usefulness is further enhanced by their prolonged duration of action (several hours).

Adverse effects. Both drugs can cause vasoconstriction, resulting in hypertension and headaches. Other cardiovascular effects include palpitations, dyspnea and transient chest pains. Gangrene can develop in patients with Buerger's or Raynaud's diseases. Patients may also experience vertigo, nausea, vomiting and diarrhea when ergonovine or methylergonovine are administered.

Table 68.2 lists the clinically significant drug interactions with ergot alkaloids.

Table 68.2
Ergot alkaloids: Drug interactions

Drug	Interaction
Vasopressors	• Vasopressors (e.g., dopamine, epinephrine, metaraminol, methoxamine, norepinephrine, phenylephrine) may increase the vasoconstriction produced by ergonovine, methylergonovine or methylergometrine

Dinoprostone (Prostin E$_2$®)

Mechanism of action and pharmacologic effects. Dinoprostone is a synthetic prostaglandin that stimulates the myometrium of the gravid uterus to contract in a manner similar to the spontaneous contractions seen during labour in the term uterus. Stimulation of the smooth muscles of the GI tract can cause nausea, vomiting and diarrhea.

Therapeutic uses. Dinoprostone tablets are used as a uterine stimulant for induction of labour at or near term in: (1) elective induction or (2) indicated induction, such as postmaturity, hypertension, toxemia of pregnancy, premature rupture of amniotic membranes, Rh incompatibility, diabetes mellitus, intrauterine deaths or fetal growth retardation. Dinoprostone vaginal gel is indicated for the induction of labour in term or near-term pregnant women who have favourable induction features, a singleton pregnancy and a vertex presentation.

Adverse effects. Vomiting, with or without nausea and diarrhea, is the most common adverse effect of dinoprostone. Fetal heart rate changes have been reported in approximately six percent of patients. Other adverse effects occur very rarely and include headache, hypertension, hypotension, hyperthermia, dizziness, chills, hiccups, flushing, tachycardia, dyspnea, bronchospasm and rash.

Table 68.3 lists the clinically significant drug interactions with dinoprostone.

Uterine Relaxants (Tocolytics)

Ritodrine HCl (Yutopar®)

Mechanism of action and pharmacologic effects. Ritodrine stimulates beta$_2$ receptors and decreases both the frequency and intensity of uterine contractions. To a lesser degree, ritodrine stimulates beta$_1$ receptors, resulting in a dose-related tachycardia.

Therapeutic uses. Ritodrine is indicated for the management of preterm labour (i.e., with > 20 weeks and < 37 weeks of gestation) in suitable patients who have intact amniotic membranes, cervical dilatation up to 4 cm, and less than 80% cervical effacement. In cases involving ruptured amniotic membranes or more advanced labour, inhibition of labour is less likely and the benefits of treatment must be carefully weighed against the potential risks of using the drug.

In the management of preterm labour, the initial intravenous treatment should usually be followed by oral administration.

Adverse effects. Ritodrine's adverse effects result mainly from its beta-adrenergic properties. These include (1) tachycardia, (2) an increase in systolic and a decrease in diastolic pressure, (3) a rise in blood glucose, insulin and free fatty acids, and (4) a decrease in serum potassium. Ritodrine also causes palpitations, tremor, nausea, vomiting, hyperglycemia, headaches, nervousness, anxiety, malaise, chest pains and tightness, and erythema

Fetal tachycardia, neonatal hypoglycemia and hypocalcemia have been reported. In addition, the fetus can be affected by maternal ketoacidosis. These effects are more prevalent following parenteral treatment with ritodrine.

Table 68.4 on the next page lists the clinically significant drug interactions with ritodrine.

Nursing Management

Table 68.5 describes the nursing management of the patient receiving oxytocic drugs. Dosage details for individual drugs are given in Table 68.6 (pages 815–816).

Table 68.3
Dinoprostone: Drug interactions

Drug	Interaction
Oxytocin	• The concomitant use of oxytocin or other oxytocics to induce abortion is generally not advised because of the increased risk of uterine rupture

Table 68.4
Ritodrine: Drug interactions

Drug	Interaction
Adrenergics	• Adrenergics may have additive effects with ritodrine
Anesthetics	• Anesthetics may have their hypotensive effects potentiated by ritodrine
Antihypertensives	• Antihypertensives may have their effects increased by ritodrine
Beta blockers	• Beta blockers inhibit the action of ritodrine; coadministration of these drugs should be avoided
Corticosteroids	• The concomitant use of corticosteroids and ritodrine may lead to pulmonary edema
Diazoxide	• Diazoxide potentiates ritodrine's hypotensive and arrhythmic effects
Dobutamine and dopamine	• Dobutamine and dopamine may have additive effects with ritodrine
Indapamide	• Indapamide potentiates ritodrine's hypotensive and arrhythmic effects

Table 68.5
Nursing management of the oxytocics

Assessment of risk vs. benefit	Patient data	• It is essential to assess both pts: fetal and maternal heart rate/rhythm must be evaluated as well as fetal position and possibility of cephalopelvic disproportion; maternal BP and R; height, consistency and location of fundus; presence of vaginal bleeding • Cautious use with hx of uterine surgery or caesarean section
	Drug data	• *Some serious drug interactions:* Confer with pharmacist • Most serious adverse effects are uterine rupture and vasoconstriction
Implementation	Rights of administration	• Using the "rights" helps prevent errors of administration
	Right route	• Give IV, IM, and by nasal, vaginal, rectal and oral routes
	Right technique	• IV administration requires knowledge of correct diluent and IV solution, correct dilution and rate of administration. Always refer to manufacturer's instructions for this route. Rate must be carefully controlled; always use an infusion pump. Administer only when continuous monitoring and emergency response staff are available
	Nursing therapeutics	• Nausea and vomiting often occur with some drugs in this class; provide supportive measures • *Emotional support:* Important whether drugs are used as adjunct to labour or to complete abortion
	Patient/family teaching	• General information regarding drug actions and administration techniques may be appropriate • For intranasal use of oxytocin, provide clear instructions for pt use (see Table 68.6)

(cont'd on next page)

Table 68.5 (continued)
Nursing management of the oxytocics

Outcomes	Monitoring of progress	*Continually monitor:*
		• Clinical response indicating tx success; uterine contractions and maternal/fetal heart rate
		• Signs/symptoms of adverse reactions; document and report immediately to physician. Particularly monitor for sustained uterine contractions, CV responses, imbalances of water or electrolytes with longer duration of tx

Response to Clinical Challenge

1. Prior to initiating this oxytocic drug, the following examinations/assessment should be completed:

• vital signs of both patients (fetal and maternal heart rate, rhythm);
• strength, frequency and duration of contractions;
• cervical dilatation.

Regarding Beth's history, it is important to determine any prior caesarean section or uterine surgery.

2. During the drip, monitoring should include frequency, strength and duration of contractions, maternal blood pressure and maternal/fetal heart rate. Discontinue if contractions exceed 1 min in length or occur more than q2–3 min, or if maternal or fetal distress occurs.

3. Oxytocin 3–10 U is ordered IM to stimulate uterine contractions and reduce bleeding. The desired site is the ventrolateral gluteal, followed by massage to promote absorption.

Further Reading

Fausett M, et al. Oxytocin labor stimulation of twin gestations: effective and efficient. *Obstet Gynecol* 1997;90(2):202–204.

Graves CR. Agents that cause contraction or relaxation of the uterus. In: Hardman JG, Li LE, Molinoff PB, Ruddon RW, Gilman AG, eds. *Goodman and Gilman's The Pharmacological Basis of Therapeutics.* 9th ed. New York: McGraw-Hill; 1995: 939–949.

Hall MH, Webster J. Obstetric and gynaecological disorders. In: Speight TM, Holdford NHG, eds. *Avery's Drug Treatment.* 4th ed. London: ADIS International; 1997:683–724.

Kramer R, et al. A randomized trial of misoprostol and oxytocin for induction of labor: safety and efficacy. *Obstet Gynecol* 1997;89(3):387–391.

Perry R, et al. The pharmacokinetics of oxytocin as they apply to labor induction. *Am J Obstet Gynecol* 1996;175(5):1590–1593.

Sultatos L. Pharmacology update. Mechanisms of drugs that affect uterine motility. *J Nurs Midwif* 1997;42(4):367–370.

Summers L. Methods of cervical ripening and labor induction. *J Nurs Midwif* 1997;42(2):71–85.

Table 68.6
Uterine stimulants and relaxants: Drug doses

Drug Generic name (Trade names)	Dosage	Nursing alert
A. Uterine Stimulants		
1. Oxytocics		
oxytocin (Pitocin, Syntocinon)	**IV:** For induction of labour: Infuse dilute solution (10 mU/mL), preferably with constant-rate infusion pump). Initial infusion rate is 0.5 mU/min; increase by 1 or 2 mU/min. q30–60min. Increase until optimal uterine response is obtained (3–4 contractions similar to normal labour in 10 min) without evidence of fetal distress. Approximately 75% of pts respond to final infusion rate ≤ 5 mU/min (For oxytocin challenge test) **IV:** Infuse dilute solution starting at the lowest pump setting (approx. 0.5 mU/min); double dose q20–30min until 3 contractions are observed q10min (max. rate, 20 mU/min) unless repetitive late deceleration or fetal bradycardia occurs earlier. If either develops, oxytocin should be discontinued immediately (For prevention of postpartum uterine atony and hemorrhage) **IV:** Give 20–40 mU/mL in an electrolyte solution at the rate of 40 mU/min or more (i.e., rate sufficient to control uterine atony) **IM:** (To control postpartum bleeding): 3–10 units (0.3–1 mL).**Intranasal:** (To promote milk ejection): 1 spray into one or both nostrils 2–3 min before nursing	•**IV:** Administer by infusion only; do not give by direct IV. Prior to infusion, rotate container to ensure thorough mixing. Use infusion pump to ensure accurate dosage. Check rate of infusion, as dosage differs for induction of labour and for postpartum bleeding. Store solution in refrigerator, but do not freeze •**IM:** Use ventrolateral gluteal and massage injection site. Have crash cart available and keep magnesium sulfate at bedside •**Intranasal:** Instruct pt to blow her nose prior to administration. She should then sit upright with head in vertical position. Holding container upright, pt should place it into her nostril, and squeeze while inhaling
ergonovine maleate (Ergotrate Maleate)	**IV:** (In emergencies, when excess uterine bleeding has occurred): 0.2 mg. **IM:** (To control uterine hemorrhage): 0.2 mg, repeated in 2–4 h if bleeding is severe. **Oral:** (To minimize late postpartum bleeding): 0.2–0.4 mg bid–qid, usually for 2 days	•**IV:** Direct IV used only in severe uterine bleeding. Dilute with 5 mL 9% NaCl. Administer over at least 1 min •**IM:** Preferred route. Dose may need to be repeated, but firm uterine contractions are generally produced within minutes of 1st dose •**PO:** Indicated within 48 h postpartum, when danger of hemorrhage is greatest •Drug should be stored in light-resistant, tightly closed container. Discard medication if discoloured. Solutions should be stored below 8°C. It is possible to keep daily stock at room temperature, but not for longer than 60 days •Hypocalcemia may antagonize response to drug. Calcium gluconate may be ordered to correct imbalance *(cont'd on next page)*

Table 68.6 (continued)
Uterine stimulants and relaxants: Drug doses

Drug Generic name (Trade names)	Dosage	Nursing alert

A. Uterine Stimulants (cont'd)
2. Prostaglandin

Drug	Dosage	Nursing alert
dinoprostone (Prostin E$_2$)	**Oral:** 0.5 mg, followed in 1 h by 2nd dose of 0.5 mg; thereafter, hourly. Single dose should never exceed 1.5 mg. For detailed dosage information, consult product information *If drug fails to elicit regular uterine contractions after 8 h, case should be classified as failed induction. Total tx period should not, in any instance, exceed 18 h* **Vaginal:** Initially, 1 mg gel placed into the posterior fornix of vaginal canal. A dose of 1–2 mg may be repeated, once, 6 h later, depending on pt's response to initial dose	• **Vaginal:** Suppositories should be refrigerated. Before administration, allow them to warm gradually to room temperature. Wear gloves when handling suppositories to prevent absorption of drug through skin. Instruct pt to empty her bladder, then insert suppository high into vagina. It is important to instruct pt to remain supine for at least 10 min after administration • Gel is stable for 24 months when refrigerated. Allow to warm to room temperature prior to administration, but do not force warming through such means such as microwave or water bath. Remove both seal from end of syringe and protective end cap. Insert end cap into the plunger stopper assembly in barrel of syringe. Using aseptic technique, prepare catheter. Attach catheter hub to syringe tip. There should be an audible click; this ensures firm attachment. When plunger is pushed, catheter should fill with sterile gel. Fill catheter just prior to administration. Instruct pt to lie in dorsal position, with cervical visualization using a speculum. Administer gel by gentle expulsion. After administration, remove catheter. Instruct pt to remain supine for 15–30 min after administration. Wash hands thoroughly after handling gel

B. Adrenergic Uterine Relaxant (Tocolytic)

Drug	Dosage	Nursing alert
ritodrine HCl (Yutopar)	**IV:** Initially, 100 µg/min; gradually increase by 50 µg/min q10min until desired result. Max. dose, 350 µg/min. Continue infusing for not < 12 h and not > 48 h after uterine contractions cease **Oral:** 10 mg approx. 30 min before termination of IV. Usual dose for 1st 24 h is 10 mg q2h; thereafter, 10–20 mg q4–6h. Max., 120 mg/day	• **IV:** If solution is discoloured or contains precipitate, do not use. CV responses are common and more pronounced during IV administration; therefore, monitor CV effects (maternal P, BP, fetal HR) • Observe pt for signs of pulmonary edema, including tachycardia > 140 beats/min, persistent R > 20 breaths/min. If pulmonary edema develops, drug should be discontinued

Pharmacology of the Respiratory System

Nurses need not be reminded of the importance of the respiratory system. Charged with the responsibility for the exchange of oxygen and carbon dioxide between blood and the environment, its normal function is essential for a healthy body. Conditions such as bronchial asthma or the common cold reduce the capacity of the respiratory system to carry out its physiological function. When this happens, drug therapy may be required.

Unit 14 discusses the use of drugs to treat these conditions. In addition, it describes the actions of antihistamines. Although the use of these drugs is not restricted to respiratory medicine, a major use for antihistamines is in the treatment of coughs and colds. For this reason, antihistamines have been included in this unit of the book.

Antiasthmatic Drugs

Topics Discussed
- Asthma, emphysema and chronic obstructive lung disease (COPD)
- Bronchodilators
- Anticholinergics
- Anti-inflammatory drugs
- Inhibitors of inflammatory-response mediators
- Leukotriene receptor antagonist
- For all drugs: Mechanism of action and pharmacologic effects, therapeutic uses, adverse effects
- Drug treatment of status asthmaticus
- Nursing management

Drugs Discussed
albuterol (al-**byoo**-ter-ol)
aminophylline (am-in-**off**-ih-lin)
beclomethasone (beck-loe-**meth**-ah-sone)
budesonide (byoo-**dess**-oh-nyde)

cromolyn (**kroe**-moe-lin)
epinephrine (ep-in-**eff**-rin)
fenoterol (fen-oh-**ter**-all)
flunisolide (flew-**niss**-oh-lyde)
ipratropium (ip-ra-**troe**-pee-yum)
ketotifen (key-toe-**tiff**-en)
metaproterenol (met-ah-pro-**ter**-eh-nole)
methylprednisolone (meth-il-pred-**niss**-oh-lone)
nedocromil (ned-oh-**kroe**-mil)
orciprenaline (or-sip-**ren**-ah-leen)
oxtriphylline (ox-**trye**-fih-lin)
prednisone (**pred**-nih-zone)
procaterol (proe-**kat**-er-all)
salbutamol (sal-**byoo**-ter-all)
salmeterol (sal-**met**-er-all)
sodium cromoglycate (kroe-moe-**glye**-kate)
terbutaline (ter-**byoo**-tah-leen)
theophylline (thee-**off**-ih-lin)
triamcinolone (try-am-**sin**-oh-lone)
zafirlukast (zah-**feer**-loo-cost)

Asthma, Emphysema and Chronic Obstructive Lung Disease

Asthma is a disease characterized by increased responsiveness of the trachea and bronchi to various stimuli and manifested by a widespread narrowing of the airways that changes in severity either spontaneously or as a result of therapy. Asthma should be considered to be predominantly an inflammatory disease with associated bronchospasm. The degree of hyperresponsiveness and narrowing of the bronchi produced by stimuli is greater in asthmatic patients than in normal individuals.

There appears little doubt that the incidence of asthma is increasing, especially among the young. Some 150 million people, or the equivalent of the population of Russia, now suffer from asthma. In the United States, the number of asthmatics has leapt by more than sixty-one percent since the early 1980s, while the death toll from the disease has doubled, to 5000 a year. In Australia, one in six people under the age of sixteen has asthma, and rates among school-age children have doubled in the past twenty years. In Britain, some three million people — one million of them school-age children — are affected by the condition, and there has been a fourfold increase in the last thirty years.

Clinical Challenge

Consider these clinical challenges as you read through this chapter. The response to the challenges appears on page 825.

You are working as an occupational health nurse in a large, industrial firm in a major city. You have observed that the incidence of asthma in employees has increased during the past three years.

Choose one of the following options to provide focus for your reading of this chapter and to offer you the opportunity to learn more about this important condition that can attack at any age and any time.

1. Prepare a proposal to research the types of asthma in the employees, the incidence and the costs related to sick time. Outline a health promotion program that could help reduce sick time and hospitalization related to asthma attacks.
2. Design an educational program for management and staff that will describe asthma, including incidence in Canada and worldwide, hypothesized underlying causes such as genetic and environmental factors and common drug treatment.
3. Research alternative treatments such as acupuncture and the current advancements being made with respect to a vaccination against asthma.

It is unclear why we see an increased incidence of asthma. It is always easy to blame the environment, but that is not the only answer. Asthma has two basic preconditions: a susceptible host and an environmental factor that induces an allergic reaction. The number of allergens or irritants — dust mites, moulds, smoke, diesel fumes — multiplies the more urban an area becomes; so it is not surprising that the disease is relatively rare in places like Papua New Guinea and sparsely populated parts of Africa, China and Indonesia. However, although air pollutants appear to aggravate the disease for some people, air pollution does not actually cause asthma. For example, the town of Portree, on the Scottish Isle of Skye, has some of the cleanest air in Britain, yet an unusually high rate of asthma. In Germany the rates of asthma in the west were higher than in the east, despite assumptions that the poorer, more polluted east would produce a less healthy population.

Persistent inflammation is a primary cause of the increased bronchial hyperresponsiveness. Mucosal edema, mucus plugging and hypersecretion may be present; the functional lung tissue is normal. Airway narrowing may reverse spontaneously or with therapy.

The exact pathogenesis of asthma remains undetermined, and many inflammatory mediators have been implicated. One such group is the leukotrienes. Leukotrienes are produced by several cell types within the lung and have been shown to cause bronchoconstriction and mucus secretion, both key features observed in asthma. Attention has focused on drugs either to inhibit the formation of leukotrienes or to block their receptors, with the hope that these medicines reduce the severity of asthma.

Type I (IgE-mediated) immune responses often play an important role in the development of asthma in children and many adults; however, when the onset of disease occurs in adulthood, allergic factors may be more difficult to identify or may be absent. Exposure to cold dry air, exercise, upper respiratory infections and other aggravating factors such as occupational exposure to provocative substances may trigger asthmatic exacerbations.

Emphysema and chronic obstructive bronchitis frequently coexist in what is commonly termed chronic obstructive pulmonary or lung disease (COPD or COLD). In emphysema, the primary pathology is parenchymal; airway collapse results from loss of elasticity and tissue destruction.

Clinically, it is difficult to assess the relative contributions of emphysema and chronic bronchitis to airway obstruction. Smoking and other environmental irritants contribute to the etiology of COPD. Response to therapy is partial at best. In some individuals, asthma, emphysema and chronic bronchitis coexist.

Drug therapy is designed to treat the factors responsible for airway obstruction. Treatment will be discussed under the categories of (1) bronchodilators, (2) anti-inflammatories, (3) inhibitors of inflammatory-response mediators and (4) leukotriene receptor antagonists.

Bronchodilators

Beta-Adrenergic Drugs

Mechanism of action and pharmacologic effects. Beta$_1$ receptors are found in the heart, and beta$_2$ receptors in the bronchioles and blood vessels. The pharmacology of these drugs is presented in detail in Chapter 29. Drugs that stimulate beta$_1$ receptors increase heart rate and force of contraction. Beta$_2$ stimulants dilate bronchioles and decrease peripheral resistance.

Examples of beta$_2$ stimulants used to treat asthma are orciprenaline/metaproterenol (Alupent®, Metaprel®), albuterol/salbutamol (Proventil®, Ventolin®), terbutaline (Brethine®, Bricanyl®), fenoterol (Berotec®), procaterol (Pro-Air®), and salmeterol (Serevent®). These drugs produce less tachycardia than isoproterenol, which was used extensively before their introduction.

Therapeutic uses. Beta$_2$ stimulants are the most effective bronchodilators and are commonly used for the treatment of asthma. These drugs are all administered by inhalation. When given in this manner, they may be used regularly to prevent attacks or periodically to stop a developing attack. Although most are also available in oral dosage forms, they are more effective and more specific for beta$_2$ receptors when inhaled. Unfortunately, the effects of beta-adrenergic drugs often decrease when they are used chronically. Beta$_2$ stimulants are contraindicated in patients with tachyarrhythmias.

Albuterol or salbutamol (Proventil®,

Ventolin®) is a very popular and effective bronchodilator. Usual doses produce little tachycardia or tremor. As with all beta$_2$ stimulants, it causes tachycardia in higher doses. Fenoterol (Berotec®) usually has a slower onset and longer duration of action than most beta$_2$ stimulants. In all other respects it is similar to these drugs. Metaproterenol or orciprenaline (Metaprel®, Alupent®) is an effective bronchodilator but produces a relatively high incidence of tremors. Terbutaline (Brethine®, Bricanyl®) is an effective drug with properties similar to those of the other beta$_2$ stimulants. Procaterol HCl (Pro-Air®) is a more recently introduced beta$_2$ agonist for the treatment of bronchial asthma. Administered orally, it is rapidly absorbed and shows bronchodilating activity for up to eight hours. When inhaled, procaterol has a rapid onset of action, commencing within five minutes and extending for up to eight hours.

Epinephrine (Adrenalin®) stimulates alpha$_1$, beta$_1$ and beta$_2$ receptors. Bronchodilatation is complemented by alpha$_1$-mediated vasoconstriction, which reduces edema and mucus production. For usual control of asthma it has largely been replaced by the more selective beta$_2$ stimulants. However, epinephrine is still used for the treatment of acute exacerbations of asthma when inhaled beta$_2$ stimulants cannot be used.

Ephedrine also stimulates alpha$_1$, beta$_1$ and beta$_2$ receptors. However, it has little place in modern medicine. Although it dilates bronchioles, the drug also increases heart rate, raises peripheral resistance and stimulates the central nervous system. In the past, products containing fixed ratios of ephedrine, theophylline and a CNS depressant were popular. There is no evidence that they are more effective than theophylline alone. Furthermore, the use of a CNS depressant in an asthmatic is strongly discouraged.

Salmeterol (Serevent®) is a unique beta$_2$ agonist. Administered by inhalation, its selectivity for beta$_2$ receptors is seventy-seven times greater than salbutamol's. As a result, salmeterol dilates the bronchioles, with less chance of increasing heart rate than salbutamol and other currently used bronchodilators. Salmeterol protects against breakthrough symptoms for at least twelve hours following inhalation of a single 50 µg dose. Compared with salbutamol, salmeterol produces three to four times greater improvement in morning peak flow, reduces significantly the frequency and severity of daytime and nighttime asthmatic symptoms, controls breakthrough symptoms better, improves the quality of patients' sleep significantly more and reduces the requirements for rescue inhalations of salbutamol.

Salmeterol does not have the same primary use as the other beta$_2$ stimulants. Inhaled beta$_2$ agonists, such as salbutamol, are recommended as level 1 care. In this situation, these drugs are used as needed. If the need for a short-acting, inhalable bronchodilator is frequent, or there are other symptoms of asthma instability, level 2 care is required, and scheduled doses of inhaled corticosteroids are added to the regimen. However, if control is still not achieved, level 3 care mandates the use of high doses of inhaled steroid and a trial of an adjunctive bronchodilator. It is in the treatment of these patients (level 3) that salmeterol should be used. This is reflected in its approved use, which states that the drug is indicated in patients with reversible obstructive airway disease who are using optimum anti-inflammatory treatment and experiencing breakthrough symptoms requiring a regular inhaled short-acting bronchodilator more than twice daily.

It must also be emphasized the salmeterol is not a replacement for anti-inflammatory therapy; its use is complementary to it. Patients must be warned not to stop or reduce anti-inflammatory therapy without medical advice, even if they feel better on salmeterol. Furthermore, as previously stated, patients must have rapid-onset, short-acting bronchodilators (i.e., albuterol/salbutamol) available at all times for relief of acute asthmatic symptoms.

If level 3 care fails to control asthma and the symptoms of instability persist, oral steroid therapy is administered reluctantly as level 4 care.

Adverse effects. Tachycardia is the major adverse effect of beta-adrenergic drugs. Although it is more common after use of drugs that stimulate both beta$_1$ and beta$_2$ receptors, it can also be seen with selective beta$_2$ agonists when large doses are used. Other adverse effects include headaches, dizziness, nausea and tremors.

Table 69.1 lists the clinically significant drug interactions with beta-adrenergic bronchodilators.

Theophylline, Aminophylline and Oxtriphylline (Choledyl®)

Mechanism of action and pharmacologic effects. Theophylline is a less effective bronchodilator than inhaled beta$_2$ stimulants. Its precise mechanism of action is still unclear. It also increases heart rate and stimulates the central nervous system.

Theophylline is sparingly soluble in water, and as a result it is usually marketed in the form of water-soluble salts. These compounds dissolve more readily in the gastrointestinal tract and are better absorbed. Two popular salts are aminophylline (theophylline ethylenediamine) and oxtriphylline (choline theophyllinate). The latter compound is sold under the trade name Choledyl®. Regardless of the salt used, theophylline is the active drug in the body.

Therapeutic uses. Oral theophylline products have been relegated to third-line therapy, chiefly due to systemic toxicity and mild bronchodilator activity. Theophylline is usually used if inhaled bronchodilator plus inhaled corticosteroid therapy has failed to control the symptoms of asthma. In this situation, theophylline can be added to existing treatments (level 3 care).

The ability to measure plasma theophylline levels has assisted in its safe and effective use.

Table 69.1
Beta-adrenergic bronchodilators: Drug interactions

Drug	Interaction
Beta blockers	• Beta blockers block the effects of beta stimulants
MAOIs	• Monoamine oxidase inhibitors potentiate the effects of beta agonists on the vascular system
TCAs	• Tricyclic antidepressants potentiate the effects of beta agonists on the vascular system

Table 69.2
Theophylline: Drug interactions

Drug	Interaction
Allopurinol	• Allopurinol can elevate theophylline serum levels
Beta stimulants	• Beta stimulants may increase the bronchodilation produced by theophylline and its salts, but they may also produce toxic synergism
Epinephrine	• Epinephrine may produce toxic synergism with theophylline and its salts
Erythromycin	• Erythromycin can elevate theophylline serum levels
Phenobarbital	• Phenobarbital can increase theophylline clearance
Phenytoin	• Phenytoin can increase theophylline clearance
Progestins	• Progestins can elevate theophylline serum levels

Therapeutic serum concentrations of theophylline are accepted as 10–20 µg/mL (55–110 µmol/L). Levels above 20 µg/mL (110 µmol/L) are associated with toxic effects.

Intravenous aminophylline is used in emergency situations. Careful individual dosing is required to prevent toxic effects. Although aminophylline has been administered in suppositories, rectal absorption is erratic. Because the margin of safety with theophylline is narrow, rectal administration is not recommended.

Theophylline-containing products are contraindicated in peptic ulcer and coronary artery disease. They should also not be used when myocardial stimulation could prove harmful.

Adverse effects. The principal adverse effects of theophylline are dose dependent and include gastric irritation, nausea, tachycardia, cardiac arrhythmias, CNS excitation, insomnia, nightmares and convulsions. Nausea is due to both gastric irritation and stimulation of the chemoreceptor trigger zone in the brain. Adverse effects occur less frequently if either oxtriphylline or aminophylline are used. However, this can be explained on the basis that these salts contain only sixty-five or eighty-five percent theophylline, respectively.

Table 69.2 lists the clinically significant drug interactions with theophylline.

Anticholinergic Drugs

Ipratropium Bromide (Atrovent Inhaler®)

Mechanism of action and pharmacologic effects. Ipratropium is an anticholinergic drug (see Chapter 28) that is administered by inhalation or nasal aerosol. It competitively blocks the action of acetylcholine at parasympathetic (cholinergic) receptors. Ipratropium is poorly absorbed and has few systemic effects.

Therapeutic uses. Ipratroprium may be given by inhalation for the treatment of bronchoconstriction associated with asthma or chronic obstructive pulmonary disease (COPD — chronic bronchitis or emphysema). For the treatment of asthma, it is a less effective bronchodilator than inhaled beta$_2$ stimulants, but has additive effects when used in conjunction with a beta$_2$ agonist. Ipratropium is an equally or more effective bronchodilator than a beta$_2$ agonist in the treatment of COPD.

It has a slower onset of action than beta$_2$ agonists, with its maximum effects appearing about two hours after inhalation. Its relatively long duration of action (approximately six hours) makes the drug suitable for maintenance therapy.

Ipratropium is a useful alternative for patients who are unusually susceptible to tremor or tachycardia from beta$_2$ agonists. Because of minimal effects on the cardiovascular system, ipratropium may be used as the initial bronchodilator in patients with heart disease, hypertension, cerebro-vascular disease or thyrotoxicosis. Tolerance does not appear to develop to ipratropium. An inhaled beta$_2$ stimulant, theophylline, cromolyn, nedo-cromil or corticosteroids may be added to ipratro-pium in patients requiring multiple-drug therapy.

Adverse effects. Ipratropium bromide is well tolerated. Its most common adverse effects are dry mouth or throat or both, headache, bad taste and/or blurred vision.

Anti-Inflammatory Drugs

Corticosteroids

Mechanism of action and pharmacologic effects. The pharmacology of these drugs is pre-sented in detail in Chapter 66. Corticosteroids are very effective anti-inflammatory drugs. In dis-cussing the effects of chronic corticosteroid therapy in asthma it is important to differentiate between inhalable steroids, which provide effective relief of inflammation for many patients with minimal or no systemic adverse effects, and the ingestion of drugs such as prednisone, which, although effec-tive as anti-inflammatories, can produce severe systemic adverse effects.

Therapeutic uses. Corticosteroids are cur-rently the most effective anti-inflammatory drug for the treatment of asthma. They may be injected, ingested or inhaled. Early treatment of severe acute exacerbations of asthma with oral cortico-steroids prevents progression of the asthma exac-erbation, decreases the need for emergency depart-ment visits or hospitalization and reduces the mor-bidity of the illness. High-dose, short-term sys-temic therapy may be needed to treat severe acute exacerbation of asthma.

Inhaled corticosteroids, such as beclometha-sone dipropionate, budesonide and flunisolide are safe and effective for the chronic treatment of asthma, when they are administered in low doses for long periods of time, or in high doses for short periods of time. These products are frequently added to inhaled beta$_2$ stimulants in level 2 care, when the beta agonist alone has failed to control the symptoms of asthma. Long-term, high-dose

regimens of inhaled corticosteroids are useful for the treatment of severe chronic asthma. Long-term inhaled corticosteroid use is associated with signif-icantly fewer adverse effects than chronic oral cor-ticosteroid therapy and reduces the need for the chronic use of oral corticosteroids.

Chronic oral corticosteroid treatment should not be used unless other forms of therapy, includ-ing high doses of inhaled steroids, have failed to mitigate the patient's asthma. Chronic oral corti-costeroids should be continued only if shown to reduce chronic symptoms substantially or reduce the frequency of severe exacerbation. Long-term oral corticosteroid therapy in severe asthma is lim-ited by the risk for significant adverse effects.

Adverse effects. The adverse effects of sys-temic corticosteroid therapy are described in Chapter 66. They include redistribution of body fat, leading to a "moon face" and a "buffalo hump," increased susceptibility to infection and reduced growth rate in children. Osteoporosis can also occur, and patients may show psychotic changes. The local effects of beclomethasone dipropionate include laryngeal myopathy and *Candida albicans* infections in the mouth and throat. The clinically relevant drug interactions for corticosteroids can be found in Table 66.2 (page 784).

Inhibitors of Inflammatory-Response Mediators

Cromolyn/Sodium Cromoglycate (Intal®)

Mechanism of action and pharmacologic effects. Sodium cromoglycate is a nonsteroid, topi-cal anti-inflammatory drug for the treatment of asthma. Its exact mechanism of action is not fully understood. However, the drug does inhibit the IgE-mediated inflammatory response in human mast cells. As well, sodium cromoglycate has cell-selective and mediator-selective suppressive effects on other inflammatory cells (macrophages, eosinophils, neutrophils and monocytes). Sodium cromoglycate also prevents bronchoconstriction induced through neuronal mechanisms.

Therapeutic uses. Sodium cromoglycate is administered via inhaler, powder or nebulizer solution, on a regular basis to prevent the onset of asthmatic symptoms. In exercise-induced asthma, it can be used when needed before exercise to inhibit bronchoconstriction. Sodium cromoglycate is not a bronchodilator and should not be used during an acute attack. Owing to its anti-inflammatory and safety profile, sodium cromoglycate is an agent of choice for the initial treatment of chronic mild to moderate asthma in children.

Adverse effects. Sodium cromoglycate has an excellent safety profile, with few adverse effects. Inhalation of the dry powder may cause local irritation.

Nedocromil (Tilade®)

Mechanism of action and pharmacologic effects. The exact mechanism of action of nedocromil sodium is not fully understood. However, nedocromil has been shown to inhibit the release of inflammatory mediators from a variety of cell types occurring in the lumen and in the mucosa of the bronchial tree. Nedocromil sodium has been shown to be four to ten times more potent than sodium cromoglycate in preventing bronchoconstriction in animal and human models of asthma. The drug is extremely potent and efficacious in preventing bronchoconstriction induced through neuronal stimuli.

Therapeutic uses. Nedocromil sodium is indicated as adjunctive therapy in the treatment of mild to moderate reversible obstructive airway disease including bronchial asthma and bronchitis, particularly where allergic factors may be present. Nedocromil sodium is intended for regular therapy, but can also be used on an occasional basis in the prevention of bronchospasm provoked by stimulants, such as inhaled allergens, cold air, exercise and atmospheric pollutants. It should not be used for relief of symptoms during an acute attack.

Adverse effects. Few minor side effects have been reported. These are, principally, headache and nausea, which are transient and seldom require discontinuation of therapy. A property of the chemical that is not perceived by all patients is a transient bitter taste.

Ketotifen (Zaditen®)

Mechanism of action and pharmacologic effects. Ketotifen has a complex pharmacologic action. Its effects include blocking histamine$_1$ (H$_1$) receptors, stabilizing mast cells and thereby reducing histamine release, and inhibiting the effects of the platelet-activating factor. In addition, ketotifen may also antagonize calcium flux in smooth muscle, and enhance beta-adrenergic mediated effects in the bronchioles. The result of these actions is that the drug may reduce the severity and duration of asthma attacks.

Therapeutic uses. Ketotifen is used as an adjunct to other drugs in the chronic prophylaxis of mild atopic (allergic) asthma in children. The efficacy of ketotifen in asthma prophylaxis in children is controversial. It does not appear to be more effective than cromolyn (Intal®), and in some trials it appears to have been no more effective than placebo therapy. However, other studies claim significant effects for the drug. Six to twelve weeks of chronic treatment with ketotifen may reduce a patient's daily requirements for theophylline, a beta$_2$ agonist or corticosteroids.

Adverse effects. Ketotifen produces few adverse effects. The most common are temporary sedation, weight gain, rash, dry mouth, dizziness, nausea and headache.

Leukotriene Receptor Antagonist

Zafirlukast (Accolate®)

Mechanism of action and pharmacologic effects. As explained in the introduction of this chapter, leukotrienes produced by several cell types within the lung cause bronchoconstriction and mucus secretion. Asthmatics are up to one hundred times more sensitive to the bronchoconstrictor effects of leukotrienes than nonasthmatic patients. Zafirlukast is a selective and competitive receptor antagonist of leukotriene D$_4$ and E$_4$ (LTD$_4$ and LTE$_4$). It is the first drug introduced into Canada to block leukotriene receptors, and it may herald a new era in asthma treatment.

Table 69.3
Zafirlukast: Drug interactions

Drug	Interaction
Acetylsalicylic acid	• ASA may increase plasma levels of zafirlukast
Erythromycin	• Erythromycin decreases bioavailability of zafirlukast. Plasma levels of zafirlukast are decreased about 40%
Terfenadine	• Terfenadine decreases plasma levels of zafirlukast. No change is seen in the plasma levels of terfenadine
Theophylline	• Theophylline can decrease plasma levels of zafirlukast. No change is noted in theophylline plasma levels
Warfarin	• Coadministration of zafirlukast and warfarin results in an approximately 35% increase in prothrombin time, compared with warfarin alone. Pts taking oral warfarin and zafirlukast should have their prothrombin times monitored closely and the anticoagulant dose adjusted accordingly

Double-blind, randomized, placebo-controlled clinical trials in patients with mild-to-moderate asthma demonstrated that zafirlukast improved daytime asthma symptoms, nighttime awakenings, mornings with asthma symptoms, rescue beta$_2$-agonist use, forced expiratory volume (FEV_1) and morning peak expiratory flow rate.

Therapeutic uses. Zafirlukast is indicated for the prophylaxis and chronic treatment of asthma in adults and children twelve years of age and older. Zafirlukast is not a bronchodilator and it should not be used for the reversal of bronchospasm in acute attacks, including status asthmaticus. Zafirlukast should be taken regularly as prescribed, even during symptom-free periods. Therapy with zafirlukast can be continued during acute exacerbations of asthma.

Adverse effects. Initial data suggest that zafirlukast has few significant adverse effects. Patients taking the drug have reported headache, infections, nausea, diarrhea and generalized pain. However, the incidence of these effects was low. Only headache, which was seen in 12.9% of patients, occurred in more than 4% of asthmatics taking zafirlukast. In addition, each adverse effect, including headache, was reported in an almost equal number of patients given placebo.

Table 69.3 lists the clinically significant drug interactions with zafirlukast.

Drug Treatment of Status Asthmaticus

An acute attack of asthma, unresponsive to the patient's usual medications, is a serious medical emergency. Patients should be hospitalized and treated intensively. Treatment should include oxygen therapy. Bronchodilators used often include a beta$_2$ agonist, such as salbutamol, in a dose of 4–8 puffs every 15–20 min, plus ipratropium bromide, in a dose of 4–8 puffs every 15–20 min. Systemic corticosteroids may also be required. These may include methylprednisolone (125 mg IV), hydrocortisone (500 mg IV) or prednisone (40–60 mg PO). Aggressive intravenous fluid treatment is also beneficial to rehydrate the patient and liquefy bronchial secretions.

Nursing Management

Table 69.4 on the next page describes the nursing management of the patient receiving bronchodilator antiasthmatic drugs. Dosage details for individual drugs are given in Table 69.5 (pages 827–832). Nursing management of the corticosteroids is described in Table 66.4 (pages 787–788).

Response to the Clinical Challenge

Discuss your responses with your instructor or colleagues. Consult Further Reading (page 827).

Table 69.4
Nursing management of the antiasthmatics

Assessment of risk vs. benefit	Patient data	• Physician should determine type of asthma and required level of drug tx. Assess for baseline respiratory and cardiac function • *Pregnancy:* Most drugs are risk category C (animal studies show adverse effects to fetus but human data are unknown or insufficient); benefits may be acceptable despite risks
	Drug data	• Staff and pts/families should follow instructions for storage of aerosol canisters: keep at room temperature, away from direct sources of heat. Check expiration date on label • Most serious adverse effects are related to cardiac overstimulation
Implementation	Rights of administration	• Using the "rights" helps prevent errors of administration
	Right route	• Usually, give PO and by inhalation. Some drugs may be given IV for urgent situations. Box 69.1 gives a sample patient teaching for proper use of an inhaler
	Nursing therapeutics	• Asthma is a serious, chronic condition that requires education and emotional support. Encourage pt/family to use self-care and lifestyle strategies to reduce attacks and to control the impact of an attack through relaxation techniques
	Patient/family teaching	• Compliance and follow-up are essential factors in successful tx; review principles of pt education in Chapter 3 • Instruct pt to rinse mouth following inhalation to minimize side effects (dry mouth, unpleasant taste) • Emphasize importance of following dosage precisely. With continued use, pts may become complacent regarding potential risks of drugs. Explain difference between drugs used as prophylaxis (continual tx) and those used to treat acute symptoms (intermittent or on-demand tx) • If pt is receiving multiple-drug tx, review order of administration and recommended time intervals between drugs • Pts/families should know warning signs/symptoms of possible toxicities of these drugs. Report immediately any cardiac signs such as rapid pulse. Discuss change in symptoms and response to drug doses with physician • Advise pts/families regarding exposure to triggers such as tobacco smoke, dust, pollens • *Discuss possibility of pregnancy:* Advise pt to notify physician and discuss potential risks
Outcomes	Monitoring of progress	*Continually monitor:* • Clinical response indicating tx success (reduction in signs/symptoms). Assess lung sounds prior to and following administration. Plasma drug levels may be ordered • Signs/symptoms of adverse reactions; document and report immediately to physician

Box 69.1
Patient teaching: Use of inhaler

✔ Insert drug canister firmly into the actuator/inhaler device.

✔ Shake inhaler and remove cap from mouthpiece.

✔ Place mouthpiece in the mouth with canister held in inverted position.

✔ Breathe out as completely as possible, and then close lips around the mouthpiece.

✔ Keep tongue flat.

✔ Press canister down firmly and breathe in slowly, deeply through the mouthpiece.

✔ Hold breath until uncomfortable; remove mouthpiece and exhale slowly.

✔ Wait at least 1 minute before repeating procedure.

✔ Remove canister, wash and dry mouthpiece daily.

Further Reading

Albuterol against acute bronchitis. *Emerg Med* 1995; 27(12):71–72.

Anderson B. An overview of drug therapy for chronic adult asthma. *Nurse Pract/Am J Primary Care* 1991;16(12):39–46.

Anticholinergic therapy in the critically ill patient with bronchospasm. *AACN Clinical Issues* 1995; 6(2):287–296.

Continuing education forum: Managing adult asthma in primary care setting. *J Resp Care Pract* 1996; 8(1):33–43.

Customized aerosol therapy. *J Resp Care Pract* 1994; 7(2):57.

Emerson CL. A randomized comparison of 100 mg vs 500 mg dose of methylprednisolone in treatment of acute asthma. *Chest* 1995;107(6):1559–1563.

Guidelines on the management of asthma. *Thorax* 1993;4:S1–S24.

Petty L. The combination of ipratropium and albuterol is more effective than either alone. *Chest* 1995; 107(5, suppl):183S–186S.

van Schayck CP. The influence of an inhaled steroid on quality of life in patients with asthma or COPD. *Chest* 1995;107(5):1199–1205.

Table 69.5
The antiasthmatics: Drug doses

Drug Generic name (Trade names)	Dosage	Nursing alert
A. Beta-Adrenergic Agonists		
albuterol/salbutamol (Proventil, Ventolin)	**Inhalation aerosol:** 1–2 puffs up to qid. More than 8 puffs/day not recommended	• **PO:** Oral medication should be administered with meals to reduce gastric irritation
	Oral: *Adults:* 2–4 mg tid–qid. *Children 6–12 years:* 2 mg tid–qid; *2–6 years:* 0.1 mg/kg tid–qid	• **Inhaler:** Ensure that pt waits 1 min between inhalations. Instruct pt in proper use of inhaler (see Box 69.1)
	IM: 500 µg (8 µg/kg body weight) q4h, prn. Max. daily dose, 2000 µg. **IV bolus:** 250 µg (4 µg/kg body weight) over 2–5 min, repeated after 15 min, prn. Max. daily dose, 1000 µg. **Continuous IV Infusion:** 5 µg/min; increase to 10 µg/min and 20 µg/min at 15- and 30-min intervals, prn	

Table 69.5 (continued)
The antiasthmatics: Drug doses

Drug Generic name (Trade names)	Dosage	Nursing alert
A. Beta-Adrenergic Agonists (cont'd)		
fenoterol (Berotec)	**Inhalation aerosol:** 1–2 puffs containing 100 µg tid–qid. Max. 8 puffs/day should not be exceeded (1–2 puffs of 200 µg tid). **Inhalation solution:** Consult Berotec product information **Oral:** *Adults:* 2.5–5 mg bid–tid	• Undiluted solution may be stored in original amber bottle at room temperature until expiration date. Diluted solution for nebulizer may be stored at room temperature for 24 h and then discarded • To prepare dose for nebulizer, withdraw ordered dose with a syringe and add to nebulizing chamber. Using a syringe, add the ordered volume of sterile, preservative-free NaCl solution to produce desired concentration. Gently shake chamber to ensure homogeneous solution and connect to air or O_2 pump, as ordered. Discard unused solution after tx. After opening drug solution, mark date on bottle and discard after 30 days
metaproterenol/orciprenaline (Alupent, Metaprel)	**Inhalation aerosol:** 1–2 puffs up to qid. **Inhalation solution:** 5–15 inhalations of 50 mg/mL (5%) solution by hand nebulizer (Devilbiss® No. 40 or 42), administered up to tid. **Intermittent positive pressure breathing:** 0.5–1 mL of 50 mg/mL (5%) solution diluted, if desired, and administered over a period of about 20 min **Oral:** *Adults/children (≥ 12 years):* Initially, 20 mg tid–qid. *Children 4–12 years:* 10 mg tid	• **Inhalation:** Dilute dose as ordered. Do not use solution if discoloured (except slightly yellow or pinkish) or containing a precipitate. Store solution at room temperature • **PO:** Give with food
procaterol (Pro-Air)	**Inhalation aerosol:** For acute symptoms, 1–2 puffs (10–20 µg) will usually relieve bronchospasm in most pts. Exercise-induced bronchospasm: 1–2 puffs (10–20 µg) at least 15 min before exertion	• Instruct pt in proper use of inhaler (Box 69.1, page 827). Explain purpose of medication regimen, e.g., if ordered for exercise-induced bronchospasm, should be used 15 min prior to activity
salmeterol (Serevent)	**Inhalation aerosol:** 50 µg bid	• Medication should be taken at 12-h intervals. Do not increase dosage. If symptoms worsen, contact physician. Medication should not be used to treat acute bronchospasm • Pts must be warned not to stop or reduce anti-inflammatory tx without medical advice, even if they feel better • Pts must have rapid-onset, short-acting bronchodilators (e.g., albuterol/salbutamol) available at all times for relief of acute asthmatic symptoms

Table 69.5 (continued)
The antiasthmatics: Drug doses

Drug Generic name (Trade names)	Dosage	Nursing alert
A. Beta-Adrenergic Agonists (cont'd)		
terbutaline (Brethine, Bricanyl)	**Inhalation aerosol:** *Adults/children (≥ 6 years):* For acute symptoms, 1–2 inhalations (0.5–1.0 mg). No more than 6 inhalations/24 h **Oral:** *Adults:* 5 mg tid. Reduce to 2.5 mg tid in the event of adverse effects	• **Inhalation:** Advise pt to rest 2 min between inhalations • **PO:** for pts with dysphagia, tablets may be crushed and mixed with food. Tablets and aerosol may be used concomitantly; monitor for toxicity
epinephrine, adrenaline (Adrenalin, Medihaler-Epi, Primatene Mist, Venonephrin)	**SC solution:** *Adults:* 0.2–0.3 mg (0.2–0.3 mL of 1:1000 solution. *Children:* 0.01 mg/kg. In severe attacks of asthma, doses may be repeated for adults and children q20min for max. of 3 doses. **SC aqueous suspension of free base** (1:200): *Adults:* 0.1–0.3 mL (max. initial dose, 0.1 mL). *Children:* 0.005 mL/kg (max. dose for children < 30 kg, 0.15 mL) **Inhalation:** *Adults/children:* 2 inhalations of 1:100 solution (0.2 mg/dose). NB: Epinephrine is not a preferred drug for this route	• Preferably, administer medication promptly after onset of bronchospasm. Fatalities have occurred with this drug because of calculation errors; therefore, check route, dose and concentration before administration • Suspension should be used only for SC route. If pinkish or brownish in colour, or containing precipitate, discard • **SC:** Rotate injection site; medication can cause tissue necrosis. Massage site afterwards to ensure absorption and decrease vasoconstriction. Shake suspension well before injection; administer promptly to prevent from settling • Instruct pt in proper technique for use of inhaler (Box 69.1, page 827). Ensure 1- to 2-min pause between inhalations. Wait 5 min after inhalation to administer other medications to prevent toxicity
B. Theophylline Products		
theophylline (Elixophylline, Bronkodyl, Theolar)	**Oral:** *Adults:* 5 mg/kg initially; then, in otherwise healthy nonsmokers: 3 mg/kg q8h; *young adult smokers:* 3 mg/kg q6h; *pts > 60 years or pts with cor pulmonale:* 2 mg/kg q8h; *pts with CHF or liver disease:* 1–2 mg/kg q12h (daily dose may be divided and given as extended-release dosage forms q12–24 h). Dose should not exceed 13 mg/kg/day or 900 mg, whichever is less **Oral:** *Children 9–16 years:* 5 mg/kg initially, followed by 12 mg/kg/day in divided doses q6h. Dose should not exceed 20 mg/kg/day in pts 9–12 years or 18 mg/kg/day in pts 12–16 years or 900 mg, whichever is less. *Children 1–9 years:* 5 mg/kg initially, followed by 4 mg/kg q6h (not to exceed 24 mg/kg/day or 900 mg, whichever is less)	• Medication should be given ATC. In case of od doses, administer in a.m. • Give with full glass of water and meals to reduce gastric irritation. Do not crush enteric-coated or timed-release tablets or capsules. Do not refrigerate elixirs, solutions, syrups or suspension; crystals may form. If medication has crystals, warm liquid to room temperature to dissolve

(cont'd on next page)

Table 69.5 (continued)
The antiasthmatics: Drug doses

Drug Generic name (Trade names)	Dosage	Nursing alert
B. Theophylline Products (cont'd)		
theophylline (Elixophylline, Bronkodyl, Theolar) (cont'd)	**IV:** *Adults:* 5 mg/kg initially over 20–30 min; then, in otherwise healthy nonsmokers: 0.43 mg/kg/h; *young adult smokers:* 0.7 mg/kg/h; *pts > 60 years or pts with cor pulmonale:* 0.26 mg/kg/h; *pts with CHF or liver disease:* 0.2 mg/kg/h. Maint. infusion rates may be decreased after 12 h **IV:** *Children 12–16 years:* 5 mg/kg initially; then, in nonsmokers: 0.5 mg/kg/h; smokers: 0.7 mg/kg/h. *Children 9–12 years:* 5 mg/kg initially, then 0.7 mg/kg/h. *Children 1–9 years:* 5 mg/kg initially, then 0.8 mg/kg/h	• **IV:** Wait 4 h after IV has been stopped before administering immediate-release oral dose. Extended-release oral dose may be given at same time that IV is discontinued • Theophylline IV solution is wrapped in moisture-barrier overwrap, which should be removed just prior to administration. Check bag for leaks by squeezing. If solution is not clear, discard. Use infusion pump for accuracy • A loading dose of theophylline should be administered over 20–30 min. Monitor plasma drug levels
aminophylline (Aminophyl)	**Oral:** *Adults:* Loading dose, 500 mg followed by 250–500 mg q6–8h. *Children:* Loading dose, 7.5 mg/kg, followed by 3–6 mg/kg q6–8h **IV:** *Adults:* Loading dose, 5.6 mg/kg infused over 30 min, followed by 0.1–0.8 mg/kg/h continuous infusion. *Children:* Loading dose, 5.6 mg/kg followed by 0.8–1.2 mg/kg/h continuous infusion	• Give ATC. In case of od doses, administer in a.m. • **PO:** Give with full glass of water and meals to reduce gastric irritation. Do not crush enteric-coated or timed-release tablets or capsules • **IV:** Wait 4 h after IV has been stopped for administering immediate-release oral dose. Extended-release oral dose may be given at same time IV is discontinued. Flush IV line prior to administration
oxtriphylline (Choledyl)	**Oral:** *Adults:* Initially, 200–400 mg. Usual daily maint. dose, 800–1200 mg. *Children 10–14 years:* Initially, 22 mg/kg in first 24 h, divided into 4 equal doses. Usual maint. dose, 400–800 mg/24 h, divided into 4 equal doses given at 6-h intervals. *Children 5–9 years:* Usual daily maint. dose, 200–400 mg/24 h, divided into 4 equal doses given at 6-h intervals. *Children < 5 years:* Total daily dose, 24–36 mg/kg/24 h, divided into 3 equal doses given at 8-h intervals	• Give ATC. In case of sustained-release tabs, where dosage interval is larger, ensure that one dose is taken in a.m. • Give with full glass of water and meals to reduce gastric irritation. Do not crush enteric-coated or timed-release tablets or capsules
C. Anticholinergic Drug		
ipratropium bromide (Atrovent)	**Inhalation aerosol:** 2 metered doses (40 µg) tid–qid. Some pts may need to 4 metered doses (80 µg) at a time to obtain max. benefit during early tx. Max. dose should not exceed 8 metered doses (160 µg), and min. interval between doses should not be < 4 h	• If drug is ordered concurrently with other inhalation medications, ipratropium should be given first. There should be a pause of 2 min between inhalations

Table 69.5 (continued)
The antiasthmatics: Drug doses

Drug Generic name (Trade names)	Dosage	Nursing alert
D. Corticosteroids		
beclomethasone dipropionate (Beclovent, Vanceril)	**Inhalation aerosol** (Beclovent®): *Adults:* Usual dosage, 200–400 µg/day, divided into 2–4 administrations (max., 1 mg/day). *Children 3–5 years:* 50 µg bid (max., 150 µg/day); *6–14 years,* 100 µg bid–qid (max., 500 µg/day) **Inhalation Rotacaps** (Beclovent®): *Adults:* Usual dosage, 200 µg tid or qid (max., 1 mg/day). *Children 6–14 years:* 100 µg bid. If needed, increase dosage to tid (max., 500 µg/day)	• Instruct pt in proper use of inhaler (Box 69.1, page 827). Bronchodilators should be administered prior to beclomethasone • Medication is delivered to lungs as pt inhales; thus, instruct pt to breathe in forcefully and deeply through mouthpiece. Pt should be instructed to rinse mouth with water after each inhalation to help prevent candidiasis. Cleansing dentures has same effect • Store medication between 2°–30°C (36°–86°F)
budesonide (Pulmicort Turbuhaler)	**Inhalation powder:** *Adults/children > 12 years:* Initially, 400–2400 µg/day, divided into 2–4 doses. Maint. dose is usually 200–400 µg bid, but higher doses may be necessary for longer or shorter periods in some pts. *Children 6–12 years:* Initially, 200–400 µg/day, in divided doses bid. Maint. tx is individualized at lowest effective dose	• Tell pts not to exceed dosage as prescribed, because of risk of hypothalamic–pituitary–adrenal axis suppression • Medication is delivered to lungs as pt inhales; thus, instruct pt to breathe in forcefully and deeply through mouthpiece. Pts should be instructed to rinse mouth with water after each inhalation to help prevent candidiasis. Cleaning dentures has the same effect • Container should not be stored in extreme heat nor broken, as contents are under pressure. Shake container before each spray
flunisolide (Bronalide)	**Inhalation Aerosol:** *Adults:* 2 inhalations bid, a.m. and evening, for total daily dose of 1 mg. Max. daily dose should not exceed 4 inhalations bid for total daily dose of 2 mg. *Children > 4 years:* 2 inhalations bid for total daily dose of 1 mg	• As for budesonide • Store medication between 2°–30°C (36°–86°F)
triamcinolone acetonide (Azmacort)	**Inhalation aerosol:** *Adults:* 2–4 inhalations tid–qid. Daily dose should not exceed 1.6 mg. *Children 6–12 years:* 1–2 inhalations tid–qid. Daily dose should not exceed 1.2 mg	• As for beclomethasone dipropionate

(cont'd on next page)

Table 69.5 (continued)
The antiasthmatics: Drug doses

Drug Generic name (Trade names)	Dosage	Nursing alert
D. Corticosteroids (cont'd)		
prednisone (Deltasone, Meticorten, Orasone)	**Oral:** *Adults:* Initially, daily dose of 5–60 mg	• Do not confuse this medication with prednisolone • Always titrate to lowest effective dose. Medication should be administered in a.m. to coincide with body's natural secretion of cortisol • **PO:** Give with meals to minimize gastric irritation. When giving liquid forms of drug, use calibrated measuring device for accuracy
methylprednisolone sodium succinate (Solu-Medrol)	**IV:** Initially, 20–100 mg over not < 10 min. Subsequent doses can be given q6h	• Reconstitute with solution provided. Rate can be 1 to several minutes for IV push. Solution for continuous infusion may appear hazy after dilution
E. Inhibitors of Inflammatory-Response Mediators		
cromolyn, sodium cromoglycate (Intal)	**Inhalation:** *Adults/children:* Initially, 1 Spincap® cartridge qid at 4- to 6-h intervals. Maintenance: 1 Spincap® q8–12 h	• After 2–4 weeks of this medication, other asthma medications may be reduced. This medication should not be used during acute asthma attack
nedocromil (Tilade)	**Inhalation aerosol:** *Adults/children > 12 years:* 2 puffs (4 mg) qid. Some pts can be maintained on 2 puffs bid	• Instruct pt re: proper technique for inhalation and care of drug/equipment (see Box 69.1, page 827) • This medication should not be used during acute asthma attack
ketotifen (Zaditen)	**Oral:** *Children ≥ 3 years:* Initially, 0.5 mg bid or 1 mg hs. Increase after approx. 5 days to 1 mg bid with a.m. and p.m. meals.	• Long-term drug tx is required with this medication. Benefits may not be realized until up to 3 months of tx
F. Leukotriene Receptor Antagonist		
zafirlukast (Accolate)	**Oral:** *Adults/children ≥ 12 years:* 20 mg bid for total daily dose of 40 mg	• Since food reduces bioavailability of zafirlukast, take drug at least 1 h ac or 2 h pc. Drug is not a bronchodilator and should not be used to treat acute episodes of asthma • Instruct pts not to decrease dose of drug or stop taking other antiasthmatics unless instructed physician

CHAPTER 70

Drugs for the Treatment of Rhinitis and Nasal Congestion

Topics Discussed
● Adrenergic vasoconstrictors
● Antihistamines
● Intranasal corticosteroids
● Intranasal histamine-release inhibitors
● For each class of drug: Mechanism of action and pharmacologic effects, therapeutic uses, adverse effects
● Nursing management

Drugs Discussed
astemizole (as-**tem**-mih-zole)
beclomethasone (beck-loe-**meth**-ah-zone)
brompheniramine (brome-fen-**eer**-ah-meen)
budesonide (byoo-**dess**-oh-nyde)
cetirizine (seh-**teer**-ih-zeen)
chlorpheniramine (klor-fen-**eer**-ah-meen)
clemastine (**klem**-as-teen)

cromolyn (**kroe**-moe-lin)
dexchlorpheniramine (dex-klor-fen-**eer**-ah-meen)
diphenhydramine (dye-fen-**hye**-drah-meen)
ephedrine (ef-**ed**-rin)
flunisolide (flew-**niss**-oh-lyde)
loratadine (lor-**at**-ah-deen)
naphazoline (naf-ah-**zole**-een)
oxymetazolone (ox-ee-met-**azz**-oh-lone)
phenylephrine (fen-il-**eff**-rin)
phenylpropanolamine (fen-il-proe-pan-**ole**-ah-meen)
pseudoephedrine (sue-doe-ef-**ed**-rin)
sodium cromoglycate (kroe-moe-**glye**-kate)
terfenadine (ter-**fen**-ah-deen)
tetrahydrozoline (tet-ra-hye-**droz**-oh-leen)
triamcinolone (trye-am-**sin**-oh-lone)
xylometazoline (zye-loe-met-**azz**-oh-leen)

Clinical Challenge

Consider this clinical challenge as you read through this chapter. The response to the challenge appears on page 836.

Rhinitis may be infectious or allergic in nature. If caused by allergic reactions, this troublesome set of symptoms may occur seasonally, as with reactions to pollen, or perennially, if caused by constant allergens such as house dust or animal dander.

As a home care nurse, you are visiting a client who complains of rhinitis and explains she experiences the symptoms periodically throughout the year. She has visited a drug store and is confused regarding the vast array of possible nasal sprays.

What advice would you give? What assessment data will you require?

An increase in nasal vascular congestion, resulting from such conditions as the common cold and inflammation of the nose and sinuses, reduces airflow. This chapter discusses the use of adrenergic vasoconstrictors, antihistamines, corticosteroids and histamine-release inhibitors in the treatment of rhinitis or nasal congestion.

Adrenergic Vasoconstrictors

Mechanism of Action and Pharmacologic Effects

Adrenergic vasoconstrictors stimulate alpha$_1$ receptors on blood vessels. When they are applied topically, their actions are restricted largely to the nasal mucosa. Administered orally, they may constrict vessels throughout the body, increasing peripheral resistance and blood pressure. Among the adrenergic vasoconstrictors currently available are ephedrine sulfate, naphazoline HCl (Privine®), oxymetazolone (Dristan®), phenylephrine HCl (Neo-Synephrine®), pseudoephedrine HCl (Sudafed®), tetrahydrozoline HCl (Tyzine®) and xylometazoline HCl (Neo-Synephrine II®, Otrivin®).

Therapeutic Uses

Adrenergic vasoconstrictors offer the patient temporary, symptomatic relief of the acute rhinitis that accompanies the common cold, hay fever, nonseasonal allergic rhinitis and sinusitis. When used topically in the form of drops or spray, they have a rapid onset of action. However, not all areas of the mucosa may be exposed to the drug. Furthermore, the topical route is more likely to produce rebound congestion, especially with chronic use.

Oral treatment may enable the vasoconstrictor to reach nasal areas not accessible if the drug is applied topically. Although the onset of action is slower following ingestion, the drug's duration of action is also longer. Oral therapy may result in a generalized vasoconstriction and an increase in blood pressure.

Adverse Effects

Applied topically, adrenergic vasoconstrictors can produce stinging, burning or dryness of the mucosa, and rebound hyperemia. Chronic abuse results in red, edematous mucosa. This results from rebound vasodilatation. As the effects of a drug wear off, previously constricted blood vessels dilate in an attempt to restore proper perfusion to the mucous membranes. The longer the vasoconstrictor is used, the more likely the patient is to experience rebound vasodilatation and red, edematous mucous membranes once the drug is stopped.

Systemic hypertension is usually not seen when the drugs are applied topically. However, systemic reactions can be seen, particularly in infants and children, if large doses are applied topically. These drugs should be used with great care in the young.

The adverse effects of oral administration include hypertension, palpitations, dizziness, nervousness and CNS stimulation. Constriction of the coronary vessels can lead to cardiac arrhythmias. Young patients and those suffering from cardiovascular disease are at greater risk.

Table 70.1 lists the clinically significant drug interactions with adrenergic vasoconstrictors.

Table 70.1
Adrenergic vasoconstrictors: Drug interactions

Drug	Interaction
Antidepressants, tricyclic	• TCAs can increase the activity of adrenergic vasoconstrictors. Because of the possibility of generalized vasoconstriction and tachycardia, vasoconstrictors should be used very cautiously in pts receiving TCAs
Monoamine oxidase inhibitors	• MAOIs can potentiate the effects of adrenergic vasoconstrictors and are contraindicated in pts receiving these drugs

Antihistamines

Mechanism of Action and Pharmacologic Effects

Antihistamines competitively block histamine$_1$ (H$_1$) receptors in the body, thereby preventing histamine from producing vasodilatation, increased capillary permeability and tissue edema. These drugs, which include astemizole (Hismanal®), diphenhydramine HCl (Benadryl®), clemastine fumarate (Tavist®), chlorpheniramine maleate (Chlor-Trimeton®, Chlor-Tripolon®), brompheniramine maleate (Dimetane®), dexchlorpheniramine maleate (Polaramine®), terfenadine (Seldane®), loratadine (Claritin®) and cetirizine (Reactine®), can be used for a variety of conditions in which the release and action of histamine play an important role. The general pharmacology of antihistamines is presented in Chapter 72. This chapter deals with their use only in the treatment of nasal congestion.

Therapeutic Uses

Antihistamines reduce the symptoms of sneezing, rhinorrhea and pruritus of the eyes, nose and throat in patients with allergic rhinitis. Their efficacy is better when the symptoms are of recent onset. Antihistamines are most effective when rhinorrhea is associated with nasal congestion. They may aggravate a dry stuffy nose, in which case patients are better treated with normal saline or a polyethylene glycol–propylene glycol solution, used alone or in combination with antihistamines.

The drugs are more effective in the treatment of seasonal allergic rhinitis than in nonseasonal, perennial allergic rhinitis. They are found in all cold preparations, but evidence for their effectiveness in this condition is not overwhelming. Antihistamines are often combined with adrenergic vasoconstrictors in many cold preparations.

Astemizole and terfenadine have been associated with rare cases of serious cardiovascular adverse events. These effects have limited the use of these drugs in recent years. (For further discussion, see Chapter 72.)

Adverse Effects

Sedation is the most common adverse effect of antihistamines. Astemizole, terfenadine, loratadine and cetirizine have minimal sedative effects. Except for patients taking these four drugs, all others should be warned of the dangers of driving a car or operating machinery during drug therapy, and informed about the additive effects of alcohol and antihistamines. Other manifestations of CNS depression are dizziness, lassitude, incoordination, fatigue, tinnitus and diplopia. Some patients, particularly children, may experience euphoria, nervousness, irritability, insomnia, tremors and an increased tendency towards convulsions.

The gastrointestinal adverse effects of antihistamines include nausea, vomiting, abdominal discomfort, constipation and diarrhea. Loss of appetite may also occur. Most antihistamines have anticholinergic properties and can cause dryness of the mouth, throat and nasal airway; tightness of the chest; palpitations; headache; and urinary retention. The drug interactions for these drugs are presented in Table 72.1 (page 847).

Corticosteroids

Mechanism of Action and Pharmacologic Effects

The general pharmacology of corticosteroids is presented in Chapter 66. They are potent anti-inflammatory drugs. Applied topically, they reduce erythema and edema in nasal passages.

Therapeutic Uses

Beclomethasone dipropionate (Beconase®, Vancenase®), budesonide (Rhinocort Aqua®, Rhinocort Turbuhaler®), flunisolide (Nasalide®, Rhinalar®) and triamcinolone acetonide (Nasacort®) are formulated for topical nasal use. Although they are officially indicated for the treatment of perennial and seasonal allergic rhinitis unresponsive to conventional therapy, many physicians use them as first-line drugs in allergic rhinitis because they have fewer side effects and are more effective than antihistamines.

These products may also be helpful in the

management of rhinitis of physical or chemical origin, and for treatment of rhinitis medicamentosa resulting from the overzealous use of topical vasoconstrictors. Polyposis originating in the nasal cavity may be controllable with topical steroids, but surgical excision is often still required.

Adverse Effects

Local reactions include a burning sensation in the nose, sneezing attacks and, on occasion, bloody nasal discharge. Patients may develop localized candida infections. If high doses of these drugs are applied to the nose, sufficient quantities may be absorbed to depress the hypothalamic–pituitary–adrenal axis and produce generalized systemic effects. Long-term use may lead to atrophic rhinitis. The drug interactions for corticosteroids are presented in Table 66.2 (page 784).

Histamine-Release Inhibitors

Cromolyn/Sodium Cromoglycate (Rynacrom®)

The pharmacology of cromolyn, or sodium cromoglycate, is discussed in greater detail in Chapter 69. The drug reduces the release of histamine following an antigen–antibody reaction. This property accounts for its prophylactic use in the treatment of seasonal rhinitis. Insufflated as a two percent solution, cromolyn affords relief to many patients afflicted with seasonal rhinitis. Other than slight local irritation, cromolyn causes few adverse effects.

Nursing Management

Table 70.2 describes the nursing management of the patient receiving decongestant drugs. Dosage details for individual drugs are given in Table 70.3 (pages 838–839) in this chapter and Table 72.3 (pages 849–851) for the antihistamines.

Response to Clinical Challenge

First, you should explore the symptoms, occurrence, known allergens and any successful attempts to avoid these. Explain the differences between allergic and infectious rhinitis. Discuss the value of medical diagnosis and treatment versus self-diagnosis and self-treatment. Emphasize the role of the phamacist in providing advice regarding the choice of products and in discussing other drugs that the client may be taking concurrently. Many community pharmacists provide a private counselling area.

Further Reading

Flonase and budesonide: two new rhinitis remedies. *Am J Nurs* 1995;95(3):57–59.

Henderson G. Budesonide in asthma. *Austr Nurses J* 1992;21(11).

Pfister SM. Drug news: ipratropium bromide nasal spray. *Nurse Pract/Am J Prim Health Care* 1996; 21(7):104–108.

Pharmacology update. Perfect timing: overview of chronotherapy. *Nurse Pract Forum* 1996;7(1):7–9.

Pseudoephedrine: safe for controlled hypertension. *Nurses Drug Alert* 1995;19(3):17–18.

Self T. Continuing education forum: treatment of rhinitis. *J Am Acad Nurse Pract* 1996;8(3):135–147.

There's a new corticosteroid for seasonal rhinitis. *RN* 1996;59(4):74.

Table 70.2
Nursing management of the decongestants

Assessment of risk vs. benefit	Patient data	• Many of these drugs are available in OTC nasal drops/sprays and tablets for self-medication. Generally, drops rather than sprays should be used for children < 6 years to ensure greater accuracy of dosage. Drug should be administered by an adult • In general, clinical data are insufficient regarding use in pregnancy and lactation; pt should discuss with physician • Public education regarding choice of drug, proper use and possible risks associated with prolonged use is an important nursing contribution to safe drug use in society
	Drug data	• Encourage pts to read labels carefully, particularly to note any contraindications to drug use, e.g., glaucoma or hypertension. Advise pts always to use the same community pharmacist and to seek advice prior to self-medication
Implementation	Rights of administration	• Using the "rights" helps prevent errors of administration

	Right technique	• **Nasal spray:** Have pt gently blow nose, ensure head is upright, insert nozzle into nostril and avoid touching side of nasal passage, if possible. Squeeze required number of sprays while inhaling. Repeat in other nostril. Tip of spray bottle should be rinsed with hot water after each use
		• **Nasal drops:** Have pt gently blow nose, squeeze bulb to load the dropper chamber with medication
		  – *To treat nasal passages:* Lie flat; aim dropper towards back of nose; squeeze bulb, counting correct number of drops. Breathe through mouth
		  – *To treat sinuses:* Tilt head back; place prescribed number of drops in one nostril; breathe through nose to help move drug into sinuses. Repeat in other nostril. Remain in this position up to 5 min Avoid touching nasal passage with the dropper, if possible. Rinse dropper with hot water and return to bottle. Do not share device with anyone else

	Nursing therapeutics	• Enhance host defences (nutrition, rest, fluids, hygiene)
	Patient/family teaching	• Instruct pt/family in proper technique • Emphasize importance of short-term use only, unless otherwise ordered by physician. Stress prevention of rebound congestion caused by overuse or prolonged use (> 5 days) • Caution pt that mild stinging or tingling may occur during administration • Explain that topical route of administration can result in some systemic absorption of drug with resulting side effects, although generally these are less pronounced with this route
Outcomes	Monitoring of progress	• Instruct pt/family in self-monitoring of symptoms

Table 70.3
Treatment of rhinitis and nasal congestion: Drug doses

Drug Generic name (Trade names)	Dosage	Nursing alert
A. Adrenergic Vasoconstrictors		
oxymetazoline HCl (Afrin, Duration, Neo-Synephrine 12-Hour)	**Topical solution/spray:** *Adults/children ≥ 6 years:* 2–4 drops or 2–3 squeezes 0.05% solution in each nostril, a.m. and hs for no more than 3–5 days. *Children 2–5 years:* 2–3 drops 0.025% solution in each nostril q 10–12 h	• Instruct pt in self-administration of nasal drops/spray
phenylephrine HCl (Coridicin Nasal Mist, Neo-Synephrine HCl)	**Intranasal:** *Adults:* 2–3 drops 0.25–1% solution or jelly q3–4h prn. *Infants:* Use 0.125% solution	• Instruct pt in self-administration of nasal drops/spray
phenylpropanolamine HCl (Propadine, Propagest)	**Oral:** *Adults:* 25 mg q4h. *Children 6–12 years:* 12.5 mg q4h	• Do not administer to children < 2 years old except on advice of physician
pseudoephedrine HCl (Eltor, Neosynephrinol, Novafed, Sudafed)	**Oral:** *Adults:* 60 mg tid–qid. *Children 6–11 years:* 30 mg q4–6h; *2–5 years:* 15 mg q4–6h	• Give 2 h before bedtime to minimize insomnia. Do not crush, break or allow pt to chew extended-release tablets. Should pt have difficulty swallowing, capsules may be mixed with jam or jelly and swallowed whole
xylometazoline HCl (Otrivin, Otrivin Pediatric Nasal Drops)	**Intranasal:** Use q8–10 h. *Adults:* 1–2 sprays (0.1% solution) or 2–3 drops (0.1%) into each nostril. *Children > 6 years:* 1–2 sprays (0.05%) or 2–3 drops (0.05%) in each nostril. *Children < 6 years:* 1 spray (0.05%) or 1 drop (0.05%)	• Instruct pt in self-administration of nasal drops/spray
B. Antihistamines		
For dosage information on antihistamines, consult Table 72.3, pages 849–851		
C. Corticosteroids		
beclomethasone dipropionate (Beconase, Vancenase)	**Intranasal:** 2 applications (100 µg beclomethasone dipropionate) into each nostril bid. A dosage regimen of 1 application into each nostril tid or qid may be preferred	• Decongestant or antihistamine may be administered prior to nasal spray

Table 70.3 (continued)
Treatment of rhinitis and nasal congestion: Drug doses

Drug Generic name (Trade names)	Dosage	Nursing alert
C. Corticosteroids (cont'd)		
budesonide (Rhinocort Aqua, Rhinocort Turbuhaler)	**Rhinocort Aqua®:** (Rhinitis): *Adults/children* ≥ *6 years:* Initially: Total daily dose, 400 µg. This dose should not be exceeded in children. Can be used od–bid. Once daily: 2 sprays (200 µg) into each nostril in a.m. Twice daily: 1 spray (100 µg) into each nostril, a.m. and p.m. Use lowest maintenance dose to control symptoms. (Tx/prevention of nasal polyps): One spray (100 µg) into each nostril, a.m. and p.m. (total daily dose, 400 µg) **Rhinocort Turbuhaler®:** *Adults/children* ≥ *6 years:* Initially, 2 applications into each nostril in a.m. (total daily dose, 400 µg). Use lowest maint. dose to control symptoms	• Instruct pt in self-administration of nasal spray
flunisolide (Nasalide, Rhinalar)	**Intranasal:** *Adults:* Initially, 2 sprays into each nostril bid. Increase to tid if needed. *Children 6–14 years:* Initially, 1 spray into each nostril tid. For both children and adults, use lowest effective maint. dose	• Pt should use decongestant or blow nose before administration to ensure proper absorption
triamcinolone acetonide (Nasacort)	**Intranasal:** *Adults/children* ≥ *12 years:* Initially, 400 µg/day, given as 2 sprays (100 µg/spray) in each nostril od. If needed, increase dose to 800 µg/day (100 µg/spray) bid or qid (i.e., 2 sprays/nostril bid or 1 spray/nostril qid). After desired effect is obtained, pts may be maintained on a dose of 1 spray (100 µg) in each nostril od (total daily dose, 200 µg/day)	• If also using a topical decongestant, inhale triamcinolone 5–15 min after other drug. Instruct pt to blow nose gently if unable to breathe freely prior to drug administration
D. Histamine-Release Inhibitor		
cromolyn, sodium cromoglycate (Rynacrom)	**Intranasal:** *Adults/children* > *5 years:* Initially, 1 mist into each nostril 6x daily. One mist delivers approx. 2.6 mg sodium cromoglycate. Maintenance: When adequate response has been obtained, frequency of inhalations may be reduced to 1 metered dose to each nostril q8–12h	• Instruct pt in self-administration of nasal spray

CHAPTER 71

Antitussives

Topics Discussed
- Nonproductive vs. productive coughs
- Cough suppressants
- Expectorants
- For each drug class: Mechanism of action and pharmacologic effects, therapeutic uses, adverse effects
- Nursing management

Drugs Discussed
codeine (**koe**-deen)
dextromethorphan (dex-troe-meh-**thor**-fan)
diphenhydramine (dye-fen-**hye**-drah-meen)
guaifenesin (gwye-**fen**-eh-sin)
hydrocodone (hye-droe-**koe**-done)

Clinical Challenge

Consider this clinical challenge as you read through this chapter. The response to the challenge appears on page 843.

As a pediatric nurse specialist, you are invited by a parents' group to give a presentation on common childhood illnesses, including the common cold and coughs.

The group provides a list of questions, including, "When should I treat a cough in my children?" and "What should I look for in a cough suppressant?"

Nonproductive versus Productive Coughs

Many over-the-counter "cough medicines" are available; however, confusion exists as to the best product for the particular patient. This is not surprising, because most cough medicines are sold on the basis of their own "unique" ingredients, rather than on an analysis of the type of cough experienced.

Nurses are well aware that patients can suffer from two types of coughs. The first, a dry, hacking, nonproductive cough, torments the patient with its incessant tickling. Yielding to the temptation for just one more cough results in more irritation and distress before the tickle and urge return again. In productive coughs, by contrast, the congested patient may woof up copious amounts of phlegm from a seemingly bottomless well. It is obvious that these two disparate, but equally pathetic, problems warrant different treatments.

Nonproductive, hyperactive coughs should be treated with a drug to stop the patient from coughing. The irritation of a nonproductive cough may be further relieved by the demulcent action of an expectorant that increases respiratory secretions.

Patients with congested, productive coughs should not receive a cough suppressant. It is bad enough to be drowning in one's own secretions without being given a drug that removes the urge to cough them up. Such patients should be assisted in their attempts to clear phlegm. Often all that is required is adequate fluids and humid air. An expectorant may also help to remove phlegm.

The multitude of cough preparations on the market makes it impossible to discuss each separately. Instead, attention will be directed to the types of drugs often used to treat coughs.

It should also be mentioned that many cough

preparations contain an antihistamine and/or a vasoconstrictor. Antihistamines are discussed in Chapter 72 and vasoconstrictors in Chapter 70; thus, they will not be considered here. There is little doubt that vasoconstrictors reduce congestion and promote easier breathing. The rationale for including antihistamines, except for diphenhydramine (which is also a cough suppressant), is less clear. It is possible that the anticholinergic activity of antihistamines allows them to provide a drying effect. Furthermore, coughs due to allergies most certainly will be helped by the inclusion of an antihistamine in the antitussive mixture.

Cough Suppressants

Mechanism of Action and Pharmacologic Effects

Cough suppressants depress the cough centre in the medulla oblongata area of the brain. As a result, the urge to cough is significantly reduced: the tormenting tickle is, at least for the moment, set to rest. Narcotics are the most effective cough suppressants. Codeine and hydrocodone (Dicodid®, Hycodan®) are often used for this purpose. Dextromethorphan is an effective non-narcotic cough suppressant found in both prescription and OTC products.

Therapeutic Uses

Cough suppressants should be used to treat non-productive, dry, hacking coughs. Codeine syrup is excellent for this purpose. Hydrocodone is also very effective, but it is more potent than codeine and thus has a greater abuse liability. Over the past decade, hydrocodone has become a popular street drug.

Dextromethorphan is popular as a cough suppressant in most OTC products. It is effective and has little dependence liability.

Diphenhydramine (Benadryl®) also suppresses the cough reflex, if given in adequate doses.

Adverse Effects

The adverse effects of narcotics are discussed in Chapter 52. Normal antitussive doses of codeine and hydrocodone are generally well tolerated. The most frequently encountered adverse reactions include nausea, vomiting, constipation and dizziness. CNS depression is particularly likely to occur if the patient is also taking an antihistamine. Patients should be warned about the dangers of operating machinery or driving a car during drug therapy. Respiratory depression occurs when large doses are taken and is more prevalent in children under the age of five. Continuous use can lead to drug dependency, particularly with hydrocodone.

The adverse effects of dextromethorphan are usually mild. They include drowsiness, nausea and dizziness. Diphenhydramine can produce significant sedation.

Table 71.1 lists the clinically significant drug interactions with cough suppressants.

Expectorants

Mechanism of Action and Pharmacologic Effects

An expectorant is a drug that increases the output of respiratory tract fluid. Guaifenesin (glyceryl guaiacolate) is the most commonly used expectorant. However, little objective evidence can be found to support its effectiveness. Guaifenesin irritates the gastric mucosa. This action may reflexly

Table 71.1
Cough suppressants: Drug interactions

Drug	Interaction
Ethanol	• Ethanol may demonstrate increased CNS depression in the presence of codeine, hydrocodone or diphenhydramine
MAOIs	• Monoamine oxidase inhibitors may require lower dosage in the presence of codeine or hydrocodone
TCAs and phenothiazines	• Tricyclic antidepressants and phenothiazines may demonstrate increased CNS depression in the presence of codeine, hydrocodone or diphenhydramine

stimulate the parasympathetic nervous system to increase respiratory secretions.

Therapeutic Uses and Adverse Effects

Guaifenesin is given to increase the flow of respiratory secretions, thereby decreasing the viscosity of phlegm and enabling the patient to clear congestion. It is also contended that the increased secretions will soothe the irritated membranes and reduce the stimulus to cough. Guaifenesin can cause drowsiness and nausea.

Nursing Management

Table 71.2 describes the nursing management of the patient receiving antitussive drugs. Dosage details of individual drugs are given in Table 71.3 (pages 843–844).

Table 71.2
Nursing management of the antitussives

Assessment of risk vs. benefit	Patient data	• Generally used for short-term self-medication. Pts should be encouraged to read labels carefully, consult pharmacist regarding potential interactions with other medications • *Pregnancy:* Risk category varies; consult physician
	Drug data	• When used as directed, generally well tolerated Most serious adverse effects occur with overdose or prolonged use
Implementation	Rights of administration	• Using the "rights" helps to prevent errors in administration
	Right technique	• **PO:** Advise parents to use calibrated device to ensure accurate doses for children
	Nursing therapeutics	• Enhance host defences (nutrition, rest, fluids, hygiene). Use symptomatic care (e.g., increase fluid intake) • Use asepsis to prevent spread of infection (including self-care for caregivers)
	Patient/family teaching	• Instruct pts/families re: hygienic measures to reduce spread of infection • Discuss supportive measures to alleviate symptoms and provide comfort • Explain difference between productive and nonproductive coughing; teach measures to stimulate coughing and to provide relief (increased fluid intake, deep breathing, lozenges for dry cough) • Explain that drugs may cause drowsiness: avoid hazardous activity until response to drug is known • Remind parents that cough syrups may appeal to small children; store safely • *Discuss possibility of pregnancy:* Advise pt to notify physician; discuss birth control methods
Outcomes	Monitoring of progress	• Remind pts/families to observe reactions to drug use and report any unusual responses

Response to Clinical Challenge

General points to address:

When should I treat a cough in my children?
- productive versus nonproductive cough
- impact of symptoms on child
- alternative measures
- value of encouraging coughing and supportive measures to reduce discomfort.

What should I look for in a cough suppressant?
- overview of action of dextromethorphan
- expected side effects
- comparison of dextromethorphan and narcotic antitussives regarding actions and side effects

Further Reading

Delirium with single dose of diphenhydramine. *Nurses Drug Alert* 1995;19(1):4–5.

Table 71.3
The antitussives: Drug doses

Drug Generic name (Trade names)	Dosage	Nursing alert
A. Cough Suppressants		
codeine	**Oral:** *Adults:* 5–10 mg q3–4h prn. *Children:* 1–1.5 mg/kg/day, divided into 6 doses	• Give with food or milk to minimize GI irritation • Not recommended for children < 2 years and only with physician's advice for children aged 2–5 years
hydrocodone bitartrate	**Oral:** Doses to be taken not < 4 h apart, pc and hs, with food or milk. *Adults:* 5 mg, not to exceed 30 mg in a 24-h period. Max. single dose, 15 mg. *Children > 12 years:* 5 mg, not to exceed 30 mg/24 h. Max. single dose, 10 mg. *Children 2–12 years:* 2.5 mg, not to exceed 15 mg/24 h. Max. single dose, 5 mg. *Children < 2 years:* 1.25 mg, not to exceed 7.5 mg/24 h. Max. single dose, 1.25 mg	• Administer in a.m. to prevent insomnia and/or disruption of sleep cycle • Give with food or milk to minimize GI irritation. Should pt have difficulty swallowing, may crush tablets and mix with fluid
dextromethorphan HCl	**Oral:** *Adults:* 10–20 mg q4h. *Children:* 1 mg/kg/day in 3–4 divided doses	• Drug has no analgesic effect and produces little or no CNS depression • To prevent dilution, do not give fluids immediately after administering. Be certain to shake suspension before administration

(cont'd on next page)

Table 71.3 (continued)
The antitussives: Drug doses

Drug Generic name (Trade names)	Dosage	Nursing alert
A. Cough Suppressants (cont'd)		
diphenhydramine HCl (Benylin)	**Oral:** *Adults:* 25 mg q4h. Max. dose, 150 mg/24 h. *Children 6–11 years:* 12.5 mg q4h or 5 mg/kg/day in 4 divided doses. Max. dose, 75 mg/day	• Give hs to benefit from sedative effects • Use cautiously in children aged 2–5 years; may cause paradoxical excitement • Give with meals or milk to minimize GI irritation. Contents of capsules may be mixed with food or water • Drug may negatively influence allergy skin tests
B. Expectorants		
guaifenesin, glyceryl guaiacolate	**Oral:** *Adults:* 200–400 mg q4h. Max. dose, 2.4 g/day. *Children 6–12 years:* 50–100 mg q4–6h. Max. dose, 600 mg/day	• To prevent dilution, do not administer fluids immediately following ingestion of liquid preparation. If sustained-released tablets are ordered, do not break, crush or allow pt to chew them

CHAPTER 72

Antihistamines

Topics Discussed
● Antihistamines: Mechanism of action and pharmacologic effects, therapeutic uses, adverse effects
● Nursing management

Drugs Discussed
astemizole (as-**tem**-mih-zole)
azatadine (az-**at**-ah-deen)
brompheniramine (brome-fen-**eer**-ah-meen)
cetirizine (seh-**teer**-ih-zeen)
chlorpheniramine (klor-fen-**eer**-ah-meen)

clemastine (**klem**-as-teen)
cyproheptadine (sye-proe-**hep**-tah-deen)
dexchlorpheniramine (dex-klor-fen-**eer**-ah-meen)
diphenhydramine (dye-fen-**hye**-drah-meen)
hydroxyzine (hye-**drox**-ih-zeen)
loratadine (lor-**at**-ah-deen)
methdilazine (meth-**dill**-ah-zeen)
promethazine (proe-**meth**-ah-zeen)
terfenadine (ter-**fen**-ah-deen)
trimeprazine (trye-**mep**-raz-een)
tripelennamine (trye-pel-**en**-ah-meen)
triprolidine (trye-**proe**-lih-deen)

Clinical Challenge

Consider this clinical challenge as you read through this chapter. The response to the challenge appears on page 847.

Jim is a 37-year-old pianist with a symphony orchestra. He has several allergies including certain foods, dust and common environmental stimuli such as paints and perfumes. When troubled by allergic reactions, including gastric and nasal symptoms, he has difficulty performing with the orchestra. Friends and family have advised him to "learn to live with the symptoms" and avoid drugs. Some friends encourage him to try natural remedies rather than nonprescription medications. Jim asks for your advice and information.

What concepts should guide your conversation?

All antihistamines, regardless of their chemical structures, have the same basic mechanism of action and the same major adverse effects.

Mechanism of Action and Pharmacologic Effects

Antihistamines reversibly block histamine$_1$ (H_1) receptors. They prevent histamine from contracting smooth muscle, dilating blood vessels, increasing capillary permeability, inducing tissue edema and stimulating mucus secretion. Not all histamine-mediated effects are blocked by these drugs; for example, antihistamines do not inhibit histamine-induced bronchiolar constriction. Nor do they prevent histamine from stimulating gastric acid secretion (an H_2 receptor-mediated effect).

Therapeutic Uses

Antihistamines are used to treat a variety of allergic disorders. However, because histamine is only one mediator of allergic reactions, antihistamines may provide only partial relief of many of the symptoms. Patients with mild symptoms of recent onset are generally more responsive to antihistamines. Patients with chronic illness derive less benefit. Antihistamines are least effective in controlling the symptoms of severe allergic or immunologic disease, including anaphylaxis.

Foremost among the conditions for which antihistamines are used are upper respiratory allergies, characterized by sneezing, rhinorrhea and pruritus of the nose, eyes and throat. Antihistamines usually relieve these symptoms, particularly if they are of recent onset. Hay fever (seasonal allergic rhinitis) responds better to antihistaminic therapy than nonseasonal, perennial allergic rhinitis. Patients with vasomotor rhinitis experience variable relief from antihistamines. Lower respiratory disorders with bronchospasm do not respond well to antihistamines.

Although most cough and cold preparations contain antihistamines, their value is still the subject of considerable controversy. Any effect antihistamines may have in drying the nose likely results from their anticholinergic properties.

Antihistamines often relieve the pruritic component of acute urticaria. Although angioedema will respond, at least partly, to antihistamines, epinephrine is the drug of choice for severe, life-threatening situations. While topical preparations are available for the treatment of allergic conjunctivitis, cases of allergic dermatitis and pruritus resulting from an insect sting respond better to oral therapy. Long-term topical antihistamine use may cause sensitization.

Antihistamines are often ineffective in the treatment of hypersensitivity reactions to drugs, foods and allergens. The serious manifestations of hypersensitivity reactions, such as hypotension and bronchoconstriction, also fail to respond to antihistamines. The flushing, urticaria and pruritus of transfusion reactions are usually reduced by antihistamine treatment.

Antihistamines are used for a number of indications that appear unrelated to their ability to block H_1 receptors. Their sedative effects have made them popular drugs in OTC sleeping preparations. Hydroxyzine (Atarax®, Vistaril®) and promethazine (Phenergan®) are used for preoperative sedation. Cyproheptadine (Periactin®) is used as an appetite stimulant; it is claimed to stimulate both linear growth and weight gain in children. Unfortunately, this effect is transient and disappears when the drug is stopped. Several antihistamines are used for their antiemetic effects, and these are discussed in Chapter 62.

Adverse Effects

The adverse effects of antihistamines are rarely serious and usually disappear within a few days of stopping treatment. Sedation is the most frequently encountered effect, and patients should be warned about the dangers of working around moving machinery or driving a car. They should also be informed of the additive effects of taking antihistamines with other CNS depressants such as ethanol, benzodiazepines and barbiturates. Other adverse effects attributable to CNS depression are dizziness, lassitude, incoordination, fatigue, tinnitus and diplopia.

Four antihistamines — astemizole (Hismanal®), cetirizine (Reactine®), loratadine (Claritin®) and terfenadine (Seldane®) — produce minimal CNS depression. For this reason, these drugs are often called second-generation antihistamines, in contrast to the older (first-generation) sedative antihistamines.

Paradoxic adverse effects of antihistamines include euphoria, irritability, insomnia and increased tendency to convulsions.

Loss of appetite is a common adverse effect of most antihistamines. Nausea and vomiting are also experienced by some patients. Other adverse effects include abdominal discomfort, constipation and diarrhea. Their anticholinergic effects cause dry mouth, throat and nasal passages. Tightness of the chest, headache, palpitations and urinary retention or dysuria can also occur.

Astemizole and terfenadine have been associat-

Table 72.1
Antihistamines: Drug interactions

Drug	Interaction
CNS depressants	• Ethanol, hypnotics, anxiolytics and other CNS depressants have additive depressant effects with most antihistamines. This interaction is probably not seen with astemizole, cetirizine, loratadine and terfenadine
Erythromycin and ketoconazole	• Together with either astemizole or terfenadine, these drugs can produce cardiac toxicities. Concurrent use is contraindicated
Fluconazole, itraconazole, metronidazole, miconazole	• Because of the chemical similarity of these drugs to ketoconazole, concomitant use with astemizole or terfenadine is contraindicated
Quinine	• Therapeutic doses of quinine can decrease the metabolism of astemizole and result in elevated plasma levels. Concurrent use is contraindicated

ed with rare cases of serious cardiovascular events, including arrhythmias. These effects can occur when either antihistamine is used in the daily recommended dose in conjunction with erythromycin and/or ketoconazole. The latter drugs inhibit the metabolism of astemizole and terfenadine, thereby predisposing patients to their cardiac toxicities. The cardiac effects of astemizole and terfenadine are also rarely seen in patients not taking either ketoconazole or erythromycin, and these adverse effects have limited the use of these antihistamines.

Table 72.1 lists the clinically significant drug interactions with antihistamines.

Nursing Management

Table 72.2 on the next page describes the nursing management of the patient receiving antihistamines. Dosage details of individual drugs are given in Table 72.3 (pages 848–851).

Response to Clinical Challenge

Essential points for discussion would include:

• Jim's beliefs regarding medication, both in terms of expected effects and compliance
• research regarding causes of allergy
• research regarding safety and efficacy of antihistamines
• risks and benefits of natural remedies, including lack of scientific testing regarding safety
• impact of symptoms on his functional ability, and lifestyle factors that may enhance/inhibit allergic reactions
• emotional support with regard to the daily disruption he experiences and the unpredictable nature of chronic allergy
• individual trial-and-error use, which is often required to find the best antihistamine
• taking medication to prevent reactions to known allergens, such as expected exposure to pets

Further Reading

Astemizole associated with Stevens-Johnson syndrome. *Nurses Drug Alert* 1995;19(10):80.
Casillas AM. Non-sedating antihistamines: an overview. *Physician Assistant* 1993;17(3):47–54.
Gordon D. Pain control: hydroxyzine doesn't 'help' opioids. *Am J Nurs* 1995;95(8):20.
Holdcroft C. Terfenadine, astemizole and loratadine: second-generation antihistamines. *Nurse Pract/ Am J Prim Health Care* 1993;18(11):13–14.
Lilley LL. Medication errors: the new antihistamines. *Am J Nurs* 1995;95(5):14.
Mathewson HS. Drug capsule: antihistamines and asthma. *Resp Care* 1996;41(3):212–214.

Table 72.2
Nursing management of the antihistamines

Assessment of risk vs. benefit	Patient data	• Drugs often used for self-medication. Pts should read label carefully or consult pharmacist • Pts with the following chronic problems should use these drugs cautiously: asthma, glaucoma, hyperthyroidism, CV disease or diabetes. Doses should be reduced for older pts • *Pregnancy:* Risk category varies; consult physician
	Drug data	• Generally, these drugs are well tolerated. First-generation drugs may cause drowsiness • May negatively influence allergy skin tests and should be stopped 4 days prior to such an evaluation
Implementation	Nursing therapeutics	• *Emotional support:* Chronic allergic reactions may be unpredictable in occurrence and severity and cause considerable disruption in pt's life • Store elixirs and parenteral preparations in light-resistant containers at room temperature
	Patient/family teaching	• Encourage pts to consult pharmacist prior to self-medication • First-generation drugs cause drowsiness: caution pts to avoid hazardous activities until reaction is known • Advise supportive measures such as fluid intake, lifestyle changes to avoid allergens, sugarless candy for dry mouth • Warn pts to avoid alcohol with first-generation drugs (increased risk for CNS depression)
Outcomes	Monitoring of progress	*Continually monitor:* • Clinical response indicating tx success (reduction in signs/symptoms)

Table 72.3
The antihistamines: Drug doses

Drug Generic name (Trade names)	Dosage	Nursing alert
astemizole (Hismanal)	**Oral:** *Adults/children > 12 years:* 10 mg od; *6–12 years:* 5 mg od; *< 6 years:* 2 mg/10 kg/day	• Give on empty stomach, 2 h pc or 1 h ac • Oral formulation is given od • Drug may negatively influence allergy skin tests and should be stopped 4 days prior to such an evaluation
azatadine maleate (Optimine)	**Oral:** *Adults:* 1 mg a.m. and p.m. In refractory or more severe cases, 2 mg bid may be used. *Children 6–12 years:* 0.5–1 mg bid	• Give with food or milk to reduce GI irritation • Drug may negatively influence allergy skin tests and should be stopped 4 days prior to such an evaluation

Table 72.3 (continued)
The antihistamines: Drug doses

Drug Generic name (Trade names)	Dosage	Nursing alert
brompheniramine maleate (Dimetane)	**Oral:** *Adults:* 4–6 mg tid–qid, or 1 sustained-release 8- or 12-mg tablet q8–12 h. *Children 6–12 years:* 2 mg q4–6h, or 1 sustained-release 8- or 12- mg tablet q12h **IM/IV/SC:** *Adults:* 5–20 mg q3–12h. Max. dose, 40 mg/day. *Children < 12 years:* 0.5 mg/kg/day, divided into 3–4 doses	• **PO:** Give with food or milk to reduce GI irritation. Extended-release tablets should not be crushed or chewed; ensure pt swallows them whole • **IV:** May be ordered in undiluted form. If dilution ordered, for each 10 mL of 10 mg/mL solution dilute with 10 mL of 0.9% NaCl. This should reduce side effects. Each dose should be given over 1 min. Diluted solution may be further diluted for intermittent infusion. Follow agency policy for direct administration • Drug may negatively influence allergy skin tests and should be stopped 4 days prior to such an evaluation
cetirizine HCl (Reactine)	**Oral:** *Adults/children > 12 years:* Initially, 5–10 mg, given od with or without food. If needed, dose may be increased to 20 mg/day. *Geriatrics:* Consider initiating tx with 5 mg/day. *Pts with reduced creatinine clearance:* Initially, 5 mg/day	• May be taken without regard to food
chlorpheniramine maleate (Chlor-Trimeton, Chlor-Tripolon)	**Oral:** *Adults:* 4 mg q4–6h, or 1 timed-release 12-mg capsule bid. *Children < 12 years:* 2 mg q6–8h **IM/IV/SC:** *Adults:* 5–40 mg. **SC:** *Children < 12 years:* 0.35 mg/kg/day, divided into 4 doses	• **PO:** Give with food or milk to reduce GI irritation. Extended-release tablets should not be crushed or chewed; ensure pt swallows them whole. Chewable tablets should not be swallowed whole • **IM/SC:** 20 mg/mL or 100 mg/mL solutions are recommended • **IV:** May be given undiluted; use only the 10 mg/mL strength. Each dose should be administered over 1 min. Follow agency policy for direct administration • Drug may negatively influence allergy skin tests and should be stopped 4 days prior to such an evaluation
clemastine fumarate (Tavist)	**Oral:** *Adults/children > 12 years:* 2 mg/day in divided doses. In refractory cases, up to 6 mg daily	• Give with food or milk to reduce GI irritation • Drug may negatively influence allergy skin tests and should be stopped 4 days prior to such an evaluation
cyproheptadine (Periactin)	**Oral:** *Adults:* 4–20 mg/day; not to exceed 32 mg/day. *Children 7–14 years:* Initially, 2 mg tid–qid. Usual maint. dosage: 4 mg bid–tid, not to exceed 16 mg/day	• As for clemastine fumarate, above

(cont'd on next page)

Table 72.3 (continued)
The antihistamines: Drug doses

Drug Generic name (Trade names)	Dosage	Nursing alert
dexchlorpheniramine (Polaramine)	**Oral:** *Adults/children > 12 years:* 2 mg tid–qid. Alternatively, a single 6-mg Repetabs® tablet may be taken a.m. and hs. *Children 6–12 years:* 1 mg tid–qid	• Drug may negatively influence allergy skin tests and should be stopped 4 days prior to such an evaluation
diphenhydramine (Benadryl)	**Oral:** *Adults:* 25–50 mg tid–qid. *Children < 12 years:* 5 mg/kg/day, in 4 divided doses over 24 h **IV/IM:** *Adults:* 10–50 mg. Max. dose, 400 mg/day. *Children:* 5 mg/kg/day, in 4 divided doses. Max. dose, 300 mg/day	• **For motion sickness:** Administer at least 30 min and preferably 1–2 h prior to travel • **PO:** Give with food or milk. Capsules may be emptied and mixed with food • **IM:** Inject into a well-developed muscle; massage well • **IV:** May be given undiluted. Inject at a rate of 25 mg/min. Follow agency policy regarding direct injection
hydroxyzine HCl (Atarax)	**Oral:** *Adults:* Initially, 25 mg tid; increase prn to 100 mg qid. *Children < 6 years:* 30–50 mg/day, divided into 3–4 doses; *> 6 years:* 50–100 mg/day, divided into 3–4 doses	• Give with food or milk. Tablets may be crushed and capsules may be emptied and mixed with food. Shake suspension well prior to administration
loratadine (Claritin)	**Oral:** *Adults/children > 12 years:* 10 mg od	• Give od on empty stomach, 1 h ac • Drug may negatively influence allergy skin tests and should be stopped 4 days prior to such an evaluation
methdilazine (Tacaryl)	**Oral:** *Adults:* 16–32 mg/day, divided into 2–4 doses. *Children > 3 years:* 4 mg bid–qid	• Give on empty stomach, 2 h pc or 1 h ac • Drug may negatively influence allergy skin tests and should be stopped 4 days prior to such an evaluation

Table 72.3 (continued)
The antihistamines: Drug doses

Drug Generic name (Trade names)	Dosage	Nursing alert
promethazine (Phenergan)	**Oral:** *Adults:* 25 mg hs or 12.5 mg qid. *Children:* 25 mg hs or 6.25–12.5 mg tid **Rectal/IM/IV:** *Adults:* 25 mg repeated in 2 h, prn. **IM:** *Children < 12 years:* No more than 1/2 adult dose	• If drug is given concurrently with opioid analgesics, supervise pt to prevent injury from increased sedation • **PO:** Give with food, milk or water to minimize GI irritation. Should pt have difficulty swallowing, tablets may be crushed and mixed with food or fluid • **IM:** Inject deep into well-developed muscle • **SC:** Injection may cause tissue necrosis • **IV:** Do not exceed concentration of 25 mg/mL; rate, at least 1 min/dose. Rapid injection may produce fall in BP. If solution appears slightly yellow it may still be used. Should solution contain precipitate, discard. Shield solution from direct light • Drug may negatively influence allergy skin tests and should be stopped 4 days prior to such an evaluation. It may also influence urine pregnancy test
terfenadine (Seldane)	**Oral:** *Adults/children > 12 years:* 60 mg bid or 120 mg od, pref. in a.m. *Children 7–12 years:* 30 mg a.m. and evening; *3–6 years:* 15 mg a.m. and evening	• Give with food or milk to reduce GI irritation • Drug may negatively influence allergy skin tests and should be stopped 4 days prior to such an evaluation
trimeprazine (Panectyl)	**Oral:** *Adults:* 10 mg/day, divided into 4 doses; or 2 doses 12 h apart (sustained-release product). *Children 6 months to 3 years:* 1.25 mg hs or tid, prn; *3–12 years:* 2.5 mg hs or tid, prn	• Give with food or milk to reduce GI irritation • Drug may negatively influence allergy skin tests and should be stopped 4 days prior to such an evaluation
tripelennamine (PBZ, Pyribenzamine)	**Oral:** *Adults:* 25–50 mg q4–6h, or 1 time-release 100-mg tablet bid–tid. *Children:* 5 mg/kg/day, divided into 4–6 doses	• Give with food or milk to reduce GI irritation • Drug may negatively influence allergy skin tests and should be stopped 4 days prior to such an evaluation
triprolidine (Actidil, Alleract, Myidyl)	**Oral:** *Adults:* 2.5 mg q4–6h (not to exceed 10 mg/24 h). *Children 6–12 years:* 1.25 mg q6–8h (not to exceed 5 mg/24 h); *4–6 years:* 937 µg q6–8h (not to exceed 3.75 mg/24 h); *2–4 years:* 625 µg q6–8h (not to exceed 2.5 mg/24 h); *4 months to 2 years:* 312 µg q6–8h (not to exceed 1.25 mg/24 h)	• Give with food or milk to reduce GI irritation • Drug may negatively influence allergy skin tests and should be stopped 4 days prior to such an evaluation

Index

(cont'd)